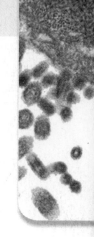

Schaechter's Mechanisms of Microbial Disease

FIFTH EDITION

N. Cary Engleberg
Professor of Internal Medicine, Division of Infectious Diseases
Professor of Microbiology and Immunology
University of Michigan Medical School
Ann Arbor, Michigan

Victor J. DiRita
Professor of Microbiology and Immunology
Associate Dean, Graduate and Postdoctoral Studies
Director, Microbial Pathogenesis Training Program
University of Michigan Medical School
Ann Arbor, Michigan

Terence S. Dermody
Dorothy Overall Wells Professor of Pediatrics and Pathology,
Microbiology, and Immunology
Director, Division of Pediatric Infectious Diseases
Director, Medical Scientist Training Program
Vanderbilt University School of Medicine
Nashville, Tennessee

. Wolters Kluwer | Lippincott Williams & Wilkins

Acquisitions Editor: Susan Rhyner
Product Manager: Julie Montalbano
Marketing Manager: Joy Fisher Williams
Designer: Joan Wendt
Compositor: SPi Global

5th Edition

Not authorized for sale in the United States, Canada, Australia, and New Zealand.
ISBN: 978-1-4511-0005-1

DISCLAIMER
Care has been taken to confirm the accuracy of the information present and to describe generally accepted practices. However, the authors, editors, and publisher are not responsible for errors or omissions or for any consequences from application of the information in this book and make no warranty, expressed or implied, with respect to the currency, completeness, or accuracy of the contents of the publication. Application of this information in a particular situation remains the professional responsibility of the practitioner; the clinical treatments described and recommended may not be considered absolute and universal recommendations.

The authors, editors, and publisher have exerted every effort to ensure that drug selection and dosage set forth in this text are in accordance with the current recommendations and practice at the time of publication. However, in view of ongoing research, changes in government regulations, and the constant flow of information relating to drug therapy and drug reactions, the reader is urged to check the package insert for each drug for any change in indications and dosage and for added warnings and precautions. This is particularly important when the recommended agent is a new or infrequently employed drug.

Some drugs and medical devices presented in this publication have Food and Drug Administration (FDA) clearance for limited use in restricted research settings. It is the responsibility of the health care provider to ascertain the FDA status of each drug or device planned for use in their clinical practice.

To purchase additional copies of this book, call our customer service department at (800) 638-3030 or fax orders to (301) 223-2320. International customers should call (301) 223-2300.

Visit Lippincott Williams & Wilkins on the Internet: http://www.lww.com. Lippincott Williams & Wilkins customer service representatives are available from 8:30 am to 6:00 pm, EST.

9 8 7 6 5 4 3 2 1

Preface

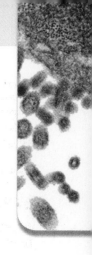

THE PREVIOUS editions of this book were designed by its original editor in chief, Moselio Schaechter, to present major concepts in microbiology and infectious diseases in a pathobiological framework and within the context of clinical cases. This format lends itself to an active form of studying and is easily adaptable to problem-based learning. It is particularly appropriate for use in revised medical curricula that feature a synthesis of basic microbiology and clinical infectious diseases or those that follow an "organ system" approach to the basic sciences.

KEY FEATURES AND APPROACH

The use of the text in these variously structured courses is facilitated by the presentation of the material in three distinct sections. Part I presents basic concepts of microbiology as well as immunology and pharmacology as these disciplines relate to infections. Part II describes the major infectious agents and the diseases that they cause. Part III illustrates how the major systems of the body are affected by infection.

This textbook is intended to be used in courses on medical microbiology or infectious diseases for medical students, allied health professionals, graduate students, or advanced undergraduates. Because the purpose of this book is to develop a conceptual framework for understanding infection, it highlights certain agents and diseases of special biological or clinical importance and does not attempt to describe the microbial world in an exhaustive fashion.

One of the most distinctive features of the previous editions has been retained: in many of the chapters on individual infectious agents, the reader will find boxed sections labeled "Paradigm." Those sections present discussions of certain general principles that are best illustrated by the agents described in that chapter but also can be applied to other organisms.

NEW TO THIS EDITION

This new edition retains the basic conceptual framework of past editions credited to Dr. Schaechter in its new title, but it has been revised to reflect many of the recent changes that have taken place in the field as well as new features to facilitate learning. Every chapter in the book has been revised and updated, many by new authors. The updated text is as current as possible, realizing that new information in the field is accumulating at such dazzling speed that it risks becoming outdated before the ink dries. Many of the illustrations are either new or have been redrawn.

This book is accompanied by online resources, which include an online e-book, an image bank, and an interactive Q&A for review. These resources can be accessed at www.thePoint.com with the code provided on the inside front cover. Although the printed text contains all of the important core information, the online resources allow for further enrichment for students.

N. Cary Engleberg
Victor DiRita
Terence S. Dermody

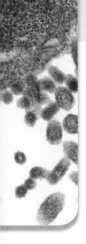

Acknowledgments

MANY COLLEAGUES and friends have helped us in the past in preparing this book. Their names appear in the previous editions. For this revision, we received invaluable advice from Tejal Gandhi, William Peterson, and David Friedman. Our heartfelt thanks go to them for their kind and thoughtful suggestions. We are particularly grateful to Keith Donnellan, who provided expert editorial assistance and helped greatly in organizing the diverse elements in the book. His support, hard work, patience, and persistence were instrumental in bringing this book to completion. We thank our product manager, Julie Montalbano, who provided thoughtful direction on format and style as well as the patience and discipline to bring the various elements of the project together in a coherent manner.

We thank Susan Rhyner, acquisitions editor, for helping to formulate the framework of the fifth edition and for her support through the course of the project. We offer special thanks to Matthew Chansky for optimizing the color artwork and maintaining a style that is both coherent and visually pleasing. We are grateful to Yvonne Poindexter and Marijean Rue for assistance in preparing the text for final submission. We also thank Andrea Ernst, Carrie Lapham, Carly Kish, and Warren Sutherland for administrative assistance during the editing of the text. Finally, our appreciation and love go to Margot, Michael, David, Kathleen, Victor, Amalia, Suzy, Roderick, and Alexander for their support and indulgence through the arduous task of making this book a reality.

Contributors

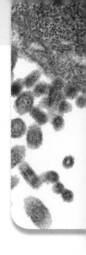

David W. K. Acheson, MD
Adjunct Faculty (Associate Professor)
Department of Microbiology and
    Immunology
Department of Epidemiology and
    Preventive Medicine
University of Maryland Medical School
Baltimore, Maryland
*Chapter 60 (with James Fleckenstein):
    Digestive System Infections*

C. Alan Anderson, MD
Professor
Department of Neurology
University of Colorado School of
    Medicine and the Denver Veterans
    Affairs Medical Center
Denver, Colorado
*Chapter 56 (with Kenneth L. Tyler):
    Prion Diseases*

Elliot J. Androphy, MD
Kampen-Norins Professor and Chair
Department of Dermatology
Indiana University School of Medicine
Indianapolis, Indiana
*Chapter 40: Human Papillomaviruses
    and Warts*

Robert L. Atmar, MD
Professor, Section of Infectious
    Diseases
Department of Medicine
Baylor College of Medicine
Chief, Infectious Diseases Service
Ben Taub General Hospital
Houston, Texas
*Chapter 37 (with Mary K. Estes):
    Rotaviruses, Noroviruses, and Other
    Viral Agents of Gastroenteritis*

Joseph T. Barbieri, PhD
Professor
Departments of Microbiology and
    Molecular Genetics
Medical College of Wisconsin
Milwaukee, Wisconsin
*Chapter 9: Damage by Microbial
    Agents*

Joel B. Baseman, PhD
Professor and Chair
Department of Microbiology and
    Immunology
University of Texas Health Science
    Center
San Antonio, Texas
*Chapter 29 (with Ken B. Waites):
    Mycoplasma: Curiosity and
    Pathogen*

Jeffrey M. Bergelson, MD
Professor of Pediatrics
University of Pennsylvania
Division of Infectious Disease
Children's Hospital of Philadelphia
Philadelphia, Pennsylvania
*Chapter 31 (with Terence S.
    Dermody): Biology of Viruses*

Karen C. Bloch, MD, MPH
Assistant Professor, Departments of
    Medicine (Infectious Diseases) and
    Preventive Medicine, Vanderbilt
    University Medical Center
Nashville, Tennessee
*Chapter 44 (with Julie E. Reznicek):
    Antiviral Treatment Strategies*

Suzanne F. Bradley, MD
Professor
Department of Internal Medicine
Divisions of Infectious Diseases and
    Geriatric Medicine & Palliative Care
University of Michigan Medical School
Program Director, Infection Control
    and Physician Scientist & Geriatric
    Research Education and Clinical
    Center
Veterans Affairs Ann Arbor Healthcare
    System
Ann Arbor, Michigan
Chapter 66: Sepsis
*Chapter 74: Fever: A Clinical Sign of
    Infection*

William J. Britt, MD
Professor
Department of Pediatrics
University of Alabama at
    Birmingham
Department of Pediatrics
Children's Health Systems
Birmingham, Alabama
*Chapter 42: Beta- and
    Gammaherpesviruses:
    Cytomegalovirus and Epstein-Barr
    Virus*

Niels Eske Bruun, MD, DMSc
Associate Professor
Director of Endocarditis and Heart
    Failure Clinics
Department of Cardiology
Gentofte University Hospital
Copenhagen, Denmark
*Chapter 67 (with Rasmus V.
    Rasmussen, Adolf W. Karchmer,
    and Vance G. Fowler Jr):
    Intravascular Infections*

Sandro K. Cinti, MD
Clinical Associate Professor
Department of Internal Medicine
Division of Infectious Diseases
University of Michigan Medical
    School
Ann Arbor, MI
*Chapter 57 (with Philip C. Hanna):
    Biological Agents of Warfare and
    Terrorism*

Jenifer Coburn, PhD
Professor
Division of Infectious Diseases
Center for Infectious Disease
    Research
Medical College of Wisconsin
Milwaukee, Wisconsin
*Chapter 25 (with John M. Leong
    and Mollie W. Jewett): Borrelia
    burgdorferi and Lyme Disease*

Laurie E. Comstock, PhD
Associate Professor of Medicine
Harvard Medical School
Associate Microbiologist, Department
    of Medicine
Brigham and Women's Hospital
Boston, Massachusetts
*Chapter 15: Bacteroides and
    Abscesses*

Peggy A. Cotter, PhD
Associate Professor
Department of Microbiology and
    Immunology
School of Medicine
University of North Carolina–Chapel
    Hill
Chapel Hill, North Carolina
*Chapter 4: Genetic Approaches to
    Studying Bacterial Pathogenesis*
*Chapter 19 (with Victor J. DiRita):
    Bordetella and Whooping
    Cough*

James E. Crowe Jr, MD
Ingram Professor of Research
Departments of Pediatrics, Pathology,
    Microbiology and Immunology
Director, Vanderbilt Vaccine
    Center
Vanderbilt University Medical
    Center
Nashville, Tennessee
*Chapter 34 (with John V. Williams):
    Paramyxoviruses: Measles,
    Mumps, and Respiratory Syncytial
    Virus*

Toni Darville, MD
Carol Ann Craumer Professor of
  Pediatrics
Chief of Infectious Diseases
Children's Hospital of Pittsburgh
Professor of Pediatrics and
  Immunology
University of Pittsburgh School of
  Medicine
Pittsburgh, Pennsylvania
*Chapter 27: Chlamydiae: Genital,
  Ocular, and Respiratory
  Pathogens*

Roberta L. DeBiasi, MD
Associate Professor of Pediatrics
George Washington University School
  of Medicine
Attending Physician, Division of
  Pediatric Infectious Diseases
Children's National Medical Center/
  Children's Research Institute
Washington, District of Columbia
*Chapter 61 (with Kenneth L. Tyler):
  Infections of the Central Nervous
  System*

Christoph Dehio, PhD
Professor
Infection Biology
Biozentrum
University of Basel
Basel, Switzerland
*Chapter 26: Cat Scratch Disease,
  Bacillary Angiomatosis, and Other
  Bartonelloses*

Mark R. Denison, MD
Professor
Departments of Pediatrics and
  Pathology, Microbiology, and
  Immunology
Vanderbilt University School of
  Medicine
Nashville, Tennessee
*Chapter 32 (with Vincent R.
  Racaniello): Picornaviruses and
  Coronaviruses*

Shira Doron, MD, MS
Assistant Professor
Department of Medicine
Tufts University School of
  Medicine
Boston, Massachusetts
*Chapter 75 (with David R. Snydman):
  Health Care–Associated
  Infections*

Roman Dziarski, PhD
Professor
Department of Microbiology and
  Immunology
Indiana University School of
  Medicine–Northwest
Gary, Indiana
Chapter 6: Innate Immunity

John R. Ebright, MD
Professor
Department of Internal Medicine
Wayne State University School of
  Medicine
Detroit, Michigan
*Chapter 24 (with Jack D. Sobel):
  Syphilis: A Disease with a History*
*Chapter 69 (with Jack D. Sobel):
  Sexually Transmitted Diseases*

Barry I. Eisenstein, MD
Executive Vice President
Research and Development
Cubist Pharmaceuticals
Lexington, Massachusetts
*Chapter 2 (with Moselio Schaechter
  and Vincent Young): The Normal
  Microbiota*

Mary K. Estes, PhD
Cullen Endowed Chair
Departments of Medicine and
  Molecular Virology and Microbiology
Baylor College of Medicine
Houston, Texas
*Chapter 37 (with Robert L. Atmar):
  Rotaviruses, Noroviruses, and Other
  Viral Agents of Gastroenteritis*

Christina Fiske, MD
Division of Infectious Disease
Department of Medicine
Vanderbilt University School of
  Medicine
Nashville, Tennessee
*Chapter 23 (with David W. Haas):
  Mycobacteria: Tuberculosis and
  Leprosy*

Kevin Flaherty, MD
Associate Professor
Department of Internal Medicine
Division of Pulmonary Medicine and
  Critical Care
University of Michigan Medical
  School
Ann Arbor, Michigan
*Chapter 62 (with Melissa Miller):
  Respiratory System Infections*

James M. Fleckenstein, MD
Associate Professor of Medicine and
  Molecular Microbiology
Infectious Disease Division
Washington University School of
  Medicine
St. Louis, Missouri
*Chapter 60 (with David W. K.
  Acheson): Digestive System Infections*

Vance G. Fowler, MD
Professor
Department of Medicine
Division of Infectious Diseases
Duke University School of Medicine
Durham, North Carolina
*Chapter 67 (with Rasmus V. Rasmussen,
  Adolf W. Karchmer, and Niels E.
  Bruun): Intravascular Infections*

Donald E. Ganem, MD
Professor
Department of Microbiology and
  Immunology
University of California, San Francisco
San Francisco, California
Chapter 43: Viral Hepatitis

Joanna B. Goldberg, PhD
Professor
Department of Microbiology,
  Immunology, and Cancer Biology
University of Virginia Health System
Charlottesville, Virginia
*Chapter 18: Pseudomonas aeruginosa:
  A Ubiquitous Pathogen*

Diane E. Griffin, MD, PhD
University Distinguished Service
  Professor
Alfred and Jill Sommer Chair
W. Harry Feinstone Department of
  Molecular Biology and Immunology
Johns Hopkins Bloomberg School of
  Public Health
Baltimore, Maryland
Chapter 33: Arthropodborne Viruses

David W. Haas, MD
Professor
Departments of Medicine,
  Pharmacology, Pathology,
  Microbiology, and Immunology
Vanderbilt University School of
  Medicine
Nashville, Tennessee
*Chapter 23 (with Christina Fiske):
  Mycobacteria: Tuberculosis and
  Leprosy*

Natasha B. Halasa, MD, MPH
Assistant Professor
Department of Pediatrics
Vanderbilt University School of
    Medicine
Nashville, Tennessee
*Chapter 45 (with H. Keipp B. Talbot):
    Vaccines and Antisera for the
    Prevention and Treatment of
    Infectious Diseases*

Philip C. Hanna, PhD
Associate Professor
Department of Microbiology and
    Immunology
University of Michigan Medical
    School
Ann Arbor, Michigan
*Chapter 57 (with Sandro K. Cinti):
    Biological Agents of Warfare and
    Terrorism*

Anne E. Jerse, PhD
Professor
Department of Microbiology and
    Immunology
Uniformed Services University of the
    Health Sciences
Bethesda, Maryland
*Chapter 14 (with Victor J. DiRita):
    Neisseriae: Gonococcus and
    Meningococcus*

Mollie W. Jewett, PhD
Assistant Professor
Burnett School of Biomedical
    Sciences
University of Central Florida College
    of Medicine
Orlando, Florida
*Chapter 25 (with Jenifer Coburn
    and John M. Leong): Borrelia
    burgdorferi and Lyme Disease*

Adolf W. Karchmer, MD
Professor
Harvard Medical School
Chief
Division of Infectious Diseases
Beth Israel Deaconess Medical
    Center
Boston, Massachusetts
*Chapter 67 (with Rasmus V.
    Rasmussen, Niels E. Bruun, and
    Vance G. Fowler Jr): Intravascular
    Infection*

Carol A. Kauffman, MD
Professor
Department of Internal Medicine
University of Michigan Medical School
Chief, Infectious Diseases
Department of Internal Medicine
Veterans Affairs Ann Arbor Healthcare
    System
Ann Arbor, Michigan
*Chapter 46: Introduction to the Fungi
    and Mycoses*
*Chapter 47: Systemic Mycoses Caused
    by Primary Pathogens*
*Chapter 48: Systemic Mycoses Caused
    by Opportunistic Fungi*
*Chapter 49: Subcutaneous,
    Cutaneous, and Superficial Mycoses*
*Chapter 50: Review of the Medically
    Important Fungi*

Gary Ketner, PhD
Professor
Department of Molecular
    Microbiology and Immunology
Johns Hopkins Bloomberg School of
    Public Health
Baltimore, Maryland
Chapter 39: Adenoviruses

Michael A Lane, MD
Assistant Professor
Department of Internal Medicine
Division of Infectious Disease
Washington University School of
    Medicine
St. Louis, Missouri
*Chapter 70 (with E. Turner
    Overton): Infections of the
    Immunocompromised Patient*

John Leong, MD, PhD
Professor and Chair
Department of Molecular Biology and
    Microbiology
Tufts University Medical School
Boston, Massachusetts
*Chapter 25 (with Jenifer Coburn
    and Mollie W. Jewett): Borrelia
    burgdorferi and Lyme Disease*

Preeti N. Malani, MD, MSJ
Clinical Associate Professor
Department of Internal Medicine
Divisions of Geriatrics and Infectious
    Diseases
University of Michigan Medical School

Ann Arbor, Michigan
*Chapter 68 (with Mark A. Zacharek):
    Head and Neck Infections*

Roshni Mathew, MD
Lucile Packard Children's Hospital
Stanford University
Stanford, California
*Chapter 72 (with Charles G. Prober):
    Congenital and Perinatal
    Infections*

Beth A. McCormick, PhD
Professor
Department of Microbiology and
    Physiological Systems
The University of Massachusetts
    Medical School
Worcester, Massachusetts
*Chapter 17: Invasive and Tissue-
    Damaging Enteric Bacterial
    Pathogens: Bloody Diarrhea and
    Dysentery*

Kevin S. McIver, PhD
Associate Professor
Department of Cell Biology &
    Molecular Genetics
University of Maryland
College Park, Maryland
*Chapter 12: Streptococci and
    Enterococci: "Strep Throat" and
    Beyond*

Stephen Melville, PhD
Associate Professor
Department of Biology
Virginia Polytechnic Institute and State
    University
Blacksburg, Virginia
*Chapter 20: Clostridia: Diarrheal
    Disease, Tissue Infection, Food
    Poisoning, Botulism, and Tetanus*

Roger W. Melvold, PhD
Chester Fritz Distinguished Professor
    Emeritus of Microbiology and
    Immunology
Department of Microbiology and
    Immunology
School of Medicine and Health
    Sciences
University of North Dakota
Grand Forks, North Dakota
*Chapter 7 (with Carl Waltenbaugh):
    Induced Defenses of the Body*

Melissa Miller, MD
Clinical Lecturer
Division of Pulmonary Medicine and
Critical Care
Department of Internal Medicine
University of Michigan Medical School
Ann Arbor, Michigan
*Chapter 62 (with Kevin Flaherty):
Respiratory System Infections*

Joseph J. Nania, MD
Consultant in Pediatric Infectious
Diseases
Phoenix Children's Hospital
Phoenix, Arizona
Cardon Children's Medical Center
Mesa, Arizona
*Chapter 65: Infections of the Bones,
Joints, and Muscles*

Lindsay E. Nicolle, MD, FRCPC
Professor
Departments of Internal Medicine and
Medical Microbiology
University of Manitoba
Winnipeg, Manitoba, Canada
Chapter 63: Urinary Tract Infections

Jennifer M. Noto, PhD
Department of Medicine
Vanderbilt University
Nashville, Tennessee
*Chapter 22 (with Richard M. Peek Jr):
Helicobacter pylori: Pathogenesis of
a Persistent Bacterial Infection*

E. Turner Overton, MD
Assistant Professor
Department of Internal Medicine
Division of Infectious Disease
Washington University School of
Medicine
St. Louis, Missouri
*Chapter 70 (with Michael
A. Lane): Infections of the
Immunocompromised Patient*

Peter Palese, PhD
Horace W. Goldsmith Professor and
Chair
Department of Microbiology
Professor, Department of Medicine
Mount Sinai School of Medicine
New York, New York
Chapter 36: Influenza and Its Viruses

Richard M. Peek Jr, MD
Associate Professor
Departments of Medicine and Cancer
Biology
Vanderbilt University School of Medicine
Nashville, Tennessee
*Chapter 22 (with Jennifer M. Noyo):
Helicobacter pylori: Pathogenesis of
a Persistent Bacterial Infection*

Brett W. Petersen, MD, MPH
Medical Officer, Poxvirus and Rabies
Branch
Division of High-Consequence
Pathogens and Pathology
National Center for Emerging and
Zoonotic Infectious Diseases
Centers for Disease Control and
Prevention
Atlanta, Georgia
*Chapter 35 (with Charles E.
Rupprecht): Rabies*

Marnie L. Peterson, PhD, PharmD
Associate Professor
Department of Experimental and
Clinical Pharmacology
College of Pharmacy
University of Minnesota
Minneapolis, Minnesota
*Chapter 11 (with Patrick M.
Schlievert): Staphylococci: Abscesses
and Toxin-Mediated Diseases*

William G. Powderly, MD
Dean, School of Medicine and Medical
Sciences
Professor of Medicine and
Therapeutics
University College Dublin
Dublin, Ireland
*Chapter 71: Acquired
Immunodeficiency Syndrome*

Charles G. Prober, MD
Professor
Departments of Pediatrics and
Microbiology and Immunology
Senior Associate Dean for Medical
Education
Stanford University School of Medicine
Stanford, California
*Chapter 72 (with Roshni Mathew):
Congenital and Perinatal Infections*

Vincent R. Racaniello, PhD
Higgins Professor
Department of Microbiology and
Immunology
Columbia University College of
Physicians and Surgeons
New York, New York
*Chapter 32 (with Mark R. Denison):
Picornaviruses and Coronaviruses*

Christian B. Ramers, MD, MPH
Assistant Professor
Departments of Global Health and
Allergy and Infectious Diseases
University of Washington School
of Public Health and School of
Medicine
Seattle, Washington
Chapter 59: Principles of Epidemiology
Chapter 76: Foodborne Diseases

Rasmus Vedby Rasmussen, MD, PhD
Department of Cardiology
Copenhagen University Hospital
Hvidovre, Denmark
*Chapter 67 (with Adolf W.
Karchmer, Niels E. Bruun, and
Vance G. Fowler Jr): Intravascular
Infection*

Julie E. Reznicek, DO
Assistant Professor
Department of Medicine
Division of Infectious Diseases
Vanderbilt University Medical Center
Nashville, Tennessee
*Chapter 44 (with Karen
C. Bloch): Antiviral Treatment
Strategies*

Charles E. Rupprecht, VMD, PhD
Chief, CDC Rabies Program
Director, WHO Collaborating Centre
for Reference and Research on
Rabies
Head, OIE Rabies Reference
Laboratory
Adjunct Professor, Emory University,
Population Biology, Ecology, and
Evolution Program
Atlanta, Georgia
*Chapter 35 (with Brett W. Petersen):
Rabies*

Moselio Schaechter, PhD
Professor Emeritus
Department of Molecular Biology and
 Microbiology
Tufts University School of Medicine
Boston, Massachusetts
Chapter 1 (with Barry I. Eisenstein):
 Establishment of Infectious Diseases
Chapter 2 (with Barry I. Eisenstein
 and Vincent Young): The Normal
 Microbiota
Chapter 3: Biology of Infectious Agents

Patrick M. Schlievert, PhD
Professor and Head
Department of Microbiology
University of Iowa Carver College of
 Medicine
Iowa City, Iowa
Chapter 11 (with Marnie L. Peterson):
 Staphylococci: Abscesses and Toxin-
 Mediated Diseases

Robert T. Schooley, MD
Professor and Head
Division of Infectious Diseases
Executive Vice Chair for Academic
 Affairs
Department of Medicine
University of California, San Diego
San Diego, California
Chapter 38: Human Retroviruses:
 AIDS and Other Diseases

Daniel S. Shapiro, MD
H. Edward Manville Jr Chair of
 Internal Medicine and Professor of
 Medicine
University of Nevada School of
 Medicine
Reno, Nevada
Chapter 73: Zoonoses

David R. Snydman, MD
Chief, Division of Geographic
 Medicine and Infectious Diseases
 and Hospital Epidemiologist
Tufts Medical Center
Professor of Medicine
Tufts University School of Medicine
Boston, Massachusetts
Chapter 75 (with Shira Doron): Health
 Care–Associated Infections

Jack D. Sobel, MD
Professor
Department of Internal Medicine
Wayne State University School of
 Medicine

Chief
Detroit Medical Center
Division of Infectious Diseases
Detroit, Michigan
Chapter 24 (with John R. Ebright):
 Syphilis: A Disease with a History
Chapter 69 (with John R. Ebright):
 Sexually Transmitted Diseases

Patricia G. Spear, PhD
John Evans Professor Emerita of
 Microbiology–Immunology
Feinberg School of Medicine of
 Northwestern University
Chicago, Illinois
Chapter 41: Alphaherpesviruses:
 Herpes Simplex Virus and Varicella-
 Zoster Virus

Dennis L. Stevens, MD, PhD
Professor
Department of Medicine
University of Washington School of
 Medicine
Seattle, Washington
Chief, Infectious Disease Section
Veterans Affairs Medical Center
Boise, Idaho
Chapter 64: Infections of the Skin and
 Soft Tissue

Michele Swanson, MD
Professor
Department of Microbiology and
 Immunology
University of Michigan Medical School
Ann Arbor, Michigan
Chapter 21 (with N. Cary Engleberg):
 Legionella: Parasite of Amebas and
 Macrophages

H. Keipp B. Talbot, MD, MPH
Assistant Professor
Departments of Medicine and
 Pediatrics
Vanderbilt University Medical Center
Nashville, Tennessee
Chapter 45 (with Natasha B. Halasa):
 Vaccines and Antisera for the
 Prevention and Treatment of
 Infectious Diseases

Kenneth L. Tyler, MD
Reuler-Lewin Family Professor and
 Chairman
Department of Neurology
University of Colorado School of
 Medicine
Neurology Service

Denver Veterans Affairs Medical Center
Denver, Colorado
Chapter 56 (with C. Alan Anderson):
 Prion Diseases
Chapter 61 (with Roberta L. DeBiasi):
 Infections of the Central Nervous
 System

Ken B. Waites, MD, FAAM
Professor
Departments of Pathology and
 Microbiology
Director, Diagnostic Mycoplasma
 Laboratory
University of Alabama at Birmingham
Staff Pathologist and Microbiology
 Consultant
Birmingham Veterans Affairs Medical
 Center
Birmingham, Alabama
Chapter 29 (with Joel B. Baseman):
 Mycoplasma: Curiosity and
 Pathogen

David H. Walker, MD
The Carmage and Martha Walls
 Distinguished University Chair in
 Tropical Diseases
Professor and Chairman
Department of Pathology
Executive Director
Center for Biodefense and Emerging
 Infectious Disease
University of Texas Medical Branch–
 Galveston
Galveston, Texas
Chapter 28: Rocky Mountain Spotted
 Fever and Other Rickettsioses

Carl Waltenbaugh, PhD
Professor
Department of Microbiology and
 Immunology
Feinberg School of Medicine
Northwestern University
Chicago, Illinois
Chapter 7 (with Roger W. Melvold):
 Induced Defenses of the Body

Jeffrey Weiser, MD
Professor
Departments of Microbiology and
 Pediatrics
University of Pennsylvania School of
 Medicine
Philadelphia, Pennsylvania
Chapter 13: Pneumococcus and
 Bacterial Pneumonia

John V. Williams, MD
Associate Professor
Departments of Pediatrics and
  Pathology, Microbiology, and
  Immunology
Vanderbilt University Medical Center
Nashville, Tennessee
Chapter 34 (with James E. Crowe Jr):
  Paramyxoviruses: Measles Virus and
  Respiratory Syncytial Virus

Vincent Young, MD, PhD
Associate Professor
Department of Microbiology and
  Immunology
University of Michigan Medical School
Ann Arbor, Michigan
Chapter 2 (with Barry I. Eisenstein
  and Moselio Schaechter): The
  Normal Microbiota

Mark A. Zacharek, MD
Clinical Associate Professor
Department of Otolaryngology Head
  and Neck Surgery
University of Michigan Medical School

Ann Arbor, Michigan
Chapter 68 (with Preeti N. Malani):
  Head and Neck Infections

PAST CONTRIBUTORS

We acknowledge several individuals
who contributed to previous editions
of this book and whose work formed a
basis for many of the updated chapters
in this edition:

Richard T. D'Aquila
George M. Baer
Neil Barg
Michael Barza
John M. Coffin
Peter Dull
Kathryn M. Edwards
Roger G. Faix
Bernard N. Fields
George Fogg
Janet Gilsdorf
Sherwood L. Gorbach
Richard K. Groger
Penelope J. Hitchcock

George S. Kobayashi
Donald Krogstad
Gerald T. Keusch
David W. Lazinski
Zell A. McGee
Gerald Medoff
Cody Meissner
James Nataro
Timothy G. Palzkill
Jeffrey Parsonnet
Jane E. Raulston
Edward N. Robinson Jr
David Schlessinger
Arnold L. Smith
John Spitznagel
David Stephens
Gregory A. Storch
Stephen E. Straus
Francis P. Tally
Debbie S. Toder
Joseph G. Tully
Ellen Whitnak
Priscilla B. Wyrick
Victor L. Yu

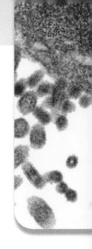

Chapter 3

Figure 3-2. Adapted from DiRienzo JM et al. The outer membrane proteins of the Gram-negative bacteria: biosynthesis, assembly, and function. *Ann Rev Biochem.* 1978;47:481.

Figure 3-8. Adapted from Blumberg P, Strominger JL. Interaction of the penicillin with the bacteria cell wall: penicillin-binding proteins and penicillin-sensitive enzymes. *Bacteriol Rev.* 1974;38:291–335.

Figure 3-9. Adapted from Kaback HR. Ion gradient coupled transport. In: Andreoli TE, Hoffman JS, Sanastil DD et al. *Physiology of Membrane Disorders.* New York, NY: Plenum Publications; 1986:287–407.

Figure 3-12. Courtesy of Drs. C. C. Brinton and J. Carnham.

Figure 3-14. Adapted from Boyd RF, Hoerl BG. *Basic Medical Microbiology.* Boston: Little, Brown; 1986.

Chapter 4

Figure 4-5. Adapted from Neidhardt et al. *Physiology of the Bacterial Cell.* Sunderland, MA: Sinauer Associates, Inc.; 1990.

Figure 4-6. Adapted from Neidhardt et al. *Physiology of the Bacterial Cell.* Sunderland, MA: Sinauer Associates, Inc.; 1990.

Chapter 5

Figure 5-2. Adapted from Gale EF et al. *The Molecular Basis of Antibiotic Action.* 2nd ed. New York, NY: John Wiley & Sons; 1981.

Chapter 6

Figure 6-4. From Knobel HR, Villinger W, Isliker H. Chemical analysis and electron microscopy studies of human C1q prepared by different methods. *Eur J Immunol.* 1975;5:78–82.

Figure 6-5. From Bhakdi S, Tranum-Jensen J. Mechanism of complement cytolysis and the concept of channel-forming proteins. *Phil Trans Roy Soc London, series B.* 1984;306:311.

Figure 6-6. Adapted and colorized from Rubin E, Farber JL. *Pathology.* 3rd ed. Baltimore, MD: Lippincott Williams & Wilkins, 1999:fig 2-30.

Chapter 7

Table 7-1. Adapted from Vivier E, Malissen B. Innate and adaptive immunity: specificities and signaling hierarchies revisited. *Nat Immunol.* 2005;6:17–21.

Figures 7-1 through 7-14. Adapted from Doan TT, Melvold R, Waltenbaugh C. *Concise Medical Immunology.* Baltimore, MD: Lippincott Williams & Wilkins; 2005.

Chapter 9

Figure 9-3. From Bell CE, Eisenberg D. Crystal structure of nucleotide-free diphtheria toxin. *Biochemistry.* 1997;36:481.

Chapter 11

Figure 11-1. From Koneman EW et al. *Diagnostic Microbiology.* 5th ed. Baltimore, MD: Lippincott Williams & Wilkins; 1997:color plate 11-1C.

Chapter 12

Figure 12-4. From Public Health Image Library-PHIL, CDC/Dr. Edwin P Ewing Jr

Chapter 13

Figure 13-1. Courtesy of Dr. Stuart S. Sagel.

Figure 13-2. From Marler LM, Siders JA, Allen SD. *Direct Smear Atlas: A Monograph of Gram-Stained Smear Preparations of Clinical Specimens.* Baltimore, MD: Lippincott Williams & Wilkins; 2001.

Figure 13-3. Modified from Kim JO et al. *Infect Immun.* 1999;67:2327–2333.

Figure 13-4. From Wood WB Jr. Studies on the cellular immunology of acute bacterial infections. *Harvey Lect* 1951–1952;47:72–98.

Figure 13-5. From Marler LM, Siders JA, Allen SD. *Direct Smear Atlas: A Monograph of Gram-Stained Smear Preparations of Clinical Specimens.* Baltimore, MD: Lippincott Williams & Wilkins; 2001.

Chapter 14

Figure 14-1. From McClatchey KD, Alkan S, Hackel E et al. *Clinical Laboratory Medicine.* 2nd ed. Philadelphia, PA: Lippincott Williams & Wilkins; 2001.

Figure 14-6. From McGee Z et al. Pathogenic mechanisms of *Neisseria gonorrhoeae*: observation on damage to human fallopian tubes in organ culture by gonococci of colony type I or type 4. *J Infect Dis.* 1981;143:413–422.

Chapter 15

Figure 15-2. Courtesy of A. Tzianabos.

Figure 15-3. Courtesy of Coy Laboratories, Ann Arbor, MI.

Chapter 17

Figure 17-1. Adapted from Taussig MJ. *Processes in Pathology and Microbiology.* 2nd ed. Oxford, UK: Blackwell Scientific Publications; 1984.

Figure 17-2. From Rubin E, Farber JL. *Pathology.* 3rd ed. Baltimore, MD: Lippincott Williams & Wilkins; 1999:fig 9-21.

Figure 17-3. Courtesy of Dr. Stanley Falkow. Panel B reproduced with permission from Jones BD, Ghori N, Falkow SJ. *J Exp Med.* 1994;180:15–23.

Chapter 18

Figure 18-2. From McClatchey KD, Alkan S, Hackel E et al. *Clinical Laboratory Medicine.* 2nd ed. Philadelphia, PA: Lippincott Williams & Wilkins; 2001.

Chapter 19

Figure 19-1. From Muse KE et al. Scanning electron microscopy study of hamster tracheal organ cultures infected with *Bordetella pertussis*. *J Infect Dis.* 1977;136:771–777.

Figure 19-3. Adapted from a figure provided courtesy of Dr. W. E. Goldman.

Chapter 20

Figure 20-2. From Schering Slide Library, Schering Corp., Kenilworth, NJ, copyright owner. All rights reserved.

Chapter 23

Figure 23-2. Redrawn after Centers for Disease Control and Prevention (CDC). Trends in tuberculosis—United States, 2008. *MMWR Morb Mortal Wkly Rep.* 2009;58:249–253.

Figure 23-3. Adapted from Myers JA. The natural history of tuberculosis in the human body. *JAMA.* 1965;194:1086.

Chapter 24

Figure 24-1. Courtesy of Dr. E. M. Walker, Department of Microbiology and Immunology, UCLA School of Medicine, Los Angeles, CA.

Figure 24-2. Adapted from Taussig MJ. *Processes in Pathology and Microbiology.* 2nd ed. Oxford, UK: Blackwell Scientific; 1984.

Figure 24-3. From Goodheart HP. *A Photoguide of Common Skin Disorders: Diagnosis and Management.* Baltimore, MD: Lippincott Williams & Wilkins; 1999.

Chapter 25

Figure 25-2. Courtesy of James Gathany, Centers for Disease Control.

Figure 25-3. Courtesy of Dr. Mollie Jewett, Dr. Cristina Fernandez-Valle, Angelika Linowski, and Stephanie Kurhanewicz, Burnett School of Biomedical Sciences, University of Central Florida.

Figure 25-4A. Courtesy of Kent Loeffler, Dr. Laura Harrington, Renee Anderson, Cornell Department of Entomology.

Figure 25-4B. Courtesy of Dr. Nancy Hinkle, Department of Entomology, University of Georgia.

Figure 25-5. Adapted with permission from a figure from the Web site of the American Lyme Disease Foundation, http://www.aldf.com/DeerTickEcology.asp

Figure 25-6. Courtesy of the Centers for Disease Control.

Chapter 26

Figure 26-2. From Goodheart HP. *Goodheart's Photoguide of Common Skin Disorders.* 2nd ed. Philadelphia, PA: Lippincott Williams & Wilkins; 2003.

Chapter 28

Figure 28-2. Redrawn after Openshaw JJ, Swerdlow DL, Krebs JW et al. Rocky mountain spotted fever in the United States, 2000-2007: interpreting contemporary increases in incidence. *Am J Trop Med Hyg.* 2010;83(1):174–182.

Figure 28-4. From McClatchey KD, Alkan S, Hackel E et al. *Clinical Laboratory Medicine.* 2nd ed. Philadelphia, PA: Lippincott Williams & Wilkins; 2001.

Chapter 29

Figure 29-1. Courtesy of Dr. Gary Shackleford.

Figure 29-2. From Koneman EW et al. *Diagnostic Microbiology.* 5th ed. Baltimore, MD: Lippincott Williams & Wilkins; 1997:color plate 16-1B.

Figure 29-3. From Hu PC et al. Surface parasitism by *Mycoplasma pneumoniae* of respiratory epithelium. *J Exp Med* 1977;145:1328.

Chapter 30

Figure 30-1. Courtesy of Dr. D. J. Krogstad.

Chapter 31

Table 31-1. Adapted from Condit RC. Principles of virology. In: Knipe DM, Howley PM, eds. *Fields Virology.* 5th ed. Philadelphia, PA: Lippincott-Raven Press; 2007:24–57.

Figure 31-1. Paramyxovirus: © Science Photo Library. Smallpox virus: Courtesy of Frederick A. Murphy, DVM, PhD, University of California-Davis, Davis, California. Influenza virus: Courtesy of Pete Palese, PhD, Mount Sinai School of Medicine, New York, New York. All other images from T. S. Baker, N. H. Olson, and S. D. Fuller. Adding the Third Dimension to Virus Life Cycles: Three-Dimensional Reconstruction of Icosahedral Viruses from Cryo-Electron Micrographs. *Microbiol Mol Biol Rev.* 1999;63:862–922.

Figure 31-2. Redrawn from Dermody TS, Tyler KL. Introduction to viruses and viral diseases. In: Mandell GL, Bennett JE, Dolin R, eds. *Mandell, Douglas, and Bennett's Principles and Practice of Infectious Diseases.* 5th ed. New York, NY: Churchill Livingstone; 2000:1536–1552.

Figure 31-3. Redrawn from Taussig MJ. *Processes in Pathology and Microbiology.* 2nd ed. Oxford, UK: Blackwell Scientific Publications; 1984.

Figure 31-4. Redrawn from Taussig MJ. *Processes in Pathology and Microbiology.* 2nd ed. Oxford, UK: Blackwell Scientific Publications; 1984.

Chapter 32

Figure 32-2. Adapted from Flint SJ, Enquist LW, Racaniello VR et al. *Principles of Virology.* 2nd ed. Washington, DC: ASM Press; 2004.

Figure 32-3. Adapted from Flint SJ, Enquist LW, Racaniello VR et al. *Principles of Virology.* 2nd ed. Washington, DC: ASM Press; 2004.

Figure 32-5. Adapted from Ogra PL, Karzon DT. Formation and function of poliovirus antibody in different tissues. *Prog Med Virol.* 1971;13:156–193.

Chapter 33

Figure 33-3. Redrawn after Lindsey NP et al.; Centers for Disease Control and Prevention. *MMWR Surveil Summ.* 2010;59:1–17.

Chapter 34

Figure 34-1. Adapted from Knipe DM, Howley PM, eds. *Field's Virology.* 4th ed. Philadelphia, PA: Lippincott Williams & Wilkins; 2001:ch 41, fig 2.

Figure 34-3. From Rubin E, Farber JL. *Pathology.* 3rd ed. Baltimore, MD: Lippincott Williams & Wilkins; 1999:fig 12-32.

Chapter 35

Figure 35-1. Courtesy of Dr. Makonnen Fedaku, Centers for Disease Control and Prevention, Atlanta, GA.

Chapter 36

Figure 36-5. Redrawn after an image contributed by James Stevens and Ian Wilson.

Figure 36-6. Images courtesy of Gina Conenello and Nicole Bouvier.

Chapter 37

Figure 37-1. Courtesy of A. Kapikian.

Figure 37-2. Adapted from Field BN et al. *Virology.* New York, NY: Raven Press; 1990.

Chapter 38

Figure 38-1. Redrawn with permission after Global Report: UNAIDS Report on the Global AIDS Epidemic 2010. http://www.unaids.org/globalreport/

Figure 38-5. Courtesy of Dr. M. Gonda.

Chapter 39

Figure 39-1A. From Stewart PL, Burnett RM, Cyrklaff M, Fuller SD. Image reconstruction reveals the complex molecular organization of adenovirus. *Cell.* 1991;67:145–154.

Figure 39-1B. Redrawn from Philipson L, Pettersson U. Advances in tumor virus research. In: *Advances in Virus Research.* vol. 18. New York, NY: Academic Press; 1971.

Figure 39-3A. From Kelly TJ Jr. Adenovirus DNA replication. In: Ginsburg HS, ed. *The Adenoviruses.* New York, NY: Plenum Publishing; 1984:278, 298.

Figure 39-3B&C. Redrawn from Kelly TJ Jr. Adenovirus DNA replication. In: Ginsburg HS, ed. *The Adenoviruses.*

New York, NY: Plenum Publishing; 1984:278, 298.

Chapter 40

Figure 40-1. Courtesy of Dr. K. V. Shah.

Figure 40-2. From Goodheart HP. *Goodheart's Photoguide of Common Skin Disorders.* 2nd ed. Philadelphia, PA: Lippincott Williams & Wilkins; 2003.

Figure 40-3. Courtesy of Dr. Benjamin Barankin.

Figure 40-4. From Rubin E, Farber JL. *Pathology.* 3rd ed. Baltimore, MD: Lippincott Williams & Wilkins; 1999:fig 17-19A.

Chapter 41

Figure 41-1. Reprinted from Grünewald K et al. Three-dimensional structure of herpes simplex virus from cryo-electron tomography. *Science.* 2003;302:1396–1398, with permission from AAAS.

Figure 41-2. Redrawn from Mettenleiter TC et al. Herpesvirus assembly: an update. *Virus Res.* 2009;143:222–234, with permission from Elsevier.

Figure 41-3. Redrawn from Fig. 28.44 in Mims CA et al. *Medical Microbiology.* Mosby, 1993, with permission.

Figure 41-4A-C. From Goodheart HP, MD. *Goodheart's Photoguide of Common Skin Disorders.* 2nd ed. Philadelphia, PA: Lippincott Williams & Wilkins; 2003, with permission.

Figure 41-4D. From Sweet RL, Gibbs RS. *Atlas of Infectious Diseases of the Female Genital Tract.* Philadelphia, PA: Lippincott Williams & Wilkins; 2005, with permission.

Figure 41-5B. From Fleisher GR, MD, Ludwig W, MD, Baskin MN, MD. *Atlas of Pediatric Emergency Medicine.* Philadelphia, PA: Lippincott Williams & Wilkins, 2004, with permission.

Figure 41-5C&D. From Goodheart HP, MD. *Goodheart's Photoguide of Common Skin Disorders.* 2nd edition. Philadelphia, PA: Lippincott Williams & Wilkins; 2003, with permission.

Chapter 42

Figure 42-1. Modified from a figure provided by Dr. Jay Nelson and Andrew Townsend, Oregon Health

Sciences University, Portland, Oregon.

Figure 42-3. Photographs provided by Dr. D. Kelly, Dept. of Pathology, Children's Hospital of Alabama, Birmingham.

Chapter 43

Figure 43-2. Adapted from Ganem D, Schneider RJ. Hepadnaviruses. In: Knipe DM, Howley PM, eds. *Field's Virology.* 4th ed. Philadelphia, PA: Lippincott Williams & Wilkins; 2001:ch 86, fig 2.

Figure 43-3. Courtesy of Dr. John Jerin.

Figure 43-4. Redrawn after Ganem D, Prince A. Hepatitis B virus infection: natural history and clinical consequences. *N Engl J Med.* 2004;350:1118–1129 with permission.

Figure 43-8. Redrawn after Lindenbach D, Rice C. Unraveling hepatitis C virus replication: from genome to function. *Nature.* 2005;436:933–938.

Chapter 44

Figure 44-2. Adapted from Freed EO, Martin MA. HIVs and their replication. In: Knipe DM, Howley PM, eds. *Field's Virology.* 4th ed. Philadelphia, PA: Lippincott Williams & Wilkins; 2001:ch 59, fig 30.

Figure 44-4. Adapted from Crumpacker C. Antiviral therapy. In: Knipe DM, Howley PM, eds. *Field's Virology.* 4th ed. Philadelphia, PA: Lippincott Williams & Wilkins; 2001:ch 15, fig 12.

Figure 44-6. Modified from Corey L et al. Intravenous acyclovir for the treatment of primary genital herpes. *Ann Intern Med.* 1983;98:914–921.

Figure 44-7. Redrawn from Straus S et al. Suppression of recurrent genital herpes with oral acyclovir. *Trans Assoc Am Phys.* 1984;97:278–283.

Chapter 46

Figure 46-2. From Koneman EW et al. *Diagnostic Microbiology.* 5th ed. Baltimore, MD: Lippincott Williams & Wilkins; 1997:color plate 19-6E.

Figure 46-4. From Koneman EW et al. *Diagnostic Microbiology.* 5th ed. Baltimore, MD: Lippincott Williams & Wilkins; 1997:color plate 19-1C.

Figure 46-5. Adapted from Koneman EW et al. *Diagnostic Microbiology.* 5th ed. Baltimore, MD: Lippincott Williams & Wilkins; 1997:fig 19-5.

Chapter 47

Figure 47-3. From Kauffman CA. Fungal infections in older adults. *Clin Infect Dis.* 2001;33:550–555.

Figure 47-4B. From Rubin E, Farber JL. *Pathology.* 3rd ed. Baltimore, MD: Lippincott Williams & Wilkins; 1999:fig 9-59B.

Figure 47-6. From Rubin E, Farber JL. *Pathology.* 3rd ed. Baltimore, MD: Lippincott Williams & Wilkins; 1999:fig 9-62.

Figure 47-8B. From Rubin E, Farber JL. *Pathology.* 3rd ed. Baltimore, MD: Lippincott Williams & Wilkins; 1999:fig 9-60.

Figure 47-9. From Rubin E, Farber JL. *Pathology.* 3rd ed. Baltimore, Md: Lippincott Williams & Wilkins; 1999:fig 9-61.

Chapter 48

Figure 48-2. From Rubin E, Farber JL. *Pathology.* 3rd ed. Baltimore, MD: Lippincott Williams & Wilkins; 1999:fig 9-54A.

Figure 48-4. Courtesy of Dr. Leonor Haley, Centers for Disease Control and Prevention, Atlanta, GA.

Figure 48-6. From Koneman EW et al. *Diagnostic Microbiology.* 5th ed. Baltimore, MD: Lippincott Williams & Wilkins; 1997:color plate 19-1C.

Figure 48-10. From Grossman ME, Roth J. Cutaneous *Manifestations of Infection in the Immunocompromised Host.* Philadelphia, PA: Lippincott Williams & Wilkins; 1995: fig 1-51.

Figure 48-11. From Rubin E, Farber JL. *Pathology.* 3rd ed. Baltimore, MD: Lippincott Williams & Wilkins; 1999:fig 9-72A.

Figure 48-13. From Rubin E, Farber JL. *Pathology.* 3rd ed. Baltimore, MD: Lippincott Williams & Wilkins; 1999:fig 9-72B.

Chapter 49

Figure 49-1. Watanakunakorn C. Photo quiz. *Clin Infect Dis.* 1996;22:765.

Chapter 52

Figure 52-2. Redrawn from Friedman MJ. Erythrocytic mechanism of sickle cell resistance to malaria. *Proc Natl Acad Sci USA.* 1978;75:1994.

Figure 52-7. Courtesy of Drs. Bartlett MS, Smith JW. Indiana University School of Medicine.

Figure 52-10. Redrawn from Ross R, Thompson D. *Proc Roy Soc London, series B.* 1910;82:411–415.

Chapter 53

Figure 53-3. Courtesy of Dr. Stanley L. Erlandsen, Washington University School of Medicine, St. Louis, MO.

Chapter 55

Figure 55-8A. From Kean BH, Sun T, Ellsworth RM. *Ophthalmic Parasitology.* New York, NY: Igaku-Shoin; 1991:212.

Figure 55-8B. Courtesy of Dr. Zaiman H, Charlottesville, VA. From a pictorial presentation of parasites. In: Sun T, ed. *Parasitic Disorders: Pathology, Diagnosis, and Management.* 2nd ed. Baltimore, MD: Lippincott Williams & Wilkins; 1999.

Chapter 56

Figure 56-2A. From the National Creutzfeldt-Jakob Disease Surveillance Unit, Western General Hospital, Crewe Road, Edinburgh, UK.

Figure 56-2B. From Rabinstein, AA. Abnormal diffusion-weighted magnetic resonance imaging in Creutzfeldt-Jakob disease following corneal transplantations. *Arch Neurol.* 2002;59:637.

Figure 56-3. From Rubin E, Farber JL. *Pathology.* 3rd ed. Baltimore, MD: Lippincott Williams & Wilkins; 1999:fig 28-109.

Figure 56-4. Adapted from Beisel CE, Morens DM. Variant Creutzfeldt-Jakob disease and the acquired and transmissible spongiform encephalopathies. *Clin Infect Dis.* 2004;38:697–704.

Figure 56-5. From Collie DA. Diagnosing variant Creutzfeldt-Jakob disease with the pulvinar sign: MR imaging findings in 86 neuropathologically confirmed cases. *AJNR* 2003;24:1560.

Chapter 57

Figure 57-1. Bush LM, Abrams BH, Beal A et al. Brief report: Index case of fatal inhalational anthrax due to bioterrorism. *N Engl J Med.* 2001;345:1607–1610. Copyright © 2001 Massachusetts Medical Society.

Figure 57-2. Jernigan JA et al. Bioterrorism-related inhalation anthrax: the first 10 cases reported in the United States. *Emerg Infect Dis.* 2001;7(6):933–944.

Figure 57-3. Public Health Image Library, Centers for Disease Control and Prevention, Atlanta, GA, http://www.bt.cdc.gov

Figure 57-4. Public Health Image Library, Centers for Disease Control and Prevention, Atlanta, GA, http://www.bt.cdc.gov

Figure 57-5. From Knipe DM, Howley PM, eds. *Field's Virology.* 4th ed. Philadelphia, PA: Lippincott Williams & Wilkins; 2001:ch 85, fig 3.

Figure 57-6. From Knipe DM, Howley PM, eds. *Field's Virology.* 4th ed. Philadelphia, PA: Lippincott Williams & Wilkins; 2001:ch 85, fig 1A.

Chapter 60

Figure 60-5. Courtesy of Dr. Pamela Sylvestre.

Figure 60-6. Courtesy of Dr. Pamela Sylvestre.

Figure 60-7. Courtesy of Dr. Pamela Sylvestre.

Chapter 61

Figure 61-2. Redrawn from Menkes JH. Viral neurological infections in children. *Hosp Pract.* 1977;12:100–109.

Figure 61-4. Courtesy of Dr. E. J. Bottone, Mount Sinai Hospital, New York, NY.

Figure 61-5. From Gilden DH. Brain imaging abnormalities in CNSA virus infections. *Neurology.* 2008;70:84.

Chapter 62

Table 62-5. Adapted from Mandell LA, Bartlett JG, Dowell SF et al. Update of practice guidelines for the management of community-acquired pneumonia in immunocompetent adults. *Clin Inf Dis.* 2003;37:1405–1433.

Chapter 63

Figure 63-1. Redrawn from Fass RJ et al. Urinary tract infection: practical aspects of diagnosis and treatment. *JAMA.* 1973;225:1509–1513.

Figure 63-3. Redrawn from Fass RJ et al. Urinary tract infection: practical aspects of diagnosis and treatment. *JAMA.* 1973;225:1509–1513.

Chapter 64

Figure 64-1. Fleisher GR, Ludwig W, Baskin MN. *Atlas of Pediatric Emergency Medicine.* Philadelphia, PA: Lippincott Williams & Wilkins; 2003:fig 11-37.

Figure 64-2. From Goodheart HP. *Goodheart's Photoguide of Common Skin Disorders: Diagnosis and Management.* 2nd ed. Philadelphia, PA: Lippincott Williams & Wilkins; 2003:fig 5-2.

Figure 64-3. From Barankin B. *The Barankin Dermatology Collection.* Baltimore, MD: Lippincott Williams & Wilkins; 2003.

Figure 64-4. From Rubin E, Farber JL. *Pathology.* 3rd ed. Baltimore, MD: Lippincott Williams & Wilkins; 1999:fig 9-11.

Figure 64-5. From Smeltzer SC, Bare BG. *Brunner and Suddarth's Textbook of Medical-Surgical Nursing.* 9th ed. Philadelphia, PA: Lippincott Williams & Wilkins; 2000:fig 51-01.

Figure 64-7. From Sweet RL, Gibbs RS. *Atlas of Infectious Diseases of the Female Genital Tract.* Philadelphia, PA: Lippincott Williams & Wilkins; 2005:fig 9-2.

Chapter 67

Figure 67-1. Adapted from Rodbard S. Blood velocity and endocarditis. *Circulation.* 1963;27:18–28.

Figure 67-2. From Rubin E, Farber JL. *Pathology.* 3rd ed. Baltimore, MD: Lippincott Williams & Wilkins; 1999:fig 11-34.

Figure 67-7A. From Rubin E, Farber JL. *Pathology.* 3rd ed. Baltimore, MD: Lippincott Williams & Wilkins; 1999:fig 11-34.

Table 67-2. Adapted from Everett ED, Hirschmann JV. Transient bacteremia and endocarditis prophylaxis. A review. *Medicine.* 1977;56:61–77, and Murdoch DR et al. Clinical presentation, etiology, and outcome of infective endocarditis in the 21st century. *Arch Intern Med.* 2009;169(5):463–473.

Chapter 73

Figure 73-3. Data from the Centers for Disease Control and Prevention, Atlanta, GA.

Contents

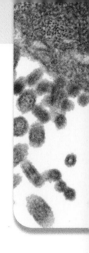

PART I

Principles

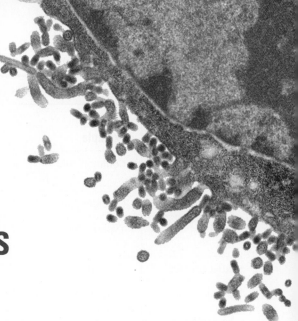

Chapter 1

Establishment of Infectious Diseases

Barry I. Eisenstein and Moselio Schaechter

BOTH STUDENTS and physicians confront a large number of facts about infectious agents and the diseases they cause. What is the best way to manage this large amount of material? Given the magnitude of the task, memorizing bits of information would be difficult and unproductive. The better approach is to develop a conceptual framework on which to hang a multitude of facts. This framework consists of two generalizations based on the features that characterize all forms of parasitism:

1. In all infectious diseases, the following events take place:
   Encounter: The agent meets the host.
   Entry: The agent enters the host.
   Spread: The agent spreads from the site of entry.
   Multiplication: The agent multiplies in the host.
   Damage: The agent, the host response, or both cause tissue damage.
   Outcome: The agent or the host wins out, or they learn to coexist.

2. Each of these events requires the breach of host defenses. The manner in which a parasite combats host defenses distinguishes it from other parasites.

ENCOUNTER

Most of us first encounter microorganisms at birth. Microbiologically speaking, we lead a sterile existence while in our mother's womb. First, the fetal membranes shield the fetus well from the microorganisms in the uterine environment. Second, the mother is not a likely source of microorganisms for the fetus. The mother's blood carries infectious agents only sporadically and in small numbers. In addition, the placenta is a formidable barrier to the transmission of microorganisms to the fetus. Such transmission is possible, however, and some diseases are transmitted to the fetus through the placenta. Examples of these so-called congenital infections are **rubella** (German measles) and **syphilis** or those caused by **HIV** or **cytomegalovirus** (**CMV**).

The first encounter with environmental microorganisms usually takes place at birth. During parturition, the newborn comes in contact with microorganisms present in the mother's vaginal canal and on her skin. Thus, the newborn faces the challenge of living in the intimate company of a bewildering number of microorganisms. The mother, however, does not send the newborn into the world totally unprotected. Through her circulation, she endows the fetus with a vast repertoire of specific antibodies. Some immunological protection is also provided by the mother's milk (colostrum), which also contains maternal antibodies. However, these acquired defenses soon wane and the child must cope on its own. The microbial challenge is renewed time and again as we come in contact with new organisms throughout our lives. Most organisms rapidly disappear from our bodies, but some are adroit colonizers and become part of the normal microbiota. A few cause disease.

Endogenous versus Exogenous Encounters

Microbial diseases are contracted in two general ways, exogenously and endogenously.

TABLE 1-1 Examples of Encounters and Disease Prevention

Type of Contact	Example	Type of Agent	Source	Strategy for Prevention	Preventive Aim
Inhalation	Common cold	Virus	Aerosol from infected persons	None	—
	Coccidioidomycosis	Fungus	Soil	None	—
Ingestion	Typhoid fever	Bacterium	Water, food	Sanitation	Lower infecting dose
Sexual contact	Gonorrhea	Bacterium	Person	Social behavior	Avoid contact
Wound	Surgical infections	Bacteria	Normal flora surroundings	Aseptic techniques	Avoid contact
Insect bite	Malaria	Protozoan	Mosquito	Insect control	Eliminate vector

Exogenously Acquired Diseases

Exogenously acquired diseases result from encounters with agents in the environment. Thus, we "catch" a cold from others, or we get typhoid fever from eating or drinking contaminated food or water. There are various ways in which disease-causing agents can be acquired from the environment: food, water, air, objects, insect bites, or humans or animals with whom we share our environment. Many agents are readily transmitted among humans through the exchange of bodily fluids—for instance, by sneezing, touching, or sexual intercourse. The way we encounter a disease agent often suggests a mode of prevention (Table 1-1); for example, infection by an agent spread through the fecal–oral route can be dramatically reduced by ensuring that wastewater and drinking water are maintained separately. Prevention has been successful for many serious epidemics, at least in the developed countries of the world. With the exception of vaccination, most preventive measures involve improving sanitation and the standard of living, rather than employing medical procedures.

Endogenously Acquired Diseases

Endogenously acquired diseases are caused by agents present in or on the body. Members of the normal collection of microbes that are normally found on our skin or mucous membranes (our **microbiota**) may cause disease, usually when they penetrate into deeper tissues. Thus, a cut can lead to the production of pus caused by the staphylococci that inhabit healthy skin. The encounter with the agent took place long before the disease—namely, at the time the skin was colonized by the staphylococci. A distinction must be made between **colonization** and **infectious disease**. Colonization simply denotes the presence of microorganisms in a site of the body that may or may not lead to tissue damage and signs and symptoms of disease. It does suggest, however, that the microorganisms have invaded that site of the body and can multiply there.

Normal Microbiota

The difference between endogenous and exogenous infections is sometimes quite sharp. However, in many other instances, the demarcation is less clear because it is difficult to define precisely which organisms constitute the **normal microbiota** (see Chapter 2). For example, some people harbor certain strains of virulent streptococci in their throat for a considerable period but only rarely come down with strep throat. Are these streptococci members of the normal microbiota? The answer is yes if *normal microbiota* refers to organisms in or on the body that are not in the process of causing disease. The answer is no if this kind of streptococcus is considered not found in the throats of approximately 95% of all healthy people. No easy way exists out of this ambiguity, and the terms *exogenous infection* and *endogenous infection* must be used tentatively. Obviously, if we cannot define precisely the composition of normal microbiota, we cannot always distinguish between endogenous and exogenous infections.

Another consideration that must also be kept in mind is that even for highly virulent microbes, exposure does not always lead to disease. For example, even at the height of deadly bubonic plague and typhus epidemics, most people were likely to have encountered the disease agent, but only about half the population became sick.

Thus, human encounters with microbes are quite varied, and disease is not inevitable in every case. Humans display an idiosyncratic pattern of response to infectious agents; even within one individual, the pattern can change with age, nutritional state, and many other factors.

ENTRY

Most of the tissues we normally think of as being inside the body are topologically connected with the outside

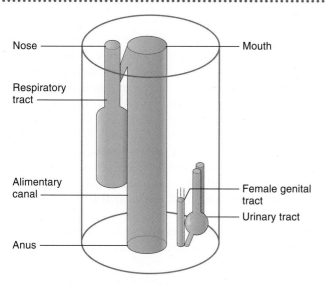

FIGURE 1-1. A schematic diagram showing the regions of the body in direct contact with the exterior. These include the outer aspects of the digestive, respiratory, and urogenital systems. These systems account for most of the organs of the thorax and abdomen. The main systems that do not have such direct connections are the musculoskeletal, nervous, circulatory, and endocrine systems. In women, the genital tract is connected to the peritoneal cavity via the fallopian tubes.

(Fig. 1-1). For instance, the surface of the lumen of the intestine, the alveoli of the lung, the bile canaliculi, and the tubules of the kidney are in direct contact with the exterior environment. In fact, this is true of almost all the organs contained within the thorax and abdomen. In principle, an insect could crawl from the mouth to the anus without penetrating any mucous membranes, although it would have to go through several valves and sphincters. In reality, these "external" sites of the body employ powerful mechanisms to keep out invading microorganisms. With the exception of much of the digestive tract and the lower reaches of the genitourinary system, these sites are normally sterile.

The term *entry* then can be used in two senses: it means either the **ingress** of microorganisms into body cavities that are contiguous with the outside environment or the **penetration** of microorganisms into deeper tissue after crossing an epithelial barrier. Both aspects of entry are discussed in detail here.

Ingress: Entry without Crossing Epithelial Barriers

Obviously, microorganisms enter the intestine by being swallowed and enter the lung by being inhaled. External microorganisms can also enter the urinary tract or the genital system. To cause disease, microorganisms do not have to enter deep into tissues but can stay only on mucosal surfaces. Examples of serious infectious diseases that occur without bacterial penetration through epithelial surfaces are **cholera** and **whooping cough**.

Inhalation

To enter the respiratory system, microorganisms face a series of aerodynamic and hydrodynamic obstacles. Microorganisms are inhaled in **aerosol droplets** or **dust particles** contained in the air we breathe. They take a circuitous path through the respiratory tract because they must navigate through complex anatomic structures such as nasal turbinates, the oropharynx, and the larynx. Accordingly, the surgical removal of the larynx (with its nooks and crannies) predisposes an individual to diseases of the lower respiratory tract. Microorganisms that arrive in the lower reaches of the respiratory tree face the powerful upward-sweeping action of the ciliary epithelium. As expected, persons in whom this ciliary elevator is impaired (e.g., heavy smokers) are more likely to get sick with pneumonia. Colonization of these sites requires that the microorganisms be able to stick to the epithelial surface.

Ingestion

When contaminated food or water is ingested, microorganisms face a powerful host defense, the acid in the stomach. The stomach is a chemical disinfection chamber where many microorganisms are destroyed. Its effectiveness in killing microbes, however, is determined by the length of time the microorganisms spend in the stomach, which in turn depends on the kind and amount of the food eaten. Even after great destruction, some bacteria and yeasts escape the stomach alive, although their original number may have been reduced a millionfold or more. In addition, the way that bacteria are ingested can influence their level of acid sensitivity because certain foods can protect the microbes from acid killing. Finally, some species have inherently greater resistance to acid and are therefore infectious at lower doses.

Bacteria, fungi, parasites, and viruses that escape the acid barrier of the stomach enter the duodenum. There they meet the enzymes of the pancreatic juice, the bile salts, and the strong sweeping force of **peristalsis**. Not unexpectedly, very few microbes can colonize the duodenum or anywhere else in the upper reaches of the small intestine. Toward the ileum, the environment is more favorable to bacterial life, but even there, the few organisms that gain a foothold must avoid being washed away. Indeed, bacteria found in this region have special mechanisms that allow them to adhere to the epithelial cells of the intestinal mucosa. As will be discussed in Chapter 2, several surface components of these bacteria serve as **adhesins**. The main adhesins are the hairlike pili (fimbriae) and the surface polysaccharides. As mentioned previously, bacteria at this site may cause disease without penetrating the mucosal epithelium. Cholera and its milder relative **traveler's diarrhea** are the manifestations of the local production of powerful toxins in the intestine that affect the epithelial cells. The bacteria that produce these toxins need not enter the host cells to cause disease.

Penetration: Entry into Tissues after Crossing Epithelial Barriers

Penetration into tissues takes many forms. Some microorganisms pass directly through epithelia, especially mucous membranes that consist of a single cell layer. To penetrate the skin, which is tough and multilayered, most infecting agents must be carried across by insect bites or await breaks in the skin surface. On the other hand, certain worms can burrow unaided through the skin and invade the host. An example is the hookworm, which can be acquired by walking barefoot on contaminated soil.

To penetrate mucosal epithelial cells, many agents first interact with specific **receptors** on the surface of the host cell. This phenomenon has been studied intensively in viruses, some of which have a complex mechanism for attachment and internalization. For instance, influenza viruses have **surface components** that bind to receptors on the surface of sensitive host cells. Binding is soon followed by the uptake of the virus particles by the cells. These two functions, **attachment** and **internalization**, are also the subjects of intensive study in relation to bacteria; many of which are able to induce their own uptake into host cells after attachment. Unlike viruses, however, not all bacteria must enter host cells to replicate; some can replicate to high levels on the mucosal epithelium.

Microorganisms can also be actively carried into tissues by white cells or macrophages that lie outside the body. For instance, macrophages that reside in the alveoli of the lungs—**alveolar macrophages**, also known as **dust cells**—can pick up inhaled infectious agents by phagocytosis. Most of the time, microorganism-containing macrophages are carried upward on the ciliary epithelium, but occasionally, infected macrophages can reenter the body and carry their load of microorganisms into deeper locations. This mechanism of **cell-mediated entry** can function in other mucous membranes as well. For example, it is thought that HIV, the virus that causes AIDS, may be sexually transmitted by the penetration of virus-laden macrophages from semen.

Insect Bites

Insect bites can lead to the penetration of viruses (viral encephalitis, yellow fever), bacteria (plague, typhus), protozoa (malaria, sleeping sickness), or worms (river blindness, elephantiasis). In the case of protozoa and worms, residence in the insect is part of their complex life cycles. The **life stage** of the parasite in the insect is often quite different from that found in the human host. Insects also spread diseases by carrying microorganisms on their surfaces and by contaminating skin or food. A particularly unsavory example of insect transmission is that of the so-called reduviid bugs, which defecate at the same time they bite. Parasites contained in the insect's feces are then introduced by scratching the bite area. A serious protozoal infection, **Chagas disease**, is transmitted in this manner.

Cuts and Wounds

Penetration from cuts and wounds is a common occurrence that often goes unnoticed because it does not usually lead to symptoms of disease. For example, brushing one's teeth or even defecating can cause minute abrasions of epithelial membranes. A small number of bacteria can then enter in the bloodstream, but they are rapidly removed by the filtering mechanisms of the lymphoreticular system. However, if internal tissues are damaged or the defense mechanisms disrupted, circulating bacteria may gain a foothold and cause serious diseases. An example is **subacute bacterial endocarditis**, a devastating disease in the preantibiotic era. The infection was usually caused by oral streptococci that invaded the heart valves damaged by a previous disease, usually rheumatic fever.

Organ Transplants and Blood Transfusions

Yet another way for organisms to penetrate into deeper tissue is through organ transplants or blood transfusions. For instance, cornea transplants have been known to result in the infection of recipients with a virus that causes a slow degenerative disease of the central nervous system, **Creutzfeldt-Jakob disease**. Kidney transplants sometimes result in infections by CMV, perhaps because of virus residing in the transplanted kidney. However, the transplanted organ is not always the source of infection. Because the immune response of transplant recipients must be suppressed to avoid graft rejection, an **endogenous virus** may take advantage of these weakened host defenses and begin to multiply.

Of the infectious agents that can be acquired through blood transfusions, none causes greater concern than HIV. However, many others, such as **hepatitis B virus (HBV)**, can also be transmitted in this manner. Screening of blood in blood banks is imperative.

Inoculum Size

Whether organisms from the microbiota of the skin or mucous membranes will cause disease depends on many factors. Among them is the size of the **inoculum**, the number of invading organisms. An encounter with a small number of organisms is unlikely to result in an infection; it usually takes many infecting agents to overcome the local defenses. An example that illustrates the importance of inoculum size is infection acquired from a contaminated hot tub. At times, the water can become a veritable culture broth with as many as 100 million bacteria (*Pseudomonas*) per milliliter. In such numbers, bacteria that are normally harmless can overcome the normal defenses of the skin and cause skin infection all over the body. Medical professionals are well aware of the importance of inoculum size in infection. Before making an incision in the skin, a surgeon prepares the area to reduce the number of bacteria that could invade a surgical wound. Infections are almost inevitable if large numbers of microorganisms are deposited in deeper tissues, either from dirty skin or from contamination by soil or other microbial-rich material. Treatment of patients with open wounds thus requires careful attention to sterile techniques, even in the modern era of powerful antimicrobial drugs.

SPREAD

The term *spread* has two shades of meaning. It suggests direct, **lateral propagation** of organisms from the original site of entry to contiguous tissues, but it can also refer to **dissemination** to distant sites. Either way, microorganisms spread and multiply only if they overcome host defenses. It should be kept in mind that spread can precede or follow microbial multiplication in the body. For instance, the parasite that causes **malaria** enters the body through a mosquito bite and is distributed throughout the bloodstream before it has a chance to reproduce. On the other hand, staphylococci that infect a cut must multiply locally before spreading to distant sites.

The role of **host defenses** in impeding the spread of microorganisms requires a fair understanding of the immune response and of the innate defense mechanisms. Host defenses are discussed in detail in Chapters 6 and 7 and are a central theme of this book. For now, it is important to keep in mind the dynamic nature of host–parasite interactions: For every host defense mechanism, microbes have developed a strategy to overcome it. The host, in turn, adapts to these new challenges, eliciting yet different responses from the agents. This intricate counterpoint is played out, sometimes over extended periods, and one of three things can happen: the host wins out, the parasite overcomes the host, or the host and parasite learn to live with one another in an uneasy truce.

Anatomical Factors

Because the pattern of spread of microorganisms from a given site is often dictated by **anatomical factors**, a knowledge of human anatomy often helps us understand infectious diseases. Consider the example of a localized infection, a bacterial abscess of the lung. The abscess could burst and allow the organisms to escape into the bronchial tree or, if the abscess is pointed outward, to the pleural cavity. Spread in one or the other direction has different consequences: in the first case, it could lead to a generalized pneumonia and in the second, to pleurisy. Another example is an infection of the middle ear, a condition more common in children than in adults. The age difference is explained in part by developmental changes that take place in the eustachian tubes with growth. These conduits are nearly horizontal in children and become more steeply inclined with age. For this and other reasons, the eustachian tubes of children do not drain as well as those of adults.

Spread of microorganisms is greatly influenced by **fluid dynamics**. Infected fluids in the interior of the body tend to flow along fascial planes. For example, infection of one site of the meninges will usually result in generalized meningitis because there are no barriers to impede the spread of the infected cerebrospinal fluid. The same is true for the pleura, the pericardium, and the synovial cavities. Of course, the most extensive liquid system of the body, the blood, is replete with defense mechanisms. All the liquids of the body (blood, lymph, cerebrospinal fluid, synovial fluid, urine, tears, etc.) contain unique antimicrobial defense factors. If these are overcome, disease results.

Active Participation by Microbes

Infectious agents are not always passive participants in the process of spread; some contribute to it by actively moving. Worms wiggle, ameba crawl, some bacteria swim. Although some of these movements appear random, others are probably in response to chemotactic signals. Spread can also be facilitated by chemical rather than mechanical action. For instance, streptococci manufacture a variety of extracellular hydrolases that allow them to break out of the walled defenses erected by the inflammatory response. These organisms make a protease that breaks up fibrin, a hyaluronidase that hydrolyzes the hyaluronic acid of connective tissue and may allow the organism to spread, and a deoxyribonuclease that reduces the viscosity of pus caused by release of DNA from lysed white cells. Some bacteria make elastases, collagenases, or other powerful proteases. Such organisms can break through natural surface barriers or spread through thick viscous pus that would otherwise impede their expansion. At a more superficial site, fungi that cause athlete's foot make keratin-hydrolyzing enzymes that help them spread through the horny layers of the skin. These factors confer clear selective advantages on the microorganisms that produce them.

MULTIPLICATION

Rarely do infectious agents cause disease without first multiplying within the body. As previously stated, the number of microorganisms we inhale or ingest (the size of the inoculum) or the number that survives initial host barriers is usually too small to produce symptoms directly. Infectious agents must reproduce before their presence is noted by symptoms (Fig. 1-2). Exceptions to the rule are agents that cause disease through production of a toxin, such as *Clostridium botulinum*, which produces the botulinum toxin that leads to botulism. This condition is an **intoxication**, not an infection.

In most infections, symptoms manifest some time after the organisms enter the host. This **incubation period** reflects the time needed for the infectious agents to overcome early defenses and grow to a certain population size. The subject of how hosts defend themselves against microbial multiplication is a lengthy and varied one. A later section in this chapter discusses how defense mechanisms sometimes go overboard and actually contribute to tissue damage in infections.

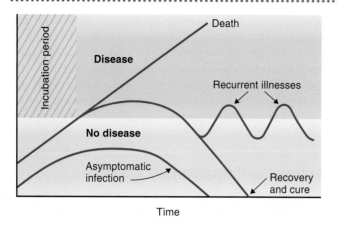

FIGURE 1-2. Microbial multiplication and clinical manifestations of disease. The number of microorganisms present in a patient must exceed a given threshold to cause disease. If the number is below that threshold, no signs and symptoms of disease will be apparent. In some cases, the numbers oscillate above and below the threshold, resulting in recurrent bouts of disease. Note that this drawing is idealized; in reality, the threshold of overt disease is not fixed but varies with the physiological state of the host.

Environmental Factors That Influence Multiplication

The physical environment of the body selects for microbes that grow within certain ranges of temperature, osmotic pressure, and pH. Those that are almost always found associated with a host tend to have a narrow **temperature optimum**. On the other hand, microbes that are also found in the environment, such as *Pseudomonas*, can grow at lower temperatures as well. Replication of some viruses, such as poliovirus, is limited to within a few degrees over normal human body temperature. Fever then may be a defense mechanism that helps restrict the disease. Fungi that cause athlete's foot do not grow well at temperatures above around 30°C and are thus found only on the cooler body surfaces. It follows that in most circumstances, these fungi cannot cause internal diseases. As with nutritional requirements, the optimal temperature range for growth is often dictated by the habits of the organism.

Subversion of Host Defenses

When a microbe causes an infection, it creates a hostile environment for itself because it impels the host to mobilize defenses that impair its growth. In most cases, the host prevails, but the existence of infectious diseases demonstrates that this is not always true and that microorganisms can thwart or evade the host defenses. Microbial countermeasures do not contribute directly to tissue damage, yet they can be thought of as virulence factors because they are essential for the microbe to be pathogenic. Generally, each species of infectious agents develops a unique spectrum of survival strategies. For every successful infection by a microbe, the question is, how does it survive in

its particular location of the body? Part of the answer is known, but by no means all of it.

Host defenses do not operate in isolation but are interrelated. The strategies that microbes use to subvert them are correspondingly complex. Two types of strategies exist: **complement and phagocytosis**, which make up constitutive defenses, and **humoral and cellular immunity**, which make up induced defenses. A microbe invading a host that has not previously encountered it will meet these defenses in that order. Many microbial countermeasures are known from in vitro experimental situations, and it is not always possible to determine if they also operate in human disease. This is the subject of intensive research that has clear therapeutic and prophylactic implications.

One type of microbial defensive strategy is making, or appropriating from the host, a protective covering. For example, some microbes produce extracellular capsules that block recognition and binding by both complement and antibodies and prevent phagocytosis by leukocytes. This is the strategy of such important mucosal pathogens as the pneumococcus or the meningococcus. Notwithstanding their protective properties, these capsules are themselves immunogenic and antigenic and thus have become the basis of vaccines used to prevent pneumonia and meningitis. Another way that bacteria avoid immune recognition is by altering their surface antigens in a genetically programmed way. Certain pathogens, such as the gonococci or the salmonellae, can modify surface structures that are recognized by the immune system.

Many microbes survive in the body because they do not cause too much damage to the host. The best adapted of them cause no disease at all, elicit no inflammatory response, and actually are a help to the host by providing nutrients in the gastrointestinal tract (e.g., vitamin B$_{12}$) or crowding out potential pathogens (on the skin and mucosal surfaces). They may even stimulate the immune system to raise useful cross-protective antibodies (e.g., protection against meningococci may be the result of the colonization by related but nonpathogenic commensal species). Among the most successful pathogens are those that cause sexually transmitted diseases. In some cases, these bacteria cause minimal disease (e.g., chlamydial infection, gonorrhea), whereas in other cases, disease comes on slowly or as part of a chronic process (e.g., syphilis). When nonpathogenic strains cause trouble, it is a result of their getting into places they do not belong, such as when the mixed microbiota of the bowel gets into the peritoneal cavity with the rupture of an appendix.

In contrast, the occasional highly pathogenic invaders with their well-developed set of toxins and other virulence mechanisms cause significant acute damage and disease but may end up killing the host (thus biting the hand that feeds them). For example, dead-end processes like lethal meningitis do not, by themselves, promote bacterial survival or transmission to a new host.

DAMAGE

There are nearly as many kinds of damage as there are infectious diseases. The type and intensity of the damage depend on the tissues and organs affected, which makes it difficult to make generalizations. An important, if not intuitively obvious, point is that damage is not always caused by activities of the invading agent alone but is often the consequence of a vehement host response. What causes damage in an infection such as pneumonia caused by pneumococci? These organisms make no known toxins, and their invasion of the lung alveoli is manifested chiefly by the extensive production of pus in the affected sites. Pus is the result of acute inflammation, the outpouring of white blood cells and liquid from the circulation. As in many other infections, the symptoms of pneumonia are due mainly to a forceful host response. In chronic infections, such as tuberculosis, the symptoms of disease can almost invariably be ascribed to the host response, with the microbe being relatively passive but able to stimulate a host response that causes the symptoms of the disease.

Mechanisms of Direct Damage

Although damage from microbial infection is often the result of the immune response, microbes are not always just innocent bystanders. Some bacteria produce extracellular factors, broadly called toxins, that are directly responsible for tissue damage. Some of these, such as the toxins of botulism and tetanus, are among the strongest poisons known. These factors cause damage in various ways: some just help bacteria spread in tissues, others lyse host cells, yet others stop cell growth, and still others exaggerate normal physiological mechanisms. By depressing or augmenting particular functions, a toxin can kill a person without directly damaging any cells. No abnormal lesions result; rather, the toxin acts by causing hyperactivity of a normal process.

One of the most dramatic manifestations of infection is cell death. This comes about in a variety of ways: direct action of cytolytic toxins, activation of cell-killing white blood cells, or induction of programmed cell death. The damage caused by the death of tissue cells is most serious when it occurs in essential organs, such as the brain or the heart. It should be noted that in some serious and even life-threatening infectious diseases, cell death is not a distinctive feature even though the agents multiply intracellularly. In the prime example, tuberculosis, the infected cells survive, yet the infection results in far-reaching and pervasive damage. However, cell death is often a prominent feature, especially of acute infections.

With many of the common Gram-negative bacteria (see Chapter 3), the host response is elicited by a major component of their surface, a lipopolysaccharide known as **endotoxin**. In small amounts, endotoxin elicits fever and mobilizes certain defense mechanisms. In large amounts, it results in shock and intravascular coagulation. Thus, the host response to the presence of these bacteria depends on the **amount** of endotoxin present.

Immune Response

The immune response is complex and has multiple functions. Because of its complexity, the immune response can go awry in many ways and cause damage. **Innate immunity** refers to immune mechanisms that are always present and available for action. These responses tend to be less specific than acquired, adaptive immunity, but since they require no prior exposure to a pathogen to be active, they represent the first line against microbial invasion. Alternatively, **adaptive immune responses** are usually classified as humoral when they lead to the production of circulating antibodies or as cellular when special immune system cells seek out and destroy infected cells. Both responses can cause damage.

Humoral Immunity

Infecting agents elicit the formation of specific antibodies. In the circulation and tissues, antibodies combine with the infecting agents or with some of their soluble products. These antigen–antibody complexes evoke an inflammatory response by facilitating the activation of a complex set of serum proteins, the **complement system**. In the presence of antigen–antibody complexes, these proteins are activated by a series of proteolytic reactions, called the **classical pathway** of activation. The complement system can also be activated by the presence of microorganisms alone, through a process called the **alternative pathway**. The products of these proteolytic cleavages are pharmacologically active compounds. Some work on platelets and white cells to produce substances that increase vascular permeability and vasodilation. The result is edema, the outpouring of fluids into tissues. Other complement factors act on white blood cells, some as chemotaxins, others to make bacteria more easily phagocytized. These activities result in the mobilization of powerful defenses against invading microorganisms and inflammation.

Antigen–antibody complexes are sometimes deposited on the membrane of the glomeruli of the kidneys, resulting in impairment of kidney function, a condition called **glomerulonephritis**. This condition is seen in the aftermath of certain streptococcal and viral infections. Similar effects also take place in blood vessels, leading to visible skin rashes.

Cellular Immunity

A different type of response is expressed via special cells of the immune system and is called **cell-mediated immunity** (**CMI**). This complex phenomenon leads to the activation and mobilization of macrophages, the powerful phagocytic cells that participate in the later stages of inflammation to clean up debris and remaining microorganisms.

CMI is associated with chronic inflammation, the histological changes that limit the spread of infections but also cause lesions in tissues. These damaging activities are characteristic of chronic infections, often caused by intracellular microorganisms and viruses. An example is chronic tuberculosis, in which the main damage to tissue is caused by CMI. The immune response is elicited by the tubercle bacilli, which are able to persist in cells for a long time. Pathological changes associated with CMI lead to the production of **tubercles** or **granulomas** and eventually to destruction of tissue cells.

It is worth repeating that although the immune responses can cause tissue damage, in most instances, the price is well worth it. This point is illustrated in people who have genetic or acquired defects in their immune systems. Unfortunately, such people are no longer a medical rarity. The advent and spread of AIDS has placed hundreds of thousands of persons in this category. Immunocompromised patients are ravaged and later killed by microorganisms that cause little or no disease in healthy persons. In the immunocompetent person, for example, active tuberculosis causes much damage, but death only occurs after many years. In the immunocompromised patient, the disease can become rampant in a much shorter period.

OUTCOME

No infectious disease, be it mild or life threatening, is simple. Various properties of the invading agent and the host lead to an intricate and ever-changing interplay. It is not always possible to discern the relative roles of the known properties, let alone those that still await discovery. To complicate matters, humans are beset by a huge number of possible invaders. New ones emerge apparently under our very eyes, to be added to the long list.

CONCLUSION

The student of medical microbiology faces a demanding challenge. The fascination of the topic may not suffice to overcome its inherent problem of tremendous detail. The conceptual framework used in this chapter, which is based on the fact that all host–parasite interactions have steps in common, may be useful in mastering many of the details of microbiology. If these steps are kept in mind, the myriad facts will fall logically into place. As indicated at the beginning of this chapter, parasite and host must encounter one another, and the parasite must enter the host, spread, multiply, and eventually cause damage. All these steps require the breaching of host defenses.

When studying the pathogenesis of infectious diseases, it is essential to remember that the outcome of microbial infection is usually the net result of offensive measures taken by the microbe and counteroffensive measures taken by the host. To intervene and to change the natural outcome of infection, one must accomplish a combination of the three goals: diagnosis, treatment, and/or prevention of the infection. If infection cannot be prevented, it must be accurately diagnosed and specifically treated. For most of the infections described in this book, the natural outcome of infection is typically altered by our understanding of the relevant events and our ability to intervene successfully.

Suggested Readings

McNeill WH. Plagues and Peoples. Garden City, NY: Anchor Books; 1976.
Mims CA. The Pathogenesis of Infectious Diseases. 5th ed. New York: Academic Press; 2001.

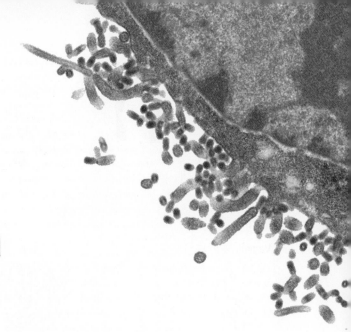

Chapter **2**

The Normal Microbiota

Barry I. Eisenstein, Moselio Schaechter, and Vincent Young

THE HUMAN body normally contains thousands of species of bacteria and a smaller number of archaea, viruses, fungi, and protozoa. Most coexist with humans without causing harm and in some cases provide great benefit. Thus, there is a **mutualistic** association where we benefit and—by having a niche in us—so do the microbes. The members of the normal microbiota change with time, but their number at any instant is still formidable. Each person possesses an individualized spectrum of species and strains. In the words of the Romans, *suum quique*, to each his own.

WHAT IS THE NORMAL MICROBIOTA?

Members of the normal microbiota are defined as microorganisms frequently found on or in the body of healthy persons (Fig. 2-1). Some of these organisms are found only in the bodies of humans or animals; others can also live freely in the environment.

A precise roll call of the organisms that constitute the normal microbiota is usually not possible, as discussed in Chapter 1. In fact, it appears that we collectively share a "core microbiota," and some of us harbor others that are perhaps more **transient**. Consider, for instance, the meningococcus or the pneumococcus, both true pathogens capable of causing meningitis, pneumonia, or septicemia. Coming and going as sporadic denizens of a person's throat, such organisms could be called transient members of the normal microbiota of that individual. Obviously, these pathogens do not usually cause trouble in most colonized individuals. Not as obvious is that disease caused by either of the two organisms does not occur without prior **colonization**. Thus, colonization is necessary, but insufficient, for meningococcal or pneumococcal disease. Long-term colonization is not a universal prerequisite for all infections, many of which develop soon after entry of the infectious agent into the body. An example is the common cold.

The problem with many of the definitions in this field is that they are not absolute. The same problems that arise in precisely identifying the normal microbiota pertain to terms such as **pathogenicity** and **virulence**. (These two terms are not identical, but the distinction between them is subtle.) As subsequent chapters will show, definitions of such terms depend not only on the properties of the infectious agent but also on the state of the defenses of the host. In addition, disease seldom results from the activities of the agent alone but often reflects the **responses of the host** as well. In many cases, the signs and symptoms of infection are actually caused by the host's inflammatory response to the infection. A good analogy: firefighters occasionally add to the property destruction resulting from a fire by producing water damage as they try to contain the flames.

In the human body, the most successful microbe is the one that can rapidly and efficiently become two microbes. In describing the nature of success among organisms, pathogenicity or virulence is not considered. In fact, the most virulent pathogens, those that kill their hosts, may be poorly adapted for survival and represent recent biological associations. After all, why would guests paying no rent want to set fire to the house in which they live? Before exploring the world of pathogens (the "misfits"), it is instructive to consider first the body's normal guests who behave well and even provide value to us—keeping in mind, though, that even the most domesticated among them can cause trouble if given the opportunity.

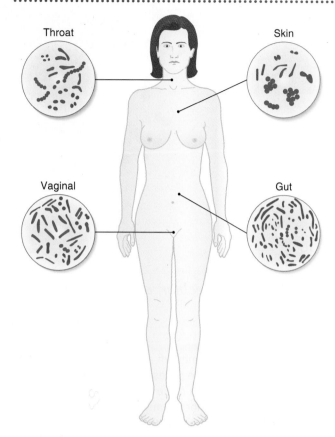

Throat

Skin

Vaginal

Gut

FIGURE 2-1. The normal bacterial microbiota in a healthy person. The typical bacteria seen in the microbe-laden sites of the body are shown in schematic fashion. Gram-positive bacteria are shown in purple, Gram-negative bacteria in red.

WHAT PARTS OF THE BODY ARE TYPICAL SITES?

Among the parts of the body colonized by the normal microbiota, the following usually contain large amounts of microorganisms:

Skin: moist areas especially, such as the groin and between the toes
Respiratory tract: nose and oropharynx
Digestive tract: mouth and large intestine
Urinary tract: anterior parts of the urethra
Genital system: vagina

Bacteria, and to a lesser extent fungi and protozoa, reside and actively proliferate at these sites. Other parts of the body contain small numbers of microorganisms, most of which are in transit and do not usually colonize. Examples include the rest of the respiratory and digestive tracts, the **urinary bladder**, and the **uterus**. Finding pathogenic microorganisms at these sites is highly suggestive of disease but not proof. At the other extreme are certain tissues and organs that are usually sterile. The presence of microorganisms at these sites is usually diagnostically significant. These sites include **blood, cerebrospinal fluid, synovial fluid**, and **deep tissues** in general.

The number of bacteria in sites that contain thriving microbial communities varies widely. In some areas, bacteria are almost as densely packed as is physically possible. For instance, the gingival pockets around teeth contain wall-to-wall bacteria. Normal feces are about one-third bacteria by weight. If the average bacterium were about 1 μm^3 in volume, the densest possible packing would result in a mass of 1×10^{12} per mL. Numbers like that are actually approached in certain parts of the body. In contrast, sites that are not quite as hospitable, such as the skin, mouth, and vagina, may harbor populations on the order of 1 to 10 million bacteria per milliliter of fluid or per gram of scrapings.

HOW DO MICROORGANISMS PERSIST IN THE BODY?

To colonize the human body, invading microorganisms must be able to resist host mechanisms that could dislodge or kill them, as well as compete successfully with other microbial species. Picture a bacterial cell entering the mouth and the problems it faces trying to remain there. Strong liquid currents will wash the organism away unless it adheres to the surface of the teeth or the mucous membranes. In addition, saliva contains antibacterial compounds, such as enzymes and antibodies, although these substances are not equally damaging toward all bacterial species. At sites of the mouth not exposed to the flushing action of saliva, such as the crevasses of the gums, the bacterial cell will find a large resident microbiota already occupying the likely adherence sites. These resident organisms also produce antimicrobial substances, such as acids derived from their metabolism of sugars that may be hostile to an incoming microbe.

Although certain body sites are normally extensively colonized, trouble from the microbes only occasionally occurs at these sites. One example is the pneumonia caused by respiratory defenses lowered by, say, a poor cough reflex following a stroke or by smoking-induced paralysis of the ciliary clearance mechanisms. Under these conditions, "aspiration pneumonia" is likely to occur. The bacteriologic etiology of such a pneumonia is highly dependent on the kinds of organisms that colonize the mouth or throat at the time of the aspiration. If the person is unlucky enough to be colonized with a virulent strain of pneumococcus, a small amount of material aspirated from the mouth or pharynx into the lungs is sufficient to cause severe pneumonia. In fact, most cases of pneumococcal pneumonia are not associated with obvious aspiration at all but rather with imperceptible microaspirations. If the oropharynx is not colonized with virulent bacteria, a significantly larger amount of aspirated material (i.e., a larger inoculum) must reach the lungs to cause disease.

Colonization involves both microbial and host factors. For example, an adhesive protein called **fibronectin** coats the mucosal surfaces of epithelial cells and has

TABLE 2-1 Issues in Bacterial Colonization

Anticolonizing Property of the Host	How Bacteria Overcome the Property
Sweep microbes away by liquid currents	Adhere to epithelial cells (e.g., gonococci stick to the mucous membrane of the urethra)
Kill microbes with host phagocytes	Avoid being taken up (e.g., the pneumococcus is surrounded by a slimy capsule that impairs uptake by neutrophils)
	Kill the phagocyte (e.g., certain streptococci produce a toxin that punches holes in the neutrophil membrane)
Starve microbes for lack of needed nutrients	Derive needed nutrients from host cells (e.g., certain staphylococci lyse red blood cells and use their nutrients hemoglobin as a source of iron)
Inhibit growth by secreting antimicrobial factors such as cationic peptides	Modify surface molecules (lipid A) to avoid cationic peptide binding

a strong predilection for Gram-positive organisms (see Chapter 3). Fibronectin is probably important in determining the nature of the bacterial microbiota in the mouth and pharynx, as suggested by the following findings. The oropharynx of individuals in poor general health, including many hospitalized patients, becomes deficient in fibronectin. With low levels of this protein, Gram-negative organisms tend to displace Gram-positives. The high incidence of Gram-negative pneumonia in hospitalized patients can be explained in part by adherence specificity.

The example of the mouth can be extended to the large intestine, vagina, perineum, skin, and other sites normally laden with microbes. It follows that colonization by new organisms is an unlikely event and that the successful colonizer must be unusually adept at resisting both host and microbial defenses. On the other hand, colonization of sites that are normally sterile or carry a sparse load of microorganisms (e.g., deep tissues and the small intestine) is not affected by microbial competition. Not surprisingly, host defenses are typically more intensive at such susceptible sites. Obviously, throughout our long history of coexistence and coevolution with the microbial world, our bodies have designated territories that are safe to share—preferably, only with well-behaved guests—and others that are off limits. Foreign devices, such as plastic catheters stuck into arteries and veins, are notorious for upsetting the delicate ecological balance between microbes and host tissues.

The attributes that permit microbes to colonize the body make a long list and, to a large extent, determine what makes each pathogenic organism distinct. Such attributes will be discussed in detail in the chapters on individual organisms. Table 2-1 lists the classes of microbial properties that allow successful colonization.

SITE PREFERENCES OF SOME INFECTIOUS AGENTS

At first glance, it may seem that microorganisms usually cause disease only in specific organs. To some extent, that statement is true: hepatitis viruses affect the liver; encephalitis and rabies viruses, the brain; and the common cold viruses, the nasal epithelium. Some bacteria, like the cholera bacillus, have strong predilections (the small intestine, in this case), whereas others, like the *staphylococcus*, may infect almost any site of the body. Such preferences are known as **tissue tropism**. In some cases, tissue tropism can be attributed to tissue-specific cellular properties, such as the presence of specific receptors on the surfaces of certain cells (e.g., fibronectin, with its affinity for Gram-positive bacteria). In other instances, physical properties—the temperature of the organ, for instance—determine the tropism.

The complexities of tissue tropism can be illustrated using the gonococcus as an example. This bacterium most often causes infection of the urethra, but it can also affect the throat, rectum, or eyes. Where the lesion occurs in this disease depends on the **site of entry** of the organism. Pharyngeal and rectal gonorrhea are the result of nonvaginal intercourse, whereas ophthalmia (eye infection) is caused by the infection of the eyes of a neonate as it passes through the birth canal of the infected mother. Thus, the gonococcus has no absolute predilection for the mucous membrane of a given organ. What about tissue other than mucosal epithelia? Some strains of gonococci survive in circulation and show a marked predilection for certain organs, such as the joints. Gonococcal arthritis is one of the most common complications of gonorrhea. Therefore, it is clear that gonococci have strong tropism for certain deep tissues, not only for epithelial membranes.

Affinity for host cell receptors is seen clearly in viruses and may explain why, in general, these agents are often tissue and organ specific. Influenza virus, for example, relies for its attachment on special glycoproteins found on the surface of respiratory epithelial cells. HIV, the virus that causes AIDS, attaches to protein receptors found selectively on certain lymphocytes and macrophages. Many research efforts, particularly in novel forms of antiviral therapy, are aimed at discovering ways to neutralize the action of receptors, thereby precluding infection by the agents that recognize them.

The temperature of an organ sometimes determines the location of the infectious agent. For example, the viruses of the common cold thrive in the nasal epithelium and not in internal organs, where high temperatures inhibit the viruses' growth. Likewise, the spirochete of syphilis is sensitive to higher-than-normal body temperatures, which induced certain physicians of the preantibiotic era to try to cure syphilis by injecting patients with the agent of malaria. Another example is the fungus that causes athlete's foot, which is confined to the skin because it does not grow at body temperature (athlete's foot of the liver is impossible).

ROLE OF THE NORMAL MICROBIOTA

The normal microbiota plays a critical role in health and disease, as illustrated by the following examples.

Common Source of Infection

Notwithstanding the benefits provided to us by our microbiota, when its constituent organisms find themselves in unaccustomed sites of the body, they may cause disease. For example, anaerobic bacteria, usually of the genus *Bacteroides*, are carried harmlessly in the intestines of normal persons, where they provide some of the capacity for us to digest complex polysaccharides. But they produce abscesses if they penetrate into deeper tissues via traumatic or surgical wounds. When *Bacteroides*-carrying fecal contents are spilled in the peritoneal cavity, as in the case of a burst appendix, the consequences can be dire. Staphylococci from the skin and nose, or streptococci and Gram-negative cocci from the throat and mouth, are also responsible for this class of infections. In fact, *Staphylococcus epidermidis*, a prevalent species on the skin, has a strong propensity to attach to plastic prosthetic surfaces and can thus cause severe bloodstream infections in patients with intravenous catheters. Likewise, *Escherichia coli*, a normal inhabitant of the gastrointestinal tract, is the most common cause of urinary tract infection. In fact, physicians see more patients with diseases resulting from the normal microbiota than from agents acquired outside the body.

These facts point out that the definition of virulence is elusive and that no microorganism is intrinsically either benign or pathogenic. Under the right circumstances, any microorganism that can grow in the body can cause disease. However, members of the normal microbiota do not all have the same pathogenic potential. Some cause disease more readily than others because they are endowed with special virulence properties. For example, when peritonitis is caused by the release of intestinal bacteria through a break in the gut wall, the resulting infection is usually caused by only a few bacterial species.

Virulence is not intrinsic to the microorganisms but depends also on the degree of immune competence of the host. Members of the normal microbiota often invade organs and tissues in immunocompromised patients. Thus, the yeast *Candida*, a harmless commensal found in about one-third of all healthy people, is a common cause of bloodstream infection in patients undergoing vigorous cancer chemotherapy. *Pneumocystis carinii*, a common inhabitant of the lungs of healthy persons, can cause a specific kind of pneumonia and is one of the principal causes of death in patients with AIDS.

Immune Stimulation

Our repertoire of antibodies (immunoglobulins) partly reflects antigenic stimulation by the normal microbiota. In general, we do not have high antibody titers to the bacteria, viruses, and fungi that inhabit our body. Nonetheless, even in low concentrations, our antibodies serve as a defense mechanism, a clear benefit from our normal microbiota. Among the antibodies produced in response to bacterial stimulation are those of the IgA class, which are secreted through mucous membranes. Although the role of these immunoglobulins is not well understood, they likely are an important first line of defense and interfere, possibly on a daily basis, with the colonization of commensal organisms in deeper tissues.

Antibodies elicited by the antigenic challenge of the normal microbiota sometimes cross-react with normal tissue components. Relevant examples are antibodies against ABO blood group antigens. People that belong to the A group have anti-B antibodies, and conversely, B-group individuals have anti-A antibodies. People in the O group make both anti-A and anti-B antibodies. None of these antibodies is found in the newborn. What is the source of antigenic stimulation for these antibodies? On reflection, the source is not obvious. Why should one make antibodies against a blood group different from one's own? Few of us come in contact with red blood cells of a different type, through transfusions of the wrong type of blood. The answer to this puzzle is that bacteria from the intestinal microbiota contain antigens that cross-react with both A and B blood antigens. These constituents are the source of antigenic stimulation. We make antibodies against foreign blood group antigens but not against those of our own group because we are immunologically tolerant to the "self" antigens but not to the "foreign" ones.

This type of **cross-reactivity** does not usually cause disease. In fact, some evidence demonstrates that cross-reactivity between bacterial antigens can be protective. For example, antibodies against various bacteria that normally reside in the bowel have been shown to cross-react with the polysaccharide capsule of meningitis-producing strains of meningococci; the presence of the antibodies is protective against this form of bacterial meningitis. By contrast, it is possible for antibodies cross-reactive to microbial antigens to play an insidiously harmful role in health. For instance, the serious disease systemic lupus erythematosus is associated with the production of antibodies against the body's DNA. Some evidence suggests that the antigens setting off the production of these antibodies are not nucleic acids but may be cross-reacting bacterial lipopolysaccharides.

In addition to the antigenic stimulation, the microbiota also plays a critical role in other aspects of immune system development. Much of our knowledge in this area comes from analyzing germfree animals (typically mice). These animals have poorly developed spleens and lymphoid tissue. Further, specific T helper cells, Th17 cells responsible for regulating mucosal immunity against microbial infection, depend on commensal microbes in order to differentiate (T helper subsets will be described in more detail in Chapter 6). Finally, the importance of just a single molecule from the normal microbiota was also demonstrated by experiments with germfree mice. Animals colonized by the commensal organism *Bacteroides fragilis* expressing a wild-type polysaccharide structure developed a healthy immune system. However, animals colonized with a polysaccharide mutant of *B. fragilis* had decreased numbers of splenic T cells, atypical thymus development, and aberrant Th1 cytokine responses.

Keeping Out Invaders

In some sites of the body, the normal microbiota helps keep out pathogens. Commensal bacteria have the physical advantage of **previous occupancy**, especially on epithelial surfaces. Some commensal bacteria produce substances that inhibit newcomers, such as antibiotics or lethal proteins called bacteriocins. It is not surprising, therefore, that colonization by a new species or a new strain is not a frequent event. As a counter to this, some enteric pathogens stimulate an inflammatory response that they can withstand and even thrive in but which diminishes the normal microbiota. This reduces occupancy of sites on the intestinal mucosa and enables the pathogen to gain a foothold.

When the normal microbiota is wiped out with antibiotics, both exogenous and endogenous microorganisms are given the opportunity to cause disease. For example, after mice are given certain antibiotics, the infecting oral dose of a *Salmonella* strain decreases almost a millionfold. Patients treated with antibiotics that are particularly effective in the gut may suffer from diarrhea caused by toxins produced from the overgrowth of a particular organism, *Clostridium difficile*. Severe infections with this bacterium result in a serious disease called pseudomembranous colitis (see Chapter 20). This organism is a minor member of the normal microbiota but can grow to a large population density when its neighbors are suppressed.

Role in Human Nutrition and Metabolism?

The normal microbiota of the intestine plays a role in human nutrition and metabolism, with the extent of its influence being extrapolated again from experiments done in animals. Obviously, humans cannot be made "germfree" at will, so most of our knowledge comes from work with animals. It is increasingly clear that the huge and metabolically active biomass residing in the large intestine plays a role in the nutritional balance of the host. Digestion of complex polysaccharides is carried out by our microbiota, and several intestinal bacteria, such as *E. coli* and *Bacteroides*, synthesize vitamin K and thus may be important sources of that vitamin for human beings and animals.

The metabolism of several key compounds involves their excretion from the liver into the large intestine and their return from there to the liver. This enterohepatic circulatory loop is particularly important for sex steroid hormones and bile salts. The compounds are excreted through the bile in conjugated form as glucuronides or sulfate but cannot be reabsorbed in that form. Members of the intestinal bacterial microbiota make glucuronidases and sulfatases that deconjugate the compounds. The extent to which these activities are physiologically important is not yet known, but they have prompted some to call the large intestine a "second liver."

Our knowledge of the metabolic capacity of the microbiota is increasing significantly through the application of DNA sequencing technology and the bioinformatics tools needed to make sense of the sequence data. The genomes of the microbiota are collectively termed the **microbiome**. From analyzing the complex collection of genomes present in the gut, it is becoming evident that the microbiome constitutes an "accessory genome" with coding capacity for many more metabolic pathways than our own genomes have.

Good and Bad Conversion of Ingested Compounds

Compounds we ingest may be chemically transformed by the varied metabolic activities of the gut microbiota. Some compounds become **carcinogens** only after being modified, which can occur through the action of microbiota in the large intestine. For example, the artificial sweetener cyclamate (cyclohexamine sulfate) is converted to the active bladder carcinogen cyclohexamine by bacterial sulfatases. Evidence does implicate the normal microbiota as a risk factor for some cancers, but the importance is difficult to assess; consequently, this is a subject of considerable scrutiny (Box 2-1). On the other hand, the microbiota also detoxifies some potential carcinogens by degrading them. Nitrosamines found in some processed foods, or generated from the use of nitrite to cure foods, can be broken down by the action of the microbiota. Similarly, carcinogenic heterocyclic amines—which can be present in cooked meat—are acted on by the normal microbiota and made less toxic.

HOW DO WE STUDY THE NORMAL MICROBIOTA?

Traditionally, our knowledge of the role of the normal microbiota in nutrition and prevention of disease has come from studying animals reared under sterile conditions—the so-called germfree animals. Rats and mice resemble humans in many physiological properties but differ in important details. Nonetheless, germfree-animal research has produced interesting information.

A small mammal can be reared in the germfree condition if it is placed in a sterile chamber after a cesarean birth. Chickens can be hatched from eggs whose shell surfaces have been sterilized. The germfree chamber is equipped with gloves and ports to allow manipulation and the exchange of food and other material without breaking the sterile barrier. Many species of animals breed under these conditions, and large colonies can be established. It is even possible to obtain germfree rats and mice from commercial suppliers.

In general, rodents thrive under germfree conditions as long as their diets are supplemented with vitamins. They even gain weight faster than do conventional animals. As expected, a germfree rodent's concentration of immunoglobulins is reduced, especially if its diet is chemically defined and does not contain antigenic compounds. One of the more interesting characteristics of germfree animals is that the histology of their intestines is quite different. The most visible difference is in the lamina propria, which has only a few lymphocytes, plasma cells, and macrophages. By contrast, in conventional animals, the same tissue is heavily infiltrated with these cells. This finding suggests that the "normal" intestine is in a constant state of chronic inflammation.

Investigators are applying principles of microbial ecology to study the diversity and community structure of various sites in the human body. The approach is to collect samples from the most heavily colonized sites—nose, mouth, gut, vagina, and skin—and carry out massive sequencing analysis. Bioinformatics methods of this **metagenome** sequencing data enables the placement of the sequences into taxonomical units without the need to culture the constituent organisms. This "Human Microbiome Project" aims to catalogue the microbiota of these sites in individuals over time to determine the healthy state, and then to correlate this state with changes in the microbiota that occur in various disease states, including in metabolic disorders, inflammatory bowel disease, and other poorly understood chronic conditions.

MEMBERS OF THE NORMAL MICROBIOTA

What types of microorganisms constitute the normal microbiota? Most are bacteria. We also carry viruses, fungi, protozoa, and occasionally worms, but in the healthy person, these microorganisms are present in smaller numbers than are the bacteria. In the early days of microbiology, it was thought that most bacteria of the body were aerobes or facultative anaerobes. For a long time, *E. coli* was believed to be one of the principal members of the fecal microbiota. This erroneous conclusion was based on the observation that most members of the normal bacteria microbiota are strict anaerobes and do not grow on media incubated in the ordinary manner in air. Only by using special techniques of anaerobic cultivation has it been realized that in the gingival pocket or in feces, strict anaerobes outnumber the others by 100 to 1 or more. Bacteria do not have to be located far from the air to find anaerobic conditions, because oxygen is not very soluble in water. Furthermore, the small amount of oxygen that diffuses into deeper tissue layers can readily be used by host cells or by actively metabolizing aerobes and facultative anaerobes. Thus, anaerobic conditions can be found a fraction of a millimeter below the surface.

Table 2-2 shows the distribution and occurrence of prominent bacteria in selected parts of the human body. It should be understood that the organisms listed, although the most frequently encountered, represent only a minute fraction of the number of genera and species represented. In the gut alone, the number of species in an individual is certainly in the hundreds and perhaps in the thousands. When counted by culture-based methods, 300 to 500 species are estimated, but data from metagenome and other culture-independent analyses indicate that the culture-based estimates are low by perhaps a factor of 10. One estimate suggests that the collective human gut microbiota—counting all the species that can colonize humans—numbers in the tens of thousands.

Newborn babies become colonized very rapidly by a varied microbial microbiota, especially in their intestines. In animals and probably in humans, organisms appear according to a specific time sequence. The earliest colonizers are *E. coli*, streptococci, and some clostridia. Within 24 hours or so, lactobacilli appear, followed within a few

TABLE 2-2 Frequent Types of Normal Bacterial Microbiota

| Site | Gram-Positive | | Gram-Negative | | Other |
	Cocci	Rods	Cocci	Rods	
Skin	*Staphylococcus*	*Corynebacterium, Propionibacterium acnes*	—	Enteric bacilli (on some sites)	—
Oropharynx	α-Hemolytic streptococci, *Micrococcus*	*Corynebacterium*	*Neisseria*	*Haemophilus*	Spirochetes
Large intestine	*Streptococcus* (enterococci)	*Lactobacillus, Clostridium*	—	*Bacteroides,* enteric bacilli	—
Vagina	*Streptococcus*	*Lactobacillus*	—	*Bacteroides*	*Mycoplasma*

days by the major anaerobes that characterize the normal intestinal microbiota.

Little is known about why species vary in their colonizing capacity and in their ability to compete with others. It seems likely that specific properties of bacteria, such as their pili, allow them to attach and survive in various microenvironments within the intestine. Thus, the microbiota is different at the base of the intestinal crypts, in the mucus that covers the villi, and in the lumen of the gut. Normally, the intestinal microbiota of one individual is remarkably constant, although this can change with antibiotic use or in certain disease states. This stability suggests that successful colonizers are equipped with powerful devices to withstand the challenge from newly ingested microorganisms.

CONCLUSION

Our knowledge about the role of the normal microbiota in health and disease is derived largely from studies with germfree animals and observation of patients on antibiotics. As we apply the principles and methods of microbial ecology to understanding the microbiota, as well as powerful sequencing and bioinformatics techniques, we are acquiring a better sense of the structure of our microbiota in health and disease. These microbes contribute significantly to maintenance of health through a variety of mechanisms: they keep out potential invaders, stimulate normal development of both local and systemic immunity, and provide a source of antigens to train the immune system. In addition, our nutritional capability is greatly expanded by hosting a large and complex microbiota. Alternatively, some members of the normal microbiota are opportunistic pathogens and may cause disease when present in tissues and organs that are not typically colonized. We cannot live in a germfree environment, and the organisms that colonize us depend on us for their survival. Consequently, it is not surprising that our microbiota has evolved to provide us a great deal of benefit.

Suggested Readings

Gonzalez A, Clemente JC, Shade A, et al. Our microbial selves: what ecology can teach us. *EMBO Rep.* 2011;12:775–784.

Relman DA. Microbial genomics and infectious diseases. *N Engl J Med.* 2011;365:347–357.

Sekirov I, Russell SL, Antunes LC, et al. Gut microbiota in health and disease. *Physiol Rev.* 2010;90:859–904.

Turnbaugh PJ, Ley RE, Hamady M, et al. The Human Microbiome Project. *Nature.* 2007;449:804–810.

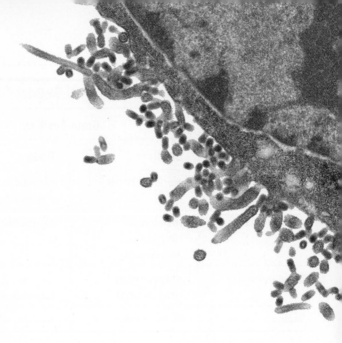

Chapter **3**

Biology of Infectious Agents

Moselio Schaechter

WHAT DO FUTURE health practitioners want to know about microbes? Mainly, how pathogenic microbes harm the host and what can be done about it. Knowing this requires more than understanding how microbes cause disease. For example, features of bacterial anatomy and metabolism have suggested targets for the successful development of powerful antibiotics. Similarly, unraveling the details of viral structures and metabolism has led to the production of protective vaccines and to antiviral therapy.

PROKARYOTIC AND EUKARYOTIC PATHOGENS

The world of pathogenic microbiology spans a large cleft in the living world—the one between the prokaryotes and the eukaryotes. Bacteria belong to the prokaryotes, whereas fungi, protozoa, and worms are eukaryotes. Prokaryotes lack nuclei and other internal membrane-bound organelles. They do not carry out endocytosis and are incapable of ingesting particles or liquid droplets. Prokaryotes differ from eukaryotes in important biochemical details, such as the composition of their ribosomes and lipids (Fig. 3-1). Prokaryotes are usually haploid, with a single chromosome and extrachromosomal plasmids; most eukaryotes have a diploid phase and many chromosomes. Microbes in a third domain of life distinct from bacteria, the Archaea, are also single celled and lacking in nuclei and internal organelles. But archaea of medical importance have yet to be identified.

Differences in organization between prokaryotes and eukaryotes have important consequences for the way they synthesize certain macromolecules. For instance, the lack of a nuclear membrane allows prokaryotes to simultaneously synthesize proteins and messenger RNA (mRNA) molecules. In other words, **translation** (protein synthesis) can be coupled to **transcription** and therefore begin rapidly on new mRNA chains. In eukaryotes, the two processes cannot be directly linked.

Transcripts of heterogeneous nuclear RNA must first be processed in the nucleus before they are transported across the nuclear membrane to the ribosomes in the cytoplasm. Only then can eukaryotic protein synthesis take place.

Table 3-1 compares the regulation of gene expression between *Escherichia coli*, a bacterium, and the best known of the unicellular eukaryotes, a yeast. A review of basic biochemistry and molecular biology may be appropriate to understand this material.

PROBLEMS OF LIVING FREELY

Unicellular free-living organisms, such as bacteria and yeasts, face constant challenges in their environment. The demands made on microbes fall into three general categories: **nutrition**, related to the intermittent availability of food; **occupancy**, related to the need to remain in a certain habitat; and **resistance** to damaging agents.

Feast or Famine

Frequently in their existence, microbes run out of nutrients. Consider a bacterium that lives in the large intestine of humans. Every so often, some 20 times a day on average, the ileocecal valve opens and nutrient-rich contents squirt from the small intestine into the cecum. There a large bacterial microbiota rapidly consumes

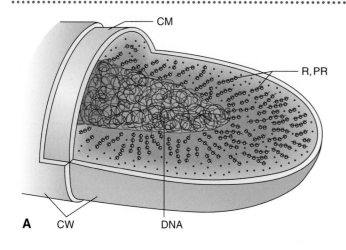

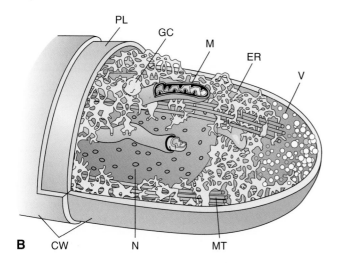

FIGURE 3-1. Ultrastructure of typical bacterial and fungal cells.
A. Inside the cell wall (CW) and membrane (CM), a bacterium is filled with ribosomes (R), polyribosomes (PR), and proteins. DNA fibrils cluster near the center of the cell in a coiled mass. **B.** The cell wall (CW) and plasmalemma (PL) of a hyphal tip surround the Golgi complex (GC), mitochondria (M), vacuoles (V), endoplasmic reticulum (ER), microtubules (MT), and nucleus (N) characteristic of the eukaryotic cell.

the nutrients, but soon, the bacteria are once again deprived of food. Clearly, the bacteria normally present at this site have adapted to a life of feast and famine. On the one hand, they can rapidly utilize nutritional substrates when they become available and compete efficiently with their microbial neighbors. On the other hand, the bacteria have adapted to the lack of nutrients during periods of starvation and are poised for action whenever nutrients again become plentiful. Two themes emerge in the evolution of such organisms: **efficiency** and **adaptability**. How these two properties are manifested in bacteria is discussed later in the chapter.

Colonization and Occupancy

Not all problems in the microbial world are nutritional. In certain environments, such as the intestinal tract, survival depends on being able to remain in a given place and avoid being swept away by liquid currents. Many species of bacteria ensure their occupancy by using mechanisms designed to stick to surfaces. For instance, bacteria attach to the surface of teeth by elaborating adhesive polysaccharides. When polysaccharides build up sufficiently, they form dental plaque (also known as a **biofilm**). Likewise, in the intestine, the abundant microbial flora that adheres to the epithelial wall is different from the one that lives free in the lumen. Because the "wall" microbiota faces different nutritional problems from the "lumen" microbiota, the selective pressures on these two populations are very different.

Resistance to Damaging Agents

Microbes often encounter chemical or physical agents that threaten their existence. Not unexpectedly, microbes have evolved mechanisms to cope with these life-threatening challenges. Among the better studied are structural devices and physiological responses that protect microbes (up to a point) from such environmental insults as membrane-damaging chemicals, heat, and DNA-damaging radiation. Microbes also use genetic strategies to withstand antibiotics and can develop resistance to insulting substances in many ways (see Chapter 5). Attempts to rid tissues of pathogenic organisms through the use of antibiotics are counteracted by the mechanisms developed by the organisms to thwart those efforts.

SMALL SIZE AND METABOLIC EFFICIENCY

The microbial world is composed of small entities, generally below the range of what the unaided human eye can see. Consequently, large numbers can be packed in small volumes. A typical bacterium is of the order of 1 μm in diameter, and, if it were shaped like a tiny block that could be neatly stacked, 10^{12} bacteria would occupy 1 cubic centimeter and weigh about 1 g. In suspension, the turbidity contributed by such small particles is so minimal that a clear fluid like urine becomes visibly cloudy only when bacteria exceed about 1 to 10 million per milliliter. Each of us currently carries a load of some **10 to 100 trillion** bacteria in the large intestine, greatly surpassing the number of eukaryotic cells.

Being small allows microbes to have high metabolic rates because the surface-to-volume ratio increases as the size of cells decreases. Ultimately, the rate of biochemical reactions is limited by diffusion; the smaller the cells, the less limiting is diffusion. Consequently, bacteria are in intimate contact with external nutrients and are capable of metabolic rates orders of magnitude higher than those of eukaryotic cells. They can grow extremely fast, and some

TABLE 3-1 Transcription and Processing of Messenger RNA (mRNA) in Typical Prokaryotes and Eukaryotes

Characteristic	*Escherichia Coli* (Prokaryote)	Yeast (Eukaryote)
Genomic Structure		
Genome organization	Single gene copies	Single gene copies plus repetitive DNA
Chromosomes	One	Many
Ploidy	Haploid	Haploid/diploid cycle
Cytoplasmic DNA	Plasmids	Mitochondria, kinetoplasts
Colinearity of gene with mRNA	Precise sequence	Introns within gene
Regulation of Gene Expression		
Type	Operon-polycistronic mRNA	Single genes
Level	Mostly transcriptional	Often posttranscriptional regulation by protein turnover, etc.
Transcription		
Relation of transcription and translation	Coupled	Uncoupled
mRNA processing	Rare; some cleavages at double-stranded functional domains	Poly(A) at 3′ end, cap at 5′ end; splicing, sites in mRNA
mRNA stability	Unstable	Range of stability; some very stable mRNAs
Translation of mRNA		
First amino acid	Formylated methionine	Methionine
Signal for start	Ribosome binding site preceding AUG codon	Binding to 5′ end, use of first AUG codon along mRNA
Initiation factors	Three	More than six
Ribosomes	30S + 50S = 70S	40S + 60S = 80S

mRNA, messenger RNA.

double once every 20 minutes under optimal conditions. One measure of the rapidity of the metabolic flux of bacteria is that small metabolites (amino acids, sugars, and nucleotides—the building blocks of macromolecules) constitute only about 1% of their total dry weight. Some eukaryotic microbes, such as yeasts and other fungi, have comparable efficiency.

The amazing speed with which these small cells convert nutrients into energy and biosynthetic building blocks requires the coordination of metabolic activities. Features of cell structure and macromolecular synthesis help us understand how individual species of bacteria maximize their chances for survival and suggest how we can intervene therapeutically against pathogenic organisms and anticipate their defenses.

COMPLEX ENVELOPES AND APPENDAGES

Going from the outside inward, bacteria are surrounded by a complex set of surface layers and appendages that differ in composition from species to species. Some of these structures are useful only in certain environments, such as the human body, and may be dispensable under laboratory conditions. These surface components often determine whether an organism can survive in a particular environment and cause disease.

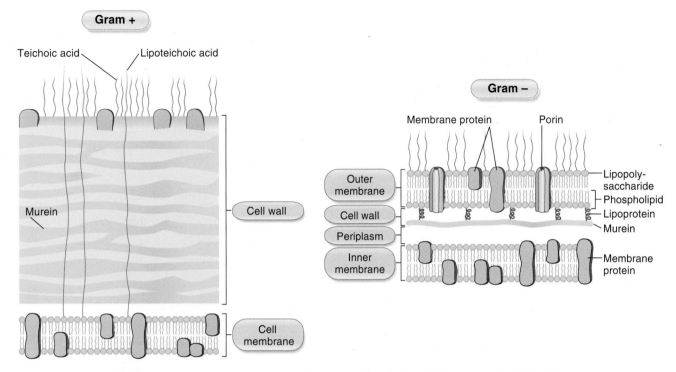

FIGURE 3-2. The envelope structure of Gram-positive (left) and Gram-negative (right) bacteria. Capsules and appendages are not shown, nor are surface proteins like the M protein of streptococci. Note the 20-fold greater amount of peptidoglycan, or murein, in the Gram-positive. The outer membrane of the Gram-negative envelope has a covering of lipopolysaccharide (LPS) molecules. The Gram-negative's outer membrane also has pores made of trimers of porin, which permit the entry of small hydrophilic molecules.

Like all cells, bacteria have an essential structure, the **cytoplasmic membrane**. Most bacteria also possess structures outside the membrane—namely, a **cell wall**—and some have an **outer membrane**, **flagella**, **pili**, and a **capsule**. These outer structures can amount to 10 to 20% of the dry weight of the cell (as in other organisms, the wet weight of bacteria is about two-thirds water). The reason for the extra layers outside the cell membrane becomes clear if one considers the stresses that bacteria must face in natural surroundings. For example, intestinal bacteria such as *E. coli* are exposed to bile salts that would dissolve an unprotected cell membrane. Bacteria use envelope layers and appendages to adhere to surfaces and for protection from phagocytes and other threats.

During colonization by microbes, the immune system of the host first senses the surface components of the invading microbes. Consequently, many of the properties of the surface constituents are relevant both to the establishment of infection and to the response of the host to the organisms. The strongest antibody response to bacterial antigens is usually directed to surface antigens.

PROTECTION OF THE CYTOPLASMIC MEMBRANE

Bacteria use three principal means to protect their cytoplasmic membrane from environmental stresses, such as low osmotic pressure or the presence of detergents.

These solutions are represented by the **Gram-positive**, **Gram-negative**, and **acid-fast** bacteria. Figure 3-2 illustrates the first two.

Gram staining (named after Dr. H. C. J. Gram, the Danish microbiologist who devised the method in 1884) divides most bacteria into two groups, nearly equal in number and importance. The staining procedure is central in microbiology and, in due course, should be learned by every medical student. In brief, Gram staining depends on the ability of certain bacteria (the Gram-positives) to retain a complex of a purple dye and iodine when challenged with a brief alcohol wash (Table 3-2). Gram-negatives do not retain the dye and can therefore be counterstained after the alcohol wash with a red dye, safranin. This distinction turns out to be correlated with fundamental differences in the cell envelopes of the two classes of bacteria.

Gram-Positive Solution

A Gram-positive bacterium protects its cytoplasmic membrane with a thick **cell wall**. The major constituent of the wall is a complex polymer **unique to bacteria**, composed of sugars and amino acids called **murein**, or **peptidoglycan** (Fig. 3-3). Murein is the critical component in maintaining the shape and rigidity of both Gram-positives and Gram-negatives but plays a larger role in protecting the cell membranes of Gram-positives.

How does murein contribute to the defense of cell integrity? Murein is composed of glycan (sugar) chains that

TABLE 3-2 Gram Stain and Acid-Fast Procedures

Gram Stain	Acid-Fast Stain
1. Stain with crystal violet (purple)	1. Stain with hot carbol–fuchsin (red)
2. Modify with potassium iodide	2. Decolorize with acid alcohol; only acid-fast remain red.
3. Decolorize with alcohol; only Gram-positives remain purple.	3. Counterstain with methylene blue: Acid-fast remain red; others become blue.
4. Counterstain with safranin: Gram-negatives become pink; Gram-positives remain purple.	

are cross-linked to one another via peptides. The overall structure of murein is similar in all cases, but some variation in chemical details occurs (Fig. 3-4). This polymeric fabric is wrapped around the length and width of the bacterium to form a sac of the size and shape of the organism. Depending on the shape of the murein sac, bacteria may be shaped like rods (**bacilli**), spheres (**cocci**), or helices (**spirilla**). The rigid murein corset allows bacteria to survive in media of lesser osmotic pressure than that of their cytoplasm. In the absence of a rigid structure to push against, the membrane bursts and the cells lyse. This can be demonstrated experimentally by removing the murein with **lysozyme**, a murein-hydrolytic enzyme present in many human and animal tissues. Treatment with lysozyme causes bacteria to lyse in a low-osmotic-pressure environment. If lysozyme-treated bacteria are kept in an isoosmotic medium, they do not lyse but become spherical. Such structures are called **spheroplasts**.

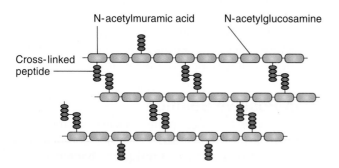

FIGURE 3-3. Structure of murein. The polysaccharide (glycan) strands consist of alternating units of *N*-acetylglucosamine and *N*-acetylmuramic acid connected to a peptide. Some of the peptides of one strand are cross-linked to those of another. Because of cross-linking, murein has a two-dimensional structure resembling a chain-linked fence.

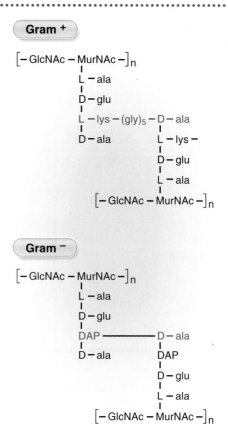

FIGURE 3-4. Typical composition of murein in Gram-positive and Gram-negative bacteria. In Gram-positives, peptide chains are cross-linked through a peptide (a pentaglycine in *Staphylococcus aureus*) between the free amino group of lysine and the terminal carboxyl group of a D-alanine residue. In the Gram-negatives, the cross-link is between diaminopimelic acid and D-alanine.

The cell wall of a Gram-positive is composed of many layers of the saclike murein. The layers are so thick that they impede the passage of hydrophobic compounds. The reason for this is that the sugars and charged amino acids of murein make the highly polar structure surrounding these cells a dense hydrophilic layer. Thus, many Gram-positives can withstand certain noxious hydrophobic compounds, including bile salts in the intestine. (The feature that makes bacteria Gram-positive—the ability to retain the dye–iodine complex—also seems to depend on the characteristic murein structure of the Gram-positive wall.)

Gram-positive walls contain other unique polymers, such as **teichoic acids**, which are chains of ribitol or glycerol linked by phosphodiester bonds (Fig. 3-5). Teichoic acids will be discussed in connection with individual groups of bacteria because some of these acids appear to play a role in pathogenesis.

Gram-Negative Solution

Gram-negatives have adopted a radically different solution to the problem of protection of the cytoplasmic membrane. These bacteria build a completely different

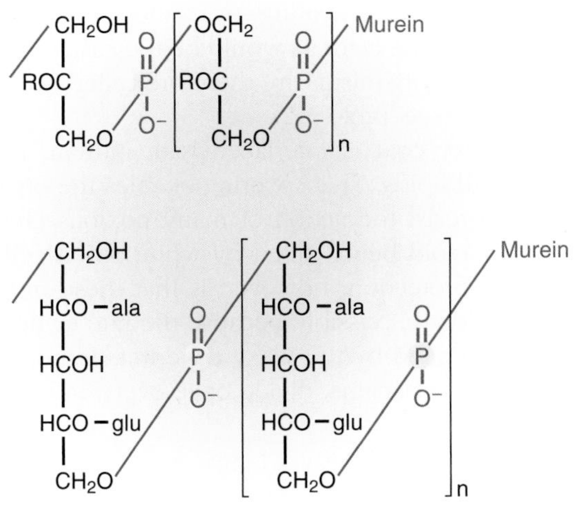

FIGURE 3-5. Teichoic acid structure. The repeating units of ribitol and glycerol teichoic acids are shown. The chains in Gram-positive organisms vary in length and amounts.

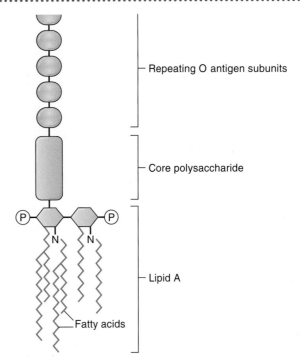

FIGURE 3-6. The structure of LPS. LPS consist of three portions. Lipid A is a phosphorylated disaccharide to which fatty acids are attached. The fatty acids vary with the organism but are always responsible for the hydrophobicity of the molecule. In a typical *Salmonella*, region I shows a characteristic series of sugars in the polysaccharide: the core polysaccharide, which consists of a variable and an invariant portion, and the O antigen, made up of repeating sugar subunits. Highly variable, the O antigen is the main reason for the different antigenic specificities among Gram-negative bacteria.

structure, an **outer membrane**, outside the murein cell wall (see Fig. 3-2). The outer membrane is chemically distinct from the usual biological membranes and is able to resist damaging chemicals. It is a bilayered structure, but its outer leaflet contains a unique component in addition to phospholipids. This component is a bacterial **lipopolysaccharide** (**LPS**), a complex molecule not found elsewhere in nature and one that deserves further attention.

LPS has three components (Fig. 3-6):

- **Lipid A**: This lipid anchors LPS in the outer leaflet of the membrane. Lipid A is an unusual glycolipid composed of disaccharides to which are attached short-chain fatty acids and phosphate groups.
- **Core**: This component consists of a short series of sugars that are nearly the same in most Gram-negative bacteria and includes two characteristic sugars, **keto-deoxyoctanoic acid** and a **heptose**.
- **O antigen**: This is a long carbohydrate chain of up to 40 sugars in length. The hydrophilic carbohydrate chains of the O antigen cover the bacterial surface and exclude hydrophobic compounds. The importance of the O-antigen chains is shown with mutants deficient in their biosynthesis. Mutants that make either no O antigen or merely shortened chains become sensitive to hydrophobic compounds such as bile salts and antibiotics to which the wild type is resistant.

Thus, exclusion of hydrophobic compounds in Gram-negative bacteria, as in Gram-positive bacteria, relies on surrounding the cells with hydrophilic polysaccharides, although these polysaccharides differ in structure and organization in the two groups. Because of its lipid nature, the outer membrane of Gram-negatives could be expected to exclude hydrophilic compounds as well. If so, nothing could cross the membrane. However,

by dealing with the problem of protecting the cytoplasmic membrane, the Gram-negative bacteria appear to have created a new one. How do they transport their nutrients? One possible solution would be to use the same active transport devices of the cytoplasmic membrane copied in the outer membrane. However, this not only would be wasteful but also probably would be incompatible with the protective role assigned to the outer membrane. Once again, bacteria have found an interesting solution. The outer membrane has special **channels** that permit the passive diffusion of hydrophilic compounds like sugars, amino acids, and certain ions. These channels consist of protein molecules with holes, aptly called **porins**. Porin channels are narrow—just the right size to permit the entry of compounds of up to 600 to 700 Da (see Fig. 3-2). The channels are small enough that hydrophobic compounds come in contact with the polar "wall" of the channel and are thereby excluded.

Certain **hydrophilic** compounds that are sometimes necessary for survival are larger than the exclusion limit of porins. These larger molecules include vitamin B_{12}, sugars larger than trisaccharides, and iron in the form of chelates. Each hydrophilic compound crosses the outer membrane by a unique permeation mechanism that uses proteins especially designed to translocate that compound. Thus, the outer membrane allows the passage of small hydrophilic compounds; excludes hydrophobic compounds, large or small; and allows the entry of some larger hydrophilic molecules by specially dedicated mechanisms.

The dual-membrane system of Gram-negative bacteria creates a compartment called the **periplasmic space**, or **periplasm**, on the outside of the cytoplasmic or inner membrane. This compartment contains the murein layer and a gel-like solution of components that facilitate nutrition. Among these components are degradative enzymes (phosphatases, nucleases, proteases, etc.) that break down large and impermeable molecules to "digestible" size. In addition, the periplasm contains so-called **binding proteins** that help soak up sugars and amino acids from the medium. It also contains enzymes that inactivate antibiotics such as penicillins and cephalosporins, the β-lactamases. The periplasm in Gram-positive bacteria, if one exists at all between the peptidoglycan and cytoplasmic membrane, is less well defined, and these microbes either secrete degradative enzymes into the medium or retain them within the cell wall.

The outer membrane barrier constitutes both an advantage and a disadvantage for Gram-negative bacteria. For example, some bacteriophages use outer membrane proteins as attachment sites for infecting their host bacteria. On the other hand, the outer membrane confers considerable resistance to many antibiotics. Broadly speaking, Gram-negative bacteria are more resistant to antibiotics, especially penicillin. In general, this complex architecture must work very well because in nature (but not necessarily in the human body) Gram-negatives outnumber Gram-positives. The peculiarly Gram-negative solution to the problem of protecting the cytoplasmic membrane has unexpected biological consequences. The LPS of the outer membrane is highly reactive in the host. The lipid A component has a large number of biological activities. It elicits fever and activates a series of immunological and biochemical events that lead to the mobilization of host defense mechanisms. In large doses, this compound, also known as **endotoxin**, can cause shock and even death (see Chapter 9). The O-antigen portion, as the name denotes, is highly antigenic. O antigens come in many varieties, each defining a species or a subspecies of Gram-negative bacteria.

Acid-Fast Solution

A few bacterial types, notably the tubercle bacillus, have developed yet another way to confront environmental challenges to the cytoplasmic membrane. Their cell walls contain large amounts of **waxes**, which are complex long-chain hydrocarbons with sugars and other modifying groups. Having such a protective cover, these organisms are relatively impervious to many harsh chemicals,

including acids. If a dye is introduced into these cells—for instance, by brief heating—it cannot be removed by dilute hydrochloric acid, as would be the case in all other bacteria. These organisms are therefore called acid fast or acid resistant (see Table 3-2).

The waxy coat is interlaced with murein, polysaccharides, and lipids. This covering enables the organisms not only to resist the action of many noxious chemicals but also to avoid being killed by white blood cells. The cost of this protection, however, is that these organisms grow very slowly, possibly because the rate of uptake of nutrients is limited by the waxy covering. Some, like the human tubercle bacillus, divide once every 24 hours.

MUREIN AND ANTIBIOTICS THAT INHIBIT ITS SYNTHESIS

The uniqueness of the bacterial murein makes it a natural target for antibiotics. Drugs that block its formation lead to lysis and death of susceptible bacteria. It is not surprising, therefore, that some of the most clinically effective antibiotics—the **penicillins**, **cephalosporins**, and **carbapenems** (collectively, the β-lactams)—act by inhibiting murein synthesis. They are among the antibiotics that are most unequivocally bactericidal and least toxic to humans. The critical steps in their mode of action are presented in Figure 3-7.

Murein, like many other polysaccharides, is synthesized from nucleotide-bound building blocks. These monomeric precursors consist of uridine diphosphate plus either *N*-acetylglucosamine (GlcNAc) or *N*-acetylmuramic acid (an unusual sugar, the 3-O-*D* lactic acid derivative of GlcNAc). The latter has a peptide chain attached to it (see Fig. 3-3). The monomeric units are made in the cytoplasm and transferred from uridine diphosphate to a **lipid carrier** in the membrane (see Fig. 3-7). Disaccharides are then linked to a growing chain of murein. This step is inhibited by the antibiotic **vancomycin**. Regeneration of the lipid carrier is inhibited by another antibiotic, **bacitracin**.

The final reaction in murein synthesis is transpeptidation. The long chains of disaccharides are cross-linked to make a two-dimensional network (see Fig. 3-3). Cross-linking requires the formation of a peptide bond between D-alanine on one chain and the free N terminus of a lysine or a diaminopimelic acid on the other chain. The link is formed with the **subterminal** D-alanine, the **terminal** D-alanine being cleaved away in the process. Thus, the reaction is the exchange of one peptide bond (that between the two D-alanines) with another—a true transpeptidation. The amino acids that make up the peptides vary in different organisms, but the D-alanine crossbridge to either lysine or diaminopimelic acid is universal. Penicillins and cephalosporins inhibit this reaction.

The reason why penicillin inhibits transpeptidation may lie in its stereochemical similarity with the D-alanine–D-alanine dimer (Fig. 3-8). In the presence of the drug, the

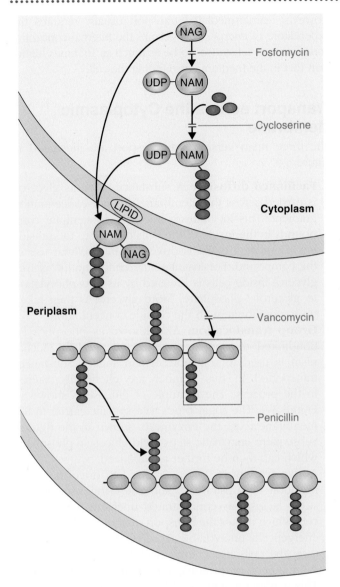

FIGURE 3-7. Biosynthesis of murein, indicating the site of action of a number of antibiotics. The successive steps occurring in the cytoplasm, at the cytoplasmic membrane, and outside the membrane (in the periplasm of Gram-negatives; in the murein layer of Gram-positives) are indicated, along with the points of attack of cycloserine, bacitracin, vancomycin, and penicillin.

FIGURE 3-8. The resemblance of part of the penicillin structure to the backbone of the D-alanine–D-alanine dimer. The *arrows* indicate the bonds broken during covalent attachment to the enzyme involved.

transpeptidase becomes confused: Instead of synthesizing an intermediate D-alanine–enzyme complex, it makes a lethal penicilloyl–enzyme complex.

Antibiotics that inhibit murein synthesis almost invariably kill bacteria by lysing them. In contrast with lysozyme, these drugs do not affect the murein itself, only its synthesis. How then do they cause lysis? When treated with these drugs, the cells continue to synthesize their cytoplasmic components and increase in mass. Because the enlarged cytoplasm is not restrained by a properly cross-linked murein sac, the cell contents extrude and the cells lyse. Cells that are not growing are not lysed by penicillin because they are not increasing in mass. Would it therefore be advisable to administer an antibiotic that

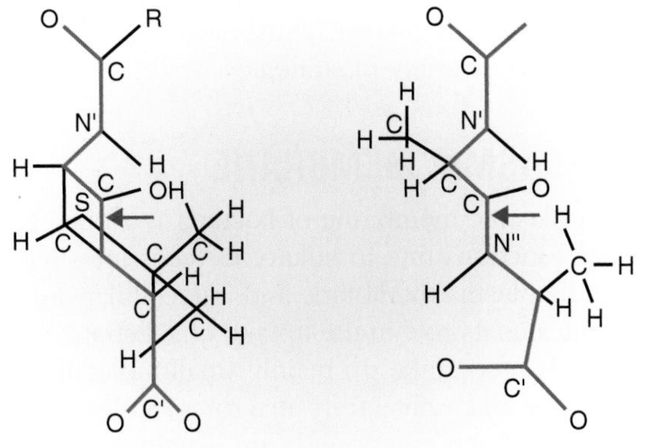

inhibits cell growth at the same time that the patient is receiving penicillin?

The simple concept that cells lyse by outgrowing their coats encounters some difficulties. First, cultures treated with penicillin usually include a small number of "persisters," bacteria that stop growing and do not lyse. Second, for some types of bacteria, penicillin is bacteriostatic, not bactericidal. These bacteria are called "tolerant." What is the explanation for persisters or tolerant bacteria? It appears that tolerant organisms are deficient in an **autolysin**, a bacterial enzyme that cleaves murein. Bacteria use such an enzyme to break open some bonds of murein at the septum, which permits the separation of daughter cells during cell division. Normally, the activity of autolysin is tightly controlled. Treatment with penicillin may arouse it to more-unrestrained action. The role of autolysin in penicillin-induced lysis is well illustrated by pneumococci, which are extraordinarily susceptible to lysis. Autolysin-defective mutants are found among penicillin-resistant derivatives; even strong detergents do not lyse these mutants. Thus, rather than a spontaneous explosion, lysis involves active steps of self-destruction.

There are exceptions to the universal use of murein to maintain bacterial cell integrity. The mycoplasmas are a group of bacteria that have no murein and consequently are not rigid and have almost no defined shape. As expected, they are resistant to penicillin. Some, like an agent of pneumonia, *Mycoplasma pneumoniae*, contain sterols in their membranes, an unusual feature among prokaryotes. It is puzzling how mycoplasmas cope well without rigid cell walls. Although these organisms are quite delicate in culture, they are common in the human body and in the environment. Other exceptions to the ubiquity of mureins exist, especially among the archaea. In addition, some bacteria, such as the anthrax bacillus, have an outside covering made up of especially tough proteins, called the S-layer. Thus, bacteria safeguard their integrity with a variety of strategies.

CYTOPLASMIC MEMBRANE

The cytoplasmic membrane of bacteria is a busy place. It assumes functions that in eukaryotic cells are divided up among the plasma membrane and intracellular organelles. Most critical is its role in the uptake of substrates from the medium. Bacteria take up mainly small-molecular-weight compounds and only rarely macromolecules and phosphate esters. Such compounds are usually hydrolyzed by enzymes in the periplasm or the surrounding medium, and the resulting breakdown products—peptides, oligosaccharides, nucleosides, and phosphate, among others—can then be transported across the cytoplasmic membrane.

The cytoplasmic membrane contains specific carrier proteins, called **permeases**, that facilitate the entry of most metabolites. In some cases, the carrier facilitates the equilibration of a compound inside and outside the cell (Fig. 3-9).

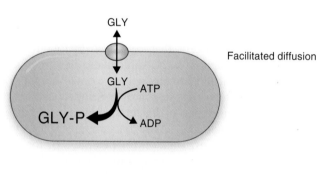

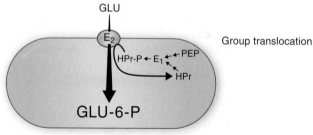

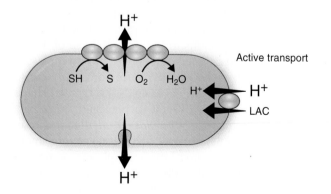

FIGURE 3-9. Mechanisms of transport. The three types of transport in *Escherichia coli* are facilitated diffusion, group translocation, and active transport with the *lac* permease.

However, carrier-mediated transport usually requires the expenditure of energy. This permits the internal concentration of certain substances to be as much as 10^5 times higher than that in the medium surrounding the cell.

Transport across the Cytoplasmic Membrane

The three main versions of transport are illustrated in Figure 3-9.

1. **Facilitated diffusion**: A substance, such as glycerol, is carried across the membrane down a concentration gradient. This mechanism does not concentrate compounds in the inside of the cells relative to the outside environment. Uptake is driven by intracellular use of the compound. For instance, the concentration of free glycerol inside cells is lowered by its phosphorylation to glycerol-3-phosphate. More glycerol is then taken up to equilibrate with the outside concentration.

2. **Group translocation**: Also known as phosphorylation-linked transport, this energy-dependent mechanism is used to transport certain sugars. Substances transported in this manner are chemically altered in the process. The example of glucose is shown in Figure 3-9. The sugar binds to a specific carrier in the membrane (e.g., the enzyme E_2 shown in the figure). Subsequent enzymatic steps yield glucose-6-phosphate, which can then be further metabolized.

3. **Active transport**: Energy is used to drive the accumulation of substrate. A substrate—for instance, the sugar lactose—is concentrated unchanged inside the cell, which makes the transport of additional molecules energetically unfavorable. To drive the transport of lactose, the cells use energy stored in an electrochemical gradient of protons, the **proton motive force**. This gradient is generated by the extrusion of protons from the cell, resulting from the oxidation of metabolic intermediates like reduced nicotinamide adenine dinucleotide or by hydrolysis of adenosine triphosphate. Lactose is accumulated intracellularly by coupling its **energetically unfavorable** transport with the **energetically favorable** reentry of protons into the relatively alkaline cytoplasm of the cell. Thus, transport of this type takes place via a **symport**, which requires the simultaneous uptake of positive hydrogen and sugar molecules.

Each type of transport system involves specific protein molecules. Some proteins aid the process by modifying or concentrating substrates in the periplasmic space of Gram-negatives. These **binding proteins** are specific for sugars, nucleotides, and so on. The periplasmic space also contains nucleotidases, nucleases, peptidases, proteases, and other hydrolytic enzymes. The actual transport process is carried out by membrane-bound carriers, or **permeases**, which are involved in all three types of transport. We do not have a physical picture of how permeases respond to the proton gradient, but we know that they assume different configurations inside and outside the cytoplasmic membrane. Thus, permeases have a high affinity for substrate on the outside and low affinity on the inside. However they work, they are essential for transport. For example, in the much-studied lactose system, cells that lack a functional permease remain impervious to the sugar, even when soaked in concentrations approaching syrup.

The three mechanisms of transport are used to different extents by different bacteria. In general, few substrates equilibrate across membranes without the expenditure of energy. Among the energy-requiring mechanisms, group translocations are used to a different extent. *E. coli*, for instance, transports a wide variety of sugars in this way, whereas strictly aerobic bacteria use it little. All in all, active transport dominates the repertoire of transport mechanisms in bacteria, especially when nutrients must be concentrated from the medium to support cell growth.

Uptake of Iron

The uptake of iron deserves special mention. Free iron is extremely scarce in the blood and many tissues because it is bound by proteins like transferrin or ceruloplasmin. It is essential for the growth of bacteria, and many species that inhabit the human body have developed ingenious mechanisms to obtain the amounts of this element they need for growth. They excrete chelating compounds, known as **siderophores**, that bind iron with great avidity. Each organism can take up its own particular form of complexed iron; individual complexes are unique enough to be less digestible for other organisms. However, in response to the competition for iron, many bacteria have multiple siderophores and uptake systems, thus trying to gain an edge on the other organisms in the same environment; some can efficiently extract iron from transferrin, an advantage at our expense.

Other Functions of the Bacterial Membrane

The cytoplasmic membrane of bacteria is also where **cytochromes** are located and **oxidative metabolism** is carried out. It thus performs the role of the mitochondria of eukaryotic cells. The membrane is also the location of nascent proteins destined either for secretion or incorporation in the membrane itself. Some bacteria secrete as much as 10% of all the proteins they make, including toxins and other virulence factors. The nascent peptide chains that have hydrophobic "signal sequences" at the N termini are translocated from ribosomes across the cytoplasmic membrane by an energy-requiring mechanism. Note that Gram-negative bacteria have the added problem of transporting proteins to the outer membrane. It is not known exactly how that takes place.

Some bacteria have also an exceptional ability to take up enormously long DNA molecules. The phenomenon was first demonstrated by genetic transformation of pneumococci and occurs among other bacteria. The mechanism of DNA uptake is less well understood, but like active transport, it depends on the proton motive force.

In spite of its versatility and range of activities, the cytoplasmic membrane of bacteria is rarely the site of useful antibiotic action (see Chapter 5). Could one possible reason for this be that the membrane's overall structure is similar to that of the eukaryotic cell membrane?

DNA AND CHROMOSOME MECHANICS

The genome of many bacteria consists of a **single circular chromosome** of double-stranded DNA. However, some species have a linear chromosome, and others have more than one. The chromosome of *E. coli* has about **5 million base pairs**, encoding about 2,000 to 3,000 genes. The total DNA sequence of hundreds of bacterial genomes is at hand, and more are being determined monthly.

Bacteria must solve a demanding topological problem in organizing their DNA because it is a long, thin molecule. If stretched out, DNA would be about 1,000 times the length of the cell. If a bacterium were to be magnified to the size of a human being, its DNA would be about a mile long. The DNA is coiled in a central irregular structure called the **nucleoid.** Its physical state is unknown and somewhat mysterious, because in the test tube, a solution 100 times more dilute is a gel. Roughly all that is known about the physical state of the bacterial DNA is that it is twisted into **supercoils** (analogous to twisted telephone coils) and that this condition is indispensable for its organization, its replication, and the transcription of a number of genes. Supercoiling depends on balancing the actions of two topoisomerases. One of these, **DNA gyrase**, introduces supercoils into circular DNA, an action counteracted by a second enzyme, **topoisomerase I**, which relaxes the supercoils by making single-strand nicks.

DNA replication has three stages: initiation, elongation, and termination. Replication takes place bidirectionally; that is, DNA synthesis starts at a precise place on the chromosome, the **replicative origin**, and proceeds away from it in both directions. The two moving polymerase complexes meet halfway around the chromosome. To replicate, the DNA helix in *E. coli* must unwind and rotate at some 6,000 rpm. One wonders how this can take place without entanglement of the tightly coiled nucleoid.

The timing of chromosome replication is a highly regulated process and is coupled to growth and cell division. At a given temperature, the *rate of DNA polymerase movement is nearly independent of the growth rate* of the cells. In *E. coli*, DNA replication takes 40 minutes, whether the cells are growing slowly or quickly. In slow-growing cells (e.g., those dividing once every 100 minutes), one round of synthesis occurs in each division cycle, and no

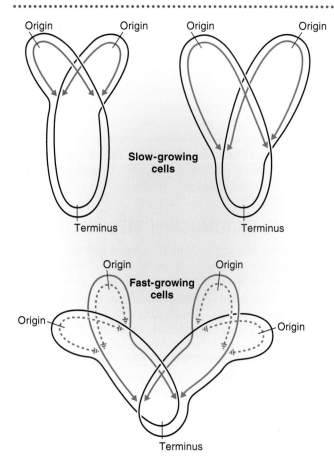

FIGURE 3-10. Replication of DNA in slow-growing and fast-growing *E. coli.* Replication begins at a specific site, the origin, and proceeds in both directions toward a terminus. The process takes about 40 minutes at 37°C. In a culture doubling every 20 minutes, the process must initiate every 20 minutes—that is, before the previous round of replication has terminated. In such cultures, the DNA is undergoing multifork replication.

DNA is synthesized during the remaining 60 minutes. In fast-growing cells (e.g., those dividing every 20 minutes), initiation of rounds of replication is adapted to produce new chromosomes as often as the cell divides (Fig. 3-10). Since each chromosome requires 40 minutes to be synthesized, replication will initiate again on a strand long before its own replication has completed. Thus, chromosome replication in bacteria is regulated by how often the process gets started—that is, by the frequency of initiation of DNA synthesis.

How do antibiotics inhibit DNA metabolism? Most inhibitors of DNA replication bind to DNA and are too toxic for clinical use. An interesting exception is **metronidazole**, a drug that is inert but can be selectively modified to an active form by some bacteria. This compound contains a nitro group that must be *partially* reduced to render the molecule active. Full reduction to the amino state makes the molecule inactive again. Partial reduction is achieved by anaerobic bacteria but only rarely by the cells of the human body or by aerobic bacteria.

Partially reduced metronidazole is incorporated into the DNA of the bacteria. This is an example of **lethal synthesis** because the metronidazole-containing DNA molecules are unstable. It follows that metronidazole and related drugs are particularly useful against anaerobic bacteria and against amoebas, which also grow anaerobically. These drugs, however, are not ideal. To a small extent, the partial reduction to active agents occurs in normal tissue, leading to possible mutagenesis and perhaps carcinogenesis.

Other DNA inhibitors act selectively by binding to specific enzymes involved in DNA supercoiling. **Nalidixic acid**, for example, inhibits DNA gyrase and is bactericidal. The more-stable fluorinated derivatives of nalidixic acid, the **fluoroquinolones**, interfere with DNA gyrase or topoisomerase and cause double-stranded DNA breaks.

GENE EXPRESSION: UNIQUENESS OF PROKARYOTIC RNA POLYMERASE AND RIBOSOMES

The bacterial cytoplasm is composed largely of proteins (about 40% of the dry weight, with about 1 million molecules per cell) and RNA (up to 35% of the dry weight in rapidly growing cells). Bacterial **ribosomes** have smaller subunits and smaller RNA molecules than do their eukaryotic counterparts. Bacterial ribosomal RNAs make up the small and large ribosomal subunits with 21 and 35 different proteins, respectively. These subunits join in the complete ribosomes, which move along mRNA molecules to synthesize proteins.

The large requirement for proteins makes **protein synthesis** the principal biosynthetic activity of rapidly growing bacteria. A large proportion of a bacterium's energy and metabolic building blocks is devoted to the assembly of the protein-synthesizing machinery, including ribosomes and RNA polymerase. Over a considerable range of growth rates, *RNA is made at a rate proportional to the number of RNA polymerase molecules* engaged in the process of transcription. Likewise, the rate of protein synthesis is proportional to the cellular concentration of ribosomes. This suggests that, as with DNA replication, the rate of polymerization of single chains of RNA or protein remains constant whether cells are growing rapidly or slowly. Thus, the synthesis of the principal macromolecules of bacteria is *regulated mainly by the frequency with which each chain is initiated* and *not* so much by altering their rate of manufacture of each molecule (i.e., the speed of **chain elongation**).

Antibiotics act selectively at **initiation** or **elongation** of macromolecular synthesis. For example, **rifampin**, a powerful inhibitor of bacterial transcription, acts at the initiation step. How does it recognize this step? The drug binds strongly to molecules of RNA polymerase that are floating freely in the cytoplasm but much less strongly to polymerase molecules that are bound to DNA. As a result, a polymerase that is bound to DNA and has initiated RNA synthesis will not be inactivated by rifampin until it completes its round of RNA synthesis and is released from the DNA. Rifampin is clinically useful, particularly in the treatment of tuberculosis and leprosy, in part because it is relatively nontoxic. The reason is that mammalian RNA polymerases do not bind rifampin.

Apart from the murein-inhibiting β-lactams and DNA inhibitors, the largest class of clinically useful antibiotics consists of those that inhibit protein synthesis. Some of these antibiotics work by binding to ribosomes, either to the large or the small subunit (Table 3-3). The reason that bacteria are selectively targeted is that the ribosome of prokaryotes is different from that of eukaryotes (Table 3-1). Among the ribosomally active antibiotics are **chloramphenicol** and **macrolides** (such as **erythromycin**), which *block the formation of peptide bonds* by binding at or near the aminoacyl transfer RNA (tRNA) binding site on the large ribosomal subunit. After some time, the previously synthesized peptidyl tRNA is released and hydrolyzed. The ribosomal subunits are then released from the mRNA and are free to rejoin other mRNA molecules to start another abortive cycle. This leads to a truncated version of the ribosome cycle (Fig. 3-11). As a result, when ribosomally active antibiotics are withdrawn, many free ribosomes are present and ready to resume normal protein synthesis. This explains why the *action of these drugs is reversible* and why they are **bacteriostatic** and not **bactericidal**. It should be pointed out that this does not necessarily diminish their usefulness. When bacteria are kept in check by bacteriostatic drugs, they are usually cleared from tissues by the host defense mechanisms.

One important group of protein synthesis inhibitors, the **aminoglycosides**, is **bactericidal.** Aminoglycosides, like **streptomycin**, **gentamicin**, and **neomycin**, are taken up by bacteria and bind to the smaller 30S ribosomal subunit. This is their critical site of action, as demonstrated by the finding that a single amino acid change in a mutated 30S ribosomal protein leads to resistance to these drugs. Binding of aminoglycosides has many effects on ribosome function; for instance, it enhances the interaction of the 30S and 50S subunits and inhibits the elongation of peptide chains. Typical of the action of this group of antibiotics is the accumulation of free ribosomes as aberrant 70S particles and not as 30S and 50S subunits. This coincides with cell death. Accumulating 70S ribosomes results in abortive attempts to initiate protein synthesis. However, these atypical ribosomes bind to mRNA and therefore block the function of normal ribosomes still unaffected by the drug. The inhibition of protein synthesis by aminoglycosides is apparently irreversible, because once the drug is taken up, it cannot be removed from the cell. Thus, cells treated with these drugs cannot recover, which is one reason why the aminoglycosides are bactericidal.

CAPSULES, FLAGELLA, AND PILI: HOW BACTERIA COPE IN VARIOUS ENVIRONMENTS

The morphological variety of bacteria is not limited to walls and membranes. Some bacteria, but by no means all, have other exterior structures such as **capsules, flagella**, and **pili**. These components are dispensable; that is, they are important for survival under certain circumstances but not others. The **capsule** is a slimy outer coating made by certain bacteria. Under laboratory conditions the capsule is not needed, and the organisms may grow well without it. Capsules usually consist of high-molecular-weight polysaccharides that make the bacteria slippery and difficult for white blood cells to phagocytize. As you will see, pneumococci, meningococci, and other bacteria that are likely to encounter phagocytes during their infective cycle are indeed encapsulated. In the laboratory, colonies of encapsulated bacteria on agar plates are viscous and shiny. Colonies of nonencapsulated organisms are usually smaller and appear dull.

Protruding through the surface layers of many bacteria are two kinds of filaments, **flagella** and **pili** (Fig. 3-12). Flagella are long, helical filaments that endow bacteria with motility. Many successful pathogens are motile, which probably aids their spread in the environment and possibly in the body of the host. Depending on the species, a single bacterial cell may have one flagellum or many flagella (Fig. 3-13). In some, the flagella are located at the ends of the cells (polar) and in others at random points around the periphery (peritrichous or "hairy all over"). This distinction is useful in taxonomy and in diagnostic microbiology. Pili (also called **fimbriae**) are involved in the attachment of bacteria to cells and other surfaces, as discussed later in the chapter.

Bacterial Chemotaxis

The movement caused by flagella is used by bacteria for **chemotaxis**—that is, movement toward substances that attract and away from those that repel. Considerable research has shown that bacterial chemotaxis is based on the following sophisticated mechanism: Flagella spin around from their point of attachment at the cell surface. Each flagellum has a *counterclockwise helical pitch*, and when there are several on one bacterium, they array themselves into coherent bundles as long as they all rotate counterclockwise. When the flagella are arranged in these bundles, they beat together, and the bacteria *swim in a straight line* (Fig. 3-14). However, when flagella rotate clockwise, they get in each other's way and cannot form bundles. As a result, the bacteria **tumble** in random fashion. The two types of motion, swimming and tumbling, account for bacterial chemotaxis. In the absence of **attractants** or **repellants**, bacteria alternate indifferently

TABLE 3-3 Antibiotics: Mechanisms of Action of Commonly Used Antimicrobial Agents

Antibiotic	Action
Cell Wall Inhibitors	
β-Lactams: penicillins, cephalosporins, carbapenems, monobactams	Interfere with cell wall cross-linking through interaction with penicillin-binding proteins (transpeptidases); autolysis
Glycopeptides: vancomycin	Interfere with incorporation of new subunits into growing murein chains
Imidazoles: fluconazole, itraconazole, voriconazole, posaconazole	Blocks synthesis of ergosterol required for fungal cell wall integrity
Echinocandins: caspofungin, micafungin	Blocks β-glucan synthesis, a major constituent of fungal cell walls
Inhibitors of Membrane Function	
Lipopeptide antibiotics: daptomycin	Forms channels in cell membranes of Gram-positive bacteria, resulting in K+ leakage and metabolic death
Polyene: amphotericin B	Bind to sterols in eukaryotic cell membranes, leading to membrane leakiness and, at high levels, lysis
Folate Antagonists	
Sulfonamides: sulfamethoxazole	Competitive inhibitor of dihydropteroate synthesis; blocks synthesis of tetrahydrofolate and sulfadiazine cell-linked metabolic pathways
Trimethoprim	Inhibition of bacterial dihydrofolate reductase
Protein Synthesis Inhibitors	
Aminoglycosides: gentamicin, tobramycin, streptomycin, amikacin, neomycin	Bind to 30S subunit of bacterial ribosome; cause translational misreading and inhibit elongation of protein chain; kill by blocking initiation of protein synthesis
Macrolides: erythromycin, azithromycin, clarithromycin, clindamycin	Bind to ribosome 50S subunit; inhibit protein synthesis at chain elongation step
Ketolides: telithromycin	
Streptogramins: dalfopristin, quinupristin	
Chloramphenicol	
RNA Synthesis Inhibitors	
Rifampin	Binds to bacterial RNA polymerase and blocks transcription (synthesis of RNA) at initiation step
DNA Synthesis Inhibitors	
Metronidazole, nitrofurans	Partially reduced nitro groups give addition products on DNA that lead to cidal strand breakage
Fluoroquinolones: ciprofloxacin, levofloxacin, gatifloxacin, moxifloxacin, gemifloxacin	Interfere with DNA replication by inhibiting the action of DNA gyrase or topoisomerase
Nalidixic acid	

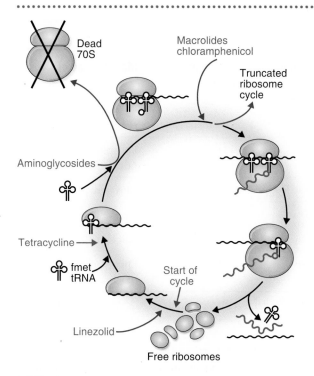

FIGURE 3-11. Antibiotic blockage of the ribosome cycle. The normal cycle of 30S and 50S subunits in and out of polysomes is recalled, with the assembly of a 70S initiation complex, elongation of the polypeptide chain as the ribosome moves across the messenger RNA, and release of all components on completion of the polypeptide. Points of blockage by antibiotics are shown. Linezolid blocks the assembly of the initiation complex; tetracycline inhibits aminoacyl tRNA binding; aminoglycosides provoke formation of "dead" aberrant initiation complexes; and chloramphenicol and macrolides block elongation, leading to premature dissociation of the active complex.

between swimming and tumbling. When an attractant is sensed, swimming lasts longer than tumbling, whereas swimming stops more quickly when a repellant is present. The net result is movement toward attractants and away from repellants. Chemotaxis has a role in pathogenesis, probably in guiding bacteria toward cellular targets or possibly away from white blood cells.

Bacterial Adhesion and Pili

Whether by active chemotaxis or by more-passive mechanisms, microbes are attracted to specific tissues. Such **tissue tropism** often involves the attachment of surface components of the organisms to **specific receptors** present on the cells of certain tissues. The bacterial structures most often involved in attachment are the **pili**, or fimbriae. These are protein filaments shorter than flagella and distributed, often in large numbers, over the surface of some bacteria. Bacteria that can conjugate have, in addition, specialized **sex pili**. These structures are rather different from the "common pili." They are much longer and link the donor (male) and recipient (female) cells during transfer of DNA by conjugation (see Chapter 4). Attachment to cells or other bacteria via pili involves the attachment at the tip of the pili followed by their retraction into the cell (a process that resembles the use of grappling hooks). Because of the importance of pili in adherence to the host, vaccine and drug discovery programs have been developed to block the function or production of pili as a way of controlling bacterial infection.

Some organisms are able to change the amino acid composition of their pili and thereby put on a succession of disguises that enables them to outflank the immune system. This process is referred to as **antigenic variation**, as is discussed in detail in Chapter 8. By a related mechanism, organisms that cause food poisoning and other illnesses, the *Salmonella*, undergo rapid changes between expression and nonexpression of genes that code for the protein of flagella. This change in flagellar synthesis is called **phase variation** and is based on the control of a gene for flagellar protein. The gene is periodically inverted on the chromosome but can be expressed in only one of the two orientations. Consequently, a population of these organisms always includes some flagellate bacteria that are selected when motility is advantageous and some nonflagellate bacteria that are selected when the innate immune system zeroes in on flagella.

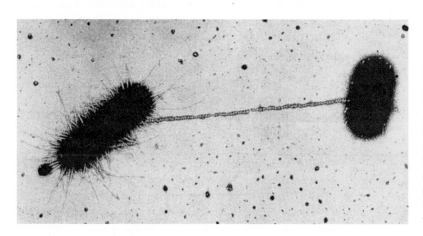

FIGURE 3-12. *E. coli* mating. The cell covered with numerous appendages (pili or fimbriae) is a genetic donor connected to a recipient cell (without appendages) by the so-called F pilus. The F pilus is a specialized structure (sex pilus) controlled by genes on the fertility, or F plasmid. The F pilus has been labeled by special virus particles that infect donor cells via the F pilus. The other pili surrounding the cell have no role in conjugation but are required by *E. coli* for colonization and pathogenicity in the intestinal and urinary tracts of humans and animals.

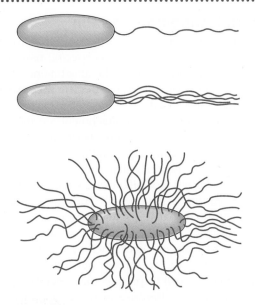

FIGURE 3-13. Arrangement of flagella in some types of bacteria.

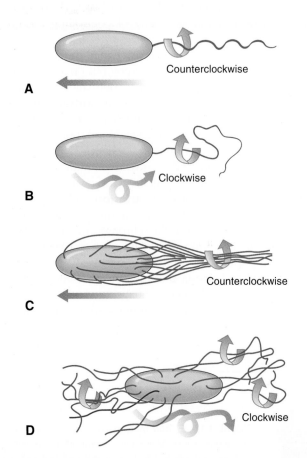

FIGURE 3-14. Flagellar arrangement and motility. A. A bacterium moving smoothly right to left when its single polar flagellum rotates counterclockwise; this is the same direction as the thread of the helix formed by the flagellin molecules in the flagellum. **B.** The same bacterium tumbles generally left to right when the flagellum rotates clockwise. **C.** With a peritrichous bacterium, counterclockwise rotation produces a coherent bundle of flagella and smooth movement. **D.** Tumbling produced by clockwise rotation is extreme.

TABLE 3-4 Glucose-Minimal Medium

Compound	Grams per Liter	Main Source of
Na_2HPO_4	6.0	Phosphorus, buffering power, osmotic strength
KH_2PO_4	3.0	Phosphorus, buffering power, osmotic strength
NH_4Cl	1.0	Nitrogen
$MgSO_4$	0.012	Magnesium, sulfur
$CaCl_2$	0.011	Calcium
Glucose	2.0	Energy, carbon-building blocks

Note: pH adjusted to 7.0.

NUTRITION AND ENERGY METABOLISM

Bacteria survive and grow in a large variety of habitats. Whatever the habitat, all bacteria must synthesize cellular constituents in a coordinated manner to grow. The required building blocks must either be provided at suitable levels in the medium or be synthesized in proper amounts by the organisms themselves. Based on their nutritional requirements, bacteria can be divided into two large groups: In one are the **photosynthetic** or **chemosynthetic** bacteria that subsist on carbon dioxide and minerals, using either light or chemical energy. The other includes all the **organisms that need preformed organic compounds**. All pathogenic microbes fall in the second group, but within it, they have many gradations of nutritional needs. Some, like *E. coli*, are satisfied with glucose and some inorganic material (Table 3-4). Other pathogenic bacteria, like their human host, are unable to make one or more essential metabolites—vitamins, amino acids, purines, pyrimidines, and so on—which must be supplied as growth factors.

Bacteria also have a wide range of responses to oxygen. At the extremes are the **strict aerobes**, which must have oxygen to grow. An example is the tubercle bacillus, which thrives in the portions of the body that are well oxygenated, such as the lungs. At the other extreme are the **strict** or **obligate anaerobes**, bacteria that cannot grow in the presence of oxygen, such as the organisms that cause botulism and tetanus. The largest number of bacteria that are medically important can grow whether or not oxygen is present. They are called **facultative anaerobes** and include *E. coli* and other intestinal bacteria.

Their various responses to oxygen mirror the ways bacteria oxidize substrates to obtain energy. Strict aerobes perform **respiration** only; in a series of coupled oxidation–reductions, the *final electron acceptor is molecular oxygen*. Strict anaerobes usually carry out

fermentation, where the final electron acceptor is an **organic molecule**. Examples of organic electron acceptors are pyruvate, which is reduced to lactate in the lactic acid fermentation, and acetyl coenzyme A, which is reduced to alcohol in ethanol fermentation. Facultative anaerobes are capable of either form of metabolism, depending on whether oxygen is present or absent. Thus, they will respire in the presence of oxygen and ferment in its absence. (To make matters more complex, some anaerobes, called anaerobic respirers, carry out respiration using compounds such as nitrate or sulfate instead of oxygen as final electron acceptors.)

Per molecule of substrate oxidized, respiration yields more energy than fermentation. Therefore, fermentative organisms must turn over more substrate to obtain the same amount of energy. The industrial microbiologist takes advantage of this for the purpose of maximizing either the yield of cell mass or the amount of metabolic products formed. Under what conditions of oxygenation would you grow yeast in a fermentation tank if the intended product were yeast cake or alcohol?

We have mentioned that *E. coli* can use glucose as its sole organic source. It can also use other compounds, such as lactose, fructose, or one of several amino acids. The list includes more than 30 known substances, but this is not particularly impressive compared with species of *Pseudomonas*, which can grow on any of several hundred organic compounds. No wonder the nearly omnivorous *Pseudomonas* have been used by genetic engineers to construct strains for use in the degradation of environmental pollutants. And no wonder *Pseudomonas* species are omnipresent in the water supply and the soil, where they can take advantage of a great variety of substrates.

Although *E. coli* and *Pseudomonas* can manage on meager solutions of glucose and a few salts, they do not disdain richer fare. When *E. coli* is given a mixture of amino acids, sugars, vitamins, and other compounds, it will use what is provided rather than making the compounds endogenously. The result is sparing of energy and biosynthetic potential and faster growth. In the laboratory, it is possible to culture bacteria in media that are truly spartan, the so-called **minimal media**, which are water solutions of glucose, ammonia, phosphate, sulfate, and other minerals (see Table 3-4). Conversely, the bacteria can be grown in a rich medium, a **nutrient broth** that contains meat extract and soluble partial hydrolysates of complex proteins. Add **agar** to these solutions and you have the corresponding **solid media**.

Some bacteria can grow only in complex media and have nutritional requirements that rival or exceed those of humans. Called **nutritionally fastidious**, these organisms include highly parasitic species found only in the rich environment of the human body. For example, staphylococci or streptococci can grow only if provided with a long list of compounds. As expected, bacteria that can get by with only a few nutrients, like *E. coli* or *Pseudomonas*,

can also exist in less-rich habitats, such as bodies of water. The ecology of an organism then usually gives good hints of its nutritional requirements.

Certain bacteria have never been cultured in artificial media and only replicate inside host cells. These bacteria, like *Chlamydia*, are known as **obligate intracellular parasites**. Other bacteria, such as *Treponema pallidum* (the causative agent of syphilis) or *Mycobacterium leprae* (which causes leprosy), should, in principle, be able to grow in laboratory media because they replicate extracellularly in the host. However, microbiologists have not figured out how to get them to do it.

GROWING AND RESTING STATES

When bacteria find themselves in a suitable environment, they grow and eventually divide. The time it takes for a bacterium to become two is called the **generation time** or **doubling time**. For example, *E. coli* requires about 20 minutes to double in a rich nutrient broth and 1 hour in a glucose-minimal medium at 37°C. For a time, the bacteria grow in an unhindered manner and are physiologically all alike. Such a steady state does not exist for long in nature, however, because the environment usually undergoes rapid changes. Growth will stop once the population reaches a certain cell density and the nutrients in the environment become exhausted or toxic metabolites accumulate.

Bacterial Growth Measurement and a Few Definitions

How is bacterial growth measured? The most direct way is to take samples at various times and count the number of bacteria under a microscope using a hemocytometer chamber. This tedious procedure has been superseded by electronic particle analyzers that detect bacteria as tiny semiconductors in an electric field. Either procedure measures the number of bacteria as physical particles. In other words, they give the body count, with no discrimination between living and dead bacteria. This is known as the **total count**. The total count can also be conveniently estimated by measuring a property proportional to the number of bacteria present—for instance, the turbidity of a liquid culture.

Often, it is important to determine the number of **living** or **viable** bacteria. This number is determined by a **colony count**, which is carried out by placing an appropriate dilution on solid growth medium. Since colonies arise from living bacteria, the number of colonies multiplied by the dilution factor is the number of **colony-forming units** (**CFUs**) originally present. Note that if bacteria grow in clumps, like staphylococci, or in chains, like streptococci, the number of CFUs is an underestimate of the total number of living bacteria present.

Law of Growth

Balanced growth can be described mathematically as follows. Let N be the number of bacteria and t the time, then

$$dN/dt = Nk$$

where k is the **growth rate constant**. By integration, we obtain the **law of growth**:

$$N_t = N_0 e^{kt}$$

where N_t is the number of bacteria at time t, and N_0 is the initial number of bacteria at $t = 0$. The law of growth describes a **geometric progression**, which holds for many situations. In some circumstances leading to cell death (for instance, sterilizing heat or antiseptic chemicals), the decrease in viable bacteria may be described by the same equation but with a negative constant. The same equation also describes the decay with time of a radioactive isotope or the kinetics of degradation of unstable mRNA molecules in cells (or the law of compound interest, which Benjamin Franklin called "the eighth wonder of the world").

Growth in the Real World

If balanced growth went unchecked, a single bacterium dividing twice an hour would produce a mass as large as that of the Earth in just 2 days. Instead, when bacteria grow to a certain density, they either exhaust required nutrients or they accumulate toxic levels of metabolites (Fig. 3-15). They may run out of the carbon source, a required inorganic compound, or essential amino acids

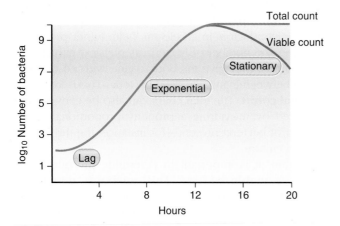

FIGURE 3-15. The growth of a bacterial culture. Bacteria in the inoculum sometimes resume growth slowly (lag phase, hours 0 to 5). They then enter the exponential phase of growth (hours 5 to 10). When foodstuff is exhausted or toxic material accumulates, they enter the stationary phase (hours 10 onward). During the stationary phase, bacterial cultures may lose their viability, as reflected in the viable count, often without losing cell integrity (maintaining a constant total count).

or vitamins. For aerobic bacteria, crowding leads to the exhaustion of oxygen, which is poorly soluble in water. Toxic metabolites may be hydrogen peroxide, which is the case for some anaerobes that lack catalase, or acids formed by fermentation, which results in a pH too low to be compatible with growth. Which of these factors actually slows down growth first depends on the strain of bacteria and on the composition of the culture medium. For example, in a well-buffered medium, *E. coli* may exhaust nutrients before the pH drops, while the converse may be true in poorly buffered media. The stage of the culture where growth stops is known as the **stationary phase**.

The explosiveness of exponential growth means that even a small number of bacteria can rapidly initiate an infection. An example of unhampered growth that leads to dangerous illness is acute bacterial meningitis in a child. Bacteria that cause this disease, such as the meningococci, grow so rapidly in the patient that the physician must intervene with great speed to avoid a fatal outcome. However, not all pathogens are fast growing. For example, tubercle bacilli divide every 24 hours or so even under optimal conditions. The disease they cause is chronic and takes considerable time to be manifested.

In the tissues of the body (as well as in the environment), bacteria are often stressed by nutritional limitations or by the damaging action of the defense mechanisms. Consequently, bacterial populations in the body are rarely fully viable. To permit them to adapt to such conditions, bacteria do not cease all metabolic activities when they stop growing. Instead, although they cease net growth, they continue some synthetic activities that permit them to make specific constituents needed for adaptation. To use a laboratory example, when *E. coli* cultures exhaust glucose, they continue to carry out a low level of protein synthesis, sufficient to adapt to the use of other nutrients, such as other sugars that may be present. Energy and building blocks are supplied by turnover of cell material not needed in the stationary phase. Major sources of amino acids are the ribosomes and preexisting proteins not greatly used under these conditions. Their breakdown products can also be utilized to supply energy. This process of feeding on itself gives bacteria adaptability and postpones death, which might otherwise occur by random degradative events in the absence of synthetic activities.

Bacteria are exposed to countless injuries and have developed special adaptive mechanisms to cope with many of them. For example, damage to the DNA of *E. coli* by ultraviolet light activates a set of genes that code for proteins capable of repairing the damage. This is known as the **SOS response**. Other protective responses are turned on when bacteria are starved for the source of carbon, nitrogen, or phosphorus; when the temperature is raised abruptly; or when anaerobic cultures are suddenly exposed to oxygen. In each case, the rapid rate at which the bacteria implement their coping mechanism is a tribute to the powers of bacterial adaptation.

Even when they are not growing, bacteria can still cause damage to their host. First, nongrowing bacteria are still immunogenic and can elicit immune responses with both beneficial and detrimental results. Second, production of toxins often starts or accelerates when bacteria enter the stationary phase. In some cases, we can fathom the reason for this timing, because toxin production may provide bacteria with nutrients. For example, some streptococci make enzymes that lyse red blood cells and proteases that degrade hemoglobin. The organisms are thus supplied with amino acids plus a source of iron. Why do these organisms make their hemolysins mainly in the stationary phase? Clearly, as long as they are growing, they must already be supplied with the necessary iron and amino acids. Why should they then expend energy to make hemolysins?

Cessation of growth of some bacterial species initiates **sporulation**. This results in the production of metabolically inert **spores** extraordinarily resistant to chemical and physical insults. During sporulation, the "mother cell" eventually lyses. The cytoplasmic contents that are released sometimes contain large amounts of toxins. This happens in tetanus, gas gangrene, and other diseases caused by sporulating bacteria.

The relationship between microbial growth and pathogenesis is far from simple but should be kept in mind when attempting to understand the etiology and course of infections.

MECHANISMS OF ADAPTATION

Both over short periods and throughout evolutionary times, bacteria are selected for their efficient and economical ways of coping with the environment. *Inefficient strains are rapidly lost in competition with others that use their resources more effectively.* Metabolic efficiency is characterized by metabolic **parsimony**; that is, bacteria tend not to make constituents they cannot use at the time. There are important exceptions to this statement, but generally, it illustrates the economy and efficiency of the bacterial way of life.

We know a great deal about the mechanisms bacteria use to adapt to changing environmental conditions. As more information is gathered, it becomes evident that a large number of mechanisms operate a certain way under specific circumstances. One example is a culture of *E. coli* growing in a minimal medium to which is added an excess of the amino acid leucine. Within seconds, the endogenous synthesis of leucine will be stopped, and the cells will use the exogenously supplied leucine exclusively. From the point of view of the economy of the bacteria, this is desirable because it saves the metabolic energy expended for biosynthesis of leucine. The same phenomenon would occur if other amino acids, purines, pyrimidines, or other metabolites were added.

Regulation of Enzyme Activity

How did the bacteria switch off the synthesis of leucine? When the enzymes of the metabolic pathway dedicated to the synthesis of leucine were studied, it was found that the first enzyme in the pathway is inhibited by leucine and will not function in its presence. This inhibition is the result of the **allosteric** properties of the enzyme— that is, its ability to change conformation by binding an effector, in this case leucine. Why was the first enzyme and not the others in the pathway affected? The reason is likely economic: stopping the flow of substrates at the very beginning of the pathway eliminates waste of unusable metabolites. This effect is known as **feedback** or **end-product inhibition**.

Regulation of Enzyme Synthesis

Feedback inhibition suffices to stop the synthesis of leucine in the leucine-fed culture. If this were all, the organisms would still synthesize the biosynthetic enzymes for leucine, at a cost of considerable energy. This is wasteful and might place the organisms at a selective disadvantage vis-à-vis more-efficient ones. To avoid such an unnecessary expenditure, the cells rapidly turn off the synthesis of the enzymes of the leucine biosynthetic pathway. How is this done? It is a characteristic of prokaryotic cells that genes for the enzymes involved in a metabolic pathway are often strung together in a multigenic segment of DNA called an **operon**. Transcription of all the genes of an operon into mRNA can be turned on or off together by throwing a single regulatory switch. At one end of the operon where transcription starts is a series of regulatory sequences that do not code for amino acids but are recognized by the regulatory mechanisms. One of these sequences is the **promoter** site, where RNA polymerase binds to initiate the synthesis of mRNA. Two such mechanisms of **regulation of gene expression** used to switch operons on and off are discussed here.

The operons involved in the biosynthesis of amino acids, such as leucine, are sometimes regulated by a mechanism called **attenuation**. This is how it works, still taking leucine as an example: A small stretch of mRNA is synthesized from the beginning of the coding sequence of the leucine operon, regardless of the presence or absence of leucine. The RNA polymerase now encounters a region called the **attenuator**, where in the presence of leucine, **transcription is terminated**. This achieves the desired effect of not making the unneeded biosynthetic enzymes. In the absence of leucine, when the biosynthetic enzymes become essential, the secondary structure of the nascent mRNA at the attenuator region is altered in such a way that transcription, and therefore translation, can proceed. Details of how this works are shown in Figure 3-16.

Another mechanism for turning on or off the synthesis of enzymes is found in the case of many enzymes involved in the utilization of sugars. Taking the utilization of lactose as an example, if this sugar is the sole carbon

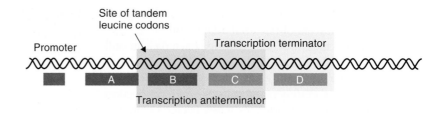

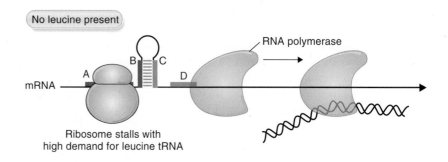

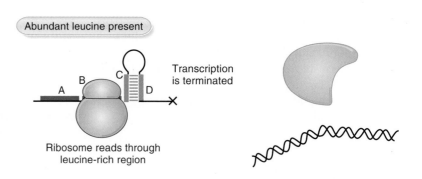

FIGURE 3-16. Regulation of enzyme synthesis by attenuation. Transcription stops when a termination stem and loop structure involving sequences C and D is formed. The middle of the drawing shows how the absence of leucine causes ribosomes to stop at sequence A and to prevent the formation of the CD stem-and-loop structure. This allows RNA polymerase to continue transcription past this region. On the bottom, when abundant leucine is present, ribosomes continue to sequence B, allowing the formation of the CD termination stem-and-loop structure. In this case, RNA polymerase cannot proceed and transcription stops.

source, the bacteria must make the enzyme β-galactosidase, which is necessary to convert lactose into glucose and galactose. In the absence of lactose, as in the case of a culture growing solely on glucose, the synthesis of β-galactosidase is unnecessary and wasteful. The synthesis of the enzyme is regulated (Fig. 3-17). At the beginning of the operon, just past the promoter, there is a regulatory sequence known as the **operator**, where a protein called the **repressor** binds. When the repressor binds to the operator, transcription cannot begin. In the presence of lactose, however, the repressor undergoes a conformational change to render it incapable of binding to the operator. Note that the lactose repressor is an allosteric protein, capable of undergoing conformational changes under the influence of an effector. The result is that when lactose is added to a culture, the repressor becomes inactive and cannot bind to the operator, thus allowing the synthesis of β-galactosidase, to proceed. β-galactosidase is an example of an **inducible enzyme**, which is made on demand, compared with a **constitutive enzyme**, which must be made at all times, such as RNA polymerase. In the case of β-galactosidase, lactose (or more precisely, one of its metabolites) is known as the **inducer**.

Overview of Regulation

Regulation of gene expression by attenuation, repression, or other mechanisms results in the relatively rapid switching on and off of gene expression. The reason is that mRNA molecules in bacteria are relatively short lived and undergo rapid turnover. Thus, after the synthesis of an enzyme is stopped, the amount of residual enzyme produced will be very small. In addition, what enzyme is left may be subject to feedback inhibition, and little of its product will be made. Note that all forms of regulation come at energy cost. Thus, feedback inhibition requires that the protein be more complex than just what is needed for catalytic activity. Regulation of enzyme synthesis by attenuation depends on the synthesis of a stretch of mRNA that will not be used if the enzymes of the operon are not made. Using a repressor to regulate an operon likewise requires the constitutive synthesis of protein repressor molecules. The energy cost of making regulatory devices is weighted against the greater disadvantage that cells would have in not being able to switch major biosynthetic pathways on and off. Thus, free-living cells like bacteria must balance their powers of efficiency and adaptability.

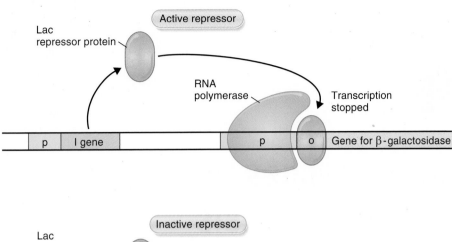

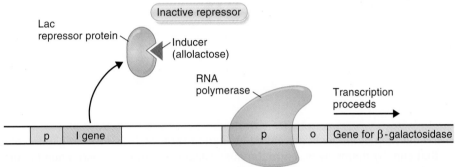

FIGURE 3-17. The operon model: regulation of β-galactosidase synthesis by repression. The repressor protein for the genes encoding enzymes for lactose utilization exists in two states: active, when the sugar inducer is absent, and inactive, when the inducer is present. The top of the figure shows that when the inducer (allolactose, a derivative of lactose) is absent, the repressor is in the active form and binds to the operator, thus preventing transcription from taking place. In the bottom of the figure, the repressor is inactivated by the inducer and cannot bind to the operator. Transcription can then proceed, and the enzyme β-galactosidase is formed.

The theme of efficiency and adaptability to environmental changes recurs throughout this book, especially in discussing how microbes cope with the changes they encounter when entering the body and certain body tissues and organs.

CONCLUSION

Bacteria share many biochemical attributes with eukaryotic cells, including the use of the same building blocks (amino acids, nucleotides, etc.) and analogous energy metabolism and polymerizing machinery. They differ, however, in their body plan, being smaller and more compactly constructed than their eukaryotic counterparts.

In addition, bacteria face the challenges of living freely in highly changing environments. They possess specialized structures that help them cope when facing scarcity of food or toxic compounds, and they are remarkably efficient in how they regulate the expression of their genes under various circumstances. They do not all use the same strategies but have a wide-ranging repertoire of ways to adapt to the environment, including the human body.

Suggested Readings

Neidhardt FC, Ingraham JL, Lin EE, et al., eds. *Escherichia coli* and *Salmonella typhimurium.* Vol. 2. 2nd ed. Washington, DC: ASM Press; 1996.

Neidhardt FC, Ingraham JL, Schaechter M. *Physiology of the Bacterial Cell.* Sunderland, MA: Sinauer Assoc.; 1990.

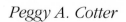

Chapter 4

Genetic Approaches to Studying Bacterial Pathogenesis

Peggy A. Cotter

TRAITS THAT RENDER bacteria pathogenic are called **virulence factors**. This term originally referred to microbial products that can, by themselves, harm the host. Classic examples of virulence factors in this context are bacterial toxins such as those discussed in Chapter 9. With increased understanding of molecular mechanisms in bacterial pathogenesis that has developed over the last few decades, the definition of the term has expanded to include any component of a microbe that is required for or potentiates its ability to cause disease. This chapter focuses on approaches that have been used to discover virulence factors and to study pathogenic mechanisms. Some basic genetic concepts are also introduced.

The number and nature of virulence factors expressed by bacterial pathogens vary as widely as the strategies the pathogens employ to establish infection and cause disease. At one end of the spectrum are organisms like *Clostridium botulinum* (see Chapter 20), a Gram-positive anaerobic bacterium with a propensity to grow in improperly prepared canned foods. A single protein toxin expressed by *C. botulinum* (botulism toxin) can cause lethal food poisoning in humans when ingested, even in the absence of the bacteria themselves. At the other end of the spectrum are bacteria like *Salmonella enterica*, serovar Typhi (see Chapter 17), which are able to adhere to, invade, and/or induce cytotoxicity in a variety of human cell types as they travel through the gastrointestinal tract, across the gut mucosa, and into deeper tissues to eventually cause a lethal systemic infection. Research into mechanisms of bacterial pathogenesis has revealed that although each organism expresses its own repertoire of virulence factors and virulence-related functions, many use similar approaches to solve common biological problems.

How are these bacterial virulence factors identified and studied in the laboratory? Researchers have traditionally used biochemical approaches, and these types of investigations continue to reveal structure–function relationships, telling us much about how toxins and other virulence factors work. Epidemiological approaches that correlate the virulence of naturally isolated strains with their clinical properties have also been extremely useful. The most commonly used approaches for identifying virulence factors and studying bacterial pathogenesis today, however, are genetic in nature. Driven by advances in molecular biotechnology, the development of broadly applicable genetic tools, and increasingly creative screening and selection strategies, these approaches have led to dramatic advances in our understanding of the molecular interactions that occur between bacterial pathogens and their mammalian hosts. Further, with rapid advances in DNA sequencing technology in the past decade, the genome sequence of a newly identified pathogen can be determined in a matter of days, and virulence traits can then be predicted based on similarity with well-established factors from other microbes.

COMPLEMENTATION APPROACHES

Genetic complementation refers to the ability of a gene to produce a functional product that overcomes a mutant phenotype, typically caused by a mutation in the same gene. Thus, when an extrachromosomal copy of gene X is expressed in a bacterium that has a mutation in the chromosomal gene X, the function normally supplied by the gene X product is expressed, and the cells are wild type. A variation of complementation has been used to identify virulence genes in a variety of pathogenic bacteria. In these cases, rather than restoring a wild-type phenotype to a mutant, the gene products expressed extrachromosomally confer one or more pathogenic traits on a nonpathogenic bacterium.

An example of such an approach was first used in the mid-1980s. Isberg et al. investigated the mechanism by which *Yersinia pseudotuberculosis* (a relative of *Yersinia pestis*, the plague bacillus) penetrates cells lining the small intestine, an early and important step in the disease caused by this organism. The researchers hypothesized that *Y. pseudotuberculosis* possesses at least one gene that encodes proteins mediating penetration (or invasion) of animal cells. They hypothesized further that expression of that gene in *Escherichia coli* would confer on that nonpathogenic, noninvasive bacterium, the ability to penetrate mammalian cells. In other words, they believed it was possible for *E. coli* to gain a function—host cell invasion—by acquiring a single gene from *Y. pseudotuberculosis*.

Their hypotheses proved to be correct and led to the identification of a gene they named *inv*, which encodes a protein, named invasin, that allows *E. coli*

(and even latex beads) to invade eukaryotic cells in culture. This basic approach was subsequently used by many other investigators to identify important virulence factors in a variety of human pathogens. To illustrate the power of the approach, the following paragraphs describe the steps Isberg et al. took and highlight the genetic and molecular biological processes involved. The basic steps are illustrated in Figure 4-1. This case study illustrates a general approach that harnesses the power of bacterial genetics for gene discovery in medically important microbes. Over time, this approach has become complemented by remarkable advances in genome sequencing technology that enable rapid identification of bacterial virulence factors. In addition to what they can teach us about infectious disease mechanisms, these factors are often targets for vaccine or drug discovery research.

Constructing Plasmid Libraries

Isberg et al. hypothesized that a single *Y. pseudotuberculosis* gene (or perhaps a cluster of linked genes) would allow *E. coli* to invade mammalian epithelial cells in culture. To test this hypothesis, they needed a collection of *E. coli* bacteria—a library composed of bacteria, each containing a unique, relatively small fragment of the *Y. pseudotuberculosis* genome (enough to contain, on average, about five genes).

The first step in constructing the genomic library was to isolate DNA from the organism of interest (*Y. pseudotuberculosis* in this case) and cut it into a large number of fragments using **restriction endonucleases**—enzymes

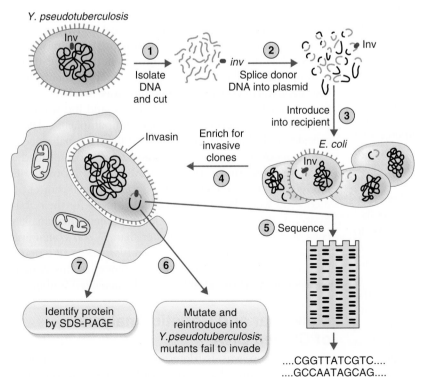

....CGGTTATCGTC....
....GCCAATAGCAG....

FIGURE 4-1. General scheme used to identify invasin.

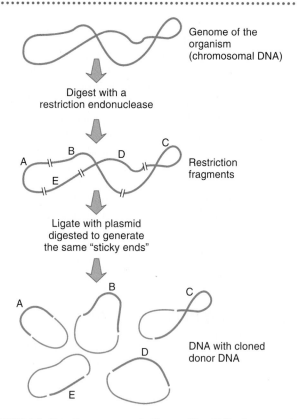

FIGURE 4-2. Creating a genomic library. The DNA of an organism is cut into restriction fragments (here labeled *A* through *E*), which are ligated with plasmid DNA that was cut with a restriction endonuclease that generates the same "sticky ends." After ligation, these recombinant plasmids are transformed into *Escherichia coli*.

that work like molecular scissors, cutting both strands of the DNA at specific sequences (Fig. 4-2). Several hundred restriction endonucleases with different specificities are available commercially. These enzymes typically recognize specific short sequences in the double-stranded DNA (four to six bases in most examples) that read the same on the top strand from 5 to 3′ as they do on the bottom strand. The enzyme cuts the DNA asymmetrically such that fragments with overhangs ("sticky ends") are generated.

Next, the large fragments of *Y. pseudotuberculosis* DNA generated by restriction endonuclease digestion were cloned into a **plasmid** so they could be introduced into *E. coli* and stably maintained. (Plasmids are small, extrachromosomal, usually circular DNA molecules capable of replicating independently within bacterial cells.) Cloning was accomplished by allowing the fragments to anneal (via their complementary sticky ends) with plasmid DNA that had been cut with a restriction endonuclease that generates the same 5′ overhangs as the one that generated the fragments in the library. Then the loosely joined molecules were covalently linked using the enzyme DNA ligase. The resulting circular plasmid molecules containing fragments of *Y. pseudotuberculosis* DNA were then introduced into *E. coli* by the mechanism of **transformation**. This process enabled bacteria to take up naked DNA from their surroundings. Strains with this ability are said to be "competent." Some bacteria are naturally competent, while others, like *E. coli*, are not but can be coaxed to take up extracellular DNA by treating them in a way that changes their surface properties before adding plasmid DNA.

The plasmid used by Isberg et al. contained a gene-encoding ampicillin resistance; therefore, the bacteria that had taken up the plasmid (transformants) could be selected by plating on agar containing ampicillin. Each colony that arose represented a single transformant that contained a plasmid with, potentially, a separate piece of the *Y. pseudotuberculosis* genome.

Positive Selection for a Virulence Trait

The next step in the process was to determine if any of the bacteria in the *E. coli* library contained plasmids with a *Y. pseudotuberculosis* gene capable of giving *E. coli* the ability to invade mammalian cells. One way to find such bacteria would be to test each member of the library (at least 1,000 different bacteria) individually for their invasion ability. Although not an impossible task, it is very labor-intensive. Isberg et al. used a clever scheme to decrease the workload. They used the invasion phenotype itself to enrich the culture for the bacteria containing the desired plasmid.

The procedure was as follows (Fig. 4-3). Pooled bacteria from the *E. coli* library were grown in liquid culture. Then aliquots were added to mammalian epithelial cells using plates with multiple wells to allow for large-scale screening. The bacteria and mammalian cells were coincubated for 1 hour, after which the bacteria were washed out of the wells and discarded. Fresh medium containing gentamicin was then added. Gentamicin is a powerful bactericidal antibiotic that cannot get into mammalian cells, which means that bacteria that remain extracellular will be killed, but those that have penetrated the tissue culture cells will live. After another hour of incubation, the gentamicin-containing medium was washed away, the mammalian cells were gently lysed, and the surviving bacteria were plated on agar containing ampicillin. Theoretically, only bacteria that penetrate the mammalian cells can be recovered in this type of genetic approach called a **positive selection**. In practice, however, the procedure is rarely completely effective. The bacteria that Isberg et al. recovered were therefore tested individually for their ability to invade mammalian cells. Most did enter mammalian cells at a rate significantly greater than *E. coli* containing the plasmid with no *Y. pseudotuberculosis* DNA (the negative control), demonstrating the usefulness of this enrichment strategy. Those clones were characterized further.

Molecular and Genetic Analysis of Cloned DNA

The next step was to determine the gene(s) responsible for conferring the invasive phenotype to *E. coli*. The

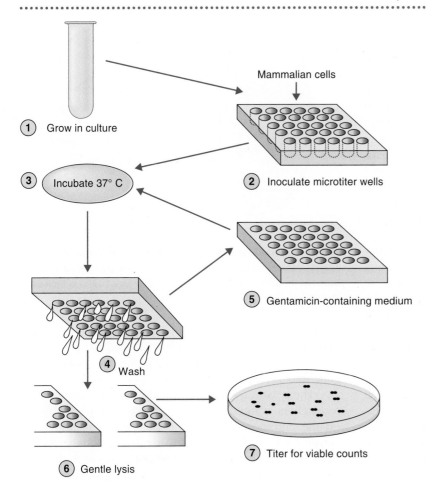

FIGURE 4-3. Enrichment for *E. coli* containing a *Yersinia pseudotuberculosis* gene conferring invasion ability. The steps in the enrichment protocol are shown.

researchers isolated plasmid DNA from the *E. coli* that were able to invade mammalian cells and characterized the *Y. pseudotuberculosis* DNA present on the plasmid. This was done by a time-consuming approach in which fragments of the cloned *Y. pseudotuberculosis* DNA were subcloned onto additional plasmids to identify smaller fragments that conferred the phenotype. The nucleotide sequence of the smallest fragment that could confer invasion was then determined.

DNA sequencing is now routine, and the complete genomes of hundreds of microbes, including many pathogens, have been determined. If a study such as this were performed today, the nucleotide sequence of just a small piece of *Y. pseudotuberculosis* DNA from the plasmid would be determined. Then the sequence corresponding to the rest of the gene(s) would be identified by computer and downloaded from a sequence database. At the time that Isberg et al. performed their study, however, DNA sequencing was quite labor-intensive. It was therefore prudent and customary to first identify the minimal DNA fragment conferring the desired phenotype before beginning a sequencing project. Inspection of the nucleotide sequence revealed an open reading frame (ORF) with the potential to encode a protein of about 103 kDa, which they named invasin (the gene designation they used was *inv*). Further biochemical analysis proved that the *inv*

gene does in fact encode such a protein and that the protein is in the outer membrane.

Recombinant Methods for Generating Chromosomal Mutations

Although compelling, the experiments described in the previous section did not prove that *inv* and its product were responsible for allowing *Y. pseudotuberculosis* to invade host cells. For the definitive proof, at least by the standards of genetics, Isberg et al. had to construct a strain of *Y. pseudotuberculosis* containing a **loss-of-function mutation** at the *inv* locus. Such a mutation would lead to complete abrogation of the *inv* function. Many varieties of these types of mutants can be created. Substitution of a single nucleotide in a gene for a different one can result in an amino acid substitution in the protein that completely abrogates its function, decreases its functionality, or even confers on the protein a new function. If a stop codon is introduced, the truncated protein produced can similarly have little, no, or different activity. Deletion mutations, in which most or all of the gene is removed from the chromosome, are nearly always loss-of-function mutations.

Isberg et al. used the following approach to create a *Y. pseudotuberculosis* strain with a loss-of-function mutation in the *inv* gene. The first step was to mutate the *inv* gene present on the plasmid on which it was identified. Using restriction endonucleases that cut the *inv* gene at locations near the 5′ and 3′ ends of the gene, the researchers replaced the majority of the ORF with a different gene, one encoding a protein that confers resistance to kanamycin, an antibiotic that kills both *E. coli* and *Y. pseudotuberculosis* (Fig. 4-4). A DNA fragment containing the mutated *inv* gene (comprising the kanamycin resistance [Km^r] gene plus about 500 bp of flanking DNA both 5′ and 3′ to *inv*) was then cloned into a plasmid with two important features: (1) it could be introduced into *Y. pseudotuberculosis* by **conjugation**, and (2) it was a **suicide plasmid** for *Y. pseudotuberculosis*, meaning that it could not replicate in *Y. pseudotuberculosis*.

Conjugation is a mechanism by which genetic material is transferred one way from a donor cell to a recipient cell in a process that requires cell-to-cell contact (Fig. 4-5). The donor cell contains a conjugative plasmid (e.g., the F plasmid of *E. coli*) with genes encoding a conjugation (or sex) pilus that forms a bridge between the donor and recipient cells. The conjugative plasmid also contains an origin of transfer and additional genes that encode proteins mediating the transfer of a single strand of DNA, beginning at the origin of transfer, from the donor cell into the recipient cell. The complementary strand is synthesized inside the recipient cell to reconstitute the complete plasmid. Conjugation is typically several orders of magnitude more efficient than transformation; therefore,

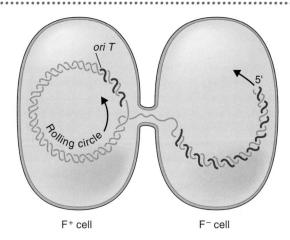

FIGURE 4-5. Transfer of F plasmid from an F⁺ to an F⁻ cell. A single DNA strand generated by replication is transferred from the donor to the recipient cell. The complementary strand is then synthesized in the recipient to reconstitute the complete F plasmid.

by cloning the mutated *inv* gene on a conjugative plasmid, the researchers greatly increased the probability of introducing the plasmid containing the mutated *inv* gene into *Y. pseudotuberculosis*.

The reason for using a suicide plasmid was that the researchers wanted to replace the wild-type *inv* gene on the chromosome with the mutated allele they had constructed on the plasmid. After using conjugation to introduce the plasmid into *Y. pseudotuberculosis*, the bacteria were plated on a medium containing kanamycin (as well as an antibiotic that would kill the conjugation donor strain but not *Y. pseudotuberculosis*). Because the plasmid could not replicate in *Y. pseudotuberculosis*, cells that had received the conjugative plasmid (**exconjugates**) would be resistant to kanamycin only if the plasmid, or at least the part of the plasmid containing the Km^r gene, had integrated into the *Y. pseudotuberculosis* chromosome. In that case the event most frequently leading to kanamycin-resistant colonies would be homologous recombination between sequences on the plasmid and sequences on the chromosome (i.e., the 5′ and 3′ ends of the *inv* gene). A single recombination event would lead to integration of the entire plasmid into the chromosome and the creation of a partially diploid strain containing one wild-type copy of *inv* and one mutant copy of *inv*. However, if two recombination events occurred, one within the 5′ region of homology and one within the 3′ region, the wild-type *inv* gene would be replaced with the mutated *inv* gene. Although not the case for most bacteria, it turns out that in *Y. pseudotuberculosis*, exconjugates resulting from double recombination events are obtained from this type of experiment much more frequently than those resulting from single recombination events.

The mutant *Y. pseudotuberculosis* strain the researchers constructed was greatly impaired for cell invasion, doing so at a frequency that was only 0.1% of that of its wild-type parental strain. To rule out any effects of inserting the antibiotic on downstream genes (called

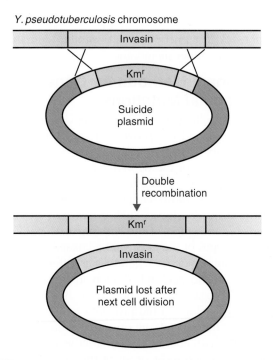

FIGURE 4-4. Replacing the wild-type *inv* gene with a kanamycin resistance (Km^r) gene. A majority of the *inv* gene contained on a suicide plasmid is replaced with a gene conferring Km^r. After mobilization of the plasmid into *Y. pseudotuberculosis*, kanamycin-resistant exconjugants, which have undergone a double recombination event, are selected.

polar effects), a wild-type copy of *inv* was introduced into the *inv* mutant on a plasmid that could replicate in *Y. pseudotuberculosis*. This **complemented** strain was able to invade mammalian cells at a rate indistinguishable from wild-type *Y. pseudotuberculosis*. Because this complementing plasmid contained only the *inv* gene and no downstream genes, the invasion defect displayed by the strain containing the insertion mutation in *inv* had to be caused by the lack of expression of a functional invasin protein.

TRANSPOSON-BASED METHODS FOR VIRULENCE GENE DISCOVERY

Transposons (Tns), first discovered in maize by Barbara McClintock in 1940, are found in all major branches of life. Basic research toward a mechanistic understanding of how Tns function led to the development of incredibly powerful genetic tools that have been used by plant, animal, and bacterial biologists.

Transposable Elements

Transposable elements ("hopping genes") are DNA segments that can insert themselves into and excise themselves from DNA molecules. These elements can therefore "hop" from one chromosomal location to another, from a chromosome to a plasmid, or vice versa. The two steps, integration and excision, are carried out by different mechanisms. There are two varieties of transposable elements: the **insertion sequence** (**IS**), which has the minimal genetic information for transposition, and **transposon** (**Tn**), which carries extra genes in addition to those required for transposition.

An IS element is a relatively small DNA sequence, about 1 to 2 kbp long, with two characteristic properties: First, it contains specific sequences located at its ends that are inverted repeats of one another and are required for the integration and excision processes (Fig. 4-6). Second,

an IS element encodes within its core region an enzyme (called **transposase**) that recognizes the inverted repeat sequences and catalyzes integration and excision of the IS element into and out of a DNA molecule. The integration process often results in duplication of a short stretch of DNA at the insertion site; therefore, an IS element is usually flanked by a small direct repeat sequence.

A Tn is more complex. It is composed of two IS elements flanking a core region that often contains genes encoding antibiotic resistance. Usually, the transposase of only one of the IS elements is functional, and the sequences of the "inner" inverted repeats have changed such that the entire Tn translocates from place to place via a reaction that is catalyzed by the functional transposase and involving the outermost inverted repeat sequences.

When a Tn inserts into an ORF, it almost always disrupts the function of the ORF, usually creating a loss-of-function mutation. If the Tn contains an antibiotic-resistant gene (as most do), it also marks its location in the chromosome by conferring antibiotic resistance. Thus, a Tn can be mapped easily, transduced (along with flanking DNA) into another bacterium, and cloned (along with flanking DNA) onto a plasmid. These features make Tns extremely useful tools, and geneticists have used and modified them extensively over the years.

Transposable Reporter Genes to Identify Commonly Regulated Traits

Tn5 is a transposon that has been widely used by researchers studying different bacterial traits, including pathogenicity. It contains a gene encoding Km^r. Originally, researchers performed Tn mutagenesis with Tn5 by introducing it into a bacterium on a suicide plasmid and then selecting for Km^r colonies that formed as a result of the Tn5 hopping from the plasmid to the chromosome. Next, pools of mutants were screened for a particular mutant phenotype (e.g., a different colony morphology or failure to grow under certain conditions), and then

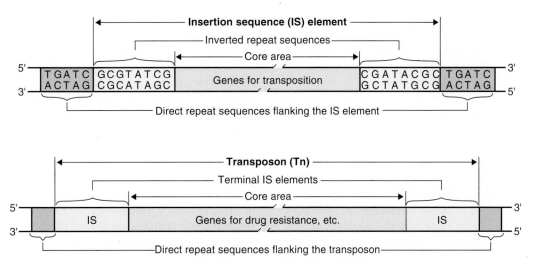

FIGURE 4-6. Insertion sequences and transposons.

the disrupted gene was mapped, cloned, and characterized by virtue of the Km^r gene. However, because Tn5 encodes a functional transposase, it is capable of translocating repeatedly; therefore, the mutations it creates are not stable. To circumvent this problem, geneticists moved the transposase gene from within Tn5 to another location on the suicide plasmid. The resulting "mini-Tn5," which lacks a functional transposase, cannot translocate again after the suicide plasmid containing the functional transposase gene is diluted out of the recipient bacterial cell. Mini-Tn5 thus creates stable mutations, facilitating mapping, cloning, and characterization experiments.

Further modification of Tn5 enabled researchers to use it to "report" information regarding the expression pattern of the gene into which it had inserted. With this new Tn5, researchers can identify genes whose expression is influenced by specific factors that might be predicted to be important during infection, like temperature or the availability of iron. Of these reporter genes, the *E. coli lacZ* gene, encoding β-galactosidase, is perhaps the most commonly used. Chromogenic substrates are available that allow bacteria expressing *lacZ* (Lac+ colonies) and those not expressing *lacZ* (Lac- colonies) to be distinguished easily on plates, allowing for efficient screening strategies, and sensitive quantitative enzymatic assays can be performed on cells grown in liquid culture. Specific antibodies for detecting the β-galactosidase protein are also available.

Mini-Tn5–*lacZ* contains a promoterless *lacZ* gene (the entire ORF from start codon to stop codon as well as enough sequence 5′ to the ATG to include the native ribosome binding site) located just inside the IS element. If mini-Tn5–*lacZ* inserts into a gene "downstream" from its promoter (i.e., such that the gene into which it has inserted is transcribed in the same direction as the promoterless *lacZ* gene), then *lacZ* transcription will be under the control of the promoter of the disrupted gene. Thus, levels of β-galactosidase activity will reflect (and thereby report) the transcription pattern of the disrupted gene. Mini-Tn5–*lacZ* can be used to identify genes that are regulated in response to specific environmental conditions. For example, to find genes that are expressed at 37°C but not 25°C, Km^r mini-Tn5–*lacZ* insertion mutants can.be plated on a medium containing X-gal (a chromogenic substrate for β-galactosidase that produces a blue product when cleaved) and incubated at 37°C. Blue colonies can then be restreaked or replica plated onto the same medium and incubated at 25°C. Those that form white colonies at 25°C would have the desired expression pattern. Many additional easily screened or selectable reporter genes have been incorporated into mini-Tn5, including *gusA* (encoding β-glucuronidase), *luxAB* (encoding luciferase), *gfp* (encoding green fluorescent protein), and genes encoding resistance to antibiotics such as chloramphenicol, tetracycline, and streptomycin.

Mini-Tn5 took another evolutionary step with the development of Tn-*phoA*. The *E. coli phoA* gene encodes alkaline phosphatase, an enzyme that is active only after transport to the periplasm. A chromogenic substrate for alkaline phosphatase analogous to X-gal, called X-P, is available. PhoA$^+$ bacteria will form blue colonies when plated on agar containing X-P, and PhoA$^-$ bacteria will form white colonies. The truncated *phoA* gene present on Tn-*phoA* lacks a promoter, a ribosome-binding site, ATG, and the nucleotides encoding the signal sequence (the first roughly 40 amino acids of the PhoA protein) used by the cellular secretion machinery to direct the alkaline phosphatase enzyme across the cytoplasmic membrane and into the periplasm. Therefore, Tn-*phoA* mutants will form blue colonies only if Tn-*phoA* has inserted into a gene such that an in-frame fusion is created and the N terminus of the fusion protein (encoded by the nucleotides at the 5′ end of the disrupted gene) contains a signal sequence for secretion across the cytoplasmic membrane. Tn-*phoA* mutagenesis is used therefore to identify genes that encode proteins secreted across the cytoplasmic membrane (and possibly also across the outer membrane of Gram-negative bacteria). Tn-*phoA* has been particularly useful in the identification of virulence factors because usually, perhaps always, they are proteins that are either surface associated or secreted. A schematic showing how Tn-*phoA* mutagenesis was used to identify virulence genes in *Vibrio cholerae* is shown in Figure 4-7. In this experiment the investigators already knew that some virulence genes in *V. cholerae* are maximally expressed at pH 6.5 in high osmolarity. So they tested PhoA$^+$ fusions for a similar pattern of expression before testing the strains in a mouse model.

Negative Selection for Identifying Essential Genes

Tn mutagenesis is most useful when the desired phenotype can be easily screened—as with the reporter Tns incorporating *lacZ* or *phoA*—or better yet, selected. In a **screen**, the entire population is examined, and the desired mutants are identified based on an observable altered phenotype, such as a difference in colony color or morphology on a specific medium, lack of production of a specific protein as determined by Western blot analysis, or an inability to adhere to mammalian cells in culture. In a **selection**, only mutants with the desired phenotype (such as resistance to a specific antibiotic) survive; therefore, a mutant that is present in a population at a frequency of 1 per 10^6 or less can be identified easily. Selection schemes are clearly much more powerful than those involving screens because they allow for the detection of very rare events with little effort. Unfortunately, it is not always possible to design a selection-based mutagenesis scheme, particularly if survival of the desired mutant is decreased. The desired selection is a **negative selection**, used to find mutants unable to grow under particular conditions.

Hensel et al. designed a clever strategy to solve this problem. They were studying the mechanisms

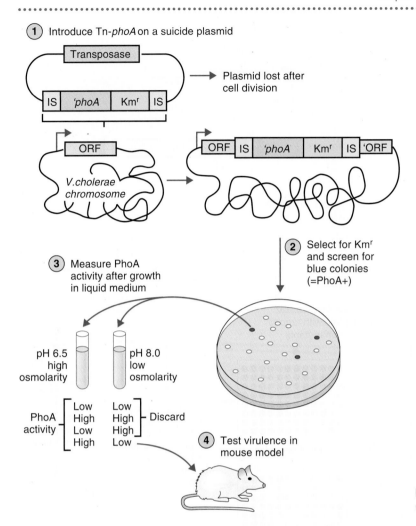

1 Introduce Tn-*phoA* on a suicide plasmid

Transposase

Plasmid lost after cell division

IS | '*phoA* | Km^r | IS

ORF

V.cholerae chromosome

ORF | IS | '*phoA* | Km^r | IS | '*ORF*

2 Select for Km^r and screen for blue colonies (=PhoA+)

3 Measure PhoA activity after growth in liquid medium

pH 6.5 high osmolarity

pH 8.0 low osmolarity

PhoA activity

Low	Low
High	High
Low	High
High	Low

Discard

4 Test virulence in mouse model

FIGURE 4-7. General Tn-*phoA* mutagenesis scheme used to identify virulence genes in *Vibrio cholerae*.

by which *Salmonella typhimurium* causes systemic infection in mice, a well-established model for typhoid fever in humans that is caused by *Salmonella typhi* (see Chapter 17). Although many *Salmonella* virulence genes had been identified, the researchers hypothesized that many more existed, some of which may not be identifiable using any of the in vitro–based schemes developed up to that time. Their desire was to determine the contribution to virulence of every gene in the *S. typhimurium* chromosome. Specifically, they were after genes that were essential for the bacterium to survive during growth within the host but not within laboratory media. Although, as previously described, it is relatively simple to perform Tn mutagenesis and collect enough mutants to be certain that every nonessential gene in the genome has been mutated (within the population), it would be extremely labor-intensive and prohibitively expensive to test each mutant individually to determine whether it had lost the ability to cause a lethal, systemic infection in mice. Hensel et al. wanted to infect mice with pools composed of hundreds of different mutants and determine which mutants were attenuated. The problem was, how do you identify the mutants that do not survive?

"Signature-Tagged" Transposons

Hensel et al. wanted to be able to create a population of random mutants, each marked to make it relatively easy to distinguish from the rest of the population. Although it is simple and straightforward to produce large numbers of random mutants using Tn mutagenesis, the individual mutants cannot be easily identified because the Tns are identical, and the mutants differ only in the chromosomal location of the Tn. To overcome this problem, the researchers created a pool of Tns that were each "tagged" with a unique 40-bp stretch of DNA (a molecular signature). The tags were synthesized in vitro as oligonucleotides with 40-bp random sequences in the center, flanked by recognition sequences for the restriction endonuclease *Hin*dIII and invariable "arms" that served as primer binding sites for amplification using the **polymerase chain reaction (PCR)** (Fig. 4-8A). The population of random tags was amplified using PCR and cloned into mini-Tn*5* present on a suicide plasmid, creating a source of tagged mini-Tn*5*s (Fig. 4-8).

Creating Transposon Pools

The tagged mini-Tn*5*s were introduced into *S. typhimurium* on a suicide plasmid by conjugation, and mutants

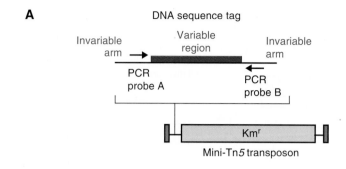

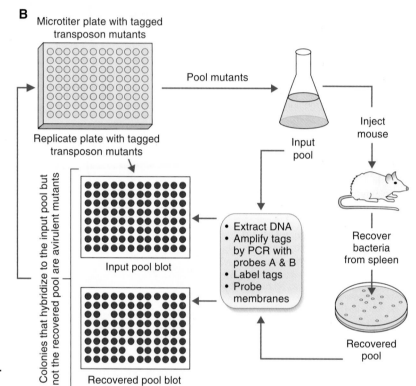

FIGURE 4-8. **Signature-tagged mutagenesis to identify virulence genes in *Salmonella typhimurium*.**

on whose chromosomes the tagged mini-Tn5s had hopped were selected on plates containing kanamycin. Each mutant was stored in a well of a 96-well microtiter dish, and a total of 1,510 individual mutants were isolated and stored.

Screening for Mutants in Animal Models of Infection

To identify mutants with this approach, Hensel et al. used the following procedure (see Fig. 4-8B). Bacteria from each well of a microtiter dish were replica-plated onto two identical membranes, the bacteria were lysed, and the DNA was denatured (to separate the two strands) and attached to the membranes by cross-linking. These membranes were saved for use later in the procedure. Bacteria from each well were also grown together in liquid medium in vitro, forming the "input pool." An aliquot of this culture was used to infect mice by intraperitoneal injection.

Three days later, bacteria recovered from the spleens of the infected mice were plated on standard laboratory medium, and about 10,000 colonies were combined,

forming the "recovered pool." Chromosomal DNA was isolated from the two pools of bacteria (the input pool and the recovered pool), and PCR was used to amplify the sequence tags. Radioactive nucleotides were used in the amplification to label the products. Because recognition sequences for the restriction endonuclease *Hin*dIII were incorporated into the sequence tags, the unique 40-bp portions of the tags could be liberated by digesting with this enzyme. The labeled, unique sequence tags generated from the input pool were incubated with one of the membranes containing DNA from each of the mutant bacteria, and the tags generated from the recovered pool were incubated with the other membrane. The incubations were carried out under conditions in which the tags could anneal with the complementary sequences present in the chromosomal DNA.

After extensive washing, the membranes were exposed to x-ray film, and the patterns obtained for the two blots were compared. The membrane incubated with labeled tags amplified from the input pool caused black spots on the film corresponding to every well of the microtiter dish. This was expected because all the mutants, and thus all the sequence tags, should have been represented in the input population. The membrane incubated with labeled tags amplified from the recovered pool caused black spots on the film corresponding to most, but not all, of the wells. A well for which a black spot was not obtained contained mutants that were not present in the recovered pool, potentially because the Tns in these mutants disrupted genes required for survival in the host. Of 12 pools tested (representing 1,152 different mutants), 40 such mutants were identified.

The DNA sequence flanking the Tn insertion in 28 of the 40 mutants was determined. Thirteen of the insertions were in previously identified *S. typhimurium* virulence genes. This result validated the usefulness of the screening approach. Six of the mutations were in genes with sequence similarity to known genes in other pathogenic bacteria but which had not previously been identified as virulence genes in *S. typhimurium*. In this class were genes for a specialized secretion system, called a **type III secretion system** (see Chapters 16 and 17) that has since been demonstrated to be required for macrophage survival of *Salmonella*. When these mutants were tested for virulence individually, they were each found to be greatly attenuated. Nine of the mutants identified in the screen were in genes with no similarity to database entries and therefore represented potentially novel virulence genes.

The power of this approach cannot be overstated. Because pools of 96 mutants could be screened simultaneously, thousands of mutants could be tested using a small fraction of the mice that would have been required if the mutants had to be evaluated individually. This represents significant savings in effort, time, and mice. In addition, because signature-tagged mutagenesis finds genes essential for survival in the host, it is an exceptional method for identifying potential new antimicrobial targets for therapeutic purposes. Signature-tagged mutagenesis has been used to discover colonization and pathogenicity traits in many microbes since it was first applied to the study of *Salmonella* infection.

PROMOTER-TRAPPING METHODS

Several approaches have been developed to identify virulence genes based on their predicted pattern of transcriptional activity during infection. The approach, called **in vivo expression technology (IVET)**, was designed to isolate promoters that are active under specific conditions. Once a promoter is identified, the genes and gene products whose expression it drives can be identified and characterized.

IVET differs significantly from most of the genetic approaches used to identify and characterize virulence genes, which require that the gene be expressed either within the pathogen itself or in a surrogate such as *E. coli* grown in or on laboratory medium. For example, the discovery of *inv* by Isberg et al. required its expression in *E. coli* growing in Luria Bertani broth. These approaches are dependent on, and limited by, the ability to mimic in the laboratory the environmental conditions that the bacteria are exposed to in the host during infection. Mahan, Slauch, and Mekalanos hypothesized that specific conditions exist in the host that laboratory conditions cannot (or do not) adequately reflect and that some virulence genes are expressed *only* under those specific conditions. To test their hypothesis, the researchers devised a genetic strategy designed to identify genes expressed in vivo but *not* in vitro. They employed this strategy to study *S. typhimurium* genes, using murine infection as the in vivo condition and MacConkey lactose agar as the in vitro condition.

Constructing Promoter Libraries

The first goal of the IVET approach was to identify *S. typhimurium* genes expressed in vivo—that is, during murine infection. It had been demonstrated previously that *S. typhimurium purA* mutants are completely avirulent. The *purA* gene encodes an enzyme required for purine biosynthesis. *S. typhimurium* can import purines from its surroundings; therefore, *purA* mutants can grow in the laboratory if purines are supplied in the medium. *PurA* mutants are completely unable to establish murine infection, indicating that purines are not readily available to *S. typhimurium* within the in vivo niches it colonizes in the mouse. Mahan et al. exploited this fact to design a **selection** scheme to identify genes expressed in vivo.

First, the researchers constructed an *S. typhimurium* strain containing a deletion mutation in the *purA* gene. It was important to use a deletion mutation, which is nonrevertible, rather than a point mutation, which could potentially revert to wild type during infection, eliminating the basis for selection. Next, Mahan et al. constructed a plasmid (pIVET1) with the following characteristics (Fig. 4-9): (1) It could be introduced into *S. typhimurium* by conjugation. (2) It was a suicide plasmid for *S. typhimurium* but not *E. coli*; that is, it could replicate autonomously in *E. coli* but not *S. typhimurium*. (3) It contained a gene encoding ampicillin resistance (called *bla*, for β-lactamase). (4) It contained a site upstream of the *purA* gene into which foreign DNA fragments could be cloned. (5) It contained a promoterless *lacZ* gene immediately downstream of *purA*, with no transcriptional termination signals between *purA* and *lacZ*. (6) It contained no sequences with homology to the *S. typhimurium* chromosome.

The researchers isolated chromosomal DNA from wild-type *S. typhimurium*, digested it with a restriction endonuclease, and ligated the resulting DNA fragments in the cloning site upstream of *purA*. The resulting plasmids were used to transform *E. coli*, and transformants were selected on agar containing ampicillin. These transformants, representing a chromosomal library of *S. typhimurium*, were pooled.

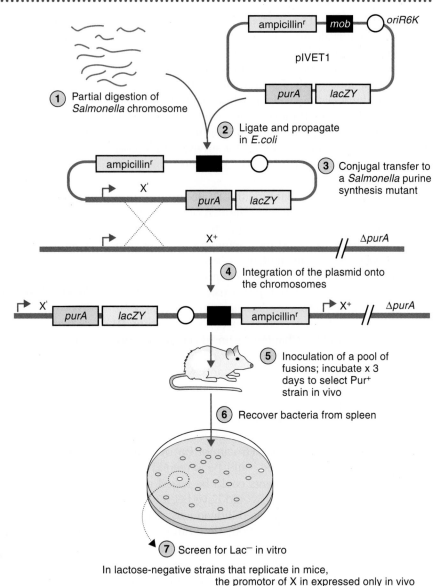

FIGURE 4-9. In vivo expression technology used to identify virulence genes in *S. typhimurium.*

In lactose-negative strains that replicate in mice, the promotor of X in expressed only in vivo

Plasmid-Based Recombination for Operon Fusion

The pIVET1 derivative plasmids were introduced into the mutated Δ*purA* strain of *S. typhimurium* by conjugation, and exconjugates were selected on agar containing purines and ampicillin. Because pIVET1 is a suicide plasmid for *S. typhimurium* with no homology to the *S. typhimurium* chromosome, ampicillin-resistant exconjugates will take place only if homologous recombination occurs between the *S. typhimurium* sequences cloned into the pIVET1 derivative and the *S. typhimurium* chromosome, resulting in integration of the entire plasmid into the chromosome (see Fig. 4-9). If the *S. typhimurium* sequences on the plasmid happen to contain a transcriptional promoter oriented in the same direction as *purA* and *lacZ*, then on integration of the plasmid, transcription from this promoter will drive transcription of *purA* and *lacZ* when it is active. Note that if the entire promoter region is present within the fragment cloned into pIVET1, transcription of the native gene on the chromosome will not be altered because these sequences will also be present upstream of the native gene. Mahan et al. pooled ampicillin-resistant exconjugates.

Selection of Promoters Active during Infection

The pooled exconjugates (containing integrated pIVET1-derivative plasmids) were injected into mice intraperitoneally. Three days later the mice were euthanized and bacteria were recovered from their spleens (see Fig. 4-9). Because *purA* mutants of *S. typhimurium* are avirulent, the only bacteria that could be recovered from a spleen 3 days postinoculation would be those in which the *purA* gene on the integrated plasmid was expressed in vivo. For such recovery to occur, the *S. typhimurium* chromosomal DNA fragment cloned into the pIVET1 plasmid either must contain a promoter oriented to directing transcription of *purA* (and *lacZ*) or must contain an internal fragment of a gene or operon oriented so that when the plasmid integrates into the gene, the upstream promoter directs expression of *purA* (and *lacZ*). Note, however, that if the fragment contains only an internal fragment of a gene or operon, the gene or operon will not be transcribed in the exconjugates because it will have been separated from its promoter by integration of the plasmid. If the gene or operon is essential for virulence, then although *purA* transcription will be restored in vivo, the strain will not survive in the mouse. Passage of the exconjugates' pool through the mouse thus provides a selection for strains with integrated plasmids that contain promoters expressed in vivo.

Because the goal of this approach was to find genes expressed in vivo and not in vitro, the next step in the analysis was to determine if any of the promoters selected on the basis of expression in vivo were not expressed in vitro. To do this, Mahan et al. plated the bacteria recovered from the mice onto MacConkey lactose agar. MacConkey lactose agar is a differential medium on which Lac⁺ bacteria form red colonies and Lac⁻ bacteria form white colonies. Most of the recovered bacteria formed red colonies. That result was expected because most genes required for *S. typhimurium* to grow in vivo (such as those encoding ribosomal proteins and RNA, RNA polymerase, cell wall constituents, and other "housekeeping" functions) are also required for growth in vitro. Five percent of the bacteria recovered from the mouse spleens formed white colonies on MacConkey lactose agar, indicating that the integrated plasmids contained promoters expressed in vivo but not in vitro. These were the clones Mahan et al. were looking for. They chose 15 strains for further characterization. To confirm that those strains contained plasmids with in vivo–induced promoters, they infected mice with each strain individually and measured β-galactosidase activity in bacteria recovered from the spleens of mice as well as from bacteria grown in a standard laboratory medium. In all cases β-galactosidase activity was greater in bacteria recovered from mouse spleens than in bacteria grown in a laboratory medium.

To identify the in vivo–induced genes, the researchers determined the nucleotide sequences of the *S. typhimurium* DNA fragments containing the in vivo–induced promoters and compared the sequences they obtained with those present in GenBank. Five genetic loci were identified. Two had no significant homology to sequences present in GenBank and therefore represented potentially novel virulence genes. Some of the genes identified with this approach were involved in quite ordinary aspects of bacterial physiology, raising the question of how we define virulence factors. Enzymes involved in amino acid, nucleic acid, or transfer RNA biosynthesis do not fit the classic definition of a virulence factor. However, expression of these enzymes occurs in vivo and is required for virulence, yet dispensable for growth in vitro. Thus, these enzymes represent "components that are required for or that potentiate the organism's ability to cause disease" and thus fit an expanded definition of a virulence factor. While a debate regarding whether factors that fall into this category represent true virulence genes will undoubtedly continue for some time, there is no question that learning that these factors are essential for *S. typhimurium* to cause a lethal infection reveals information regarding the types of environments it encounters within the host to do so. Furthermore, given their requirement for growth during infection, the genes identified by IVET also represent attractive therapeutic targets.

A variation of IVET, termed differential fluorescence induction (DFI), was subsequently developed. The basic features of library construction and pooling of strains are similar to IVET, but the key feature of DFI is its use of fluorescence as a reporter. The method was designed to identify promoters specifically upregulated by pathogens that can survive within professional phagocytic cells, which represent a major defense against infection (see Chapter 6). A number of important pathogens, such as *S. typhi* (see Chapter 17), *Legionella pneumophila* (see Chapter 21), and *Mycobacterium tuberculosis* (see Chapter 23), to name just a few, can survive within professional phagocytes. An updated approach, DFI uses **fluorescence-activated cell sorting** (**FACS**) of pooled libraries of bacteria in which promoter DNA has been randomly fused to a fluorescent reporter gene, such as *gfp*, which encodes green fluorescent protein (Fig. 4-10). Promoters that are activated by bacteria within the phagocyte cause the phagocyte to become highly fluorescent, which causes it to be sorted from the rest of the nonfluorescent population. The basic elements of DFI are shown in Figure 4-10.

ANTIBODY-BASED APPROACHES

In addition to performing their primary and critically important functions in clearing current infections and preventing new ones, our adaptive immune responses also provide powerful tools for studying bacterial pathogenesis. Antibodies are particularly useful because they are easily obtained from serum, and a plethora of reagents and protocols that take advantage of their specificity and binding characteristics have been developed. Indeed, because pathogen-specific antibodies are induced to very high levels in response to infection, relatively simple yet highly sensitive antibody-based protocols are used routinely in clinical laboratories to diagnose many bacterial and viral infections. Pathogen-specific antibodies have also been extremely useful for identifying, purifying, and characterizing virulence factors. An antibody-based approach designed to identify virulence genes expressed exclusively in vivo is described here.

In vivo–induced antigen technology (IVIAT) uses the host antibody response to identify proteins expressed by the bacteria during infection but not during growth in

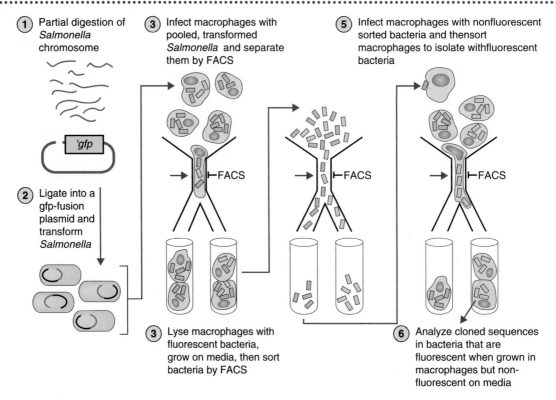

① Partial digestion of *Salmonella* chromosome

② Ligate into a gfp-fusion plasmid and transform *Salmonella*

③ Infect macrophages with pooled, transformed *Salmonella* and separate them by FACS

③ Lyse macrophages with fluorescent bacteria, grow on media, then sort bacteria by FACS

⑤ Infect macrophages with nonfluorescent sorted bacteria and thensort macrophages to isolate withfluorescent bacteria

⑥ Analyze cloned sequences in bacteria that are fluorescent when grown in macrophages but non-fluorescent on media

FIGURE 4-10. Differential fluorescence induction technique used to identify genes expressed by *S. typhimurium* during intracellular survival in macrophages.

standard laboratory conditions. Although similar to IVET in that its goal is to identify factors expressed *only* in vivo, IVIAT does not rely on the use of animal models. This represents a significant advantage because animal models that reproduce, at least to some extent, the natural course of infection do not exist for many human pathogens. The rationale behind IVIAT is as follows: On exposure to a particular pathogen, production of a large population of pathogen-specific antibodies is induced. Each antibody in the population recognizes a single epitope and there-fore, most likely, a single factor expressed by the bacteria during the course of infection. As discussed earlier, most factors expressed during infection are also expressed dur-ing growth in vitro. Antibodies that recognize such factors should be present in the population of induced antibod-ies. However, if, as hypothesized, some bacterial factors are expressed *only* during infection, antibodies that rec-ognize these in vivo–induced antigens should also be pre-sent in the population of induced antibodies. The goal of IVIAT is to isolate this population of antibodies and use it to identify the in vivo–induced antigens. One of the first studies using this approach helped identify virulence genes in *M. tuberculosis*, the causative agent of tuberculo-sis (TB), which kills about three million people annually (see Chapter 23).

Preparing Convalescent Sera

The first objective of the IVIAT approach is to isolate a population of antibodies that recognize bacterial factors

expressed only during infection. In the TB work, sera were collected and pooled from 25 TB patients. The pooled convalescent serum theoretically contained antibodies recognizing all *M. tuberculosis* factors expressed in vivo and capable of stimulating the immune system to produce antibodies. To remove antibodies that recognized factors expressed by *M. tuberculosis* in vitro, a lysate of *M. tuber-culosis* grown on Lowenstein-Jensen agar was prepared and immobilized on a nitrocellulose membrane, and the membrane was incubated with the pooled serum. Anti-bodies that bound to the factors present on the membrane were removed when the membrane was removed from the serum sample (Fig. 4-11). This absorption procedure was repeated multiple times, resulting in depletion of antibodies recognizing in vitro–expressed antigens from the pooled serum and leaving behind the antibodies that recognize *M. tuberculosis* factors expressed in vivo but not in vitro. For reasons that will become apparent in the following sections, a lysate of *E. coli* was also prepared, bound to nitrocellulose, and used to deplete the serum of anti–*E. coli* antibodies.

Phage-Based Expression Libraries

The next objective of the IVIAT approach is to use the absorbed serum to identify in vivo–induced factors. Because the genes encoding these factors are, by defini-tion, not expressed during growth in vitro, the researchers needed to activate transcription of these genes artificially. They accomplished this by constructing an **expression**

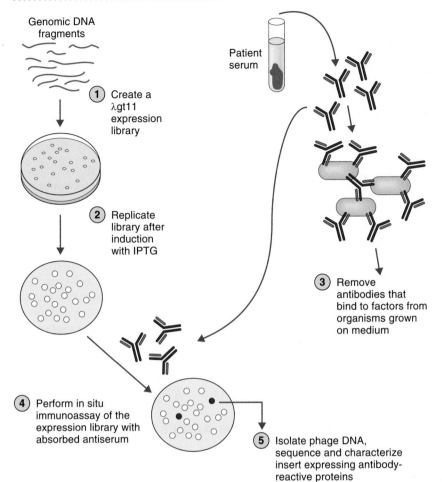

Genomic DNA
fragments

1. Create a
λgt11
expression
library

2. Replicate
library after
induction
with IPTG

4. Perform in situ
immunoassay of the
expression library with
absorbed antiserum

Patient
serum

3. Remove
antibodies that
bind to factors from
organisms grown
on medium

5. Isolate phage DNA,
sequence and characterize
insert expressing antibody-
reactive proteins

FIGURE 4-11. In vivo–induced antigen technology used to identify in vivo–induced antigens in *Mycobacterium tuberculosis*.

library. The goal of constructing an expression library is to express all or part of every protein that the bacterium is capable of producing in at least one member of the library. A commonly used expression library is **bacteriophage λgt11**.

Bacteriophages, or simply phage, are viruses that infect bacteria. When some phages, called **temperate phages**, infect bacteria, they can take one of two pathways of growth. In one pathway, they incorporate their genomes into that of their host and replicate in a benign, quiescent state in which most of their genes are not expressed or are expressed at low levels. Bacteria in which phage are replicating this way are called **lysogens**, and many pathogenic bacteria are actually lysogens in which important virulence factors are expressed from the phage genome. An example of this is *Corynebacterium diphtheriae*, which produces a potent toxin by virtue of being lysogenic for a toxin-encoding phage (see Chapter 9). Under conditions of DNA damage and possibly other stresses, lysogens can be induced, and the phage **lytic growth** program is activated. During lytic growth, phage take over the host cell transcription and translation machinery to express phage genes and proteins at very high levels, assemble 100 or more phage particles per bacterial cell, and then lyse the

bacterial cell and infect neighboring cells. On a lawn of bacteria growing on an agar plate, a single phage can form a **plaque** (a clearing zone resulting from the lysis of infected bacteria) containing 10^8 to 10^9 phage particles in a matter of hours.

The expression phage λgt11 is a modified form of the well-studied temperate phage λ. This modified phage has been engineered to contain a *lacZ* gene with a unique restriction endonuclease cleavage site just downstream of the transcription and translation initiation sites. Moreover, the promoter driving expression of *lacZ* in λgt11 is inducible by isopropyl-β-D-thiogalactopyranoside (IPTG). *M. tuberculosis* chromosomal DNA was isolated and fragmented to an average size of about 3 kbp and inserted into λgt11 DNA using restriction enzymes and DNA ligase. The recombinant λ chromosomes were packaged into phage particles in vitro and used to infect lawns of *E. coli*. The first several hours of infection were allowed to proceed in the absence of IPTG. Under these conditions, phage genes were expressed, but *lacZ* and any fusion proteins resulting from insertion of *M. tuberculosis* DNA were not expressed. For the last few hours of the infection process, IPTG was added to the medium. The presence of IPTG results in high levels of transcription from the *lacZ* promoter. If inserting *M. tuberculosis* DNA into *lacZ* results in the formation of an in-frame fusion between *lacZ* and an *M. tuberculosis* open reading frame, a fusion protein is synthesized at high levels, and when λ lyses the bacterial cells to infect neighboring cells, the fusion protein is released.

The λgt11 expression library system has been developed such that every step is very efficient. It is relatively easy to construct a library of expression phages in which every open reading frame of the bacterial genome is represented as a fusion protein in at least one member of the library. Because the infection process is so efficient and tiny plaques can contain high levels of the fusion proteins, it is also easy to set up conditions such that thousands of plaques can be produced on a single lawn of *E. coli* growing on an agar plate, which can then be screened for expression of the desired protein.

Screening Expression Libraries with Sera

The next step in the process was to identify recombinant λ phage expressing the in vivo–induced *M. tuberculosis* genes. Lawns of *E. coli* were infected with the phage library such that about 1,000 plaques formed on each plate. Then a nitrocellulose membrane saturated with IPTG was placed on top of the lawn. The IPTG-induced transcription of the *lacZ* promoter and therefore expression of the LacZ fusion proteins resulting from insertion of *M. tuberculosis* open reading frames, and proteins that were released from the bacterial cell bound to the nitrocellulose membrane. The membranes with their bound proteins were then incubated with the absorbed serum. Any proteins recognized by antibodies present in the serum would be bound by those antibodies. The membranes were washed to remove unbound antibodies and then incubated with antihuman antibodies to which the enzyme horseradish peroxidase (HRP) was conjugated. After additional washing steps, the membrane was incubated with a substrate for HRP that produces a dark brown product when cleaved. The position of any brown spots on the membrane therefore indicated the position of λ phage expressing fusion proteins recognized by the absorbed serum. Because the serum was depleted of antibodies that recognize *M. tuberculosis* proteins expressed in vitro and *E. coli* proteins, the fusion proteins should have represented *M. tuberculosis* proteins expressed only in vivo. The IVIAT approach is obviously very useful for identifying genes whose products can stimulate an immune response and which therefore might be valuable components in vaccine development.

With the advent of accessible and inexpensive methods using mass spectrometry for protein identification and the determination of genome sequences from hundreds of pathogenic bacteria, more direct approaches based on the IVIAT method are available. Extracts of proteins from pathogenic species can be separated from one another in a gel by electrophoresis and then transferred to nitrocellulose. Pooled sera are then used to bind to antigens in the extract much the same as described for the expression library approach above. Proteins identified by the antibodies in the sera can then be directly identified by mass spectrometry, enabling researchers to rapidly identify the genes encoding those proteins from the sequenced genome.

GENOMIC APPROACHES

As previously mentioned, DNA sequencing technology is now so fast and efficient that determining the complete nucleotide sequence of entire genomes is quite routine. For most bacterial pathogens, the genomic sequence of at least one strain is known and publicly available, and for some organisms the sequences of several strains have been determined, allowing comparative analyses. The availability of genome sequence information has revolutionized all aspects of microbiology: many diagnostic tests are now based on genomic sequence information; epidemiological studies are much more sensitive and sophisticated; and the ability to identify, clone, and mutate genes specifically, accurately, and efficiently has increased the pace of research enormously.

Transcriptome Analysis

With the availability of genomic sequence information and the advent of **microarray** technology, it is now possible to measure the relative transcription level of every gene in a bacterial chromosome at the same time. Moreover, gene expression patterns (or transcriptomes) in bacteria grown under various environmental conditions can be compared simultaneously so that genes that are differentially expressed in response to specific conditions can be identified. Thus, while some of the approaches described in the preceding sections allow the identification of individual genes expressed preferentially or exclusively in vivo, microarray-based approaches have the potential of identifying *all* the genes with that expression pattern. A typical analysis was performed by researchers studying *V. cholerae* pathogenesis.

DNA Microarrays

The researchers wanted to identify in vivo–induced genes in *V. cholerae* on a genome-wide scale. Their goal was to identify all the *V. cholerae* genes transcribed at a higher rate when the bacteria were colonizing the human intestine than when growing under standard laboratory conditions. The first step was to construct a microarray of the *V. cholerae* genome. A fragment of every open reading frame identified from the nucleotide sequence of the *V. cholerae* genome (which happens to be composed of two separate circular chromosomes) was amplified by PCR and placed (or printed), using a special robot, onto a discrete spot on a microscope slide coated with polylysine to which the DNA molecules would bind and be

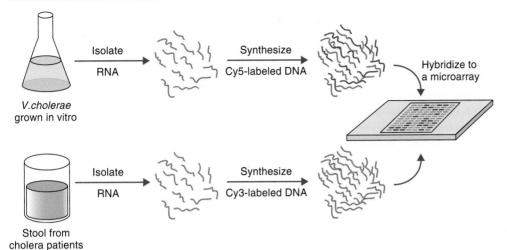

FIGURE 4-12. Microarray scheme used to compare the transcriptomes of *V. cholerae* grown in vitro and in vivo.

immobilized (Fig. 4-12). Using this technique, thousands of individual DNA fragments, each corresponding to a different gene, were spotted onto a single square inch area of the slide such that the identity of the gene present in each location was known.

RNA Isolation

The next step was to isolate total cellular RNA from bacteria grown under the two conditions to be compared. For the in vitro–grown sample, *V. cholerae* was grown in a standard laboratory medium to stationary phase. To obtain bacteria grown in vivo, the researchers obtained stool samples from cholera patients in Bangladesh. As discussed in Chapter 16, *V. cholerae* causes severe diarrhea that is characterized by "rice water" stools. Merrell et al. found that not only did these stools contain incredibly high numbers of bacteria (10^8 to 10^9 per mL, which is similar to the density obtained after overnight growth in a standard laboratory medium) but also they were nearly all *V. cholerae*. Sufficient in vivo–grown *V. cholerae* bacteria could therefore be obtained rather easily to isolate enough RNA to do several experiments.

Complementary DNA Synthesis and Fluorescent Labeling

Next the researchers synthesized complementary DNA (cDNA) from the RNA samples. For the RNA isolated from in vitro–grown bacteria, the cDNA was synthesized using deoxycytidine triphosphate (dCTP) conjugated to Cy5, a fluorescent dye that emits red light; for the RNA isolated from in vivo–grown bacteria, the cDNA was synthesized using dCTP conjugated to Cy3, a fluorescent dye that emits green light.

Probing DNA Microarrays

The Cy3- and Cy5-labeled cDNA samples were then mixed together and incubated with the microarray, first under denaturing conditions to separate all the DNA strands and then under renaturing conditions to allow the

Cy3- and Cy5-labeled cDNA molecules to hybridize with cDNA molecules immobilized on the glass slide. The slide was then washed to remove all unbound cDNA molecules and analyzed using a special microarray fluorescence scanner. For every spot on the microarray, the level of green and red fluorescence was recorded, and the data were reported as a ratio of the two. A high green-to-red ratio resulted when more Cy3-labeled cDNA was present in the sample, indicating a higher level of expression of that particular gene in the bacteria recovered from the stool samples than in the bacteria grown in vitro. Reciprocally, a low green-to-red ratio indicated a higher level of expression in the in vitro–grown bacteria than in those recovered from the cholera patients. A ratio of one, or very close to one, indicated approximately equal expression in the in vitro– and in vivo–grown bacteria.

This analysis identified 237 differentially regulated genes: 44 that were expressed more highly in the bacteria recovered from the stool samples and 193 that were expressed more highly in the in vitro–grown bacteria. Some of the in vivo–induced genes were the same as those identified using other approaches, including those involved in the ability of *V. cholerae* to mount an acid-tolerance response, and some were previously unidentified *V. cholerae* genes. Genes that were repressed in vivo included many involved in chemotaxis.

While microarrays remain a powerful and well-used tool to analyze gene expression at a global level, newer transcriptomics methods have taken advantage of the remarkable advances in nucleotide sequencing technology, generally termed "**massively parallel sequencing**" or "**deep sequencing**." With these new sequencing technologies, researchers can sequence many small, overlapping fragments of the genome and generate millions of nucleotide sequencing reads in a single experiment. Using computational methods, the overlapping reads can be assembled into a single genome sequence that has effectively been analyzed thousands of times in that experiment. If the source is the RNA from a microbe grown under different conditions (such as in an infection model), the RNA can be converted into cDNA using an enzyme called reverse transcriptase. After the RNA has been converted into DNA, the DNA can be used in massively parallel sequencing experiments, and the abundance of any particular sequence in the mixture is related to the amount of that particular RNA that was present in the sample. Direct comparison of the numbers of every transcript in the cell can be made very rapidly, enabling researchers to determine patterns of gene expression under conditions of interest, including during infection.

The use of deep sequencing approaches to determine transcriptomes directly has led to a much greater appreciation of how much of the genome of pathogens (and nonpathogens as well of course) is made up of sequences that encode small, noncoding RNAs (**ncRNAs**) other than transfer RNAs and ribosomal RNAs. These ncRNAs, which play important roles in regulating gene expression through a variety of mechanisms are considered potential targets for therapeutic development.

Proteome Analysis

All the approaches described in this chapter so far have focused on identifying and characterizing genes involved in pathogenesis. However, it is not the genes that allow pathogenic bacteria to grow in or on host tissues to cause disease; it is their protein products. Although protein levels in bacteria frequently reflect gene transcription levels, biological influences that affect the stability, half-life, posttranscriptional, cotranslational, and degradative modifications of proteins cannot be deduced from transcriptional analyses. Therefore, major goals toward understanding mechanisms of pathogenesis have been to identify and characterize directly the entire protein profile (or **proteome**) expressed by pathogenic bacteria. A comparison of the proteome expressed by bacteria grown in vitro with that of those recovered from an infected host, analogous to the transcriptome comparison described earlier, should be especially informative. Significant advances in two-dimensional polyacrylamide gel electrophoresis technologies, coupled with increased ability to recover proteins and determine their amino acid sequences using highly sophisticated mass spectrometry and mass peptide fingerprinting technologies, have made such analysis possible, and combining both genetic and proteomic techniques has a major advance in this field.

Analyzing the Host Response

Just as bacteria alter their gene expression profiles in response to the environments they encounter during the course of infection, their mammalian hosts also activate and repress different classes of genes in response to bacterial infection. Host gene transcription responses to different pathogens in various tissues and cell types of hosts—both human and from experimental animal models—have been analyzed extensively. Sometimes researchers discover very similar gene expression responses to killed bacteria and to common bacterial components, such as lipopolysaccharide. Of interest to questions of infection and immunity, however, is that qualitative and quantitative differences in responses to various live bacterial pathogens were observed. One potential outcome envisioned for this work is to identify specific infections based on the distinct "signature" responses of the host. If true, bacterial infections could be diagnosed in the future by analyzing the gene expression profile in cells obtained from a peripheral blood specimen rather than culturing the organism from the primary site of infection.

CONCLUSION

The experimental "case studies" described in this chapter demonstrate how a combination of genetic, biochemical, molecular, and cell biological approaches can be used to identify and characterize bacterial virulence genes and their products, improving the understanding of the mechanisms of microbial pathogenesis. Such information is crucial to the development of new diagnostic tests, vaccine strategies, and therapeutic agents.

Suggested Readings

Boldrick JC, Alizadeh AA, Diehn M, et al. Stereotyped and specific gene expression programs in human innate immune responses to bacteria. *PNAS.* 2002;99:972–977.

Deb DK, Dahiya P, Srivastava KK, et al. Selective identification of new therapeutic targets of *Mycobacterium tuberculosis* by IVIAT approach. *Tuberculosis (Edinb).* 2002;82:175–182.

Fraser CM, Rappuoli R. Application of microbial genomic science to advanced therapeutics *Annu Rev Med.* 2005;56:459–474.

Hensel M, Shea JE, Gleeson C, et al. Simultaneous identification of bacterial virulence genes by negative selection. *Science.* 1995;269:400–403.

Isberg RR, Voorhis DL, Falkow S. Identification of invasin: a protein that allows enteric bacteria to penetrate cultured mammalian cells. *Cell.* 1987;50:769–778.

Mahan MJ, Slauch JM, Mekalanos JJ. Selection of bacterial virulence genes that are specifically induced in host tissues [comments]. *Science.* 1993;259:686–688.

Pallen MJ, Loman NJ, Penn CW. High-throughput sequencing and clinical microbiology: progress, opportunities and challenges. *Curr Opin Microbiol.* 2010;13:625–631.

Peterson KM, Mekalanos JJ. Characterization of the *Vibrio cholerae* ToxR regulon: identification of novel genes involved in intestinal colonization. *Infect Immun.* 1988;56:2822–2829.

Valdivia RH, Falkow S. Fluorescence-based isolation of bacterial genes expressed within host cells. *Science.* 1997;277:2007–2011.

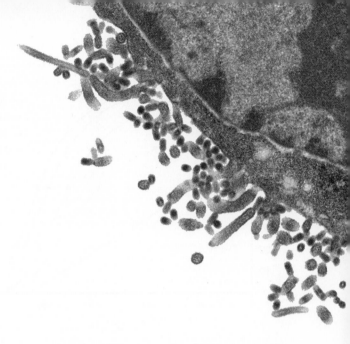

Chapter **5**

Biological Basis for Antibacterial Action

Cary Engleberg and Victor DiRita

KILLING MICROORGANISMS is relatively simple as long as it is not selective. Among the substances that can kill microorganisms are heat, radiation, and strong acids. Targeting specific microbes while sparing host cells and tissues is much more difficult. According to Paul Ehrlich, a pioneer of modern chemotherapy, what we want is a "specific chemotherapy" to kill the microbes and not ourselves. Paradoxically, we depend on the microbial world to provide us with many of the chemotherapeutic agents that we need to kill bacteria.

HOW AND WHEN WERE ANTIBIOTICS DISCOVERED?

One way organisms in the environment—soil, water, or areas of the human body—attempt to gain an advantage over other organisms is by secreting specific chemicals. Some secrete antibiotics, and others employ more subtle methods of competition. Chapter 3 described how microorganisms secrete iron-chelating compounds and are capable of reabsorbing their own iron-bearing products. In this manner, microbes reduce the iron concentration to levels that do not permit the growth of other organisms unable to scavenge iron more efficiently. Thus, in complex environments, competition for nutrients combines with the action of antibiotic substances to produce a balanced microbial ecology.

In the last 30 years, we have taken advantage of this natural warfare for our own purposes, borrowing antibiotics from one organism to combat others. The result has been a medical revolution of immense proportions. Figure 5-1 shows the increase in human longevity since the introduction of antibiotic therapy. Now, because we take for granted the use of antibiotics, it is difficult to recapture the early impact of modern chemotherapy. Ask older family members how they feared the loss of a loved one from pneumonia or postoperative infection, or talk to older physicians about how powerless they were when treating children with meningococcal meningitis or subacute bacterial endocarditis.

However, there is a price to pay for our therapeutic progress. The selective pressure exerted by antibiotics on

bacteria is so great that within one human generation, many bacteria have responded by becoming resistant, often to several antibiotics.

The first important antimicrobial agents were not true antibiotics but synthetic **antimetabolites**. Ehrlich's seminal work derived from his findings that dyes used in histochemistry became bound to cell-specific receptors. "Why then," he asked, "should not such dyes be made toxic for specific organisms?" As validation of Ehrlich's intuition, workers in the mammoth German chemical industry systematically synthesized thousands of compounds and tested them for biological effects. In 1934, Domagk found that one of those compounds, prontosil, cured a fatal streptococcal infection in mice. It was then shown that prontosil was inactive in pure cultures of bacteria in vitro but was hydrolyzed in vivo to the active drug **sulfanilamide**. Cures with this first sulfa drug, or **sulfonamide**, were soon reported. These findings gave impetus to the efforts to purify penicillin, a true antibiotic produced by the mold *Penicillium* and first detected by Alexander Fleming in 1928. A new era had arrived; the search for new antimetabolites and antibiotics has continued ever since.

WHAT IS THE BASIS FOR SELECTIVE ANTIMICROBIAL ACTION? THE EXAMPLE OF SULFONAMIDES

Early on, researchers discovered that extracts from yeast contain a substance that antagonizes the action of

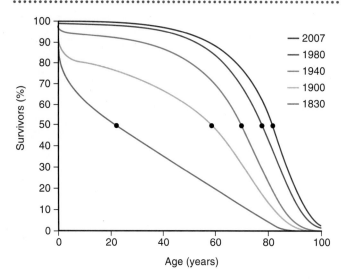

FIGURE 5-1. Survival of human populations, by year. The average life expectancy, that is, the age to which half of the population survives, is indicated by the black dots. This 50% survival level remained at 25 years until 1830. Between 1830 and 1940, the impact of sanitation, public health, and immunization extended life expectancy. Antibiotics (along with better nutrition and health education) added an average of another 8 years in the subsequent 40 years. Note that more recent medical breakthroughs have not extended the life expectancy very much.

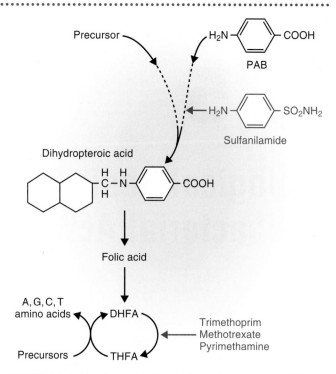

FIGURE 5-2. Inhibition of folic acid synthesis (by sulfa) and function (by other antibacterial drugs). The addition of sulfanilamide instead of *p*-aminobenzoic (PAB) acid to dihydropteroic acid inhibits the synthesis of folic acid. In addition, the resulting analog functions as a "lethal product."

sulfonamides. When purified, the substance was found to be *p*-aminobenzoic acid (PAB; Fig. 5-2), a component of folic acid. The similarity in the structure of PAB and sulfanilamide is obvious. Following this lead, hundreds of thousands of antimetabolites have been tested for possible therapeutic value. In the sulfa class alone, thousands of derivatives with small and large modifications have been studied; about 25 are still in use.

The competition between sulfonamide and PAB in bacteria is illustrated in Figure 5-3. When more sulfonamide is added, proportionally more PAB is required to counteract its action. This type of antagonism is called **competitive inhibition**. The mechanism of action was clarified when the function of PAB became better known. Because PAB is a constituent of folic acid (see Fig. 5-2), it was inferred that sulfa drugs inhibit the synthesis of that vitamin and thus the coenzymes that contain it. The main coenzyme is tetrahydroformyl folic acid, which functions in reactions that add a carbon unit to synthesize nucleosides and certain amino acids (see Fig. 5-2). Therefore, researchers reasoned that folic acid should suppress the action of sulfa drugs and, further, that if bacteria were given enough folic acid to satisfy their growth requirements, no amount of a folic acid inhibitor synthesis could suppress their growth. In contrast to PAB, antagonism of sulfas by folic acid is **noncompetitive**. This expectation was subsequently confirmed (see Fig. 5-3).

The effectiveness of sulfa drugs against bacteria depends on the different ways body cells and bacteria synthesize and use folic acid. Body cells require **preformed**

folic acid, which explains why they are unaffected by sulfonamides. Sulfonamides inhibit the *synthesis* of the compound, not its *utilization*. On the other hand, the folic acid we require must be present in the circulation and tissues. Why then cannot bacteria use this and escape sulfonamide action? The reason seems to be that many bacteria that make folic acid lack a system for the uptake of preformed folic acid and cannot benefit from its presence in

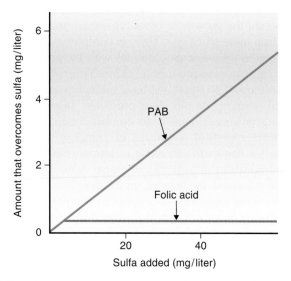

FIGURE 5-3. PAB overcomes sulfa addition competitively; folic acid, noncompetitively.

the environment. These bacteria must synthesize their own folic acid, which makes them susceptible to sulfa drugs. Folic acid everywhere, and not a molecule to save them!

WHAT LIMITS THE EFFICACY OF ANTIMICROBIAL DRUGS?

The mechanism of action of a drug is only one of the properties that determine its potential usefulness. This book describes many others, including pharmacodynamics, cost, and the likelihood of patient compliance. Briefly considered here are three kinds of limitations on the efficacy of antimicrobial drugs that are related directly to their modes of action: the speed with which the drugs work, the sensitivity of the microbial target, and the side effects on the host.

Speed of Action

The practical efficacy of drugs sometimes depends on how fast they stop bacteria in their tracks. The case of sulfanilamide is instructive: when the drug is added to a culture of susceptible bacteria, growth is inhibited after about two to four generations. The reason for the delay is that each bacterium contains enough preformed folic acid to meet the demands of up to 16 daughter cells. Only after 16 cells are formed does the drug become effective. Inhibition by sulfonamides then is dependent on the continued growth of the bacteria.

Other things being equal, **bactericidal** agents, which kill microorganisms rapidly, are preferable to **bacteriostatic** ones, which inhibit growth reversibly (Fig. 5-4). Organisms that remain alive in the presence of a drug can still harm the host, either by continuing to produce toxins or by becoming resistant to the drug and eventually resuming growth. Bactericidal drugs have been clearly

shown to work better when the body's defenses are insufficient to clear the invading agents. Important examples are bacterial endocarditis, bacterial meningitis, and infections in patients with low numbers of circulating neutrophils (agranulocytopenia). Nevertheless, the preference for bactericidal agents depends on the circumstances. For example, an inhibitor of protein synthesis, such as erythromycin, is bacteriostatic but stops the synthesis of protein toxins abruptly. In contrast, penicillin kills bacteria but not immediately: during the lag before the drug exerts its lytic effect, the organisms continue to produce toxins. Therefore, in experimental infections of mice with an agent of gas gangrene, *Clostridium perfringens*, a static drug protected the animals better than a cidal one. Thus, in practical terms, static antibiotics can be more useful in some circumstances. Ultimately, inhibition of bacterial growth gives the defense mechanisms of the body an opportunity to get rid of the organisms.

The distinction of **static versus cidal** should not be taken as absolute. First, a drug may act differently in different organisms. For example, the modified aminoglycoside, spectinomycin, is static for *Escherichia coli* and cidal for gonococci. Second, some drugs show odd kinetics of action that make them difficult to classify. For example, rifampin rapidly kills 99% of *E. coli* cells in vitro but is static for the remaining 1%, perhaps because these bacteria are particularly resistant during a phase of their cell cycle. In other cases, a combination of two static drugs may achieve a cidal action. Despite these ambiguities, the criterion of static versus cidal is generally useful in considering the outcome of drug therapy. In the future, drugs may be developed that work in other ways, for example, inhibiting virulence factors (e.g., toxins or adhesins). Because such drugs would not affect the growth of microorganisms in vitro, their action would only be manifested during infection in vivo.

Sensitivity of the Target

The efficacy of antimicrobial drugs depends on the degree of sensitivity of the intended target organisms. Every agent is effective against a defined range or **spectrum** of organisms. Broad-spectrum antibiotics, which are effective against a wide range of bacteria, might be thought to be preferable to drugs with narrow spectra. However, several practical considerations, such as cost and the risk of selecting resistant bacteria, argue against the widespread use of broad-spectrum antibiotics. These drugs should be reserved for appropriate situations, such as when the etiological agent cannot be determined before therapy begins or for immunocompromised patients who may be subject to simultaneous infection by several agents.

The spectrum of microbial susceptibility depends not only on the organisms but also on the conditions of the infection. For example, aminoglycosides are taken up poorly by bacteria under anaerobic conditions. Thus, these drugs are ineffective against anaerobes. Also, the level of a drug achievable at the site of infection limits its usefulness. For example, nitrofurantoin is concentrated in the urine

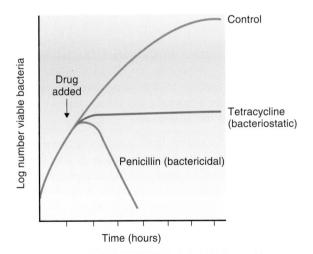

FIGURE 5-4. Effect of bacteriostatic and bactericidal drugs on the growth of bacteria. Note that certain bacteriostatic drugs may not inhibit growth for some time. In the case of sulfa drugs, the lag is the result of the time required to use up preformed folic acid in the bacteria.

and is effective in many cases of uncomplicated urinary tract infections. However, the rapid excretion of this drug prevents it from achieving effective levels in blood or tissues. Consequently, susceptible organisms outside the urinary tract are not affected by nitrofurantoin.

Side Effects

An important limitation is that antimicrobial drugs may have side effects on the host. With antimicrobial chemotherapy, the object is to optimize the **therapeutic index**, the ratio between the effective and the toxic dose. It is important to keep in mind that the degree of selectivity chosen depends on the plight of the patient. Certain inhibitors of folic acid metabolism, like methotrexate, are very toxic in humans but are useful as anticancer or anti-inflammatory agents.

Infectious agents that do not penetrate into deep tissues are special cases in therapy. Topical applications for skin infections are less likely to produce side effects. This lack of side effects permits extensive use of agents that can harm host cell membranes, such as the antibacterial drug polymyxin and the antifungal antibiotic nystatin. Drugs against intestinal worms, which are topologically located outside body tissues (see Fig. 1-1), are also less likely to cause side effects.

Occasionally, an astute clinical observation can turn a side effect to an advantage. Some derivatives of sulfonamides act as a diuretic and cause blood acidosis and alkaline urine. Although these effects are weak, they led to the synthesis of an important group of modern diuretics. Similarly, some sulfa drugs produce hypoglycemia, which led to the development of new drugs for the treatment of diabetes.

HOW ARE ANTIBIOTICS SELECTIVE?

In the case of sulfa drugs, selectivity is based on the fact that, unlike humans, bacteria must synthesize their own folic acid. Any step in metabolism, whether unique to microorganisms or not, is a potential target for antimicrobial action. All that is needed is selective toxicity. In the same pathway as that affected by sulfonamides, the drug **trimethoprim** blocks the function rather than the synthesis of folic acid (see Fig. 5-2). Trimethoprim inhibits the enzyme dihydrofolate reductase, which catalyzes the reduction of dihydrofolate to tetrahydrofolate. This enzyme is necessary for human cells as well as for bacteria, but the amount needed to cause 50% enzyme inhibition is 0.005 mM for bacteria, 0.07 mM for protozoa, and 250 mM for mammals. Thus, the drug can be used against bacteria and protozoa at concentrations that do not harm humans.

This example of efficacy is based on the relative insensitivity of the host compared with bacterial targets. In another example, both host cells and bacteria are sensitive to tetracycline. However, unlike mammalian cells, bacteria concentrate the antibiotic. As a result, tetracycline is effective against even intracellular organisms (e.g., chlamydiae).

The armamentarium of antimicrobials includes drugs that affect the synthesis or function of every class of microbial macromolecules. Extreme selectivity is achieved when the biochemical target is absent in the host cells. The best examples are the β-lactam antibiotics (e.g., penicillin), which affect the biosynthesis of the murein layer of the bacterial cell wall (see Chapter 3). No comparable structure exists in mammalian cells, which are therefore totally insensitive to the action of these antibiotics. Nonetheless, even β-lactams can have undesirable side effects. Some individuals cannot take them because they have a strong allergic reaction. Also, administration of broad-spectrum β-lactams can result in the destruction of the normal intestinal microbiota. This effect can lead to colitis, overgrowth by fungi, and other complications. Even a nearly perfect antibiotic comes with a price.

HOW DO MICROBES CIRCUMVENT THE ACTION OF ANTIBIOTICS?

The destructive power of antibiotics is so pervasive that within a few years of their introduction, resistant organisms can supplant susceptible ones. At what point in the action of antibiotics does resistance come into play? The action of antimicrobial drugs can be broken into a sequence of three steps: First, the drugs must associate with the bacteria and penetrate their envelope. Second, they must be transported to an intracellular site of action. Third, they must bind to their specific biochemical target. Resistance to drugs can occur at each step. Microorganisms, like sophisticated biochemists, have developed a multitude of ways to become resistant. Resistance poses a serious problem when it arises in a pathogenic microbe capable of causing damage to human hosts. Following are the clinically relevant mechanisms of resistance:

- Synthesis of enzymes that break down the drug molecule
- Chemical modification of the drug that interferes with its function
- Prevention of access to the target site by inhibiting uptake
- Prevention of access to the target site by increasing export of the drug from the microbial cell
- Modification of the target site

All these mechanisms have been recognized in clinical pathogens, but the most common is the last one. Some of the examples introduced in Chapter 3 are treated more fully in the following paragraphs. A more extensive list of mechanisms of antibacterial resistance is shown in Table 5-1.

β-Lactams and Enzymes that Inactivate Them

Chapter 3 summarized the effects of penicillins, cephalosporins, and carbapenems on cell wall formation and their consequences for bacterial survival. This group of drugs is large, and for various reasons, their efficacy varies greatly.

TABLE 5-1 Most Common Mechanisms of Resistance to Antibacterial Agents

Agent	Plasmidborne	Resistance Mechanism
Penicillins, cephalosporins, carbapenems	Yes	*Modification of the drug:* hydrolysis of β-lactam ring by β-lactamase
Methicillin	No	*Target modification:* acquisition of a resistant penicillin-binding protein (not in β-lactamase)
Tetracyclines	Yes	*Efflux pump* transports the drug out of cell
Aminoglycosides (gentamicin, tobramycin, amikacin, streptomycin, etc.)	Yes	*Modification of the drug* by R-plasmid–encoded enzyme; reduced affinity for the ribosome and reduced transport into the cell
Sulfonamides	Yes	*Target modification:* sulfanilamide-resistant dihydropteroate synthase
Trimethoprim	Yes	*Target modification:* trimethoprim-resistant dihydrofolate reductase
Erythromycin	Yes	*Target modification:* methylation of 23S ribosomal RNA
Chloramphenicol	Yes	*Modification of the drug:* Acetylation of hydroxyl groups by chloramphenicol transacetylase; interference with transport into cell
Oxazolidinones (linezolid)	No	*Target modification:* mutations in 23S ribosomal RNA
Quinolones (nalidixic acid, ciprofloxacin, etc.)	No	*Target modification:* mutations in genes encoding DNA gyrase and topoisomerase IV
Vancomycin	Yes	*Target modification:* change in binding site in the peptidoglycan target
	No	*Restricted access to drug target*
Daptomycin	No	*Restricted access to drug target*

These antibiotics contain a β-lactam ring (Fig. 5-5). Particular side chains located on the β-lactam ring permit the drugs to penetrate the outer membrane of Gram-negative bacteria, thus extending the list of susceptible organisms. In effect, these drugs become "broad-spectrum antibiotics" by virtue of modification of their β-lactam rings. Other modifications may allow these drugs to be more easily absorbed or more resistant to stomach acid, thus making them effective oral chemotherapeutic agents.

An example of drug development is the transformation of cephalosporin. The original drug is more resistant to inactivating enzymes but less potent than is penicillin. The addition of new side chains created a so-called second generation of cephalosporins with greater potency, especially against Gram-negative anaerobes. The third- and fourth-generation cephalosporins, synthesized with further modifications of the side chains, have a somewhat expanded spectrum of activity (see Fig. 5-5). Cephalosporins in this class have two important advantages: First, they extend the spectrum of activity to organisms that were resistant to most of the previous cephalosporins, including *Pseudomonas*, an opportunistic pathogen, and *Haemophilus influenzae*, an important pathogen in pulmonary infections and meningitis. Second,

unlike the previous cephalosporins, they penetrate well into the central nervous system. This ability has made them especially useful in the treatment of Gram-negative meningitis. Like third- and fourth-generation cephalosporins, carbapenems typically have a very broad spectrum of activity, including most Gram-positive, Gram-negative, and anaerobic bacteria.

The bactericidal action of the β-lactam antibiotics requires the following steps:

1. Association with the bacteria
2. Penetration through the outer membrane and the periplasmic space (only in Gram-negatives)
3. Interaction with penicillin-binding proteins (PBPs) on the cytoplasmic membrane
4. Activation of an autolysin that degrades the cell wall murein

The principal mechanism of resistance to the β-lactams is the elaboration of inactivating enzymes, the **β-lactamases**. So far, more than 300 β-lactamases have been identified, a small number of which account for most of the clinically encountered resistance. They can be divided into major categories, including the penicillinase, cephalosporinases, extended-spectrum beta-lactamases or ESBLs (which confer

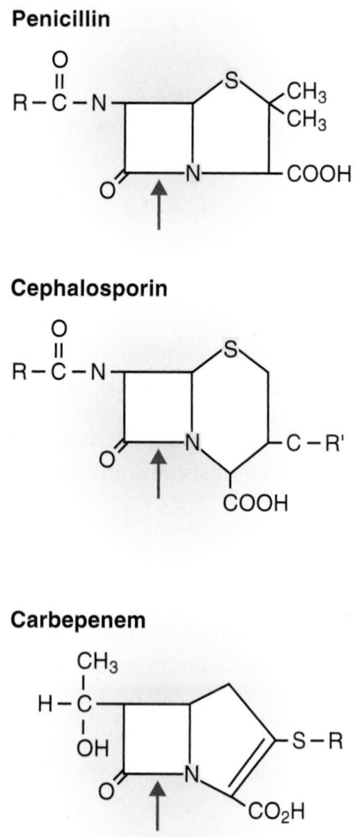

Penicillin

Cephalosporin

Carbepenem

FIGURE 5-5. Core structure of penicillin, cephalosporin, and carbapenem. The R groups specify the particular antibiotic; *arrows* indicate the bonds broken during function and during inactivation by β-lactamases, respectively.

resistance to both penicillins and cephalosporins), and carbapenemases (which may confer resistance to all beta-lactam antibiotics).

In general, Gram-positive bacteria such as the staphylococci produce extracellular β-lactamases. Because these enzymes are secreted into the medium, they destroy the antibiotic before it comes in contact with the bacterial surface. Gram-positive bacteria often make β-lactamases in large amounts after induction by the corresponding antibiotic. Adding more of the drug only induces formation of greater amounts of enzyme, and as a result, resistance usually cannot be overcome even with massive doses. In Gram-negatives, β-lactamases are found in the periplasm or bound to the inner membrane. They are often constitutively produced; that is, they are produced at a constant rate that does not increase with addition of greater amounts of the drugs. Therefore, resistance in these organisms can sometimes be overcome with higher doses of the antibiotic.

β-lactamase–dependent resistance to penicillins and cephalosporins is widespread among pathogenic bacteria. It has become so common in staphylococci, both those acquired in hospitals and in the community, that infecting strains of these organisms must be considered

penicillin-resistant unless proven otherwise by antibiotic susceptibility tests.

Development of β-lactam resistance among Gram-negative bacteria differs from that of Gram-positives. With few exceptions, such as the gonococcus, Gram-negative organisms are resistant to the first drug of this group, the original penicillin G. However, when challenged with newer drugs to which they are susceptible, the Gram-negatives have eventually developed resistance. For example, before 1974, *H. influenzae* was universally susceptible to the penicillin derivative ampicillin. This antibiotic was considered the drug of choice in treatment of *H. influenzae* infections. However, in 1975, it became apparent that 10 to 20% of the isolates of *H. influenzae* elaborate an ampicillin-degrading β-lactamase. This enzyme is encoded on a highly promiscuous plasmid, which probably accounts for the rapid spread of ampicillin resistance in this organism.

A similar reversal has occurred with gonococcus. This organism was once universally susceptible to penicillin, although higher levels of the drug have been gradually required over the last 30 years. In 1976, highly penicillin-resistant strains were isolated in two widely separated areas of the world. The gene coding for the relevant β-lactamase is carried on a **transposon** that transfers to other strains of gonococci and to other aerobic Gram-negatives. Thus, for the past 30 years, penicillin has ceased to be the universal agent for the treatment of gonorrhea.

These examples illustrate the role of transferable genetic elements in the spread of β-lactamase resistance. The role of plasmids and transposons in the transfer of resistance has increased in importance since the early days of the antibiotic era. The early resistant strains harbored chromosomal resistance genes that were only later replaced by strains with plasmidborne resistance. This trend for the genes to become associated with a mobile genetic element has facilitated the development of resistance in previously susceptible organisms. During the past few years, transferable genes encoding broadly active carbapenemase enzymes have spread globally. These include a family of carbapenemases from *Klebsiella pneumoniae* that were first detected in North America (**KPCs**) and a novel metallo-beta-lactamase that spread from New Delhi, India (**NDM**-1, also known as PCM for *p*lasmid-encoding *c*arbapenem-resistant *m*etallo-beta-lactamase). The presence of these enzymes in Gram-negative organisms severely limits the choice of therapy for infected patients. As a consequence, physicians are often forced to resort to using intravenous **colistin**, a polymyxin antibiotic, for serious infections. This agent, which had previously been abandoned because of its inherent toxicity for the kidneys and nervous system, has recently seen a resurgence of use for highly-resistant Gram-negative infections. If broadly active beta-lactamase genes find their way into other important susceptible pathogens, such as the meningococci and certain streptococci, it would be a serious blow to our ability to treat some important and common infectious diseases.

Other mechanisms of resistance to β-lactams are also important. In Gram-negative bacteria, β-lactams must be able to pass through outer membrane pores to make contact with the antimicrobial targets, **penicillin-binding proteins (PBPs)**. Resistance can occur in some Gram-negative organisms when spontaneous mutations in the outer membrane **porins** lead to exclusion of β-lactams to the periplasmic space. Alternatively, many Gram-positive organisms have become resistant by altering the PBPs themselves so they fail to bind β-lactams. This type of β-lactam resistance has been most important in the emergence of penicillin-resistant *Streptococcus pneumoniae* and methicillin-resistant *Staphylococcus*. Most strains of *S. aureus* are already resistant to penicillins by virtue of a β-lactamase. However, acquisition of an altered PBP in many strains has resulted in resistance to all penicillins and cephalosporins, including ones that were specifically designed to resist the staphylococcal β-lactamase, like methicillin. For this reason, these strains have the blanket designation of **methicillin-resistant *Staphylococcus aureus* (MRSA)**. They are responsible for some of the worst outbreaks of hospital-acquired infection in recent history. These strains must be treated with antimicrobials from another class, such as the cell wall–inhibiting cyclic glycopeptide, vancomycin, or newer antistaphylococcal drugs, such as linezolid or daptomycin. Unfortunately, resistance to all these agents has also been reported (as discussed later).

Finally, some strains of pneumococci and staphylococci are inhibited rather than killed by certain levels of β-lactams. This form of partial resistance is called **tolerance**. In the case of tolerant pneumococci, the drugs are bacteriostatic and not bactericidal because these strains lack sufficient levels of the suicidal **autolysin**. Bacterial tolerance might explain some of the relapses that occur following treatment of staphylococcal and streptococcal infections. However, compared with drug inactivation by β-lactamases, tolerance accounts only for a small percentage of clinically important resistance.

Vancomycin: Resistance by Target (Cell Wall) Modification

Vancomycin, a glycopeptide antibiotic in constant clinical use since the 1950s, has been a mainstay of therapy for resistant Gram-positive infections. Since this antibiotic is given intravenously, it is most commonly used in hospitalized patients, many with nosocomial (hospital-acquired) infections. Vancomycin has been particularly valuable against MRSA strains for which it has been, until recently, the only useful drug available.

Since the late 1980s, many strains of *Enterococcus* have acquired resistance to vancomycin by acquisition of a set of plasmidborne genes. These genes act in concert to produce an altered peptidoglycan precursor. Instead of the usual D-alanine–D-alanine terminus, these modified precursors have D-alanine–D-lactate. The normal D-alanine–D-alanine is the target for vancomycin, whereas D-alanine–D-lactate is not. Bacteria with this modified terminus are resistant to vancomycin (Fig. 5-6).

Patients infected with strains of **vancomycin-resistant *Enterococcus* (VRE)** are extremely difficult to treat because these strains are usually also resistant to

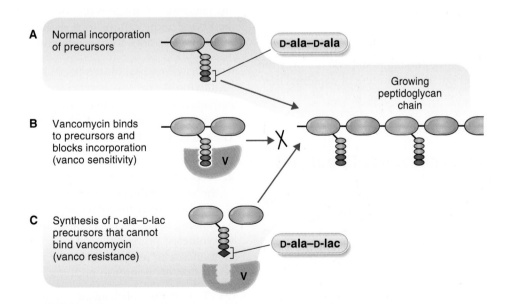

FIGURE 5-6. Mechanism of vancomycin resistance. A. Normally, peptidoglycan precursors composed of two sugars and a five-amino-acid peptide are exported from the bacterial cell and added to a growing peptidoglycan chain as the cell wall enlarges. **B.** Vancomycin inhibits peptidoglycan chain elongation by binding to the D-ala–D-ala terminal peptides on the precursor. **C.** The basis of vancomycin resistance in *Enterococcus* is the production of precursors with D-lactate in the position of the terminal D-ala. This blocks the binding of vancomycin and allows the precursor to be incorporated.

β-lactams and aminoglycosides. Fortunately, enterococci are not aggressively invasive pathogens. However, since the recognition of VRE, microbiologists have expected that their plasmidborne vancomycin resistance genes would eventually be transferred to the more virulent *S. aureus*. This concern was realized in the early part of this century. Strains of **vancomycin-resistant *S. aureus* (VRSA)** have now been identified in patients who were coinfected with MRSA and VRE and on long-term treatment with vancomycin. As of this writing, the VRSA isolates have been contained and have not circulated in the general population. Instead, vancomycin-intermediate *S. aureus* (VISA) strains are becoming increasingly common. These strains do not carry the genes that modify the peptidoglycan precursor. Rather, they elaborate overabundant, modified peptidoglycan that impedes the access of vancomycin to its target. Strains that develop these characteristics have increased minimal inhibitory concentrations (MICs) to vancomycin and are becoming increasingly responsible for clinical failures of therapy.

Daptomycin: Reduced Access to the Drug Target (Cell Membrane)

Daptomycin is the first of the lipopeptide antibiotics, composed of a 13-member peptide with a 10-carbon lipid tail. This lipophilic structure permits daptomycin to bind to the cell membrane of Gram-positive bacteria and to form a disruptive ion channel that causes depolarization and rapid cell death. This novel mechanism of action allows daptomycin to be active against *Staphylococcus* and *Enterococcus* species that are resistant to vancomycin and other antimicrobials. At the time of this writing, daptomycin resistance remains uncommon, but when it does occur in *S. aureus*, it is most common among VISA strains. Presumably, a minority of VISA strains possess peptidoglycan layers thick enough to impede not only the influx of vancomycin but also the access of daptomycin to the cell membrane. Since daptomycin is a relatively large molecule that cannot pass through porin channels, the drug is inactive against all Gram-negative bacteria.

Quinolones: Resistance by Target and Efflux Alteration

The quinolone antibiotics act by inhibiting the action of bacterial topoisomerases, including **DNA gyrase** (in Gram-positive bacteria) and **topoisomerase IV** (in Gram-negatives). Quinolones kill bacteria by trapping the topoisomerases in the act of cutting DNA and thus promoting the formation and persistence of double-strand breaks in the bacterial chromosome. Nalidixic acid was the first quinolone used clinically and was effective for treating urinary tract infections caused by Gram-negative bacteria. More recently developed **fluoroquinolone** antibiotics are used to treat infections caused by both Gram-negative and Gram-positive bacteria, and these agents are now widely used. Resistance to fluoroquinolone antibiotics is mainly the result of mutations in the genes encoding the target enzymes DNA gyrase and topoisomerase IV, which cause reduced binding of the drugs. Another important source of resistance is the elimination of quinolones from the bacterial cell by **efflux pumps**. A role for efflux in resistance has been demonstrated in both Gram-negative bacteria, such as *Pseudomonas aeruginosa*, and Gram-positive bacteria, such as *S. aureus*.

Antiribosomal Antibiotics

The effectiveness of the second-largest class of antibacterial agents, the antiribosomal antibiotics, is based on structural differences between the ribosomes of bacteria and those of eukaryotic cells; in eukaryotic cells, ribosomes have larger RNA molecules and more protein components. Typical drugs of this group, including streptomycin and erythromycin, bind to bacterial but not mammalian ribosomes. The difference is not always absolute and does not completely explain the selective toxicity of all the drugs of this class. First, some antibiotics like tetracycline target mammalian and bacterial ribosomes in vitro. Second, mammalian cells have bacterial-like ribosomes in their mitochondria, and these are sensitive to many of the drugs of this class. Researchers believe that some of these drugs are not toxic because they cannot pass through the plasma membrane. Recent additions to the antiribosomal antibiotics are the **oxazolidinones**, including linezolid. These agents bind to the 50S subunit of bacterial ribosomes to prevent the assembly of the translational complex and the initiation of protein synthesis.

Other toxic side effects of these antibiotics cannot be anticipated from their mechanisms of action. Examples are chelation of magnesium by tetracyclines with attendant bone and tooth malformation in children, or toxicity of aminoglycosides for the renal tubules and inner ear.

Aminoglycosides: Resistance by Transport or Drug Inactivation

Perhaps the most complex mechanism of action of all antiribosomal antibiotics is that of the aminoglycosides. Their action results from the following steps:

1. Penetration of the outer membrane of Gram-negatives
2. Association with a two-stage active transport system in the cell membrane. (This system is one way and irreversible, unlike that of tetracycline or most metabolites.)
3. Binding to the 30S ribosome subunit to inhibit protein synthesis, primarily at or near the initiation step, and to increase "miscoding" by the ribosomes and the production of "nonsense proteins"

Two major mechanisms of resistance to aminoglycosides have been recognized in Gram-negative bacteria. Obligate anaerobic bacteria may inactivate the transport of aminoglycosides. However, a more common mechanism in clinically important isolates involves **modifying enzymes**. Various aminoglycoside-modifying enzymes may modify these antibiotics by the addition of acetyl, adenyl, or phosphoryl groups to the drug molecules rendering them inactive. Several distinct enzymes have been identified in coliforms, pseudomonads, and staphylococci. Each one can inactivate more than one but usually not all aminoglycosides. Thus, a given strain can become resistant to, say, gentamicin and tobramycin but remain fully susceptible to amikacin. Usually, the aminoglycoside-inactivating enzymes are encoded by genes carried on plasmids or transposons, and more than one enzyme may be carried by one plasmid.

Tetracyclines: Resistance by Drug Excretion

Resistance to antiribosomal antibiotics can take many forms because these drugs must go through many steps to reach their targets. Tetracyclines, for example, must do the following:

1. Bind to the cytoplasmic membrane, which, in the case of Gram-negatives, requires passage through the outer membrane and the periplasmic space.
2. Be transported across the cytoplasmic membrane by an active transport mechanism. This transport mechanism involves two components: an initial rapid uptake and a second phase of slower uptake.

Resistant strains do not accumulate tetracycline within the cell. The reason is not, as might be expected, failure to take up the drug. Rather, the intracellular concentration is kept low by an exit mechanism that actively excretes the drug. Tetracycline resistance has been found in almost all bacteria, including Gram-positives, Gram-negatives, aerobes, and anaerobes.

Macrolides: Resistance by Target (Ribosome) Modification

The macrolide antibiotics and their derivatives are represented in clinical medicine by **erythromycin, clindamycin, azithromycin,** and **clarithromycin**. Like tetracyclines, macrolides can be transported out of the bacterial cell by efflux pumps, creating a low level of resistance. However, a more significant degree of resistance occurs by a particularly interesting mechanism of drug target alteration—methylation of the 23S ribosomal RNA. This modification renders the 50S ribosomal subunits resistant to the drugs. The **methylase** involved is usually made from a plasmid gene under highly regulated conditions: little enzyme is formed during growth in the absence of a macrolide, but it is rapidly induced in the presence of a macrolide.

Oxazolidinones: Resistance by Target Modification

Unlike most of the antibiotics previously mentioned, oxazolidinone antibiotics such as **linezolid** are not derived from naturally occurring antimicrobial substances. They are entirely synthetic, much like the sulfonamides described earlier in this chapter. Consequently, preexisting resistance genes such as those that encode β-lactamases, aminoglycoside-modifying enzymes, or ribosomal methylases

do not exist. Nevertheless, resistant bacteria have been identified and isolated. In all cases so far, resistance has been the result of point mutations in the 23S RNA of the 50S ribosomal subunit. These mutations presumably block the binding of linezolid to the ribosome.

Linezolid and daptomycin (described above) were developed to address the growing problem of resistance among Gram-positive bacterial pathogens. Other recent entries into the antimicrobial armamentarium that address this problem include tigecycline, a modified tetracycline, and ceftaroline, a cephalosporin with activity against MRSA.

Targeting Virulence Mechanisms: Novel Approaches to Antimicrobial Discovery

The approach favored for decades in developing antimicrobial compounds has been to target the growth of microbes during infection. Resistance to growth-inhibiting antibiotics and the rapid spread of resistance genes to previously susceptible microbial populations are serious concerns among physicians and within the general population. An active area of research and development for identifying new antimicrobial compounds is in targeting virulence mechanisms so as to block their function during infection. Many virulence traits—including specialized secretion mechanisms, regulatory pathways, assembly, structure, and function of extracellular organelles and toxins—are conserved across pathogenic species, providing the possibility of broad-spectrum efficacy of compounds targeted at these traits. Because such compounds would not be aimed at the growth of the microbe, but only at the mechanisms that contribute to disease, theoretically, there would be greatly reduced selective pressure for resistance. While antivirulence drugs have not yet made it into the clinic, promising lead compounds that reduce pathogenicity in relevant animal models of infection have been identified. Thus, basic research into virulence mechanisms of pathogens discussed in succeeding chapters is likely to pay off with new therapeutic agents.

SELECTIVITY AND LIMITATIONS OF ANTIFUNGAL AGENTS

Moving up the phylogenetic tree to the eukaryotic pathogens, the differences between host and parasite begin to narrow. For example, most of the antibiotics that inhibit fungal ribosomes are also active against human ribosomes and are therefore too toxic to use. In general, therapeutic agents against fungi, viruses, and animal parasites are often quite toxic. Nevertheless, antifungal agents with selective toxicity do exist.

Especially interesting examples are the **polyenes** (see Chapter 50), which bind more avidly to ergosterol in the membranes of fungi than to cholesterol in the membranes of higher eukaryotes. The margin of safety is often considerable. For example, yeasts are about 200-fold more sensitive to the polyene antibiotic **amphotericin B** than are cultured human cells. Nevertheless, the efficacy of amphotericin B is limited by toxicity to blood cells and damage to membranes of kidney cells. To some extent, this toxicity has been limited by conjugating the drug to lipid complexes.

The **imidazoles** are another group of agents with greater specificity for a fungal target than for a similar target in the host. The target is cytochrome P450 demethylase, which is involved in sterol synthesis. These antifungal agents can be used topically to treat local infections or systemically to treat invasive disease. Similarly, **echinocandins** are inhibitors of another component of the fungal cell wall, β-glucan, which is not present in human cells.

IF ONE ANTIBIOTIC IS GOOD, ARE TWO BETTER?

A potent argument for counteracting drug resistance in microorganisms can be made for the administration of several antibiotics at once. Mutations conferring resistance to some antibiotics occur with frequencies of 10^6 to 10^9 per generation. Thus, because of the rapid growth of bacteria in human infection, outgrowth of resistant mutants can easily take place and become a significant clinical risk. However, two antibiotics given simultaneously can theoretically reduce the chance that a bacterium will completely evade antibiotic destruction. For example, assume that resistance to drug A arises with a frequency of 10^6 per generation. If drug B has a similar frequency of resistant mutants and is given simultaneously, the chance of a single bacterium becoming resistant to both antibiotics is $10^6 \times 10^6$, or 10^{12}, which is vanishingly small.

An excellent example of this concept currently in practice is combination therapy with sulfamethoxazole and trimethoprim. Although both drugs act on one-carbon metabolism, their sites of action are different, and resistance to one does not influence resistance to the other. Other example is the obligatory combination of drugs used to treat tuberculosis and HIV infection. Treatment of active tuberculosis with a single agent is invariably associated with clinical failure and the emergence of drug-resistant strains. Similarly, HIV is typically treated with three-drug regimens to avoid rapid emergence of resistant viruses. Multidrug therapy for these diseases is therefore considered essential.

The use of drugs in combination is not without problems. In fact, three outcomes are possible:

1. **Synergism**: The effectiveness of the drugs together is greater than that of either drug alone. For example, enterococci are naturally tolerant to penicillins and resistant to gentamicin. However, when penicillin is given along with gentamicin, the bacteria become permeable to gentamicin, which exerts a bactericidal effect in the cytoplasm.
2. **Antagonism**: The action of one drug reduces the effectiveness of the other. Thus, when tetracycline is given with penicillin, it blocks protein synthesis, preventing the cell growth required for penicillin to cause lysis. The result is dominance by the weaker bacteriostatic drug.
3. **Indifference**: Each drug works no better and no worse alone or in combination.

Further cautions are warranted with multiple drug administration. Drugs can show **synergism in toxicity** as well as in antimicrobial action (an example is the heightened damage to the kidney by the joint administration of vancomycin and an aminoglycoside). Finally, in a hospital setting, the main sources of drug resistance are the members of the resident microbiota (not bacterial flora). Therefore, the decision to administer multiple drugs and which ones to choose should be governed by the spectrum of multidrug resistance of the dominant organisms in that hospital.

ARE SUPERGERMS A THREAT?

Some of the genes that lead to antibiotic resistance are chromosomal and thus are inherent in the genome of the species. But many resistance genes are plasmidborne and are probably acquired from other bacteria (see Table 5-1).

Resistance genes, both chromosomal and on plasmids, predate the use of antibiotics. Such genes have been found in strains stored before the introduction of the drugs or in isolates from areas where antibiotics have never been deliberately introduced. The selective pressure of the widespread use of antibiotics has resulted in an increasing frequency of resistant bacteria. In broad terms, the spread of resistance genes increases with the use of drugs in a particular geographic area or medical center. Multiple resistance genes may accumulate in a given strain by the effective mechanism of gene transposition. This process could lead to the emergence of "supergerms," microorganisms resistant to a large number of antimicrobial agents. Near-supergerm status has been achieved by occasional isolates resistant to 15 or more antibiotics. Particular examples are strains of enterococci resistant to most available antibiotics. In contrast, meningococci, group A streptococci, and the spirochete of syphilis remain nearly as susceptible to penicillin today as they were when the drug was first used. The reasons for this persistent susceptibility are not clear.

CONCLUSION

The countermeasures taken against resistant organisms include continued development of more effective antibiotics (such as the cephalosporins) and identifying completely new targets (such as with antivirulence compounds). Certainly, the war between effective therapy and drug resistance is unlikely to abate, but the battles must continue to be fought and won. The alternative would be to give up what many physicians and historians of science regard as a key difference between modern medicine and the Dark Ages.

Suggested Readings

Barczak AK, Hung DT. Productive steps toward an antimicrobial targeting virulence. *Curr Opin Microbiol.* 2009;12:490–496.

Bush K, Miller GH. Bacterial enzymatic resistance: β-lactamases and aminoglycoside modifying enzymes. *Curr Opin Microbiol.* 1998;1:509–515.

Hogan D, Kolter R. Why are bacteria refractory to antimicrobials? *Curr Opin Microbiol.* 2002;5:472–477.

Hooper DC. Clinical applications of quinolones. *Biochem Biophys Acta.* 1998;1400:45–61.

Levy S. Active efflux mechanisms for antimicrobial resistance. *Antimicrob Agents Chemother.* 1992;36:695–703.

Levy S. *The Antibiotic Resistance Paradox.* New York, NY: Plenum; 1992.

Moellering RC. Linezolid: the first oxazolidinone antimicrobial. *Ann Intern Med.* 2003;138:135–142.

Nordmann P, Naas T, Poirel L. Global spread of carbapenemase-producing *Enterobacteriaceae. Emerg Infect Dis.* 2011;17(10):1791–1798. http://dx.doi.org/10.3201/eid1710.110655

Tenover FC, Moellering RC. The Rationale for revising the clinical and laboratory standards institute vancomycin minimal inhibitory concentration interpretive criteria for *Staphylococcus aureus. Clin Infect Dis.* 2007;44(9):1208–1215.

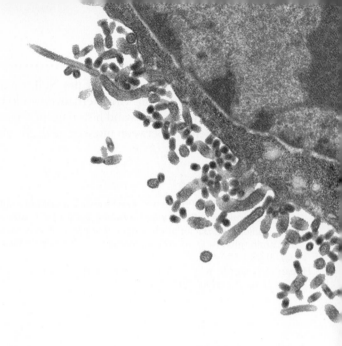

Chapter 6

Innate Immunity

Roman Dziarski

WE HAVE A UNIQUE ability to shape our environment. Largely, our sanitary lifestyle determines the extent to which we encounter exogenous microorganisms, including potential pathogens. Our health is influenced by such external factors as cleanliness and nutrition. Thus, defenses against infectious diseases begin with the way we affect our environment and one another. For example, children who live in crowded, inadequately ventilated housing and eat a diet lacking in protein are more likely to contract infectious diseases such as tuberculosis than are other children. The reason is twofold: poor nutrition diminishes the effectiveness of body defenses, and crowding makes the encounter with tubercle bacilli more frequent. The adults in such households may already have tuberculosis and, in close quarters, become ready sources of contagion. Defenses against such events are clear: good nutrition, adequate housing, and treatment of the ill. While these favorable conditions occur readily in affluent societies, they have to be fostered with care and sacrifice in the developing countries of the world.

Physicians share with others their concern for defense against infectious diseases. Good food in sufficient quantity, uncontaminated water, and protection from insects and rodents—these are the primary business of the sanitary engineer and the social scientist. Other activities are mainly medical, such as immunizations and treatment of human carriers or patients likely to contribute to the spread of disease (see Chapter 56). This chapter focuses on the body's own defense mechanisms.

FUNCTIONS AND COMPONENTS OF THE INNATE IMMUNE SYSTEM

Throughout life, the body surfaces tolerate a rich and complex microbiota that is usually harmless and often helpful but can cause opportunistic infections. In contrast, domains of the body just a few micrometers beneath the epidermis or the mucous membranes are usually free of microorganisms. Host defenses intensify as microorganisms encounter the skin and mucous membranes. This and the next chapter explore how the body maintains this microbial gradient, from microorganism-associated surfaces to aseptic intercellular and intracellular tissue domains. The question is important because a breakdown of the gradient is usually what infection is about.

Innate immunity is the host's first line of defense against infections. It is present in all metazoans, and in plants and invertebrate animals, it is the only (and very effective) defense against infections. Vertebrates, including humans, have not only innate immunity but also adaptive immunity (also known as acquired immunity), which is the second line of defense (see Chapter 7).

Following are the functions of innate immunity:

- Recognize microbes that are encountered by the host
- Prevent infection of the host by either eliminating the microbes or allowing them to exist on body surfaces as normal microbiota that is not harmful (and is often beneficial)
- Initiate adaptive immune responses and influence the nature of those responses based on the type of the invading microorganism
- Serve, in some cases, as an effector mechanism for adaptive immune response

As shown in Table 6-1, the components of the innate immune system that perform these functions are either **cellular**, consisting of various types of cells, or **humoral**,

TABLE 6-1 Components of the Innate Immune System

Component	Main Function
Cellular	
Skin and mucous membranes (epithelial cells)	Mechanical and chemical defenses
Phagocytic cells (neutrophils, macrophages)	Ingest and kill bacteria and fungi
Proinflammatory cells (macrophages, mast cells, eosinophils, basophils, platelets)	Induce host defenses and inflammation
Natural killer (NK) cells	Kill virus-infected cells and tumor cells
Antigen-presenting cells (dendritic cells, macrophages)	Recognize, process, and present antigens to lymphocytes Initiate adaptive immune responses
Humoral	
Antimicrobial peptides	Kill microorganisms
Complement	Enhances phagocytosis (opsonization) Induces inflammation Kills some microorganisms
Cytokines	Activate innate and adaptive defenses
Chemokines	Attract leukocytes
Kinins	Induce inflammation
Acute phase proteins	Enhance cellular and humoral defenses
Enzymes	Kill and digest microorganisms
Inflammation	
Increased blood supply (erythema)	Brings more antimicrobial cells and proteins to the site of infection
Increased vascular permeability (edema)	Brings more antimicrobial proteins to the site of infection
Chemotaxis (induration)	Infiltration of infection site with white cells

consisting of various secreted soluble peptides, proteins, and other mediators. The interaction of these components in the body with the invading microbes often, but not always, leads to a constellation of responses called **inflammation**. The purpose of inflammation is to amplify the body's defenses by increasing blood supply to the site of infection and by bringing more antimicrobial proteins and white cells to fight the infection.

This chapter discusses how the innate immune system functions and how it protects us from infections.

SKIN AND MUCOUS MEMBRANES

Before microorganisms can enter the normally aseptic regions of the body, they must pass through the barriers of the skin, the conjunctivae of the eyes, or the mucous membrane of the respiratory, alimentary, or urogenital tracts. Each barrier has its own protective mechanisms, which can be broadly classified as mechanical, chemical and molecular, and microbial (Table 6-2).

Mechanical barriers are highly effective, especially in the skin, which is covered with a thick layer of **keratinized epithelium**. The mucous membranes of the mouth, pharynx, esophagus, and lower urinary tract are composed of several layers of epithelial cells, whereas those of the lower respiratory, gastrointestinal, and upper urinary tracts are delicate single layers of epithelial cells, often endowed with specialized functions. Membranes of the alveoli and the intestine are thin because they serve as exchangers of gases, fluids, and solutes. Although all epithelia have protective **tight junctions** that do not allow passage of microorganisms, these epithelia can be traumatized, especially when subjected to high pressure or abrasions. In fact, trauma occurs daily in the colon

TABLE 6-2 Defenses on the Skin and Mucous Membranes

Component	Main Function
Mechanical	
Keratinized epithelium in the skin	Offers protection against microorganisms
Desquamation of stratified epithelium	Removes microorganisms attached to its surface
Epithelial cells joined by tight junctions	Offer protection against microorganisms
Mucus-coated hair in the nose	Traps particles
Mucus-coated ciliated epithelium	Removes particles from the respiratory tract
Mucus-coated intestinal epithelium	Keeps the bulk of bacteria away from intestinal epithelium
Coughing and sneezing	Expel particles
Flow of urine	Cleanses the urethra
Chemical and Molecular	
Low pH in the stomach	Kills many bacteria, fungi, or parasites, and inactivates many viruses
Antimicrobial peptides (constitutive and induced)[a]	Kill many microorganisms
Defensins (skin, intestine, mucous membranes)	Kill bacteria and fungi
Phospholipases (in intestinal Paneth cells and tears)	Kill bacteria
Dermcidin (in sweat glands)	Kills bacteria and fungi
Ribonucleases (on the skin)	Kill bacteria and fungi
Fatty acids (from sebaceous glands of the skin)	Inhibit bacterial growth
Enzymes	
Lysozyme (in tears, sweat, saliva, and serum)	Hydrolyses bacterial cell wall peptidoglycan
Amidase (in the skin and serum)	Hydrolyses bacterial cell wall peptidoglycan
Microbial Antagonism	
Normal microbiota bacteria and fungi	Compete for nutrients with potential pathogens
	Produce antimicrobial factors (bacteriocins)

[a]See Table 6-3.

during defecation and in the mouth during vigorous toothbrushing.

Many mucous membranes are covered by a protective layer of **mucus** that provides a mechanical and chemical barrier yet permits proper function. Mucus is a giant cross-linked gel-like structure made up of glycoprotein subunits. It entraps particles and prevents them from reaching the mucous membrane. Mucus is hydrophilic and allows diffusion of many substances produced by the body, including antimicrobial peptides and enzymes such as **lysozyme** and **peroxidase**. Its viscous properties enable it to bear substantial weight and yet be readily moved by the motion of the cilia of the underlying cells.

To afford additional protection, skin and mucous membranes are rich in chemical and molecular antimicrobial factors (see Table 6-2). Some of these factors are constitutive (always present), such as low pH in the stomach, fatty acids on the skin, and lysozyme, a bacteriolytic enzyme in tears, sweat, and saliva.

The most potent antimicrobial factors are **antimicrobial peptides** (Table 6-3). One of the most active peptides is **phospholipase A$_2$ (PLA$_2$)**, which is an enzyme that destroys bacterial cytoplasmic membrane. **Defensins** are cysteine-rich small peptides (3 to 5 kDa), which are ubiquitous in all vertebrates and invertebrates and which, in humans, are subdivided into two families, α-defensins and β-defensins, based on their structure. Six α-defensins and four β-defensins have been well characterized in humans, but recent analysis of the human genome revealed 34 defensin genes, which highlights the significance of this

TABLE 6-3 Antimicrobial Peptides

Peptide	Location	Active Against
Phospholipases A$_2$ (PLA$_2$ most active)	PMN primary granules Intestinal Paneth cells Tears Serum	Gram-positive bacteria Gram-negative bacteria together with BPI
α-Defensins	PMN primary granules Intestinal Paneth cells	Bacteria, fungi, some parasites and viruses
β-Defensins	Induced in epithelial cells (skin, respiratory tract, genitourinary tract)	Bacteria and fungi
Ribonucleases	Constitutive and induced in epithelial cells (skin, genitourinary tract, intestinal tract) PMNs, monocytes	Bacteria and fungi
Dermcidin	Sweat glands	Bacteria and fungi
BPI	PMN primary granules	Gram-negative bacteria
Cathelicidins (CAP18 in humans)	PMN secondary granules	Bacteria and fungi
Serprocidins (serine proteases: elastase, cathepsin G, proteinase 3)	PMN primary granules	Bacteria and fungi
Lysozyme	Phagocyte granules Tears, saliva Serum Intestinal Paneth cells	Gram-positive bacteria (hydrolyses peptidoglycan)

BPI, bactericidal permeability-increasing protein; CAP, cationic antimicrobial protein; PMN, polymorphonuclear leukocyte.

family of antimicrobial peptides. Defensins, like most other antimicrobial peptides, are highly cationic, enabling them to bind to the negatively charged cell walls of bacteria and fungi and to kill them by pore formation and permeabilization of their cell membranes.

Many antimicrobial peptides are constitutively present on the skin and mucous membranes, such as PLA$_2$, α-defensins, and ribonucleases (RNases) in the intestinal Paneth cells. Other antimicrobial peptides, such as β-defensins and RNases, are present in low levels on epithelial surfaces of the skin and mucous membranes, and their increased production can be induced by high numbers of bacteria or by proinflammatory cytokines released from macrophages following exposure to bacteria.

The enzyme **lysozyme** is present in large amounts in tears, sweat, saliva, and serum. It hydrolyses **peptidoglycan**, the main structural component of bacterial cell walls. Lysozyme acts mainly on Gram-positive bacteria, although many bacterial species have evolved resistant modifications of their cell wall chemistry. Gram-negative bacteria, however, are resistant because their peptidoglycan substrate is shielded by their outer membranes. In this case, lysozyme can work synergistically with other antimicrobial peptides or complement. Damage to the outer membrane of Gram-negative bacteria can allow lysozyme

to access its substrate. **Amidase** is another enzyme in the skin and serum that hydrolyses bacterial cellwall peptidoglycan, although in contrast to lysozyme, it does not have a direct bacteriolytic activity. However, peptidoglycan-lytic enzymes are important not only in killing bacteria but also in removing proinflammatory peptidoglycan from the tissues. Many antimicrobial peptides and bacteriolytic enzymes are also present in the granules of phagocytic cells (which will be discussed later) and can be released from the granules into the surrounding tissues by a process called **exocytosis**.

The innate immune system prevents colonization of the skin and mucous membranes by potential pathogens but allows colonization by limited numbers of the nonpathogenic bacteria and fungi of the normal microbiota. The **normal microbiota** is unique for each area of the body (see Chapter 2) and is beneficial to the host because it protects the skin and mucous membranes from colonization by pathogenic microorganisms. Called **microbial antagonism**, this protection is likely accomplished by competition for nutrients with potential pathogens and by production of antimicrobial factors (bacteriocins) by the normal microbiota. However, in immunocompromised patients, the normal microbiota can cause opportunistic infections that are quite severe or even life threatening.

The barrier function of skin and mucous membranes is seldom breached except by injuries, such as burns, cuts, or wounds. Once microorganisms have traversed the skin, they encounter powerful defenses in the underlying soft tissues. However, these defenses do not work at full capacity under all conditions. For instance, abrasions or lacerations impair the local vascular and lymphatic circulation and interfere with soluble and cellular defense mechanisms, thus rendering the underlying connective tissue vulnerable. When this occurs, substantially fewer microorganisms are required to cause infection. For example, many chronically debilitated patients suffer from decubitus ulcers (bed sores) that become contaminated and are constantly infected with normally harmless organisms on the skin. When an injury introduces foreign bodies, such as splinters or particles of soil, the impairment of the defensive mechanisms is even more profound. Moreover, pathogenic microorganisms have developed many virulence mechanisms (discussed in subsequent chapters) that allow them to escape the body defenses, either by evasion or by resistance mechanisms.

When a microorganism crosses the protective epidermis of the skin or the epithelia of mucous membranes, it encounters the next line of defense mechanisms: phagocytic cells, proinflammatory cells, natural killer (NK) cells, and antigen-presenting cells. Once in the body, microorganisms are also confronted by humoral defenses, of which complement is the most powerful. We will discuss all these defense mechanisms in this chapter.

RECOGNITION STRATEGIES OF THE INNATE IMMUNE SYSTEM

One of the central questions in immunology is how the immune system is able to recognize the invading (and potentially dangerous) microbes and discriminate between potentially dangerous microorganisms and nondangerous materials in the host or the environment (clothing, food, etc.). During its long evolution and coexistence with microorganisms, the innate immune system developed three recognition strategies: detection of microbes through pattern recognition receptors, detection of danger signals from damaged tissues, and detection of a missing self (host).

The first and most frequently used strategy is recognition through receptors specific for microbial molecules that are not present in the host. These are called **pattern recognition receptors** because they recognize characteristic structures present in microbes but not in mammals (Table 6-4). These structures are found in microbial products that are essential for survival of the microbes and thus cannot be easily changed, dispensed with, or substituted. Several pattern recognition receptors are located on the cell membrane of phagocytic cells, lymphocytes, endothelial cells, and epithelial cells (although not all these cells express all pattern recognition receptors).

One family of pattern recognition receptors is called **toll-like receptors** (**TLRs**) because of their homology to a fruit fly *Drosophila* receptor called toll. As shown in Table 6-4, TLRs recognize many essential microbial molecules, including essential cell wall components (lipopolysaccharide, lipoproteins, lipoteichoic acid, peptidoglycan), flagella, bacterial DNA (which has unmethylated cytidine phosphate guanosine nucleotide motifs not found in mammalian DNA), fungal cell walls, and viral double-stranded or single-stranded RNA. TLRs that recognize bacterial surface components are usually present on the surface of host cells, because they encounter extracellular bacteria. TLRs that recognize viral or bacterial nucleic acids are usually present in endosomes, where bacterial or viral nucleic acids are found after phagocytosis or endocytosis.

Another pattern recognition receptor, **CD14**, recognizes some of the same molecules as TLR4 and TLR2 (*CD* stands for "cluster of differentiation" and refers to cell surface molecules characterized by different stages of differentiation for various types of leukocytes). The TLRs and CD14 allow the host cells (especially macrophages and dendritic cells) to recognize most microbes (bacteria, fungi, viruses), alert the host to their presence, start proinflammatory defense response, and then start adaptive immune responses. Other pattern recognition receptors, such as the **scavenger receptor**, **mannose receptor**, and **CLR** (named for **C-type lectin receptor** specific for **β-glucan**), are present primarily on phagocytic cells, recognize various bacterial or fungal surface molecules, and allow the host cells to phagocytize them.

Some pattern recognition receptors are cytosolic, which allows them to detect pathogens present in the cell cytoplasm. These receptors can detect viruses, which are synthesized and assembled in the cytoplasm. The need for cytosolic recognition of bacteria stems from the ability of some bacteria (e.g., *Shigella* and *Listeria*) to enter the host cells and escape into the cytoplasm, a strategy that allows these bacteria to avoid recognition and destruction by phagocytic cells and other extracellular antimicrobial mechanisms. The largest family of cytoplasmic pattern recognition receptors is called **NLR** (**NOD-like receptors**), because it includes proteins with a common structural feature, nucleotide oligomerization domain (NOD). These receptors are further subdivided based on their additional structural features (see Table 6-4). The main two groups are **NLRC** (NLRs with caspase recruitment domain) and **NLRP** (NLRs with pyrin domain). NLRC1 and NLRC2, also known as **NOD1** and **NOD2**, recognize fragments of peptidoglycan from bacterial cell walls and allow the cells to produce proinflammatory cytokines, which enhance antimicrobial responses. Other NLRC receptors, as well as NLRP receptors, recognize various microbial components (Table 6-4) and form multiprotein complexes called **inflammasomes**, which activate a proteolytic enzyme, caspase-1. Caspase-1 is required for secretion of a proinflammatory cytokine interleukin-1β (IL-1β), which is synthesized as an inactive form (pro-IL-1β) and needs to be cleaved by caspase-1.

TABLE 6-4 Pattern Recognition Receptors

Receptor	Recognition of	Main Effect
Cell Membrane		
TLR2 (plus TLR1 or TLR6)	Lipoproteins (many bacteria) Peptidoglycan (all bacteria) Lipoteichoic acid (Gram-positive bacteria) Lipoarabinomannan (*Mycobacterium*) Zymosan (fungal cell wall)	Activation of macrophages and dendritic cells to secrete proinflammatory mediators, mature and initiate adaptive immune response
TLR4	Lipopolysaccharide (Gram-negative bacteria), its recognition requires another cell surface molecule, MD-2	Similar to TLR2
TLR5	Flagella (many bacteria)	Similar to TLR2
CD14	Lipopolysaccharide (Gram-negative bacteria) Peptidoglycan (all bacteria) Lipoteichoic acid (Gram-positive bacteria)	Activation of macrophages to secrete proinflammatory mediators
CLR (dectin-1)	β-Glucan (fungi)	Phagocytosis by macrophages and inflammation
Scavenger receptors	Negatively charged polymers (bacteria and fungi)	Phagocytosis by macrophages
Mannose receptor	Mannose-containing polymers (bacteria and fungi)	Phagocytosis by macrophages
N-formylmethionyl peptide receptor	Bacterial proteins	Chemoattraction of PMNs and macrophages
Endosomes		
TLR3	Double-strand RNA (viruses)	Similar to membrane TLRs Induces expression of a viral-inhibitory protein, interferon
TLR7 and TLR8	Single-strand RNA (viruses)	Similar to TLR3
TLR9	DNA (bacteria and viruses)	Similar to TLR3
Cytoplasmic		
NLRC1 and NLRC2 (NOD1 and NOD2)	Peptidoglycan (bacteria)	Activation of macrophages and epithelial cells to produce proinflammatory mediators
NLRC3, NLRC4, and NLRC5	Flagella (many bacteria)	Induction of secretion of proinflammatory cytokine IL-1β (formation of inflammasome, a protein complex that activates caspase-1, which cleaves pro-IL-1β)
NLRP1, NLRP2, and NLRP3	Toxins (bacteria) RNA (bacteria and viruses) Uric acid crystals (humans)	Similar to NLRC3
RLR	RNA (viruses)	Induces expression of a viral-inhibitory protein, interferon

continued on page 72

TABLE 6-4 Pattern Recognition Receptors *(continued)*

Receptor	Recognition of	Main Effect
Secreted		
Soluble CD14	Lipopolysaccharide (Gram-negative bacteria)	Activation of CD-14 negative cells (e.g., endothelial cells) to secrete proinflammatory mediators
Lipopolysaccharide-binding protein	Lipopolysaccharide (Gram-negative bacteria)	Activation of macrophages to secrete proinflammatory mediators
Mannose-binding lectin (MBL) (collectin)	Mannose-containing polymers (bacteria and fungi)	Activation of complement
Surfactant proteins (collectins)	Bacteria, fungi, viruses	Opsonization (enhancement of phagocytosis)
Serum amyloid P (pentraxin)	Bacteria	Activation of complement, opsonization
C-reactive protein (pentraxin)	Bacterial polysaccharides	Activation of complement, opsonization
PGRP-1, PGRP-2, PGRP-3, and PGRP-4	Peptidoglycan (all bacteria)	Bactericidal Hydrolysis of peptidoglycan (amidase)

CD, cluster of differentiation; CLR, C-type lectin receptor; IL, interleukin; NLRC, NOD-like receptor with caspase recruitment domain; NLRP, NOD-like receptor with pyrin domain; NOD, nucleotide oligomerization domain; PGRP, peptidoglycan recognition protein; PMN, polymorphonuclear leukocyte; RLR, RIG (retinoic acid-induced gene-1)-like receptor; TLR, toll-like receptor.

Another family of cytoplasmic receptors is called **RLR** for **RIG-like receptors** (RIG stands for retinoic acid–induced gene-1). They recognize viral RNA and induce synthesis of the antiviral substance interferon. Interferon is released from the virus-infected cells and inhibits the growth of viruses in other host cells.

Several of the pattern recognition receptors are **secreted** or soluble (see Table 6-4). Some of these molecules enable or enhance responses of the host cells to microbial products. For example, soluble CD14 and lipopolysaccharide-binding protein (LBP) enhance responses to bacterial lipopolysaccharide. Other secreted pattern recognition receptors enhance phagocytosis or activate complement (phagocytosis and activation of complement are discussed later in this chapter).

The clinical significance of these pattern recognition receptors has been only recently realized by identification of patients who suffer from severe recurrent pyogenic bacterial infections resulting from genetic defects in signal transduction pathways activated by **TLRs**. Another genetic defect recently discovered is a mutation in an intracellular recognition protein, **NOD2**. The mutation is present in many patients with **Crohn disease**, a chronic inflammatory bowel disease associated with the inability to properly control the responsiveness to bowel bacteria.

The second recognition strategy of the innate immune system is to detect danger signals produced by tissue damage, which would be found in tissue-damaging infections or other injuries to tissues. For example, in gout, uric acid crystals released from damaged cells activate NALP3, which results in overproduction of proinflammatory IL-1β and painful inflammation. This condition can be treated with an IL-1 antagonist.

The third recognition strategy of the innate immune system is to detect a missing or changed self. This strategy is used by the specialized NK cells, which can recognize the host's own cells (self) that do not express a normal set of major histocompatibility complex (MHC) class I molecules. The functions of these cells will be discussed later in this chapter.

CONSEQUENCES OF RECOGNITION: EFFECTOR MECHANISMS

The consequences of recognition by the innate immune system depend on the type of tissue and the recognition system (cells or soluble factor; see Table 6-1). Constitutive innate immunity is an immediate response based on presynthesized antimicrobial factors and effector cells ready to act. Keratinocytes, epithelial cells, and several specialized cells (e.g., Paneth cells present in the crypts in the intestine or cells in sweat and sebaceous glands) produce many antimicrobial peptides (see Table 6-3). When a microbe comes in contact with the skin or mucous membranes, it is confronted by mechanical barriers and antimicrobial factors. When a microbe escapes these mechanisms and penetrates the skin or mucous membranes, it is phagocytized and killed by phagocytic cells (neutrophils and macrophages) present in blood and tissues. The presence of microbes on the skin or mucous membranes or in tissues also triggers **induced innate immunity**, which amplifies and supplements the initial constitutive response. This response consists of the following:

- **Increased production of antimicrobial peptides** by keratinocytes, epithelial cells, and specialized cells in the tissues; this action enhances the killing of microorganisms.
- **Secretion of numerous mediators of inflammation**, such as cytokines, chemokines, and vasoactive products, by macrophages, mast cells, eosinophils, basophils, and platelets; this action induces inflammation.
- **Activation of complement**, which enhances phagocytosis (opsonization), chemotactic attraction of phagocytic cells, inflammation, and direct killing of some microorganisms
- **Activation of clotting cascade and generation of bradykinin**, a nonapeptide that has proinflammatory effects and whose action increases vascular permeability, vasodilation, hypotension, pain, and smooth muscle contraction
- **Chemotactic attraction of phagocytic cells and lymphocytes** to the site of infection
- **Acute phase response**, which involves greatly increased production of many defense proteins and proinflammatory mediators, collectively known as acute phase proteins (which include C-reactive protein, LBP, serum amyloid P, and fibrinogen). Acute phase response is induced in the liver by proinflammatory cytokines, such as IL-1 and IL-6 and tumor necrosis factor-α (TNF-α), produced by proinflammatory cells (mainly macrophages) in response to infection.
- **Inflammation** induced by a combined action of the previously mentioned mediators (as discussed later in this chapter)

These responses have various sensitivities to microbial stimulation depending on the local need of a given tissue. The extent of the response is also usually proportional to the need—that is, the location and the extent of the infection. For example, external tissues (skin and mucous membranes) constantly come in contact with microorganisms, which are usually controlled by constitutively produced antimicrobial peptides. Therefore, these tissues respond only to high numbers of microorganisms; responsiveness to low numbers of microorganisms would induce constant unnecessary inflammation. By contrast, the immune cells in tissues that are normally sterile (have no microorganisms), especially macrophages and leukocytes, are highly sensitive to very low amounts of microbial products. The reason for this high responsiveness is the need for detection of low numbers of microorganisms in normally sterile blood and tissues, because any appearance of microorganisms in the tissues indicates that these microorganisms breached the first line of defense (skin and mucous membranes) and need to be immediately eliminated. Epithelial cells from skin and mucous membranes, however, are highly responsive to cytokines produced by macrophages because cytokine production means that an infection is already being established in the tissues.

Severe clinical manifestations of infection include fever, inflammation, and **septic shock**. They are the price we pay for high responsiveness to microorganisms to fight the infection. Although usually very effective and self-limiting, this high proinflammatory response unfortunately sometimes results in death of the patient because of an irreversible septic shock.

COMPLEMENT

The complement system has many components (Table 6-5), mediates a large number of biological effects, and interacts with other complex systems, such as blood clotting and adaptive immune responses. Complement derives its name from the original belief that it complements, or completes, the action of antibodies. Only later did researchers realize that it plays a crucial role in body defenses even in the absence of antibodies. The complement system is normally barely "on" and must be **activated** to become a significant part of the defense mechanisms (Fig. 6-1). Once activated, it functions to enhance the antimicrobial defenses in several ways:

- Makes invading microorganisms susceptible to phagocytosis (opsonization)
- Lyses some microorganisms directly
- Activates antimicrobial systems of phagocytes
- Produces substances that are chemotactic for white blood cells
- Promotes the inflammatory response

The complement system can be activated in one of three ways. The three activation pathways are known as **classical**, **lectin**, and **alternative** (see Fig. 6-1). Each pathway starts out separately, but the three eventually converge to make the same products. The classical pathway is usually set in motion by the presence of antigen–antibody complexes. It is the most prominent pathway and was described first, hence its name. The lectin and alternative pathways are elicited independently of antibodies, often by microbial surface components like mannose-containing polysaccharides (lectin pathway) or bacterial lipopolysaccharides (alternative pathway). In either case, activation results from proteolytic cleavage of inert larger proteins. Some important steps in activation by either pathway depend on the function of protein complexes made by binding several of the cleaved fragments.

TABLE 6-5 Components of the Complement System[a]

Component	Role in the Complement Cascade
Classical Pathway	
C1q	Binds to Fc region of Ig in antigen–antibody complexes; this binding leads to the activation of C1r
C1r	C1r is cleaved on activation to generate a serine protease that cleaves C1s
C1s	C1s is cleaved to produce a serine protease that cleaves C4 and C2
C4	Is split by C1s into C4a and C4b; C4b binds to the surface membrane and becomes part of the C3 convertase
C2	Binds to C4b and is cleaved by C1s into C2a, which is a serine protease component of the C3/C5 convertase, and C2b that diffuses away
C3 (also part of the lectin and alternative pathways)	Cleaved by C4b2a into the anaphylatoxin C3a and C3b, which is an opsonin and is also part of the C3/C5 convertases
Lectin Pathway	
MBL (mannose-binding lectin)	Binds to mannose-containing carbohydrates on bacterial and fungal cells, analogous to C1q in the classical pathway, and associates with MASP-1 and MASP-2
MBL-associated proteases-1 and MBL-associated proteases-2 (MASP-1 and MASP-2)	Serine proteases that associate with MBL and activate C4 and C2 by cleaving them, similar to C1s
Alternative Pathway	
Factor B (B)	Analogous to C2 in the classical pathway
Factor D (D)	A serine protease that activates factor B by cleaving it
Properdin (P)	Binds to the C3–C5 convertase of the alternative pathway and stabilizes it
Membrane Attack Complex (MAC)	
C5	Cleaved by the convertase complex; C5a is an anaphylatoxin, and C5b is the anchoring protein for C6
C6	Binds to C5b and this complex becomes the anchor for C7
C7	Binds to the C5bC6 complex and then C5bC6C7 inserts into the membrane and becomes an anchor for C8
C8	Attaches to C5bC6C7 and produces a stable membrane-associated complex that can bind C9
C9	Polymerizes at the site of the C5–C8 complex; this completes formation of the fully lytic MAC
Complement Receptors	
Complement receptor type 1(CR1, CD35)	Accelerates dissociation of the C3 convertases, enhances phagocytosis of C3b- or C4b-coated microorganisms—present on red blood cells—and mediates clearance of immune complexes

TABLE 6-5 Components of the Complement System*ᵃ* *(continued)*

Component	Role in the Complement Cascade
Complement receptor type 2 (CR2, CD21)	Activates B cells, cell surface receptor for Epstein-Barr virus
Complement receptor type 3 (CR3, CD11b/CD18)	Adhesion protein (integrin family), important in phagocytosis of iC3b-coated microorganisms
Complement receptor type 4 (CR4, CD11c/CD18)	Adhesion protein (integrin family), important in phagocytosis of iC3b-coated microorganisms
C3a receptor	Release of vasoactive products from mast cells
C5a receptor	Release of vasoactive products from mast cells, chemotactic attraction of phagocytic cells

ᵃThe proteins that regulate complement activity are listed separately in Table 6-6.
CD, cluster of differentiation.

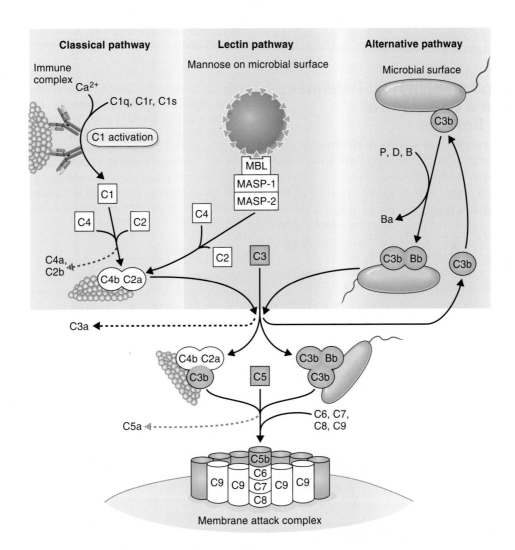

FIGURE 6-1. Activation of complement through the classical, lectin, and alternative pathways.

Nomenclature

The complement system has more than 35 proteins, most of which are present in plasma and a few that are part of cell membranes. Complement proteins constitute 15% of plasma globulins, which amounts to more than 3 g/L. The nomenclature of complement components is complicated by their sheer numbers and by the chronology of their discovery. The major components of the classical pathway are designated by the letter *C* followed by a number, for example, **C3** (see Table 6-5). When the component is cleaved in the process of activation, its fragments receive an additional letter, *a* or *b*. Thus, **C3a** and **C3b** are the products of proteolytic cleavage of C3. The *a* usually designates a small soluble peptide, whereas the *b* denotes a larger peptide that may bind to cell surfaces. Cleavage products often bind to form an active enzyme, for example, C4b2a. Components of the lectin pathway are designated by abbreviations and numbers (such as **MASP-1**), and components of the alternative pathway are designated by letters (such as **B**, **D**, **P**), except for C3b, which is used by all three pathways. What an alphabet soup it is!

Role of Complement in Host Defenses: Overview of the Functions of Complement Proteins

Activation of the complement system is involved in several important aspects of host defenses. Two activities of complement are specifically directed toward enhancing phagocytosis, which is probably the most effective of the innate defenses against microorganisms. These activities are the recruitment of white cells by **chemotactic proteins**, such as C5a (Fig. 6-2), and the facilitation of phagocytosis by proteins called **opsonins** (Fig. 6-3).

Complement activation also induces acute inflammation by generating **anaphylatoxins** (C3a and C5a), which act by causing release of vasoactive mediators from mast cells. This activity can be considered beneficial,

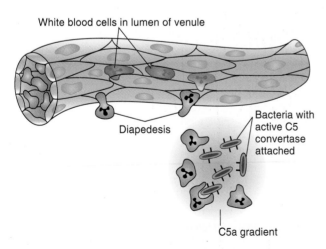

FIGURE 6-2. Chemotactic action of C5a diffusing from bacteria toward a postcapillary venule.

White blood cells in lumen of venule

Diapedesis

Bacteria with active C5 convertase attached

C5a gradient

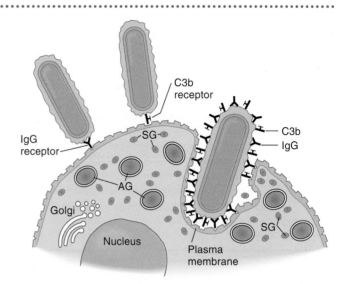

FIGURE 6-3. Opsonization enhances phagocytosis. This schematic representation shows how *Escherichia coli* is opsonized with immunoglobulin (IgG) and complement component C3b. The Fc and C3b ligands on the bacteria attach to the phagocyte through specific receptors. The mechanism of this interaction probably resembles that of a zipper or perhaps Velcro. Thus, sequential binding leads to the ingestion of the bacteria by the phagocytic membrane until the vesicle formed is pinched off as a new organelle inside the phagocyte. Meanwhile, degranulation (the fusion of granules with the phagocytic vesicle) forms a chamber in which bacteria are destroyed. The secondary granules (SG) and the azurophil granules (AG), also known as primary granules, fuse their membranes with that of the nascent phagosome, thus making a phagolysosome. Because phagocytes tend to be "sloppy" eaters, there is some "drooling," and the enzymes and surfactant proteins enter the surrounding fluid, contributing to the tissue changes of inflammation.

insofar as the inflammatory response helps fight invading microorganisms. However, they can also have negative, possibly quite severe, effects. In persons with hypersensitivity disorders, the inflammatory response damages sensitive tissues, especially by causing leukocytes to secrete their lysosomal enzymes in inappropriate ways (see Chapter 7).

Other components of complement make the so-called **membrane attack complex** (**MAC**), which is responsible for the lysis of Gram-negative bacteria, enveloped viruses, and foreign cells. They may even lyse infected tissue cells that appear alien because they display viral or other foreign proteins in their cell membranes. This activity is particularly important in killing bacteria that resist phagocytosis, such as meningococci and gonococci. Indeed, genetic deficiencies of the proteins involved in the formation of the MAC result in increased susceptibility to infections by these particular organisms.

Crucial Step in Complement Activation: Cleavage of C3

The three pathways of complement activation converge at a key biochemical step, the **cleavage of component C3** (see Fig. 6-1). From that point, the remaining steps of all three pathways are the same. The enzymes responsible for this activity, **C3 convertases**, yield fragments C3a and C3b. Both components are pharmacologically active. **C3a**, which diffuses into the surrounding fluid, is an **anaphylatoxin**. **C3b**, which has an active thioester group that covalently binds to hydroxyl groups of carbohydrates or proteins on the antigen (e.g., bacterium), is an **opsonin**. C3b binds to **complement receptor type 1 (CR1)** on phagocytic cells and thus greatly enhances binding of the opsonized bacteria to phagocytic cells (see Fig. 6-3). C3b also binds to CR2 on B cells and enhances B-cell activation and production of antibodies in the adaptive immune response. In addition, C3b becomes part of the C3 convertase of the alternative pathway and a part of C5 convertase (as discussed later in the chapter and shown in Fig. 6-1).

C3 Convertase of the Classical Pathway

Activation of complement by the classical pathway is usually initiated by the presence of antigen–antibody complexes and thus is set off as the result of an adaptive immune response. The immune complexes are recognized by a protein complex called **C1**, composed of three proteins, **C1q**, **C1r**, and **C1s**. C1q is made up of six subunits, each shaped like a tulip (Fig. 6-4). The globular "head" of C1q binds to the Fc portion of antibodies in antigen–antibody complexes (the *c* in *Fc* stands for "constant" or "crystallizable"). One IgM molecule is sufficient for C1q binding, but two closely adjacent IgG molecules are needed. For this reason, IgM is a very potent C activator, whereas only high concentrations of IgG can activate C. C1q binds only to antibodies bound to antigens, which prevents C activation by free antibodies always present in the serum, and ensures that only antigen–antibody complexes activate the classical pathway. Following binding to the antigen–antibody complex, C1q converts C1r into a protease that carries out the next step in the pathway, the cleavage of C1s. The activated enzyme C1s in turn cleaves **C2** and **C4** into fragments **C4b2a**, which bind covalently to the antigen and become the **C3 convertase** of the classical pathway (see Fig. 6-1), and C4a and C2b fragments that are released.

C3 Convertase of the Lectin Pathway

The lectin pathway is activated by binding of the **mannose-binding lectin** (**MBL**), which is a C1q analog, to mannose-containing polysaccharides, frequently present in the cell walls of many bacteria and fungi. This results in activation and complexing of MBL with the MBL-associated proteases **MASP-1** and **MASP-2**, which then cleave **C4** and **C2** to generate **C4b2a**, which is the same **C3 convertase** as in the classical pathway (see Fig. 6-1). From that point, the activation of the lectin pathway proceeds the same as the classical pathway.

C3 Convertase of the Alternative Pathway

How is the alternative pathway activated? C3 is constantly cleaved at a very low level even without complement activation. Such cleavage generates C3b in plasma, but normally specific inhibitors inactivate most of these fragments. In the presence of microorganisms, some C3b fragments survive by binding covalently to their surfaces. Such **surface-bound C3b** is protected from inactivation and can participate in subsequent complement reactions. This C3b binds **factor B**, a protein homologous to C2, to form **C3bB** complex. **Factor D** then cleaves factor B from the C3bB complex to yield **C3bBb** complex, which is **C3 convertase** of the alternative pathway. Binding of **factor P** (properdin) to **C3bBb** stabilizes this enzyme. **C3bBb** then complexes with another C3b fragment to yield another enzyme (**C3b3bBb**) that splits C5 (see Fig. 6-1).

Late Steps in Complement Activation: The Membrane Attack Complex

Once C3b is formed by either pathway, the downstream steps in complement activation can take place (see Fig. 6-1). C4b2a3b of the classical and lectin pathways or C3b3bBb of the alternative pathway cleaves C5 to produce two important fragments, C5a and C5b. **C5a**, like C3a, is an **anaphylatoxin**. In addition, C5a is a powerful **chemoattractant** for phagocytes. The other fragment, **C5b**, is involved in making the final product of the complement cascade, the **membrane attack complex**. This armor-piercing weapon can punch holes in bacteria and, in some cases, in tissue cells (Fig. 6-5). The MAC damages

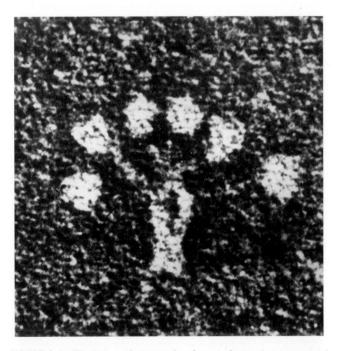

FIGURE 6-4. Electron micrograph of complement component C1q × 500,000. In this lateral view of C1q, six terminal subunits are connected to a central subunit by fibrillar strands. Mannose-binding lectin, which has a similar function to C1q in activation of the lectin pathway, has a similar structure.

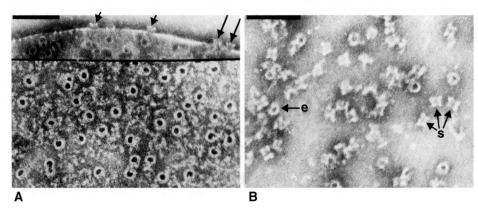

FIGURE 6-5. Membrane attack complex (MAC) seen under the electron microscope. A. MACs inserted into complement-lysed red blood cell membranes. On top portion, MACs are shown in their lateral projections (*arrows*). **B.** Isolated MACs in a detergent solution: a MAC on end (e) and MACs on their side (s).

cells and bacteria by inserting donut-shaped multimers of C9 (which are assembled with the help of components C5b, C6, C7, and C8) into their membranes. The resulting hole makes cells permeable to ions and metabolites. Water enters the cells and raises their pressure, which eventually causes the cells to lyse.

Regulation of Complement Activation

The complement system is programmed to destroy. It must therefore be strictly regulated. On one hand, the complement activation pathway can amplify itself: Each active

enzyme can split and activate many complement molecules. On the other hand, fortunately, each activated component has its inhibitor (Table 6-6). The inhibition usually involves one of three mechanisms: (1) a suicide substrate mechanism, in which an inhibitor forms a covalent bond with the active site of the enzyme (e.g., C1 inhibitor binds to C1r and C1s); (2) proteolytic digestion of the active fragments into smaller inactive fragments (e.g., digestion of C4b and C3b by factor I); or (3) inhibition of association of complement components (e.g., inhibition of MAC formation by CD59). Without inhibition, all complement

TABLE 6-6 Proteins that Regulate Complement Activity

Component	Function
Soluble Serum Proteins	
C1 inhibitor (C1 INH)	Inhibits enzymatic activity of C1r and C1s of the classical pathway and MASPs of the lectin pathway by suicide substrate mechanism
C4-binding protein (C4bp)	Binds to C4b and enhances the decay of C4b2a classical and lectin pathway C3 convertase
Factor H (H)	Binds to C3b and enhances the decay of the alternative pathway C3 convertase
Factor I (I)	Proteolytically inactivates C4b and C3b
Anaphylatoxin inactivator (ANA-IN)	Proteolytically inactivates the anaphylatoxins, C3a and C5a
S-protein (S; vitronectin)	Inhibits insertion of the MAC into the lipid bilayer by binding to the C5b-7 complex
Membrane Proteins	
Complement receptor type 1 (CR1, CD35)	Accelerates dissociation of both C3 convertases
Membrane cofactor protein (MCP)	Cofactor for factor I–mediated cleavage of C3b
Decay accelerating factor (DAF, CD55)	Accelerates dissociation of both C3 convertases
Protectin (membrane inhibitor of reactive lysis, MIRL, CD59)	Binds to C9 and prevents MAC formation
Homologous restriction factor	Blocks MAC insertion into the surface of cells

in the body would eventually be activated and massive inflammation would ensue. The adjacent host cells are also protected from the damage by activated complement components by several membrane proteins that inhibit complement activation or inactivate the activated components (see Table 6-6). These plasma and membrane inhibitors ensure that the activation of complement occurs locally and is limited to the microbial surface at the site of infection.

The importance of complement and its appropriate regulation is demonstrated by genetic deficiencies of complement components. Patients lacking complement components that participate in the activation cascade suffer from more frequent and more severe bacterial infections. The impact of MAC deficiencies on susceptibility to infections with *Neisseria* was mentioned earlier in the chapter. Patients with C3 deficiencies suffer from infections with pyogenic bacteria, such as *Streptococcus pneumoniae, Staphylococcus aureus,* and *Haemophilus influenzae.* MBL and the lectin activation pathway were discovered by studying a group of children with recurrent pyogenic bacterial infections and failure to thrive. Their serum could not opsonize a yeast, *Saccharomyces cerevisiae* (which has mannose polymers in its cell wall), with C3; the serum was found to be deficient in MBL.

Deficiencies in complement inhibitors often result in overactivation of complement and inflammatory diseases. The genetic deficiency of C1 esterase inhibitor permits activation of the classical and lectin pathways with the uncontrolled production of anaphylatoxins. The result may be **hereditary angioedema**, a potentially fatal condition that causes laryngeal edema and airway obstruction. Another serious hereditary disease, **paroxysmal nocturnal hemoglobinuria**, manifests as bouts of intravascular hemolysis caused by complement-induced host cell lysis. This condition results from a deficiency of the inhibitory proteins CD55 (DAF) and CD59 (MIRL) on the surface of red blood cells. In healthy individuals, CD55 and CD59 are linked to the cell membrane through glycosylphosphatidylinositol (GPI). Patients with this disease lack one of the enzymes needed for the synthesis of this GPI anchor. Since each red blood cell binds as many as 1,000 molecules of C3b per day, lack of functional inhibitory proteins on the red cells in these patients results in red cell lysis.

Microbial View of Complement

Complement killing by insertion of the MAC affects not only bacteria but also **enveloped viruses**. Not surprisingly, sensitive microorganisms have evolved countermeasures, some of which are discussed in Chapter 8. An interesting example of microbial defenses against complement is provided by herpes simplex virus. One of the glycoproteins of herpes simplex virus, glycoprotein C, contains a region that has an amino acid sequence similar to that of part of CR1. This amino acid sequence allows glycoprotein C to bind complement component C3b, thereby interfering with the rest of the complement cascade and with complement-mediated killing of the virus.

Several viruses have evolved to take advantage of complement receptors to enter host cells. Epstein-Barr virus uses CR2 to enter B cells and epithelial cells. Some viruses (e.g., HIV) or bacteria (e.g., *Mycobacterium*) not only have developed resistance to the lytic action of complement but also activate complement and use the C3b that deposits on its viral or bacterial surface to enter host cells through C3b receptors.

Leukocyte Chemotaxins: Sounding the Alarm

We have already seen that a product of complement activation, C5a, is an attractant for neutrophils and monocytes. It is not the only one; chemically distinct **chemotaxins** are also made by bacteria and by host cells. Prominent among the latter are the leukotrienes, which are lipid products of cell membrane metabolism, and IL-8 and numerous other chemokines (discussed later), products of monocytes and macrophages.

The chemotaxins made by bacteria have an interesting origin. Many bacterial proteins "mature" after their synthesis, when a peptide is clipped off from their N terminus. The first amino acid in the peptide is *N*-formylmethionine, the initiator amino acid in prokaryotic protein synthesis. Eukaryotic cells do not use this device. The clipped peptide is recognized by the host as a strong chemoattractant for phagocytes. Its activity depends on its amino acid sequence and can be remarkably potent. *N*-formylmethionyl-leucyl-phenylalanine, for example, s active at concentrations of 10^{-11} molar. That is an extremely sensitive way for the host to detect bacterial proteins.

Chemotaxins enhance and direct the motility of phagocytic cells. As these compounds diffuse from their source, a concentration gradient is formed in the surrounding tissues. If the tissues are inflamed, neutrophils are already poised for action on the vascular endothelia. When neutrophils sense the chemotaxins, they travel along the gradient, cross the endothelial cells, and move into the tissues toward the microorganisms. This chemical homing mechanism guides the neutrophils precisely and efficiently to their targets.

Opsonization and Opsonins

Phagocytic cells alone can phagocytize bacteria, but without enhancing cofactors, this process is inefficient. In the presence of substances called **opsonins**, neutrophils and macrophages will phagocytize many more bacteria. The term *opsonin* is related to the Latin word *opsonium*, which means "relish," an apt term for making bacteria more appetizing to phagocytes.

Several substances normally serve as opsonins, including the **C3b** component of complement and IgG antibodies (see Tables 6-4 and 6-5). C3b binds covalently to the surface of bacteria and forms a ligand that is recognized by receptors on neutrophils, monocytes, and macrophages. Microorganisms coated with C3b become anchored to the surface of phagocytes, which facilitates their uptake (see Fig. 6-3). Three receptors for C3b and its various cleavage products are located on white blood cells: **CR1**, **CR3**, and **CR4** (see Table 6-5).

PHAGOCYTES

Of all the innate antimicrobial defenses of the body, the most potent is the cellular response. It consists of the influx of neutrophils, eosinophils, and monocytes into infected tissues. The properties of these and other white blood cells are listed in Table 6-7.

Neutrophils

Neutrophils are actively motile phagocytic cells produced in the bone marrow (see Table 6-7). They differentiate

from stem cells over a period of about 2 weeks. Together with eosinophils and basophils, they are also known as **polymorphonuclear leukocytes** (**PMNs**) because of their segmented nucleus or as **granulocytes** because of their granules. They produce four kinds of granules—primary, secondary, tertiary, and secretory vesicles—of which the first two kinds, azurophil (primary) and specific (secondary) are the largest and most easily visible under the microscope. These granules have many antimicrobial factors (see Tables 6-3 and 6-8). When PMNs mature, in numbers of about 10^{10} per day, about 5% enter the peripheral blood and circulate for an average of 6.5 hours. Half of these neutrophils enter the capillary bed where they **marginate**—that is, they adhere to the endothelium of venules. In response to distress signals from the tissues (complement components, the chemokine IL-8, and cytokines such as IL-1 and TNF-α), the endothelium in the involved region expresses a set of adhesion molecules that bind more firmly to the neutrophils. When summoned by chemotaxins, the neutrophils cross the endothelium by **diapedesis** through the cell

TABLE 6-7 White Blood Cells

Cell	Source	Function
Neutrophil	Bone marrow stem cells to peripheral blood	Adherence, chemotaxis, diapedesis Phagocytosis Degranulation Antimicrobial action, oxidative and nonoxidative
Eosinophil	Similar to neutrophil	Antiparasitic action, nonoxidative and oxidative
Basophil	Similar to neutrophil	Release of proinflammatory vasoactive mediators
Monocyte	Bone marrow stem cells Promonocyte to peripheral blood	Adherence, chemotaxis, diapedesis Phagocytosis Antimicrobial action Secretion of cytokines
Macrophage	Monocytes of the peripheral blood	See monocytes
		Synthesis of many important molecules, including cytokines (TNF-α, IL-1, IL-6, IL-12, IL-15, and others), chemokines (IL-8 and others), complement components, plasminogen activator and other proteases, lysozyme, cell membrane components, including major histocompatibility complex (MHC) class I and class II molecules Functions in adaptive immunity through antigen recognition, antigen processing, antigen presentation, and regulation of immune responses
T lymphocyte	Bone marrow stem cells via thymus	Helper, effector, and regulatory functions in adaptive immune response
B lymphocyte	Bone marrow stem cells	Antibody production in adaptive immune responses
NK cell	Bone marrow stem cells	Killing of virus-infected cells and tumor cells

IL, interleukin; TNF, tumor necrosis factor.

TABLE 6-8 Antimicrobial Substances Associated with the Azurophil and Specific Granules of Neutrophils

Granule Type	O$_2$-Independent	O$_2$-Dependent	Other
Azurophil (primary)	α-Defensins (HNP1–4) PLA$_2$ Azurocidin (CAP37) BPI Elastase Cathepsin G Proteinase 3 Lysozyme	Myeloperoxidase[a]	
Specific (secondary)	Cathelicidin (CAP18) Lactoferrin Lysozyme	NADPH oxidase[b] cofactors	Bacterial chemotaxin receptors C5a receptors Collagenase Gelatinase Vitamin B$_{12}$–binding protein

[a]Myeloperoxidase together with Cl$^-$ and hydrogen peroxide form a potent antimicrobial system.
[b]This enzyme complex forms with fusion of specific granule membranes with the cytoplasmic membrane. Specific granules contribute the cytochrome component of the complex and the flavoprotein, while neutrophil cytoplasmic membrane contributes NADPH oxidase to the complex. BPI, bactericidal permeability-increasing protein; CAP, cationic antimicrobial protein; HNP, human neutrophil peptide (an abbreviation used for four α-defensins found in human neutrophils).

junctions, traverse the basement membrane, and enter the extravascular tissue spaces (see Fig. 6-2).

Neutrophils and monocytes can be enticed into foci of infection by gradients of many chemoattractants, such as the C5a complement component, formylated bacterial proteins, and chemokines. But what ensures that these phagocytes will arrive precisely where they are needed?

The answer to the question is that neutrophils and monocytes, as well as the endothelial cells to which they must adhere, become sticky (see Fig. 6-2). The molecular explanation is simple: It is the result of sugars on gly-cosylated surface proteins. These glycoproteins on the endothelial cells are **selectins** (which mediate weak binding) and **integrin ligands** (which mediate strong binding, e.g., intercellular adhesion molecule-1, ICAM-1). They bind to **integrins** on the phagocytes (e.g., leukocyte function-associated antigen-1, LFA-1). However, stickiness introduces a problem: Blood cells that originate in the marrow must enter the bloodstream and be able to circulate there without sticking too firmly. For their part, the endothelial cells lining the blood vessels must avoid becoming too sticky to allow circulation of the blood cells. At the proper time, however, both leukocytes and endothelial cells must be able to stick to each other. The transition from loosely adherent to tightly adherent is critical for the leukocytes when they leave the circulation and move through the tissues. Clearly, leukocytes and endothelial cells are subject to regulatory mechanisms that induce stickiness of these cells at the proper time. Complement components such as C5a, chemokines such as IL-8, and cytokines such as IL-1 and TNF-α play such directive and regulatory roles, attracting leukocytes and stimulating endothelial cells, upregulating their stickiness, and causing them to produce additional cytokines and prostaglandins.

The importance of glycoprotein receptors for endothelial cells that are present on neutrophils is illustrated in people with congenital defects in these proteins. Neutrophils of these patients are unable to pass through the vascular endothelium and fail to orient, bind, and ingest particles. Such defective neutrophils are unable to form pus. Patients with this condition are said to have congenital **leukocyte adhesion deficiency** (**LAD**) and suffer recurrent, often fatal infections. Neutrophils of LAD patients do not pass through endothelia because their receptors fail to bind to the endothelial cells and they are also deficient in ingesting bacteria. The reason for these multiple defects is a mutation in CD18, which is a component of three types of leukocytes' integrins: one adhesion molecule (LFA-1, a dimer composed of CD11a and CD18) and two complement receptors (CR3 and CR4, which are CD11b:CD18 and CD11c:CD18 dimers, respectively).

In a healthy person, sticking of leukocytes to endothelial surfaces is most intense in the submucosa of the alimentary tract. The large intestine has an enormous microbial population just one cell layer away from the host's aseptic tissues. This abundant microbiota generates large amounts of chemotaxins that recruit the bulk of the normally available neutrophils. Thus, the submucosa of the gut is in a constant state of low-level inflammation, which keeps the microbiota of the lumen in check. When the bone marrow fails to make neutrophils in reaction to toxic chemicals or radiation or for other reasons, infections emanate from the gut.

Monocytes and Macrophages

Slower to arrive at the sites of microbial invasion are the **monocytes**. These circulating members of the mononuclear family eventually settle in tissues and become known as resident **tissue macrophages**. Although monocytes and macrophages share a common progenitor with neutrophils, their kinetics of maturation and appearance are substantially different. Unlike the neutrophils, monocytes continue to differentiate after they leave the bone marrow. Most importantly, monocytes and macrophages function in both innate and adaptive immune responses, a point that will be elaborated later in this chapter and in Chapter 7.

In general, monocytes and macrophages come into play slowly, often hours after neutrophils have been actively combating invading microorganisms. Neutrophils play a role in recruiting mononuclear cells because they release a granule protein (**azurocidin** or CAP37) that is a potent attractant specific for monocytes. The delay in monocyte activity is seen in patients who become neutropenic from chemicals or radiation. If the neutropenia develops slowly, there is time for monocytes to replace the disappearing neutrophils. The risk of infection is much smaller in these patients than in those with an abrupt onset of neutropenia.

Tissue or resident macrophages exist throughout the body and have different names and functions, depending on the tissue. Thus, they are called **Kupffer cells** in the liver, **alveolar macrophages** in the lungs, **osteoclasts** in the bone, and **microglia** in the brain. All these tissue macrophages phagocytize invading microorganisms. Tissue macrophages contribute greatly to the inflammatory response by releasing IL-1, which enhances sticking of neutrophils to the capillary endothelia, and TNF-α, which activates newly arrived neutrophils. In addition, tissue macrophages release an activator of the acute phase reaction (IL-6) and many chemokines (including IL-8) that attract neutrophils. These macrophages are replenished by the arrival and differentiation of monocytes from the bone marrow.

Eosinophils

Eosinophils parallel neutrophils in lifestyle and function. Although they are not efficient in phagocytosis, they can readily **exocytose** (release to the outside) their granules. Their target is usually animal parasites rather than bacteria. Indeed, the increase of these cells in the circulation, **eosinophilia**, is the hallmark of multicellular parasitic diseases such as schistosomiasis or trichinosis. The cytoplasmic granules of the eosinophils carry large amounts of an enzyme known as **eosinophil peroxidase**, as well as specific cationic proteins. These compounds have the power to kill certain parasites. Thus, eosinophils have an anti-infectious armamentarium similar to that of neutrophils but specifically targeted to certain protozoa and worms, which are too large to be phagocytized by neutrophils.

How do Phagocytes Kill Microorganisms?

Once near their microbial target, neutrophils and other phagocytes can begin their antimicrobial action (see Figs. 6-3, 6-6, and 6-7). To start the process, they must

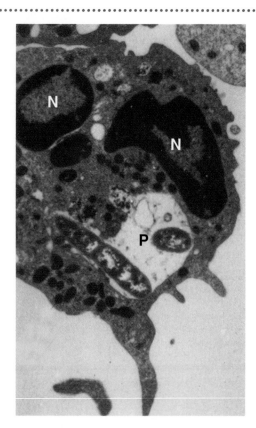

FIGURE 6-6. Phagocytosis of *E. coli* by a neutrophil visualized by transmission electron microscopy. Shown here are lobes of the segmented nucleus (N) and two bacteria engulfed and seen within a phagosome (P).

attach and ingest the microorganisms, either spontaneously or with the aid of **opsonins** (substances that enhance phagocytosis, as described earlier in this chapter). The membranes of neutrophils contain the receptors for chemotaxins and opsonins. After chemotaxins bind to these membranes, the receptor molecules are internalized and replaced with new ones. What makes chemotaxis so effective is that neutrophils are extraordinarily motile. Neutrophils move by recombining their cytoplasmic microfilaments and their microtubules. **Actin** and **myosin** in microfilaments are affected by the protein **gelsolin** (which invites the comparison of neutrophils with muscle cells). The result is a morphological alteration of the cell shape. During chemotaxis, the portion of the cell that faces upstream in the chemotactic gradient forms a structure called a **lamellipodium**, where the cytoplasm is densely packed with microfilaments. The portion of the cell that faces downstream in the gradient forms a knob-like structure, the **uropod**.

Engulfing of bacteria or other particles of suitable size takes place by formation of a pouchlike structure, the **phagosome**, which invaginates, displacing the nucleus and the granules toward the uropod (see Figs. 6-6 and 6-7). The cytoplasmic granules soon discharge their contents into the phagosome by fusion of their membranes (a process called degranulation),

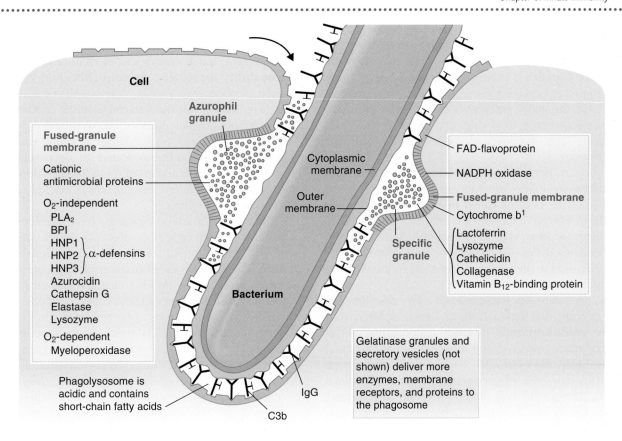

FIGURE 6-7. Fusion of the phagosome and the granules. Fusion between the membranes of the specific granules and the cytoplasmic membrane, together with proteins from the cytosol, completes the enzyme complex that generates reduced oxygen species, including H_2O_2, which then forms antimicrobial hypochlorite from chloride by the action of myeloperoxidase. Fusion of specific and azurophil granules with the phagosome also activates oxygen-independent mechanisms and delivers many antimicrobial proteins to the phagosome.

forming a new structure known as the **phagolysosome**. The phagolysosome quickly pinches off from the plasma membrane and becomes a separate cytoplasmic organelle. By the time the pinching off is completed, the fusion of the granules is well under way, and bacteria are already coated with antibacterial proteins. Thus, like poisonous snakes that disable their prey before swallowing them, neutrophils kill bacteria before they completely ingest them.

Bacteria become enfolded into the plasma membrane of the neutrophils by a zipper-like action, with the receptors on the phagocyte surface progressively attaching to the ligands on the bacterial surface (see Figs. 6-3 and 6-7). This binding stimulates two mechanisms that lead to the killing of bacteria. One mechanism is set in motion by a vigorous burst of oxidative metabolism that leads to the production of hydrogen peroxide and other compounds lethal to microorganisms (see Fig. 6-7). This is **oxygen-dependent killing**. The second mechanism also results in the discharge of toxic compounds from the granules into the phagosome. This is known as **oxygen-independent killing**. The granules of these cells may be considered enlarged lysosomes, packed with large

amounts of powerful hydrolytic enzymes and other active substances. They are contained within unit membranes (see Fig. 6-7). **Azurophil**, or **primary granules**, contain a variety of enzymes and several cationic proteins that are also powerfully antibacterial (see Tables 6-3 and 6-8). **Specific**, or **secondary**, **granules** contain a cytochrome, the iron-binding protein **lactoferrin**, bactericidal cathelicidin, and other proteins.

Oxygen-Dependent Killing

How does the oxidative process kill microorganisms? The mechanism is complex and involves several radicals and chemical species. A highly active, multicomponent **NADPH oxidase** rapidly reduces molecular oxygen to superoxide, O_2^-, which in turn becomes H_2O_2 in the following reaction:

$$2O_2^- + H_2O \rightarrow H_2O_2 + O_2$$

The components of the NADPH oxidase include several proteins. Two of them, the cytochrome **Phox 91** (*Phox* stands for "phagocyte oxidase") and **Phox 22** are inserted into the cytosolic membrane by fusion of the specific granules with the phagosome. There they are joined by the cytosolic proteins **Phox 47** and **Phox 67** to form the completed oxidase. Separating NADPH oxidase components into different subcellular compartments ensures that the active enzyme is assembled only inside the phagolysosomes following phagocytosis and prevents generation of toxic oxygen products outside the phagolysosome.

Hydrogen peroxide, while bactericidal, does not work alone in killing microorganisms within phagocytes. Rather, an enzyme called **myeloperoxidase** uses peroxide to convert chloride ions into the highly toxic **hypochlorous ions**, the same chemical found in common bleach (see Fig. 6-7 and Table 6-8). Myeloperoxidase is delivered to the phagolysosome by fusion with the azurophil granules.

The importance of these oxidative processes in neutrophil microbicidal action is illustrated in children with **chronic granulomatous disease**, a congenital defect caused by mutations involving the NADPH oxidase Phox proteins, most often Phox 91. Such defects render their phagocytes incapable of producing the reduced oxygen products. These cells can phagocytize and degranulate, but they fail to kill the ingested bacteria. Interestingly, microorganisms that lack catalase, such as the streptococci, obligingly release H_2O_2 into the phagocytic vacuole when phagocytized, thereby committing suicide. Thus, pneumococci (a species of streptococci) do not cause disease any more frequently in such patients than they do in normal persons. The incidence of chronic granulomatous disease is about four per million. Mutations involving Phox 91 make up 65% of the cases of chronic granulomatous disease and are X chromosome linked (the remaining 35% of patients lack other components of NADPH oxidase complex). These patients develop subcutaneous abscesses, lung abscesses, hepatic abscesses, lymphadenitis, pneumonias, and osteomyelitis.

Oxygen-Independent Killing

Oxygen-independent killing mechanisms are also triggered by the binding of opsonized bacteria to the plasma membrane of neutrophils (see Fig. 6-7 and Table 6-8). Specific and azurophilic granules fuse with phagosomes within 30 seconds of phagocytosis and deliver to the phagosomes several bactericidal proteins. Specific granules deliver **cathelicidin** (CAP18), lysozyme (the enzyme that disrupts the cell wall of many bacteria), and lactoferrin (an iron-binding protein that effectively reduces the amount of iron available to the microorganisms). The azurophil granules discharge into phagosomes **antimicrobial cationic proteins** (such as α-**defensins** and **azurocidin**), **phospholipase A_2**, and **neutral proteases** (cathepsin G, elastase, and proteinase 3). Each of these substances has a unique antimicrobial spectrum, and they usually damage microbial membranes either through direct insertion into the membranes (e.g., **defensins**) or through enzymatic activity (proteases and PLA_2). They also act synergistically; for example, sensitivity of Gram-negative bacteria is much greater to a mixture of **bactericidal permeability-increasing protein** (**BPI**) and PLA_2 than to each peptide individually. The activity of these proteins may account for the survival of some children with chronic granulomatous disease. The oxygen-independent mechanisms also account for bacterial killing under the highly anaerobic conditions found in deep abscesses. However, combined action of both oxygen-dependent and oxygen-independent mechanisms is needed for most efficient bacterial killing.

Deficiencies in cationic proteins have been described in patients with chronic skin infections and abscesses. A genetic disease known as the **Chediak-Higashi syndrome** is caused by the formation of large granules in neutrophils, which are poorly functional and substantially reduce the killing power of these cells.

How do various kinds of bacteria differ in their sensitivity to the two bactericidal mechanisms of neutrophils? In general, organisms found in the gut, such as Gram-negative rods, are readily killed by the oxygen-independent mechanism. Gram-positive bacteria, like those found on the skin and in the upper respiratory epithelia, tend to be resistant to oxygen-independent killing and are killed chiefly by the oxygen-dependent pathway. Does this reflect the abundance of oxygen in the skin and its absence in the gut?

Killing by Monocytes and Macrophages

Together, monocytes and macrophages serve to mop up what is left at the scene of the battle between microorganisms and neutrophils. They phagocytize the microorganisms and the debris left by neutrophils. Their mechanisms of chemotaxis, phagocytosis, and microbial killing resemble those of the neutrophils. **Nitric oxide**, a simple chemical made by macrophages in some animal species as the result of activation by interferon-γ and TNF-α, plays an important role in the killing of microorganisms by macrophages in mice. However, human monocytes and macrophages do not make nitric oxide in any significant amounts; thus, the contribution of nitric oxide to microbial killing by these cells is negligible. In humans nitric oxide is made in small amounts by fibroblasts, some neurons, and cells of the vasculature, where nitric oxide may perform some vasoactive and transmitter functions.

An important point is that monocytes and macrophages, unlike the neutrophils, continue to differentiate after they leave the bone marrow and become activated when properly stimulated. In addition, these versatile cells synthesize several complement components and cytokines. Activated macrophages phagocytize more vigorously, take up more oxygen, and secrete a large quantity of hydrolytic enzymes. In general, they are better prepared to kill microorganisms and, appropriately, have been called the "angry" macrophages. Macrophage activation is elicited by substances made in response to the presence of microorganisms, like complement fragment C3b and interferon-γ. They are also activated by a variety of other compounds, such as endotoxin of Gram-negative bacteria. Some bacteria, fungi, and protozoa can grow within unstimulated macrophages, but in general, they are killed when these cells become activated. Perhaps the most important property of macrophages is their participation in the recognition of antigens and induction of adaptive immune responses, which is discussed later in this chapter.

INFLAMMATION: COMPLEX RESPONSE TO INFECTION AND INJURY

The combined action of the various defense mechanisms discussed so far in this chapter results in **inflammation**, which further amplifies both innate and adaptive immune defenses. Inflammation is a process that occurs in vascularized tissues in response to injury. Early signs of inflammation are confined locally and include pain, swelling, or both and a sense of heat and throbbing of the injured part. The inflamed site appears red, shiny, hot, and painful to the touch as the result of alterations in local blood vessels and lymphatics. These rapid changes, which are called **acute inflammation**, are dynamic and undergo predictable and continued evolution. The tissues may return to normal or become scarred. The outcome depends on the extent of damage done by trauma, by the infecting microorganisms, or by the inflammatory response itself. If acute inflammation does not cure the problem, it may change character and become a **chronic inflammation**.

Many **mediators** induced by various mechanisms cause inflammation (Table 6-9). They include **complement-generated split products**; **histamine** released from mast cells, basophils, and platelets; lipid mediators (**prostaglandins** and **leukotrienes** generated from arachidonic acid and **platelet-activating factor** generated from phospholipids in the cell membranes of mast cells and other cells); and **kinins** (mainly bradykinin) generated in plasma during activation of the clotting system.

Cytokines (literally, "cell movers") are 10- to 25-kDa polypeptides secreted from microbe-activated proinflammatory cells (primarily macrophages and lymphocytes). They have multiple proinflammatory effects. Produced locally in small amounts, the cytokines **tumor necrosis factor** (**TNF-α**), **IL-1**, and **IL-6** locally activate other proinflammatory cells and endothelial and epithelial cells, enhance their defensive activity, and induce production of more cytokines and chemokines. When produced in large amounts, these cytokines enter circulation and have endocrine-like effects. They induce fever, increased lipolysis in adipose tissues, mobilization of amino acids from muscles (to be used in synthesizing

defense proteins), and synthesis of acute phase proteins in the liver (which enter circulation and enhance body defenses). The cytokines mentioned here also enhance the function of antigen-presenting cells and lymphocytes that participate in adaptive immune responses. Excessive production of cytokines (especially TNF-α) and other mediators of inflammation induce **septic shock**, which can be fatal.

Many microbe- or cytokine-activated host cells, including macrophages and endothelial and epithelial cells, produce numerous **chemokines**, which are cytokines with chemotactic properties. More than 100 chemokines and chemokine receptors have been identified to date, which is a testimony to the complexity of chemotactic events and their importance for host defenses. Classified into two families based on a structural motif of two cysteines separated by one amino acid (CXC) or two adjacent cysteines (CC), chemokines are named **CXCL** or **CCL** (*L* stands for "ligand") and numbered consecutively. Similarly, chemokine receptors are named CXCR or CCR (*R* stands for "receptor") and numbered. Chemokines are usually chemotactic for many cell types, but in general, most of the chemokines of the CXC group (which includes the well-known chemokine IL-8) are chemotactic for neutrophils. Chemokines of the CC group are primarily chemotactic for T lymphocytes, although some are also chemotactic for eosinophils, basophils, monocytes, and other cells. High induction of CXC chemokines by various bacteria is responsible for accumulation of large amounts of **pus** (which is primarily composed of PMN exudate and bacteria) at the site of infections.

The combined action of the mediators of inflammation results in the following:

- **Increased blood supply** (manifested as erythema or redness), which brings more antimicrobial cells and proteins to the site of infection
- **Increased vascular permeability** (manifested as edema or swelling caused by accumulation of fluid), which brings more antimicrobial proteins to the site of infection
- **Chemotaxis** (manifested as induration or hardening of the lesion caused by accumulation of cells), which causes infiltration of the site of infection with phagocytic cells and lymphocytes attracted to the site of infection by chemotactic factors

Inflammation is essential for defenses against infections; therefore, patients with infections should generally *not* be treated with anti-inflammatory agents. However, excessive or uncontrolled inflammation, or inflammation induced by noninfectious causes, may produce substantial damage to the tissues and needs to be treated. Such a condition is called hypersensitivity. Because hypersensitivities often result from exaggerated adaptive immune responses, they will be discussed in Chapter 7.

TABLE 6-9 Mediators of Inflammation

Mediator	Source	Main Effect
C3a (peptide)	Complement	Anaphylatoxin, causes histamine release from platelets and mast cells, which increases vascular permeability
C5a (peptide)	Complement	Chemotaxis of PMNs Anaphylatoxin causes histamine release from mast cells and platelets
Histamine (decarboxylated histidine)	Mast cells Basophils Platelets	Increased vascular permeability Vasodilation
Prostaglandins (lipids)	Arachidonic acid from membranes of mast cells and other leukocytes, by cyclooxygenase pathway	PGE_2, PGI_2 (prostacyclin): vasodilation, edema TXA_2 (thromboxane A_2): vasoconstriction
Leukotrienes (lipids)	Arachidonic acid from membranes of mast cells and other leukocytes, by lipoxygenase pathway	LTB_4: chemotaxis LTC_4, LTD_4, LTE_4: vasoconstriction, increased vascular permeability
Platelet-activating factor (lipid)	Mast cells Basophils PMNs, Macrophages Endothelial cells	Release of vasoactive products from platelets Increased vascular permeability Adhesion of PMNs to endothelial cells
Bradykinin (peptide)	Plasma	Increased vascular permeability Vasodilation
Cytokines (Peptides)		
TNF-α	Macrophages	Endothelial cell and PMN activation Inflammation Fever Shock Fat and protein catabolism Acute phase protein synthesis in liver
IL-1	Macrophages Endothelial cells	Endothelial cell activation Inflammation Fever Acute phase protein synthesis in liver
IL-6	Macrophages Endothelial cells T cells	Acute phase protein synthesis in liver Fever B-cell growth and differentiation
Chemokines (Peptides)		
CXC family[a] (includes IL-8)	Macrophages Endothelial and epithelial cells	Chemotactic attraction of PMNs
CC family[a]	Macrophages Endothelial and epithelial cells	Chemotactic attraction of T lymphocytes

[a]More than 50 chemokines are divided into two families based on a structural motif of two cysteines separated by one amino acid (CXC) or two adjacent cysteines (CC).
IL, interleukin; PMN, polymorphonuclear leukocyte; TNF, tumor necrosis factor.

NATURAL KILLER CELLS

NK cells are large granular lymphocytes that have cytotoxic activity for other cells. In this aspect, they resemble cytotoxic T cells. However, NK cells are neither T cells nor B cells because they do not have the markers characteristic of T or B lymphocytes. They also do not have the T- or B-cell antigen receptors and the associated signal transduction molecules that make B- and T-cell antigen specific (see Chapter 7). Therefore, they do not recognize antigens through the types of receptors that T and B cells use, and they do not need to be selected and generated in adaptive immune responses directed to specific antigens. The name NK thus stems from their readiness to kill other cells without the need for time-consuming antigen-driven selection in adaptive immune response. NK cells constitute 5 to 20% of mononuclear cells in peripheral blood and spleen but are rare in other lymphoid organs.

NK cells kill virus-infected cells before these cells can produce mature infective viral particles. This function is important because viruses can only grow inside the living host cells, using their biochemical machinery to produce more viruses. Once the virus enters the host cell, however, it is not visible and thus not susceptible to extracellular host defenses. Therefore, virus-infected cells must be destroyed before they can make more infective viruses. Cytotoxic T cells can do this by using T-cell antigen receptors that recognize viral peptides bound to host MHC class I antigens exposed on the surface of infected cells (see Chapter 7). How can NK cells discriminate between virus-infected and uninfected cells? NK cells can also kill some tumor cells and other damaged cells. How can they discriminate between malignant and nonmalignant cells, or healthy and damaged cells?

NK cells use the previously mentioned missing or changed-self strategy to detect virus-infected cells, tumor cells, and damaged cells. NK cells have, on their surface, two types of receptors. The first type is the **natural killer receptors (NKRs)**. NK cells have several types of NKRs, but in general, these receptors are lectins that bind to various glycoproteins present on many cells in the body. Thus, many host cells are potential NK targets. Some NKRs recognize cell surface proteins produced in response to stress, which allows NK cells to recognize damaged or unhealthy cells, including virus-infected cells and some tumor cells. An example of such a stress-response protein is **MIC** (named for its resemblance to MHC class I molecules). Engagement of NKRs triggers the killing of target cells. However, this would induce the killing of not only unhealthy cells but also many healthy cells in the body. Therefore, NK cells have a second type of receptors, the **killer inhibitory receptors (KIRs;** also called killer Ig-like receptors, e.g., CD158), which prevent the killing action of the NKRs. KIRs bind to self MHC class I molecules on target cells. Because all healthy cells in the body express MHC class I molecules (see Chapter 7), KIRs inhibit killing of normal healthy cells by NK cells. However, virus-infected cells or some tumor cells often have missing or changed MHC class I molecules and therefore do not engage KIRs but still have stress proteins or other glycoproteins that engage NKRs. In the absence of inhibition by KIRs, NKRs trigger the killing of these target cells (Fig. 6-8). Allogeneic transplanted cells have different MHC class I molecules than the transplant recipient (see Chapter 7) and may also be killed by NK cells; KIRs of NK cells recognize self, but not foreign MHC molecules. What a clever way to dispose of unwanted infected cells, other unhealthy cells, tumor cells, or foreign cells!

NK cells are stimulated by the macrophage-derived cytokines IL-15 and IL-12. **IL-15** is a growth factor for NK cells, and **IL-12** induces **interferon-γ** production in NK cells and enhances their cytolytic activity. Interferon-γ in turn activates macrophages to produce more IL-12 and inhibits growth of viruses in host cells. The activity of NK cells is also enhanced by **IL-2**, produced by helper T cells in adaptive immune response (see Chapter 7), and by **interferon-α** and **interferon-β**, two other types of interferon produced by virus-infected cells.

NK cells, similarly to T cells, also express **CD2** molecule, which binds to CD58 (also called leukocyte function-associated antigen-3, or LFA3), which is expressed on many cells in the body. CD2–CD58 binding stabilizes interaction between killer cells and target cells and enhances the effectiveness of killing. NK cells also have **FcγRIIIa receptors** (CD16), which bind the Fc portion of IgG when complexed with the antigen. This allows NK cells to function as killer cells in the so-called **antibody-dependent cell-mediated cytotoxicity (ADCC)**, which is the killing of target cells coated with the IgG antibody. This type of killing is also sensitive to inhibition by KIRs, which ensure that only unhealthy cells are killed.

Although the recognition mechanisms of target cells by NK cells and cytotoxic T cells are different, the **mechanism of killing** by both cell types is the same. NK cells, similar to cytotoxic T cells, have granules filled with **granzymes** and **perforin** (see Chapter 7). On engagement of the target cells, the content of the granules is released onto the surface of the target cell. In the low Ca^{+2} environment of the granules, perforin is a monomeric protein, but in the presence of high extracellular Ca^{+2}, it aggregates and inserts itself into the membrane of target cells in a manner very similar to the assembly of the MAC of the complement. This destroys the permeability of the membrane and allows granzymes (also released from the granules) to enter the target cells. **Granzymes** are serine proteases that cleave and activate intracellular caspases in target cells, which triggers target cell death by **apoptosis** (programmed cell death).

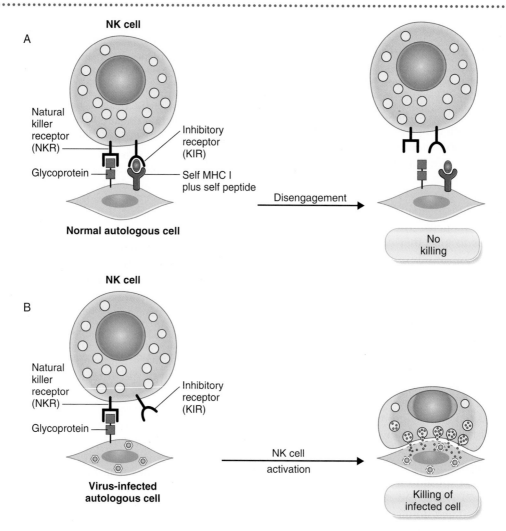

FIGURE 6-8. Function of NK cell killing and inhibitory receptors. Activating receptors (NKRs) on NK cells engage glycoproteins or stress-response proteins on autologous host cells. Inhibitory receptors (e.g., KIRs) engage major histocompatibility complex (MHC) class I–peptide complexes on autologous host cells. **A.** Engagement of inhibitory receptors is dominant and prevents NK cell activation and killing. **B.** If a virus-infected host cell expresses NKR ligands but does not express MHC class I peptide complexes, inhibitory receptors on NK cells are not engaged and binding of activating NKRs to stress-response proteins or glycoproteins on host cells activates NK cells and induces killing of virus-infected cells. This scheme is a simplification because in reality NK cells express multiple stimulatory and inhibitory receptors, and the balance between all stimulatory and inhibitory signals determines whether the NK cells kill the targets.

INITIATION OF ADAPTIVE IMMUNE RESPONSES BY INNATE IMMUNITY

From the examples cited in the previous sections, it is obvious how tightly the functions of the innate and adaptive immune systems are intertwined and how they complement each other and depend on each other for full activity. This section considers another important concept: The innate immune system is required for the initial recognition of antigen and initiation of the adaptive immune response.

The main function of innate immunity is to provide immediate protection against infections and to defend the host and eliminate less severe infections with low-virulence microorganisms. In infections with more pathogenic

microorganisms, that can evade or resist the elimination by the innate immune system, the adaptive immunity must develop to eliminate these infections (adaptive immunity will be discussed in detail in Chapter 7).

Another important function of the innate immune system is to recognize, process, and present antigens to lymphocytes, the cells required to initiate adaptive immune responses. This function is performed by **antigen-presenting cells**, such as **dendritic cells** (e.g., **Langerhans cells** in the skin) and **macrophages**. These cells use pattern recognition receptors, like TLRs (see Table 6-4), to recognize the antigen (the antigen could be the entire microorganism or isolated microbial products). This interaction induces uptake of the antigen by dendritic

TABLE 6-10 Sequence of Events in Initiation of Adaptive Immunity to Extracellular Antigens by Innate Immunity

Sequence of Events

Microbial antigen

↓

Recognition by dendritic cell through pattern recognition receptors (e.g., TLRs)

↓

Uptake of the antigen

↓

Migration of dendritic cells into the lymph nodes and maturation into antigen-presenting cells

↓

Expression of T-cell costimulatory molecules on dendritic cells (B7, also known as CD80/CD86)

↓

Processing of the antigen and loading of antigenic peptides into MHC class II molecules

↓

Presentation of the antigenic peptide–MHC complex to T helper cells

↓

Secretion of T-cell–activating cytokines

↓

Activation, proliferation, and differentiation of antigen-specific T cells

↓

Generation of effector cells specific for the antigen

↓

Elimination of the antigen

MHC, major histocompatibility complex.

cells or macrophages, stimulates them, and induces their migration into the lymph nodes adjacent to the site of infection (Table 6-10). The dendritic cells or macrophages mature into functional antigen-presenting cells. This maturation involves expression of T-cell costimulatory molecules on dendritic cells or macrophages (mainly **B7**, also known as **CD80/CD86**), which are absolutely required for the activation of helper T cells (see Chapter 7).

Antigens that are not recognized by dendritic cells or macrophages through the pattern recognition receptors (and do not stimulate these cells) are unable to induce maturation of these cells and expression of this costimulatory molecule. Such antigens, therefore, are not immunogenic or very poorly immunogenic. This mechanism ensures that the adaptive immune response is triggered by potentially dangerous microbial products recognized by pattern recognition receptors. The dendritic cells process the antigen, digesting the antigen into peptides, loading the peptides into MHC class II molecules, and expressing the MHC class II–peptide complexes on the surface of the antigen-presenting cells. The complexes are then presented to helper T cells that have the T-cell antigen receptor specific for a given combination of the antigenic peptide and MHC class II molecules. This interaction induces activation, proliferation, and differentiation of antigen-specific helper T cells, which are required for the initiation of the adaptive immune response to the antigen. (The entire process of the adaptive immune response will be discussed in more detail in Chapter 7.)

The type of antigen and the way the antigen is recognized and processed by dendritic cells dictates the direction of the adaptive immune response. The example given in Table 6-10 describes the response to an extracellular antigen, which typically would be presented to Th1 cells as an MHC class II–bound peptide. This antigen would also be available to B cells, would be processed by B cells, and would activate Th2 cells, which would then induce B-cell antibody response to this antigen (see Chapter 7).

If the antigen comes from an intracellular pathogen present in a macrophage or dendritic cells but is not readily available as an extracellular antigen to B cells, the antigen would be processed only by the macrophages and dendritic cells (but not by B cells) and would primarily induce Th1 cells (but not Th2 cells). Macrophages and dendritic cells, on contact with the antigen, secrete cytokines that direct maturation of the helper T cells into Th1 cells, Th2 cells, or the third type of helper T cells, Th17 cells. These three types of T helper cells secrete different cytokines and induce different types of responses: Th1 cells induce cell-mediated responses that primarily activate macrophages through interferon-γ, Th2 cells help B cells to differentiate into antibody-secreting plasma cells, and Th17 cells produce IL-17 and IL-22 and induce fibroblasts and epithelial cells in tissues to produce chemokines that induce local inflammation, recruit PMNs, and induce production of antimicrobial peptides (see Chapter 7).

If the antigen is a virus whose proteins are being synthesized by host cells, peptides derived from these viral proteins are delivered to MHC class I molecules, which triggers generation of cytotoxic T cells. Cytotoxic T cells recognize viral antigenic peptides bound to MHC class I molecules (see Chapter 7).

Thus, the way the antigen-presenting cells respond to the antigen, process the antigen, and present the antigen to T cells determines what type of adaptive immune response is induced: Antibody production is induced by extracellular antigens that activate B cells and Th2 cells, Th17 response is induced by extracellular antigens that activate macrophages and dendritic cells to induce differentiation of T cells into Th17 cells, Th1 cell-mediated response is induced by intracellular pathogens delivered to MHC class II molecules, and a cytotoxic T-cell response is induced by intracellular viral antigens delivered to MHC class I molecules.

Another way the innate immune system affects the generation of adaptive immunity is through activation of complement. Activation of complement can enhance adaptive immune responses because B cells have CR2 receptors for the C3b complement split product. Thus, coating an antigen with C3b enhances its delivery to the B cells in the spleen and lymph nodes and enhances B-cell–antigen interaction and B-cell–antibody response to the antigen.

INNATE IMMUNITY AS AN EFFECTOR MECHANISM OF ADAPTIVE IMMUNITY

Some components of the innate immune system are also used as effector mechanisms of adaptive immunity. Cell-mediated responses generate cytokine-secreting Th1 cells, which secrete large amounts of **interferon-γ** (also known as **macrophage-activating factor**, or MAF), whose primary function is to activate macrophages. Activated macrophages become very efficient in killing pathogens, such as *Mycobacterium tuberculosis*, which can normally survive and grow in nonactivated macrophages. Interferon-γ is produced by Th1 cells generated in the adaptive immune response to *Mycobacterium*. Thus, macrophages function as effector cells for the T-cell responses to *Mycobacterium*. Many other examples of close cooperation between the effector mechanisms of innate and adaptive immunity have been already given, such as activation of complement by antibodies, which enhances phagocytosis and induces inflammation, antibody-dependent killing by NK cells, or induction by Th17 cells and local production of PMN-attracting and activating chemokines that enhance elimination of bacteria in tissues. Thus, innate immunity is

indispensable not only for early protection against infections but also for the development of adaptive immune responses and for some of the effector functions of adaptive immunity.

CONCLUSION

It is apparent that innate immunity is *not* a static constitutive defense that has little specificity, handles all microbial invaders in the same way, and is separate from adaptive immunity (as was earlier believed, thus its old name, nonspecific resistance). Innate immunity is a complex and dynamic web of microbial recognition systems that are specific for various microorganisms and swiftly generate various antimicrobial responses precisely tailored to the microbial invader that challenges the host. Moreover, innate immunity is intricately connected with adaptive immunity because it serves as the recognition system for the antigens and is required for efficient initiation of adaptive immune responses. It also often directs which type of adaptive immune response is induced and in some cases serves as the effector mechanism of adaptive immunity.

Suggested Readings

Dunkelberger JR, Song WC. Complement and its role in innate and adaptive immune responses. *Cell Res.* 2010;20:34–50.

Flannagan RS, Cosío G, Grinstein S. Antimicrobial mechanisms of phagocytes and bacterial evasion strategies. *Nat Rev Microbiol.* 2009;7:355–366.

Greer JP, Foerster J, Rodgers GM, et al. Section 3: granulocytes and monocytes. In: *Wintrobe's Clinical Hematology.* 12th ed. Philadelphia, PA: Lippincott Williams & Wilkins; 2008.

Kawai T, Akira S. The roles of TLRs, RLRs and NLRs in pathogen recognition. *Int Immunol.* 2009;21:317–337.

Klempner MS, Malech HL. Phagocytes: normal and abnormal neutrophil host defenses. In: Gorbach SL, Bartlett JG, Blackow NR, eds. *Infectious Diseases.* 3rd ed. Philadelphia, PA: Lippincott, Williams & Wilkins; 2004:14–39.

Kumar V, Abbas AK, Fausto N, et al. *Robbins and Cotran Pathologic Basis of Disease.* 8th ed. Philadelphia, PA: Saunders Elsevier; 2010.

Murphy K, Travers P, Walport M. *Janeway's Immunobiology.* 7th ed. New York: Garland Science; 2008.

Parham P. *The Immune System.* 3rd ed. New York: Garland Science; 2009.

Chapter 7

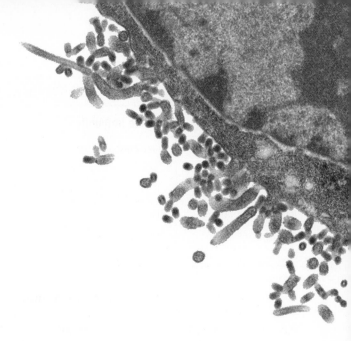

Adaptive Immunity

Carl Waltenbaugh and Roger Melvold

WE LIVE in a world populated by microorganisms with the ever-present potential for microbial attack. Although physical (e.g., skin and membranes) and chemical (e.g., microbicidal molecules secreted by some skin cells) barriers are usually very effective in preventing the entry of microbes into the body, sometimes they are not enough. If these physical and chemical barriers are breached, microbes invade and a "state of war" ensues, the outcome of which may determine our very survival or extinction. The immune system becomes actively involved in resisting and eliminating infection. Humans use two immune systems to combat invasion by infectious organisms: the innate immune system, discussed in Chapter 6, and the adaptive immune system (also known as the acquired immune system). This chapter focuses on the constituents and functions of the adaptive immune system.

INNATE VERSUS ADAPTIVE IMMUNE SYSTEMS

The innate immune system uses a limited number of genetically encoded receptors (e.g., pattern recognition receptors and toll-like receptors) to detect foreign organisms. In contrast, the adaptive immune system employs subsets of an elite set of leukocytes called **lymphocytes**, which have the capacity to generate a large number of antigen-specific cell surface receptors by random gene rearrangement. Bone marrow–derived lymphocytes (**B lymphocytes** or **B cells**) generate **B-cell receptors** (**BCRs**), and thymus-derived lymphocytes (**T lymphocytes** or **T cells**) generate **T-cell receptors** (**TCRs**). Further diversity is added by some degree of flexibility in the precision of the cutting and joining of these genes (**junctional diversity**) and, in the case of BCRs, the accumulation of small mutations (**somatic hypermutation**) as the B cells undergo periods of intense proliferation. The number of possible receptors becomes immense, with estimates exceeding 10^{15} possible specificities.

Another key difference between the two systems is the way they respond to attack. Unlike cells of the innate immune system, those of the adaptive immune system, once stimulated to respond, have the ability to recall previous exposures to the same stimulus and to modify their response accordingly, a process called **memory**. Additional features that distinguish innate and adaptive immune responses are summarized in Table 7-1.

CELLS AND MOLECULES OF THE ADAPTIVE IMMUNE SYSTEM

Cells of the innate immune system are morphologically distinct. In contrast, lymphocytes of the adaptive immune system generally look alike, although they vary in size from small (4 to 7 μm), to medium (7 to 11 μm), to large (11 to 15 μm). Lymphocytes are broadly categorized according the antigen-specific receptors they generate by gene rearrangement and the organs in which they develop. They may be likened to the soldiers of the adaptive immune system, and like soldiers, they often display combinations of additional surface molecules that, in essence, serve as molecular "badges of rank." Some of these badges are useful for identifying a lymphocyte's function and its role in immune defense. Even the most basic appreciation of adaptive immune mechanisms depends on understanding the role that soluble molecules and molecular badges play in immune function. These molecules include **immunoglobulins**, BCRs, TCRs, **cluster of differentiation** (**CD**) molecules, **human leukocyte antigen** (**HLA**) molecules, **cytokines**, and **complement**.

TABLE 7-1 Hallmarks of Innate and Adaptive Immune Responses

	Innate Immunity	Adaptive Immunity
Receptors	Germline encoded	Generated by somatic genetic recombination, junctional diversity, and somatic mutation
Receptor distribution	Expressed by a variety of cell types	Clonally expressed on lymphocytes
Receptor repertoire	Limited	Vast
Memory	None	Both the magnitude and quality of a response to an epitope is altered by previous exposures to that same epitope

Synthesized by B cells, **immunoglobulins** also serve as the BCRs. When activated, some B cells differentiate further into **plasma cells** that produce and secrete large quantities of immunoglobulin. **Immunoglobulin** is a generic term for a diverse group of globular molecules found in the blood and tissue fluids. They include immunoreactive molecules of the gamma (γ) globulin group of serum proteins, so named because they migrate slowly in the γ region of an electrophoretic field. An **antibody** is an immunoglobulin that specifically binds to a known **ligand** or epitope. An **epitope** is the smallest molecular structure recognized by a specific receptor. An **antigen**, such as a microbe, may be viewed as a collection of (sometimes) repeating and/or unique epitopes. For purposes of clarity, the term *immunoglobulin* is used in this chapter in reference to the general structural characteristics of these molecules, and the term *antibody* is used in reference to their functional activities.

T cells also use a set of cell surface receptors, the TCRs, that recognize and bind to antigen but are distinct from antibodies. Other molecules (or "badges") such as **CD3**, **CD4**, and **CD8** associate with and assist the TCRs in antigen recognition. More than 250 cell surface CD molecules serve as useful indicators of the functional capacities of leukocytes and other cells of the body.

HLA molecules are the products of distinct genetic loci within the major histocompatibility complex (MHC), which encodes proteins of three different types called MHC class I, II, or III molecules. Cytokines are protein molecules that act as soluble messengers between cells that affect cell behavior. *Complement* is a collective term for a set of serum proteins involved in both innate and adaptive defense mechanisms. The role of the classical, lectin, and alternative complement pathways in innate immune defenses has already been discussed (Chapter 6).

Immunoglobulins: Structure and Synthesis

The basic structural element for all immunoglobulins is the **immunoglobulin monomer**. It contains four polypeptides: two *identical* light (L) and two *identical* heavy (H) glycoprotein chains linked by disulfide bonds (Fig. 7-1). There are five types of heavy chains, termed α (alpha), δ (delta), ε (epsilon), γ (gamma), and μ (mu), as well as two types of light chains, termed κ (kappa) and λ (lambda). The amino acid sequence of the heavy chain of an immunoglobulin determines the serological **class** or **isotype** of the immunoglobulin molecule. A single immunoglobulin molecule is composed of one or more monomers (Table 7-2).

Heavy and light chains can be further divided into **regions** or **domains**, homologous portions containing approximately 110 amino acids and an intrachain disulfide bond (see Fig. 7-1). Light chains contain two regions, a **variable** (V_L) and a **constant** (C_L) domain. Heavy chains contain a single variable (V_H) and three or four constant (C_H1, C_H2, C_H3, and sometimes C_H4) region domains. Constant regions of the heavy and light chains determine immunoglobulin isotype. Variable regions are so named because they exhibit great variation in amino acid sequence in immunoglobulin molecules produced by various B cells. The amino acid sequence determines the conformation structure of an individual V_H or V_L region. Disulfide bonds link a single heavy chain with a single light chain, and the combination of the V_H and V_L regions forms a pocket that constitutes the epitope-binding region of the immunoglobulin molecule. Disulfide bonds also link the heavy chains to form an immunoglobulin monomer. Following are some landmarks of immunoglobulin monomers (see Fig. 7-1):

- **Fab** (*ab* stands for "antigen binding") fragment is produced by papain cleavage of the monomer and contains only a single epitope-binding site (V_H,C_H1,V_L,C_L).
- **Fc** (*c* stands for "constant" or "crystallizable") fragment is produced by papain cleavage of the monomer to produce a fragment containing C_H2, C_H3, and (for IgA and IgE) C_H4 portions of the heavy chains. Epitope engagement by the epitope-binding site of the intact immunoglobulin monomer causes conformational changes in the Fc region that may trigger a number of biologic activities, including activation of the classical pathway of complement and binding to specific cell surface receptors on neutrophil, lymphocytes, macrophages, and dendritic cells.
- **F(ab′)₂** is produced by **pepsin cleavage** of the immunoglobulin monomer to yield a fragment containing two linked epitope-binding sites.

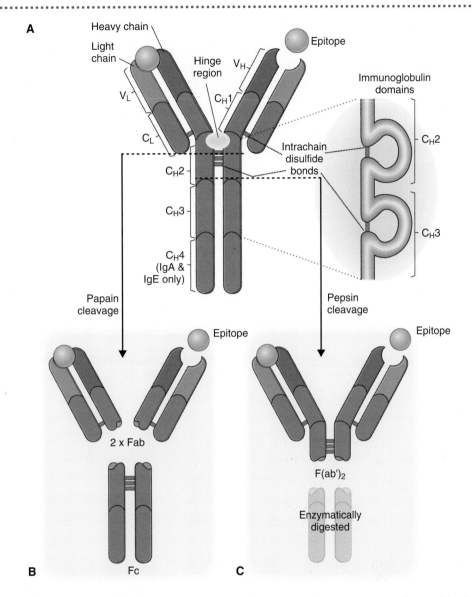

FIGURE 7-1. Immunoglobulin landmarks. A. The immunoglobulin monomer contains two identical heavy and two identical light polypeptide chains. The polypeptides are organized into variable or constant domains, each containing approximately 110 amino acids and an intrachain disulfide bond (see inset). A light chain contains a single variable (V_L) and a single constant (C_L) region domain. Each heavy chain contains a single variable (V_H) and three or four constant region domains (C_H1, C_H2, C_H3 and, for IgA and IgE, C_H4). Disulfide bonds link a single light chain to a single heavy chain and link the heavy chains. Some isotypes are built from two or five monomers to form dimers or pentamers (see Table 7-2). Together, $V_L V_H$ form a combinatorial epitope (or antigen)-binding pocket. **B.** Enzymatic cleavage of the immunoglobulin monomer by papain yields three fragments: two Fab fragments and one Fc fragment. Disulfide bonds link peptides within each fragment. Each Fab fragment is monovalent, containing a single epitope-binding site. **C.** Pepsin cleaves the monomer's heavy chains below the disulfide bonds to create two Fab' fragments (the prime mark ' indicates extra amino acids) linked by disulfide bonds, $F(ab')_2$. The $F(ab')_2$ fragment has valency of two, retaining the two epitope-binding sites of the original immunoglobulin monomer.

- **Hinge region** is a proline-rich region between the C_H1 and C_H2 domains that allows flexibility of the Fab portions of the monomer.

Many other immune and nonimmune-related proteins have been found to share a degree of structural homology with immunoglobulins, including a certain degree of sequence homology and the presence of intrachain disulfide bonds. These proteins are collectively identified as members of the **immunoglobulin supergene family** or **Ig superfamily**.

Immunologists estimate that a typical adaptive immune system in a single individual has the ability to

TABLE 7-2 Immunoglobulin Isotypes

Isotype	Heavy Chains[a]	Heavy Subclass	Associated Chains	Formula[a]	Number of Monomers[b]	Subclass	Valence	MW	Diagram
IgM	μ			2 Hμ[c] 2L	1		2	180,000	T7-2a
			J chain	5 [2 Hμ 2L] + J	5		10	900,000	T7-2b
IgG	γ			2 Hγ 2L	1		2	150,000	T7-2c
		γ_1		2 Hγ_1 2L	1	IgG$_1$	2	150,000	
		γ_2		2 Hγ_2 2L	1	IgG$_2$	2	150,000	
		γ_3		2 Hγ_3 2L	1	IgG$_3$	2	150,000	
		γ_4		2 Hγ_4 2L	1	IgG$_4$	2	150,000	
IgA[d]	α			2 H α 2L	1	IgA	2	170,000	T7-2d
			J chain and SC	2 [2 Hα_1 2L] + J + SC	2	sIgA	4	390,000	T7-2e
IgD	δ	δ		2 Hδ 2L	1		2	180,000	T7-2f
IgE	ε	ε		2 Hε 2L	1		2	190,000	T7-2g

[a]Each monomer contains two identical heavy (H$_{isotype}$) and two identical (κ–κ or λ–λ) light (L) chains.
[b]A single monomer is expressed on the B-cell surface; IgM is secreted as a pentamer by plasma cells.
[c]The carboxyl-terminal portion of the μ chain cytoplasmic tail differs significantly from the μ chain present in the pentameric secreted form of IgM.
[d]IgA is synthesized as a monomer or dimer. Special epithelial cells add SC to the dimer and transfer it to the external surface.
MW, molecular weight; SC, secretory component.

recognize and respond to more than 10^{15} epitopes. Two major theories have been proposed to account for the genetic basis of immune recognition. The **germline theory** holds that a unique gene encodes each immunoglobulin and TCR. This theory is untenable because the number of unique genes would need to be several thousand times greater than the entire human genome. Alternatively, the **somatic mutation theory** states that a single germline gene undergoes multiple mutations to generate diversity. This scheme would require an unimaginable mutation rate. The adaptive immune system has, in fact, developed an elegant solution, **chromosomal**

rearrangement of separate gene segments, which also employs some elements of both the germline and somatic mutation theories.

DNA chromosomal rearrangement is responsible for a significant portion of immunoglobulin diversity. This rearrangement is accomplished by the removal of nucleotides (both at the DNA and RNA levels) to bring together genes that were previously separated. Light- and heavy-chain gene clusters on chromosomes 2 (κ light chains), 22 (λ light chains), and 14 (heavy chains) encode the basic building blocks for this process. For a pre-B cell to generate a light κ or λ chain, 1 of 35 (V_Lκ) or 30 (V_Lλ)

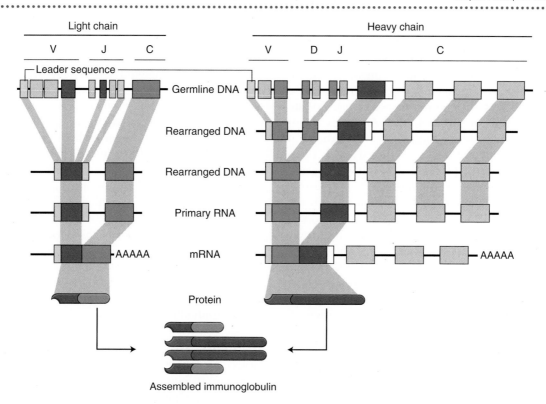

FIGURE 7-2. Immunoglobulins, genes, rearrangement, and synthesis. Immunoglobulin-diverse regions result from DNA chromosomal rearrangement. Light chains are generated by the random selection of 1 of 35 $V_L\kappa$ (30 $V_\kappa\lambda$) and its accompanying leader sequence, 1 of 5 $J_L\kappa$ (4 $J_L\lambda$), and 1 constant ($C_H\kappa$ or $C_H\lambda$) region gene segment. Heavy chains are generated by the random selection of 1 of 45 V_H and its accompanying leader sequence, 1 of 23 D_H, and 1 of 6 J_H gene segments. Rearranged DNA is transcribed into primary RNA, intervening sequences are edited out of messenger RNA (mRNA), and polypeptides are synthesized and assembled within the Golgi apparatus.

variable (V_L) genes recombine with 1 of 4 ($J_L\kappa$) or 5 ($J_L\lambda$) light chain–joining (J_L) segments and a single constant ($C_L\kappa$ or $C_L\lambda$) segment (Fig. 7-2). Thus, κ light chains are a union of three genes ($V_L\kappa J_L\kappa C_L\kappa$), as are λ light chains ($V_L\lambda$-$J_L\lambda$-$C_L\lambda$). Likewise, a pre-B cell must combine 1 of 65 heavy-chain variable (V_H) segments with 1 of 27 diversity (D_H) segments and 1 of 6 joining (J) segments and a single constant region ($C_H\mu$, $C_H\delta$, $C_H\gamma$, $C_H\alpha$, or $C_H\varepsilon$).

A cautionary note on terminology: *Variable genes* refer to the DNA level, one of the types of genes that are rearranged to encode *variable regions* that are part of the immunoglobulin polypeptides. Although both maternal and paternal immunoglobulin alleles are inherited, a single B cell can express only one $V_L J_L C_L$ combination and one $V_H D_H J_H$ combination to the exclusion of all others. The restriction of light- and heavy-chain expression to a single member of the chromosome pair encoding them, either maternal or paternal, is termed **allelic exclusion**. Heavy and light chains may be expressed from both paternal chromosomes, from both maternal chromosomes, or from one each.

Now for the math. Because combinations apparently are generated at random, this process can generate 175 κ-chain variable regions (35 $V_L\kappa \times 5$ $J_L\kappa$) and 120

λ-chain variable regions (30 $V_L\lambda \times 4$ $J_L\lambda$) and amino acid sequences for at least 295 different light-chain variable regions (sum of the κ and λ variable regions). Heavy-chain gene recombination can generate at least 6,210 different heavy-chain variable regions (45 $V_H \times 23$ $D_H \times 6$ J_H). Both the V_L and V_H regions of the immunoglobulin molecule contribute to the epitope-binding site so that 1.8×10^6 ($295 \times 6{,}210$) binding specificities can be generated by recombination alone. Diversity of several orders of magnitude are also added by an enzyme, **terminal deoxyribonucleotidyl transferase (TdT)**, that removes or adds nucleotides between the V, D, and J genes in a process known as **junctional diversity**. The net effect is that junctional diversity greatly increases V region diversity so that at least 10^{10} specificities can be generated. While undergoing rapid proliferation following activation, B cells can also accumulate small mutations in the V, D, and J genes of their light- and heavy-chain genes.

Because of its particular combination of V_L and V_H regions and allelic exclusion, an individual B cell synthesizes immunoglobulin of only a single specificity. Initially, B cells synthesize and display monomeric IgM (and IgD) on their cell surfaces. B cells, however, have the ability to change the immunoglobulin isotype they produce to IgG, IgE, or IgA, a process known as the **isotype switch**, and by doing so influence the ultimate nature of the humoral immune response. Immunoglobulins may be likened to the "ballistic missiles" of the adaptive immune system: their V regions form a specific "warhead," and their constant regions constitute the "rocket" portion of the molecule. Although a single B cell can manufacture a single type of warhead, it can be placed on different rockets. As we will see, often T cells stimulate B cells to proliferate, switch isotype, and differentiate into immunoglobulin-secreting (plasma) cells. The intracellular machinery of the stimulated B cell is such that immunoglobulins of only a single isotype can be produced at a given time. The isotype ultimately determines whether an antibody activates complement, is secreted into a lumen or onto a mucous membrane, or is immobilized by certain tissues of the body. Isotype switching permits the adaptive immune system to direct antibodies with identical specificity toward a variety of immune responses.

The immunoglobulin heavy chains encoded by C_H genes (μ, δ, γ, ε, or α) determine the isotype (IgM, IgD, IgG, IgE, or IgA, respectively) of the immunoglobulin monomer. The nature of the constant region (particularly the Fc region) of the immunoglobulin determines what type of interaction will occur with other cells and molecules of the immune system. Large-sized immunoglobulins (e.g., IgM) are confined to the bloodstream, while those of lower molecular weight (IgG and IgE) can leave the vasculature and enter the tissues. IgG is the only isotype that can cross the placenta and enter the fetal circulation. Maternally derived IgG provides the primary immunologic protection for newborns until their own immune systems become sufficient at about 6 months of age. IgM and IgG can activate the complement system. IgA can dimerize, and specialized secretory epithelial cells can internalize dimeric IgA, transport it across the cell, and release it to the exterior in saliva, tears, breast milk, and mucus secretions. Secreted IgA (sIgA) is extremely important in immunologic functions involving the alimentary and respiratory tracts and can provide some immunologic protection to nursing infants.

T Cell–Associated Molecules

As distinct cell surface antigen-specific receptors, TCRs are members of the immunoglobulin supergene family. The TCR is a heterodimer composed of an $\alpha\beta$ or $\gamma\delta$ polypeptide pair. Similar to immunoglobulin, each membrane-bound polypeptide contains a single variable domain but only a single constant region domain. In addition, an $\alpha\beta$ TCR associates with transmembrane molecules (CD4 or CD8) that stabilize the interaction of the TCR with its ligand and with the CD3 complex responsible for transmembrane signal transduction once the variable region of the TCR is engaged. Unlike antibodies that can readily bind soluble or particulate antigen, TCRs can only bind enzymatically cleaved fragments of larger peptides

presented as peptide–MHC (pMHC) complexes. This is discussed later in the chapter when antigen presentation is considered.

TCRs are generated by gene rearrangement and recombination, in a manner similar to that seen in immunoglobulins, to produce heterodimers consisting either of a smaller α chain and a larger β chain ($\alpha\beta$ TCR) or a smaller γ chain and a larger δ chain ($\gamma\delta$ TCR). The variable regions of the TCR α and δ chains are encoded by uniting V_H and J_H genes. The variable regions of β and δ chains are encoded by uniting V_H, D_H, and J_H genes (Fig. 7-3). The constant region genes (Cα and Cβ or Cγ and Cδ) encode the constant domains for each TCR heterodimer. Junctional diversity, a process mediated by TdT, contributes greatly to the number of possible specificities, similar to that seen for immunoglobulins. However, unlike immunoglobulins, TCRs do not increase their diversity by incorporation of small mutations during T-cell proliferation.

Cell Surface and Soluble Molecules

Molecules encoded by the MHC, also known as HLA, are important to immune function (Table 7-3). Small proteolytic cleavage peptides (p) are loaded by the cell into MHC class I or class II molecules (pMHC class I or class II) for display at the cell surface. The display of pMHC complexes is "scrutinized" by the TCRs.

MHC class I molecules are found on the surfaces of all nucleated cells (Fig. 7-4). These single-chain, 45-kDa glycoproteins are found on the cell surface in association with 12-kDa $\beta2$ microglobulin. Codominantly expressed genes at each of the three MHC class I loci—**HLA-A**, **HLA-B**, and **HLA-C**—are highly polymorphic, with more than 100 possible alleles at each locus. Up to six MHC class I molecules (if all three loci are heterozygous) are displayed on the surface of each nucleated cell. All MHC class I molecules fold to produce a cleft that holds a peptide of eight to nine amino acids in length. Peptides, the fragments resulting from proteasome degradation of cytoplasmic proteins, are transported into the endoplasmic reticulum, where some are loaded into nascent MHC class I molecules. MHC class I molecules, peptides, and $\beta2$ microglobulin are exported via exocytotic vesicles, where they are displayed on the cell surface. This combination of peptide, MHC class I, and $\beta2$ microglobulin is often termed **pMHC class I**. In general, endogenous peptides such as intracellular bacterial or viral proteins synthesized within the cell's cytoplasm are loaded into MHC class I molecules.

MHC class II molecules are $\alpha\beta$ heterodimers (see Fig. 7-4) displayed on the surfaces of a relatively small number of cells: dendritic cells, macrophages, B cells, thymic epithelial cells, and some activated T cells. It needs to be stressed that the use of the terms α and β for MHC class II molecules is distinct from the use of α and β for TCRs, and the two should not be confused with one another. Human MHC class II polypeptides are encoded by genes within the HLA-DP, HLA-DQ,

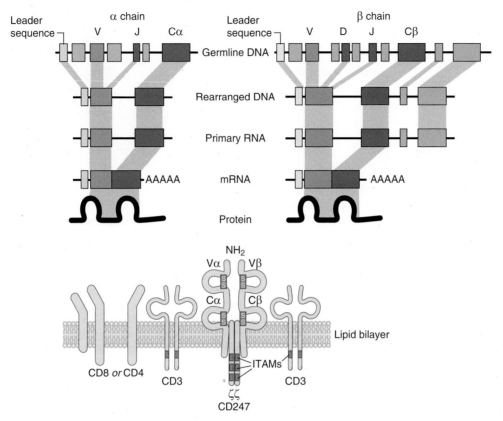

FIGURE 7-3. T-cell receptor (TCR): genes, rearrangement, and synthesis. The α and β poly-peptides of the TCR complex contain a single variable (Vα and Vβ) and a single constant (Cα and Cβ) region. A V region gene segment combines with a joining (J) segment and a C region to be transcribed into mRNA and translated into an α polypeptide chain within the endoplasmic reticulum. Recombination of the β-chain DNA is similar to that of the α chain but also includes a diversity (D) gene segment. The γδ TCR has a similar construction but uses distinct gene sets for the γ and δ chains. The cell surface TCR complex is composed of an αβ heterodimer pair, associated CD3 (γ, δ, and ε) and a CD247 ξ-chain homodimer, and CD4 or CD8 molecules. The short cytoplasmic tail of the TCR lacks signaling sequence or immunoreceptor tyrosine activation motifs. The CD3 and CD247 molecules supply these.

and HLA-DR regions. Contained within each region are α and β loci (DPα, DPβ, DQα, DQβ, etc.). MHC class II polypeptides only associate with other class II peptides encoded within the same region. The combination of α (32 to 38 kDa) and β (29 to 32 kDa) chains forms a peptide-binding grove that can accommodate peptides of 18 to 20 amino acids or more in length (**pMHC class II**). Like MHC class I genes, a large number of allelic forms are known to exist for each locus. Genetic variation among MHC class II molecules, as well as αβ association,

TABLE 7-3 Molecules of the Major Histocompatibility Complex[a]

HLA Class	Nomenclature	Distribution	Functions
I	HLA-A, HLA-B, HLA-C	All nucleated cells	Presentation of intracellularly derived antigens
II[b]	DPα, DPβ, DQα, DQβ, DRα, DRβ1, DRβ2, DRβ4	Dendritic cells, macrophages, B cells, and some activated T cells	Presentation of extracellularly derived antigens
III	C2, C4, Bf	Secreted, not expressed on cell surfaces	Some components of the complement system

[a]Also known as human leukocyte antigen (HLA) molecules.
[b]Class II molecules α and β are encoded by the α and β loci, respectively. Thus, DPA encodes the DPα chain, DPB the DPβ chain, DQA the DQα chain, and so on.
Bf, regulatory factor B.

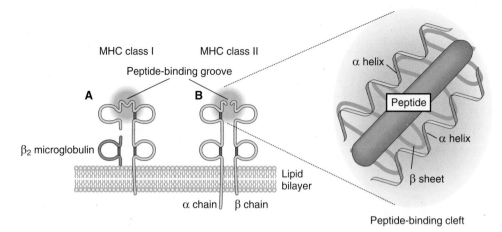

FIGURE 7-4. Hallmarks of major histocompatibility complex (MHC) class I and class II molecules. Molecules of the human MHC are also known as human leukocyte antigens. **A.** MHC class I molecules are single-chain 45-kDa polypeptides displayed on the surfaces of all nucleated cells in association with 12-kDa β2 microglobulin. MHC class I molecules contain three immunoglobulin-like domains, two of which have intrachain disulfide bonds. A peptide-binding cleft is formed between the first and second domains (see insert). **B.** MHC class II molecules are expressed as α and β heterodimers. Each polypeptide contains two immunoglobulin-like domains. The amino terminus portion of each molecule contributes to the peptide-binding portion of the heterodimer (see inset).

creates a wide range of subtly varying binding grooves for which peptides compete. Peptides that load into MHC class II molecules are generally of exogenous origin. Antigens (microbes or their products) present in the extracellular fluid are engulfed (phagocytosis), contained within phagocytic vesicles that fuse with lysosomal vesicles to form phagolysosomes that enzymatically degrade the ingested material to produce peptides that may be loaded into nascent MHC class II molecules.

MHC class III molecules are several components of the complement system—namely, C2, C4, and regulatory factor B (Bf).

Cluster of differentiation molecules populate the surfaces of a wide variety of cell types and serve as indication of the functional capacities of leukocytes and a number of other cells. It is beyond the scope of this book to describe more than just a few of the more than 250 CD molecules that have been so far identified. Fortunately, a basic understanding of the underlying mechanisms of the adaptive immune response requires knowing only a few of these:

- **CD3 complex** contains several molecules associated with the TCR (see Fig. 7-3). It is composed of six polypeptides (2 CD3ε + 1 CD3γ + 1 CD3δ + 1 CD247 ζ–ζ homodimer) that function to both support the TCR and is involved in transmembrane signaling when the TCR is engaged.
- **CD4** is a single-chain member of the immunoglobulin supergene family and is expressed on the surfaces of approximately two-thirds of mature T cells. CD4 molecules recognize a nonpeptide-binding portion of MHC class II molecules. CD4+ T cells, also known as helper

T (Th) cells, are "restricted" to the recognition of pMHC class II complexes.

- **CD8** is a two-chain cell surface molecule composed of homodimers (αα) or heterodimers (αβ) and expressed by about one-third of mature T cells. CD8 molecules recognize the nonpeptide-binding portion of MHC class I molecules. CD8+ T cells, "restricted" to the recognition of pMHC class I complexes, are also known as cytotoxic T (Tc) and suppressor T (Ts) cells.

Mature αβ T cells express CD4 or CD8 cell surface molecules; CD4 associates only with MHC class II, and CD8 only with class I. A useful mnemonic to remember these restricted associations is the **rule of eight**:

$$CD4 \times MHC\ class\ II = "4" \times "2" = 8$$

and

$$CD8 \times MHC\ class\ I = "8" \times "1" = 8$$

T cells of the γδ lineage often express neither CD4 nor CD8, and their restriction, if any, is unclear.

Cytokines are chemical messengers. Involved in all aspects of innate and adaptive immune responses, cytokines are low-molecular-weight soluble molecules that function to initiate growth, differentiation, and maturation of cells and to promote or inhibit inflammation and tissue repair. Originally termed lymphokines and monokines to reflect their production by lymphocytes or monocytes, it is now recognized that these same substances may be produced by a wide variety of leukocytes and nonleukocytes. Chemoattractant cytokines known as **chemokines** stimulate leukocyte movement and migration. Whether or not certain cytokines or chemokines are expressed on microbial encounter strongly influences the nature and strength of the immune response.

Various cell surface molecules, called **adhesion molecules**, provide stable cell-to-cell contact. Because the immune system polices the body for invaders, adhesion molecules establish a temporary, yet stable, contact that allows leukocytes to scrutinize other cells, leukocytes and nonleukocytes alike. Stable contact for a period between cells, provided by adhesion molecules, is critical to the ability of cell surface receptors and ligands to interact. They are classified as widely distributed **integrins** that initiate adhesion interactions and **selectins** and **addressins** that have a limited leukocyte distribution and function to activate leukocytes and facilitate leukocyte migration.

LYMPHOCYTE DEVELOPMENT AND RECEPTOR SELECTION

The immune system must be able to distinguish its own molecules, cells, and organs (**self**) from those of foreign origin (**nonself**). The innate immune system does this elegantly by expressing germline-encoded pattern recognition receptors on cell surfaces, receptors that have been selected over time to recognize structures on potentially invasive organisms (see Chapter 6). The adaptive immune system, on the other hand, uses antigen-specific receptors (TCRs and BCRs) that are somatically created anew and randomly within each individual (indeed, within each lymphocyte) by gene recombination *prior to* encounter with an antigen. This also means that no two individuals, even identical twins, have identical adaptive immune systems. Three distinct categories of receptors are randomly generated: those that recognize peptide epitopes that will never be encountered, those that recognize peptides produced by potential pathogens or peptides of nonself origin, and those that recognize peptides produced by the self. Recognition of self peptides by the immune system could lead to a "coup," with the immune system attacking the very body it is intended to protect and defend. Fortunately, the adaptive immune system has developed an elegant solution against this threat, and it occurs within the thymus where self- and nonself-recognizing TCRs are sorted out.

T Cells

T-cell precursors originate in the hematopoietic tissues of bone marrow from which they migrate by the circulation to the thymus. These thymocytes, as they are now called, do not express a TCR, nor do they express either CD4 or CD8 molecules; thus, they are called **double-negative (DN) cells**. DN cells proliferate in the thymic subcapsular region, where most differentiate and express low levels of newly generated αβ TCR and *both* CD4 and CD8 molecules, and are termed **double-positive (DP)** cells. Some cells develop γδ TCRs and may or may not express CD4

and CD8 molecules. Thymocytes that generate a γδ TCR appear to exit from the thymus early, before undergoing any selection. Their functions are not fully understood. On the other hand, the αβ DP cells migrate deeper within the thymus, fated to die within 3 to 4 days unless their TCRs recognize an MHC class I or class II molecule on thymic dendritic cells, a process known as **positive selection**. Thymocytes that generate γδ TCRs appear to exit from the thymus early, before undergoing this selection.

Although the mechanism of positive selection is not fully understood, it is known that partial recognition of MHC class I by CD8 molecules or MHC class II by CD4 molecules must occur. Cells that "pass muster" and recognize self MHC molecules will survive, and those that do not will die. A DP thymocyte that engages MHC class I may become a CD8+ T cell, and one that recognizes MHC class II may become a CD4+ T cell. Because MHC class I and class II molecules are not displayed on cell surfaces unless their binding cleft contains a peptide (pMHC), only peptides of self origin are seen by the DP thymocytes. Thymocytes that show strong interaction with self pMHC complexes are selectively induced to undergo programmed cell death or apoptosis, a process known as **negative selection**. Thymocytes that survive both positive and negative selection migrate from the thymus as T cells and are destined to populate the lymphoid tissues and organs.

The thymus is a tough training academy: less than 2% of all thymocytes are estimated to "graduate" as T cells. By applying both positive and negative selection of thymocytes, the adaptive immune system is assured of a population of naive T cells that will react with nonself peptides presented by self MHC molecules and in which T cells reactive to self peptides have largely been eliminated.

B Cells

Only B cells and plasma cells synthesize immunoglobulins. Arising from pluripotent hematopoietic stem cells in the fetal liver and bone marrow, B cells are divided into two distinct lineages, B-1 and B-2 cells. They do not migrate to the thymus but remain in the bone marrow during development.

Because they are the first to embryologically develop, B-1 cells are a self-renewing population that predominate the plural and peritoneal cavities. Although the function of B-1 cells is not fully understood, as a population they constitutively secrete IgM antibodies of limited diversity that react strongly with carbohydrates. A large portion of serum IgM in normal individuals is of B-1 origin and is often referred to as "natural antibody." As a cellular class, B-1 cells may bridge innate and adaptive immunity by producing antibodies that react with carbohydrates expressed by infectious organisms.

In contrast, conventional or B-2 cells arise during and after the neonatal period, are continuously replaced from the bone marrow, and are widely distributed throughout

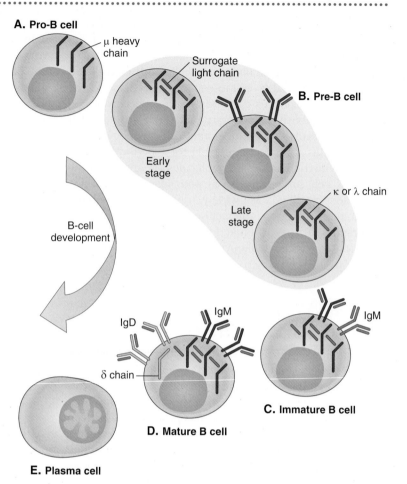

FIGURE 7-5. B-cell developmental stages. The stages of B-cell development reflect changes in gene activity within the cell and its ability to synthesize, display, and secrete immunoglobulin. **A.** A pro-B cell synthesizes μ heavy chains; this polypeptide is confined within the cell. **B.** Pre-B cells are the next developmental stage (shaded), beginning with an early stage in which μ and surrogate light chains are synthesized and the μ-surrogate light chain monomer may be displayed on the cell surface. The final pre-B cell stage occurs when κ or λ light chains replace surrogate light chains. **C.** Immature B cells synthesize and display IgM monomers on their cell surfaces. **D.** Each mature B cell displays both IgM and IgD of *identical specificity* on its cell surface. **E.** Plasma cells represent the end stage of differentiation of B-lineage cells and function as "factories," synthesizing and secreting large amounts of immunoglobulin.

the lymphoid organs and tissues. Somatic gene rearrangements are more extensive in B-2 cells than in B-1 cells, giving them a broader repertoire of immunoglobulin specificities and affinities. Unstimulated B-2 cells, unlike B-1 cells, produce low levels of immunoglobulins that increase only when they are activated by helper T cells that cause them to differentiate into antibody-secreting cells. B-2 pathway-committed cell precursors graduate though several levels that involve changes in gene activity (Fig. 7-5):

- *Pro-B cells use enzymes encoded by recombination activation genes, Rag-1 and Rag-2.* Rag-1 and Rag-2 are responsible for chromosomal rearrangement of V, D, and J genes to form the V_H domain. Following union with the μ heavy-chain gene, the cytoplasmically confined immunoglobulin μ heavy chain is synthesized.
- *Early-stage pre-B cells synthesize a transitional or surrogate non-κ, non-λ light chain.* The surrogate light chain associates with the μ heavy chain to form a monomer-like structure that decorates the surface of the cell. **Late-stage pre-B cells** synthesize κ or λ light chains that replace the surrogate light chain, and the cell expresses true IgM monomers.
- *Immature, or naive, B cells are so called because their BCRs (IgM monomers) have not engaged the appropriate epitope.* If the BCR of a naive B cell engages an

epitope within the bone marrow environment, the cell is destroyed by apoptosis. Surviving cells exit the bone marrow and enter the circulation. On leaving the bone marrow, the naive B cells are fated to have a short half-life unless they receive additional signals from lymph node stromal cells that allow them to further develop. Within the lymph node, B cells begin to synthesize both δ heavy chains and μ heavy chains and display both IgD and IgM monomers with identical specificity on their cell surface.

- *Mature B cells coexpress IgM and IgD cell surface monomers.* Activation for the vast majority of mature B-2 cells requires both epitope binding and T-cell interaction for further differentiation.
- *Plasma cells are derived from differentiated mature B cells and secrete immunoglobulin.* All the immunoglobulin secreted is exported, and the cells cease using it as a membrane receptor. Plasma cells can be viewed as "munitions factories," producing large quantities of immunoglobulin during their short lifespan of less than 30 days.

LYMPHOCYTE ACTIVATION

Unlike the innate immune system, the adaptive immune system recognizes epitopes using a very diverse array of randomly generated TCRs and BCRs. Because of the initial paucity of lymphocytes bearing the appropriate epitope-specific TCR or BCR, epitope-specific lymphocytes must clonally proliferate to make enough cells and cell products to deal with a perceived threat. Consequently, adaptive immune responses develop slowly compared with responses of the innate system. In the process of randomly generating receptors, the adaptive immune system can make receptors that recognize nonpathogens or receptors that recognize self molecules. A system of checks and balances minimizes the potential for adverse immune responses that rely on different cell types for recognition, regulation, and effector function. T cells play a central role as arbiters of immune function; therefore, the manner in which T cells recognize and are activated by epitopes is highly regulated.

Cells of the innate immune system are the gatekeepers of the adaptive immune response. In large part, adaptive immune responses are initiated by components of the innate system resulting in T-cell activation and clonal expansion. Effector responses of the adaptive immune system often end by activating and focusing the cells and/or molecules of the innate system on targets selected by lymphocytes.

Self-Recognition

"Who are you, friend or foe?" A simple question, you would think, but one that is critical to our survival in the microbial world in which we live. The body must be able to distinguish self molecules and cells from those of nonself or foreign origin. This is not a problem for the innate immune system, in which genomically encoded pattern recognition receptors have been selected over evolutionary time to recognize a limited number of epitopes widely expressed by microbes but not by cells of the body. For the adaptive immune system, it is another matter altogether. In large part, self-reactive TCRs fail to "graduate" from the thymus (occasional self-reactive T cells "slip by" to become autoreactive). However, this only begs the question, "How do you recognize an epitope that you have never seen?" Enormous numbers of TCRs and BCRs are generated in anticipation that at least some of them will be specific for an epitope of nonself origin. But the peril with this approach is that without some means of identification, molecules of self origin that were not seen during lymphocyte development could possibly trigger a response. The adaptive immune system's solution is elegant. This is also where the innate and adaptive immune systems interact. Phagocytic cells, such as dendritic cells and macrophages, sample their environment by phagocytosis and pinocytosis, proteolytically degrade what they find, and load the peptide fragments into MHC class I (forming pMHC class I) or MHC class II (forming pMHC class II) molecules in a process that immunologists call **antigen presentation**.

Antigen Presentation

Specialized cells located at potential microbial portals of entry into the body (e.g., skin and mucous membranes)

serve as sentinels. These are **dendritic cells** named for their elongated, branchlike projections and comprise less than 1% of the cells in these tissues. Known at this stage as immature dendritic cells, they are voracious eaters, ingesting large amounts of soluble and particulate matter by phagocytosis or macropinocytosis. **Phagocytosis** involves the engagement of cell surface receptors (e.g., Fc receptors, heat shock proteins, and low-density lipoprotein-binding scavenger receptors; see Chapter 6) associated with specialized regions of the plasma membrane called **clathrin-coated pits**. Receptor engagement induces actin-dependent phagocytosis and receptor internalization to form small **phagosomes** or endocytic vesicles.

Immature dendritic cells also sample large amounts of soluble molecules present in the extracellular fluids by **macropinocytosis**, a process in which cytoplasmic projections (**cytoplasmic ruffles**) encircle and enclose extracellular fluids to form endocytotic vesicles. Macropinocytosis does not require clathrin-associated receptor engagement. Enzyme-containing cytoplasmic vesicles (**lysosomes**) fuse with the endocytic vesicles derived from phagocytosis or macropinocytosis (Fig. 7-6). Within this newly formed **phagolysosome**, ingested material is enzymatically degraded into short peptides. For the most part, the process of ingestion and enzymatic degradation has little consequence immunologically, but that can rapidly change.

If an immature dendritic cell senses an invasive threat, it begins to mature, and maturation comes rapidly. Dendritic cells detect threats either directly or indirectly through the same cell surface receptors used by the innate immune system. **Direct sensing** occurs through engagement of pattern recognition receptors, which recognize **pathogen-associated molecular patterns** (**PAMPs**) on viruses, bacteria, fungi, and protozoa (see Chapter 6). Engagement of other receptors (e.g., those that detect antibodies or complement molecules bound to microbes) are responsible for **indirect sensing** of perceived threats. Although the physiological mechanisms for dendritic cell maturation remain to be clarified, threat sensing is known to cause the dendritic cells to migrate to nearby lymph nodes, decrease their phagocytic and macropinocytic activity, and upregulate MHC class II synthetic activity. MHC class II α and β polypeptides, together with an invariant chain, are assembled as a complex within the endoplasmic reticulum. Vesicles bud off from the endoplasmic reticulum to fuse with the peptide-containing, acidic phagolysosomes. The invariant chain disintegrates in the acidic environment of the newly formed vesicle, allowing phagolysosome-derived peptides to possibly occupy the peptide-binding groove of the MHC class II molecule. The pMHC class II complex is transported to the cell surface for display and possible recognition by CD4+ T cells.

Not all pathogens enter cells through phagocytosis or macropinocytosis. Some avoid phagocytes and endocytic vesicles entirely and directly enter the cytoplasm of the host cell (see Fig. 7-6). As part of normal physiological

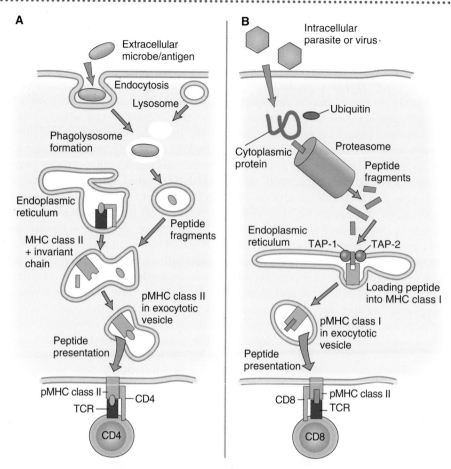

FIGURE 7-6. Antigen presentation pathways. The manner by which a microbe or its products enter an antigen-presenting cell (APC) strongly influences the nature of the immune response. **A.** APCs capture microbes or their products from the extracellular environment by phagocytosis or macropinocytosis and contain them within endocytic vesicles (phagosomes). Phagosomes fuse with enzyme-laden lysosomes to form a phagolysosome for degradation of the microbial material into proteolytic fragments. Vesicles containing the MHC class II–invariant chain complex bud off from the endoplasmic reticulum to fuse with the peptide-containing phagolysosome. The invariant chain disintegrates within the acidic environment, allowing the peptide to load into the vacated peptide-binding groove of the MHC class II molecule. Exocytotic vesicles containing peptide-loaded MHC (pMHC) class II are transported to the cell surface for display and recognition by the TCRs of CD4+ T cells. **B.** Some microbes avoid endocytic vesicles altogether to enter the cytoplasm. Ubiquitin covalently attaches to many of these proteins, marking them for enzymatic degradation by the proteasome. Proteolytic peptide fragments are transported into the endoplasmic reticulum by a heterodimer composed of transporters associated with antigen processing (TAP-1 or TAP-2) for possible loading into nascent MHC class I complexes. Exocytotic vesicles containing pMHC class I are transported to the cell surface for display and recognition by the TCRs of CD8+ T cells.

processes, nucleated cells constantly degrade and recycle cytoplasmic proteins. Cytoplasmic proteins targeted for destruction are covalently tagged with **ubiquitin**, a highly conserved protein with 76 amino acids. The underlying mechanisms for selecting molecules for ubiquitination are not known. The binding of one or more ubiquitin molecules to a protein targets it for destruction by the **proteasome**, a large proteolytic complex with the cytoplasm. Postproteasome peptides of 6 to 24 amino acids are transported to the endoplasmic reticulum by a heterodimer, composed of **transporter associated with antigen processing** (**TAP-1** and **TAP-2**). The TAP heterodimers allow peptides to enter the endoplasmic reticulum and be loaded into MHC class I (pMHC class I). Special transport exocytotic vesicles containing pMHC class I molecules bud from the Golgi and are rapidly transported to the cell surface for display to CD8+ T cells.

T-Cell Activation

T cells largely direct the adaptive immune response. Unlike receptors within the innate immune system, TCRs cannot recognize soluble molecules. The nature of the adaptive immune response is strongly influenced by how epitopes are presented by antigen-presenting cells (APCs). The interface between an APC and a naive T cell is called the **immunologic synapse**.

The initial step in building the immunologic synapse occurs when the TCR recognizes pMHC. The weak interaction of the TCR with pMHC is stabilized by the interaction of CD4 or CD8 molecules. CD4 and CD8 molecules bind to the "constant" nonpeptide-binding portions of pMHC class II and class I, respectively (remember the **rule of eight**). Formation of the pMHC–TCR–CD4 (or CD8) complex provides an initial or first signal through the TCR-associated CD3 complex to the T cell. This first signal is necessary, but not sufficient, to stimulate a naive T cell to proliferate and differentiate. A second signal provided by one or more **costimulatory molecules** is required for T-cell activation. The first and second signals initiate intracellular signaling cascades that cause the activation of one or more transcription factors leading to specific gene transcription. Without costimulation, T cells either become selectively unresponsive, a condition known as **anergy**, or undergo apoptosis.

The immunologic synapse both stabilizes T cell–APC interaction and promotes the migration of molecules within the T-cell membrane. The cytoplasmic tails of certain of those molecules contain **immunoreceptor tyrosine–based activation motifs** (ITAMs), which initiate a signaling cascade on close proximity. The CD3 (2 CD3ε + 1 CD3γ + 1 CD3δ + 1 CD247 ζ–ζ homodimer) complex contains ITAM-bearing molecules. The cytoplasmic tails of the TCR lack ITAMs. TCR engagement leads to signal transduction through the CD3 complex, and the activation of transcriptional factors leads to cytokine synthesis, T-cell proliferation, and differentiation. The nature of the immune response largely depends on the manner in which the APCs initiate the immunologic synapse.

The initial encounter of T cells with antigen is called **priming**, and the nature of this encounter is crucial to the development of the subsequent adaptive immune response. As shown earlier, CD8+ T cells interact with pMHC class I, and CD4+ T cells recognize pMHC class II. Primed CD4+ T cells are called **T helper** cells because they are instrumental in "helping" other leukocytes respond (Fig. 7-7). CD4+ Th cells can mature along one of two pathways. In one developmental pathway, CD4+ T cells generally respond to intracellular pathogens by recruiting and activating phagocytic cells. These T cells are known as **Th1 cells**. To avoid detection by cells of the adaptive immune response, some pathogens circumvent phagolysosomes either by directly entering the cytoplasm (e.g., viruses) or by exiting the phagolysosome before they can be enzymatically harmed (e.g., *Listeria monocytogenes*). But the microbial ruse is not perfect, because some infected cells die, prompting dendritic cells to scavenge their cellular debris and display the proteolytic peptides, including those derived from microbes. T cells that develop along the other pathway are known as **Th2 cells**, and they generally

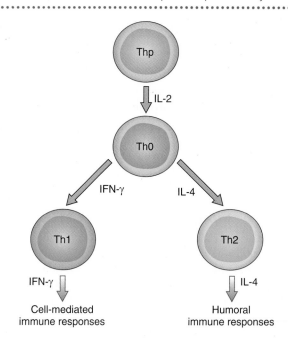

FIGURE 7-7. Th1 and Th2 maturational pathways. Initial epitope engagement through the immunologic synapse induces naive CD4+ T cells to undergo several rounds of proliferation, resulting in their maturation into pathway-uncommitted Th0 cells. Cytokine and costimulatory signals from antigen-presenting and other cells determine whether Th0 cells will differentiate along a Th1 or Th2 pathway. In the presence of interleukin-12 (IL-12), Th0 will differentiate into interferon-γ-secreting Th1 cells. Th1 cells are mediators of cell-mediated immune responses. If Th0 cells initially encounter IL-4, they will differentiate into Th2 cells and secrete IL-4, which mediates B-cell differentiation, isotype switching, and transformation into plasma cells. Animal models show polarization of Th1 and Th2 cytokine secretion and cellular function. Human Th1 and Th2 cells show cytokine polarization, but the degree of polarization of Th1–Th2 function is less dramatic.

respond to extracellular pathogens by stimulating B cells to differentiate into antibody-secreting plasma cells.

Antigen naive CD4+ **Th precursor (Thp) cells**, on activation by engagement of an epitope through the immunologic synapse, are stimulated to secrete a variety of cytokines and express cell surface cytokine receptors, thus becoming pathway-uncommitted **Th0 cells**. The developmental pathway that the Th0 cell follows depends primarily on the nature of signals provided by the APC. In the presence of microbe-derived lipopolysaccharide, the APC may secrete interleukin-12 (IL-12). Consequently, Th0 causes cells to further differentiate into Th1 cells, of which some actively secrete cytokines such as interferon-γ (IFN-γ) and others increase leukocyte recruitment and activation. In some cases, the presence of IL-4 may lead Th0 to follow the Th2 differentiation pathway. Among the functional roles of Th2 cells is the production of cytokines responsible for the growth and stimulation of B cells as well as their differentiation into plasma cells.

As noted, some pathogens, such as viruses, avoid contact with endocytic vesicles entirely by directly entering and replicating within the host cell cytoplasm. Naive CD8+ T cells recognize pMHC class I (first signal) displayed on the surface of an infected cell. On encountering an appropriate pMHC class I on an infected cell, CD8+ cells proliferate and differentiate into cytolytic effector cells called **cytotoxic T lymphocytes (CTLs)**. Fully differentiated CTLs contain two types of cytolytic granules, **perforin** (a pore-forming protein) and **granzymes** (serine proteases), which are used to deliver a fatal blow to a cell expressing the appropriate pMHC class I complex.

B-Cell Activation

In contrast to TCRs, BCRs recognize and bind soluble molecules. The BCR complex of mature B cells contains membrane-bound IgM and IgD monomers associated with Igα and Igβ molecules (Fig. 7-8). Similar to CD3 complex, the cytoplasmic tails of Igα and Igβ molecules contain ITAM motifs. Cross-linking of BCRs leads to the initiation of the downstream intracellular signaling cascade. Because all the immunoglobulins on a given B cell have the same specificity, an antigen must contain multiple identical epitopes for cross-linking to occur. A microbe

may bind to a BCR, but additional copies of that epitope may not be present. B cells use a fail-safe mechanism that requires signaling by both the BCR and a C3b complement receptor. Engagement of the C3b receptor serves as a second signal for B-cell activation.

BCR binding initiates endocytosis, enzymatic degradation, and subsequent display of peptide fragments as pMHC class II complexes. In addition, the B cell expresses costimulatory molecules, thus allowing the B cell to function as an APC for TCR recognition by a CD4+ T cell. T–B cell communication is necessary for the B cell will gear up its cellular machinery for the production of antibodies. T-cell signaling induces the B cell to proliferate, differentiate, and in the presence of additional T-cell–derived cytokines (such as IL-4), differentiate into an antibody-secreting plasma cell.

FUNCTIONS OF THE ADAPTIVE IMMUNE SYSTEM

Not only must the adaptive immune system recognize invasive organisms or their products as nonself, but also it is critically important for host survival that action be taken to minimize the microbial threat. As in any state

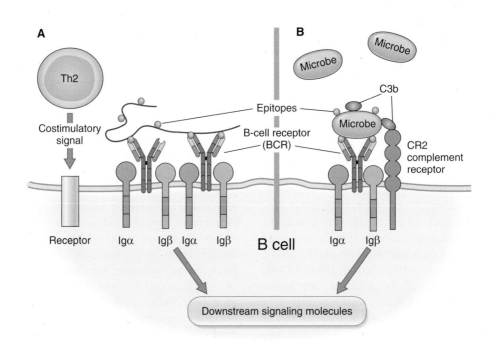

FIGURE 7-8. B-cell activation. B cells recognize soluble or cell-bound epitopes through their B-cell receptors (BCRs) without antigen presentation. **A.** Multiple epitopes on an antigen engage and cross-link several BCRs. Immunoreceptor tyrosine–based activation motifs present on BCR-associated molecules Igα and Igβ phosphorylate and provide a first signal to the B cell. A second (cytokine) signal is provided by a CD4+ Th2 cell that, together with the first signal, begins a downstream signaling cascade that leads to B-cell activation. **B.** Microbes recognized by the innate immune system may also trigger B-cell activation. Activated fragments of the third component of complement (C3b) bind to a microbe. Bound C3b fragments are themselves bound by a CR2 complement receptor on the surface of the B cell to provide a first signal. Binding of microbe epitopes by the BCR provides a second signal through the Igα and Igβ BCR-associated molecules. Both signals combine to initiate a downstream signaling cascade leading to B-cell activation.

of war, it is important first and foremost to prevent the enemy from spreading. The innate immune system does this by surrounding, phagocytizing, and enzymatically degrading or otherwise preventing the spread of would-be invaders throughout the body. Two arms of the adaptive immune system also are dedicated to preventing microbial dissemination.

One arm is called the **humoral immune response**, named for the fluids or humors of the body that prevent or defend against microbial attack. Humoral responses can be likened to the arrows or missiles of the immune system. Locally produced by B cells and plasma cells, they may travel great distances to reach their target epitopes. Antibodies recognize and bind to microbial epitopes to prevent microbial spread by immobilization (**agglutination**), prevention of microbial attachment to host cells (**neutralization**), promotion of microbial phagocytosis and clearance (**opsonization**), and targeting of microbial destruction by soluble molecules (**complement**) or by leukocytes (**antibody-dependent cell-mediated cytotoxicity [ADCC]**).

The other arm of the adaptive immune response is called **cell-mediated immunity**. Like hand-to-hand combat, leukocytes encounter invaders "face-to-face" to destroy invading cells. Cell-mediated adaptive immune responses are controlled and regulated by T cells either to directly cause the destruction of invading CTLs or to direct other leukocytes to perform the deed; the latter action is called delayed-type hypersensitivity (DTH).

Humoral Immunity

Humoral immunity is based on the actions of two sets of soluble molecules, antibodies and complement. Although the production of both depends on cellular activity, it is the binding of these soluble molecules that initiates the humoral immune responses of the adaptive immune system. One response, neutralization, is a direct result of the binding by antibodies, while the other responses—opsonization, complement activation (more specifically, the classical pathway of complement activation), and ADCC—involve the use of antibodies to "tag" cells or molecules for destruction by other elements of the immune system.

Antibody–Antigen Reactions

Antigen–antibody (Ag-Ab) interactions are some of the most specific noncovalent biochemical reactions known and can be represented by the following simple formula:

$$Ag + Ab \rightleftarrows AgAb$$

Although the reaction is driven to the right, notice that **antigen–antibody interactions are reversible**. The strength of interaction (i.e., how far the reaction is driven to the right) is termed its **affinity**. Immunoglobulin populations within an individual show a wide range of affinity. **Valence** (the number of epitope-binding sites on an immunoglobulin molecule) varies from 2 for monomeric

forms of all isotypes, to 4 for secretory IgA, to 10 for pentameric IgM. The term **avidity** is often used to describe the collective affinity of multiple binding sites on an antibody molecule.

The **precipitin reaction** is the term applied to the interaction of soluble antigen with soluble antibody, resulting in a precipitate. Although discovered in the late 19th century, it was not until the 1930s that scientists were able to quantify the amount of antibody present in serum using this reaction. Understanding antigen–antibody reactions requires an understanding of the **quantitative precipitin reaction**.

In the classical series of experiments by Heidelberger and Kendall, rabbits were immunized with capsular polysaccharide (antigen) from *Streptococcus pneumoniae*. Several weeks later, the sera from the immunized rabbits were prepared and used as the antibody source (antisera). Known amounts of antigen (in a constant volume) were mixed with an equal, constant volume of antiserum and incubated (Fig. 7-9). Precipitate formed in several tubes and was separated (by centrifugation) from the supernatant, and the amount of total nitrogen in the precipitate was determined. In these experiments, a polysaccharide antigen was used, and because the antigen did not contain nitrogen, any nitrogen detected had to originate from the antibody (i.e., protein). This experiment demonstrated that an **antibody is a protein** and that antigens and antibodies react in a **predictable** manner. The degree of antigen–antibody cross-linking results in lattice formation and can be used to describe the three distinct zones of the quantitative precipitin curve:

- **Zone of antigen excess**: The antigen–antibody complexes are too small to precipitate. The net result is the formation of soluble complexes.
- **Equivalence zone**: Optimal precipitation occurs in this area of the curve. Large, visible precipitating complexes are formed. It is this property, the formation of a visible precipitate, that is the basis for many immunologically based diagnostic tests.
- **Zone of antibody excess**: Not enough antigen is present to form a precipitate. The net result is formation of soluble complexes.

The principles of the quantitative precipitin curve apply to all antigen–antibody reactions and form the basis for many modern clinical diagnostic tests.

Agglutination

Antibodies can also bind to and cross-link cells or particles, causing an aggregate formation in a reaction known as **agglutination**. Agglutination has the effect of throwing a molecular net over microbial invaders, greatly hindering their mobility and spread throughout the body before they encounter the tissue, cells, and fluids of the body (Fig. 7-10A). Antibodies of the IgM and IgA isotypes are particularly adept at this because they contain 10 and 4 binding sites, respectively; but sufficient concentrations

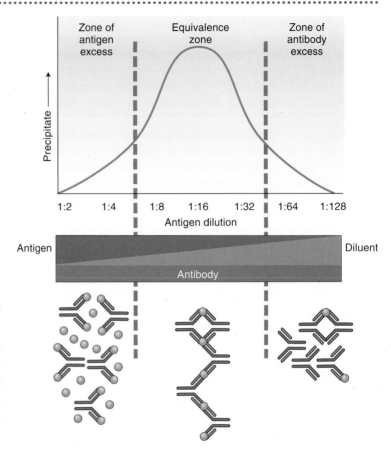

FIGURE 7-9. Quantitative precipitin curve. Antigen composed of multiple epitopes (*green* spheres) is diluted in a mild salt solution (diluent) in a test tube and expressed as a ratio (1:2, 1:4, 1:8, etc.). Identical amounts of antibody are added to each test tube. After a brief incubation period, precipitation is seen in some of the tubes. Optimal precipitation (equivalence zone) occurs when antigen and antibody react to form large latticelike complexes. Much smaller complexes, too small to precipitate, are formed where there is a relative abundance of antigen to antibody (zone of antigen excess) or a relative abundance of antibody to antigen (zone of antibody excess).

of IgG isotype antibodies will also agglutinate particles. Antibodies can also agglutinate nonmicrobial cells, as demonstrated by the agglutination seen when antibodies are used for ABO typing of erythrocytes.

Neutralization

Neutralization describes the process of antibodies binding to microbial epitopes or soluble molecules (e.g., toxins) in a manner that inhibits the ability of the microbes or molecules to bind to host cell surfaces. Many microbes and all viruses inflict damage when they bind to host cell surfaces to facilitate entry. Likewise, most toxin molecules bind to host cell surface structures before entry and exertion of their toxic effects. In both cases, the binding to host cell surfaces is specific. The binding structures on the microbe or toxin are shaped to fit together with specific host cell surface structures. For example, rhinoviruses (the common cold viruses) bind to the intracellular adhesion molecule 1 found on the surfaces of respiratory epithelium.

Antibodies generated against the microbes (or toxins) often include some that can bind and block the microbial structures that interact with the host cell surface, effectively preventing the microbe (or toxin) from entering the cell (see Fig. 7-10B). This form of immunoglobulin-mediated protection is called neutralization because it neutralizes the infective capacity of the invader. Neutralizing antibodies are usually of the IgG

and IgA isotypes. It is the presence of neutralizing antibodies generated during the initial infection that provides the greatest protection against subsequent reinfection by the same organism.

Opsonization

Sometimes, the binding of an antibody (usually IgG) to a microbial surface is enough to "whet the appetite" of a phagocyte, making the microbe an attractive "meal." In essence, antibodies bind to structures and mark them for subsequent destruction by phagocytic cells. Phagocytic cells such as macrophages, dendritic cells, and neutrophils bear surface receptors (FcRs) for the Fc portion of immunoglobulin. By binding an epitope, an antibody molecule makes several conformational changes that include changes in the Fc region (see Fig. 7-1). The FcRs on phagocytic cells recognize and bind conformationally changed Fcs but not immunoglobulins that have not bound an epitope. The binding of a microbe-associated epitope–antibody complex by the FcRs tethers the bound invader to the phagocytic cell and stimulates it to engulf and destroy the microbe (see Fig. 7-10C). In fact, initial microbe binding and engulfment stimulates the phagocytic cell to increase its search for other such "tagged" microbes. The immunoglobulin serves as an **opsonin** (an agent that stimulates phagocytosis), and the increased phagocytic activity that ensues is termed **opsonization**.

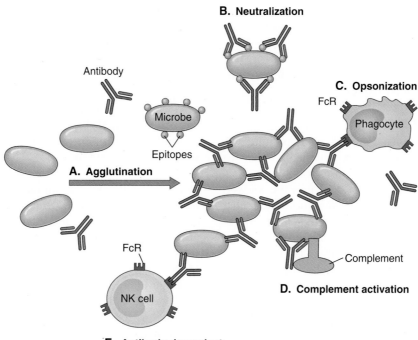

FIGURE 7-10. Humoral immune effector functions. A. Agglutination: Recognition of microbial surface epitopes by antibodies causes a cross-linked lattice formation analogous to the equivalence zone of the quantitative precipitin curve (see Fig. 7-9). This process prevents system-wide spread of the microbes. The order of efficacy is IgM >> IgA > IgG. **B.** Neutralization: In some instances, antibodies are specific for epitopes on the microbe, epitopes that would normally interact with molecules on the surface of the host cell. Antibodies that prevent molecule-to-molecule interaction between microbe and host cells are termed neutralizing antibodies. **C.** Opsonization: Antibody binding to microbial epitopes causes a conformational alteration in the Fc portion of the antibody molecule. Specialized Fc receptors (FcR) on phagocytes recognize and bind to the altered Fc portion of the antibody molecule, initiating phagocytosis of the FcR–antibody–microbe complex for enzymatic degradation by the phagolysosome. A fragment of the third component of complement (C3b) can also function as an opsonin, binding both to a microbial surface and to a specialized complement receptor (CR2) on the surfaces of phagocytes and signaling enzymatic destruction by phagocytosis and the phagolysosome. **D.** Complement activation: Antibody binding to a microbial surface may initiate the classical pathway of complement activation to initiate complement-mediated lysis and/or the binding of C3b as an opsonin. **E.** Antibody-dependent cell-mediated cytotoxicity: Antibody binding to microbial epitopes causes a conformational alteration in the Fc portion of the antibody molecule. FcRs on natural killer (NK) cells recognize and bind to these altered Fcs on the antibody. The microbe–antibody–FcR complex triggers the NK cell to release perforin and granzymes that facilitate the pore formation in the microbe, leading to its death.

Complement Activation

The **classical pathway of complement activation** is one in which antibodies mark a structure for destruction by facilitating the attraction and subsequent binding of components of the complement system. Unlike the alternative pathway of complement activation, the classical pathway must be initiated by the action of a product unique to the adaptive immune system. In this case, the antibodies (usually of the IgM and IgG isotypes) facilitate the sequential binding of the C1, C2, C3, and C4 components of the complement system (see Fig. 6-1). Completion of the classical complement pathway results

in production of the opsonin C3b, release of proinflammatory fragments **C2b** and **C4a** and assembly of the **membrane attack complex** (see Chapter 6 for more details).

Antibody-Dependent Cell-Mediated Cytotoxicity

The binding of an antibody to an invasive organism can act as a "tag" to attract not only phagocytic cells but also cytolytic cells. Cells such as **natural killer (NK) cells** and **eosinophils** bear FcRs that aid in the detection of infectious organisms as large as worms. Like phagocytic cells, they use these receptors to identify invasive organisms identified by IgG or IgA antibodies; but rather than engulfing them, they use cytolytic and inflammatory mechanisms to kill the tagged organisms (see Fig. 7-10E). These cytolytic mechanisms are discussed later in this chapter. The process is termed **antibody-dependent cell-mediated cytotoxicity (ADCC)**.

Cell-Mediated Immunity

The actions of both the innate and adaptive immune systems are like warfare waged against (potentially) invasive organisms. Humoral immune responses, both antibodies and complement activation pathways, may be viewed as the arrows and missiles of the immune system that are aimed or lobbed at a distant enemy. Often these responses are used as preemptive strikes, attacking a potential enemy before it has the ability to breach epithelial, endothelial, or cell membrane barriers. Agglutination, neutralization, opsonization, complement-mediated lysis, and ADCC all serve to curtail the potential spread of an infectious organism once it has established a beachhead. Yet, as Sun-tzu said, "Warfare is the Way of deception," and microbes are not beyond employing pathogenic stealth.

Cell-mediated immune responses are directed to curtail microbial stealth by determining whether infectious agents are sheltered within host cells and thus are beyond the "reach" of humoral immunity. Cell-mediated responses resemble "hand-to-hand combat" and take two basic forms: DTH mediated by CD4+ Th1 cells and cell-mediated lysis mediated by CD8+ CTLs. Cell-mediated immunity is a life-or-death struggle at close quarters. In the case of DTH, some T cells act as scouts and senior officers, identifying sites of infection, calling in reinforcements (mostly macrophages and other leukocytes), and ordering them to kill the infectious foe or the host cell that harbors the foe. CTLs, on the other hand, directly engage in cell-to-cell combat to actively destroy their infectious opponent or the host cell in which it is hiding.

Delayed-Type Hypersensitivity

Previously activated CD4+ Th1 cells patrol the body, looking for host cells displaying the same pMHC class II combination that originally triggered their activation (e.g., a *Mycobacterium tuberculosis* peptide-bearing MHC class II complex). If, during its recirculation through body tissues, a previously activated Th1 cell reencounters the appropriate pMHC class II displayed on a host cell, it reactivates to synthesize and secrete cytokines that attract and activate macrophages (Fig. 7-11). Thus, the T cells from the adaptive immune system can recruit, direct, and activate elements of the innate immune system. Activated macrophages become blind, enraged killers that attack not only infectious agents and infected cells but also normal uninfected cells in the vicinity. When activated by Th1 cells, macrophages increase their production and release of destructive enzymes and reactive oxygen intermediates that injure adjacent cells. They also begin to secrete cytokines that attract other leukocytes, especially neutrophils, to the site of infection. Together, the activated macrophages and neutrophils rampage through the site of infection, assaulting both infected and normal cells and removing cellular debris.

DTH responses can be a double-edged sword. Because the activated macrophages are not "antigen specific," they are perfectly capable of destroying friend and foe alike, normal tissue along with infected cells. Excessively active or chronic DTH responses can create permanent damage that impairs normal function and, in some cases, is fatal. For example, much or most of the injury to the lungs of tuberculosis patients stems from the damage inflicted by the activated macrophages of the DTH response against *M. tuberculosis* rather than by the infectious agent itself.

Cytotoxic T Lymphocytes

Only a small proportion of the cells of the body express MHC class II molecules, although all nucleated cells express MHC class I molecules. Previously activated

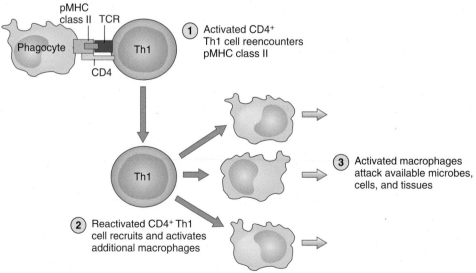

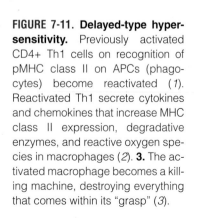

FIGURE 7-11. Delayed-type hypersensitivity. Previously activated CD4+ Th1 cells on recognition of pMHC class II on APCs (phagocytes) become reactivated (*1*). Reactivated Th1 secrete cytokines and chemokines that increase MHC class II expression, degradative enzymes, and reactive oxygen species in macrophages (*2*). **3.** The activated macrophage becomes a killing machine, destroying everything that comes within its "grasp" (*3*).

① Activated CD4+ Th1 cell reencounters pMHC class II

② Reactivated CD4+ Th1 cell recruits and activates additional macrophages

③ Activated macrophages attack available microbes, cells, and tissues

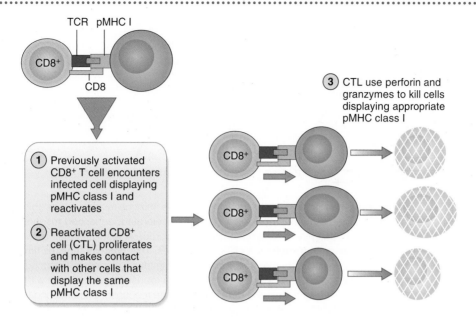

FIGURE 7-12. Cytotoxic T lymphocyte (CTL) activation. Activated CD8+ T cells circulate throughout the tissues of the body as CTLs, scrutinizing the pMHC class I molecules displayed by nucleated cells (*1*). On recognition of the appropriate pMHC class I complex, a series of events are initiated by the CTL that ultimately leads to the lysis of the infected "target cell" (*2*). Although contact between the CTL and the target cell lasts only a few minutes, the CTL delivers a fatal "kiss of death" to the target cell in the form of perforin granules and granzymes (*3*). The perforin granules polymerize to form pores in the cell, creating an electrolyte imbalance and through which granzymes enter. Both perforins and granzymes conspire in the demise of the target cell by osmotic lysis and apoptosis, respectively.

CD8+ CTLs circulate throughout the body, "sampling" for the initial activating pMHC class I combination. If the CTL encounters that combination on the surface of another cell, it recognizes that it has contacted an infected cell (Fig. 7-12). CTLs bind directly to infected cells and destroy them using one or more mechanisms. They release perforins that puncture the cell membranes, effectively lysing them. CTLs also release granzymes that enter the cytoplasm through the perforin-created holes. Granzymes induce the infected cell to commit suicide by destroying its own DNA, a process known as apoptosis. CTLs alter their membranes in the area of contact to make themselves resistant to the perforins and granzymes being released. Finally, CTLs may engage receptors on the surfaces of the infected cells, inducing the infected cells to undergo apoptosis. Apoptosis is an important protective mechanism because, in destroying its own DNA, the infected cells also destroy the nucleic acids of the infectious organisms within it, thus preventing the spread of infection. Furthermore, apoptosis is a noninflammatory process that does not promote destruction of uninfected adjacent cells.

IMMUNOLOGIC MEMORY

An important feature that distinguishes the adaptive immune system from the innate immune system is the presence of **immunologic memory**. Simply put, once an infectious organism stimulates an adaptive response, subsequent encounters with that organism produce mild or even unapparent effects because of the rapid and enhanced action of antibodies or effector T cells. Antigen-specific cells that have been clonally expanded and have undergone some activation during previous encounters with antigen (**memory cells**) can be rapidly mobilized in much greater numbers, thus shortening the response time to antigen. Whether generated against infectious organisms or other types of antigens, these **secondary responses** are typically faster and more vigorous than the primary responses stimulated by the initial exposure (Fig. 7-13). In addition, the antibody isotypes generated against a repeatedly encountered antigen change over time. IgM is the predominant isotype seen in primary responses, while secondary responses include mostly IgG, with IgA and IgE also present. As the antibody isotypes change with repeated stimulation by a given antigen, the binding affinity of the antibodies also increases because of the incorporation of small mutations in the DNA encoding the variable regions of the light and heavy chains. B cells with mutations that result in tighter binding actually proliferate more rapidly and come to dominate the response. The deliberate initial exposure to an infectious organism, in a form unable to cause full-blown disease, can thus provide protection against a subsequent

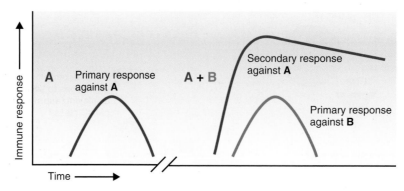

FIGURE 7-13. Immunologic memory. The hallmark of the adaptive immune response is its ability to recall a previous encounter with a microbe and mount an accelerated, enhanced response against it. Initial activation of antigen-naive lymphocytes with microbe A results in their activation, proliferation, and response of microbe-specific lymphocytes. This process requires time, hence the lag time between initial encounter and a discernible immune response. Reencountering the same microbe days, months, or years later results in a robust, rapid response with a significantly shorter lag time—a heightened and persistent immune response. Encountering the antigenically distinct microbe B at the time of the reencounter with microbe A results in a primary response similar to that seen for the initial encounter with microbe A.

exposure with a fully virulent form of that organism. This, of course, is the basis of **vaccination**.

Although immunological memory is primarily associated with enhancing the response to subsequent exposures to an infectious organism or other antigen, that is not always the case. In some cases, responses to future exposures can be diminished, a state known as **tolerance**. This phenomenon is important in preventing the immune system from producing superfluous (and potentially injurious) responses against harmless organisms and molecules in the environment, as well as against the body's own cells and molecules.

WHAT HAPPENS IF A GOOD SYSTEM GOES AWRY?

The function of the innate and adaptive immune systems is to recognize and attack the nonself while leaving the self relatively undisturbed. The innate immune system readily makes this distinction by expressing a finite number of receptors expressed by a wide variety of potentially pathogenic organisms. Because its receptors are somatically generated, the adaptive immune system is faced with a much more daunting task of distinguishing nonself from self. Selection mechanisms eliminate overtly self-reactive T and B cells during lymphocyte development. However, the adaptive immune system often encounters self molecules that were not present at the time of receptor selection, such as molecules that arise during and after puberty. If these mechanisms fail to distinguish self from nonself, serious and potentially fatal consequences may result. Fortunately, the adaptive immune system has evolved several mechanisms to deal with potentially self-reactive lymphocytes.

Tolerance and T-Cell Regulation

Normally, the immune system's offensive machinery is reserved for use against external threats. Part of the selection process during T-cell development (i.e., positive selection) requires that a thymocyte recognize self. Selective nonresponsiveness or **tolerance** requires that when recognizing self, the adaptive immune system must adopt a nondestructive strategy. Several tolerance mechanisms have evolved to minimize potential harm caused by post-developmental selection-autoreactive cells.

One mechanism, anergy, has already been discussed briefly. Basically, anergy is a state of lymphocyte non-responsiveness that occurs following pMHC engagement (T cells) or free epitope engagement (B cells). T cells require interaction with both pMHC *and* a costimulatory second signal. B cells, too, require a second signal following BCR engagement. Failing to receive a second signal, lymphocytes become unresponsive to the combined restimulation by both first *and* second signals. Anergized cells are not killed but remain in circulation and cannot, under normal circumstances, be reactivated.

In addition to Th1 and Th2, a third subset of effectors known as **Th17 cells** produce several potent proinflammatory cytokines including IL-17A, IL-17F, IL-21, and IL-22. Th17 cells, which depend upon IL-23 to maintain their function, are important effectors providing protection against a number of human bacterial and viral infections. Th17 cells may also participate in the development of autoimmune tissue inflammation including diseases such as psoriasis, rheumatoid arthritis, multiple sclerosis, asthma, and inflammatory bowel disease.

Another CD4+ population, called **regulatory T (Treg) cells**, plays a critical role in controlling the intensity of effector immune responses. Two main subsets of Treg have been described: **natural Tregs**, which arise in the thymus and are distributed throughout the body where they constitutively express FoxP3 as well as both CD25 and CD4 on their surfaces, and **inducible Tregs**, which develop from conventional CD4+ T cells upon exposure to specific conditions such as costimulatory signal blockade, certain cytokines, or drugs. These actions appear to help control autoimmune responses. Perhaps more importantly, both Treg subsets play a major role during infection by curtailing excessive effector immune activity that would otherwise result in collateral tissue damage. Despite extensive evidence for in vivo Treg activity, exactly how Tregs limit effector responses in vivo is still poorly understood. Long-lasting interactions with Tregs impair the ability of dendritic cells to activate effector T cells. Tregs also inhibit effector T cells by cell–cell interaction and by the production of anti-inflammatory cytokines such as TGF-β and IL-10. Tregs have been shown to prevent immune-mediated lung damage in *Pneumocystis* pneumonia, liver damage in chronic *Schistosoma mansoni* infection, and maternal *Toxoplasma gondii* infection during pregnancy. Because Tregs limit the severity of the immune response, many pathogens have evolved strategies to favor development of Treg activity in the host. Consequently, Tregs are implicated in the persistence of a number of diseases including malaria, leishmaniasis, human immunodeficiency virus-1 (HIV-1), hepatitis B virus, hepatitis C virus, *Helicobacter pylori*, *M. tuberculosis*, and *Chlamydia trachomatis* infections in humans. Lack of or severely limited Treg activity is associated with the development of a number of autoimmune diseases. Suppressor T cells are CD8+ and inhibit the activation and proliferation of CD4+ T cells, including Th1 cells. Certain subpopulations of both CD8+ and CD4+ T cells can inhibit specific antibody production by B cells. One possible mechanism for minimizing unwanted reactivity might involve cytokines produced by Th1 and Th2 cells that can mutually inhibit one another. Th1-produced IFN-γ inhibits the maturation of Th0 cells into Th2 cells, and Th2-produced IL-4 inhibits the differentiation of Th0 cells along the Th1 pathway. Thus, efficacy and pathology of immune responses to infectious organisms may well lie in the balance between effector (e.g., Th1, Th2, or Th17; CTL) and regulatory (e.g., Treg, Ts) activity.

Immunodeficiency

Unlike the nervous, visual, olfactory, and similar systems, the immune system is one of the few systems in the body that humans do not directly sense. No one wakes up in the morning and says, "My immune system feels great!" or "My immune system is feeling a little out of sorts." We generally perceive that something is wrong with our immune systems only when we are subjected to multiple, recurrent infections or when our immune systems overtly misperceive self and nonself. The immune system employs a great deal of redundancy, with a number of mechanisms available to fight a given threat. As a result, should one mechanism be ineffective or fail altogether, others can still clear the infections. Under these normal circumstances, the immune system functions reliably.

Sometimes, however, the system fails dramatically, leaving the individual open to potentially fatal infections or the unhealthy effects of an imbalanced immune system. Such defects in the immune system—**immune deficiencies** or **immunodeficiencies**—occur infrequently but can have severe consequences. Although some are extremely dramatic in their effects, those tend to be relatively rare; subtle immune deficiencies with less dramatic effects are more common. **Primary immune deficiencies** occur as intrinsic defects, usually genetically inherited but sometimes also due to random errors during development. Thus, although individual immunodeficiency diseases are rare, there are so many of them that collectively they represent a significant health problem. **Secondary immune deficiencies** are cases of reduced immune function caused by environmental factors (e.g., malnutrition, infection, malignancy, and therapeutic treatments for other diseases).

Immune deficiency diseases have several characteristics. Some are common to numerous forms of immunodeficiency, while others are associated with only a few such deficiencies. Among the most common are unusually frequent infections, chronic infections, an inability to clear infectious agents from the body, and diminished effectiveness of standard treatments.

The types of responses that are affected usually categorize primary immunodeficiencies, and each such category can include several defective mechanisms. Among the best known of these diseases are those that cause the many different forms of **severe combined immunodeficiency disease** (**SCID**). Most of these involve defects in the stem cells that give rise to most or all of the cellular elements of the immune system, including T and B cells. Individuals with SCID display varying degrees of reduced antibody-mediated and cell-mediated responses.

Defects in antibody-dependent responses may result from defective development of B cells (e.g., Bruton hypogammaglobulinemia), an inability to undergo the isotype switch (e.g., immunodeficiency with hyper-IgM), an inability to interact with T cells (common variable immunodeficiency), or a variety of defects in the genes encoding the immunoglobulin light or heavy chains or other molecules critical to normal function. However, individuals with B cell defects typically have normal cell-mediated immunity. Deficiencies in T-cell function include defects in T-cell development (e.g., DiGeorge syndrome), an inability to express MHC class I or class II molecules (e.g., bare lymphocyte syndrome), an inability to load antigenic peptides into MHC class I (e.g., TAP-2 deficiency), and a variety of other defective molecules involved in specific T-cell functions. Because T cells are critical to the normal

TABLE 7-4 Hypersensitivity Reactions

Type	Common Name	Initiated by	Immune Response	Inflammatory Mechanism(s)	Reaction Time
I	Immediate hypersensitivity or allergy	Allergens: pollens, parasites (e.g., dust mites), etc.	IgE-mediated degranulation of mast cells or basophils	Histamine and vasoactive amine release	Seconds to a few hours
II	Antibody-dependent cytotoxicity	Antibodies binding to molecules displayed on host cell surfaces, membranes, or extracellular matrices	Conformational change in Fc portion of antibody activates complement or FcR binding by phagocytes	Complement or cell-mediated lysis of cells	Hours to days
III	Immune-complex disease	Antibodies binding to soluble molecules	Extracellular deposition of antigen–antibody complexes	Activation of the classical complement pathway	Hours to days
IV	Delayed-type hypersensitivity	Intracellular microbes (e.g., *Mycobacterium tuberculosis*, *Leishmania* spp.)	Cell-mediated immune response to intracellular organisms	Macrophage and neutrophil activation and infiltration in infected tissues	1–4 d

function of B cells, individuals with T-cell defects often also display defective antibody-mediated responses.

Defects in cells other than lymphocytes can also diminish immune function. Defects in phagocytic cells, for example, can reduce their ability to ingest and destroy microbes (e.g., chronic granulomatous disease). As a result, innate immunity is lessened, as is the ability of the phagocytes to interact with T cells for initiation of adaptive responses. In addition, individuals bearing defects in the genes encoding various components of the complement system may face severe infectious problems because of the importance of these molecules in both innate and adaptive immunity.

In most cases, efforts to improve the outcomes for immunodeficient patients involve protection, appropriate antibiotic treatments, and replacing the missing molecules or cells on a repeating basis. Recently, attempts have been made to replace defective cells with cells from the patients that have been genetically engineered to function normally and provide a self-sustaining population that does not need regular replacement.

Hypersensitivity Reactions

Like any weapon or tool, the immune system can harm its user if not properly controlled. Its destructive capacity, meant to be directed against infectious agents or intruding toxins, can damage the body when it becomes too vigorous, too sustained, or misdirected. The state in which an immune system inflicts damage on the body is called **hypersensitivity**. Unlike autoimmunity, hypersensitivity need not be a response against the self but

often results from an "innocent bystander" destroying normal cells and tissues in the vicinity of a "free fire zone," where the immune system is aggressively battling infectious agents. The four recognized types of hypersensitivities are described in the following paragraphs and in Table 7-4.

Type I or immediate-type hypersensitivity manifests itself seconds to a few hours after an appropriate stimulus. Commonly known as **allergy**, this hypersensitivity state results from cross-linking surface-bound IgE antibodies on mast cells (and some basophils), triggering the release of vasoactive amines. Humoral immune responses against relatively harmless substances (e.g., pollens, food, etc.) lead to the secretion of specific IgE antibodies by plasma cells. Mast cells and some basophils express an ε-specific heavy-chain Fc receptor (FcR$_\varepsilon$). Unlike other FcRs specific to other heavy chains, the FcR$_\varepsilon$ binds epitope-free IgE molecules. Mast cells and some basophils decorate their cell surfaces with IgE molecules of various specificities. These IgE molecules then serve as epitope-specific receptors. Encounter with the appropriate antigen containing multiple recognized epitopes causes IgE cross-linking, triggering the release of cytoplasmic granules from the cell. The granules contain various pharmaceutical mediators that trigger the changes in the skin, vasculature, airways, or gut that are associated with allergy. Severe, life-threatening manifestations of allergy can lead to **anaphylaxis** and shock.

Type II hypersensitivities are those caused by the activation of complement, via the classical pathway, by antibodies (usually IgG but sometimes also IgM) bound to cell surfaces, membranes, or intracellular matrices. The antibodies may be directed against normal self molecules (autoimmunity) or against nonself molecules that attach themselves to membranes or matrices in the body. In either case, the location of the bound antibodies focuses the inflammatory response initiated by complement activation to that site and can lead to temporary or permanent damage. Damage can also be incurred by the interaction of the bound antibodies with FcRs of phagocytic cells or cells capable of ADCC. Goodpasture syndrome, myasthenia gravis, and Graves disease are all examples of type II hypersensitivities.

Type III hypersensitivities, like those of type II, are caused by the activation of complement via the classical pathway. However, the antibodies involved are binding to soluble molecules rather than surfaces. As a result, antigen–antibody complexes can form, and if they become large enough, they can precipitate out of solution (see Fig. 7-9) and become deposited on tissues. The most common sites of deposition are the kidney glomeruli (the filtering apparatus of the kidney), the endothelial surfaces of blood vessels, the skin, and the synovial membranes of joints. Once deposited in tissues, the antibodies bound within the complexes interact with and activate complement, leading to inflammation focused on the site of deposition. Again, the damage inflicted may be temporary or permanent. Poststreptococcal glomerulonephritis and systemic lupus erythematosus (SLE) are examples of type III hypersensitivities.

Type IV hypersensitivities do not involve antibodies but are due to inflammatory reactions arising from purely cell-mediated immune responses. Usually, these are CD4+-mediated DTH responses, but sometimes, they also involve the action of CD8+ CTLs. Among the most common examples of this hypersensitivity type are positive skin tests for tuberculosis (the Mantoux test); inflammations caused by contact with poison ivy, poison sumac, and other plants; and the inflammations (contact sensitivity) resulting from contact with certain chemicals or metals (e.g., nickel).

Autoimmunity

Despite the checks and balances that are built into the adaptive immune system, it sometimes mistakes self epitopes for nonself. The loss of self-tolerance mechanisms leads to a condition known as **autoimmunity**, a state in which the immune system attacks the body's own normal molecules, the very cells and tissues that it was designed to protect. Unfortunately, autoimmune diseases occur all too frequently.

Microbial epitopes sometimes bear structural similarities to molecules expressed by host cells. In attempting to curtail the spread of an infectious organism, the adaptive immune system may respond to these structurally similar epitopes, a process known as **molecular mimicry**. Strong host defenses to a particular microbial epitope can also inflict damage to host cells that display

similar epitope-bearing structures. A classic example of this mechanism is **rheumatic fever**, which can lead to life-threatening heart disease. Pharyngeal infection with *Streptococcus pyogenes* is the common cause of "strep throat." Group A β-hemolytic stains of *S. pyogenes* produce large quantities of **M protein**. The adaptive immune response readily makes IgM and IgG antibodies to M protein. Unfortunately, antibodies to M protein can cross-react with similar structures found on the sarcolemma of cardiac muscle and on the heart valves. Antibody binding to the sarcolemma and heart valves initiates inflammation of these tissues that can result in fatal damage to the tissues. Chronic strep throat infections can be life threatening. This is the main reason that pediatricians promptly treat children with strep throat with antibiotics, thereby minimizing development of adaptive immune response to this organism and preventing autoimmune sequelae. Autoimmune type 1 diabetes mellitus is another example of molecular mimicry. T cells of individuals infected with *Coxsackie virus* or *cytomegalovirus* may develop responsiveness to glutamate decarboxylase responses, a pancreatic islet β-cell enzyme that is a major target for autoreactive T cells.

Other autoimmune diseases that collectively are known as **reactive arthritis** may be attributable to molecular mimicry. These include **ankylosing spondylitis**, an inflammatory disease of the lower spine, in which prior *Klebsiella* infection leads to immune cross-reactivity with a certain MHC class I (HLA-B27) molecule in susceptible individuals. *Klebsiella* has been implicated as the causative agent in **Reiter disease**, marked by arthritis in the lower-limb joints and involvement of the gastrointestinal, genital, and urinary tracts. Molecular mimicry has also been implicated in **myasthenia gravis**, a disease in which the nerve ending–muscle junction is impaired, and **hypoglycemia**, in which the insulin receptor is affected.

In some cases, autoimmune disease results from the loss of regulatory T or suppressor T cells. Evidence suggests that the ability of Treg and Ts cells to prevent responses by self-reactive cells is lost with time. Therefore, as people age, the opportunity for self-reactive lymphocytes to escape regulation also increases. Autoimmune diseases such as **systemic lupus erythematosus (SLE)** are thought to result from impaired regulation, and affected individuals produce antibodies against nucleic acids and chromosomal proteins.

Some autoimmune diseases result from an altered immune response to an initial infection. Initial infection can expose normally sequestered antigens to immune scrutiny. The phenomenon, called **epitope spreading**, appears to originate with an immune response to an infectious disease, and the collateral damage to normal tissues makes sequestered antigens available to the adaptive immune system. Epitope spreading has been suggested as a contributing mechanism to SLE, inflammatory bowel disease, multiple sclerosis, and some forms of diabetes.

WELL PATIENTS, OR HOW INNATE AND ADAPTIVE IMMUNE RESPONSES MAINTAIN HEALTH

Immune system responses to microbial infection are vital for the protection of the body. The adaptive immune system is designed to attack infectious organisms that enter the body. Often, microorganisms resist attack by the immune system by evading or subverting and redirecting the immune response. Sometimes, it is just as important that the immune system not respond to an antigen. For instance, the mucosal surfaces are constantly awash in nonself molecules and microorganisms associated with our environment and with the food and fluids that we consume. Immune defenses must focus on potentially infectious microorganisms and their products but ignore or selectively diminish responses to others.

From the human perspective, the microbial world has four classes of citizens: (1) those that do not inhabit the human body; (2) those that live on or in the body, benefiting one or both partners and harming neither; (3) those that that live on or in the body in a state of truce, neither benefiting nor harming either partner; and (4) those with the potential for causing harm to the human body. Members of the fourth category are known as **pathogens**. The disease-causing potential for a pathogen often depends on circumstances. Some pathogens invade the human body as part of their life cycle. Others are **opportunistic** pathogens and become a threat only when the immune system is weakened. Products of some microbes, such as the *Vibrio cholera* toxin, can be life threatening, and the development of specific, neutralizing antibodies against the toxin are crucial for protection. Many people enjoy a healthy, active life, unaware of the critical, life-sustaining role played by their immune systems. In fact, most of us become aware of immune dysfunction by the inability of our bodies to resist infection.

Effective Immune Responses to Pathogens

Immune responses vary in their effectiveness against particular types of pathogens. Which responses will be effective in providing protection is determined by the physical nature of the pathogen in question as well as its "lifestyle." Pathogens or their toxic products vary in the ways that they enter the body, the cells or tissues that they infect once they are within the body, and the ways in which they move through the body and reproduce. All these factors participate in determining which types of immune responses will be most effective against them.

Viral infections trigger both innate and adaptive immune responses. Infected cells synthesize and secrete cytokines that heighten the resistance of neighboring uninfected cells while rendering themselves more "available" to the immune system to trigger the initiation of protective responses by NK cells and phagocytic cells. NK cells are lymphocytes that bridge both the innate and adaptive immune systems (see Chapter 6) able to detect cells that have subnormal expression of MHC class I molecules and to kill them by direct contact. This is an important ability because, as will be seen shortly, some viruses attempt to escape the notice of the immune system (especially CTLs) by reducing the number of MHC class I molecules on the surface of the cells they infect. Following the activation of the innate immune system by viral infection, humoral and cellular adaptive responses arise.

During **primary infections** (the initial exposure to a particular virus), adaptive cell-mediated responses, primarily involving CTLs, clear the viral infection by destroying the cells within which the viruses are replicating. The generation of antiviral antibodies, although not effective in clearing active infections (because replicating viruses are sequestered within cells and not accessible to antibodies), is extremely important because antibodies minimize or prevent reinfection through neutralization. Even if reinfection is not completely prevented by neutralizing antibodies, the infected cells remain few and can be destroyed readily by increased cell-mediated responses. These reinfections may be dealt with so rapidly that symptoms do not become evident.

Extracellular bacteria remain in the body fluids and intercellular spaces, while intracellular bacteria enter and reproduce within cells. Various immune responses are effective against each of these two categories of bacteria. Free-living extracellular bacteria, such as *Staphylococci* and *Streptococci*, are readily exposed to antibodies and complement. As a result, they are vulnerable to destruction and clearance by phagocytic cells (via recognition and binding by pattern recognition receptors) and by all the pathways of complement activation. Recognition and binding of the bacteria by antibodies also increases their clearance through opsonization.

Intracellular bacteria (e.g., *Mycobacterium* spp. and *Legionella pneumophila*) are exposed to complement and antibodies en route to the cells they are to infect. Once inside the cell, they are no longer available to the actions of antibodies and complement. The portal of entry for many intracellular bacteria is the phagosome. Thus, destruction of these intracellular bacteria often requires activation of the infected phagocytes by CD4+ T cells through DTH. Because CD4+ T cells can only recognize pMHC class II complexes, this is only effective if the infected cells express MHC class II molecules. This activation causes the phagocytes to increase their metabolic activity and synthesis of bactericidal molecules, allowing them to kill or inhibit the growth of the microbes residing in the phagosomes.

Cells infected by intracellular bacteria can sometimes also be killed by CTLs. As described earlier, some intracellular bacteria (e.g., *Listeria monocytogenes* and *Rickettsia* spp.) can escape from phagosomes and move into the cytoplasm. Once in the cytoplasm, some of the bacterial proteins are degraded by proteasomes; their proteolytic fragments are loaded onto MHC class I molecules and displayed on the cell surface in pMHC class I complexes. These pMHC class I complexes can be recognized by CTLs that go on to destroy the infected cell.

Immune responses to infectious **protozoa** are much like those seen for bacteria. Free-living protozoa are sometimes vulnerable to antibody-mediated opsonization or antibody-initiated complement lysis, while intracellular protozoa are destroyed primarily by cell-mediated responses (usually DTH). While fungal infections trigger both antibody and DTH responses, it is the latter that are responsible for resistance and clearance of infectious **fungi**. Immune responses can even be generated against larger pathogenic invaders such as flatworms (flukes and tapeworms) and roundworms (such as nematodes, hookworms, and *Ascaris* spp.). Tapeworms are generally localized in the gastrointestinal tract, while various species of flukes infect a variety of tissues such as blood, liver, lung, and intestine. Roundworms usually infect either the blood or the gastrointestinal tract. Infections by flatworms and roundworms can trigger inflammatory responses involving IgE and DTH that may provide some degree of protection against subsequent reinfection, although not as effectively as is seen against bacteria or viruses.

Evasion and Subversion of the Immune Response

Infectious organisms do not lie down and surrender when confronted by the immune system. After millions of years of interactions with their hosts, they have developed numerous methods for countering immune responses, ranging from simple evasion ("camouflage") to deliberately destroying cells and molecules of the immune response ("assassination").

Various forms of camouflage allow some microbes to sneak beneath the radar of the immune system. For example, the larval and adult forms of some blood flukes (*Schistosoma*) can cover themselves with molecules from host cells, passing themselves off as the self. Others (e.g., *Plasmodium* spp.) practice a form of invisibility by entering erythrocytes. Mature erythrocytes, being enucleate and lacking MHC class I or class II molecules on their surface, are ignored by T lymphocytes. Finally, many microbes can reduce the expression of some of their surface molecules, making them less visible to the immune system.

Many infectious organisms evade the immune response by altering the antigen molecules on their surfaces. In some cases (e.g., the bacterium *Neisseria gonorrhoeae* and protozoans within *Trypanosoma* spp.), microbes carry numerous, slightly varying, copies of genes to encode some of their critical surface antigens. Periodically, they alter their surface antigens by altering the gene being transcribed (using chromosome rearrangement mechanisms similar in concept to those generate immunoglobulin diversity). Some organisms (e.g., influenza virus and HIV) use error-prone polymerases to replicate their DNA, leading to an elevated rate of accumulated small mutations—a process known as **antigenic drift**. Influenza virus, HIV, and others can also change their surface antigens in more drastic ways through a process known as **antigenic shift**. Antigenic shift occurs when viruses from different sources infect the same cell and recombine. For example, in regions of the world where domestic birds and mammals are in close contact, an avian influenza virus (e.g., from a duck) and a mammalian influenza virus (e.g., from a pig) can infect a single cell (e.g., in the pig). Once within the same cell, the duck-derived and pig-derived influenza genomes can recombine to form hybrid progeny containing parts of the two genomes. These hybrid forms may infect not only the parental avian and mammalian species but other species as well (e.g., humans). Often, the hybrid viruses are so different from their progenitors that individuals who developed protective immune responses against the original forms have little protection against the new hybrid forms. Thus, in all these cases, the immune system must start anew, developing responses to the newly expressed antigens, only to find that by the time they become effective, the organism has generated yet other new antigens.

Some infectious organisms have developed the ability to interfere with the immune responses generated against them. For example, many intracellular bacteria can prevent fusion between the phagosome in which they are taken up and lysosomes containing the enzymes that would otherwise kill and degrade them. Some pathogens secrete factors that interfere with the proliferation of nearby lymphocytes, while others produce enzymes that degrade complement molecules or immunoglobulins in their vicinity. Even organisms as simple as viruses have developed several means to protect themselves from the immune system by inhibiting the presentation of virus-derived peptide fragments into MHC class I molecules and their expression on the surface of the infected cell (Fig. 7-14). Finally, some organisms can remodel the immune response to make it less detrimental to the organism. For example, microbes that are susceptible primarily to cellular responses may promote antibody-dominated responses or vice versa.

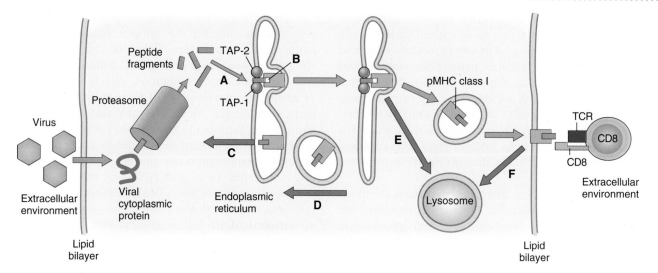

FIGURE 7-14. Viral evasion of pMHC class I presentation. Some viruses (e.g., some herpes-viruses, adenoviruses, cytomegaloviruses, and HIV) are able to disrupt different stages of the normal MHC class I presentation pathway (*light blue arrows*). Points of viral intervention (*dark blue arrows*) include the following: (*A*) Prevention of peptide entry into the endoplasmic reticulum via TAP-1 and TAP-2. (*B*) Inhibition of peptide exit from TAP-1 and TAP-2 into the endoplasmic reticulum. (*C*) Diversion of pMHC class I complexes from the endoplasmic reticulum back into the cytoplasm. (*D*) Return of pMHC class I complexes from the Golgi to the endoplasmic reticulum. (*E*) Diversion of pMHC class I complexes from exocytotic vesicles to the lysosomes. (*F*) Diversion of cell surface pMHC class I complexes to the lysosomes.

CONCLUSION

The adaptive immune system builds upon and amplifies the foundation established by the innate immune system. It adds several defensive features including (1) random generation of antigen-specific receptors with far greater variety than is available in the innate system; (2) a variety of destructive mechanisms (including those of the innate system) that focus on narrowly defined targets, which vary among different infectious agents; and (3) memory, which allows it to modify its response to stimuli that are encountered repeatedly. In concert with the innate immune system, the adaptive immune system provides a versatile and coordinated set of defensive responses capable of dealing with the invasive styles of a broad array of infectious agents.

Suggested Readings

Abbas AK, Lichtman AH. *Cellular and Molecular Immunology.* 5th ed. Philadelphia, PA: WB Saunders; 2003.

Doan T, Melvold R, Waltenbaugh C. *Concise Medical Immunology.* 1st ed. Baltimore, MD: Lippincott Williams & Wilkins; 2005.

Janeway CA Jr, Travers P, Walport M, et al. *Immunobiology: The Immune System in Health and Disease.* 6th ed. Philadelphia, PA: Garland; 2004.

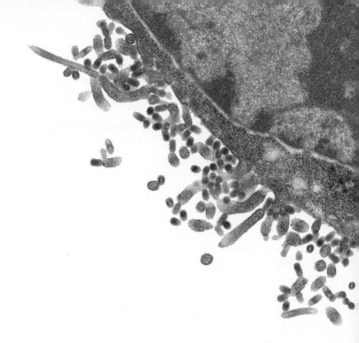

Chapter **8**

The Parasite's Way of Life

Victor J. DiRita

IN VIEW of our long acquaintance with infectious diseases, it is not surprising that we tend to take an anthropomorphic view of our relationship with our microbial neighbors. Analogies to war are common, as in references to a microbial "attack" or "invasion" repelled by host "defense systems." In reality, what drives microbes is not aggression but survival and reproduction. To succeed, many microbes have evolved the ability to persist in the body, only incidentally causing disease, making them more analogous to unwanted houseguests than to invaders. Whether as aggressive pathogens or harmless commensals, microbial agents face many problems in their association with the host. To survive, microbes must do the following:

- Avoid being washed away (colonize the surfaces of host cells).
- Find a nutritionally compatible niche.
- Survive innate and adaptive defenses.
- Transmit to a new host.

Every successful commensal or pathogen has evolved a specific repertoire of strategies to face these challenges. Those strategies are discussed in detail in the chapters on individual agents. This chapter presents an overview of the mechanisms involved.

SURFACE COLONIZATION

Picture a microbe entering the mouth and imagine the obstacles it faces trying to remain there. Strong liquid currents will wash it away unless the organism can adhere to the surface of the teeth or mucous membranes. At places not exposed to the flushing action of saliva, such as the crevices of the gums, the organism encounters a large **resident microbiota** that already occupies potential adherence sites outmaneuvering the resident microbes.

Colonization of microbes to host surfaces involves both microbial and host factors. Microbes elaborate substances or organelles that are involved in the adherence and are known as **adhesins** (Table 8-1). In many cases, adhesins bind to special **receptors** on host surfaces. Both adhesins and receptors are usually highly specific for the species of microbes and the host.

Adhesive molecules in some Gram-negative bacteria are positioned on the tips of long, slender structures called fimbriae or pili. **Fimbrial adhesins** interact with structural constituents of host epithelial cells, often glycolipids. In other Gram-negative bacteria, adhesins are found directly on the cell surface and not on protrusions. An example of such an adhesin is **invasin**, a protein that recognizes normal cellular receptors on host cells called **integrins**. Integrins are receptors primarily involved in other processes, such as the adherence of white blood cells to endothelial surfaces, but bacteria usurp integrins for another use. Binding of bacteria to integrins results in intimate association between the bacteria and the host cell membrane. Such appropriation of normal host functions by microbes is a recurrent theme in pathogenic microbiology. The interplay between adhesins and host cell receptors is different in Gram-positive bacteria. A receptor for certain Gram-positive bacteria is the protein **fibronectin**, which normally coats the mucosal surfaces of epithelial cells. Fibronectin plays an important role in selecting the bacterial microbiota in the mouth and pharynx. The oropharynx of individuals

TABLE 8-1 Bacterial Adhesins

Gram-Negative Bacteria	Gram-Positive Bacteria
Pili (fimbriae)	Surface proteins
Surface proteins (nonfimbrial)	Capsules
Capsules	

in poor general health, including many hospitalized patients, is deficient in fibronectin. In part because the fibronectin-denuded mucosal cells reveal receptors for Gram-negative fimbrial adhesins, Gram-negative organisms tend to displace Gram-positive bacteria in these patients. The greater incidence of pneumonia caused by Gram-negative bacteria in hospitalized patients can be explained in part by such adherence specificity.

The mouth, large intestine, vagina, perineum, skin, and other sites are normally laden with bacteria. Because the bacterial populations at these sites are fairly stable, it follows that colonization by new organisms is unlikely. The successful colonizer must be adept at outmaneuvering the resident microbes. On the other hand, microbial competition is not an important factor in colonization of sites that are normally sterile or carry a sparse load of microbes, such as all the deep tissues or the small intestine.

Obviously, in our long history of coexistence and coevolution with the microbial world, our bodies have learned what territory is safe to share and what is off limits; and we have managed to share this space preferentially with well-behaved guests. Foreign devices, like plastic catheters inserted into arteries and veins, may upset the delicate ecological balance between microbes and host tissues, partly because they allow bacteria and fungi to bypass the normal defenses and partly because they potentiate growth by organisms with the special ability to stick well to plastics (e.g., strains of *Staphylococcus epidermidis*, which are otherwise harmless skin residents; see Chapter 11).

FINDING A NUTRITIONALLY COMPATIBLE NICHE

To microbes, the human body would seem to be a rich nutritional environment. Body fluids such as plasma contain sugars, vitamins, minerals, and other substances that bacteria, fungi, and animal parasites can use for growth. Still, bacteria grow sparsely on fresh plasma in a test tube, primarily because of the presence of antimicrobial substances, such as lysozyme, constituents of the complement system, and antibodies. In addition, some nutrients are in short supply in body fluids. Plasma and most other body fluids, for example, contain very little **free iron**. The metal is highly insoluble and must be combined with iron-binding proteins for transport. The lack of free iron significantly limits the growth of bacteria in the body because bacteria

need iron for the synthesis of their cytochromes and other enzymes. The body may sequester iron even further in response to microbial invasion. When a sufficient number of organisms enters the body, iron-binding proteins are poured into plasma and tissue fluids, and the normally low amount of available iron is further reduced. Many bacteria respond to this challenge by excreting compounds that bind iron with high affinity (**chelators**). After capturing an iron molecule, these compounds deliver the iron to specific bacterial receptors (see Chapter 3). Other bacteria possess surface molecules that can "steal" iron from the iron-binding proteins of the host. Certain bacteria (e.g., some streptococci) scavenge intracellular iron by making toxins that destroy host cells, such as red blood cells.

Some microbes use specific nutrients found only in certain sites of the body. Thus, mouth strains of streptococci are adept at using dietary sucrose, which gives them a growth (and colonization) advantage over bacteria that do not have that ability. Even more startling is the example of brucellosis in cattle, which is caused by the microbe *Brucella abortus*. Brucellosis is a systemic disease in humans and other animals. In addition, brucellosis causes abortion in cattle and a few other animal species. The reason for this species-specific abortion is that the placentas of cattle and some other animals, but not humans, contain a four-carbon sugar, **erythritol**, for which the organisms have a special affinity. An example of how finely tuned the physiology of *B. abortus* is to the presence of erythritol in the placenta is that this sugar increases the production of iron-scavenging molecules, which are also critical for growth in the animal, more than does any other sugar on which the microbe is capable of growing.

The spectrum of nutritional requirements of microbes that live in the body reflects their ecological habits. For instance, many of the bacteria found mainly in the human body, such as staphylococci or certain streptococci, have complex nutritional requirements and need several amino acids and vitamins for growth. Organisms found both in the body and in soil or water are usually much less picky and can fulfill their organic requirements with simple carbon compounds. Examples are *Escherichia coli* and many pseudomonads that can grow in the laboratory in "**minimal media**." Another connection between physiology and ecology is illustrated by a bacterium's oxygen requirements. Many of our most heavily colonized sites—for instance, the periodontal spaces and the colon—are anaerobic. Not surprisingly, the bacteria found in those sites are overwhelmingly anaerobic, with very few strict aerobes present.

SURVIVING THE CONSTITUTIVE AND INDUCED DEFENSES

Many bacteria that enter the body do not survive because of the physical barriers and inhospitable microenvironments that they encounter. These factors are the host's first lines of defense against infection. However, over millennia of coevolution with their bacterial neighbors, mammals have also developed second lines of defense to deal with microbes that manage to evade the first-line defenses. How do microbial agents overcome these powerful defense mechanisms? How do they avoid the action of complement and phagocytosis or evade antigenic recognition by the host immune system?

Defending Against Complement

The most effective way to protect against the antimicrobial action of complement is to prevent its activation. Bacteria prevent complement activation in several ways (Table 8-2). One is by **masking** surface components that activate the alternative pathway. Lipopolysaccharides of Gram-negative bacteria, teichoic acids of Gram-positive bacteria, and other structural components of microbes are potential complement activators. Meningococci and pneumococci are examples of bacteria that prevent complement activation by secreting capsules that cover these activators (Fig. 8-1).

Some organisms take advantage of the host's own mechanism for avoiding complement activation. Most host cells incorporate **sialic acid**, a sugar that inhibits complement activation, into their surface molecules. Many bacteria achieve the same protection by incorporating sialic acid into their capsular polysaccharides. When they grow in tissues, gonococci add sialic acid to the terminal sugar of their lipopolysaccharide, which makes them resistant to complement lysis. Meningococci employ a different strategy to avoid complement

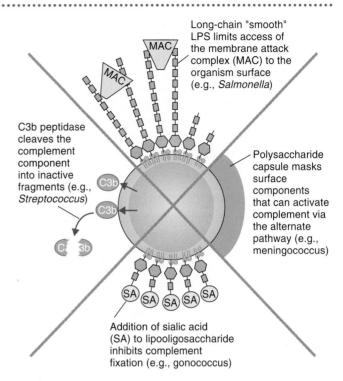

FIGURE 8-1. **Mechanisms microbes use to prevent harmful effects of complement.**

activation: they become coated with **circulating IgA antibodies**, a class of immunoglobulins that do not activate the complement cascade (a "wolf in sheep's clothing" strategy). The IgA coating prevents other kinds of antibodies capable of setting off complement activation by the classical pathway from reaching the surface of the organisms.

Certain viruses have also evolved mechanisms to prevent complement activation. For example, herpes simplex virus has an **envelope glycoprotein** that binds **complement component C3b**, thus inhibiting activation by the alternative pathway (see Chapter 41). Cells infected with vaccinia virus secrete a virally encoded protein that shares amino acid homology with a complement control protein (C4bp). C4bp binds to the C4b fragment. By mimicking the action of the host C4bp, the virus limits complement activation by the classical pathway and causes the accelerated decay of C3 convertase. Mutants of vaccinia virus that lack the protein produce smaller, more rapidly healing skin lesions in experimental animals.

Some Gram-negative bacteria, such as *Salmonella* and *E. coli*, do not prevent formation of the complement **membrane attack complex** but rather hinder its access to its target, the bacterial outer membrane. **"Smooth" strains**, which have a long O-antigen polysaccharide chain, do not allow access of the membrane attack complex to their outer membrane, while **"rough" mutants**, which have little or no O antigen, are readily killed by it. The presence or absence of the O antigen correlates well

TABLE 8-2 Some Microbial Anticomplement Strategies

Activate Masking Substances
- Coat with capsule (e.g., *Streptococcus pneumoniae*)
- Coat with IgA antibodies (e.g., *Neisseria meningitidis*)
- Cap lipooligosaccharide with sialic acid residues (e.g., *Neisseria gonorrhoeae*)

Apply Appropriate Inhibitor of Activation to Surface
- Bind factor H (e.g., *Escherichia coli*, *Borrelia*, group B streptococci)
- Bind decay-accelerating factors (e.g., *Schistosoma* spp.)
- Mimic component C4b-binding protein (C4bp) (e.g., vaccinia virus)

Cover-Up Target of Membrane Attack Complex (e.g., *E. coli*, *Salmonella* spp.)
Inactivate Complement-Derived Mediators
- Inactivate chemotaxin C5a (e.g., group A streptococcus, *Pseudomonas aeruginosa*)
- Activate surface of plasminogen to plasmin and cleave C3b (e.g., *Staphylococcus aureus*)

with pathogenicity. Smooth strains tend to be virulent, while rough strains are not. However, capsules and other protective surface structures come with a price: most of them are highly antigenic and in time elicit the production of anticapsular antibodies that enable the activation of complement by the classical pathway. Notice that these organisms defend themselves better against the more immediate host defense, activation of complement by the alternative pathway, than against later events, the formation of antibodies.

Subverting Phagocytosis

Microbes employ a number of strategies to avoid being killed by phagocytes. The host attempts to overcome these microbial countermeasures, and in turn, those efforts are answered by yet other microbial tactics. A point must be made at the outset: being phagocytized by a cell is not necessarily a bad thing for the microbe. Some microbes are able to grow within host cells, where they are shielded from antibodies and certain antimicrobial drugs. Such is the allure of intracellular growth that some microbes have evolved mechanisms to induce their uptake into cells of the host.

The following paragraphs present a few examples of strategies used by microbes to withstand the killing power of phagocytic cells. Various aspects of phagocytosis are affected, from the arrival of the phagocytes at the scene to the killing powers of phagocytic cells (Table 8-3).

Inhibiting Phagocyte Recruitment and Function

As previously discussed, some microbes prevent the activation of complement. In doing so, they prevent the secondary release of neutrophil chemotaxins and opsonins, thus reducing the risk of encountering those cells as well as their function. Other organisms (e.g., *Bordetella pertussis*; see Chapter 19) directly inhibit neutrophil motility and chemotaxis by producing a toxin that increases cyclic adenosine monophosphate (AMP) to inhibitory levels. Group A streptococci produce a **C5a peptidase** that specifically inactivates this chemotactic product of the complement cascade.

Microbial Killing of Phagocytes

Some pathogenic bacteria produce exotoxins called **leukocidins** to kill neutrophils and macrophages. Leukocidins are soluble products that work at a distance and thus may protect bacteria before the phagocytes come near them. In many cases, however, microbes kill after they are ingested. In this strategy, the phagocyte commits suicide by carrying out phagocytosis (see Chapter 9). Typical leukocidin producers are highly invasive bacteria, such as pseudomonads, staphylococci, group A streptococci, and the clostridia that cause gas gangrene. Yersiniae produce proteins that are injected directly into host cells and interfere with cellular activation (see Chapter 17 paradigm), and through a similar injection mechanism, shigellae kill phagocytic cells.

Avoiding "NETS"

Neutrophils—potent early responders to invading microbes—can release complexes of DNA, histones, and enzymes called "**neutrophil extracellular traps**" (**NETS**) that can bind to and kill bacteria. Many bacteria have evolved the ability to secrete nucleases that destroy the NETS and enhance survival of the microbe.

Escaping Ingestion

A notable microbial counterdefense to phagocytosis is the capsule. One of the more captivating visual experiences in microbiology is to watch a preparation of live neutrophils and encapsulated pneumococci under the microscope: each time a neutrophil attempts to embrace a pneumococcus, the slimy bacterium squeezes away with what looks like total indifference, and repeated attempts are no more successful. The picture changes when a small amount of capsule-specific antiserum is added: the neutrophils have no trouble engulfing the opsonized pneumococci. Anticapsular antibodies thus provide protective immunity against infection by encapsulated bacteria. However, bacteria have evolved measures to counter opsonization, either by complement components or by specific antibodies. Any mechanism that inhibits activation of complement or synthesis or activity of antibodies will reduce the probability of opsonization.

Staphylococci, streptococci, and probably other bacteria have evolved a mechanism to reduce opsonization even when antibodies are present: they make a surface component, **protein A**, that binds to IgG molecules by the "wrong" end, the Fc portion. These antibodies therefore cannot act as opsonins because their orientation on the surface of the bacteria is reversed from what is required to bind to the Fc receptors on phagocytic cells. It is not known to what extent this antiphagocytic mechanism plays a role in actual infections.

How Microbes Survive Inside Phagocytes

Microbes have many ways to survive once they are taken up by host cells:

- **Inhibition of lysosome fusion with phagosomes**: When lysosomes fuse with phagosomes, they release powerful microbicidal substances (see Chapter 6). Inhibiting this fusion clearly benefits intraphagosomal microbes, such as the agents of tuberculosis, psittacosis, and Legionnaires disease. How this inhibition is accomplished is an active area of investigation, and it is likely that compounds secreted or present on the surface of the microbes modify the phagosome membrane and alter the trafficking processes that would normally fuse the phagosome with the lysosome.
- **Escape into the cytoplasm**: The shigellae, *Listeria monocytogenes*, and the rickettsiae cross the membrane of the phagocytic vesicle, the phagosome, and enter the cytoplasm. Because lysosomes do not

TABLE 8-3 Microbial Strategies to Evade Phagocyte Function

Antiphagocyte Activity	Mechanism	Example
Avoid Being Phagocytized		
Diversion (to nonproductive use)	Activate complement C5a Leucoaggregation Pulmonary sequestration	Streptococci. Gram-negative enterics
"Playing hard to get"	Slimy capsule on organisms	Pneumococci, meningococci, *Haemophilus influenzae*, *Bacteroides fragilis*, many others
—	M protein	Group A streptococci
—	Pili	Gonococci
Humiliation	Release adenylate cyclase, leading to high levels of cyclic adenosine monophosphate; all phagocyte functions depressed	*Bordetella pertussis* (toxin)
Paralysis	Make cells unresponsive to chemotactic factors	*Capnocytophaga*
—	—	Tubercle bacilli
—	Induce inhibitors of migration	Leprosy bacilli
—	Inactivate chemotaxins (C5a)	*Pseudomonas* (elastase)
After Being Phagocytized		
Murder	Membrane lysis	Streptococci (streptolysins O and S) *Pseudomonas* (exotoxin A) *Staphylococcus aureus* (α-toxin)
Indifference (resist lysosomal enzymes)	—	*Salmonella enterica* var. *typhimurium* *mycobacteria* spp.
—	Protection by surface lipophosphoglycan	*Leishmania* spp.
Disabling (inhibit phagosome— lysosome fusion)	— Redirect phagosomal trafficking Remove host proteins from the phagosomal membrane	Tubercle bacilli *Legionella pneumophila* *Toxoplasma gondii*
Disabling (inhibit oxidative killing)	Inhibit respiratory burst	Virulent salmonellae
—	—	*Legionella pneumophila*
—	Catalase breaks down H_2O_2	*Listeria monocytogenes*
—	—	*S. aureus*
Escape (from phagosome into cytoplasm)	Pore-forming hemolysins Phospholipase	*L. monocytogenes Shigella* Rickettsiae Influenza viruses

release their contents in the cytoplasm, the microbes are protected from lysosomal enzymes in that site. This escape is accomplished by destroying the phagosomal membrane. *L. monocytogenes* secretes a pore-forming toxin, **listeriolysin**, which is required for the phagosomal escape. A phospholipase may also be responsible for weakening the phagosomal membrane.

- **Resistance to lysosomal enzymes**: Some microbes are innately resistant to the lysosomal enzymes and survive in the phagolysosome,. the vesicle formed by fusion of the lysosomes with the phagosomes. An example is the protozoa called *Leishmania*, which causes several severe tropical diseases. Resistance of *Leishmania* to lysosomal enzymes may be a result of resistant cell surfaces and to the excretion of enzyme inhibitors. Note that the pH of the phagolysosome may be as low as 4, which means that leishmaniae can thrive in an extreme environment.

- **Inhibition of the phagocytes' oxidative pathway**: Some microbes, such as *Legionella*, inhibit the hexose monophosphate shunt and oxygen consumption in neutrophils, thus reducing the respiratory burst used by these cells for killing engulfed microbes. Others, such as some staphylococci, produce a powerful catalase that breaks down the hydrogen peroxide necessary for oxidative killing.

Intracellular Life

Many bacteria, protozoa, and fungi have adapted to intracellular existence within the host. This lifestyle is obviously obligatory for viruses but not for organisms capable of free existence. The advantages of a free existence are clear: while inside host cells, the organisms are protected from antibodies and some antimicrobial drugs. However, intracellular residence is not without peril and requires ingenious forms of adaptation. An intense subject of current research, intracellular existence requires the expression of specific microbial genes and the usurpation of normal cell functions. The following paragraphs describe some issues associated with intracellular existence.

Penetration

Penetration of the host cell by a microbe is not a problem when the cell is a professional phagocyte, such as a neutrophil or macrophage. However, taking up microbes is not a normal activity for other types of cells. Thus, penetration is often induced by microbial activities, including binding to specific receptors and sending signals to the interior of the cell that stimulate uptake by rearrangements of the cellular cytoskeleton.

Surviving Host Cell Defenses

As previously mentioned, microbes have developed a repertoire of strategies to avoid or resist antimicrobial factors such as the lysosomal contents. So successful are some parasites that they grow within dedicated antimicrobial cells, such as

macrophages. Members of *Ehrlichia* thrive even within the most powerfully antimicrobial of cells, the neutrophils.

Transmission to Other Cells

When the growth of microbes results in the lysis of the host cell, transmission through the blood or body fluids can take place directly. Other organisms do not impair the cell's integrity, but they can spread from cell to cell directly, without exposing themselves to the extracellular environment. Several viruses spread by causing infected cells to fuse with uninfected, neighboring cells. The histopathology associated with these viral infections (e.g., herpes simplex virus, varicella zoster virus, and respiratory syncytial virus) are notable for the formation of **syncytia** and **multinucleated giant cells**.

Some bacteria can also spread directly from one cell to another. This type of spread is accomplished by making intricate use of the host cytoskeleton. For example, *Shigella* species and *L. monocytogenes* induce polymerization of actin at one of their ends, which results in the formation of a cytoskeletal scaffold at that end (Fig. 8-2). In the electron microscope, this scaffold can be visualized as a cometlike trail behind the bacterium, with actin polymerizing at the "head" and depolymerizing throughout the "tail." As actin is rapidly polymerized and de-polymerized at the tip of the bacterium, the organisms are pushed ahead and can be observed microscopically to be moving through the host cell cytoplasm. If the bacteria reach the cell membrane, they push out fingerlike projections, each containing one bacterium. These projections extend into adjacent cells, where they are eventually engulfed and snipped off. The microbes are now within two sets of membranes: one from the original cell and the other from the neighboring cell. Through production of membrane-damaging enzymes, they cross these membranes into the cytoplasm of a new host cell.

Subverting the Immune Responses

As with their ability to evade phagocytosis, microbes have many ways to avoid clearance by other arms of the immune system. Some of these are aimed broadly at the general immune responsiveness of the host, whereas others more specifically target the precise host response to a specific pathogen.

Immunosuppression

Some infectious agents protect themselves by inducing a general suppression of the host's immune responses. The outcome is that the host becomes susceptible to all kinds of agents and the threat to survival is heightened. Patients infected by immunosuppressive agents may suffer from several concurrent infections, which expands considerably the complexities of their clinical problems. The ability of infectious agents to cause immunodeficiency has reached its known limit with AIDS. Immunodeficiency in this disease is especially profound because HIV, the AIDS

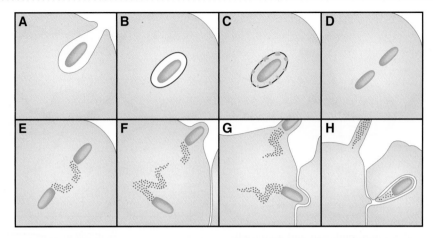

FIGURE 8-2. Actin-dependent intracellular motility and intercellular spread. A. The bacterium is ingested by conventional phagocytosis and resides briefly in a membrane-bound phagosome. **B,C.** The ingested bacterium lyses the phagosomal membrane surrounding it. **D.** After escaping into the cytoplasm, the organism may divide. **E.** Actin polymerizes at one pole of each bacterium. **F.** Continued actin polymerization forms scaffolding that propels the bacteria through the cytoplasm in random directions. **G.** Both bacteria encounter the cell membrane and continue to move outward; one is pushing toward a second cell, the other into an extracellular space. **H.** The second cell has ingested one of the bacteria, its actin tail, and some of the cell membrane and cytoplasm from its neighbor. Eventually, this bacterium will be released into the cytoplasm of the second host cell.

virus, infects the CD4+ (inducer-helper) subset of lymphocytes (see Chapter 6), leading to the collapse of the immune system (see Chapter 38).

The regulatory interactions of the immunocompetent cells may go awry even when lesser changes are introduced into the network. Long before AIDS, it was known that infection with measles virus is immunosuppressive. It had been noticed, for example, that tuberculosis was more common in a community after a widespread measles outbreak. Immunosuppression has been found to follow other viral infections as well, like hepatitis B and influenza. These viruses function more subtly than HIV, impairing the function of lymphoid or myeloid cells without causing major structural changes.

In some cases, immune suppression results from inhibition of the synthesis or of the function of selected cytokines that stimulate the proliferation and differentiation of lymphocytes. Cytokines, themselves the secreted products of inflammatory and immunodirected cells, act to amplify the inflammatory response (see Chapter 6). Mycobacteria, certain viruses, and some multicellular parasites have been shown to affect different steps in the cytokine cascade, perhaps thereby enhancing the pathogen's persistence in the host.

Another mechanism for immune suppression carried out by some bacteria and many viruses is to target the process of antigen presentation carried out by infected cells. To revisit the mechanism of antibody formation or stimulation of a cellular response (see Chapter 7), recall that antigen-presenting cells display on their surfaces the peptides derived from antigens they engulfed. Such peptides are "presented"—that is, reach the cell surface—in association with major histocompatibility complex (MHC) class I or class II molecules. These complexes are recognized by T cells, setting in motion the processes of cell-mediated immunity or specific helper functions to enhance antibody production. Some pathogens specifically disarm MHC class I or class II function, thereby removing a major process for amplifying the immune response.

Diversion of Lymphocyte Function: Superantigens

Certain bacteria and viruses have evolved a particularly insidious strategy to subvert the immune response. Instead of suppressing immune functions, they actually stimulate them but in a manner that squanders these important defensive tools in a nonproductive way. An example are toxins made by certain streptococci, called **superantigens**, which stimulate a **nonspecific T-cell response**. A large subpopulation of T cells is stimulated by superantigens, but these cells have specificities that are mostly unrelated to streptococcal antigens. This misdirection of the immune response not only keeps the host from mounting a proper response but also unleashes a toxic cascade of cytokines.

Superantigens take a shortcut, binding directly to both the MHC molecule (but not at the antigen-binding groove) and the T-cell receptor (but not at the antigen recognition sites; Fig. 8-3). Because it is not dependent on specific antigen recognition, superantigen binding occurs on the surface of many more antigen-presenting cells than is usual and thus leads to the diversion of these cells to nonproductive uses. As an example of why these compounds are known as superantigens, consider that

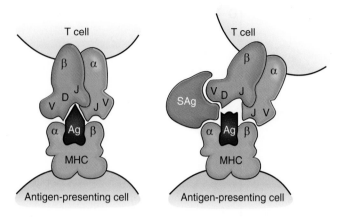

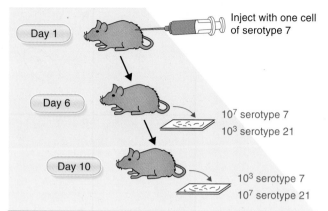

FIGURE 8-3. A comparison of antigen-mediated and superantigen-mediated T-cell activation. Both antigens and superantigens bring antigen-presenting cells and T cells together. Antigens, in conjunction with major histocompatibility complex (MHC) class II molecules, interact with the specific antigen-binding domain of the T-cell receptor (TCR). In contrast, superantigens form a bridge between the two molecules that does not involve the antigen-binding groove. Instead, they bind to a portion of the TCR, the Vβ domain. Every T cell has a TCR with one of numerous Vβ types. Each superantigen binds preferentially to one Vβ type and can activate any T cell carrying that type, regardless of the specificity of the TCR for antigen.

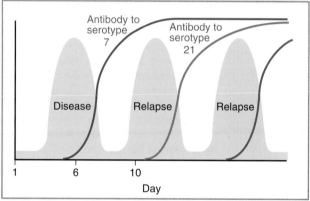

FIGURE 8-4. An experimental infection in which the development of type-specific antibodies against *Borrelia* sp. is associated with the emergence of new antigenic types. The emergence of each new type is associated with a relapse of disease; thus, the common name for these *Borrelia* infections—"relapsing fever." The rapid emergence of the new antigenic types is mediated by successive DNA rearrangement.

normally 1 in 10,000 antigen-presenting cells is stimulated by processed antigens, whereas the figure for superantigens is as high as 1 in 5. The result is an overwhelming, but wholly inappropriate, immune response that can be lethal. The advantage, if any, to the microbe that produces such a response is unclear.

Masquerading by Changing Antigenic Coats

Certain protozoa, bacteria, and viruses are adept at frustrating immune recognition by changing their surface antigens. The classic cases are trypanosomes, gonococci (the agents of relapsing fever), and influenza viruses (see Chapter 14 paradigm).

Trypanosomes One of the best-studied examples of **antigenic variation** is seen with the protozoan that causes sleeping sickness, *Trypanosoma brucei*. The organism affects humans and domestic animals and infects the blood and interstitial fluids. Thus, the organisms are exposed to circulating antibodies. Trypanosomes are covered with a thick protein coat called **variable surface glycoprotein**, which undergoes periodic antigenic changes during the infection. These parasites have several hundred genes that encode for various antigens, but they express only one at a time (see Chapter 50). When antibodies against one type are made, the number of parasites in the blood of an infected host drops, but they are soon replaced by a new antigenic type. There can be many successive waves of antigenically different parasites in a single host. Thus, protective immunity does not function in the long term against this master of disguise.

Gonococci Like the trypanosomes, some bacteria can also switch their surface antigens. For example, gonococcus undergoes periodic changes in **pilin**, which is the protein that makes up its pili, the apparent means of attachment of host cells (see Chapters 3 and 14). This enables multiple new gonococcal infections because the immune response an infected individual may raise to one antigenic type does not protect against a variant that may cause a subsequent infection. The borreliae also undergo antigenic variation of their major surface antigen in a manner that is analogous to the trypanosomes (Fig. 8-4). Thus, the surface of these organisms displays a highly variable antigenic profile to the host immune system, causing relapsing fever every time a new antigenic type emerges.

Influenza Viruses The tendency of influenza to reappear in a population on a regular basis is due in part to the great ability of the influenza virus to change its antigenic composition. This is also the major obstacle to developing a truly effective vaccine against this pathogen. Unlike the processes of antigenic variation in trypanosomes and gonococci, antigenic changes in influenza viruses do not emerge repeatedly within individual hosts. Instead, the novel antigenic types develop gradually in a population of viruses over the course of an epidemic season. Minor changes are called **antigenic drift** and occur every 2 or 3 years. Major antigenic changes, called **antigenic shifts**, take place every 10 years or so. These changes involve two surface proteins: a **hemagglutinin** that serves to bind to cell surface receptors and a **neuraminidase** that changes these receptors. How these proteins are involved in attachment and penetration of the virus is discussed in Chapter 36.

Proteolysis of Antibodies

Certain bacteria—gonococci, meningococci, and *Haemophilus influenzae*—and some dental pathogenic streptococci make extracellular proteases that specifically inactivate antibodies of the secretory IgA class. They cleave IgA molecules at the hinge region to yield complete but relatively ineffective fragments. The proteases are present in active form in tissues and fluids infected by the bacteria that produce them. Nonpathogenic relatives of these organisms are protease negative. The absence of proteases in nonpathogenic bacteria suggests, although it does not prove, a role for IgA proteases in pathogenesis. Other mechanisms, perhaps more subtle, exist for destroying immunoglobulins. For example, staphylococci produce **staphylokinase**, which cleaves host plasminogen into plasmin at the bacterial cell surface. This serine protease then degrades both immunoglobulin G and the complement protein C3b (see Table 8-2), which enables the microbe to avoid opsonization and phagocytosis.

In some instances, it is known that when an organism cleaves IgA, the antigen-binding fragment (Fab) remains attached. The attached Fab fragment makes the antigens unavailable for binding by intact antibody molecules. This phenomenon has been called **fabulation** (after "Fab") and may serve to protect organisms from antibodies. Fabulation may be more widely used by pathogens than is currently known.

Latency

The more long-lived an infection, the more lasting must be the mechanisms for microbial evasion of host defenses. This tenet is well illustrated in herpes infection. To limit access from circulating defenses, herpes viruses do not usually enter the extracellular fluid but pass from cell to cell over cytoplasmic bridges. Intracellular herpesviruses reside within certain cells but do not proliferate; therefore, such a virus can avoid a host response and remain in a state called **latency** (see Chapters 41 and 42). A latent virus is not affected by antibodies, cell-mediated immunity, or interferon and can survive for a long time in an immunocompetent host without symptoms emerging. Later, often when the host's defenses have subsided, the virus may reactivate to cause disease and perhaps even cancer. Latency is not restricted to viruses, as the tubercle bacillus *Mycobacterium tuberculosis* (see Chapter 23) can also become latent within the host for long periods of time.

Slightly distinct from latency is a state of chronic infection, in which the microbe remains in an active infectious state at low level within the host. Some pathogenic bacteria remain in chronic association with the host, often with limited host response that is insufficient for clearing the infection. An important example is *Helicobacter pylori*, which causes gastric ulcers and probably is responsible for gastric adenocarcinomas (see Chapter 22).

TRANSMISSION TO A NEW HOST

Infectious agents are carried into a new host through food, drinks, aerosols, bites, or sexual contact or by introduction into a wound from the skin or soil. Although these modes of transmission may seem passive, many infectious agents contribute actively to their transmission to new hosts. They do this by taking on traits specific for transmission or by producing molecules that cause the host to participate in transmissions.

Many microbes **differentiate** into a **transit form**, a stage in their life cycle that helps them survive in the environment and in reservoirs or, if vectorborne, in insects. Among the animal parasites, transit forms usually differ greatly in structure and function from those that cause disease in the host, as in the case of worms or the protozoa that cause malaria. Note that living reservoirs and vectors shield infectious agents from deleterious environmental factors and obviate the need for the transit form to be highly resistant. In certain bacteria, such as the chlamydiae, the transit form (in this case called the elementary body) becomes encased in a tough envelope composed of highly cross-linked proteins (see Chapter 27). The chlamydia elemental body is thus reminiscent of the bacterial spore, the environmentally "tough" life form par excellence. In other bacteria, changes are more subtle and are revealed at the level of selective expression of certain genes, such as those involved in entering the stationary phase of growth.

An active area of investigation is how infectious agents know where they are—that is, how they express different sets of genes outside and inside the body. The problems of transit are minimized when contact between hosts is direct and the agent is not subjected to prolonged exposure to the environment. In this context, it is logical that many sexually transmitted agents do not appear to have developed tough transit forms. For example, the gonococci, the treponemes of syphilis, and HIV are particularly sensitive to drying and chemicals (chlamydiae may be an exception).

Microbes can actively **potentiate** their spread from one host to another, thus providing themselves with new feeding grounds. Examples are organisms that cause diarrhea (e.g., *Vibrio cholerae* and pathogenic strains of *E. coli* or *Shigella*), which is an effective way of spreading large amounts of bacteria-laden intestinal contents in the environment. Agents that induce coughing (e.g., *M. tuberculosis*) lead to their dispersal via aerosols, and those that produce exudative lesions on the skin (e.g., *Streptococcus pyogenes*) are transmitted through the contamination of objects or skin.

Some of the mechanisms developed by microbes for actively enhancing their transmission seem fiendishly clever. For example, the agent of plague, *Yersinia pestis*, is transmitted from an infected human to another by a flea bite. These bacteria greatly increase the efficiency of this transmission by making the flea feel hungry. How do the bacteria enhance the flea's appetite? The plague bacilli reproduce within the digestive tract of infected fleas, eventually causing blockage. To ward off starvation, the "blocked fleas" feed repeatedly and, during each feeding, regurgitate some of the contaminated material, thus increasing the chances of infecting a new host. Not all pathogens that are transmitted by insects use such a mechanism, but it should not be surprising that many microbes alter an arthropod vector's behavior to enhance their own survival and transmissibility.

CONCLUSION

The ways of microbes that must make a living by interacting with hosts are as complex and varied as the mechanisms that have evolved in hosts to avoid infection. The story of microbial diseases is one of progressively escalating rounds of response and counterresponse from each side, the microbe and the host. The measures taken by each can be general or very specific; for every constitutive immune mechanism that hosts have to protect themselves, there is a microbe out there with the capacity to avoid it. Likewise, although the development of specific immunity is generally very effective for protecting against second infection, some microbes have developed impressive ways to steer clear of that response. The exquisite specificity of these responses points to coevolution of hosts and microbes. Given that microbes can go through multiple generations in a very short time and that they are constantly subject to new selection pressures, it is not surprising to find remarkable variation among pathogenic species.

Suggested Readings

Coombes BK, Valdez Y, Finlay BB. Evasive maneuvers by secreted bacterial proteins to avoid innate immune responses. *Curr Biol.* 2004;14:R856–R867.

Cossart P, Sansonetti PJ. Bacterial invasion: the paradigms of enteroinvasive pathogens. *Science.* 2004;304:242–248.

Deitsch KW, Lukehart SA, Stringer JR. Common strategies for antigenic variation by bacterial, fungal and protozoan pathogens. *Nat Rev Microbiol.* 2009;7:493–503.

Gouin E, Welch MD, Cossart P. Actin-based motility of intracellular pathogens. *Curr Opin Microbiol.* 2005;8:35–45.

Rautemaa R, Meri S. Complement-resistance mechanisms of bacteria. *Microbes Infect.* 1999;1:785–794.

Schwarz-Linek U, Hook M, Potts JR. The molecular basis of fibronectin-mediated bacterial adherence to host cells. *Mol Microbiol.* 2004;52:631–641.

Urban CF, Lourido S, Zychlinsky A. How do microbes evade neutrophil killing? *Cell Microbiol.* 2006;8:1687–1696.

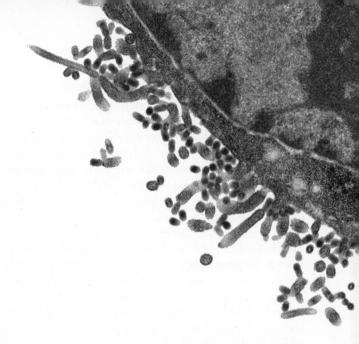

Chapter **9**

Damage by Microbial Toxins

Joseph T. Barbieri

INFECTIOUS diseases inflict many kinds of damage to host tissues and organs. Advances in our understanding of the action of microbial toxins, coupled with our progress in understanding the molecular biology of the human cell, provide a framework to understand the molecular basis for microbial pathogenesis and the host response to infection. Damage during the infectious processes may be caused by the direct action of the microbial pathogen or by the host response to infection. These actions are often interrelated, and both are usually active during an infection. This chapter presents an overview of the cellular damage that occurs during infection and provides detailed descriptions of the major classes of microbial toxins.

MECHANISMS THAT DAMAGE THE HOST DURING INFECTIONS

Cell Death

The most dramatic effect of a microbial infection is the death of cells in host tissues. The pathology associated with cell death depends on the type and number of cells involved and the speed of the infectious process. If the infected cells are a component of an essential organ, such as the heart or the brain, the outcome is likely to be serious and could be fatal. For example, myocarditis, an infection of the heart muscle, is a fulminating and deadly disease when caused by the coxsackievirus. This virus is also thought to kill the insulin-producing cells of the islets of the pancreas and may be one cause of infantile diabetes. During a microbial infection, two mechanisms lead to cell death: cell lysis and programmed cell death.

Lysis of host cells occurs in three ways:

- The microorganism produces a toxin that affects the integrity of the cell membranes. In patients with **gas gangrene**, membrane-damaging toxins produced by one of the anaerobic clostridia lyse red blood cells.
- The microorganism multiplies within the host cell, leading to cell lysis from the inside. This is seen in **Rocky Mountain spotted fever**, which derives its name from the skin rash produced when endothelial cells of small vessels are killed by the intracellular growth of

rickettsiae with the release of peroxide that damages membranes.

- The microorganism multiplies in the host cell, but the infected cells are eradicated by cytotoxic lymphocytes or natural killer cells as the result of triggering **cell-mediated immunity**. This is observed when microorganisms that do not cause cell lysis directly, such as many viruses or mycobacteria, grow intracellularly.

The alternative mode of cell death is programmed cell death, or **apoptosis**. This process is a normal part of the mammalian cell cycle that ensures the maintenance of healthy cells. Some microorganisms, such as *Shigella* (the agent of dysentery), usurp this process when invading the host cell. This may explain why *Shigella* survives after being taken up by phagocytes. Some viruses, such as herpes simplex virus and HIV, may stimulate cells to undergo premature apoptosis. In contrast, viruses, like the Epstein-Barr virus, block apoptosis and thereby immortalize the host cell.

Pathological Alterations of Metabolism

Certain infections do not kill cells directly but result in some of the most severe diseases, such as **tetanus**, **botulism**, **cholera**, and **whooping cough**. The pathology of each of these diseases is the result of a bacterium-produced toxin that alters a key aspect of metabolism in ways that resemble the action of hormones or other pharmacological effectors.

Mechanical Causes of Damage

If present in sufficient numbers, infectious agents can obstruct vital passages. Although rare, such mechanical obstructions do occur in children with an overload of worms in their intestines. A heavy infestation with the large roundworm *Ascaris* (15 to 35 cm long and about 0.5 cm thick) can cause occlusion of the intestinal lumen. A single worm may also migrate into the common bile duct and obstruct the passage of bile.

Often, mechanical obstruction results not from the microorganism but from the inflammatory response of the host. In **elephantiasis**, an enormous swelling of limbs or the scrotum is caused when small worms, called filariae, become lodged in lymphatics. The worms stimulate a tissue reaction that occludes the vessels, causing swelling and tissue hypertrophy. Almost any duct or tubelike organ, thick or thin, can be obstructed during an infection, sometimes with life-threatening consequences. Inflammation of the epiglottis may impede the passage of air; infection of the meninges can cause hydrocephalus (a dilatation of the cerebral ventricles resulting from obstruction of the flow of cerebrospinal fluid); infection of the prostate can obstruct the flow of urine from the bladder; and an inflammatory reaction to the eggs of the liver fluke may result in severe disturbances of the portal circulation.

Damage Caused by Host Responses

The symptoms of infectious diseases are typically the product of the microbial pathogen and the host's response to infection. The host response is rarely so finely tuned that only the infection is controlled. In gonorrhea, the gonococci set off the host response, an inflammation that accompanies copious pus production (pus comprises the products of dead immune cells) and swelling and accounts for disease symptoms. Likewise, in many chronic infections, like tuberculosis, damage to tissues is caused by chronic inflammation.

The host response to infection is often owing to both **inflammation** and the **immune response**. The importance of these mechanisms cannot be overemphasized. Both operate in acute and chronic diseases and can manifest either locally or systemically. The mechanisms involved in inflammation are discussed in detail in Chapter 6, and those involved in immunopathology are discussed in Chapter 7. The role of inflammation and the immune response on cell damage will be further emphasized in chapters on individual diseases, where they may occupy center stage.

Examples of host responses to infection leading to harmful outcomes for the host include (1) the accentuated inflammatory response that places patients with a brain abscess at risk of dying, (2) the overwhelming activation of the **complement** system that kills patients suffering from septicemia, (3) an autoimmune response that causes rheumatic fever, and (4) cell-mediated immunity responsible for manifestations of chronic tuberculosis. In circumstances like these, medical intervention is required to attenuate the inflammatory response to infectious disease. Although the overexpression of the host response contributes greatly to the immediate signs and symptoms of disease, it also helps the host survive. This is illustrated by tuberculosis, a chronic disease that some patients live with for many years. However, if the host response is defective, as in AIDS, tuberculosis can progress rapidly to a lethal infection.

BACTERIAL TOXINS

Traditionally, bacterial toxins have been understood as being protein molecules that kill a host cell. The term has become defined more broadly now to describe a range of proteins that alter the normal metabolism of host cells with deleterious effects on the host. Toxins are often responsible for the major symptoms of a bacterial infection. Knowledge of how toxins work fosters an understanding of the pathophysiology of many infectious diseases and, in some instances, reveals important information about normal cellular processes of the host. The role of many toxins in causing disease has been studied in detail and will be described in chapters on specific bacterial pathogens. Here, the discussion focuses on the basic concept of how bacterial toxins damage the host. Although many toxins have been associated with bacterial diseases, toxins have not been implicated as important components of diseases caused by fungi, protozoa, or worms. Bacterial toxins are categorized by their site of action in the host. **Exotoxins**, **type III cytotoxins**, and the more recently recognized **type IV to VII cytotoxins** modulate intracellular targets (Fig. 9-1); **endotoxin**, **membrane-damaging toxins**, and **superantigens** act on the cell surface (Fig. 9-2); and **exoenzymes** modulate targets in the extracellular matrix.

Toxins that Modulate Intracellular Targets

Toxins that modulate intracellular targets modify host targets through covalent mechanisms. Exotoxins are organized into three distinct domains that can bind surface receptors and stimulate the translocation of a catalytic domain into the cytosol of the host cell. In contrast, bacteria directly inject type III cytotoxins into the host cell.

Exotoxins

Exotoxins are proteins usually secreted by the bacterium into the surrounding medium by the type I secretion system (an autotransport system built into the toxin) or the type II secretion system (an apparatus within the bacterial cell membrane), which transport toxins out of the bacterial cell. Occasionally, exotoxins are bound to the surface or synthesized in the cytoplasm of the bacterium and released on lysis of the cell. Exotoxins circulate throughout the host, attach to receptors on the surface of sensitive

Exotoxins (AB)   **Type III cytotoxins**

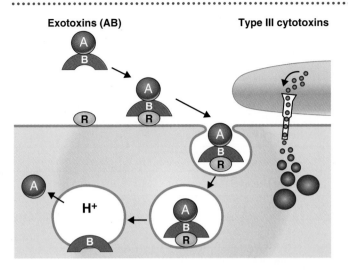

FIGURE 9-1. Bacterial toxins that modify intracellular host proteins. Most bacterial exotoxins bind to receptors on the surface of host cells and travel into the intracellular environment using the host's endocytotic pathway. Upon maturation, the endosome acidifies, stimulating a conformational change in the **B** domain, which inserts into the endosome membranes to generate a pore that translocates the **A** domain into the cytosol. Type III cytotoxins are synthesized in the cytosol of the bacterium and are delivered into the host cell by the type III secretion system. Thus, the bacterium provides the **B** domain function. Once inside the cell, type III cytotoxins subvert host cell physiology by direct cytotoxicity or by modulation of the host actin cytoskeleton. Recent studies have identified type IV to VII secretion systems for delivery of cytotoxins outside the bacterium.

cells, and possess the ability to become internalized into the host cell and then delivered into the intracellular compartment of the host cell (see Fig. 9-1). Bacterial exotoxins vary in their specificity; some act only on specific cells, while others affect a wide range of cells and tissues. Some bacteria make a single toxin, while other bacteria produce numerous toxins (Table 9-1). Some bacteria, like the pneumococci, make no known toxins and probably cause disease by toxin-independent mechanisms.

For each toxin-producing pathogen, it is ideal to know whether the toxin is important in the infectious process. Answering the following questions can help make that determination:

- Does the toxin alone, in purified form, damage the host, using animals or cultured cells as experimental hosts?
- Is virulence quantitatively correlated with toxin production?
- Can a specific antibody (antitoxin) prevent or alleviate the manifestations of the disease?
- If toxin production is impaired in the pathogen, is the disease process affected?

When a toxin contributes to the infectious process, the following questions need to be answered:

- What is the toxin's mechanism of action?
- Why does the toxin damage certain cells or tissues?
- Does the pathogen make other toxins? Do these toxins interact during an infection?

These questions are easiest to answer when a single toxin is responsible for the symptoms of the disease, which is the case in cholera, diphtheria, tetanus, and botulism. In contrast, many pathogenic bacteria, such as staphylococci, streptococci, pseudomonads, and bordetellae, make several toxins. In such multifactorial situations, the importance of any one toxin is difficult to assess.

Toxins share with antibiotics an ambivalent position in the life of the pathogen that produces them. On the one hand, toxins are dispensable because they are not required for bacterial growth. On the other hand, toxins may be essential for the survival and spread of the bacteria within the host. Reflecting their dispensability, the genes that encode toxins are frequently contained within DNA elements that are themselves dispensable: **plasmids** and **temperate bacteriophages**. The locations of these genes on mobile DNA molecules ensure that the ability to produce toxin can rapidly spread to nontoxigenic bacteria. Conversely, these genetic

Pattern recognition receptors   **Pore-forming toxins**   **Superantigens**

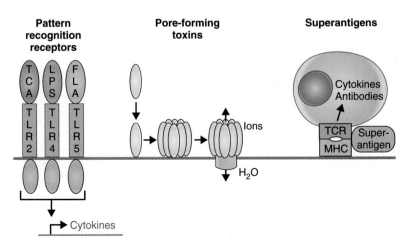

FIGURE 9-2. Toxins that act on the surface of host cells. Pattern recognition receptors include lipoteichoic acid (TCA), the endotoxin lipopolysaccharide (LPS), and flagella (FLA), which bind to specific toll-like receptor (TLR) proteins. Binding to the TLR stimulates intracellular signal transduction, which results in the production of cytokines that activate both the innate and adaptive immune systems. Pore-forming toxins bind to the host's cell membrane and polymerize to form a pore that allows ions and water to pass. Superantigens bind to the MHC and T-cell receptor (TCR) to stimulate an antigen-independent production of antibodies and cytokines.

TABLE 9-1 Major Toxinogenic Organisms

Organism (Toxin and AB Organization Component)	Effect	Mechanism
Bacillus anthracis		
Anthrax toxin 2A + B	Required for other toxins	Receptor-binding domain
Protective antigen B		
Edema factor A	Edema	Adenylate cyclase
Lethal factor A	Pulmonary edema	Protease
Bordetella pertussis		
Adenylate cyclase toxin AB	Inhibits, kills white cells	Adenylate cyclase
Pertussis toxin AB5	Many hormonal effects	ADP ribosylation of G protein
Tracheal cytotoxin	Kills cilia-bearing cells	Unknown
Clostridium botulinum		
Botulinum toxin AB	Neurotoxin	Inhibits synaptic vesicle fusion to the plasma membrane at the neuromuscular junction; flaccid paralysis
Clostridium difficile		
Enterotoxin	Hemorrhagic diarrhea	Acts at membrane
Toxin A and Toxin B	Cytoplasmic; cells lose filaments	Deamidation of Rho GTPase
Clostridia spp.		
α-toxin	Necrosis in gas gangrene; cytolytic, lethal	Phospholipase C
β-toxin	Necrotic enteritis	Unknown
Enterotoxin	Food poisoning; diarrhea	Cytotoxin; damages membranes
Clostridium tetani		
Tetanus toxin AB	Neurotoxin	Inhibits synaptic vesicle fusion with the plasma membrane nerve terminals at inhibitor synapses; spastic paralysis
Corynebacterium diphtheriae		
Diphtheria toxin AB	Kills cells	ADP-ribosylates elongation factor 2
Escherichia coli (enterics)		
Heat-labile enterotoxin AB5	Diarrhea	Identical to cholera toxin
Cytotoxin	Hemorrhagic colitis	Like shiga toxin
Heat-stable enterotoxin	Diarrhea	Activates host guanylate cyclase
Legionella pneumophila		
Cytotoxin	Lyses cells	Unknown
Type IV cytotoxins	Inhibit endosome maturation	Interfere with Rab protein function

TABLE 9-1 Major Toxinogenic Organisms (*continued*)

Organism (Toxin and AB Organization Component)	Effect	Mechanism
Listeria monocytogenes		
Listeriolysin	Membrane damage	Like streptolysin O
Pseudomonas aeruginosa		
Exotoxin A	Kills cells	Like diphtheria toxin
Type III cytotoxins	Modulate host cell physiology	Inhibit actin cytoskeleton
Salmonella		
Type III cytotoxins	Modulate host cell physiology	Alter actin cytoskeleton
Shigella dysenteriae		
Shiga toxin	Kills cells	Inactivates 60S ribosomes
Staphylococcus aureus		
α-toxin	Hemolytic, leukocytic, paralysis of smooth muscle	Pore-forming toxin
β-toxin	Cytolytic	Sphingomyelinase
δ-lysin	Cytolytic	Detergent-like action
Superantigens		
Enterotoxins	Food poisoning (emesis, diarrhea)	Activate host antibody and cytokine synthesis by an antigen independent mechanism
Toxic shock syndrome toxin	Fever, headache, arthralgia, neutropenia, rash	Activates host antibody and cytokine synthesis by an antigen-independent mechanism
Exfoliating toxin	Sloughing of skin ("scalded skin syndrome")	Protease
Streptococcus pneumonia		
Pneumolysin	Cytolysin	Similar to streptolysin O
Streptococcus pyogenes		
Streptolysin O	Cytolysin	Pore-forming toxin
Erythrogenic toxin	Fever, neutropenia, rash of scarlet fever	Mediated through IL-1
Vibrio cholerae		
Cholera toxin AB5	Diarrhea	Hormone-independent activation of adenyl cyclase
Yersinia enterocolitica		
Heat-stable enterotoxin	Diarrhea	Activates host guanylate cyclase
Type III cytotoxins	Modulate host cell physiology	Regulate actin cytoskeleton

ADP, adenosine diphosphate; GABA, gamma-aminobutyric acid; IL, interleukin.

elements may be lost by "curing" the bacteria of plasmids or prophages. Some toxins are produced continuously by growing bacteria; others are synthesized when the bacteria enter the **stationary phase**. The latter is often also true for antibiotics and other "secondary metabolites," which are produced as growth stops or slows down. In some instances, producing toxin only when the growth rate slows makes sense, because the toxin may help the bacterium obtain nutrients that have become scarce. Thus, high levels of diphtheria toxin are produced only when the diphtheria bacilli are iron starved. Because little free iron exists in normal tissues, it is believed that pathogenic bacteria obtain iron from cells killed by the toxin.

Sporulating bacteria sometimes release toxins during **spore formation**. In this process the bacterial cells in which the spores are formed eventually lyse, leading to the liberation of cytoplasmic proteins—including accumulated toxins. Sporulating bacteria that make potent exotoxins include the organisms that cause botulism, gas gangrene, and tetanus, which are of the genus *Clostridium*, and the organism that causes anthrax, which is of the genus *Bacillus*. In a heterogeneous environment, such as a contaminated wound, some organisms are growing and others are sporulating. In such an environment, toxins will be produced continuously during the course of the infection.

Bacterial toxins work at extraordinarily low concentrations and are among the strongest poisons for humans. One gram of tetanus, botulinum, or shiga toxin can kill about 10 million people; thus, 1 pound could theoretically kill all humankind. In contrast, humans are about a 100-fold more resistant to the action of diphtheria toxin.

Structure-Function Organization of Exotoxins

Many exotoxins are proteins with an **A** domain and a **B** domain (Fig. 9-3). The B domain binds to the cell membrane and delivers the A domain into the host cell. The **A** domain possesses enzymatic activity that is specific for each toxin. One example of an enzymatic reaction catalyzed by bacteria toxins is the adenosine diphosphate (ADP) ribosylation of host proteins, resulting from the covalent transfer of ADP ribose from the coenzyme nicotinamide adenine dinucleotide (NAD) to target proteins. These **ADP ribosyltransferases** are exemplified by diphtheria toxin, cholera toxin, and exotoxin A of *Pseudomonas aeruginosa*. Other exotoxins express different enzymatic activities and may act as proteases, glucosyltransferases, or deamidases.

Exotoxins are organized in various ways. An exotoxin can be a single **AB** protein in which the **A** and **B** domains are covalently joined, as observed in diphtheria toxin, or it can be a complex of six proteins noncovalently bound with the stoichiometry of **AB5**, as seen in cholera toxin. Some exotoxins, such as anthrax toxin, are synthesized by bacteria as independent proteins that associate on the host cell membrane (**2A + B**). Anthrax toxin is a tripartite toxin with two A domains produced:

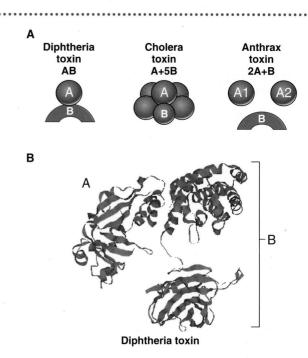

FIGURE 9-3. AB organizations of bacterial exotoxins. A. The three common structural organizations of bacterial exotoxins, in which the **A** domain is the catalytic domain and the **B** domain is the binding domain. Diphtheria toxin is an **AB** toxin, with the **A** and **B** domains covalently aligned within a single protein. Cholera toxin is an **AB5** toxin, with six peptides noncovalently bound in a complex. Anthrax toxin is a 2**A** + **B** toxin, in which the proteins are expressed as independent proteins that associate on the host cell membrane. **B.** Diphtheria toxin has a three-dimensional structure. The **B** domain is divided into two domains, which are involved in two sequential steps in the intoxication process: receptor binding and translocation of the **A** domain into the host cell.

one **A** domain is an adenylate cyclase (termed the edema factor), and the second **A** domain is a protease (termed the lethal factor).

Exotoxins are synthesized as protoxins that must be activated on binding to the host cell membrane. Diphtheria, cholera, tetanus, and shiga toxins must be activated to become toxic. Activation usually involves a proteolytic cleavage and reduction of a disulfide bond that often holds the **A** and **B** domains together.

After binding to the cell membrane, exotoxins are typically internalized into the cell by a **receptor-mediated endocytosis** mechanism. During this process the **A** domain is translocated across the cell membrane and into the intracellular compartment of the host cell, where this enzymatic domain modifies host components. Although host proteins are the typical targets for modification, shiga toxin inhibits host protein synthesis by modifying RNA.

While diphtheria and cholera toxins are members of the ADP-ribosylating family of exotoxins, the botulinum and tetanus toxins are neurotoxins, which are zinc proteases. The molecular aspects of these exotoxins are described in the following paragraphs.

Diphtheria Toxin   The diphtheria toxin inhibits cell physiology by blocking host cell protein synthesis. After binding to a cell membrane receptor (a derivative of a host growth factor receptor), diphtheria toxin is cleaved at a protease-sensitive site between the **A** and **B** domains, which remain covalently associated by disulfide linkage. The diphtheria toxin–receptor complex then enters the cell by receptor-mediated endocytosis, just like hormones and many enveloped viruses. Once inside the endosomal vesicle, the acidic conditions within the vesicle promote insertion of a portion of the **B** domain into the endosomal membrane, which forms a pore to facilitate passage of the **A** domain into the cytosol. Thus, the **B** domain contributes three functions for the delivery of the **A** domain into the cytosol: receptor binding, transport into the endosome, and a translocation function for the A domain into the cytosol. During translocation, the disulfide bond is reduced, and the **A** and **B** domains separate, allowing the **A** domain to enter the cytosol. The **A** domain ADP-ribosylates elongation factor 2 (EF-2), a factor in eukaryotic protein synthesis that catalyzes the hydrolysis of guanosine 5′-triphosphate (GTP) required for the movement of ribosomes on messenger RNA. The A domain remains active for a long time inside cells, which in part accounts for its potency, because internalization of a single A domain is sufficient to kill a cell.

ADP ribosylation of EF-2 by diphtheria toxin

$$EF\text{-}2 + NAD^+ \rightarrow ADP - \text{ribosylated } EF\text{-}2 + \text{nicotinamide} + H^+$$

EF-2 is the only known substrate for diphtheria toxin. The reason for this specificity is that EF-2 contains a rare modification in one of its histidine residues, and this is the site at which diphtheria toxin ADP-ribosylates EF-2. Mutant mammalian cells lacking this modified histidine are resistant to diphtheria toxin. The addition of ADP ribose inactivates EF-2 and kills cells by irreversibly blocking protein synthesis.

Cholera Toxin   The cholera toxin, which does not kill the target cell, modulates normal cell functions by elevating the intracellular level of **cyclic adenosine monophosphate (cAMP)**. As a secondary messenger, cAMP regulates numerous cellular functions. The target tissue for cholera toxin is the epithelium of the small intestine. Cholera toxin is composed of six noncovalently associated proteins comprising one **A** domain and five identical **B** domains (**AB5**). The **B** pentamer binds specifically to the ganglioside, GM1a, on the intestinal epithelial mucosa. On internalization, the **A** domain of cholera toxin ADP-ribosylates a G protein, which upregulates host adenylate cyclase and produces more intracellular cAMP.

ADP ribosylation of G-protein by cholera toxin

$$\text{G protein } + NAD^+ \rightarrow ADP - \text{ribosylated G protein}$$
$$+ \text{ nicotinamide} + H^+$$

The adenylate cyclase complex is membrane bound in intestinal cells and includes the G protein and the adenylate cyclase. G proteins exist in two conformations: a GTP-bound form that binds and activates adenylate cyclase and a guanosine 5′-diphosphate (GDP)-bound form that is inactive. The GTP-bound form has a short half-life because the G protein possesses GTPase activity that cleaves GTP to GDP. The activity of adenyl cyclase is determined by the nucleotide state of the G protein. Cholera toxin promotes the "active" GTP-bound form of the G protein by the ADP ribosylation of one of its arginine residues. ADP-ribosylated G protein is locked in the active conformation that stimulates adenylate cyclase. The elevated intracellular synthesis of cAMP provokes the movement of massive quantities of ions and water across the intestinal membrane and into the lumen of the gut that is characteristic of the "watery" diarrhea associated with cholera.

Activation of adenylate cyclase by ADP ribosylation of G proteins is a strategy adopted by a number of other diarrhea-producing pathogens, including the heat-labile enterotoxin of *Escherichia coli*. Other toxins, such as pertussis toxin produced by *Bordetella pertussis*, the agent of whooping cough, raise cAMP in leukocytes through the ADP ribosylation of a G protein that is different from the G protein ADP-ribosylated by cholera toxin. The different effects of cholera toxin and pertussis toxin on the host illustrate the importance of the site of bacterial colonization and the targeting of specific host proteins for ADP ribosylation.

Numerous bacterial toxins possess the ability to add an ADP-ribose group host proteins. The specificity of toxins is realized by the observation that each toxin ADP-ribosylates a unique host protein. Thus, while diphtheria toxin and cholera toxin both catalyze the ADP-ribosylation reaction, the pathology that each toxin elicits is unique because each toxin ADP-ribosylates a unique host protein: diphtheria toxin targets EF-2, and cholera toxin targets a G protein.

Botulinum and Tetanus Toxins   Because they act on the nervous system, the botulinum and tetanus toxins are collectively called **neurotoxins**. Botulinum toxin is the most potent protein toxin to humans and recently has been implicated as a potential agent of **bioterrorism**. Tetanus toxin produces irreversible muscle contraction, yielding spastic paralysis, while botulinum toxin blocks muscle contraction, yielding flaccid paralysis. These neurotoxins are produced by anaerobic spore-forming bacteria of the genus *Clostridium*. Tetanus and botulinum toxins, like diphtheria toxin, are single proteins that contain **A** and **B** domains. Their actions as neurotoxins are based on the specific binding of the B domain to receptors on the surface of neurons and the targeting of neuron-specific host proteins. The **A** domain is a protease that cleaves intracellular proteins responsible for the fusion of intracellular synaptic vesicles with the plasma membrane. The specific pathology associated with each neurotoxin is based on its ability to migrate to unique locations in the nervous system to inactivate specific steps in neuronal signaling. Both neurotoxins enter peripheral nerve cells through receptor-mediated endocytosis. Once inside the endosome, the A domain of botulinum toxin is delivered into the cytoplasm to inactive vesicle fusion at the peripheral nerve ending, which inhibits the release of **stimulatory neurotransmitters**, such as **acetylcholine**, resulting in flaccid paralysis. Tetanus toxin migrates up the axon, across the interneuronal junction, and into inhibitory neurons, where its **A** domain inactivates vesicle fusion at the interneuronal junction to inhibit the release of **inhibitory neurotransmitters**, resulting in spastic paralysis. In tetanus and botulism, the excitatory and inhibitory effects of motor neurons become increasingly unbalanced, which can lead to death from decreased ventilation.

Tetanus is caused by the introduction of the **tetanus bacilli** into the host, typically through the penetration of a foreign object, such as a rusty nail. Although the bacillus rarely moves from its location in a wound, tetanus toxin is released by the bacterium and travels to the central nervous system to produce the symptoms of tetanus, which are distanced from the site of infection. Thus, tetanus is a good example of a disease resulting from a single toxin acting on a distant target. Botulism occurs from the production of botulinum toxin on the infection of the intestine of an infant by *Clostridium botulinum* (**infant botulism**) or from the ingestion of botulinum toxin made in food contaminated by *C. botulinum* and stored under anaerobic conditions, such as improperly sterilized canned foods. The latter is therefore a true intoxication; it does not require the presence of the bacterium to cause symptoms and pathology.

Type III Cytotoxins

Some pathogenic bacteria can secrete **type III cytotoxins** (see Fig. 9-1) directly into the host cell by a **contact-dependent** mechanism when the bacterium directly contacts the host cell. The proteins that collectively comprise the type III secretion system (T3SS) have been termed the **injectisome** and are considered potentially good targets for development of broad therapeutics against a wide range of pathogens. The stimuli provided by the host cell to initiate the T3SS are not well characterized but may include temperature, oxygen tension, and salt concentration. On contact with the mammalian cells, the bacterium uses T3SS apparatus to generate a pore in the host cell membrane that delivers the type III cytotoxin directly into the cytosol of the host cell. Type III cytotoxins are delivered efficiently and are not likely to contact neutralizing antibodies. Numerous bacteria, including *Salmonella*, *Shigella*, *Pseudomonas*, the cholera bacilli, and the plague bacilli, deliver type III cytotoxins into host cells (see Chapter 17 paradigm). Type III cytotoxins vary in their mechanism of action but often interfere with the ability of the host to respond to infection by direct cell killing or through the modulation of the actin cytoskeleton. A functional actin cytoskeleton is required for the efficient phagocytosis of pathogens by macrophages and other phagocytes.

Type IV to VII Cytotoxins

While the type III cytotoxins are the prototypes for bacterial delivered toxins, recent studies have identified additional bacterial secretion systems that deliver cytotoxins across the bacterial outer membrane and into either the environment or directly into host cells, termed type **IV to VII secretion** systems. The type IV secretion system is a multiprotein complex that was originally shown to transfer DNA between bacteria through conjugation and subsequently to transport cytotoxins into host cells. Type IV secretion contributes in the pathogenesis of several intracellular bacterial pathogens, including *Legionella*, *Brucella*, and *Coxiella*. The type V secretion system has autotransporter features. IgA1 protease, which cleaves mammalian IgA, is secreted through a type V system similar to that produced by several genera of bacteria. More recently, type VI secretion system has been described in *Vibrio cholerae* and *Pseudomonas aeruginosa*, while a type VII secretion system was identified in the mycobacteria and some Gram-positive bacteria. Current studies are addressing the properties of the expanding mechanisms utilized by bacteria to deliver cytotoxins across the outer membrane. As with T3SS, these specialized secretion systems may be attractive targets for development of novel therapeutics against bacterial pathogens.

Toxins that Act at the Host Cell Surface

Surface-acting toxins bind to the cell membrane and modulate host cell physiology without having to enter the intracellular compartment of the cell. Modulation can affect host cell signaling or through the direct damage to the cell membrane.

Endotoxin

Endotoxin is the **lipopolysaccharide (LPS)** of the outer membrane of Gram-negative bacteria (see Fig. 3-2) and plays an important role in the diseases caused by those organisms. At low concentrations, endotoxin elicits a series of **alarm reactions**: fever, activation of complement by the alternative pathway, activation of macrophages, and stimulation of B lymphocytes. At high concentrations, it produces **shock** and even death. The term *endotoxin* is misleading on two counts: endotoxin is not internalized, and it exerts a toxic effect only at high concentrations. Recent studies have highlighted the importance of endotoxin in the host response to infection. Endotoxin is one of several structural components of microorganisms that

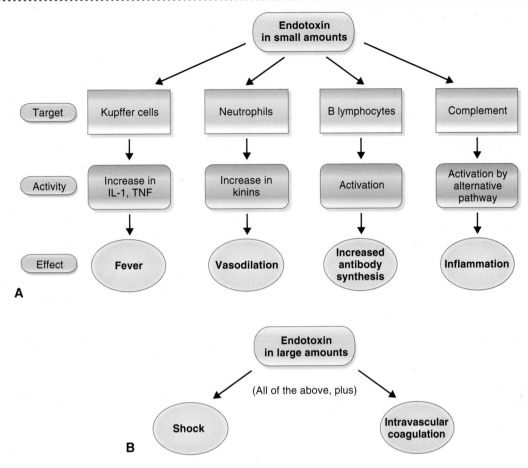

FIGURE 9-4. The action of endotoxin at low and high concentrations.

stimulate our innate immune system as an early indication of infection. These structural components have been referred to as **pattern recognition receptors** (see Fig. 9-2) and are highly conserved among microorganisms. Pattern recognition receptors include endotoxin from Gram-negative bacteria, lipoteichoic acid from Gram-positive bacteria, lipoglycans from the mycobacteria, and mannans from yeast. Early activation of our **innate immune system** by pattern recognition receptors provide us with a rapid and effective response to infection and is the catalyst for activating our **adaptive immune system**, which is responsible for long-term resistance to infection.

Chemistry of Endotoxin   As discussed in Chapter 3, bacterial LPS is composed of three parts: a glycolipid called **lipid A**; a **core** of sugars, ethanolamine, and phosphate; and the **O antigen**, a long side chain of species-specific, often unusual sugars (see Fig. 3-6). Lipid A is the biologically active component, while the other components serve as carriers. Lipid A alone is water insoluble and inert, but its activity is restored when complexed with large-molecular-weight carriers, such as proteins. The

structure of lipid A is unusual: it contains uniquely short fatty acids (12, 14, and 16 carbons in length).

Endotoxin has different pharmacological effects when delivered at low or high concentrations (Fig. 9-4): in small amounts, endotoxin sets off a series of alarm reactions, and in large amounts, **shock** is induced. The extent to which these complex events overlap depends not only on the amount of endotoxin but also on the route of injection and the previous exposure of the host to this substance.

The primary targets for endotoxin are mononuclear phagocytes (peripheral blood monocytes, macrophages of the spleen, bone marrow, lung alveoli, peritoneal cavity, and Kupffer cells), **neutrophils**, **platelets**, and **B lymphocytes**. These cells possess specific endotoxin receptors, called **toll-like receptors** (**TLRs**). There are several TLRs that recognize different pattern recognition receptors. The binding of the pattern recognition receptors to TLRs stimulates a signal transduction cascade within the cell. This results in the production of proteins known as **cytokines**, which induce "alarm reactions" such as fever, activation of complement, activation of macrophages, and stimulation of B lymphocytes (see Fig. 9-2).

Fever In the words of the pioneering immunopathologist Lewis Thomas, endotoxin acts like propaganda: it tells the body that bacteria are present. Endotoxin in small amounts is **pyrogenic**; that is, it elicits **fever**, a common sign of infection. About 100 ng (0.1 μg) of endotoxin injected intravenously in an adult human volunteer will produce a measurable pyrogenic response. Note that this amount comes from about 10 million enteric bacteria, which is not a particularly large number of microbes; the normal intestinal microbiota contains perhaps 1 million times more bacteria. If all the endotoxin in the intestine were to enter the bloodstream, and if fever followed an absurdly linear response, body temperature would rise to about 1 million degrees. Obviously, the amount of endotoxin that spills over from the intestine into the circulation is quite small. Nonetheless, endotoxin serves as a constant low-level stimulation of the immune response in healthy people, without pathological manifestations. Low titers of antibodies to endotoxin are found in most healthy persons.

Fever induced by endotoxin during activation of the innate immune system is caused by the release of cytokines from mononuclear phagocytes. The best-characterized cytokines are **interleukin-1** (**IL-1**) and **tumor necrosis factor** (**TNF-α**), which set off a complex series of events known as the **acute phase response** (see Chapter 6). Lipoteichoic acids of Gram-positive bacteria also stimulate the innate immune system with the subsequent release of IL-1 and TNF.

Activation of Complement Endotoxin activates complement by the alternative pathway (see Chapter 6). At a low endotoxin concentration, the most likely consequence to bacteria is the production of the **membrane attack complex** (**MAC**), plus phagocyte chemotaxis and opsonization. Neutrophils are activated and, because of the opsonizing effect of C3b, become available for phagocytosis. Complement activation also leads to the production of **anaphylatoxins** (C3a, C5a), which increase capillary permeability and release of lysosomal enzymes from neutrophils (degranulation). Thus, endotoxin elicits an inflammatory response.

Activation of Macrophages Endotoxin activates **macrophages** to increase the production of lysosomal enzymes, enhance the rate of phagocytosis, and secrete hydrolases. Once activated, macrophages become superscavengers, ingesting large numbers of invading microorganisms. Their high activation state extends to killing certain cancer cells, partly by direct attachment and partly by releasing proteins such as TNF. The ability of endotoxin, through macrophages, to limit the growth of certain tumors has been recognized for some time and is the subject of continued investigation. Endotoxin derivatives belong to a class of potential anticancer agents known as **biological response modifiers** and as such are viewed as potentially promising therapeutic tools.

Stimulation of B Lymphocytes By inducing the release of IL-1, endotoxin induces B lymphocytes (but not T lymphocytes) to divide. B lymphocytes mature into antibody-producing cells, thus adding to long-term resistance to infection by increasing the concentration of antibodies in circulation. In this capacity, endotoxin is an **immunological adjuvant**.

Shock The full panoply of endotoxin activity is more emphatically displayed when it is administered in large amounts. Fully activated endotoxin produces a condition known as **bacterial sepsis** (Fig. 9-5). Fortunately rarely seen, bacterial sepsis overwhelms the body with bacteria, often Gram-negative bacteria such as *E. coli*, *P. aeruginosa*, or meningococci (see Chapters 14, 19, and 64). The result is a frequently lethal condition known as **endotoxic shock**, which manifests as a serious drop in blood pressure (**hypotension**) and **disseminated intravascular coagulation** (DIC). Cytokines, nitric acid, and small-molecule inflammatory mediators called **eicosanoids** are key mediators in endotoxin-induced hypotension; hypotension is considerably reduced by the administration of anticytokine antibodies prior to the injection of endotoxin. An earlier view was that decreased resistance of peripheral vessels results from a buildup of vasoactive amines (histamine and kinins). Considerable effort has been made at understanding the molecular basis for endotoxic shock to develop new methods for intervention.

DIC is the deposition of thrombi in small vessels, with consequent damage to the areas deprived of blood supply. The effect is most severe in the kidneys and leads to cortical necrosis. Other organs affected include the brain, lungs, and adrenals. In some cases of menin-

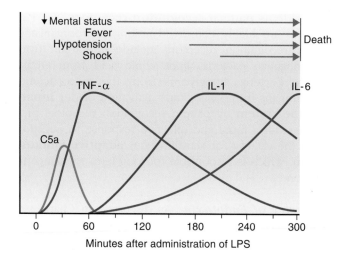

FIGURE 9-5. Release of mediators of sepsis following the experimental injection of lipopolysaccharide (LPS). Tumor necrosis factor α (TNF-α) triggers the release of interleukin 1 (IL-1). These cytokines act synergistically to induce the damaging effects of sepsis. Other cytokines, such as IL-6, are released as a consequence of this synergy. IL-6 does not produce shock, but the level of IL-6 release is highly correlated with death from septic shock.

gococcal infection, adrenal insufficiency due to infarction leads to rapid death, a condition known as the **Waterhouse-Friderichsen syndrome**. Endotoxin contributes to coagulation of blood in three ways: clotting factor XII (the so-called Hageman factor) is activated to set off the intrinsic clotting cascade; platelets release the contents of their granules, which are involved in clotting; and neutrophils release proteins known to stabilize fibrin clots.

Endotoxin represents the calling card of Gram-negative bacteria. Binding of endotoxin to the TLRs on macrophages stimulates the production of a series of alarm reactions that rapidly help to fend off the invading pathogen. These include the mobilization of neutrophils, the activation of macrophages, and the stimulation of B lymphocytes. Stimulation by pattern recognition receptors also initiates the adaptive immune system of the host, leading to long-term resistance to microbial infections. In large amounts, endotoxin induces shock and widespread coagulation. In summary, recognition of endotoxin is a mechanism our bodies use to activate our immune response against Gram-negative bacterial pathogens. But the unregulated nature of this response may lead to detrimental effects.

Membrane-Damaging Toxins

Some toxins harm the host cell by causing membrane damage. They act either as **lipases** or by inserting themselves in the membrane to form pores. **Lecithinase** is a lipase toxin produced by *Clostridium perfringens*, which causes gas gangrene. Lecithinase lyses cells indiscriminately because its main substrate, phosphatidylcholine (lecithin), is ubiquitous in mammalian membranes. Microbes that elaborate lipase toxins thus eliminate potential host defenses and at the same time create a necrotic, nutritionally rich anaerobic milieu in which the microorganisms thrive.

Membrane-damaging toxins are often generally termed **hemolysins**, because they can cause lysis of red blood cells. Red blood cell lysis may not be the principal activity of these toxins in pathogenesis but is a convenient assay to characterize these toxins in the laboratory. One class of membrane-damaging toxins is **pore-forming toxins**, which insert directly into the host membrane to generate pores (see Fig. 9-2). Pore-forming toxins make the membranes permeable to water, which flows into the cytoplasm to swell the cell and, if excessive, lyse the cell. Even at toxin concentrations too low to cause cell lysis, cellular functions are damaged by perturbations of the permeability barrier that allow leakage of potassium ions needed for protein synthesis and cell viability. Thus, pore-forming toxins effectively inhibit the function of phagocytes, the host's first line of defense.

The pattern of ion leakage and subsequent damage is the same for many pore-forming toxins. Working nonenzymatically, these toxins use a mechanism similar to the MAC of complement (see Chapter 6). The pores formed by the complement complex as well as by the pore-forming bacterial toxins consist of fortified protein structures unusually resistant to proteases and detergents. This resistance likely contributes to the stability of the toxin at the cell surface. An example of a toxin that works in this manner is the **α-toxin** of *Staphylococcus aureus*. This toxin is a **homogeneous pore former**; that is, each pore has the same number of protein molecules (see Fig. 6-5 for similar-looking channels produced by the MAC of complement).

The **heterogeneous pore-forming toxins** constitute another class of membrane-damaging toxin. These toxins make pores that vary in size and number of monomer toxin molecules. The prototype of this class is **streptolysin O**, a toxin produced by certain streptococci. Streptolysin O (*O* stands for "oxygen labile") binds to cholesterol in the cell membrane. Streptolysin O lyses red blood cells but not neutrophils or macrophages. Nevertheless, this toxin contributes indirectly to white blood cell death because it acts preferentially on the membranes of lysosomes, releasing their hydrolytic enzymes. This results in damage to the cytoplasmic contents of the white blood cell, leading to the suicidal type of cell death termed **apoptosis**. In addition, the lysosomal enzymes released from killed neutrophils damage the surrounding tissue. The heterogeneous pore formers demonstrate that pores made by toxins need not be well defined to cause widespread damage.

Superantigens

A unique aspect of the action of several virulence factors is their ability to subvert the normal antibody response of the host. Acting as so-called **superantigens**, some toxins stimulate the production of large amounts of antibodies, not directed against the superantigen, by complexing MHC molecules of an antigen-presenting cell with the T-cell receptor on lymphocytes to stimulate antigen-independent activation of the lymphocyte (see Fig. 9-2). Such antibody production is wasteful and inefficient in combating infection. This intriguing aspect of how microbes can ultimately turn a normal response by the host into one that causes significant host damage is described in Chapter 8.

Virulence Factors that Act in the Extracellular Matrix

In contrast to toxins that modify proteins in the intracellular compartment of the host cell or act on the cell surface, numerous virulence factors, **exoenzymes**, act in the extracellular matrix of the cell. These virulence factors include degradative enzymes that function as **spreading factors** by facilitating dispersal of infecting organisms. Some Gram-positive bacteria secrete a **hyaluronidase** that breaks down hyaluronic acid, the ground substance of connective tissue, and also secrete **deoxyribonuclease** (**DNase**), which thins pus made viscous by the DNA released from dead white blood cells. Other bacteria make proteins that bind and activate host plasminogen. For example, **streptokinase** produced by *Streptococcus pyogenes* activates plasminogen and converts it to plasmin, a serum protease that in turn attacks fibrin clots. In this way, streptokinase eliminates fibrin barriers that might interfere with invading streptococci. Similar roles have been suggested for the **collagenases** and **elastases** produced by other organisms. These enzymes are also produced by the uninfected host, but their activities are normally under control to keep them from becoming meat tenderizers.

Immune Protection against Exotoxins

Because exotoxins are foreign proteins and stimulate an immune response when produced in the host, **immune protection** is a possible response to the toxin. For some diseases, such as tetanus, the clinical disease itself does not confer immunity to subsequent infections, probably because the toxin is produced in amounts too small to induce an effective response. On the other hand, vaccination and treatment with **antitoxins** have been used successfully against tetanus and other diseases. Of course, injecting the toxin itself is dangerous and does not result in active immunization. Fortunately, some exotoxins can be chemically modified to eliminate their intrinsic toxicity while retaining immunogenicity. Such chemically inactivated toxins are termed **toxoids** and are commonly used to vaccinate against several diseases, including diphtheria and tetanus (as part of the widely used DTP vaccine). Undergoing a series of vaccinations through the first 5 years of life, with boosters every 10 years, enables humans to mount an immune response sufficient to maintain immunity to natural infection with the microbes that cause diphtheria and tetanus. As may be anticipated, infection by the microbes can occur in individuals immune only to the toxin, but serious clinical symptoms of the diseases are not observed.

Passive immunization involves administration of an antitoxin, usually produced in horses or other animals, to individuals who have been exposed to toxin-producing pathogens, like the diphtheria and tetanus bacilli. One problem with antitoxin administration is the possibility of **serum sickness**, an immune reaction against foreign proteins. In the nonimmune individual, antitoxin must be administered rapidly to be effective against infection resulting from the tetanus or diphtheria bacilli, because once exotoxins are bound to host cell, they are rapidly internalized and become unavailable to antibody molecules.

Recombinant DNA technology can refine some of the procedures used to generate an immunogen that elicits a protective immune response to an exotoxin. Vaccines directed against tailor-made domains of the exotoxin are being developed. The B domains of AB exotoxins seem to be particularly promising candidates, because antibodies which prevent binding of a toxin block the initial steps of toxin action. In the absence of the A domain, the B domains are innocuous and can be administered with little risk to the host. Vaccination with a recombinant form of the **B** domain of anthrax toxin is an approach being pursued to develop a safe and effective vaccine against intoxication by the microbe responsible for anthrax. In addition, recombinant DNA techniques have allowed the development of humanized monoclonal antibodies that target specific epitopes of bacterial toxins, such as botulinum neurotoxin. In vivo studies indicate that multiple-monoclonal antibodies clear bacterial toxins via an **immune clearance** mechanism.

Not all toxin-mediated diseases respond to vaccination. For example, some of the approved vaccines against cholera elicit only limited protection. An effective cholera vaccine must elicit secreted IgA antibodies in the intestine that are active against the microbe, blocking its ability to colonize and intoxicate the host. Cholera vaccines administered by injection give poor or short-lived protection, in part because an effective IgA antibody response is not achieved. However, live strains of oral vaccine, made of the disarmed pathogen, stimulate intestinal antibody production of the IgA class similar to what natural infection does. These strains hold promise for generating long-lived protection against cholera.

Bacterial exotoxins are also being used to target drugs to specific cell populations, by coupling a specific antibody to an A domain of an exotoxin. The antibody seeks out the specific cells, and the A domain is delivered to kill the cell. Although there have been successes in treating cancers this way, nonspecific toxicity and potential adverse side effects are issues that have to be addressed with this therapeutic approach. Nonetheless, the idea of using toxins to this advantage remains appealing.

CONCLUSION

Advances in our knowledge of toxin action and host cell physiology provide a foundation for understanding the molecular basis of infectious disease. Pathology associated with disease is often a combination of the toxicity of the toxin and the host response to the infectious agent. Toxins are categorized based on their site of action, targeting the intracellular compartment of the host, the host cell surface, or the extracellular matrix. Toxins have specific modes of action that are responsible for the unique pathology associated with an individual infectious agent, such as cell death caused by the action of diphtheria toxin or elevated cAMP resulting from the action of cholera toxin. Often, toxins can be detoxified (toxoids) and administered as protective vaccines.

Suggested Readings

Aktories K, Barbierie JT. Bacterial cytotoxins: targeting eukaryotic switches. *Nat Rev Microbiol.* 2005;3:397–410.

Alouf JE, Freer J, eds. *Sourcebook of Bacterial Toxins.* San Diego, CA: Academic Press; 1991.

Barbieri JT, Burns D. Bacterial ADP-ribosylating exotoxin. In: Burns D, Barbieri JT, Iglewski B, Rappuoli R, eds. *Bacterial Protein Toxins*. Washington, DC: ASM Press; 2003.

Bhakdi S, Tranum-Jensen J. Alpha-toxin of *Staphylococcus aureus*. *Microb Rev*. 1991;55:733–751.

Bryant CE, Spring DR, Gangloff M, et al. The molecular basis of the host response to lipopolysaccharide. *Nat Rev Microbiol*. 2010;8:8–14.

Hallman M, Ramet M, Ezekowitz RA. Toll-like receptors as sensors of pathogens. *Pediatr Res*. 2001;50:315–321.

Johnson HM, Russell JK, Ponzer C. Superantigens in human disease. *Sci Am*. 1992;266:92–101.

Moss J, Iglewski B, Vaughan M, et al. Bacterial toxins. *Handbook of Natural Toxins*. Vol 8. New York: Marcel Dekker; 1995.

Schiavo G, Benfenati F, Poulain B, et al. Tetanus and botulinum-B neurotoxins block neurotransmitter release by proteolytic cleavage of synaptobrevin. *Nature*. 1992;359:832–835.

PART II

Infectious Agents

Chapter **10**

Introduction to the Pathogenic Bacteria

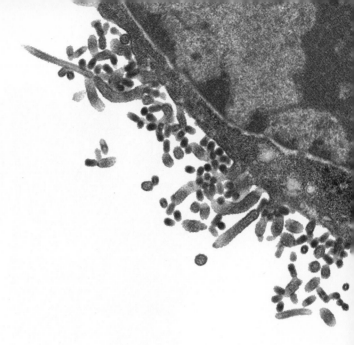

Victor J. DiRita

THOUSANDS OF SPECIES of bacteria, both harmless and pathogenic, are found in association with the human body. Although you need to know only the principal bacteria, even they make up a long list. However, knowing the taxonomy of bacteria may help you make important diagnostic and treatment decisions. For example, among other things, it is helpful to know that staphylococci and streptococci both belong to a group called the Gram-positive cocci, that *Escherichia coli* is classified among the Gram-negative enteric bacteria, and that the tubercle bacillus belongs to the acid-fast bacteria.

This chapter uses a simplified, practical scheme to divide the main pathogenic bacteria, rather than the organizational scheme used in the science of bacterial taxonomy (Fig. 10-1). In broad terms, medically interesting bacteria belong to one of two large categories:

1. The "typical" bacteria—the rods and cocci (spheres) that lack unusual morphological features. These "garden variety" bacteria can be subdivided into the Gram-positive and Gram-negative bacteria, and each of those categories can be further divided into rods and cocci.
2. Those that do not fall in the first category.

Like all other forms of life, each bacterium is named by its genus, as in *Escherichia*, and species, as in *coli*. Conventionally, after its first use in a text, the genus name is shortened to the first letter, as in *E. coli*. Many bacteria also have common names, usually related to the main disease they cause—for example, the meningococcus (*Neisseria meningitidis*) and the tubercle bacillus (*Mycobacterium tuberculosis*). Sometimes the origin of the genus and species names is interesting and useful to know. Many bacterial names honor famous microbiologists; for instance, *Escherichia* is named after the German pediatrician Theodor Escherich and *Salmonella* after the American veterinarian Daniel Elmer Salmon. Other names are descriptive; *pyogenes* (as in *Streptococcus pyogenes*), for example, indicates that the bacteria promote pus production.

A confusing aspect of bacterial taxonomy is that considerable variety usually exists within a species. Thus, a *Staphylococcus aureus* isolated from one patient may be distinctly virulent, whereas another strain of the same bacterium may not be. These isolates are called **strains**. This point is well illustrated by the many strains of *E. coli*, which include the strain commonly used in molecular biology research, known as K12, as well as less benevolent strains that cause infection of the intestine, the urinary bladder, or the meninges. All are *E. coli*, but each is a different strain expressing different pathogenic factors.

"TYPICAL" BACTERIA

The **Gram stain** property reflects fundamental differences among bacteria; these differences lie mainly in their permeability properties and surface components. The chief differences that the Gram stain illustrates are presence of an outer membrane in the Gram-negative bacteria and of a thick **murein** layer in the Gram-positive bacteria (see Chapter 3). These organisms can also be divided into rods and cocci, yielding four categories in which to classify them (Fig. 10-2).

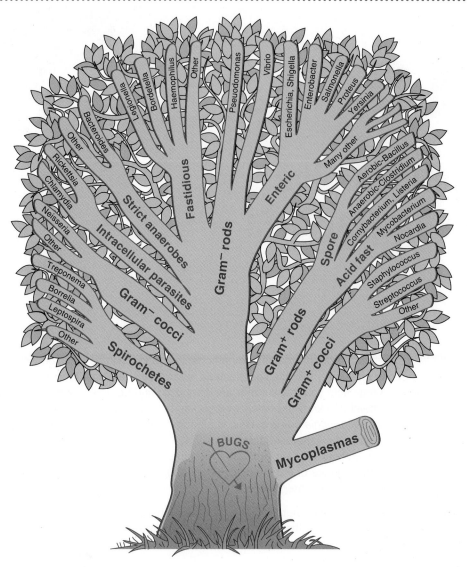

FIGURE 10-1. The major groups of medically important bacteria. This illustration is a practical representation of the principal groups of pathogenic bacteria. It is meant to be a study aid, not a taxonomic or phylogenetic tree.

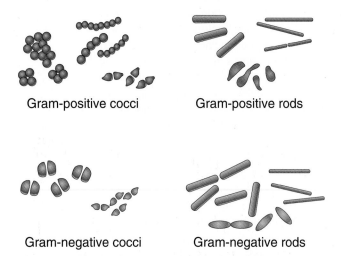

Gram-positive cocci

Gram-positive rods

Gram-negative cocci

Gram-negative rods

FIGURE 10-2. The "Big Four" typical bacteria. Many of the chapters on individual infectious agents include sections called paradigms. These sections highlight points of general relevance to the understanding of microbial pathogenesis.

Because the Gram stain reflects such fundamental differences among bacteria, Gram-positive bacteria differ more from Gram-negative bacteria than cocci differ from rods. For instance, the Gram-positive streptococci are closely related to the lactobacilli, which are Gram-positive rods; however, the streptococci are quite distinct from Gram-negative cocci, such as the gonococci. Gram-positive bacteria accept the Gram stain and appear dark violet, whereas Gram-negative bacteria do not accept the stain and appear red (see Chapter 3 and Table 3-2).

The four categories presented in Figure 10-2 are fairly evenly represented among the **normal microbiota** of the mouth, the pharynx, and the large intestine; major pathogens, however, are represented in fewer numbers. The Gram-positive cocci and the Gram-negative rods are the most common agents of infection, followed by the Gram-negative cocci and the Gram-positive rods.

Gram-Positive Cocci

The two most medically relevant genera of Gram-positive cocci are *Streptococcus* and *Staphylococcus*. Species within each genus are among the most successful human pathogens and, consequently, are the targets of vigorous research efforts to understand and combat them.

Streptococci

Streptococci grow in chains of spherical cells—like strings of pearls—and constitute a large and diverse group. Streptococci are subdivided according to the changes they produce when grown on agar-containing blood. Thus, **β-hemolytic** streptococci (or "beta strep"), which cause most streptococcal infections, lyse red blood cells signified by a clear area around the colonies. The **α-hemolytic** streptococci produce a different change and cause blood-containing media around the colony to turn green. Other streptococci do not change the blood at all. Many streptococci strains are nonpathogenic and are found in the environment as well as in the normal human intestine. Some strains are used in production of yogurt and cheese.

Streptococci do not carry out respiration, only fermentation. Fermentation is characteristic of anaerobic bacteria, and indeed some streptococci are strict anaerobes. However, most of the pathogenic species of streptococci grow in air and are thus described as **oxygen-tolerant anaerobes**. Streptococci usually grow in small colonies on agar. Streptococci produce many extracellular proteins, some of which are virulence factors that confer on the organisms the ability to destroy tissues and damage host cells.

The main pathogens in the *Streptococcus* genus are the β-hemolytic strains. These strains are further subclassified into groups by the presence of different cell wall polysaccharides. Of all the groups (A through T), the most important strains in human disease are those of group A. The full taxonomic name of these organisms is *S. pyogenes*, but they are often referred to as "group A strep." They cause "strep throat," infections of soft tissues, and other serious infections. These infections can cause serious complications, such as rheumatic fever or glomerulonephritis. α-Hemolytic streptococci include one important pathogen, *S. pneumoniae* (the principal agent of bacterial pneumonia), and other, mainly opportunistic, species.

Staphylococci

The two main pathogenic species of *Staphylococcus* are *S. aureus* and *S. saprophyticus*; however, opportunistic infections by staphylococci that are part of the normal microbiota, such as *S. epidermidis*, can also occur. Under the microscope, staphylococci look like arrays of buckshot or bunches of grapes (*staphylo* comes from the Greek word for grapes). They are more robust than streptococci and are able to withstand many chemical and physical agents; these qualities make it difficult to eradicate them from the human environment. Their colonies on agar are larger than those of the streptococci.

Staphylococci are found in many sites of the body, especially on the skin. They are the most likely organisms to cause pus in wounds and may produce serious infections in deep tissues, such as osteomyelitis (infection of the bone marrow) or endocarditis (infection of the heart valves). Like the streptococci, they secrete a large number of extracellular enzymes and toxins. One enzyme, **coagulase**, clots plasma and is useful in distinguishing the most pathogenic species of the genus, *S. aureus*, from others because only *S. aureus* produces the enzyme.

Gram-Negative Cocci

Gram-negative cocci include several genera of medical importance, the most significant of which is *Neisseria*. This genus includes many organisms found in the mouth and pharynx of healthy people and two important pathogens, **gonococcus** (*N. gonorrhoeae*) and **meningococcus**. Like all Gram-negative bacteria, their outer membranes contain **endotoxin** (**lipopolysaccharide**). The gonococcus causes gonorrhea, and the meningococcus causes meningitis and severe **septicemia**.

Gram-Positive Rods

Abundant in the environment, this group includes bacteria that only infrequently cause diseases, at least in the developed regions of the world. One disease, diphtheria, was deadly among children until vaccination nearly eradicated it. The agent of diphtheria is called *Corynebacterium diphtheriae* and has many relatives called the **diphtheroids**. The diphtheroids are common inhabitants of the skin and mucous membranes and can cause opportunistic infections. (Notice that *diphtheria* has two *h*'s.)

In the human environment, the most common Gram-positive rods are **spore forming**. They are the largest of the typical bacteria, with 5 to 10 times the volume of an average *E. coli*, and can measure 3 to 5 μm in length. They are divided into two genera: the **aerobic** *Bacillus*, containing only one important pathogenic species, *B. anthracis*, which causes anthrax, and the **strict anaerobes**, which are members of the genus *Clostridium*. This genus includes several medically important species such as *C. botulinum*, which cause botulism; *C. tetani*, the agent of tetanus; and several other species that produce gas gangrene (most commonly *C. perfringens*). Symptoms of these diseases are caused by powerful exotoxins. Among the most commonly encountered clostridial disease is one associated with antibiotic use: pseudomembranous colitis caused by *C. difficile*. Another important pathogen among the Gram-positive rods is *Listeria monocytogenes*, which occasionally causes serious infections in infants and in adults who are immunocompromised and in pregnant women.

Gram-Negative Rods
Enteric Bacteria

The Gram-negative rods are a large group of bacteria that includes many important pathogens. The **enteric**

bacteria are among the most clinically important of the Gram-negative rods. The exemplar is *Escherichia coli*, the typical bacterium *par excellence*. The enteric bacteria (or family Enterobacteriaceae) comprise many genera, including *Salmonella*, species of which cause typhoid fever and food poisoning, and *Shigella*, which causes bacillary dysentery. All enteric bacteria grow readily on laboratory media, make colonies typically less than 1 mm across on agar, and do not form spores or have distinct cell arrangements. Many, but not all, are motile. They are divided into two main groups: those that ferment lactose (*E. coli* and others) and those that do not (*Salmonella* and *Shigella*). Although many pathogens are not lactose fermenters, the characteristic is not universal, and many exceptions exist. Relatives of the enteric bacteria include the yersiniae, which cause plague and certain intestinal infections.

Among their more distant relatives are Gram-negative rods that differ in metabolism and somewhat in morphology. These are in various families outside the Enterobacteriaceae, including the genus *Vibrio* (containing *V. cholerae*, the cholera bacillus) and the genus *Pseudomonas*. Pseudomonads, as the members of the *Pseudomonas* genus are sometimes called, are often found in aqueous environments, such as rivers, lakes, swimming pools, and tap water; these environments are thus frequent sources of human infection. Other clinically important Gram-negative rods outside the Enterobacteriaceae are *Campylobacter jejuni*, a common agent of infectious diarrhea, and *Helicobacter pylori*, which causes gastritis, gastric ulcers, and gastric cancer.

"Fastidious" and Small Gram-Negative Rods

Besides the organisms already mentioned, the Gram-negative rods include an important and heterogeneous group of genera. They can be lumped, somewhat arbitrarily, into a group that may be awkwardly described as the "fastidious" and small Gram-negative rods because they have complex nutritional requirements and tend to be smaller than, for example, *E. coli*. Included in this group are the following genera: *Haemophilus* (which causes pneumonia and meningitis), *Bordetella* (whooping cough), *Brucella* (brucellosis), *Francisella* (tularemia), *Bartonella* (cat scratch fever), and *Legionella* (Legionnaires disease, a form of pneumonia).

Strictly Anaerobic Gram-Negative Rods

An important group of Gram-negative rods is distinguished by its strictly anaerobic way of life. Clinically, the most noteworthy of these organisms belongs to the genus *Bacteroides*. These bacteria are common in the human body and are the most frequent members of the intestinal microbiota, where they may serve as a critical stimulus for proper tissue development within the intestine and break down some polysaccharides in the human diet. They are also found in the gingival pockets that surround the teeth. Although the bacteria are usually harmless, members of this genus may cause serious disease when deposited in deep tissues, such as in peritonitis, the abdominal infection that results from the release of intestinal contents into the peritoneum. These organisms usually do not cause disease alone but are found in association with other bacteria, thereby causing mixed or polymicrobial infections. They will not reproduce if incubated aerobically, and their growth requires special anaerobic techniques.

"NOT SO TYPICAL" BACTERIA

A taxonomic hodgepodge, the "not so typical" bacteria include organisms that have special shapes, sizes, or staining properties. Other than their medical importance, they do not have many features in common. Thus, each group stands alone.

Acid-Fast Bacteria

This group is almost synonymous with the genus *Mycobacterium*, which includes the **tubercle bacillus**, *M. tuberculosis*, and the **leprosy bacillus**, *M. leprae*. The name "Mycobacterium" contains the root word for fungus (*myco*) because the organisms sometimes form branches that vaguely suggest the fungi. There acid fastness refers to the ability of these organisms to resist decolorization by acids, a trait that is exploited in specialized staining procedures (see Chapter 3). The Gram stain is not useful for identifying these bacteria because they do not take up the Gram stain dyes. They are surrounded by a waxy envelope that can only be penetrated by dyes if the bacteria are heated or treated with detergents. All mycobacteria grow slowly (perhaps taking days or even weeks to form a colony on agar media) and are resistant to chemical agents but not to heat.

The special staining procedure used for acid-fast bacteria is called the **Ziehl-Neelsen technique**. Its most frequently used modification consists of treating smears with a solution of a red dye (fuchsin) that contains detergents. After washing, the smear is treated with a solution of 3% hydrochloric acid that removes the dye from all bacteria except the acid-fast organisms. The preparation is then exposed to a blue dye that counterstains all other bacteria, white blood cells, and so on. Tubercle or leprosy bacilli, which stain red in this procedure, are clearly visible against the blue background.

Several species of mycobacteria found free living in the environment can cause opportunistic infections, especially in immunocompromised patients. These environmental species used to be called **atypical acid-fast bacilli**. Among the most commonly encountered of these bacteria are members of a complex known as *Mycobacterium avium-intracellulare*.

Even more akin to fungi in morphology are relatives of the mycobacteria called the actinomycetes. These organisms take up the Gram stain and are Gram-positive, although some are also weakly acid-fast. They form true branches and long filaments with complex structures, a feature that places them among the most highly differentiated of the prokaryotes. There are two pathogenic genera: *Nocardia*, which are aerobic, and *Actinomyces*, which are strict anaerobes. Bacteria of these genera cause certain forms of pneumonia and soft tissue infections. A generally nonpathogenic genus, *Streptomyces*, includes organisms that make important antibiotics (streptomycin, tetracycline, etc.)

Spirochetes

These bacteria are helical, having the shape of a spring (not a screw). They include the agent of syphilis, *Treponema pallidum*, the species name of which refers to the fact that these organisms are so thin ("pale") that they do not take up enough dye to be readily seen under the microscope. Unstained, they can be seen with a phase contrast or a dark-field microscope. The spirochetes of syphilis are not readily cultivated in the laboratory.

Other spirochetes include the genus *Leptospira*, which causes a disease called icterohemorrhagic fever, and *Borrelia recurrentis*, the agent of relapsing fever. Another spirochete in the *Borrelia* genus, *B. burgdorferi*, causes Lyme disease (named after the town of Old Lyme, Connecticut), which is one of the most important spirochetoses in both eastern and western United States.

Chlamydiae

The chlamydiae are small, strictly intracellular bacteria that cannot be grown in artificial media. They are among the smallest cellular forms of life but have a fairly complex life cycle. Their morphological form when they are growing inside cells differs from their form when they are in transit between cells. *Chlamydia trachomatis* is the most common cause of sexually transmitted disease (chlamydial urethritis) and other more unusual infections. *C. pneumoniae* is an agent of pneumonia in young adults and has been linked to atherosclerosis. These organisms set up housekeeping within phagocytic vesicles of their host cells and obtain their energy from them.

Rickettsiae

Like the chlamydiae, the rickettsiae are small, intracellular bacteria that are also obligate parasites. Among the diseases these bacteria cause are epidemic typhus and Rocky Mountain spotted fever. Included in this group is the genus *Ehrlichia*, bacteria that infect white blood cells in humans and animals. Each species is transmitted by the bite of different arthropod species (lice, fleas, ticks, etc.), with the exception of *Coxiella burnetii*, the agent of Q fever, which may also be acquired by inhalation. Rickettsiae are small, rod-shaped bacteria that lack distinctive growth cycle stages.

Mycoplasmas

Perhaps most evolutionarily distant from all other bacteria, mycoplasmas lack a rigid cell wall. They are almost plastic in structure, grow slowly on laboratory media, and have special nutritional requirements. The most unique of these is the need for sterols, which are not required by any other group of bacteria. Mycoplasmas lack murein and consequently are resistant to penicillin and other cell wall antibiotics. The oldest known human pathogenic mycoplasma is *Mycoplasma pneumoniae*, which causes a form of pneumonia. Others, such as *Ureaplasma urealyticum* have been implicated in various diseases.

Mycoplasmas resemble the laboratory-produced forms of regular bacteria—the so-called **L forms**—which lack cell walls. Regular bacteria take on the same amorphous appearance as the mycoplasma when their cell walls are removed with lysozyme or when murein synthesis is inhibited with penicillin. Cell lysis usually occurs, but if the L forms are placed in a hypertonic medium, they can be grown in colonies that resemble those of the mycoplasmas. However, the similarity is only superficial. L forms usually revert to the regular bacterial form when they are removed from lysozyme or penicillin. Mycoplasmas, on the other hand, do not.

Mycoplasmas also differ in terms of their degree of relatedness to all other bacteria as measured by DNA hybridization. Further, they are thought to have the smallest genomes among free-living organisms. Because of this, they have been the subject of a significant amount of research regarding the evolution of genome structure and function. In 2010 a group of scientists claimed the creation of the first "synthetic" microbe by replacing the natural chromosome of a mycoplasma cell with a laboratory-synthesized chromosome.

CURRENT CONCEPTS REGARDING THE MICROBIOTA

Many microorganisms can be seen under the microscope but cannot be cultured. Some are suspected of causing important diseases, but the point has been difficult to establish without pure cultures. New technologies have allowed scientists to make some progress in this area. For example, *Tropheryma whippelii*—the agent of the rare Whipple disease, which is characterized by diarrhea and intestinal bleeding but can have systemic manifestations such as lymphadenopathy—was identified by PCR and 16S rRNA sequence analysis several years before it could be cultured in the laboratory (see Chapter 58). This approach demonstrates the limits of Koch postulates, which include culturing the potential pathogen in the laboratory. With rapid advances in DNA sequencing technology and bioinformatics, scientists are developing important new methodologies to study complex microbial populations and identify both beneficial and pathogenic species, without the need to isolate and culture them in the laboratory.

Cloning techniques have been useful in studies of bacteria that are well known but cannot be cultivated, such as the treponeme of syphilis or the mycobacterium of leprosy. The genes of these agents have been introduced into surrogate organisms, such as *E. coli*, and many of the protein gene products have been studied, especially with regard to their immunological properties.

More and more possible agents of disease are being recognized and studied because of the disruption in immune system function caused by HIV and other agents of immunosuppression. Bacteria, viruses, fungi, protozoa, and worms that were previously unknown or known to be present only in animals or the environment have now joined the list of potential or known human pathogens. The combination of new technologies and the changes in the human immune condition will undoubtedly lead to the discovery of many more agents of infectious diseases. At the same time, with progress in sanitation and vaccination, the importance of many of the classic infectious pathogens is waning. The list of important pathogens is constantly changing.

CONCLUSION

Over the hundred or so years that microorganisms have been studied in the laboratory, they have exhibited remarkable genetic constancy. The staphylococci or streptococci of today fit their original descriptions from the end of the 19th century. Likewise, a microbiologist from Robert Koch's laboratory would have no problem correctly identifying a modern strain of *Vibrio cholerae* or tubercle bacilli. On the other hand, important changes have occurred with alarming speed. Virtually all the pathogenic bacteria have become significantly more resistant to every new antibiotic that has been introduced in the last five decades. For example, pathogenic staphylococci are now almost universally resistant to penicillin, although in the 1950s, when the drug came into general use, their ancestors were sensitive to it. Furthermore, we are now in an era in which the threat of biological weapons based on human pathogens is very real, and our understanding of how some of those microbes cause disease and how to protect populations from them is scant. Finally, there is the growing understanding of exactly how the normal microbiota contribute to human health, in many cases by altering the host environment in which pathogens can thrive or be kept under control. Thus, the study of microbial pathogens and microbial biology in general remains a rich target area for research and innovations that will have a significant impact on human health.

Suggested Readings

Gibson DG, Glass JI, Lartigue C, et al. Creation of a bacterial cell controlled by a chemically synthesized genome. *Science.* 2010;329:52.

Jorgensen JH, Pfaller MA. *A Clinician's Dictionary of Pathogenic Microorganisms.* Washington, DC: ASM Press; 2004.

Lipkin WI. Microbe hunting. *Microbiol Mol Biol Rev.* 2010;74:363.

Maza LM, Pezzlo MT, Shigei JT, et al. *Color Atlas of Medical Bacteriology.* Washington, DC: ASM Press; 2004.

Chapter 11

Staphylococci: Abscesses and Toxin-Mediated Diseases

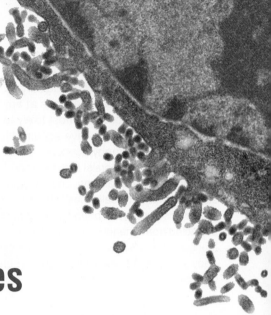

Patrick M. Schlievert and Marnie L. Peterson

KEY CONCEPTS

Pathogens: Staphylococci are Gram-positive cocci that form grapelike clusters. They include *Staphylococcus aureus, Staphylococcus epidermidis, Staphylococcus saprophyticus* (which almost exclusively causes urinary tract infections), and numerous others.

Encounter: Organisms grow on the surface of humans and survive on inanimate surface. During a lifetime, approximately 90% of humans are colonized with at some point with *S. aureus* in their external nares or skin.

Entry: Carriage of staphylococci usually occurs after direct, skin-to-skin contact with another carrier. Infection may also occur after penetration of a contaminated object through the skin.

Spread and Multiplication: Commensal staphylococci (e.g., *S. epidermidis*) are colonizers of normal skin and rarely cause deeper infection unless they are physically introduced into deeper tissues in association with an intravenous catheter or other artificial device. Virulent staphylococci (i.e., *S. aureus*) may cause skin infections, from which organisms may disseminate to almost any organ or tissue.

Damage: *S. aureus* is pyogenic ("pus forming"), except in toxic shock syndrome, which may occur with nonpyogenic infection. Staphylococci cause skin and soft tissue infections (such as furuncles, abscesses, and necrotizing fasciitis), pneumonia, food poisoning, and toxin-induced diseases (toxic shock and scalded skin syndromes). If the organisms enter the bloodstream, they may cause osteomyelitis, kidney abscesses, or endocarditis.

S. aureus produces microbial surface components recognizing adhesive matrix molecules (MSCRAMMs), including peptidoglycan, teichoic acids, protein A, clumping factor, and others. They also secrete virulence factors such as hemolysins, leukocidins, superantigens, and other exotoxins.

Diagnosis: Staphylococci have a characteristic appearance on Gram stain, and they are easily isolated on most laboratory media.

Treatment: Most strains produce β-lactamase (an enzyme that breaks down penicillin). Consequently, antistaphylococcal penicillins or cephalosporins are used. However, some strains express penicillin-binding protein 2a, which also makes the organism resistant to the abovementioned agents (methicillin-resistant *S. aureus* or MRSA). Drainage of abscesses and supportive therapy for hypotension and shock are also critical, nonantimicrobial elements of care.

Prevention: There is no vaccine against staphylococci.

STAPHYLOCOCCUS AUREUS (Gram-positive cocci) are the most common of the **pyogenic**, or pus-producing, bacteria that cause human diseases. They colonize the anterior nares of 30 to 40% of individuals and may be present on other mucous membranes and the skin. The organism also causes more-frequent and varied types of diseases than perhaps any other human pathogen (see box, *Diseases Caused by Staphylococci*). The bacteria can produce focal abscesses at almost any site in the body, from the skin (furuncles or "boils") to the lungs (pneumonia), bones (osteomyelitis), kidneys, and heart (endocarditis). In addition, many strains of the bacterium secrete potent exotoxins that can cause signs of illness at sites distant from the bacterial infection. These illnesses include **toxic shock syndrome** (TSS), caused by toxic shock syndrome toxin-1 (**TSST-1**) and staphylococcal enterotoxin serotypes A through X; **staphylococcal scalded skin syndrome** (SSSS), caused by exfoliative toxin serotypes A and B; and **staphylococcal food poisoning** (SFP), caused by ingestion of staphylococcal enterotoxin serotypes A through E and I. Staphylococcal enterotoxin F was renamed TSST-1 because of its association with TSS and its lack of ability to cause food poisoning. TSS is a serious condition that results from focal infections at any body site by toxin-producing *S. aureus*, but vaginal mucosal and respiratory infections are most likely to lead to the illness. SSSS, another serious illness, occurs most often in neonates who have acquired focal infections, often of the upper respiratory tract, by exfoliative toxin-producing staphylococci.

   S. aureus can persist in the human host and cause illness because it produces numerous cell surface virulence factors, exotoxins, and enzymes. The secreted and cell surface virulence factors produced by staphylococci act locally mainly to help them withstand phagocytosis by neutrophils. For example, **clumping factor** (also known as bound coagulase) binds fibrin and helps the organism form walled-off abscesses protected from phagocytes. In addition, some factors act systemically to disrupt the normal immune system function (e.g., TSST-1). As a result, staphylococci are among the most adaptable of the pathogenic bacteria. They are difficult to eliminate from the human environment, and they are responsible for many community- and hospital-associated infections.

DISEASES CAUSED BY *STAPHYLOCOCCUS AUREUS*

Skin and soft tissue infections
    Furuncles, carbuncles, paronychia (nail infections)
    Wound infections (traumatic, surgical)
    Cellulitis
    Impetigo (also caused by streptococci)
    Bacteremia (frequently with metastatic abscesses)
Endocarditis
Central nervous system infections
    Brain abscess
    Meningitis (rare)
    Epidural abscess
Pulmonary infections
    Embolic
    Aspiration
Musculoskeletal infections
    Osteomyelitis
    Arthritis
Genitourinary tract infections
    Renal abscess
    Lower urinary tract infection
Toxin-related diseases
    Toxic shock syndrome
    Necrotizing pneumonia
    Scalded skin syndrome
    Extreme pyrexia syndrome
Food poisoning (gastroenteritis)

CASE

Necrotizing Pneumonia and Purpura Fulminans

Mr. K., a 21-year-old previously healthy college student, developed mild symptoms of a head cold, including cough. Four days later, his condition deteriorated, and he developed fever, chills, and shortness of breath (dyspnea), followed by nausea and vomiting. He was brought to the emergency department.

Physical examination revealed a fever of 37.9°C (100.1°F), heart rate 172 beats per minute, blood pressure 91/72 mm Hg but quickly deteriorated to 81/36 mm Hg, and respiratory rate 32 breaths per minute. Initial examination showed significant respiratory distress, no rash, supple neck, no heart murmur, decreased breath sounds in the right lower lung field, no abdominal tenderness, and no focal neurological findings. The laboratory reported that his white blood cell count was low. A Gram stain of organisms grown on blood agar plates from sputum cultures after intubation showed Gram-positive cocci in clusters (Fig. 11-1). Methicillin-resistant *Staphylococcus aureus* (MRSA) was cultured from sputum samples after intubation. Blood cultures were negative. The *S. aureus* strain produced the superantigen enterotoxin C (in vitro 80 μg/mL), and it produced Panton-Valentine leukocidin and alpha toxin (hemolysin). The organism was shown to be susceptible to clindamycin, trimethoprim/sulfamethoxazole, tetracycline, linezolid, rifampin, and vancomycin.

Mr. K. underwent intubation in the emergency department, started receiving intravenous fluids and electrolytes to maintain blood pressure and antibiotics, and he was transferred to the intensive care unit. Despite aggressive treatment, his condition continued to worsen, his skin became mottled, and he developed purpura over his lips and legs that progressed to cover his entire body in 12 hours. An example of purpura is shown in Figure 11-2.

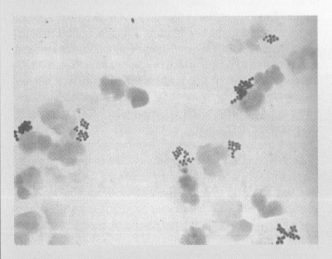

FIGURE 11-1. Gram stain of *Staphylococcus aureus*. Gram stain purple and appear as clusters of grapes (*staphylo* is derived from the Greek word for grape clusters).

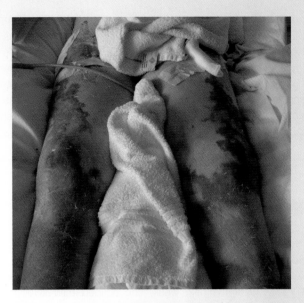

FIGURE 11-2. Purpuric rash of the legs associated with *Staphylococcus aureus*. Skin purpura is a result of shock and activation/dysregulation of the clotting cascade systemically.

Mr. K. succumbed within 24 hours after being examined in the emergency department. Postmortem examination revealed diffuse purpura of the skin and necrotizing pneumonia caused by community-associated MRSA, which were also isolated from postmortem lung cultures.

This case raises several questions:

1. What was the source of the organisms that infected Mr. K.?
2. What might have contributed to development of the pulmonary abscess due to *S. aureus*?
3. What are the roles of the demonstrated exotoxins made by the causative bacteria?
4. Why did Mr. K. die if the *S. aureus* did not invade his bloodstream?
5. What does community-associated MRSA mean?
6. What is the appropriate antimicrobial and therapeutic approach?

See Appendix for answers.

The case of Mr. K. illustrates several features of recent serious *S. aureus* infections. It is likely that Mr. K. was colonized with a community-associated methicillin-resistant *S. aureus* (CA-MRSA). As many as 40% of humans carry *S. aureus* nasally. Usually, nasal *S. aureus* does not cause illness in the vast majority of individuals colonized nasally, except occasionally adjacent soft tissue infections (e.g., boils). Boils are the most common manifestation of *S. aureus* disease. It is likely that Mr. K. had become physically run-down as a college student, it could be that he has allergies, or it could be that he was recovering from an upper respiratory tract viral infection. Any of these could have

continued on page 152

compromised his immune system's ability to fight off the CA-MRSA when it made its way to his lungs. *S. aureus* strains typically form walled-off lesion such as occurred in Mr. K.'s lower right lung. This is due to the organism making large numbers of cell-associated virulence factors that cause clotting and adherence to human tissues. Once established as an infection site, the CA-MRSA secreted virulence factors, such as cytolysins (Panton-Valentine leukocidin and alpha toxin) that locally damaged lung tissue, and the superantigen enterotoxin C that systemically caused massive production of proinflammatory cytokines with tumor necrosis factor leading to hypotension, shock, and ultimately death. Mr. K.'s illness progressed very rapidly with production of skin purpura as a result of shock and activation of the clotting cascade systemically; this intravascular coagulation also contributed significantly to the rapid progression to death.

CASE

Soft Tissue Infection and Toxic Shock Syndrome

A 20-year-old college athlete, Ms. G., had arthroscopic knee surgery. Over the next week, she noticed mild swelling, increasing pain, and a small amount of redness at the incision site. Within 3 weeks, the incision site had nearly completely healed, but the patient's knee remained swollen and painful. In addition, she was febrile (41.3°C) and had developed vomiting and diarrhea. She came to the emergency department for treatment. Examination revealed a "toxic-appearing" young woman who had a sunburnlike rash on her face, mild skin peeling above the eyes, and red eyes and lips (Fig. 11-3A). Her blood pressure was 70/50 mm Hg, indicating she was hypotensive, and she had elevated white cells in the blood and a significantly reduced number of platelets.

Ms. G. was admitted to the intensive care unit for management of her fever and hypotension. Throat, anterior nares, and vaginal cultures were negative for *S. aureus* and *Streptococcus pyogenes*, but because the surgical incision site had healed, it was not cultured originally. Over the next day, her condition worsened, despite being treated with nafcillin, gentamicin, and supportive care (fluid and electrolytes and vasopressors to maintain blood pressure), and she developed gangrenous toes (Fig. 11-3B). A needle was inserted into the site of the previous knee surgery, and 300 mL of serous fluid was removed that cultured positive for *S. aureus* (a strain that made the superantigen TSST-1). The bacterium also was methicillin resistant. The treatment therapy was changed to include vancomycin plus rifampin and clindamycin, and intravenous immunoglobulin (which contains antibodies to neutralize TSST-1). Two weeks after recovery, the patient's hand showed extensive peeling (Fig. 11-3C).

This case raises several questions:

1. What was the source of the organisms that infected Ms. G.?
2. What contributed to the development of the subcutaneous abscess?
3. Why is the incision site not highly inflamed?
4. What properties of TSST-1 led to the patient's symptoms?
5. What are the properties of the organism that prevented it from being cleared by nafcillin?

See Appendix for answers.

The case of Ms. G. illustrates several features typical of *S. aureus* toxin-mediated diseases. The initial lesion was a subcutaneous abscess that was overlooked because of its minimal inflammatory features. This is not surprising, because the primary site of *S. aureus* infection is often trivial or inapparent in TSS. The lack of inflammation makes it difficult to identify the infection site, but the clinical features are clearly typical of staphylococcal TSS. It is important in such patients to maintain blood pressure adequately to prevent development of gangrene, as happened with Ms. G.'s toes. She lost the tips of two toes as a consequence of her prolonged hypotension. The patient's causative bacterium was methicillin resistant, which emphasizes the need to find the infection site and determine antibiotic susceptibility. Vancomycin and rifampin are synergistic against MRSA, and clindamycin was added to reduce production of exotoxins by the organism (in addition to antimicrobial effects). Intravenous immunoglobulin has been shown experimentally to reduce the case fatality rate of streptococcal TSS, and it is being used to treat both staphylococcal and streptococcal TSS. Its mechanism of action is likely to be neutralization of the causative exotoxins including TSST-1.

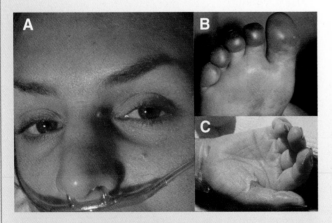

FIGURE 11-3. Toxic shock syndrome. A. Appearance of the rash associated with staphylococcal toxic shock syndrome (TSS). **B.** Gangrenous toes associated with prolonged hypotension in TSS. **C.** Desquamation of the skin that occurs during the resolution of TSS.

THE PATHOGEN: STAPHYLOCOCCI

Staphylococcus aureus is a large (1 µm in diameter) Gram-positive coccus that grows in grapelike clusters. It is one of the hardiest of the non–spore-forming bacteria and can survive for long periods on dry, inanimate objects. It is also relatively heat resistant. These properties permit *S. aureus* to survive in almost any environment in which humans coexist.

The genus *Staphylococcus* includes several species (Table 11-1). The most ubiquitous *Staphylococcus* species is *S. epidermidis*, which is found on the skin of most people and only infrequently causes disease in otherwise healthy individuals. The organism causes numerous infections in hospitals and in patients with implanted artificial devices (e.g., intravenous catheters, vascular grafts, and artificial joints). *S. aureus* generally causes more serious infections, including pneumonia, bone and joint infections, endocarditis, sepsis, and severe life-threatening TSS. The species name *aureus* means "golden" and refers to carotenoid pigmentation of *S. aureus* colonies (other species colonies are white, but occasionally, *S. aureus* colonies are also white). *S. saprophyticus* is unique in that it causes only urinary tract infections. A fourth species, *S. lugdunensis*, is an uncommon cause of aggressive endocarditis. The genus *Staphylococcus* contains other species that occasionally cause disease; those species are described in standard microbiological texts. The four species specified here suffice for the purposes of this book as they are most commonly associated with human diseases.

It is relatively easy to identify staphylococci in the laboratory. All members make large, creamy colonies on nutrient agar, and in a Gram stain (Fig. 11-1), they look like clusters of grapes (*staphylo* is derived from the Greek word for grape clusters). *S. aureus* is best distinguished from other species of the genus by using the **coagulase test**. Free coagulase, a secreted enzyme that clots plasma, is made by *S. aureus* but not by the other staphylococci.

Occasional strains fail to produce free coagulase, but *S. aureus* also makes clumping factor (bound coagulase) that causes plasma to clump around the organisms in a diagnostic slide test.

Within a species of staphylococci, individual strains can be identified by differences in their resistance to a panel of antibiotics and by using a procedure called phage typing, or more commonly, pulsed field gel electrophoresis. Phage typing, which is rarely done today, involves determining the sensitivity of a strain to a variety of standard bacteriophages. **Pulsed field gel electrophoresis** involves isolating staphylococcal DNA, treating the DNA with restriction enzymes that cut the DNA only rarely, and then resolving those DNA fragments in agarose gels. The newer molecular techniques for typing staphylococci based on the DNA sequence of the bacterial chromosome provide greater discrimination than phage typing between outbreak-related and non–outbreak-related strains, and as shown in the cases cited in this chapter, showed the relatedness of the organisms.

ENCOUNTER

Staphylococci share their environment with that of human beings. They live on people and survive on inanimate objects and surfaces (fomites), such as bedding, clothing, and doorknobs. Humans are the major reservoir for *S. aureus*. The organisms frequently colonize the anterior nares and are found in approximately 30% of healthy individuals. However, studies of individuals over time have found that up to 90% of people are eventually colonized in the nares with *S. aureus* at some point in their lives. The organisms can also be found transiently on the skin, oropharynx, vagina, and in feces. Staphylococci are well equipped to colonize the skin because they grow at high salt and lipid concentrations. They make enzymes, referred to as **lipases** and **glycerol ester hydrolases**, that degrade skin lipids.

TABLE 11-1 Properties of Various Species of *Staphylococcus*

Species	Frequency of Disease	Coagulase	Color of Colonies	Mannitol Fermentation	Novobiocin Resistance
Staphylococcus aureus	Common	+	White to gold	+	−
Staphylococcus epidermidis	Common	−	White	−	−
Staphylococcus saprophyticus	Occasional	−	White	−	+
Staphylococcus lugdunensis	Uncommon	−	White	−	−
Others	Different responses by individual species	—	—	—	—

The ability of *S. aureus* to colonize the skin and mucosal surfaces has been associated with bacterial cell surface proteins—the MSCRAMMs (microbial surface components recognizing adhesive matrix molecules)—that bind to a variety of host extracellular matrix proteins. **Fibronectin-binding proteins (FnbpA** and **FnbpB)** have been identified on the surface of *S. aureus*. Fnbp's allow the bacteria to invade epithelial and endothelial cells and to attach to exposed fibronectin in wounds, which may make FnbpA and FnbpB important virulence factors for the invasion of deeper tissues. *S. aureus* also has MSCRAMMs for **collagen binding**, called CNAs. They are important components of connective tissue, bones, and joints. Other MSCRAMMs, called clumping factors A and B, are present for **fibrinogen binding** and experimentally have been shown to be important in clot formation and endocarditis. These proteins are responsible for the clumping seen in the slide coagulase test.

Staphylococci spread from person to person, usually through direct contact or aerosols associated with upper respiratory viral or bacterial infections. It is important to remember that *S. aureus* is an important secondary pathogen associated with patients recovering from influenza and parainfluenza (croup) infections. Infants may become colonized with *S. aureus* shortly after birth, acquiring the organism from people in their immediate surroundings. Some people will become carriers for prolonged periods, while others will harbor the organisms only intermittently. For unknown reasons, people in certain occupations, including physicians, nurses, and other hospital workers, are more prone to colonization. Also, certain patient groups, including diabetics, patients on hemodialysis, and chronic intravenous drug abusers, have a higher carriage rate than does the general population.

ENTRY

S. aureus and most other bacteria do not usually penetrate into deep tissues unless the skin or the mucous membranes are damaged or actually cut. Skin damage may be caused by burns, accidental wounds, lacerations, insect bites, surgical intervention, or associated skin diseases. If present in very large numbers, some bacteria, including *S. aureus*, are able to enter spontaneously and cause disease. This scenario occurs in cases of poor hygiene or prolonged moisture of the skin, which permit the growth of large numbers of organisms. It is not known if these infections are caused by spontaneous penetration or if the organisms enter through inapparent cuts and abrasions.

SPREAD AND MULTIPLICATION

The survival of *S. aureus* in tissues depends on several factors: the number of entering organisms, the site involved, the speed with which the body mounts an inflammatory response, and the immunological status of the host. When the inoculum is small and the host is immunologically competent, infections by these and other organisms are usually stopped. Nonetheless, staphylococci possess a particularly complex but effective pathogenic strategy, and even healthy persons may be unable to combat *S. aureus*. Luckily, the area of inflammation most often remains localized, and the organisms can be contained.

DAMAGE

Most local staphylococcal infections lead to the formation of a collection of pus called an **abscess**. Abscesses in the skin are called boils or, in medical parlance, **furuncles**. Multiple interconnected abscesses are called **carbuncles**. Alternatively, staphylococci can spread in the subcutaneous or submucosal tissue and cause a diffuse inflammation called **cellulitis**. In most cases, these skin infections are caused by *S. aureus* and not by the other staphylococcal species.

The development of an abscess is a complex process that involves both bacterial and host factors (Fig. 11-4). The early events are characteristic of an **acute inflammatory reaction**, with a rapid and extensive influx of leukocytes (e.g., neutrophils). Chemotactic factors, derived both from bacteria and complement, are made in large amounts. However, some staphylococci not only survive this onslaught but are even capable of killing and lysing many of the neutrophils that have entered the infection area by the production of cytolysins. The lysed neutrophils pour out large amounts of lysosomal enzymes, which damage surrounding tissue.

The combination of MSCRAMMs and an intense host response to the organisms results in the area being surrounded with a thick-walled fibrin capsule. The center of the abscess is usually necrotic and contains debris consisting of dead neutrophils and epithelial cells, dead and live bacteria, and edema fluid. An abscess, then, is a well-defined area in tissue that contains pus. From the point of view of the host, it represents a containment of invading organisms in one site. However, from the point of view of the staphylococci, it represents a walled-off site protected from the host immune attack. The site may also be the source of toxins produced and secreted by the organism such as TSS toxin-1, staphylococcal enterotoxins, and staphylococcal enterotoxin–like molecules, which can result in TSS.

Staphylococcal infection involves a massive struggle between the white blood cells and the invading organisms (see Fig. 11-4). Despite an impressive array of virulence factors, *S. aureus* does not always win the struggle; neutrophils usually gain the upper hand. The importance of neutrophils in containing staphylococcal infections is evident in children with the hereditary defect in phagocyte function called **chronic granulomatous disease**. This potentially fatal disease is characterized by frequent and serious infections with *S. aureus*. Neutrophils of these patients are unable to make sufficient hydrogen peroxide to set off the oxidative killing pathway. In these children, the balance between staphylococci and phagocytes is clearly shifted toward the microorganisms.

S. aureus produces an unusually large number of virulence factors that either prevent the bacteria from being phagocytized or help them to survive in phagocytes after they are ingested. These factors include soluble enzymes, toxins, and cell-associated constituents. This formidable list invites speculation: why are so many virulence factors needed? Perhaps these factors do not individually impart virulence but act in concert to permit the pathogen to cause disease. Or perhaps different factors are important in different sites of infection. More detailed study of these molecules is needed to answer these puzzling questions.

What are the main factors that allow staphylococci to defend themselves against neutrophils? First, the cell surface of staphylococci plays an important defensive role. More than 90% of *S. aureus* strains that cause disease are surrounded by a **capsule** that may inhibit phagocytosis, but its role in virulence is far less clear than the capsules of meningococcus or pneumococcus. By far the most common capsular serotypes are 5 and 8. Staphylococci also make a slime layer that provides protection from host neutrophils. **Peptidoglycan** in the cell wall of *S. aureus* activates complement by the alternative pathway, thus contributing to the inflammatory response.

Lipoteichoic acid in peptidoglycan also interacts with toll-like receptors (particularly **toll-like receptor-2**) on the surface of macrophages, causing these phagocytic cells to release proinflammatory cytokines. Note that in this regard, staphylococcal lipoteichoic acid resembles the endotoxin of Gram-negative bacteria. Endotoxin activates the alternative pathway of complement and interacts with toll-like receptor 4 on macrophages to cause proinflammatory cytokine release. **Lipoteichoic acids** and **teichoic acid** are polymers of ribitol and glycerophosphates (see Chapter 3), which also appear to be involved in complement activation and possibly in the adherence of these organisms to mucosal cells.

A fourth wall component, **protein A**, has an unexpected property: it binds to the Fc terminus of immunoglobulin G. This binding incapacitates the antibody function of these molecules because their antigen-binding end, the Fab portion, is dangling away from the surface of the organisms. As a result, the number of Fc residues available for attachment to phagocytes is reduced, thereby reducing opsonization. Protein A is also released into the environment surrounding bacterial growth, where it may bind free antibodies in the same manner (see Fig. 11-4).

In addition to these components, *S. aureus* secretes many enzymes and toxins that are almost certainly directed

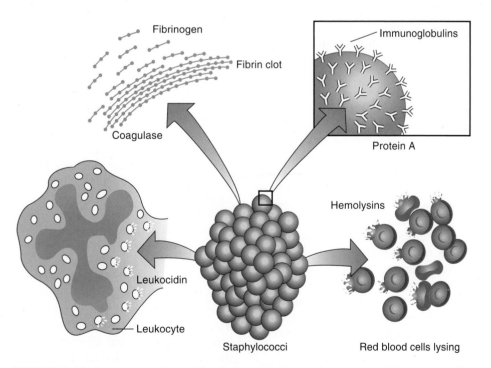

FIGURE 11-4. Virulence properties of *Staphylococcus aureus* in pus and abscess formation. The development of an abscess is a complex process that involves both bacterial and host factors. *S. aureus* infections causes a rapid and extensive influx of leukocytes (e.g., neutrophils). Chemotactic factors, derived both from bacteria and complement, are made in large amounts. *S. aureus* secretes coagulase that causes formation of clots. Protein A is released where it may bind antibodies reducing opsonization. *S. aureus* lyse neutrophils and red blood cells that have entered the infection area by the production of cytolysins (leukocidins and hemolysins). The lysed neutrophils pour out large amounts of lysosomal enzymes, which damage surrounding tissue.

toward the struggle with phagocytes. **Catalase** converts hydrogen peroxide to water and may help counteract the neutrophils' ability to kill bacteria by the production of oxygen free radicals. **Coagulases** convert fibrinogen to fibrin and may help prevent the organisms from being phagocytized, since white cells penetrate fibrin clots poorly.

Several **pore-forming toxins** are important virulence factors of *S. aureus*. The molecules damage not only phagocytic cells but also other cells (e.g., vascular endothelium, renal endothelium, neurons, and myocardial cells). These toxins exert their effect by creating channels in cell membranes that significantly disturb cellular homeostasis. The α-, γ-, and δ-toxins have been traditionally referred to as **hemolysins (cytolysins)** because they lyse red blood cells contained in blood agar plates. However, this effect on red cells does not appear to play a role in human infection. α-Toxin, γ-toxin, and a related toxin called **Panton-Valentine leukocidin** are particularly effective in damaging neutrophils. Another non–pore-forming hemolysin is called β-toxin; this protein toxin is a sphingomyelinase (also called hot–cold hemolysin) that prepares red blood cells at 37°C for lysis at 4°C. The role of β-toxin in human disease is unclear but appears to be important in biofilm formation, sometimes called biofilm ligase, especially during endocarditis.

Several other proteins made by *S. aureus* probably enhance its virulence by damaging tissues. Many strains make a **hyaluronidase**, which hydrolyzes the matrix of connective tissue and perhaps facilitates bacterial spread along tissue planes. Most strains also make lipases, proteases, deoxyribonucleases (DNases), and other enzymes that may also act as **virulence enhancers**.

In addition to tissue-damaging factors, *S. aureus* produces substances that make them difficult to treat with antibiotics. Two highly clinically significant examples of these substances are **β-lactamase**, a powerful enzyme that hydrolyzes the classical penicillins, and production of **penicillin-binding protein 2a** (**PBP2a**), which confers resistance to all penicillin- and cephalosporin-class antibiotics. The bacteria carrying PBP2a are referred to as **methicillin-resistant S. aureus** or **MRSA**. β-Lactamase is found in about 90% of *S. aureus* strains and is responsible for the resistance to penicillins that was identified in the late 1940s and spread rapidly around the world. PBP2a mediates continued peptidoglycan synthesis in the presence of all types of penicillin and cephalosporin antibiotics as a result of an alteration in the binding site and decreased affinity for these antibiotics. Today, up to 70% of hospital-associated *S. aureus* strains and 30% of community-associated strains may be methicillin resistant owing to PBP2a. Currently, PBP2a is encoded by as many as eight different staphylococcal cassette chromosome methicillin resistance (*mec*) DNAs contained within the chromosome.

Most local staphylococcal diseases are self-limiting by spontaneously draining through the skin; they do not typically result in metastatic infections. In healthy individuals, organisms that escape from a local abscess are usually destroyed by the clearance mechanisms of the blood and the lymphatics. When staphylococci become implanted in deep tissues, they tend to colonize tissues that have been previously damaged by physical trauma, disease, or surgical intervention. Otherwise, the site of metastatic infection seems random and is probably dictated by the clearing capacity of the organ and the amount of blood flowing through it. The main sites of metastatic abscesses are the highly vascularized organs: bones, joints, lungs, and kidneys. Immunocompromised patients frequently have multiple staphylococcal metastases, which can lead to serious and often fatal diseases.

Once implanted in deep tissue and able to survive, *S. aureus* elicits an inflammatory reaction similar to that of a skin abscess. In the words of Pasteur, osteomyelitis is a "boil of the bone." The consequences of abscess formation in deep sites depend on their location. Nowhere is it more devastating than in the heart, lung, or brain. However, if the function of the organ is not directly compromised, staphylococcal abscesses can persist for a considerable period and cause relatively mild symptoms. These symptoms may tax the diagnostic acumen of the physician.

Damage Caused by Other Species of Staphylococci

S. epidermidis, the common inhabitant of the normal skin, rarely causes disease. However, infections with *S. epidermidis* and other coagulase-negative staphylococci are found with increasing frequency in patients with implanted artificial devices, such as prosthetic joints or intravenous catheters. When defense mechanisms are impaired, *S. epidermidis* can cause serious infections, like septicemia and endocarditis. A potential virulence factor of these organisms is the peptidoglycan, and the same exopolysaccharide **slime layer** that is present in *S. aureus* has been found in more than 80% of disease-causing isolates of *S. epidermidis*. It is thought that this slime layer allows the organisms to stick to the surface of plastics used in various devices.

S. saprophyticus, another coagulase negative organism, may be the most highly specialized of the staphylococci in terms of pathogenicity because it is almost entirely associated with urinary tract infections, particularly cystitis in young women. The reason for this specialization is not yet known, but it seems likely that this organism has unique properties that allow it to bind the epithelium of the urethra or the bladder. Uncommonly, the coagulase-negative *S. lugdunensis* is now recognized as the cause of an aggressive endocarditis. The virulence properties of the organism that lead to this infection are unclear.

Staphylococcal Toxin Diseases

In contrast to the classical complicated infections already discussed, staphylococci cause three definite toxin-related diseases. The symptoms of each of these diseases are clearly caused by toxins, even in the absence of bacteria. The first disease is called **staphylococcal scalded skin syndrome (SSSS)**, a life-threatening disease that mainly affects neonates. SSSS is characterized by extensive sloughing of the skin. Two exotoxins, known as **exfoliative toxins A** and **B**, cause these symptoms. Their role in human disease has been clearly established because the administration of specific antitoxin prevents the skin lesions in humans or mice. Exfoliative toxins are highly tissue-specific serine proteases that cause separation of the layers of the epidermis at the **desmosomes**. Exfoliative toxin production by *S. aureus* does not contribute to systemic infections by the bacteria.

A second disease definitively caused by exotoxins, called **toxic shock syndrome (TSS)**, is characterized by fever, skin rash, hypotension, peeling of the skin on recovery, and the dysfunction of several essential systems as was the case in Ms. G's illness (see Fig. 11-3). However, TSS can occur in the absence of one or more of those defining symptoms. The disease was originally associated with the use of highly absorbent tampons, which appear to introduce oxygen into the vagina and stimulate toxin production by the organisms. Oxygen is absolutely essential to the production of TSS-inducing toxins, and the vagina in the absence of tampons is anaerobic. TSS still occurs in association with tampon use, though less frequently as a result of the use of lower-absorbency tampons, but also commonly follows staphylococcal infections of any other type, and it occurs in men as well as women. Ms. G presented with the typical signs of TSS; she was of menstrual age and also used tampons. However, her case of TSS was associated with an abscess associated with recent arthroscopic knee surgery. Of particular importance is the increasing association of TSS with lung infections and necrotizing pneumonia, particularly in strains of bacteria that are methicillin resistant.

The exotoxins involved in TSS include **toxic shock syndrome toxin-1**, the cause of all menstrual TSS cases and one-half of nonmenstrual cases, and **staphylococcal enterotoxins**, particularly enterotoxin serotypes B and C. These three exotoxins are produced by the bacteria in high concentrations, and that may be why they cause TSS. The toxins have been referred to as **superantigens** because of their novel way of interacting with T lymphocytes and macrophages (see Fig. 8-3). Superantigens cross-link one chain (β-chain) of the T-cell antigen receptor with major histocompatibility complex class II molecules on macrophages. The effect of this interaction is a massive release of cytokines from macrophages and T cells that mediate TSS. For example, interleukin 1 (endogenous pyrogen) released from macrophages causes the fever of TSS. Tumor necrosis factor-α released from macrophages and tumor necrosis factor-β released from T cells cause capillary leak and therefore hypotension. Finally, interferon-γ and interleukin 2 release from T cells accounts for the rash of TSS patients. It is also important to remember that the massive release of interferon-γ

in TSS appears to prevent formation of protective neutralizing antibodies against the superantigens. Thus, TSS patients mostly remain susceptible to recurrent TSS, particularly women who continue to use tampons after TSS episodes. In addition, superantigens appear to subvert the formation of inflammation through an undefined mechanism when the organism is in abscesses. Thus, for example, surgical incision sites may not show the characteristic inflammation associated with staphylococcal infections. The staphylococcal superantigens are structurally related to the streptococcal scarlet fever toxins, which also cause TSS.

Recently, a new syndrome has been described and is associated with a superantigen related to TSST-1. This illness called extreme pyrexia syndrome is characterized by acute onset of fevers exceeding 108°F. Because of the exceptionally high fevers in spite of heroic efforts to reduce body temperature, all patients thus far described have succumbed. The high fevers in these patients are consistent with the exceptional pyrogenicity of this and other superantigens.

Finally, **staphylococcal enterotoxin serotypes A through E** and **I** are major causes of **food poisoning** when ingested. These exotoxins can cause disease even in the absence of the organism. They cause intensive intestinal peristalsis, apparently by working directly on the vomiting control center of the brain. They are heat stable, resist proteases, and are not necessarily destroyed by cooking, even though the staphylococci that produced them are killed. These toxins cause signs and symptoms that mimic the disease when administered to laboratory animals. Note that the same strain of *S. aureus* can cause several of the diseases mentioned.

All of the virulence factors, whether cell associated or secreted, are under the control of global genetic regulators. As in many other bacteria, these regulators include two-component regulatory systems, such as **accessory gene regulator**, **staphylococcal respiratory response**, and others (see Chapter 19 paradigm).

DIAGNOSIS

Recognizing staphylococcal infections is not usually a difficult diagnostic problem, and they are among the most frequent infections seen both in the community and in the hospital. A localized abscess in a seriously ill patient should be aspirated and the contents examined by Gram stain and culture to identify the staphylococcal species as well as the antibiotic susceptibility patterns. Clusters of large Gram-positive cocci point to staphylococcal infection. The patient's blood should also be cultured to determine if the organisms have invaded the bloodstream. Both *S. aureus* and coagulase-negative staphylococci are commonly isolated in blood cultures; however, the latter is most often a contaminant and is considered pathogenic only under special circumstances. The coagulase test serves to distinguish the two species.

TREATMENT

Antibiotics to treat *S. aureus* infections target multiple pathways that are essential for bacterial survival, including bacterial cell-wall synthesis (e.g., β-lactams, glycopeptides), folic acid metabolism (sulfonamides), and bacterial protein synthesis (e.g., macrolides, lincosamides, and aminoglycosides) (Table 11-2).

A staphylococcal abscess should be drained, and an appropriate antibiotic should be administered. The bacteria will probably be resistant to penicillin but sensitive to semisynthetic penicillins, such as nafcillin—that is, **methicillin-sensitive *S. aureus* (MSSA)**. Semisynthetic penicillins and cephalosporins that are resistant to staphylococcal β-lactamase will kill these bacteria. **Methicillin-resistant *S. aureus* (MRSA)** has appeared with increasing frequency, first in hospitals and more recently in the community. Infections with MRSA require treatment with vancomycin, which until recently was the last available drug for some highly resistant strains. Other antibiotics active against MRSA include aminoglycosides, macrolides, clindamycin, Synercid (quinupristin/dalfopristin), daptomycin, tetracyclines, linezolid, doxycycline, tigecycline, and/or trimethoprim/sulfamethoxazole, which may be useful second-line agents in the treatment of certain kinds of staphylococcal infections (particularly in penicillin-allergic patients), although some strains are resistant to them as well. Fluoroquinolones had been used to treat MRSA infections. Unfortunately, resistance to these antibiotics has also developed rapidly; 60 to 70% of MRSA isolates are also quinolone resistant.

TABLE 11-2 Antistaphylococcal Therapies and Resistance Mechanism(s)

Classification	Antimicrobial Agents	Mechanism of Action	Main Resistance Mechanism(s)
β-Lactam	Methicillin, oxacillin, nafcillin, cephalosporins	Inhibit cell wall biosynthesis	β-lactamase (penicillinase); modified penicillin-binding protein PBP2a (*mec*A)
Glycoprotein	Vancomycin	Inhibits cell wall synthesis by inhibiting the incorporation of newly synthesized precursors in the cell wall peptidoglycan	Thickened cell wall that traps vancomycin (increased and structurally varied pentapeptides); change of binding site (D-ala-D-ala to D-ala-D-Lac)
Lipopeptide	Daptomycin	Depolarization of the membrane	Decreased access to the cell membrane
Macrolides	Erythromycin, clarithromycin, and azithromycin	Reversibly binds to 23S ribosomal RNA (rRNA) of the 50S subunit of bacterial ribosome inhibiting RNA-dependent protein synthesis	A methylase that dimethylates an adenine within the 23S ribosomal binding site of the macrolides (*erm*; inducible) An efflux pump [*mef* (E)] that expels the macrolides
Lincosamide	Clindamycin	Binds to the 50S ribosome and inhibits protein synthesis	*erm*; cross-resistance to macrolides
Oxazolidinone	Linezolid	Binds to 23S rRNA of the 50S ribosomal subunits and prevents formation of the 70S initiation complex	Mutation in the 23S rRNA
Streptogramin	Quinupristin/dalfopristin	Inhibit protein synthesis	*erm*; cross-resistance to macrolides and clindamycin
Aminoglycoside	Gentamicin, tobramycin, amikacin	Binds to the 30S ribosome and inhibits protein synthesis	Aminoglycoside-modifying enzymes
Tetracycline	Tetracycline, minocycline, doxycycline, tigecycline	Binds to the 30S ribosome and inhibit protein synthesis	Efflux transporters
Sulfonamides	Trimethoprim/sulfamethoxazole	Inhibit folic acids biosynthesis	Single amino acid substitution in dihydrofolate reductase

The ability of the antibiotic to inhibit protein synthesis should also be considered in the selection of antimicrobial agents to treat infections caused by toxin-producing Gram-positive pathogens. One antibiotic that deserves special mention is clindamycin. This inhibitor of protein synthesis has become a useful antibiotic in the treatment of exotoxin diseases of staphylococci because of its ability to prevent exotoxin synthesis prior to inhibiting the growth of the organisms. The choice of drugs should be based on the antibiotic sensitivity of the infecting strain and the special characteristics of the patient.

Unfortunately, in the last few years, a handful of patients in the United States have been identified with high-level vancomycin resistance in the presence of methicillin resistance. **Vancomycin-resistant *S. aureus* (VRSA)** has acquired the genes that encode vancomycin resistance from resistant *Enterococcus* species in patients infected with both pathogens. Newer antimicrobial agents, such as linezolid, Synercid, and daptomycin, generally have activity against staphylococci that are resistant to multiple antibiotics. These newer antibiotics are generally reserved for such cases and when vancomycin cannot be used. Nevertheless, if multidrug-resistant staphylococci emerge as major clinical entities, we may one day face the daunting problem of common and potentially dangerous staphylococcal infections with no effective antibiotics at our disposal.

Some physicians have advocated the use of intravenous immunoglobulin in the treatment of superantigen-mediated TSS. These antibody preparations are obtained from large pools of human volunteers, many of whom have preexistent antibodies to superantigens. There is published evidence of reductions in fatality rates with use of intravenous immunoglobulins for the treatment of streptococcal TSS.

PREVENTION

Over the years, vaccines have been developed for the treatment of recurrent, recalcitrant staphylococcal infections and to prevent the carrier state. Success has been limited, probably because circulating antibodies play a relatively minor role in these infections. Currently, there is no FDA-approved *S. aureus* vaccine, and attempts to develop vaccines continue today.

CONCLUSION

Staphylococci are potent pathogens, are widely found in the human environment, and may cause a variety of infections. They are hardy organisms that can survive under adverse conditions. They possess a large number of virulence factors that allow them to cause serious diseases by various mechanisms. The most common diseases caused by these versatile pathogens are pyogenic infections, sometimes leading to the formation of abscesses in deep tissues. They can also cause distinct disease entities by making specific toxins. Staphylococci have acquired antimicrobial resistance promptly after the introduction of new antibiotics. Currently, many strains are resistant to multiple antibiotics, and the prospect of the emergence of a strain resistant to all available antibiotics is a serious concern.

Suggested Readings

Brosnahan AJ, Schlievert PM. Gram-positive bacterial superantigen outside-in signaling causes toxic shock syndrome. *FEBS J.* 2011;278(23):4649–4667.

Herold BC, Immergluck LC, Maranan MC, et al. Community-acquired methicillin-resistant *Staphylococcus aureus* in children with no identified predisposing risk. *JAMA.* 1998;279:593–598.

Hiramatsu K, Cui L, Kuroda M, et al. The emergence and evolution of methicillin resistant *Staphylococcus aureus. Trends Microbiol.* 2001;9:486–493.

Lin YC, Peterson ML. New insights into the prevention of staphylococcal infections and toxic shock syndrome. *Expert Rev Clin Pharmacol.* 2010;3(6):753–767.

Lowy F. *Staphylococcus aureus* infections. *N Engl J Med.* 1998;339:520–532.

Novick RP. Autinduction and signal transduction in the regulation of staphylococcal virulence. *Mol Microbiol.* 2003;48:1429–1449.

Schwarz-Linek U, Hook M, Potts JR. The molecular basis of fibronectin-mediated bacterial adherence to host cells. *Mol Microbiol.* 2004;52:631–641.

Thwaites GE, Edgeworth JD, Gkrania-Klotsas E, et al. UK Clinical Infection Research Group. Clinical management of *Staphylococcus aureus* bacteraemia. *Lancet Infect Dis.* 2011;11(3): 208–222.

Chapter **12**

Streptococci and Enterococci: "Strep Throat" and Beyond

Kevin S. McIver

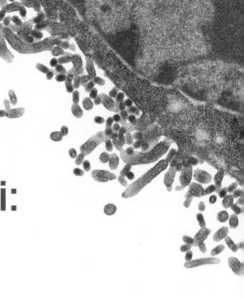

KEY CONCEPTS

Group A Streptococci

Pathogen: Gram-positive cocci that grow in pairs or chains and ferment carbon sources to produce lactic acid. They are classified by their hemolytic patterns on blood agar, serologic reaction of cell wall antigens, and speciation based on metabolic and DNA sequence differences.

Encounter: Streptococci reside in a human reservoir.

Entry: Group A streptococci (GAS) are strict human pathogens that colonize the nasopharynx and the skin as portals of entry. They may also exhibit asymptomatic carriage at these sites.

Spread: Streptococci are transmitted by contact between humans who carry the organism or have disease.

Multiplication: Extracellular growth of the organisms occurs on mucous membranes, in skin, or in deeper tissue.

Damage: GAS elaborate numerous extracellular toxins and surface virulence factors that mediate evasions of the immune response and cause extensive tissue damage and spread from the initial site of infection. GAS infection can also result in immune-related diseases (e.g., acute rheumatic fever, glomerulonephritis), which persist even after the organism has been cleared from the body.

Diagnosis: GAS can be cultured from the throat or detected by rapid immunoassays.

Treatment and Prevention: GAS remains susceptible to penicillin. Treatment prevents locally invasive infection, rheumatic fever, and transmission to other susceptible hosts. There is no vaccine currently available.

Group B Streptococci: Group B streptococci (GBS) are also strict human pathogens and are a leading cause of neonatal sepsis and meningitis.

"Viridans" Streptococci: "Viridans" streptococci are a-hemolytic species inhabiting the oral cavity that can seed the bloodstream and cause endocarditis under certain conditions.

Enterococci

Pathogen: Enterococci are Gram-positive cocci that grow in pairs or chains and ferment carbon sources to produce lactic acid. They can grow in bile and in relatively high salt concentrations.

Encounter: Enterococci are commensal organisms in the gastrointestinal tract of healthy individuals as well as many other animals. They can act as opportunistic pathogens of compromised patients in nosocomial infections.

Entry: Gastrointestinal or by contamination of indwelling catheters by infected hands.

Spread: Enterococcal infections are local but may cause transient bacteremia.

Multiplication: Extracellular growth of the organisms occurs in the genitourinary tract or in abscesses (in association with other bacteria).

Damage: They possess a hemolysin for human RBCs but cause relatively weak pathogens. Bacteremia may result in endocarditis.

Diagnosis: Routine cultures grow nonhemolytic or weakly hemolytic colonies on sheep blood agar.

Treatment and Prevention: Enterococci are intrinsically resistant to many antibiotics and often require synergistic antibiotic combinations to successfully treat infection. Vancomycin-resistant enterococci are an increasing problem in hospitals because physicians are running out of effective antibiotics to treat them.

THE STREPTOCOCCI and enterococci are a heterogeneous group of bacteria that colonize and infect humans and animals. In humans, they cause diseases as diverse as streptococcal pharyngitis ("strep throat"), cellulitis, neonatal meningitis, brain abscess, endocarditis, and life-threatening necrotizing fasciitis (the "flesh-eating" bacteria). Because they cause the most widespread disease in humans, ***Streptococcus pyogenes***, also known as the **group A streptococcus** (**GAS**), are best understood in terms of mechanisms of disease. The pneumococcus (*Streptococcus pneumoniae*) is another important streptococcal species that is addressed in Chapter 13.

CLASSIFICATION OF STREPTOCOCCI AND ENTEROCOCCI

The nomenclature for the streptococci and enterococci can be confusing because there are three different methods of classification:

- **Hemolytic pattern**: When streptococci and enterococci are grown on blood agar media in the clinical laboratory, the colonies may be surrounded by an area of partial hemolysis that appears greenish (α-hemolysis), the absence of a zone (γ-hemolysis or nonhemolysis), or a clear zone of complete hemolysis (β-hemolysis) as shown in Figure 12-1.
- **Group-specific antigens (Lancefield classification)**: Rebecca Lancefield first used **serological reactivity** to extracted cell wall antigens from various streptococci/enterococci to divide them into groups lettered A through U. Many streptococcal species cannot be assigned to any group because there are no antisera that react to their cell wall antigens.
- **Species**: Various species of streptococci can be determined by performing **biochemical tests** that analyze the metabolism and presence of enzymes in the bacterium. Newer molecular techniques can differentiate species on the basis of **DNA sequences**.

In the clinical laboratory, all three methods may be employed to characterize an isolated streptococcus. Although they react with group D antisera, the enterococci are now considered to be a separate genus. In Table 12-1, you will find a list of clinically relevant streptococci and enterococci with their classification and common disease associations.

GROUP A STREPTOCOCCI
ENCOUNTER

Historically, the group A streptococci (GAS; *S. pyogenes*) have been the most important pathogens to humans in the streptococcal family. Serious GAS infections have become less common in the developed world, but sporadic outbreaks of highly virulent strains remind us that GAS has the potential to be a significant reemerging pathogen. Morbidity and mortality as a result of GAS infection are still common in the developing world, leading to over 500,000 deaths worldwide per year. The spectrum of diseases caused by GAS is influenced by the strain type, host factors, and portal of entry. Some of the most important clinical manifestations of GAS infection are shown in Figure 12-2.

GAS is ubiquitous in the human population and is distributed worldwide. Disease is most common in school-aged children between 5 and 15 years old, and like V., primarily presents as **acute pharyngitis**, or "**strep throat**." The other common site of infection is in the skin and soft tissues, resulting in a group of infections called **pyoderma**. Pyoderma is most prevalent in

CASE • V., a 5-year-old girl, had a sore throat, headache, and fever for 5 days. Her mother then brought her to the pediatrician because she developed a red, rough "sandpaper-like" rash on her arms. She had swollen, tender cervical lymph nodes, and her oropharynx was red with a grayish-white exudate covering both tonsils. Her throat swab was positive for presence of GAS antigen using a rapid enzyme immunoassay (rapid strep test), and the culture grew a b-hemolytic streptococcus 24 hours later. However, on the basis of the immunoassay, a 10-day course of penicillin was prescribed. After the second day on antibiotics, V. felt much better, and her mother decided to stop giving her the penicillin so she could have it for other illnesses in the future. Three weeks later, V. was having trouble keeping up with her classmates on the playground, had pain in her knees, and was again having fevers. After hearing a loud heart murmur on physical examination, her pediatrician obtained an echocardiogram that demonstrated mitral valve regurgitation and extensive damage to the valve leaflets.

This case raises several questions for you to consider:

1. Streptococcal pharyngitis is a common self-limited disease. Why do physicians always treat this disease?
2. What bacterial process caused the rash?
3. Why were 2 days of antibiotics insufficient treatment, even though V. felt better?
4. Did the GAS directly spread to the heart and cause the damage to the heart valves?

See Appendix for answers.

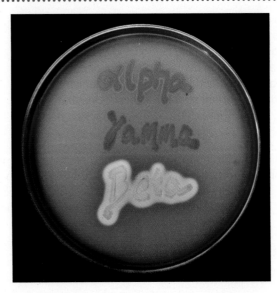

FIGURE 12-1. Hemolytic classification of streptococci. Ability to produce a zone of hemolysis on blood agar is an important phenotype used to classify streptococcal species in the clinical laboratory. A representative of each type of hemolysis is shown in the figure. Partial lysis is called **α-hemolysis** (e.g., *S. sanguinis*) and results in the leakage of hemoglobin from the lysed cells producing a greenish colorization (viridans streptococci). Lack of lysis is called **γ-hemolysis** or **nonhemolysis** (e.g., *E. faecalis*). **β-hemolysis** (e.g., *S. pyogenes*) represents complete lysis and heme degradation producing a clear zone around the streptococcal colony. There are clinically relevant streptococci represented by all three types of hemolysis (Table 12-1).

preschool children and is seen more frequently in tropical climates or during periods of hot, humid weather. GAS can occasionally cause foodborne outbreaks but is not associated with gastrointestinal disease. The delayed non-suppurative (immune-based) sequelae of GAS infection, acute glomerulonephritis (AGN) and acute rheumatic fever (ARF), are more commonly encountered in developing countries, probably because of frequency of disease and poor access to medical care.

GAS are usually found in the nasopharynx and on the skin of humans. As many as 20% of school-aged children may carry GAS for weeks at a time in the pharynx during the winter months, although many do not have symptoms of infection. V. probably acquired her infection from a schoolmate who may have had a clinical, subclinical, or asymptomatic infection. Person-to-person spread is mediated by **respiratory droplets** or by **direct contact** in the case of skin transmission. People with nasal colonization are able to transmit the organisms more efficiently than are people with skin or pharyngeal colonization.

ENTRY

For streptococcal pyoderma infections, the bacterium must gain entry into deeper layers of skin through direct implantation after a break or trauma (e.g., abrasions, chickenpox lesions, bites, wounds, and eczema), because GAS cannot penetrate intact skin. In many cases, the damage to the skin can be quite subtle, and even a minor scratch

TABLE 12-1 Hemolytic Patterns of Streptococci and Enterococci Important for Human Disease

Classification	Genus/Species	Hemolysis	Human Disease
Group A	*S. pyogenes*	β	Pharyngitis, skin and soft tissue infections, toxic shock, necrotizing fasciitis, acute rheumatic fever, scarlet fever, cellulitis
Group B	*S. agalactiae*	β, γ	Neonatal meningitis and sepsis
Group C/G	*S. dysgalactiae*	β	Respiratory and deep tissue infections
Group D: *Enterococcus*	*E. faecalis, E. faecium*	α, γ, β[a]	Nosocomial infections, urinary tract infections, endocarditis
Group D: Bovis group	*S. bovis, S. infantarius*	α, γ	Endocarditis
Viridans, Mitis group	*S. mitis, S. sanguinis, S. gordonii*	α	Endocarditis, systemic infection in neutropenic patients
Viridans, Mutans group	*S. mutans, S. sobrinus*	α, γ, β[a]	Dental caries and endocarditis
Viridans, Salivarius group	*S. salivarius, S. vestibularis*	α	Opportunistic pathogen in compromised hosts
Viridans, Anginosus group	*S. milleri, S. anginosus, S. intermedius*	α, γ, β[a]	Abscesses, endocarditis
	S. pneumoniae	α	Pneumonia, sepsis, meningitis, otitis media

[a]Rare hemolysis pattern.

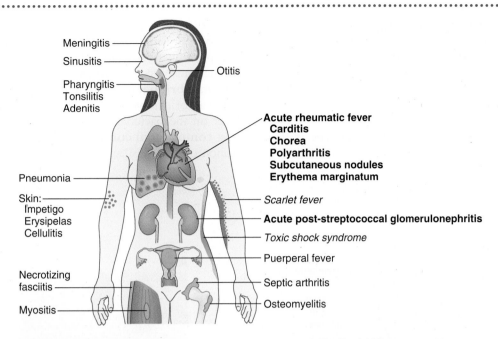

FIGURE 12-2. Diseases caused by group A streptococci (GAS). GAS cause a wide spectrum of diseases throughout the human body. The suppurative diseases (*labeled in black*) are caused by direct damage by the organism and the secreted enzymes of GAS. The nonsuppurative sequelae of GAS infection (*labeled in bold*) are late manifestations caused by an autoimmune response. The toxin-mediated diseases (*labeled in italics*) are caused by streptococcal exotoxins that are secreted into the bloodstream.

can serve as a portal of entry. In streptococcal pharyngeal infections, the bacterium is thought to bind to the mucous membranes of the pharynx using **adhesins** on the bacterial cell surface to prevent it from being swept away by fluid secretions. **M protein** has been implicated as an important adhesin to keratinocytes, the main cell type in the outer layers of the skin. The **hyaluronic acid (HA) capsule** may allow GAS to bind to the host HA receptor CD44 found on the surface of pharyngeal epithelial cells and skin keratinocytes. GAS also adhere to host extracellular matrix (ECM) molecules found surrounding host tissue such as fibronectin and laminin using ECM adhesins such as the cell wall–associated **lipoteichoic acid, streptococcal fibronectin-binding proteins (SfbI, Protein F, Fba)**, and **serum opacity factor**.

Once GAS enters a host, it must evade phagocytosis and the immune response to multiply and establish an effective infection. The pathogen elicits two major **antiphagocytic factors**, the aforementioned **M protein** and **HA capsule**. In addition, GAS are able to produce several proteins to degrade chemotaxins that recruit neutrophils to the site of infection, inactivate or degrade antibodies, and block antimicrobial peptide function.

SPREAD AND MULTIPLICATION

GAS usually remain localized to the site of initial infection, but an increase in aggressive life-threatening diseases of the deeper tissues was noted in the 1990s. In the orophar-

ynx, infections are usually self-limiting and localized to the pharynx and tonsils, accounting for the erythema and exudate associated with V.'s strep throat. Rarely, the infection can cause a peritonsillar abscess (quinsy) or spread to adjacent structures such as the mastoid air cells or middle ear.

Benign GAS infections of the superficial layers of skin result in crusty honey-colored lesions called **impetigo**, which are most common in children living in hot, humid climates. Infections in deeper layers of skin cause **erysipelas** and **cellulitis**.

On rare occasions (1–3 per 100,000 in the United States), GAS reaches the fascial planes between the skin and muscle. This may occur as a result of a traumatic breach through the skin (wound or insect bite). In such cases, the infection may spread rapidly and proximally from the initial site of infection. GAS secretes several enzymes that may promote spread along tissue planes resulting in life-threatening diseases such as **necrotizing fasciitis** and **myositis**. These enzymes include proteases, hyaluronidase, deoxyribonucleases (DNases), and **streptokinase**. Streptokinase can bind to human **plasminogen** to form a catalytic complex that converts plasminogen to plasmin, which is then bound on the GAS surface. Plasmin-coated GAS can degrade and spread through fibrin, a major component of blood clots and barrier to microbial spread. GAS also secretes **streptolysins S and O**, hemolysins that lyse the membranes of various host cells. Lysis of red blood cells by these hemolysins is the basis for the β-hemolysis pattern seen on blood agar media. It is thought these hemolysins also contribute to the extensive tissue damage seen in invasive GAS infections. Thus, the products secreted by GAS support the dissemination of the pathogen.

M Protein

M protein, a central player in GAS pathogenesis, is a fibrillar, coiled-coil surface protein covalently attached to the cell wall of the pathogen (Fig. 12-3). As mentioned above, M protein plays a role in adhesion to keratinocytes and prevents opsonization by complement through two mechanisms. First, M protein binds the host cell plasma protein, **fibrinogen**, which interferes with the alternative pathway of complement deposition by forming a dense layer on the bacterial surface. Second, M protein binds host **complement control proteins** that inhibit the formation of opsonins by the complement cascade. Despite

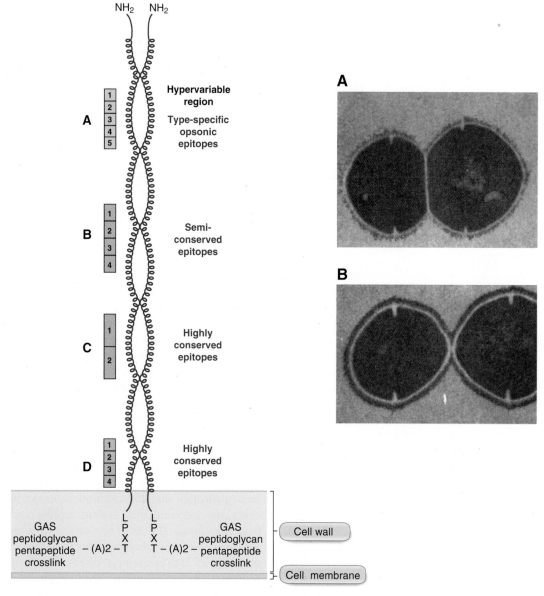

FIGURE 12-3. M protein of GAS. M protein molecules are fibrillar, typically 500 amino acids long, and are covalently anchored to the peptidoglycan cell wall at the carboxy-terminus of the protein. Each M protein is primarily α-helical in structure, contains as many as four blocks of repeating amino acid sequences (*A–D*), including the hypervariable amino-terminal region (*A*) that represents the epitope for type-specific antibodies. Two α-helical fibrils of M protein are wound around each other in a coiled-coil conformation that extends away from the GAS surface. The proximal portion of the molecule (*C* and *D*) binds the complement control protein factor H and the distal portion (*B*) is able to bind fibrinogen, allowing protection from nonspecific opsonization by the alternative pathway of complement. **Inset A.** Electron micrograph of GAS after growth in liquid culture showing a fuzzy hairlike layer on the surface composed of M protein and lipoteichoic acid. The hyaluronic acid capsule cannot be seen because it is in a dehydrated and collapsed state resulting from the fixation process. **Inset B.** Electron micrograph of GAS after exposure to blood plasma. The fuzzy layer appears dense owing to fibrinogen bound to M protein and inhibits complement-mediated phagocytosis.

these antiphagocytic properties, antibodies formed against the hypervariable amino-terminal regions of M protein (Fig. 12-3) are able to effectively opsonize the organism and are protective against infection. Unfortunately, there are more than 100 M protein serotypes, and protective immunity is type specific. In fact, DNA sequence analysis of the hypervariable region of the M protein gene (*emm*-typing) currently used by the Centers for Disease Control (CDC) indicates that there are **over 200 distinct M-types**. Although this was probably not the first GAS infection for V., the strains of her previous infections expressed M proteins different from those of her current infection, so antibodies generated from her previous exposures could not protect her against reinfection.

Hyaluronic Acid Capsule

The HA capsule is another **antiphagocytic structure** on the streptococcal surface. HA is found in great abundance in human connective tissue. Therefore, streptococci enveloped in an HA capsule have camouflaged themselves in a host antigen that does not elicit an immune response. Indeed, outbreaks of severe GAS infections are often associated with highly encapsulated strains of bacteria that appear mucoid when cultured on blood agar media. Interestingly, this capsule interferes with adherence of GAS to epithelial cells, and the organism may need to shed the capsule during the early stages of infection. This may be achieved by digesting the capsule with hyaluronidase secreted by the bacteria.

DAMAGE

GAS characteristically evokes an intense inflammatory response in tissues. Although it has mechanisms to avoid the immune response, the large variety of secreted substances cause considerable damage to host tissues. The digestive enzymes that enable the GAS to spread to deeper tissues do much of the damage. GAS are able to grow in nonimmune whole blood where they can secrete toxins (**septicemia**) or the toxins alone can enter the bloodstream from infected tissue sites and cause systemic effects (**toxemia**).

Streptococcal Toxins

V. had a localized infection in her throat but developed a rash in distant parts of her body. This rash is the hallmark of **scarlet fever**, a toxemia almost exclusively associated with pharyngeal infections. The three toxins responsible for scarlet fever are the **streptococcal pyrogenic exotoxins (SPE) A**, **B**, and **C**. In addition to causing the rash seen in scarlet fever, SPE-A and SPE-C are also bacterial **superantigens** that can nonspecifically activate a large subset of T cells. The resulting massive release of proinflammatory cytokines by the activated T cells results in a sepsis-like clinical picture with shock and multiorgan failure. This **streptococcal toxic shock syndrome (STSS)** is very similar to the toxic shock syndrome (TSS) caused by *Staphylococcus aureus* (see Chapter 11). Epidemiologically, SPE-A has been most closely linked with STSS, but GAS also make several other superantigens.

Immunologically Mediated Disease

Although most GAS infections are mild, self-limited diseases, the immune system's intense inflammatory reaction to an infection may cause a group of diseases called the **nonsuppurative sequelae** (non–pus-forming secondary manifestations). The most feared sequela of GAS infection is **acute rheumatic fever**, a significant cause of valvular heart disease in the preantibiotic era and now in developing countries. Pharyngitis is the only type of streptococcal infection that can lead to ARF. The clinical manifestations of ARF (known as the Jones Criteria) appear 1 to 4 weeks following strep throat and may include **carditis, polyarthritis**, **chorea** (a neurological tic disorder resulting in uncontrollable dancelike movements), **subcutaneous nodules**, and a distinctive rash called **erythema marginatum**. The most common manifestations are carditis and polyarthritis. Eventually, all these acute manifestations resolve.

The primary reason streptococcal pharyngitis is treated with antibiotics is to prevent ARF and the permanent heart damage that may follow the acute carditis. People who have had ARF are susceptible to further exacerbations when they acquire subsequent streptococcal pharyngitis. The ongoing inflammation in the heart can lead to extensive **mitral** and/or **aortic valvular scarring** and **stenosis**. This manifestation, called "**rheumatic heart disease**," adversely affects the function of the heart (Fig. 12-4), leading ultimately to death from heart failure if the affected valves are not replaced. Furthermore, the turbulent flow of blood across a scarred or deformed valve can predispose to bacterial endocarditis. Fortunately, ARF and rheumatic heart disease can be prevented by eradicating the bacteria with antibiotics before a fulminant immunological response is mounted. This is the most critical reason for diagnosing and treating strep throat aggressively. Studies have shown that treatment with a full course of penicillin initiated up to 9 days after the onset of sore throat can effectively prevent ARF. Failure to complete a full course of treatment may result in ARF, as in the case of V. Patients like V. who develop ARF are usually given **prophylactic antibiotics** until well into adulthood or even for life to prevent repeat streptococcal infections that will inevitably worsen any ongoing heart damage.

Although the precise pathogenic mechanism of ARF is not known, the most compelling evidence suggests that ARF may be an **autoimmune disease** in which the body's own tissues are attacked by the immune system in a misguided attempt to eradicate the streptococci. GAS possess a number of surface constituents that appear

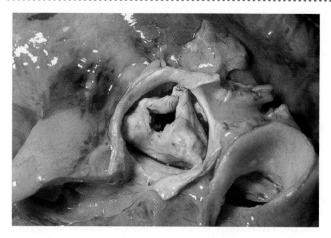

FIGURE 12-4. Aortic stenosis due to Acute Rheumatic Fever (ARF). ARF is a nonsuppurative sequela that may follow a GAS pharyngeal infection leading to inflammatory lesions of the heart (carditis), joints (arthritis), subcutaneous tissues (nodules), and CNS (chorea, tics). Although acute in nature, GAS reinfections can trigger recurrent ARF and lead to chronic rheumatic heart disease (RHD) evidenced by mitral or aortic valve damage, cardiac enlargement, and heart failure. The image shows an example of aortic stenosis representative of RHD where the normally three distinct leaflets of the aortic valve (center) have thickened and fused into two. The result is a defective, leaky valve that, if not replaced, can lead to heart failure.

immunologically identical to host tissue components. In particular, there is immunological cross-reaction between GAS antigens (such as certain M proteins) and tissues in the heart, synovium, and neurons in the brain. Such GAS M-types (called **rheumatogenic strains**) are more frequently associated with ARF; however, only a minority of people infected by a rheumatogenic strain go on to develop ARF. After years of research to elucidate the basis of ARF, the precise pathogenesis of this disease remains unclear. It is likely complex and depends on both host and bacterial factors.

The other important nonsuppurative sequela of GAS infection is **acute poststreptococcal glomerulonephritis (APSGN)**, which is caused by only a few M-types. Unlike ARF, APSGN may follow either a pharyngitis or pyodermal infection. Also unlike ARF, treatment with antibiotics does not affect the occurrence of this complication. In some outbreaks, the attack rate of APSGN has been as high as 40%, suggesting that susceptibility is common, if not universal. The pathogenic mechanism of APSGN is also incompletely understood, but it is thought that **immune complexes** consisting of streptococcal proteins and antibodies are deposited in the glomerular basement membrane and lead to complement fixation with subsequent renal injury. Like ARF, APSGN usually occurs 1 to 4 weeks after an infection. Patients with APSGN have blood and elevated protein in their urine, and they may go on to renal failure and require dialysis.

DIAGNOSIS

The various streptococcal skin infections have characteristic appearances, and the diagnosis is usually made presumptively, on clinical grounds. Impetigo, an infection of the most superficial skin layers, appears as a cluster of small vesicles on a pink base that breaks down to honey-colored crusts. Erysipelas is a raised, bright red patch of skin with a sharply demarcated but rapidly advancing margin. Deep infections such as myositis and necrotizing fasciitis are accompanied by excruciating pain and often some evidence of overlying skin necrosis. These disorders should be treated aggressively with both IV antibiotics and surgery without delay, given their rapid spread and the likelihood that culture results will not be available in time to make an impact on therapy.

The diagnosis of streptococcal pharyngitis, on the other hand, is more confounding. Despite efforts to develop clinical criteria specific for strep throat, the condition cannot be reliably distinguished from viral pharyngitis, which is also extremely common in children. To determine the cause of pharyngitis, physicians perform **rapid strep tests** on a throat swab in the office and then culture the organism on blood agar plates. The rapid strep tests rely on detection of the group A carbohydrate antigen from organisms obtained from the throat swab. They are very specific, so a positive test indicates the presence of GAS. Since they are not as sensitive as throat cultures, strep throat is not ruled out until a negative throat culture is found several days later. Neither one of these tests can distinguish asymptomatic GAS throat carriage with a concurrent viral pharyngitis from a true GAS infection. In a case of ARF and APSGN, diagnosis requires evidence of a preceding GAS infection. Because the organisms may no longer be present, serologic titers to GAS antigens can be used to establish a previous infection. The most common are the **antistreptolysin O titer**, **anti-DNase B titer**, and **Streptozyme® screen** (an agglutination test that detects a mixture of five secreted streptococcal enzymes).

TREATMENT AND PREVENTION

Fortunately, resistance to **penicillin** has never been detected in GAS, so penicillin remains the antibiotic of choice for patients who are not allergic to it. A course of 10 days of oral penicillin is standard therapy. As V.'s case demonstrates, compliance with the full course of treatment is a major problem, and shorter courses are not sufficient therapy to prevent ARF. An alternative therapy is a single-dose injection of long-acting penicillin (**benzathine penicillin**) that persists in the bloodstream for an adequate period. Although this addresses the compliance issue, the injection is painful. For individuals allergic to penicillin, **erythromycin** or other **macrolide antibiotics** are appropriate; however, erythromycin-resistant GAS have been found in the community.

Prevention of GAS infection is difficult because it is continuously circulating in the human population. Avoiding crowded living conditions and practicing good hygiene are the most effective public health measures to prevent GAS infections. In the school-aged population, early recognition and treatment of pharyngeal and skin infections can decrease spread to other children. At least 24 hours of antibiotic therapy should be completed before a child is allowed to return to school. There is active research to develop a vaccine against GAS, but currently there is no such vaccine available to physicians.

GROUP B STREPTOCOCCI

Group B streptococci (GBS; *Streptococcus agalactiae*) are aerobic Gram-positive diplococci that are β-hemolytic on blood agar plates. As common inhabitants of the lower gastrointestinal and female genital tracts, GBS generally do not cause significant disease in healthy people. Because GBS are particularly pathogenic organisms in **newborn infants**, colonization of the bacteria in a pregnant woman can lead to a life-threatening infection if the baby acquires the organism during vaginal delivery. The colonization rate in pregnant women ranges from 15 to 40%, and currently pregnant women are screened for GBS at **35 to 37 weeks of gestation** by the collection of vaginal and rectal swabs. If a woman has a positive GBS screen, **intrapartum antibiotics** are given to the mother to reduce the risk of transmission to the infant. Despite these measures, GBS is still a leading cause of **neonatal sepsis** and **meningitis**. The mortality rate in infants is approximately 5%, and many surviving infants with neonatal infection have long-term problems such as seizures, deafness, developmental delay, and motor deficits. In pregnant women, GBS can cause urinary tract infection, endometriosis, and amnionitis. The other major population susceptible to severe GBS infection is the elderly, especially those with chronic diseases such as diabetes mellitus, liver disease, renal disease, or malignancy. Fortunately, like GAS, GBS are still susceptible to penicillin, the first-line therapy for these organisms.

Like GAS, GBS evades opsonization and phagocytosis by the elaboration of a **polysaccharide capsule**. There are nine capsular serotypes, but type III is responsible for the majority of the cases of neonatal sepsis and meningitis in the United States. In general, the capsular polysaccharides are poor antigens for stimulating a protective immune response. Therefore, there has been great interest in developing a protein-carbohydrate conjugate vaccine, similar to the *Haemophilus influenzae* type b and pneumococcal vaccines, for use in females of childbearing age.

OTHER PATHOGENIC STREPTOCOCCI

There are many other streptococcal species that may also cause diseases in humans (Table 12-1). **Groups C and G streptococci** (*S. dysgalactiae*) are β-hemolytic on blood agar plates and can cause pathology similar to the closely related GAS. Disease manifestations include respiratory and deep tissue infections and the nonsuppurative sequela of AGN, but *not* ARF. The group C/G pathogens share several virulence factors with GAS, including M proteins, adhesins, and streptokinase. The **α-hemolytic *Streptococcus pneumoniae*** is another major pathogenic streptococcus described in Chapter 13.

The **viridans streptococci** are a diverse collection of primarily α-hemolytic species found in the oral cavity that produce a greenish discoloration upon growth on blood agar ("viridis" is Latin for green). *S. mutans* and *S. sobrinus* are important components of **dental plaque** that produce lactic acid during metabolism of sugars, causing **dental caries**. Most viridans streptococci, including *S. mitis*, *S. sanguinis*, *S. gordonii*, *S. mutans*, and *S. sobrinus* can also intermittently seed the bloodstream and lead to endocarditis in people with defective heart valves, including those who have had ARF. *S. milleri* is another viridans streptococcus in the anginosus group that is anaerobic and is often involved in **polymicrobial** abscesses of the brain, liver, and abdominal cavity.

Another medically significant group comprises **nutritionally variant streptococci** that are difficult to grow in the laboratory because they require supplemental cofactors for growth in artificial media. They can cause a destructive form of endocarditis that results in more complications than do infections with other streptococci.

ENTEROCOCCI

Initially characterized as group D streptococci, the enterococci have been reclassified in their own genus, *Enterococcus*. In humans, two species, **E. faecalis** and **E. faecium**, are the most medically important because they cause urinary tract infections, wound infections, endocarditis, intra-abdominal abscesses, and bacteremia. Enterococci are part of the normal flora of the gastrointestinal and genitourinary tracts, and they are distinguished from the streptococci by their resistance to bile and the high salt concentrations found in the intestine. For years, they were regarded as harmless colonizing bacteria. However, as various antibiotic classes were used with much more frequency, the enterococci demonstrated their amazing adaptability by developing resistance to every type of antibiotic. Thus, in the 1990s this usually harmless commensal bacterium became one of the most feared **nosocomial (hospital-acquired) infections**, because it developed resistance to the last-line antibiotic against Gram-positive organisms, vancomycin. Transmission is primarily via the hands of health care workers, but also can involve inanimate objects (fomites) such as bed rails, computer keyboards, draperies, and instruments.

Despite having low overall virulence, enterococci possess some virulence traits such as biofilm formation and cytolysin production. One of the reasons that these organisms have emerged as significant problems in hospitals is that they possess remarkable **intrinsic resistance** to several classes of antibiotics. Antibiotics like penicillins usually kill bacteria because they disrupt their cell wall synthesis. In enterococci, however, penicillins are merely **bacteriostatic** (i.e., they inhibit growth but do not kill the bacteria), and cephalosporins are not active at all. Enterococci are also intrinsically resistant to aminoglycosides by resisting their penetration into the cytoplasm. However, bacterial killing can be achieved by using a combination of a penicillin and an aminoglycoside. In this combination, the penicillin damages the cell wall and facilitates the entry of the aminoglycoside. This situation, in which the combination of two antibiotics produces a greater effect than the sum of their individual activities, is called **antibiotic synergy**.

The enterococci are also capable of genetic transfer via conjugative elements (transposons, plasmids) and bacteriophage, which may lead to uptake of novel resistance genes or **extrinsic resistance**. In this way, enterococci may acquire absolute resistance to penicillins or aminoglycosides that negates the benefits of antibiotic synergy. In addition, the most prevalent vancomycin resistance gene cluster in **vancomycin-resistant enterococci** (**VRE**) is found on exogenously acquired plasmids and transposons. In fact, the few isolates of vancomycin-resistant *Staphylococcus aureus* that have been identified thus far arose after transfer of resistance genes from coinfecting VRE.

VRE are a major problem in many hospitals, because physicians have limited options to treat them. Most VRE are *E. faecium*; *E. faecalis* infections are more common clinically but are less likely to have vancomycin resistance. Unfortunately, many VRE strains are also highly resistant penicillins and aminoglycosides so that even antibiotic synergy is not sufficient to kill them. Because of the problem of VRE and other resistant Gram-positive bacteria, newer antibiotics have been developed to address these pathogens. These include **linezolid**, a bacterial protein synthesis inhibitor; **daptomycin**, a novel bacteriocidal lipopeptide that inserts into the bacterial membrane and causes cytoplasmic leak; **tigecycline**, a tetracycline derivative; and **dalfopristin–quinupristin**, a combination of two synergistic agents that also inhibit bacterial protein synthesis but has limited use because of toxicity and emerging resistance. Although all these drugs are welcome additions to the antimicrobial armamentarium, bacterial isolates with resistance to each of them have already been observed. Good infection control measures and prudent antibiotic use in hospitals are the best ways to prevent the proliferation of VRE strains in medical centers.

CONCLUSION

Streptococci are a diverse group of Gram-positive pathogens that cause a wide variety of infections in humans. GAS can cause disease by direct damage, by elaborating potent toxins, and by causing the immunological sequela. GBS is an important pathogen to both mother and child in the peripartum period. While both of these organisms remain susceptible to penicillins, the previously innocuous enterococci have emerged as significant nosocomial pathogens, primarily due to their ability to acquire antibiotic resistance as new classes of antibiotics are introduced and abused in hospital settings. Enterococci may also act as reservoirs for antibiotic resistance in the commensal microbiota.

Suggested Readings

Bisno AL, Brito MO, Collins CM. Molecular basis of group A streptococcal virulence. *Lancet Infect Dis.* 2003;3:191–200.

Carapetis JR, Steer AC, Mulholland EK, et al. The global burden of group A streptococcal diseases. *Lancet Infect Dis.* 2005;5:685–694.

Cunningham MW. Pathogenesis of group A streptococcal infections. *J Clin Microbiol.* 2000;13:470–511.

Hancock LE, Gilmore MS. Pathogenicity of enterococci. In: Fischetti V, et al., eds. *Gram Positive Pathogens.* 2nd ed, ASM Press; 2006:299–311.

Phares CR, Lynfield R, Farley MM, et al. Epidemiology of Invasive Group B Streptococcal Disease in the United States. *JAMA.* 2008;299:2056–2065.

World Health Organization. *Rheumatic Fever and Rheumatic Heart Disease.* WHO technical report series 923. Geneva, Switzerland: World Health Organization; 2004:1–122.

Swift HF, Wilson AT, Lancefield RC. Typing group A hemolytic streptococci by M precipitin reaction in capillary pipettes. *J Exp Med.* 1943;78:127.

Chapter **13**

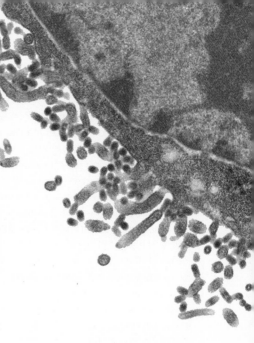

Pneumococcus and Bacterial Pneumonia

Jeffrey N. Weiser

KEY CONCEPTS

Pathogen: *Streptococcus pneumoniae* (aka pneumococcus) is an α-hemolytic streptococcus.

Encounter: Pneumococcus commonly colonizes the human nasopharynx and is transmitted between individuals by contact and respiratory droplet spread.

Entry: Bacteria are introduced into the nasopharynx; colonization precedes infection or disease.

Spread and Multiplication: Pneumococci resist phagocytic clearance by expression of a polysaccharide capsule. Organisms may spread to other parts of the respiratory tract or into the bloodstream.

Damage: Infection is characterized by an acute inflammatory response, resulting in respiratory tract infections, including otitis media, sinusitis, chronic bronchitis, and pneumonia, as well as invasive infections such as bacteremia and meningitis.

Diagnosis: The diagnosis is suspected when Gram-positive diplococci are seen in sterile tissue and body fluids. Infection is usually confirmed with culture.

Treatment: Usually treatable with a wide variety of antibiotics; however, pneumococci have developed increased resistance to penicillin and other commonly used antibiotics.

Prevention: Immune protection depends on antibody to the pneumococcal capsule (opsonins) and neutrophils (phagocytes). However, pneumococci express multiple capsular types; consequently, multiple capsule types are combined for use in vaccines.

STREPTOCOCCUS PNEUMONIAE, the pneumococcus, referred to by Sir William Osler as "the captain of the men of death," remains a leading cause of serious infection, particularly bacterial pneumonia, worldwide. It commonly colonizes the mucosal surface of the nasopharynx without causing disease, unless host factors allow it to gain access to normally sterile sites such as the lung, where it is able to trigger an acute inflammatory response. The presence of a thick layer of surface polysaccharide, however, inhibits otherwise effective host clearance functions involving complement- and antibody-mediated phagocytosis. Progress in treating disease caused by this major pathogen has been eroded by the acquisition and widespread dissemination of antibiotic resistance.

CASE • In January, Mr. P., a 68-year-old grandfather and a heavy smoker, noted that he had nasal congestion, muscle aches, and a low-grade fever. He felt that his symptoms were resolving until he abruptly developed a shaking chill, cough, and severe pain on the right side of his chest that worsened with breathing. The cough was productive of rust-colored (blood-tinged) sputum. When he was seen in the emergency department 2 days later, he appeared acutely ill and had a temperature of 40°C. His respiratory rate was rapid at 30 breaths per minute. His breathing was shallow, with diminished breath sounds over the right side of the thorax, indicating consolidation of the air spaces of the lung. This pattern of breathing, in which the patient is reluctant to move one side of the chest because of inspiratory pain, is a condition known as splinting and indicates inflammation of the pleura (lining of the thoracic cavity and lungs) or pleurisy.

The laboratory reported that Mr. P.'s white blood cell count was 23,000/μL³, indicative of a leukocytosis (an increase in the number of circulating white blood cells that often characterizes bacterial infection). A chest radiograph revealed a dense infiltrate in the right lung (Fig. 13-1). A Gram stain of the sputum showed many neutrophils and lancet-shaped Gram-positive diplococci (Fig. 13-2). Blood was obtained for culture, and treatment for a **community-acquired pneumonia** was begun with the fluoroquinolone antibiotic, levofloxacin. Both the blood cultures and sputum cultures were positive for the pneumococcus, *Streptococcus pneumoniae*. Because the isolate was found to be sensitive to penicillin, the antibiotic regimen was revised. Two days later, Mr. P. was much improved, and after 8 more days of penicillin therapy, he recovered completely.

Mr. P.'s case illustrates many of the classical features of pneumococcal pneumonia: abrupt onset of severe symptoms, ill appearance of the patient, rust-colored sputum, homogeneous involvement of an entire lobe of a lung (lobar

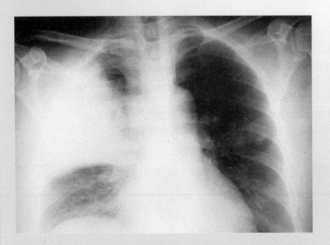

FIGURE 13-1. Chest radiograph showing homogeneous consolidation involving the right upper and middle lobes (lobar pneumonia). The air spaces of the lobes are filled with liquid.

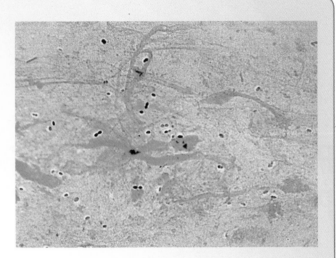

FIGURE 13-2. Gram stain of sputum revealing many neutrophils and lancet-shaped Gram-positive diplococci.

consolidation), leukocytosis, and rapid response to antibiotics. **Bacteremia**, the presence of bacteria in the bloodstream, occurs in about 25% of the cases and is indicative of more severe illness. Pneumococcal pneumonia is a dramatic illness that can be life threatening in a patient who may have been well only a few days earlier. It was one of the most common causes of death in the preantibiotic era.

Today, as a result of penicillin (and other antibiotics), it is less often fatal. However, penicillin, once considered a "miracle," must now be used in much higher doses and is ineffective for some strains and some manifestation of pneumococcal disease. Nevertheless, pneumococcal pneumonia remains the most common form of community-acquired bacterial pneumonia and continues to be fatal in up to 5% of all patients, with higher mortality rates in elderly or debilitated patients and those with bacteremia, even when they are treated with an antibiotic to which their organism is sensitive. Pneumococcal disease frequently follows a viral infection of the upper respiratory tract, particularly influenza, as illustrated in Mr. P.'s case by the preceding "flulike" illness that was resolving as his pneumonia began. Because of his age, Mr. P. should have previously received immunization against both influenza and the pneumococcus. Either of these might have prevented the development of pneumococcal pneumonia.

This case raises several questions:

1. Where did Mr. P. acquire this organism? What host factors might have contributed to the pneumococcus gaining entry into his lungs?

2. What possibilities should be considered if the initial antibiotic treatment was not effective in this case?

3. If Mr. P.'s own immune response was not sufficient to control this infection, why might immunization have ameliorated or prevented these events?

See Appendix for answers.

STREPTOCOCCUS PNEUMONIAE

CHARACTERISTICS

The pneumococcus is classified in the genus *Streptococcus*, based on its morphology and purely fermentative energy metabolism. It is one of many species of aerobic streptococci that tolerate ambient levels of oxygen, a characteristic that is critical to its niche on the surface of the airway. Other closely related species such as *S. oralis*, *S. sanguis*, and *S. mitis* coinhabit the same environment in the human nasopharynx, but compared with the pneumococcus are uncommon causes of infection. The pneumococcus, like other streptococci, lacks the enzyme catalase; therefore, its normal metabolism generates copious amounts of **hydrogen peroxide**. This substance inhibits the growth of competitive members of the microflora and, together with the cholesterol-binding toxin **pneumolysin**, accounts for much of its ability to damage host tissue and inhibit effective clearance by the infected host. In addition, like other Gram-positive bacteria, pneumococcal cells are surrounded by a thick cell wall, fragments of which are recognized by the innate immune system and are responsible for stimulating much of the inflammatory response associated with pneumococcal infection. In the stationary phase of growth, pneumococci express the enzyme **autolysin**, which degrades its own cell wall. The continuous self-destruction, or autolysis, further contributes to the release of these inflammatory mediators.

Exterior to the cell wall is a **capsule** that imparts a mucoid or "smooth" appearance to colonies on agar. (In 1944, Avery, McCarty, and MacLeod reported that an extract consisting of DNA derived from smooth pneumococcal strains was able to transform "rough" to smooth strains. This was among the earliest evidence that DNA is the carrier of genetic information.) Capsules are composed of porous zones of polysaccharide that completely envelop the cell (Fig. 13-3). Thick polysaccharide capsules,

much like carbohydrate O antigens on the surface of the lipopolysaccharide of some Gram-negative bacteria, do not activate complement efficiently in the absence of a specific antipolysaccharide antibody and thus serve to shield the underlying components of the bacterial cell surface (see the paradigm).

Expression of a capsule is particularly important for an organism to survive in the bloodstream, where the activity of complement is most pervasive (see Chapter 6). The presence of a capsule therefore enables the pneumococcus to cause infection beyond where it normally resides in the respiratory tract. For bacteria to pass through the blood–brain barrier and reach the central nervous system, for example, it generally requires a sustained (rather than transient) presence of bacteria in the bloodstream or bacteremia. This is what occurs in **meningitis**, which is inflammation in the meninges, the three membranes that envelop the brain and spinal cord. The importance of capsule is demonstrated by the pathogens that are the most common causes of this life-threatening infection: like the pneumococcus, all are encapsulated. Nonencapsulated pneumococci rarely cause disease.

Capsular polysaccharides tend to be highly immunogenic and are often the dominant or serotype-determining antigen on the organism. Because they are the target of selective pressures from the immune response, there is considerable structural and thus antigenic variation among pneumococcal capsular polysaccharides. The basis for antigenic differences among serotypes lies in the chemical structure of the capsular polysaccharide. Various pneumococcal strains express capsules with distinct sugar constituents or the same array of sugars linked in various ways. There are more than 90 known pneumococcal capsule structures or types. Even though these structures are antigenic, they allow for extracellular bacterial survival in the nonimmune host until a specific bactericidal and/or opsonic antibody to these polysaccharides can be generated to enhance clearance of the pathogen. Capsules can be visualized by the addition of an antibody that causes an antigen–antibody precipitation in the normally transparent zone occupied by the capsule (**Quellung reaction**). This has been used in the past for selection of type-specific serum therapy and is currently used for epidemiological studies. Antibodies to the capsules play a major role in protection against subsequent infections by pneumococci of the same serotype but have minimal impact on pneumococci of antigenically different capsular types.

ENCOUNTER

Pneumococcal pneumonia is the most common form of **bacterial pneumonia** acquired in the community (as opposed to hospital-acquired pneumonias; see Chapter 59). It is estimated that approximately 500,000 cases of pneumococcal pneumonia occur each year in the United States.

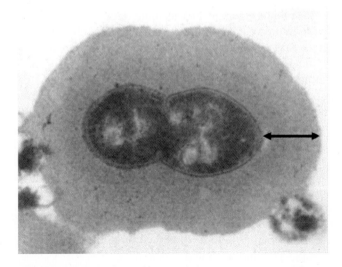

FIGURE 13-3. Immunoelectron micrograph showing a diplococcus. The *arrow* points to the thick layer of capsular polysaccharide surrounding the cell (original magnification, ×41,200).

PARADIGM BOX

BACTERIAL CAPSULES AS DEFENSES AGAINST OPSONIZATION AND PHAGOCYTOSIS

The antiphagocytic capsule that characterizes virulent strains of pneumococcus is also found in a number of other extracellular pathogens. Examples of encapsulated organisms include the following:

Bacteria

- *Streptococcus pneumoniae* (pneumococcus)
- *Streptococcus pyogenes* (group A streptococcus)
- *Streptococcus agalactiae* (group B streptococcus)
- *Staphylococcus aureus* (some strains)
- *Neisseria meningitidis* (meningococcus)
- *Haemophilus influenzae* (except nontypable strains)
- *Klebsiella pneumoniae*
- *Escherichia coli* (some strains)
- *Bacteroides fragilis*

Fungi

- *Cryptococcus neoformans*

Prominent examples of encapsulated bacteria are *Haemophilus influenzae* type B and *Neisseria meningitidis* (the meningococcus), which, together with the pneumococcus, are the most frequent causes of bacterial meningitis after the newborn period. Nonencapsulated pneumococci are readily opsonized and phagocytized; consequently, they are avirulent. More than 10,000 nonencapsulated pneumococci must be injected into the peritoneal cavity to kill a mouse, but only about 10 encapsulated bacteria are required—a 1,000-fold difference in virulence.

How does encapsulation protect the pathogen from antibacterial defenses? One of the main host defense mechanisms against bacterial infection involves the complement system, which can be directly bactericidal through the generation of the lytic membrane attack complex. The complement system is highly efficient in eliminating most extracellular bacteria. Other organisms, like the pneumococcus, are not killed by complement alone but require phagocytosis by neutrophils or macrophages, the professional phagocytes. Recognition by professional phagocytic cells, however, requires signaling through opsonization, a process whereby complement components with or without antibodies are activated on the bacterial cell surface. A successful pathogen circumvents these mechanisms by completely enveloping its cell surface in a thick layer of hydrophilic polysaccharide, or capsule. The polysaccharide does not activate complement efficiently in the absence of a specific antibody and thus serves to protect the underlying components of the bacterial cell surface. In other words, the capsule provides the pneumococcus with "stealthlike" capability.

How then is the host able to vanquish this formidable opponent? Not all capsular polysaccharides are totally effective in shielding underlying structures from recognition by complement and antibodies. Moreover, other components of the innate immune system contribute to host defense and to opsonizing pneumococci. Eventually, the capsular material, itself antigenic, will elicit a specific anticapsular antibody response that promotes opsonophagocytic clearance and tips the balance in favor of the host.

Worldwide, it is estimated that more than a million deaths occur annually as a result of this disease, making it one of the leading infectious causes of mortality. The incidence is highest in certain subgroups, including children younger than 5 years, adults older than 40 years, African Americans, and Native Americans. Although the reason for this distribution is not known, poverty and a debilitated state of health are risk factors. Certain diseases also predispose to pneumococcal infections, including sickle cell anemia, alcoholism, Hodgkin disease, multiple myeloma, HIV infection, and the absence of a functional spleen. Pneumococcal infections are also distinctly seasonal, with the highest incidence occurring in the winter and early spring, often in the setting of recent upper respiratory viral infection, as illustrated in the case of Mr. P. Most cases are sporadic, but outbreaks do occur, particularly in residential institutions, army barracks, and work camps, where people live in crowded conditions. In addition, the pneumococcus is a leading cause of other infections involving the respiratory tract, including acute otitis media (infection of the middle ear space), acute sinusitis, and chronic bronchitis. Several million cases of otitis media occur each year in the United States, making the disease the single most common reason for medical visits among children. It is estimated that 40% of acute bacterial otitis media is caused by the pneumococcus. Bacteremic infection can also introduce the organism into other normally sterile sites, resulting in pneumococcal infections of the peritoneal cavity (in the presence of increased fluid, called ascites), joints, or heart valves that cause peritonitis, septic arthritis, and endocarditis, respectively. As previously noted, the pneumococcus is one of the encapsulated pathogens that causes meningitis, an especially devastating disease. There are more than a thousand cases of pneumococcal meningitis per year in the United States.

The environmental **reservoir** of *S. pneumoniae* is humans colonized by the organism, rather than animals or the inanimate environment. Interestingly, if the physician had asked Mr. P. whether he had been exposed recently to another person with pneumonia, the answer would probably have been "no." By far, the majority of individuals who harbor pneumococci never experience symptoms, because the organism most often exists in a commensal relationship with its human host. Pneumococci have a particular predilection for the human respiratory tract, although the precise reasons for this marked tropism are unknown. The initial step in the host–pathogen interaction is **colonization** on the mucosal surface of the nasopharynx. The outcome of colonization can be clearance of the organism, asymptomatic persistence for several weeks to months (the **carrier state**), or progression to disease. The outcome is determined by the intrinsic virulence of the colonizing strain and the efficiency of host defense mechanisms. Some serotypes of *S. pneumoniae* are more virulent than others. Certain serotypes can cause severe disease, whereas others colonize the nasopharynx of asymptomatic persons but seldom are responsible for disease. The interval between colonization and the onset of disease is variable (and ordinarily undefinable in clinical practice), but there is some evidence to suggest that disease is most likely to occur shortly after colonization.

Several aspects of *S. pneumoniae* colonization have been elucidated by longitudinal studies in which nasopharyngeal cultures were obtained at regular intervals from healthy individuals. Pneumococci are carried by up to two-thirds of normal preschool children. In general, the incidence of colonization declines with increasing age; rates of colonization in adults average only 10%. One individual may become colonized many times, usually with different serotypes. This occurs because in immunocompetent individuals, colonization generates a serotype-specific immune response that limits reacquisition of an isolate of the same serotype. Sometimes one individual is simultaneously colonized by more than one pneumococcal serotype.

Transmission from a sick person, or more commonly from an asymptomatic carrier, occurs through **droplets** of respiratory secretions that remain airborne over distances of a few feet. Infecting organisms can also be carried on hands contaminated with secretions. Transmission occurs directly from person to person and appears to be highly efficient considering the high rates of colonization in settings such as family groups and day care centers. Because healthy carriers far outnumber symptomatic individuals, most of the links in the chain of person-to-person transmission are invisible. In contrast, an agent such as measles is also transmitted person to person by a respiratory route, but asymptomatic colonization does not take place, and each link in the chain is evident as disease.

ENTRY

Disease occurs when the organism spreads from its site of residence in the nasopharynx and becomes established in normally sterile parts of the airway, usually as a conse-

quence of multiple host factors. Ordinarily, the lungs are protected by elaborate mechanisms, including the tortuous pathway that air and inhaled particles must follow to reach the lungs, the **epiglottis** that protects the airway from aspiration, the **cough reflex**, the presence of a layer of sticky **mucus** that is continuously swept upward by the **cilia** of the respiratory epithelium, and **alveolar macrophages** that phagocytose bacteria and foreign particles. These mechanisms are highly effective in preventing progression from colonization of the upper respiratory tract to infection of the lower respiratory tract. However, a number of factors can interfere with these mechanisms, including aspiration that can occur with loss of consciousness, cigarette smoking, alcohol consumption, viral infections, or excess fluid in the lungs. Likewise, otitis media is often a consequence of eustachian tube dysfunction leading to aspiration of nasopharyngeal contents into the normally sterile middle ear space.

How do these considerations relate to the case of Mr. P.? The source of the infecting organisms was certainly another individual who may have been entirely healthy, for example, his grandchildren. The decline in adult pneumonia following widespread vaccination of young children indicates that they are a major source of infecting pneumococci for adult populations. His smoking history and recent viral infection may have depressed his defense mechanisms by weakening his cough reflex, damaging the mucociliary escalator, and decreasing the activity of alveolar macrophages. It is possible that Mr. P. had the misfortune to acquire one of the more virulent pneumococcal serotypes.

SPREAD, MULTIPLICATION, AND DAMAGE

Much of the current understanding of the pathogenesis of pneumococcal pneumonia is derived from studies carried out in the 1940s by W. Barry Wood and his colleagues, who produced pneumonia by injecting pneumococci suspended in mucin into the bronchi of anesthetized mice. These animals were sacrificed at various intervals, and histological sections of the lungs were examined. Four zones of the pneumonic process were identified, corresponding to four stages of the inflammatory process (Fig. 13-4).

In the first stage, the alveoli fill with **serous fluid** containing many organisms but few inflammatory cells. Recent studies suggest that components of the pneumococcal cell wall stimulate the outpouring of fluid and the subsequent inflammatory response. The fluid that fills the alveoli serves as a culture medium for multiplying organisms and a means of spreading the infection, both into adjacent alveoli through the pores of Kohn and to nearby areas of the lung via the small airways. While this outpouring of fluid may have minimal effects in some organs, it threatens the basic function of the lung—namely, gas exchange.

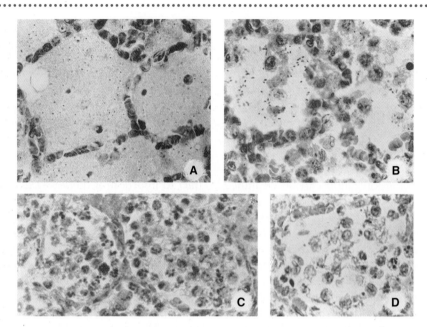

FIGURE 13-4. Four zones or stages of lung involvement in pneumococcal pneumonia. Pneumonia was induced in rats by intrabronchial installation of live pneumococci suspended in mucin. **A.** Alveoli filled with clear exudate (original magnification, ×430). **B.** Early consolidation: Organisms are plentiful, and some are engulfed by neutrophils (original magnification, ×430). **C.** Late consolidation: A closely packed cellular infiltrate is present, and phagocytosis of organisms has occurred (original magnification, ×530). **D.** Resolution found at center of lesion: Macrophages are present, and the exudate is beginning to clear (×430).

In the second stage, called **early consolidation**, the alveoli are infiltrated by neutrophils and red blood cells. Strong **chemotactic signals**, produced by the pneumococci and by the alternative pathway of **complement**, lead to the recruitment of large numbers of neutrophils and a typical acute inflammatory process. The stage is now set for the classic struggle between bacteria and phagocytes. On the one hand, pneumococci resist phagocytosis because of the presence of capsules. On the other hand, if the pneumococci are ingested by the neutrophils or macrophages, they are rapidly killed. The extent of successful phagocytosis determines the outcome of the infection.

Fortunately, the immune system employs various mechanisms that make even the heavily encapsulated pneumococci more "ingestible" to the neutrophils. If the patient has had previous contact with pneumococci of the invading serotype, he or she will have developed type-specific anticapsular antibodies that interact with complement to opsonize the organisms and facilitate their uptake. If the individual lacks specific adaptive immunity, the organisms may be opsonized by nonspecific or innate immunity. Complement components that bind to the bacterial surface in the absence of antibodies (activated mostly by the alternative pathway) are particularly important in protecting the host. Binding of complement components differs among pneumococcal serotypes, which may explain in part why some serotypes are more virulent than others.

An additional protective mechanism of the innate immune system involves interaction of a serum component, **C-reactive protein** (**CRP**), with cell surface phosphorylcholine, a conserved feature on pneumococcal teichoic acid (C substance or C polysaccharide). Binding of CRP to the bacterial surface leads to activation of the complement cascade through the classical pathway. Because levels of CRP rise dramatically in the sera of patients with many inflammatory diseases, not just pneumococcal infection, it is referred to as an **acute phase reactant**. Individuals with lower-baseline unstimulated serum levels of CRP appear to have an increased risk of invasive pneumococcal disease.

In the case of Mr. P., phagocytic cells, mainly neutrophils, failed to contain the pneumococci early on, and the infection progressed to adjacent areas until it involved an entire lobe of his right lung. What accounted for his fever and ill appearance? Although Mr. P.'s lung involvement was serious, the resulting impairment of gas exchange does not fully explain why he became so sick. It is likely that the systemic manifestations were the result of the host inflammatory response triggered by pneumococcal components, particularly cell wall fragments produced locally or entering the circulation, rather than being a direct effect of any bacterial toxin or other secreted product.

The third stage of pneumococcal pneumonia is called **late consolidation**. At this stage, the alveoli are packed with victorious neutrophils and only a few remaining pneumococci. On a macroscopic level, the affected areas of the lungs are heavy and resemble the liver in appearance, a state that early pathologists called **hepatization**. In the fourth and final stage, or **resolution**, neutrophils are replaced by scavenging macrophages, which clear the debris resulting from the inflammatory process. One of the remarkable aspects of pneumococcal pneumonia is that in most cases, the architecture of the lung is eventually restored to its normal condition. This restoration is different from what takes place in many other forms of pneumonia, in which recovery is accompanied by necrosis and normal lung tissue is replaced by fibrous scar tissue.

Pneumococcal pneumonia may lead to both local and distant complications. The most common local complication is **pleural effusion**—the outpouring of fluid into the pleural space—which occurs in about one-quarter of all cases. Usually, the pleural fluid effused is a sterile exudate, stimulated by the adjacent inflammation. However, in about 1% of cases, pneumococci can be isolated from this site. Infection of the pleural space is called **empyema** and is a purulent condition that may require drainage of the infected fluid.

Distant complications of pneumococcal pneumonia result from spread of the organisms via the bloodstream. In the early stages of pneumonia, the organisms may enter the lymphatic vessels that drain the infected area of the lungs, pass into the thoracic duct, and from there enter the bloodstream. The organism can be documented by positive blood cultures in about 25% of all cases of pneumococcal pneumonia. However, transient pneumococcemia probably occurs much more often. When bacteremia is present, the organisms may cause infection at secondary sites such as the meninges, as discussed earlier. Had Mr. P. not responded quickly to antibiotic therapy, he would have been at risk for such complications. Spread to the bloodstream is usually a complication of pneumonia, although in young children, there may also be direct seeding of the bloodstream by organisms resident in the nasopharynx (a process called occult bacteremia).

Host defenses against pneumococcal bacteremia depend largely on the lymphoreticular system to remove circulating bacteria from the bloodstream. **Humoral factors**, including antibodies, complement, and perhaps CRP, assist macrophages in the spleen, liver, and lymph nodes in carrying out their filtering function. The critical filtering function of the spleen is demonstrated by the fulminant, rapidly progressive pneumococcal bacteremia that sometimes strikes individuals with anatomic or functional asplenia (e.g., postsplenectomy or in sickle cell disease).

DIAGNOSIS

Pneumococcal infection is often suspected because of the clinical scenario, because it is a leading cause of lobar pneumonia, acute otitis media, chronic bronchitis, and

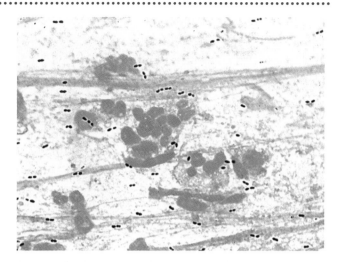

FIGURE 13-5. Classic appearance of a Gram stain of sputum from a patient with pneumococcal pneumonia. The smear shows lancet-shaped diplococci with many polymorphonuclear leukocytes, and no other prominent bacterial morphology is present.

acute sinusitis. In the case of pneumonia, the first step in obtaining a microbiological diagnosis is the examination of expectorated sputum. When **Gram stain** of sputum contains neutrophils and more than 10 lancet-shaped Gram-positive **diplococci** per oil immersion field, the diagnosis of pneumococcal pneumonia is likely (Fig. 13-5). In the case of Mr. P., the results of the Gram stain of sputum confirmed the clinical suspicion and justified the use of initial therapy with an antipneumococcal antibiotic, such as levofloxacin.

In Mr. P.'s case, final identification was made by a culture of his sputum, purulent material expectorated from his lungs. The culture was performed by streaking the specimen on **blood agar**. Pneumococcal colonies are surrounded by an area of **α-hemolysis**, a green-brownish discoloration caused by hydrogen peroxide production without the clearing from lysis of the red blood cells that characterizes β-hemolysis. Because most of the other streptococcal species normally present in the heavily colonized upper respiratory tract are also α-hemolytic, pneumococci must be differentiated from less pathogenic contaminants by other properties. These properties include sensitivity to a compound called **optochin** and solubility in bile salts. Because pneumococci are fastidious organisms with exacting growth requirements, they are not always cultured from sputum of patients with pneumococcal pneumonia. Thus, a negative sputum culture does not rule out pneumococcal pneumonia.

Unfortunately, the interpretation of a positive sputum culture is not always straightforward. A positive finding may indicate the cause of the patient's pneumonia. However, it may also be the result of contamination of the sputum specimen as it passes through the mouth of a colonized individual, in which case the clinical context is important and therapy is often empiric. In contrast to sputum cultures, growth of *S. pneumoniae* from Mr. P.'s blood could be considered definitive proof of the etiology of the disease. In recent years, interest has increased in the use of specific antisera to detect the capsular antigen directly in sputum, blood, or urine, thus obviating the need for culture. Unfortunately, these techniques are not positive in many cases of pneumococcal pneumonia.

TREATMENT AND PREVENTION

Penicillin revolutionized the treatment of pneumococcal infection. Other antibiotics, such as macrolides or selected fluoroquinolones with activity against pneumococci, are available for patients who are allergic to penicillin. Despite the dramatic effectiveness of penicillin, the mortality rate in pneumococcal pneumonia remains unacceptably high. Treatment fails because of rapid progression of the infection or underlying debility of the patient. Recent work on the pneumococcal cell wall has suggested another possible explanation. Lysis of pneumococcal cells by antibiotics releases breakdown products of the cell wall that stimulate an abrupt increase in inflammation. The ultimate effect of antibiotic therapy is to cure the infection, but the short-term effect of increased inflammation may be deleterious to some patients.

Recently, the worldwide spread of antibiotic resistance in pneumococci has emerged as a major concern. Resistance to penicillin was first recognized in the 1960s. During the 1980s, antibiotic resistance became widespread in a number of European countries, and by the 1990s, a major increase in antibiotic-resistant pneumococci in North America was apparent. Rates of resistance vary widely among communities but are generally highest where antibiotics are used most frequently. Approximately three-fourths of the penicillin-resistant strains have only an intermediate level of resistance and can still be treated with penicillin or related drugs unless the infection occurs in the central nervous system, where the penetration of penicillin is insufficient. The remaining one-fourth of strains, however, have high-level resistance (minimum inhibitory concentration ≥ 2 μg per mL) and must be treated with other antibiotics. Unfortunately, the penicillin-resistant strains are often also resistant to other β-lactams, as well as unrelated antibiotics that might have served as alternatives. In particular, rates of resistance to other common classes of oral antibiotics, such as macrolides and sulfas, are now generally high.

The mechanism of penicillin resistance does not involve the production of β-lactamase, an enzyme that breaks down penicillin and accounts for penicillin resistance among staphylococci. Instead, the resistant pneumococci have accumulated mutations in the enzymes that cross-link the cell wall and are normally bound and inactivated by penicillin. These altered **penicillin-binding proteins** allow for continued cell wall synthesis but no longer bind or are affected by penicillin. Moreover, pneumococci with altered penicillin-binding proteins become more resistant to other β-lactam antibiotics, including cephalosporins, so that these modified forms of penicillin may be no more effective than penicillin itself. The genetic information encoding these altered proteins appears to have been acquired from other species of streptococci that may reside in the oropharynx. The emergence of resistance, therefore, appears to be a result of the strong selective pressure caused by the presence of antibiotics coupled with the natural ability of the organism to adapt by taking up and integrating DNA found in its environment in a process known as **transformation**.

The physicians caring for Mr. P. initially selected treatment with levofloxacin because of the currently low rates of resistance to this agent and the possibility of a high level of a penicillin-resistant strain in the clinical setting of a life-threatening community-acquired pneumonia. Once the microbiology laboratory excluded the possibility of a high level of resistance to penicillin, it was appropriate to complete his therapy with penicillin.

The adaptability of the pneumococcus, as demonstrated by its ability to develop drug resistance, has also made it a challenging target for vaccine development. A vaccine would be especially useful for people at highest risk for pneumococcal disease, such as young children, the elderly, and individuals with underlying conditions that predispose them to infection or severe disease. The antigenic diversity of the pneumococcus, however, is a significant barrier to developing a vaccine based on the polysaccharide capsular antigens. Nonetheless, most cases of pneumococcal pneumonia are caused by a limited number of serotypes. Accordingly, a vaccine based on those serotypes was approved for use in 1977. This vaccine now contains the capsular polysaccharides of the 23 most common serotypes and is recommended for the elderly and individuals with predisposing conditions. Unfortunately, patients with Hodgkin disease or multiple myeloma, who are especially at risk, often do not make an adequate antibody response to the vaccine. Because it is a complex vaccine targeting a population with highly variable and often complicated health problems, the impact on the overall morbidity and mortality caused by this organism remains controversial. Likewise, young children respond poorly to polysaccharide vaccines (see Chapter 45 for a discussion of vaccination of children against *H. influenzae*).

Rising rates of antibiotic resistance have spurred efforts at improving prevention, particularly among children. In 2000, a **pneumococcal conjugate vaccine**, based on the successful approach for *H. influenzae* type B, was introduced in the United States for use in children. This vaccine now contains up to 13 of the most common serotypes found in that age group linked to a protein carrier that results in a more effective antibody response because, unlike vaccines consisting strictly of polysaccharide antigens, the presence of a protein recruits T cells to help. The pneumococcal conjugate vaccine reduces carriage of the serotypes in its formulation and has thus far been shown to be highly efficacious against invasive pneumococcal disease and somewhat effective at preventing overall cases of pneumonia and otitis media. Therefore, immunization of Mr. P's grandchildren could have prevented them from carrying the pneumococcus that spread to Mr. P. There is concern that selective pressure is increasing the prevalence of nonvaccine serotypes (serotype replacement) and over time may render the conjugate vaccine less effective in preventing pneumococcal infection.

CONCLUSION

The pneumococcus is a Gram-positive streptococcus that commonly colonizes the human nasopharynx and is a leading infectious cause of morbidity and mortality. The expression of a capsule makes the organism more resistant to opsonization and phagocytosis by antibodies and complement. In susceptible hosts, this characteristic enables the pneumococcus to overcome the acute inflammatory response when it gains access to normally sterile sites such as the lung. Antibiotics continue to have a major impact on pneumococcal disease, although rising rates of resistance are increasingly limiting treatment options. Prevention is currently based on vaccines made from the capsular polysaccharide of the most common serotypes.

Suggested Readings

Kadioglu A, Weiser JN, Paton JC, et al. The role of *Streptococcus pneumoniae* virulence factors in host respiratory colonization and disease. *Nat Rev Microbiol.* 2008;6:288–301.

Klugman KP, Feldman C. *Streptococcus pneumoniae* respiratory tract infections. *Curr Opin Infect Dis.* 2001;14:173–179.

Swartz MN. Attacking the pneumococcus—a hundred years' war. *N Engl J Med.* 2002;346:722.

Tomasz A. The pneumococcus at the gates. *N Engl J Med.* 1995;333:514–515.

Tuomanen E, Mitchell T, Morrison D, Spratt B, eds. *The Pneumococcus.* Washington, DC: ASM Press; 2004.

Weiser JN. The pneumococcus: why a commensal misbehaves. *J Mol Med.* 2010;88:97–102.

Whitney CG, Farley MM, Hadler J, et al.; Active Bacterial Core Surveillance of the Emerging Infections Program Network. Decline in invasive pneumococcal disease after the introduction of protein-polysaccharide conjugate vaccine. *N Engl J Med.* 2003;348:1737–1746.

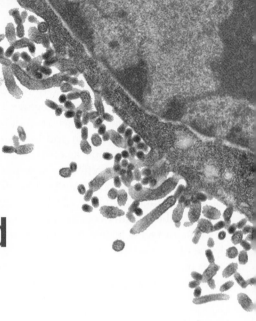

Chapter 14

Neisseriae: Gonococcus and Meningococcus

Ann E. Jerse and Victor DiRita

KEY CONCEPTS

The Pathogens: *Neisseria gonorrhoeae* (the gonococcus) and *Neisseria meningitidis* (the meningococcus). Gram-negative diplococci that do not appear to have a niche outside of the human host

Encounter: May be carried asymptomatically in the genital tract (gonococcus) or nasopharynx (meningococcus)

Entry: *N. gonorrhoeae* is sexually transmitted in men and women and can lead to pelvic inflammatory disease in women and epididymitis in men.

N. meningitidis is spread from person to person by respiratory droplets and may cause septicemia and meningitis.

Spread and Multiplication: Both microbes colonize the mucosa by means of a pilus and replicate there. Gonococci produce an IgA protease as protection against antibody surveillance on the mucosal epithelium. Surface structures of both pathogens can undergo both phase variation and antigenic variation, enabling them to avoid immune detection. Both can enter the bloodstream, but only meningococci produce a capsule that protects them from attack by neutrophils. Some gonococci are serum resistant and thus can spread in the blood.

Damage: Localized gonococcal infection can damage the genitourinary epithelium, cause urethral discharge of pus, and lead to urinary pain. Meningococcal septicemia has life-threatening consequences, including disseminated intravascular coagulation and meningitis.

Diagnosis: A characteristic Gram stain from the genital tract or cerebrospinal fluid can be diagnostic for gonococcal and meningococcal infection, respectively. *Neisseria* species require chocolate agar for culture. CSF and blood cultures are used to diagnose meningococcal infection. Polymerase chain reaction–based identification is widely used for screening.

Treatment and Prevention: Both meningococcal and gonococcal require antibiotics; resistance is a concern with gonococci. A meningococcal vaccine consists of a mixture of all capsule types except serogroup B. Vaccines against serogroup B meningococcus target protein antigens. Gonococcal vaccines have not been developed due to the number of variable surface antigens.

THE GRAM-NEGATIVE cocci, in contrast with the great variety of pathogenic Gram-negative bacilli, contain only one genus of organisms that frequently cause disease. This genus, *Neisseria*, has two important species pathogenic for humans: *Neisseria gonorrhoeae*, the agent of **gonorrhea**, and *N. meningitidis*, a major cause of **septicemia** and **meningitis**.

The gonococcus (*N. gonorrhoeae*) usually causes an uncomplicated, localized **cervicitis** and **urethritis**. In addition, it can cause upper genital tract or disseminated infection. It is estimated that about 700,000 new cases of gonorrhea occur every year in the United States, with fewer than half reported to the Centers for Disease Control (CDC). Of the infectious diseases that must legally be reported to the U.S. Public Health Service, only genital chlamydial infections are identified more frequently. Gonococcal infections and their complications are responsible for more than $1 billion per year in direct and indirect health care costs in the United States.

GONOCOCCAL INFECTIONS: SITES AND TYPES

- Lower tract infections
  - Cervicitis
  - Urethritis (male and female)
  - Abscess formation in glands adjacent to the vagina, such as Skene duct or Bartholin glands
- Upper tract infections
  - Endometritis (uterine infection)
  - Epididymitis
  - Pelvic inflammatory disease (PID; infection of the fallopian tube [salpingitis], the ovary, or adnexal tissues)
- Other (nonreproductive tract) localized sites
  - Proctitis (rectal gonorrhea)
  - Pharyngitis
  - Ophthalmia neonatorum (bilateral conjunctivitis in infants born of mothers infected with gonococci)
  - Extension of the infection to areas contiguous with the pelvis causing peritonitis or perihepatitis (Fitz-Hugh-Curtis syndrome)
- Disseminated gonococcal infection (DGI)
  - Dermatitis–arthritis–tenosynovitis syndrome: fever, polyarthritis, and tenosynodermatitis (vesicles or pustules on a hemorrhagic base) caused either by immune complexes or by whole gonococci
  - Monoarticular septic arthritis (one infected joint)
  - Rarely, endocarditis (infection involves heart valves) or meningitis (infection of the central nervous system)

The gonococcus attaches through pili and other adherence ligands to the mucosal epithelia of the male urethra or female cervix, where it can elicit a brisk inflammatory response. Ascent of the organism into the female upper reproductive tract results in infection and inflammation of the uterus and fallopian tubes, called **pelvic inflammatory disease (PID)**. This condition may result in scarring of the upper female genital tract and adjacent organs and chronic pelvic pain. Tubal scarring can lead to **ectopic pregnancy** (development of the embryo in the fallopian tube rather than the uterus) and/or infertility. In men, ascent of the gonococcus into the upper reproductive tract is less frequent but can cause **epididymitis**. Rarely, a localized gonococcal infection can invade the bloodstream and cause an acute dermatitis–arthritis–**tenosynovitis** syndrome (the last complication being an inflammation of the tendons and joints) called **disseminated gonococcal infection (DGI)**. The complement membrane attack complex consisting of late complement components can lyse most neisseriae, so individuals with complement deficiencies are predisposed to systemic spread of both gonococci and meningococci. Nevertheless, DGI and gonococcal arthritis can be seen in patients without complement deficiency.

Meningococci are also piliated and colonize human upper respiratory mucosal surfaces. Meningococci are surrounded by a capsule that enhances the ability of the organism to resist host defense mechanisms, such as complement-mediated killing in the bloodstream. This allows meningococci to grow to high numbers in the blood. Meningococci also shed large amounts of outer membrane material. These membrane blebs contain lipopolysaccharide (LPS) (**endotoxin**), also called **lipooligosaccharide (LOS)** because the *Neisseria* lacks an O antigen. LPS induces release into the bloodstream or cerebrospinal fluid (CSF) of potent biological mediators, such as tumor necrosis factor-α (TNF-α) that elicits the systemic signs of meningococcemia, disseminated intravascular coagulation (DIC), and shock. Meningococci have a predilection for the central nervous system, where they can cause the serious complication of bacterial meningitis.

NEISSERIAE
BIOLOGY

The gonococcus and the meningococcus belong to the genus *Neisseria*, the main group of Gram-negative cocci associated with human disease. The neisseriae include a number of nonpathogenic organisms often found on the mucous membranes of healthy people, especially in the nasopharynx. Another Gram-negative coccus, *Moraxella catarrhalis*, causes respiratory tract infections, especially in immunocompromised patients. Sometimes considered to be an obligate aerobe, *Neisseria* spp. are in fact facultative

CASE

Pelvic Inflammatory Disease

Ms. C., a 14-year-old female, came to the emergency room with an acutely painful abdomen. Her temperature was 38.5°C, and laboratory tests indicated an elevated white blood cell count and sedimentation rate. Before results of urinalysis and a pregnancy test were returned, a pelvic examination revealed a purulent cervical discharge. A culture was sent, and a Gram stain of the discharge was prepared and examined (Fig. 14-1). Abdominal tenderness was apparent during the bimanual examination.

Ms. C. reported that her last menses was 4 days ago. When asked about her sexual behavior, she told the resident physician that she had intercourse for the first time 2 years ago. That relationship ended a few months ago, and she recently began "going steady" with a new friend. She and her partners have never used condoms or any other forms of birth control.

This case raises several questions:

1. What test should be ordered for the cervical specimen? What will the stained preparation most likely reveal?

2. Assuming that Ms. C. has PID, how did she acquire the infection?

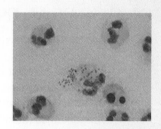

FIGURE 14-1. Gram stain of urethral pus. Notice the neutrophils with associated gonococci.

3. Is it significant that this patient has just finished her menses?

4. If the patient has PID, what other causative organisms, other than gonococci, should be considered?

5. If the patient has PID, would the proper use of male condoms have prevented the infection? Could any other forms of birth control and/or disease prevention have prevented transmission?

6. What other benefits would Ms. C. realize if she and her partner used condoms consistently and correctly? (See Chapter 69 for additional discussion of PID.)

See Appendix for answers.

---

anaerobes that can use nitrite as an electron acceptor and grow anaerobically. They have typical Gram-negative cell envelopes containing outer membrane proteins and endotoxin although, as noted, they do not have repeating O-antigen subunits and thus are classified as having LOS and not the LPS observed in many Gram-negative bacteria. These organisms are fragile and may not survive for long outside of their human hosts. The only source of infection for Ms. C. is another infected person (and not objects such as toilet seats).

When initially cultured from patients, *Neisseriae* grow best in an atmosphere with increased CO_2 (which can be provided by a "candle jar," a closed canister that uses a burning candle to convert O_2 to CO_2). A complex medium containing boiled blood, iron, and vitamins ("chocolate agar") also facilitates optimal growth.

Substantial differences exist in the pathogenic potential of different strains of gonococci. A given strain may cause uncomplicated **cervicitis** or **urethritis**, complications such as PID, or DGI. Host factors such as complement are also thought to be important in the severity and clinical presentation of the disease. Strains of meningococci also differ in their pathogenic potential.

ENCOUNTER AND ENTRY

Humans are the only known reservoir for gonococci. They do not persist free in the environment or spontaneously infect other animals; an estradiol-treated mouse model has improved our ability to study gonococcal infections in the laboratory after years of being unable to colonize mice productively with this pathogen.

Both men and women can carry gonococci without demonstrating symptoms, although the prevalence of **asymptomatic carriage** is greater among women. Asymptomatic carriers of either sex are a major problem in the control of gonorrhea because, without symptoms, they are less likely to be diagnosed or receive treatment and more likely to engage in sexual activity.

As part of its insidious pathogenic profile, the gonococcus has evolved to maximize its transmissibility. Consequently, it is important to test and to treat the known sexual contacts of a patient with gonorrhea. Such **case-contact tracing** and treatment is especially important in PID because the male sexual partners of PID patients are more likely to be asymptomatic and therefore may not seek therapy on their own. Consequently, a cured PID patient may be discharged from the hospital only to return to an infected sexual partner and become infected again.

Once gonococci are introduced into the vagina or the urethral mucosa of either gender, they attach to epithelial cells of the distal urethra or cervix and multiply. Several surface structures of the gonococcus facilitate attachment and anchor the organisms to the urethral or vaginal

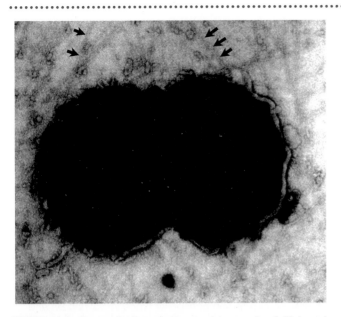

FIGURE 14-2. Transmission electron micrograph of *Neisseria gonorrhoeae*. Notice the presence of pili—long, thin strands of protein—emanating from the surface of the organisms and outer membrane blebs.

epithelial cells. Gonococci possess **pili** (Fig. 14-2), other **surface proteins**, and **lipooligosaccharide** that help them attach to host cells.

Sophisticated genetic mechanisms enable the bacteria to express or not express many of its surface adherence components (a phenomenon called **phase variation**; see the paradigm) or to control their structure (**antigenic variation**). Pili and gonococcal surface proteins are immunodominant; that is, they are well recognized by the immune system. However, they are also highly variable in structure, which makes them ineffective targets and explains why antibodies to these components do not protect against different gonococcal strains or reinfection.

Gonococci may or may not be taken up by neutrophils, depending on the type of outer membrane proteins they express. Some of the outer membrane proteins are called **colony opacity-associated (Opa) proteins**. Organisms that lack these proteins are not engulfed by neutrophils. Gonococci lacking Opa proteins are commonly associated with PID, DGI, and arthritis.

PARADIGM BOX

ALTERATION OF GENE EXPRESSION BY DNA REARRANGEMENTS

The basic strategies that pathogenic microbes use for immune avoidance, subversion, or disruption are found in highly unrelated species. In some cases, immune evasion involves activities or molecules that are expressed continuously. Examples include **sialylation of lipopolysaccharide** or other surface structures to mimic the host, production of **IgA1 protease**, and occupancy of an intracellular environment and remodeling of host immune processes to avoid detection or clearance by the immune system. In some cases, evasion of specific host immune responses (e.g., antibodies) involves a process called **antigenic variation**. Antigenic variation results in changes in the composition or structure of predominant surface molecules. These changes allow an organism to avoid recognition by specific antibodies arising during the course of infection. Rather than occurring in response to specific antibodies, variation is achieved by genetic rearrangements that take place randomly and at a high frequency within the bacterial population. Consequently, new variants are selected for and emerge by virtue of their escape from antibody-mediated immune mechanisms. In many cases, the repertoire of new antigenic types that can be expressed is so great that protective immunity rarely develops. Thus, chronic and repeated infections are hallmarks of diseases caused by these agents, such as gonorrhea.

Antigenic variation occurs in microorganisms as diverse as African trypanosomes (which cause African sleeping sickness), *Borrelia* species (which cause relapsing fever), and *N. gonorrhoeae*. In these microbes, antigenic variation can result from the reassortment and recombination of duplicated gene segments. This mechanism is analogous (but not identical) to the way in which diversity is generated within immunoglobulins of animals.

Having evolved to grow exclusively within human hosts, gonococci are a paradigm for organisms that have evolved special mechanisms to adjust to life in immunocompetent individuals. Efforts to develop a gonococcal vaccine have involved a great deal of work to understand the molecular mechanisms of gonococcal antigenic variation. For example, the gonococcal chromosome contains a single copy of the complete **pilin** gene (pilin is the structural protein that is polymerized to form pili). This gene is called *pilE*, for "pilin expression locus." In addition, the gonococcal chromosome contains 10 to 15 copies of variant-encoding pilin genes. All of these copies are truncated at their 5′ ends and lack transcriptional promoter elements, as well as the sequences specifying the *N*-terminus part of pilin. These copies are called *pilS* loci, for "silent (nonfunctional) loci." Antigenic variation occurs when the genetic information from the nonfunctional alleles is transferred to the complete pilin gene locus by homologous recombination. Figure 14-3 depicts this process as an antigenic switch from a β-pilin type to an α-pilin type.

continued on page 182

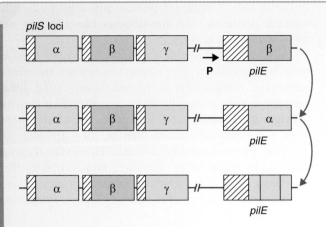

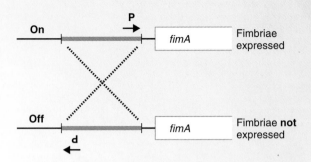

FIGURE 14-4. Phase variation of *Escherichia coli* fimbriae by inversion of a DNA segment containing a promoter.

FIGURE 14-3. Antigenic variation of pili in *N. gonorrhoeae.*

Pilin diversification depends not only on the mere number of *pilS* genes but also on the fact that small stretches of *pilS* sequence can be recombined into the expression locus resulting in chimeric pilin types. Such an event is depicted in Figure 14-3 as the formation of a *pilE* hybrid between the α- and γ-alleles. Note that this process occurs through a mechanism called gene conversion, in which the *pilS* alleles act as donors of new genetic information but are not altered themselves. The result is a virtually infinite variety of pilin serotypes that can be expressed using only a limited number of *pilS* alleles.

Another form of altered gene expression arising from DNA rearrangements results in **phase variation**. In this process, the expression of a particular gene product is turned on or off at high frequency. Oscillation between on and off states occurs by two basic mechanisms. One mechanism involves the site-specific **inversion** of a DNA segment that bears a gene promoter. An example of this mechanism is the phase variation of type I fimbriae expression in *Escherichia coli* (Fig. 14-4). In the "on" state, the promoter element is oriented so that transcription of the fimbrial subunit

gene, *fimA*, can take place. Inversion of the element (shown in blue) orients the promoter in a direction divergent to that of *fimA* (i.e., the off state). Analogous inversion systems control the expression of flagellar types in *Salmonella* and pilus expression in other Gram-negative pathogens.

The second mechanism of phase variation is associated with the somewhat unusual occurrence of short nucleotide repeats at the 5′ ends of genes. Such repeats can readily be gained or lost as a consequence of strand misalignment during normal DNA replication and repair. Events of this sort, termed **slipped strand mispairing**, occur at frequencies much higher than point mutations and disrupt the integrity of the gene's translational reading frame. *N. gonorrhoeae* employs this mechanism to change the expression of its virulence-associated Opa proteins. Multiple copies of complete *opa* genes (which each encode different Opa antigenic variants) are scattered throughout the genome. Each gene copy contains repeats of the sequence CTCTT within the 5′ end of its reading frame. Gain or loss of these elements alters the translational reading frame of the gene and determines whether the intact protein can be made. For example, Figure 14-5 shows a protein expressed from a gene

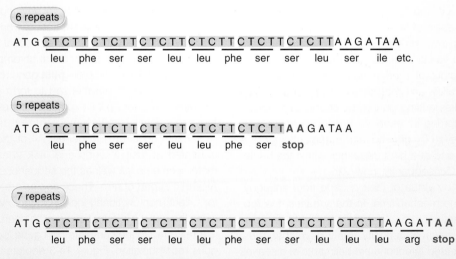

FIGURE 14-5. Representation of the phase variation mechanism of the gonococcal *opa* genes. The sequences have been modified and shortened to demonstrate the mechanism succinctly.

carrying six copies of the element. If a CTCTT sequence is gained or lost within this stretch, the reading frame is altered and translation is terminated prematurely. In this way, gonococci can turn on or off the expression of any of *opa* genes independently.

A similar mechanism is known to control the expression of many other gonococcal and meningococcal surface proteins and to oscillate expression of the biosynthetic genes for gonococcal and meningococcal LPS, resulting in its structural variability. Analogous phase variation mechanisms have been shown to operate in a number of important surface molecules in other Gram-negative pathogens. In each of these other instances, different repetitive elements are found. The only common feature is that the number of nucleotides of the repeat element is not three, nor is it divisible by three. Because the genetic code operates through trinucleotide codons, deletion or addition of a three base pair repeat would not change the reading frame.

Another way that slipped strand mispairing can disrupt gene expression is when it occurs in the promoter element of a gene. Binding by RNA polymerase to initiate transcription requires precise positioning of the enzyme onto the DNA, often by recognizing two elements that are spaced appropriately to enable polymerase to recognize the promoter. In some instances, the spacing between these elements may change due to slipped strand mispairing, thereby reducing the efficiency with which RNA polymerase binds and, consequently, the amount of expression of that gene.

Phase variation can represent a simplified form of antigenic variation in which a specific protein antigen is either expressed or not (as opposed to multiple different antigenic types of a protein), but gain or loss of molecules also has important functional consequences unrelated to immune pressure. The widespread distribution of this form of phase variation among microbes suggests that it is biologically important and that there is an evolutionary advantage to existing as a heterogeneous population.

SPREAD AND MULTIPLICATION

After colonizing the mucosal cell surface, gonococci multiply rapidly and are shed in large numbers into the genital secretions of infected men and women. Movement into the urethra or through the cervix can be aided by menses, secretions, or urethral or uterine contractions.

Genital mucosal secretions contain three types of IgG and both IgA1 and IgA2. IgG found in secretions may indicate leakage of the antibody from serum onto the mucosal surface, whereas most of the IgA is actively secreted into the lumen of the genital tract. Gonococci produce an extracellular **protease** that specifically cleaves IgA1 but not IgA2 in the hinge region. This property is also present in other bacteria that inhabit mucosal epithelia, such as *Haemophilus influenzae* and certain streptococci. How this protease contributes to pathogenicity is not known. The protease also may have activity on gonococcal surface proteins and may help the organisms escape phagocytosis by removing the Fc end of the immunoglobulin from gonococcus-bound IgA molecules. Because the Fc region is the portion recognized by phagocytes, the organisms may be less likely to be taken up by white blood cells when this portion of the immunoglobulin molecule is removed.

Gonococci also can enter epithelial cells. What is known about invasion of epithelial cells by gonococci is assumed from studies with in vitro organ culture of human fallopian tubes and from primary human cervical epithelial cells. Two major types of cells compose the epithelial mucosal surface of human fallopian tubes: ciliated cells and nonciliated cells. The nonciliated cells have fingerlike processes, called microvilli, on their luminal surface. When gonococci are exposed to fallopian tube sections, several events occur:

- **Attachment**: Gonococci attach to the microvilli of nonciliated cells.
- **Ciliary stasis**: Motility of the ciliated cells slows and ultimately ceases. Ciliary activity is thought to be important in moving the fertilized egg from the fallopian tube to the uterus and in providing a flushing mechanism for clearing mucus and bacteria from the mucosal surface.
- **Death of ciliated cells**: Ciliated cells die and are selectively sloughed from the epithelial surface (Fig. 14-6). This step does not require intact organisms and can be elicited by gonococcal LPS or gonococcal peptidoglycan fragments (parts of the cell wall).
- **Internalization**: Through a cascade of events initiated by the gonococcus, the microvilli of nonciliated cells, acting as pseudopodia, engulf the bacteria. Gonococci are then internalized by these "nonprofessional" phagocytes by a process termed parasite-directed endocytosis.
- **Intracellular replication**: Gonococci are transported to the interior of the cell within phagocytic vacuoles. These vacuoles coalesce to form larger vacuoles, within which gonococci multiply. Inside the nonciliated cells, gonococci are sheltered from antibodies, professional phagocytes, and antibiotics that do not enter human cells well.

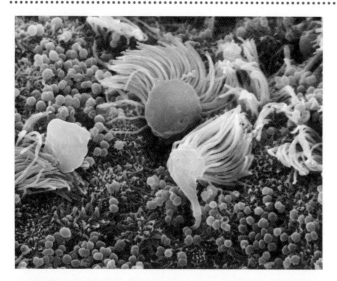

FIGURE 14-6. Scanning electron micrograph of human fallopian tube tissue 20 hours after infection with *Neisseria gonorrhoeae*. Notice that gonococci attach almost exclusively to the surface of nonciliated cells. The damage occurs to ciliated cells. Ciliated cells sloughed from the surface of the mucosa appear at the left and center of the photomicrograph, whereas intact ciliated cells are seen at the top and right.

- **Intracellular traffic**: The gonococci can be transported to the base of the nonciliated cells where the bacteria-laden vacuoles fuse with the basement membrane.
- **Exocytosis**: The phagocytic vacuoles discharge gonococci into the subepithelial connective tissue. From there, the organisms probably either cause local inflammation or enter blood vessels to cause disseminated disease.

In primary cervical cells, pilus-mediated association with complement receptor 3 (CR3) may lead to stimulation of cellular uptake of the gonococci, which induce a series of downstream events, ultimately leading to epithelial cell colonization. The pilus–CR3 association may also serve to diminish the inflammatory response by these cells. This may be in part what accounts for a more asymptomatic colonization of the cervix than is observed when gonococci colonize the epithelium of the male urethra, where CR3 is not expressed and infections can be more inflammatory.

DAMAGE

Gonococci are not known to secrete exotoxins; thus, damage to host tissues is most likely caused by LPS and other components of the bacterial cell wall, such as peptidoglycan. Both LPS and peptidoglycan are known to induce the production of TNF-α by a variety of human cells, and TNF-α has been shown to cause the sloughing of ciliated cells from human fallopian tube mucosa. In addition to the death of ciliated cells, as demonstrated in the fallopian tube model, nonciliated epithelial cells containing gonococci may lyse, releasing cellular tissue

factors that mediate further inflammation. The inflammatory response in the male urethra is probably responsible for local symptoms such as pain on urination (**dysuria**) and urethral discharge of pus. It is noteworthy that these symptoms do not distinguish gonococcal urethritis from that caused by other genital pathogens, like the chlamydiae (see Chapter 27). However, the urethral discharge in gonorrhea tends to be more copious, thick, and greenish yellow, and the pain is more intense. Although, as noted, women with gonococcal cervicitis are more often asymptomatic than are men with urethritis, women can experience dysuria, dyspareunia (pain on intercourse), discharge, or genital discomfort.

Survival of Gonococci in the Bloodstream

Normal human serum is capable of killing circulating organisms of many Gram-negative species, including *N. gonorrhoeae*. This natural protective effect depends on complement activation and IgG and IgM antibodies. In the case of the gonococcus, the targets for antibodies are LOS; the major outer membrane protein, called **protein I**; and other proteins exposed on the surface of the organisms. Thus, for gonococci to survive in the bloodstream, they must be able to evade this defense mechanism.

However, gonococci, and especially those strains associated with DGI, can be serum resistant. Gonococci can become serum resistant when LOS is altered by the addition of a terminal sialic acid molecule on the short, core carbohydrate chain. Because sialic acid is a negatively charged molecule and a surface component of cells, this modification may camouflage the organisms and protect them from the antibodies responsible for serum killing. Serum resistance in strains associated with DGI can also occur by binding both C4b-binding protein and factor H, two negative regulators of complement activation (see Chapter 6 for details on the complement system).

The surface constituents of DGI strains are different from those of their serum-sensitive counterparts. However, the serum-resistant strains may be more sensitive to penicillin and have specific nutritional requirements. It is not clear whether these properties directly contribute to the ability of the organisms to disseminate or whether these properties are closely linked genetically.

Host factors also affect the outcome of gonococcal infections. For example, individuals deficient in the final components of the complement cascade that form the membrane attack complex are predisposed to recurrent systemic infections with both gonococci and meningococci.

The manifestations of DGI include pustular skin lesions with a surrounding red areola, tenosynovitis, and frank infections of the joints (**suppurative arthritis**). Often, despite appropriate diagnostic attempts, cultures of blood, joint fluid, or skin lesions are sterile. There are several reasons for this phenomenon. First, gonococci may be present but in numbers too low to be detectable in culture. Second, the nutritional requirements of these organisms may be unusual, and they may be inhibited or not grow using normal culture conditions. Third, in cases of tenosynovitis, fragments of cell wall peptidoglycan (murein) or perhaps immune complexes consisting of gonococcal antigens and host antibodies, rather than viable gonococci, may be deposited in synovial tissue and cause local inflammation. The latter possibility is supported by experiments in rats showing that purified gonococcal peptidoglycan, when injected into joints, induces arthritis. If this phenomenon were to apply to humans, active joint infection need not be present at the site of intense inflammation.

Outcome of Gonococcal Infection

What is the outcome of gonorrhea? Data from the era prior to use of antibiotics suggest that the symptoms of urethral infection in males usually subside in several weeks without treatment. However, repeated infections, if untreated, can lead to scarring and stricture of the urethra. Such sequelae of gonococcal infection are now rare because most men seek medical attention once urethritis becomes apparent. Symptoms of cervicitis include cervical discharge (reported as vaginal discharge), bleeding, and pain. Paradoxically, local urogenital infections are asymptomatic in approximately 30% of women and are often heralded by the complications of the infection. Chronic fallopian tube inflammation can lead to scarring and stricture, resulting in such long-term sequelae as chronic pelvic pain; ectopic pregnancy; recurrent PID caused by chlamydiae, anaerobes, and other organisms; and infertility. For unknown reasons, DGI occurs predominantly in women. Gonococcal arthritis remains a common type of joint infection in sexually active adults.

The outcome of gonococcal infection depends not only on the gender of the patient but also on the timeliness of medical attention. Prompt treatment decreases the risk of ascending or disseminated infection and the resulting sequelae.

Meningococcal Infections

Gonococci and meningococci are close taxonomic cousins; the two organisms share about 90% of their DNA sequences, and both possess similar virulence factors including pili, outer membrane proteins, and LPS. Both organisms can colonize mucous membranes without causing symptoms; it is estimated that in endemic areas, 5 to 10% of the population carries meningococci. While gonococci and meningococci each cause purulent infections, infection usually results in a contrasting spectrum of diseases. Whereas gonococcal infections are most often local and rarely lethal (even upon spread to the bloodstream), meningococcal infection of the bloodstream is a systemic and life-threatening disease. Why do these two species cause such different illnesses? As previously mentioned, a major factor is that the meningococcus is heavily **encapsulated**, which plays an important role in the pathogenicity of this organism.

While isolated cases, case clusters, or large epidemics of meningococcal disease can occur, the more usual outcome of exposure to the meningococcus is colonization of the nasopharynx with no local symptoms or systemic consequences. Based on organ cultures of nasopharyngeal epithelium, the cascade of events (attachment, ciliary stasis, death of ciliated cells, etc.) at upper respiratory mucous membranes appear to be similar for the meningococcus in the nasopharynx and the gonococcus in the fallopian tube (as described earlier). Patients susceptible to meningococcemia or meningococcal meningitis are often deficient in bactericidal anticapsular antibodies or in activity of the complement cascade. Individuals with capsule-specific antibodies or antibodies directed at other surface components, presumably produced in response to cross-reacting antigens or past colonization, resist the ability of the meningococcus

MENINGOCOCCAL INFECTIONS

Meningococcal meningitis
Meningococcal bacteremia
Meningococcemia (purpura fulminans and the Waterhouse-Friderichsen syndrome)
Respiratory tract infection
Pneumonia
Epiglottitis
Otitis media
Focal infection
Conjunctivitis
Septic arthritis
Urethritis
Purulent pericarditis
Chronic meningococcemia

to invade and multiply in the bloodstream. By providing a serologic correlate of protection, these observations were instrumental in developing the currently licensed vaccines made of purified capsular polysaccharide or capsular polysaccharide conjugated to protein.

If they are not killed by bactericidal activity or phagocytes in the bloodstream, meningococci multiply rapidly, reaching blood titers that are among the highest known for any bacterium. It is possible, for example, to observe the organisms directly on a smear of the buffy coat of blood (the layer containing the white cells when whole blood is centrifuged). Other bacterial septicemias rarely result in bacteria visible in buffy coat stains.

The entry of meningococci into the human bloodstream can lead to devastating systemic disease marked by **purpura fulminans** and **disseminated intravascular coagulation (DIC)** with generalized skin manifestations (petechiae and ecchymoses), meningitis, shock, and death. These systemic signs are the direct result of the ability of the meningococcus to survive and multiply in the bloodstream. DIC is accompanied by shock, fever, and other responses to endotoxin or other cell components mediated by cytokines such as TNF-α and interleukin-1. In meningococcal sepsis and meningitis, the likelihood of death or neurologic damage is proportional to levels of endotoxin and the elevation in serum and CSF of TNF-α concentrations. Because TNF-α is a chemical mediator of our host defense system, this observation gives weight to Lewis Thomas' observation: "Our arsenals for fighting off bacteria are so powerful… that we are in more danger from them than from the invaders. We live in the midst of explosive devices. We are mined."

As noted, meningococcal disease is effectively prevented by vaccines containing capsular polysaccharide. A notable exception is disease caused by serogroup B meningococci. The capsule of serogroup B strains is a homopolymer of sialic acid that is identical to human sialic acid polymers, is poorly immunogenic, and does not normally elicit protective antibodies.

In contrast, when gonococci reach the bloodstream of most individuals, they are usually killed by host defense mechanisms. Even serum-resistant strains do not grow appreciably in the circulation, although they may survive long enough to reach other organs. Although gonococcal meningitis is reported on rare occasions and gonococcal endocarditis was common in the preantibiotic era, gonococcal bacteremia is now seldom fatal.

DIAGNOSIS

The finding of neutrophils containing Gram-negative diplococci in cervical or urethral secretions is presumptive evidence of gonococcal infection. Positive microscopic findings justify beginning antibiotic therapy before the results of cultures are known in the appropriate clinical setting. The Gram stain of urethral exudate of men is more sensitive than the Gram stain of cervical exudate in

women. A cervical Gram stain may be negative, despite a positive culture result. A positive Gram stain of cervical secretions is confirmatory evidence of active gonorrhea in a symptomatic woman, but routine Gram stains of secretions from asymptomatic women are not clinically useful.

Because the social implications of gonorrhea can be as serious as the medical consequences, the physician must confirm the clinical findings by culturing or using genetic probes. It is also important to monitor how the laboratory identifies these organisms. There are two reasons to culture: (1) to be completely certain of the identity of the infecting microorganism and (2) to obtain the isolate for antimicrobial susceptibility testing. Nucleic acid–based detection tests are increasingly used for purposes of screening asymptomatic patients at risk.

Gonococci grow on several kinds of media that allow presumptive identification within a day. The most commonly used medium is called "chocolate agar" because it contains heated blood and has the appearance of milk chocolate. Special varieties of this medium are known as **Thayer-Martin medium** and **Martin-Lewis medium**; each contains unique antibiotics to inhibit other bacterial species and yeasts found in the genital tract. Specimens taken from the cervix, urethra, and other sites should always be cultured on chocolate agar with antibiotics (e.g., Thayer-Martin or Martin-Lewis medium) to inhibit the normal microbiota. It is noteworthy that an occasional strain of gonococci is sensitive to the antibiotics used in the Thayer-Martin medium. For this reason, fluids that are normally sterile (e.g., CSF, blood, and synovial fluid) should be cultured on chocolate agar without antibiotics to allow recovery of antibiotic-sensitive gonococcal strains.

All members of the genus *Neisseria* and related genera possess a cytochrome oxidase that can catalyze a color change in the presence of a specific reagent. If a Gram-negative diplococcus is oxidase positive in this test, it is a member of *Neisseria* or a close relative. To distinguish *N. gonorrhoeae* from the other species of this genus, the microbiological laboratory determines the pattern of fermentation of various sugars. Unlike other neisseriae, gonococci utilize glucose but not maltose or sucrose, and meningococci utilize both glucose and maltose. Although Gram stain and culture remain the mainstays of diagnostics for meningococcal infection, polymerase chain reaction–based testing is also now available in clinical labs.

TREATMENT

A relatively high proportion of gonococci now bear a plasmid that encodes a β-lactamase, an enzyme that destroys penicillin. Gonococci bearing the resistance plasmids can cause serious locally invasive diseases, like PID, as well as DGIs. As a consequence of widespread penicillin resistance, the recommended initial therapy for gonorrhea is no longer penicillin but a β-lactamase-resistant cephalosporin—cefixime or ceftriaxone—given orally or intramuscularly, respectively. Single-dose oral therapy is effective and offers the distinct advantage of observed therapy. Both quinolones (ciprofloxacin, ofloxacin, and levofloxacin) and cefixime are available for this purpose, but gonococci resistant to quinolones have spread from Southeast Asia to North America and are no longer recommended for empiric treatment. Isolation of strains resistant to extended-spectrum cephalosporins has been reported, raising concern that gonococcus is attaining "superbug" status. Patients infected with *N. gonorrhoeae* are often coinfected with *Chlamydia trachomatis*. This has led to the recommendation that patients treated for gonococcal infection should also receive an antichlamydial agent such as azithromycin or doxycycline. Additionally, infection with *N. gonorrhoeae* is a proven risk factor for HIV transmission, and treatment for gonococcal infection among some groups has led to a concomitant decrease in rates of HIV transmission.

Treatment of meningococcal infection by intravenously administered antibiotics, such as ceftriaxone or penicillin, and other supportive therapy is indicated. Although reports of meningococcal isolates with decreased susceptibility to penicillin have been reported, the clinical significance of this level of resistance remains uncertain.

PREVENTION

Despite effective antimicrobials and active public health measures, an estimated 700,000 cases of gonococcal infection occur annually in the United States. Prevention efforts must be based on a multipronged approach that includes the following:

- Behavioral interventions, including condom use and decreasing the number of sexual partners
- Early diagnosis and treatment
- Partner notification
- Screening and case finding
- Vaccine development and use

Vaccine development has proven to be difficult because gonococci, as solely human pathogens, have a long-standing and sophisticated relationship with their hosts. These organisms have managed to survive the host immune response, as discussed in the paradigm, by antigenic variation, phase variation, and the occupation of protective intracellular environments. Acquired immunity following infection is inadequate, and repeat infections are common among individuals with repeat exposures. New approaches to prevention are being actively pursued. Topical microbicides for intravaginal and intrarectal use are being developed to safely and effectively prevent sexually transmitted diseases, including HIV.

Prevention of meningococcal infections is primarily approached with two strategies: treatment with antibiotics such as rifampin or ciprofloxacin of close contacts of cases and targeted mass vaccination in outbreak settings where indicated. A polysaccharide conjugate vaccine, MCV4,

for prevention of meningococcal disease resulting from serogroups A, C, Y, and W-135 has been licensed for use in individuals aged 2 to 55 and is recommended for adolescents. The B serogroup capsule includes polysialic acid, which is found on human glycoproteins as well. Thus, vaccinating against the capsule could lead to antibodies against our own proteins. Promising candidates for broadly protective serogroup B meningococcal vaccine, based on noncapsular antigens, have been developed. One of these, MenZB™, which targets outer membrane proteins, is being used in New Zealand for individuals under the age of 20. Undoubtedly, more noncapsular vaccines against serogroup B meningococcus will be introduced in the near future.

CONCLUSION

Gonococci and meningococci are found only in humans and are often carried asymptomatically. Both gonococci and meningococci have developed mechanisms to attach to and avoid loss from host cells, cause ciliary stasis, and invade cells. They are able to traverse epithelial cells and either cause local inflammation or disseminate to other parts of the body. Meningococci have an exceptional ability to survive in the bloodstream and cause systemic infections that often have disastrous consequences. In principle, effective vaccines may be developed, which could control and prevent disease. Recent progress has been made in vaccine development against meningococcal infection, but challenges remain for prevention of infection by *N. gonorrhoeae*.

Suggested Readings

Britigan BE, Cohen MS, Sparling PF. Gonococcal infection: a model of molecular pathogenesis. *N Engl J Med*. 1985;312:1683–1694.

Centers for Disease Control and Prevention. Sexually transmitted diseases treatment guidelines, 2002. *MMWR Recomm Rep*. 2002;51(RR-6):1–78.

Edwards JL, Butler EK. The pathobiology of neisseria gonorrhoeae lower female genital tract infection. *Front Microbiol*. 2011;2:1–12.

Figueroa JE, Densen P. Infectious diseases associated with complement deficiencies. *Clin Microbiol Rev*. 1991;4:359–395.

Jerse AE, Wu H, Packiam M, et al. Estradiol-treated female mice as surrogate hosts for neisseria gonorrhoeae genital tract infections. *Front Microbiol*. 2011;2:107.

Merz AJ, So M. Interactions of pathogenic neisseriae with epithelial cell membranes. *Annu Rev Cell Dev Biol*. 2000;16:423–457.

Oster P, Lennon D, O'Hallahan J, et al. MeNZB: a safe and highly immunogenic tailor-made vaccine against the New Zealand Neisseria meningitidis serogroup B disease epidemic strain. *Vaccine*. 2005;23:2191–2196.

Rosenstein NE, Perkins BA, Stephens DS, et al. Meningococcal disease. *N Engl J Med*. 2001;344:1378–1388.

Sadarangani M, Pollard AJ. Serogroup B meningococcal vaccines-an unfinished story. *Lancet Infect Dis*. 2010;10:112–124.

Stephens DS. Gonococcal and meningococcal pathogenesis as defined by human cell, cell culture, and organ culture assays. *Clin Microbiol Rev*. 1989;2:S104–S111.

Swanson J, Koomey M. Mechanisms for variation of pili and outer membrane protein II in *Neisseria gonorrhoeae*. In: Berg D, Howe M, eds. *Mobile DNA*. Washington, DC: ASM Press; 1989:743–761.

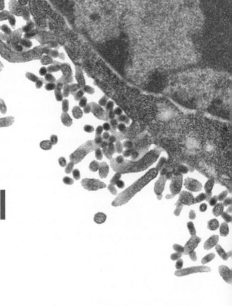

Chapter 15

Bacteroides, Intra-Abdominal Infection, and Abscesses

Laurie E. Comstock

KEY CONCEPTS

Pathogen: Bacteroidales are an order of bacteria containing several genera including *Bacteroides*, *Parabacteroides*, *Prevotella*, and *Alistipes* which include species that are members of the human colonic microbiota. Bacteroidales species are collectively the most abundant Gram-negative bacteria of the human colonic microbiota reaching densities greater than 10^{10} bacteria/g of colonic contents.

Encounter: Bacteroidales are commensal/symbiotic bacteria of the human intestine but become opportunistic pathogens if they gain access to the otherwise sterile peritoneal cavity following leakage of colonic contents.

Entry: Among the numerous intestinal Bacteroidales species, *Bacteroides* and *Parabacteroides* species are most commonly isolated from clinical infections, with *Bacteroides fragilis* comprising approximately 50% of clinical, intestinally derived Bacteroidales isolates.

Spread and Multiplication: Large numbers of bacteria can enter the sterile peritoneal cavity if the bowel wall is breached through rupture, appendicitis, or abdominal surgery. Infection often begins with peritonitis and bacteremia, which can be followed by intra-abdominal abscess formation.

Damage: Abscess formation is facilitated by the zwitterionic capsular polysaccharides that initiate a host response contributing to abscess formation.

Diagnosis: Imaging methods, such as ultrasound or computed tomography, are used to identify and localize abscesses. Anaerobic culture or PCR methods can identify particular species and determine antibiotic sensitivities.

Treatment: Abscesses are treated by drainage and antibiotics; antibiotics therapy effective against both facultative anaerobes and strict anaerobes is necessary, with particular attention to the resistance profile of Bacteroidales species.

Prevention: Rapid and effective antibiotic treatment in cases where there is concern for potential polymicrobial infection in the peritoneum.

THE PATHOGENS: *BACTEROIDALES*

This chapter focuses mainly on one of the most frequently isolated genera of bacteria from intra-abdominal abscesses, the *Bacteroides*, but also includes the intestinally derived opportunistic pathogens of the *Parabacteroides* genus, which are also members of the Bacteroidales order (Fig. 15-1 and Table 15-1). Until recently, many species within the order Bacteroidales were incorrectly classified phylogenetically. Most intestinal Bacteroidales species were originally considered to be in the genus *Bacteroides*; however, sequencing of the 16S ribosomal RNA genes has demonstrated that these species segregate into five different families, four of which include intestinal species and are listed in Figure 15-1. Due to this historical classification, and the fact that *B. fragilis* is the most frequently isolated intestinally derived clinical organism from this order, other non–*B. fragilis* intestinal Bacteroidales species (such as *Parabacteroides* spp.) are commonly referred to as belonging to the *B. fragilis* group, even if they are not part of the *Bacteroides* genus or even of the same family.

CASE • Ms. A., an 18-year-old college freshman, was admitted to the hospital with diffuse abdominal pain, diarrhea, and nausea without vomiting. Her pain was localized to the right side of the abdomen. Physical examination revealed tenderness in the lower quadrant of her abdomen, principally over McBurney point. She received a first-generation cephalosporin antibiotic (cefazolin) and was taken to the operating room, where her ruptured appendix was removed. Cultures of the peritoneal cavity in the neighborhood of the appendix grew a mixture of bacteria, typical of those found in stool. On the second day after the operation, her temperature spiked to 38.6°C. Blood cultures obtained preoperatively grew *Escherichia coli*.

Ms. A. improved postoperatively and completed a 7-day course of cephalosporin. Because she had no further symptoms and her blood cultures were negative, the antibiotic was stopped. However, 36 hours later, her temperature

was 38.8°C and she felt diffuse pain over the site of the appendectomy. A CAT scan of her abdomen revealed a retroperitoneal abscess. Cultures obtained after drainage of the abscess grew *Bacteroides fragilis*. She was again treated with antibiotics. This time, metronidazole was used for 14 days, and Ms. A. had an uneventful recovery.

This case raises several questions:

1. How did the two episodes of Ms. A.'s disease differ with regard to pathogenesis and the kind of bacteria involved?

2. Why did *B. fragilis* survive the first course of antibiotic treatment?

3. Was Ms. A. treated properly? What could have been done to lessen the likelihood of abscess formation?

4. How does *B. fragilis* facilitate intra-abdominal abscess formation?

See Appendix for answers.

ENCOUNTER AND ENTRY

The human colon is one of the most densely packed microbial ecosystems on earth containing upward of a thousand different species and collectively reaching densities of 10^{11} to 10^{12} microbes per gram of colonic contents. The most abundant bacterial species of this microbial ecosystem are Gram-positive members of the phylum Firmicutes and Gram-negative bacteria of the phylum Bacteroidetes, most contained within the order Bacteroidales. Proteobacterial species such as *Escherichia coli* are also present, although at lower concentration. Despite the incredible diversity of microbes present in this ecosystem, few of these endogenous intestinal species are equipped to survive in extraintestinal sites and therefore few have the capacity to become opportunistic pathogens.

Due to the incredible microbial load of the intestine, no other body site is more prone to contamination by a large number of endogenous bacteria than the peritoneal cavity. Breach of the intestine can occur from a number of adverse events including blunt trauma, a penetrating

wound, a ruptured appendix, intestinal disease, and abdominal surgery. The majority of intra-abdominal infections result from the rupture of **infected appendices** or **intestinal diverticula**, the abnormal outpouchings of the colon. In the United States, more than 250,000 cases of appendicitis and some 350,000 cases of diverticulitis are reported each year. Of these infections, about 15% perforate. The prevalence of diverticula increases with aging, as does diverticulitis as the cause of intra-abdominal infection. In the case of Ms. A., obstruction of outflow from the appendix led to inflammation and eventually to perforation, another common cause of peritoneal contamination with intestinal contents.

SPREAD AND MULTIPLICATION

Spillage of microbe-laden colonic contents into the peritoneal cavity initiates an infection that often begins with peritonitis and bacteremia, followed in some cases by intra-abdominal abscess formation. This **biphasic disease** process occurred in the case of Ms. A. The resulting intra-abdominal infection dramatically illustrates what happens

PARADIGM BOX

POLYMICROBIAL INFECTIONS

The contamination of deep tissues with endogenous microbial residents, such as that of the intestine or the oropharynx, often results in infection caused by a mixture of bacteria that are part of the normal microbiota of the original site. Examples are **peritonitis**

caused by a ruptured appendix and a **pulmonary abscess** caused by aspiration of oropharyngeal bacteria. From such sites, it is usually possible to isolate many different combinations of bacteria. These infections are exceptions to a "one germ, one disease" concept. That is, they are usually **polymicrobial** rather than monomicrobial.

Bacteroidales (order)
    Bacteroidaceae (family)
        Bacteroides fragilis
        Bacteroides thetaiotaomicron
        Bacteroides ovatus
        Bacteroides caccae
        Bacteroides uniformis
        Bacteroides vulgatus
        Bacteroides intestinalis
        Bacteroides xylanosolvens
        Bacteroides stericoris
        Bacteroides eggerthii
        Bacteroides nordii
        Bacteroides dorei
        Bacteroides fingoldii
        Bacteroides cellulosilyticus
        Bacteroides coprocola
        Bacteroides coprophilus
        Bacteroides plebeius
        Bacteroides salyersae
        Bacteroides massilensis
    Porphyromonadaceae (family)
        Parabacteroides johnsonii
        Parabacteroides distasonis
        Parabacteroides merdae
        Tannerella forsythia
        Porphyromonas gingivalis
    Prevotellaceae (family)
        Prevotella copri
        Prevotella melaninogenica
        Prevotella intermedia
        Prevotella bivia
        Prevotella disiens
    Rikenellaceae (family)
        Alistipes putredenis
        Alistipes shahii
        Alistipes onderdonkii
        Alistipes fingoldii

FIGURE 15-1. Bacteroidales species commonly found in the human body. Those in blue font are normal members of the human intestinal microbiota. Species in *red* font are present in the oral cavity and are usually associated with pathogenic states. *Prevotella bivia* and *Prevotella disiens* are associated with female genital tract infections.

when microorganisms are introduced in large numbers into the wrong place. The spillage of a few milliliters of intestinal content into the peritoneal cavity delivers trillions of bacteria to a normally sterile site. The ensuing infections are polymicrobial and include **strict anaerobes** and **facultative anaerobes** (such as members of the Enterobacteriaceae family), probably interacting in complex metabolic ways. Animal studies have documented a need for synergy between various microorganisms for

TABLE 15-1 Intestinal Bacteroidales Species Most Frequently Isolated from Extraintestinal Infections, in Descending Order of Frequency

Bacteroides fragilis
Bacteroides thetaiotaomicron
Bacteroides ovatus
Bacteroides vulgatus
Parabacteroides distasonis
Bacteroides uniformis
Bacteroides caccae
Bacteroides stercoris
Bacteroides eggerthii
Parabacteroides merdae

abscess formation. The inoculation of a single species of intestinal bacteria seldom leads to infection, but infection by a mixture of facultative and strict anaerobes produces acute inflammation and abscess formation.

Because the bacterial inoculum is potentially diverse, a large number of factors are involved in determining which species become dominant in the infection. Many intestinal bacteria can grow in the peritoneal fluid, which is not particularly antibacterial. Before the content of the colon spills, the peritoneal cavity is well oxygenated, and highly oxygen-sensitive anaerobes are killed. After the spillage, the first organisms that become numerically dominant are facultative anaerobes, especially *E. coli.* However, many of the less oxygen-sensitive strict anaerobes survive and can be isolated from both the fluid and surface of mesothelial cells. Although *Bacteroides* and *Parabacteroides* are strict anaerobes, they are not killed by exposure to oxygen.

Because *B. fragilis* is found in approximately 50% of intestinally derived Bacteroidales infections and is the most important of the anaerobic bacteria associated with abscess formation, most of the studies have been conducted using *B. fragilis* as a model for intestinally derived opportunistic Bacteroidales pathogens. It has been shown that not only is *B. fragilis* aerotolerant but it can also grow in extremely reduced (nanomolar) concentrations of oxygen. *B. fragilis* has an extensive, highly regulated oxidative stress response system, including several enzymes typically absent from strict anaerobic organisms that protect the organism from oxygen radicals. These include a **superoxide dismutase**, which detoxifies oxygen radicals, and a **catalase**, which breaks down hydrogen peroxide. The organism synthesizes many new gene products in response to oxidative stress. As the peritoneal cavity has a higher Po_2 than the colon, products contributing to the organism's tolerance of air are likely important for survival of *B. fragilis* when it is initially released into the peritoneal cavity.

Upon entry into the peritoneal cavity, intestinal organisms find themselves first in a liquid environment that could, in principle, lead to their dissemination throughout the cavity. However, the omentum and the loops of the small intestine drape themselves around areas of inflammation and serve to contain the infection. Although this takes time, the abscesses that eventually develop are usually well localized. Lymphatic drainage and the effect of gravity also influence the location of abscesses. These factors likely influenced the location of Ms. A.'s abscess at a retroperitoneal site, even though the original bacterial spill was near her appendix.

Other properties that evolved for intestinal fitness of these bacteria may also contribute to their success as opportunistic pathogens. The intestinal Bacteroidales obtain energy by fermenting carbohydrates. They are able to use the complex plant polysaccharides that the host cannot digest. Some Bacteroidales species are also able to cleave host-derived glycans present in the colon such as mucin, hyaluronate, chondroitin sulfate, and sialylated glycans and are able to use these glycans as a food source. Neuraminidase, an enzyme that cleaves terminal sialic acid from host carbohydrates, is required for *B. fragilis* to produce abscesses in an animal model. It is not known if other enzymes involved in cleaving host glycans contribute to the virulence of the *Bacteroides* when they are released to the peritoneal cavity, but this feature may allow these bacteria to use host-derived glycans as a source of nutrients in extraintestinal sites.

Many enteric Gram-negative bacteria synthesize a **lipopolysaccharide** (**LPS**) that is endotoxic. The LPS of *B. fragilis* contains a lipid A component that has a significantly different structure compared with that of *E. coli*. This structural difference accounts for the **low endotoxicity** of *B. fragilis* LPS compared with that of *E. coli* and many other Gram-negative organisms.

A very important trait of *B. fragilis* that facilitates abscess formation is production of its capsular polysaccharides. *Bacteroides* and *Parabacteroides* species synthesize a large number of capsular polysaccharides, some species synthesizing 11 or more per strains. The synthesis of many of these polysaccharides is subject to **phase variation**, characterized by a reversible on-off phenotype. Phase variation

of these polysaccharides is regulated at the transcriptional level by DNA inversion of promoter regions that drive expression of the polysaccharide biosynthesis genes and by regulatory products encoded by each polysaccharide locus. Whether synthesis of such an extensive number of phase-variable surface polysaccharides contributes to virulence of this organism is not known. What is clear is that the structural motif present on at least one of these polysaccharides, **polysaccharide A** (**PSA**), is essential for *B. fragilis* to induce abscesses in animal models. The repeating unit of PSA is **zwitterionic** in that it contains residues with **both positive and negative charges**. This structural motif induces a host immune response, mediated by activation of CD4+ T lymphocytes, which leads to abscess formation in the peritoneal cavity. In addition, the capsular polysaccharides of *B. fragilis* are involved in the attachment of the organisms to the peritoneal mesothelium, the first cell boundary likely encountered in the peritoneal cavity following release from the colon. Also, the capsular polysaccharides inhibit complement-mediated killing, a feature critical to the ability of these bacteria to disseminate via the blood.

DAMAGE

Following leakage of bacteria, an immediate host response is mounted. Much of the contaminating bacteria are removed by the diaphragmatic lymphatics. Phagocytes are mobilized rapidly to the infected site and, to a point, dispose of large numbers of bacteria and debris. Because of the many phagocytes that migrate to the site of peritoneal contamination, the minimal infecting dose that results in disease in humans is possibly quite high, perhaps several milliliters of intestinal content, judging from experiments with laboratory animals.

If the peritoneal defenses are unable to eradicate spilled intestinal content, an abscess usually develops. Bacterial contamination triggers an increase in vascular permeability, resulting in the influx of plasma and **fibrin deposition**. Fibrin accumulation is enhanced as a result of reduced abdominal fibrinolytic activity during intra-abdominal infection. Bacteria that are adherent to or near the peritoneal mesothelium become trapped in fibrin matrices that develop to delimit the necrotic material and

PERITONITIS IN THE PREANTIBIOTIC ERA

The magician Houdini died of peritonitis. Houdini was known for his astounding feats of escape while enchained and enclosed in containers submerged in water. He possessed amazing physical strength and could control many muscles, including, it is said, some normally not under voluntary control. His fame was the cause of his demise. Houdini received an unexpected blow to his abdomen from a bystander intent on testing his legendary muscular powers. The magician's large intestine ruptured, and he died a few days later. Had Houdini lived today and been in the hands of a competent physician, he would have been treated with antibiotics and surgical repair and would have had a good chance of surviving.

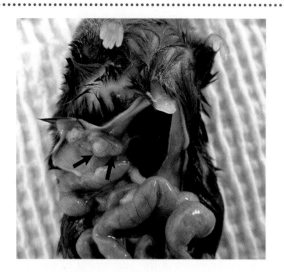

FIGURE 15-2. Intra-abdominal abscesses of the mouse abdominal wall following intra-abdominal challenge with *Bacteroides fragilis*. This photograph, taken 6 days after infection, shows fully formed abscesses that have become extensively vascularized. (Photo by A. Tzianabos.)

residual bacteria. These areas become surrounded by a thick, fibrous collagen-containing capsule (Fig. 15-2). Inside the capsule are live and dead white blood cells, bacteria, and cell debris. In general, these abscesses resemble those caused by staphylococci (see Chapter 11). Inside peritoneal abscesses, the dominant *B. fragilis* is often accompanied not only by facultative anaerobes but also by other strict anaerobes, such as clostridia or anaerobic streptococci (i.e., *Peptostreptococcus*).

Intra-abdominal abscesses exact a high toll on the host because they can extend to nearby sites and cause necrosis of adjacent tissue. In addition, they serve as a focus of bacterial contamination from which organisms can enter the bloodstream. The resulting bacteremia may produce septic shock or cause metastatic infections and abscesses at distant sites.

DIAGNOSIS

Intra-abdominal abscesses should be suspected in patients with prior history of appendicitis, diverticulitis, abdominal surgery patients, or other predisposing conditions who present with abdominal pain. Various imaging procedures, including computed tomography and ultrasonography, are used to confirm and localize the abscesses.

Proper chemotherapy of mixed bacterial infections requires determining the bacterial species involved and their antibiotic sensitivity. Very little has changed in the methodology of characterizing clinical Bacteroidales isolates, and more rapid and efficient genetic-based methods are clearly needed. Currently, anaerobic cultures are performed using an incubator in the form of a glove box, a device in which the atmosphere can be made anaerobic by flushing with a mixture of nitrogen, carbon dioxide, and hydrogen (Fig. 15-3). Speciation is performed by different techniques in different laboratories, but few utilize differences in 16S rRNA gene sequences, which would greatly increases the accuracy of speciation. As recent susceptibility profiling has shown different resistance

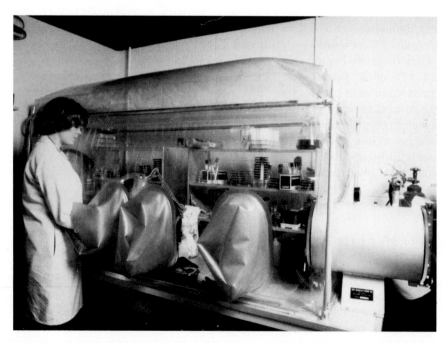

FIGURE 15-3. An anaerobic glove box used for the culture of strictly anaerobic bacteria. This device is used for large-scale work and for experimentation. The port on the right is used to introduce and remove material from the chamber. It has two doors (not visible) and can be independently flushed free of oxygen.

trends in different Bacteroidales species, it is important to accurately speciate these isolates. Antibiotic susceptibility profiling also currently requires that the organisms are cultured. As many of the genes involved in antibiotic resistances are characterized, a more rapid PCR-based analysis of resistance profiles should be possible.

TREATMENT AND PREVENTION

Left untreated, peritonitis is often fatal. Measures can be taken to minimize the risk of intra-abdominal infection and abscess formation if contamination from the colon is suspected. In Ms. A.'s case, the appendix had perforated and bacterial contamination of the peritoneal cavity was confirmed. When contamination is known or even suspected, appropriate antibiotic therapy is necessary. Physicians must be aware of the need for the proper antibiotic regimen, including effective treatment for *Bacteroides*, at the time of the contamination to reduce the likelihood of subsequent abscess formation. The antibiotics should be broad spectrum and designed to prevent bacteremia resulting from facultative anaerobes and abscesses caused by *Bacteroides*. Several antibiotics, including **metronidazole**, **β-lactam–β-lactamase inhibitor combinations**, and the **carbapenems**, have good activity against Bacteroidales. However, the target in these infections is seldom a single bacterial species but a mixed population with different sensitivities. Thus, a combination of antibiotics or an antibiotic effective against both aerobes and anaerobes is indicated. For Ms. A., the cephalosporin first administered was effective against *E. coli* but not against *B. fragilis*. Her second treatment recognized the need for an appropriate choice, and she also received metronidazole, an effective drug against this organism.

Although several antibiotics are still effective treatments for Bacteroidales infections, antibiotic resistance continues to be a significant problem. Members of *Bacteroides* possess sophisticated genetic systems that transfer genes for drug resistance not only among the *Bacteroides* species but also to species of other genera. These antibiotic resistance genes are often encoded on mobile genetic elements such as **conjugative transposons** or conjugative plasmids, enabling their transfer to other organisms. The transfer of these elements is likely facilitated in their natural colonic environment because the organisms are present in high numbers. The gene conferring resistance to clindamycin is harbored on conjugative elements of *Bacteroides*. Clindamycin, once the drug of choice against Bacteroidales, is now reported to be ineffective in as many as 42% of clinical isolates.

The National Survey for the Susceptibility of *Bacteroides fragilis* Group was initiated in 1981 to monitor the emergence of antibiotic resistance among intestinally derived clinical Bacteroidales species. The latest data (reference 1 of suggested reading) demonstrate that the carbapenems and the β-lactam–β-lactamase inhibitor combination piperacillin/tazobactam were the most active agents against these bacteria. The study also revealed that resistance profiles were often species dependent with some Bacteroidales species being largely resistant to one treatment to which isolates of other species were mostly susceptible. Antibiotic resistance was found to be greater in non–*B. fragilis* Bacteroidales species, compared to *B. fragilis*. In addition, the first strains with resistance to metronidazole were detected; however, the resistance rate is very low and metronidazole is still a drug of choice for these infections.

If intra-abdominal abscesses do form because either antibiotic treatment was not effective or leakage from the bowel was not previously identified, dual therapy—namely, drainage of the abscess and administration of antibiotics—is usually required. In addition, the anatomical defect that allowed spillage from the intestine must be repaired. Thus, a combined medical and surgical approach is often necessary in cases of intra-abdominal infection. Percutaneous drainage of intra-abdominal abscesses, guided by computed tomography, is a viable alternative to surgical drainage when the abscess is localized with no evidence of generalized peritonitis.

OTHER BACTEROIDES AND BACTEROIDALES-ASSOCIATED DISEASES

In addition to intra-abdominal abscesses, *Bacteroides* and *Parabacteroides* are also isolated from other clinical sites, usually as part of a polymicrobial infection. These include the blood of patients with intra-abdominal infection, secondary abscesses resulting from the hematogenous spread from a primary intra-abdominal abscess, infections of the diabetic foot, soft tissue infections, and suppurative infections of the genital tract.

An increasing number of *B. fragilis* strains have been demonstrated to contain a gene encoding an enterotoxin termed *Bacteroides fragilis* toxin (BFT) a metalloprotease that disrupts the tight junctions of epithelial cells by cleaving E-cadherin. Although *B. fragilis* strains that harbor *bft* are part of the gut microbiota of apparently healthy individuals, these strains are associated with acute diarrheal disease of livestock and humans, and the toxin may mediate colitis. In addition, BFT has been shown to induce cellular proliferation that may contribute to oncogenic transformation and colon cancer.

Two other frequently isolated genera of anaerobic Gram-negative rods were originally classified as part to the *Bacteroides* genus but belong to other Bacteroidales genera. Unlike the *Bacteroides*, *Porphyromonas* and *Prevotella* form characteristically pigmented colonies on blood agar. *Prevotella melaninogenica*, named for its production of a black pigment, is commonly found in the human gingival flora and is often associated with periodontal diseases. Although this organism is also found in other sites, it is most commonly associated with infections of oral origin, including aspiration pneumonia (see Chapter 62) and rather serious infections following human bites. The Bacteroidales species *Tannerella forsythia*, *Porphyromonas gingivalis*, and *Prevotella intermedia* are also important oral pathogens involved in periodontal disease. In contrast, the Bacteroidales species *Prevotella bivius* and *Prevotella disiens* are common vaginal isolates associated with bacterial vaginosis, pelvic infections, and peritonitis.

CONCLUSION

The *Bacteroides* and *Parabacteroides* species are abundant members of the colonic microbiota of humans and other mammals and can become opportunistic pathogens if they gain access to the peritoneal cavity or other normally sterile body sites. The predominant pathogen of the genera, *B. fragilis*, synthesizes a capsular polysaccharide containing both positive and negative charges. This zwitterionic motif stimulates an immune response in the host that leads to intra-abdominal abscess formation. Although the diseases caused by Bacteroidales can be cured, the organisms still present challenges to therapy and, above all, to prevention. Although mechanisms are in place to reduce intra-abdominal abscess formation, none presently available can totally prevent these infections.

Suggested Readings

Snydman DR, Jacobus NV, McDermott LA, et al. Lessons learned from the anaerobe survey: historical perspective and review of the most recent data (2005–2007). *Clin Infect Dis.* 2010;50(suppl 1):S26–S33.

Tzianabos AO, Kasper DL. Role of T cells in abscess formation. *Curr Opin Microbiol.* 2002;5:92.

Wexler HM. *Bacteroides*: the good, the bad, and the nitty-gritty. *Clin Microbiol Rev.* 2007;20(4):593–621.

Zaleznik DF, Kasper DL. Intraabdominal infections and abscesses. In: Braunwald E, Fauci AS, Isselbacher KJ, et al., eds. *Harrison's Online*. New York: McGraw-Hill; 2004.

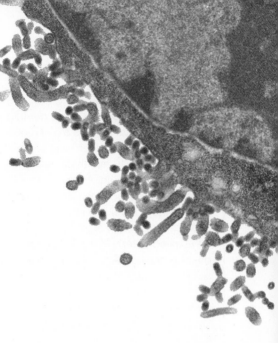

Chapter **16**

Enteric Bacteria: Secretory Diarrhea

Victor J. DiRita

KEY CONCEPTS

Pathogens: Enteric bacteria that cause secretory (watery) diarrhea include members of Enterobacteriaceae and Vibrionaceae.

Encounter and Entry: Pathogens are usually transmitted to humans in contaminated food and water.

Spread: In the gastrointestinal tract, organisms face formidable defenses. Pathogen access to the small and large intestine requires passage through the highly acidic stomach. The more heavily contaminated the food and water, the more likely an infectious dose will survive, infect the intestines, and produce disease.

Multiplication: In the small intestine, organisms adhere to the epithelial cells of the tract via pili (fimbriae) or surface adhesins.

Damage: Some pathogens (*Vibrio cholerae* and enterotoxigenic *Escherichia coli*) elaborate toxins that reduce sodium absorption and increase chloride secretion of the intestinal cells, which leads to watery diarrhea.

Diagnosis: The microbial cause of most sporadic cases of most mild diarrheal infections is typically not determined. In outbreaks or in life-threatening infections, special microbiological or genetic techniques can be used to identify the pathogen in many cases.

Treatment: Secretory diarrheas are effectively treated with oral rehydration therapy.

Prevention: The development of effective vaccines for enteric pathogens, including cholera, has been difficult. No fully satisfactory vaccines are available.

DIARRHEA, usually no more than a bothersome but brief illness in industrialized nations, is a leading cause of infant and childhood mortality in developing countries and remains a major target for control by the World Health Organization (WHO). Diarrheal disease is noted by WHO as being the second leading cause of death (after pneumonia) for children under the age of 5, killing millions of children annually and contributing to malnutrition and growth retardation in those who survive the illnesses.

Secretory or **watery diarrhea** is caused by the loss of electrolytes and fluids from the small intestine. An extreme example is cholera, which can cause fatal dehydration in hours, usually in small children. Traveler's diarrhea is a generally milder form of watery diarrhea. It most commonly affects adults. Infections of the intestinal tract can lead to local tissue damage or inflammation and cause bloody diarrhea or **dysentery** (see Chapter 17).

Bacteria, viruses, and protozoa that cause diarrheal disease are grouped together as **enteric pathogens**. Several traits endow these agents with the ability to cause secretory diarrhea, and these virulence factors vary in their mode of action. The array of factors particular to each organism determines the characteristics of the clinical illness.

CASE • Mr. D., a 33-year-old fully immunized, rather nervous accountant who is blood group O positive and taking H2 blockers for ulcer disease; his 29-year-old healthy wife; and their 10-month-old baby boy returned from a 2-week trip to South America. The next morning Mr. D. passed a semisolid stool, which was quickly followed by a large watery bowel movement. Within an hour, he passed another large watery stool, now opaque gray–white in color. He vomited several times and became slightly sweaty. After passing another large watery stool, Mr. D. called his physician, who advised him to go to the emergency department. When he arrived there, Mr. D. was afebrile but had a rapid heart rate with a feeble pulse and low blood pressure. He complained of muscle cramps and dizziness. All these signs and symptoms were consistent with a significant loss of extracellular fluids. Laboratory studies showed a normal leukocyte count, a slightly elevated level of serum sodium, a normal serum potassium level, and an elevated blood urea nitrogen level, also consistent with dehydration.

A diagnosis of cholera was suspected. Mr. D. was immediately given 2 L of fluid intravenously and then started on oral rehydration solution. His stool volumes progressively diminished over 48 hours, and he was discharged. Because of the suspected diagnosis, special media were used, and the stool culture grew *Vibrio cholerae*, serogroup O1, biotype E1 Tor. Mrs. D., a native Peruvian, had two loose bowel movements on the second day of her husband's illness. Her stool culture grew only *Escherichia coli*.

Two weeks later, Baby D. stopped feeding and developed watery diarrhea. His rectal temperature was 38°C. His parents brought the infant to the pediatrician. The baby had signs and symptoms of dehydration, with fluid loss estimated at approximately 7% of body weight. He was admitted to the hospital. Neither leukocytes nor red blood cells were seen in the stool. Baby D. was rehydrated with an oral rehydration solution. His fever abated and appetite returned, although the diarrhea persisted. The preliminary laboratory report stated that the stool cultures contained "normal fecal flora"; 2 days later, the laboratory identified enteropathogenic *E. coli* (EPEC) by polymerase chain reaction (PCR) test for the characteristic adherence factor. Baby D. improved and was discharged after 4 days, having lost 1 pound in weight. One month later, he returned to his normal growth curve.

This case raises several questions:

1. Why did the physician caring for Mr. D. think of cholera?

2. Are all enteric bacteria capable of causing disease, or are some more frequently pathogenic than others? Which enteric pathogens cause diarrhea, and where do they come from?

3. What are the clinical manifestations caused by enteric pathogens? Why do the organisms cause different intensity of symptoms in individuals?

4. What factors are involved in colonization? What factors are involved in causing symptoms?

5. What is the proper therapy for watery diarrhea?

6. Can these diseases be prevented?

See Appendix for answers

Mr. D. and his son developed two different secretory diarrheal diseases. Mr. D. had acquired cholera during travel; Baby D. was infected with an EPEC, probably acquired after returning home. Among the most common bacterial pathogens in the United States are strains of *E. coli* present in the intestine of humans or animals. Other important causes of watery diarrhea include *Shigella sonnei* and *Salmonella* (see Chapter 17). In addition, viruses (most commonly, rotavirus) and protozoa (*Giardia, Cryptosporidium,* and *Cyclospora*) can cause watery diarrhea.

THE PATHOGENS: DIARRHEAL DISEASES

Most diarrhea episodes can be traced to a specific pathogen; however, clinical laboratories do not routinely use all available diagnostic methods. Strains of the predominant isolate under aerobic culture conditions, *E. coli*, cannot usually be classified as either pathogenic or nonpathogenic by the usual laboratory studies. As many as 40% of patients under 2 years of age have rotavirus (see Chapter 37), and many preschool children in day care are infected with *S. sonnei* or protozoa (see Chapter 53).

Although infants in the United States may have 1 or 2 readily treated diarrhea episodes per year, infants and children in developing countries may have as many as 10 or more. Many of these infants and children advance to life-threatening dehydration. Limited access to medical care in some countries means that many potentially treatable cases end in death.

Most of the bacteria that cause diarrheal disease belong to a large family of Gram-negative rods, the **Enterobacteriaceae**; some belong to the **Vibrionaceae** family (Tables 16-1 and 16-2). The Enterobacteriaceae include members of the normal microbiota of the intestine as well as frank pathogens. Members of both families may cause a wide spectrum of disease including diarrhea, urinary and respiratory tract infection, sepsis, and meningitis. Members of the Enterobacteriaceae family are differentiated on the basis of serological and metabolic properties. The family Vibrionaceae also includes many nonpathogenic

TABLE 16-1 Main Genera of Pathogenic Enterobacteriaceae and Vibrionaceae

Genus	Main Reservoirs	Principal Diseases
Enterobacteriaceae		
Escherichia	Ileum and colon of vertebrates	Diarrhea, dysentery, urinary tract infections, septicemia, neonatal meningitis, others
Shigella	Human colon	Diarrhea, dysentery
Salmonella	Gastrointestinal system of animals and humans	Diarrhea, bloody diarrhea, typhoid (enteric) fever, aortitis, osteomyelitis, other focal infections
Proteus	Colon of vertebrates, water, soil	Urinary tract infections, septicemia, pneumonia
Klebsiella, Enterobacter, Serratia, Citrobacter	Colon of vertebrates, water, sewage	Pneumonia, septicemia; special problems in debilitated or immunocompromised patients
Yersinia	Rodents, pigs, water	Plague, bloody diarrhea, diarrhea, pseudoappendicitis, mesenteric adenitis syndrome
Vibrionaceae		
Vibrio (alginolyticus, vulnificus)	Marine water ecosystems	Watery diarrhea (certain species associated with phytoplankton); can cause skin infections or septicemia
Campylobacter	Gastrointestinal system of animals	Diarrhea, bloody diarrhea, septicemia (certain species only)

+, principal manifestation; ±, occasional manifestation.

TABLE 16-2 Gram-Negative Rods that Cause Diarrhea, Bloody Diarrhea, and Dysentery

Rod	Diarrhea	Bloody Diarrhea	Inflammatory Diarrhea or Dysentery	
			Ileitis	*Colitis*
Enterobacteriaceae				
ETEC	+			
EPEC	+		±	
EAggEC	+			
EIEC		+		+
EHEC		+		+
Shigella		+	±	+
Nontyphoidal *Salmonella*	+	±	+	±
Salmonella typhi			±	
Yersinia enterocolitica	+	+	+	
Others	+			
Vibrionaceae				
Vibrio cholerae	+			
Vibrio parahaemolyticus	+	+	±	±
Campylobacter jejuni	+	+	±	+

EAggEC, enteroaggregative *E. coli*; EHEC, enterohemorrhagic *E. coli*; EIEC, enteroinvasive *E. coli*; EPEC, enteropathogenic *E. coli*; ETEC, enterotoxigenic *E. coli*.

species as well as organisms that cause epidemic cholera, sporadic diarrhea, and local skin or bacteremic infections.

Cholera is the paradigm of secretory diarrhea and is caused by *Vibrio cholerae*, a member of the Vibrionaceae. One particular serological type, *V. cholerae* O1, has been responsible for yearly epidemics in the Indian subcontinent for centuries and, for at least the last two centuries, periodic global pandemics. The O1 in its name indicates that it contains a **lipopolysaccharide (LPS)** antigen that belongs to the O1 serogroup. The O1 group contains two biotypes, the **classical** and **El Tor** types. Until 1961, the El Tor type was considered an avirulent commensal when it was found to cause the seventh recorded pandemic in the early 20th century. Beginning in Indonesia, El Tor cholera rapidly spread in Asia, reaching Europe and Africa in the early 1970s and Latin America in 1991. Although the disease rapidly disappeared from Europe, it has become endemic in Africa and Latin America (Fig. 16-1). In late 2010 and early 2011, an epidemic swept through Haiti, following a massive earthquake there in early 2010. DNA sequence analysis of the strain responsible suggested it was introduced into Haiti accidentally, apparently originating in a cholera-endemic country from which aid workers had traveled as part of a large international earthquake relief effort.

A small endemic focus of cholera, known since 1973, exists along the Gulf Coast of the United States, and a few cases of cholera occur yearly as a result of eating shellfish harboring the organism. In the United States, cholera is transmitted primarily by eating contaminated raw or partially cooked shellfish harvested from that area of the Gulf of Mexico. Cholera rarely occurs in other areas of the United States because of the high level of environmental sanitation and protected drinking water supplies.

In contrast to *V. cholerae*, which is never a member of the normal human microbiota, *E. coli* is the most abundant **facultative anaerobe** in normal human feces. However, it is outnumbered by at least 1,000 to 1 by **strict anaerobes** like the *Bacteroides* (see Chapter 15). Most fecal *E. coli* are avirulent and do not cause disease; some human strains have been cultivated in the laboratory for so long that they have lost the ability to colonize humans. These strains include *E. coli* K12, the strain that occupies center stage in molecular biology and gene cloning and is perhaps the best understood cellular form of life.

E. coli is an umbrella designation for a number of rather varied pathogenic and nonpathogenic strains. There are at least five distinguishable groups of *E. coli* now known to cause enteric disease (Table 16-3). With one exception (the non–sorbitol-fermenting *E. coli* serotype O157:H7), routine stool cultures cannot distinguish pathogenic from nonpathogenic *E. coli*. The problem in distinguishing "bad" *E. coli* from "good" *E. coli* is that all strains share the same basic taxonomic and biochemical features, although they may have different virulence factors. How then are these strains distinguished? The classic way

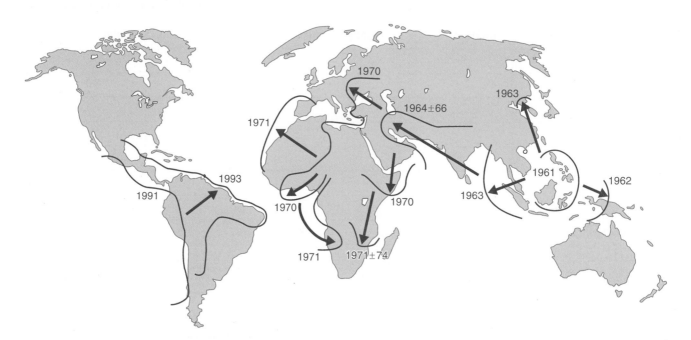

FIGURE 16-1. The spread of the seventh cholera pandemic from Southeast Asia. This pandemic was caused by the El Tor biotype of *Vibrio cholerae*, which has a higher asymptomatic carriage rate than the classical biotype. In the 1990s, a new type emerged from El Tor by acquiring a novel LPS antigen, O139, instead of O1. Prior infection with El Tor provides no immunity to *V. cholerae* O139 (Bengal). Infections with this new strain appeared in Bangladesh in the 1990s and have spread to India and other countries; this may represent the beginning of the eighth pandemic of cholera.

TABLE 16-3 Classification of Pathogenic *Escherichia coli* and Representative Serotypes

Group	Symptoms	Epidemiology
Enterotoxigenic (ETEC)	Watery diarrhea (traveler's diarrhea)	Worldwide, adults and children
Enteropathogenic (EPEC)	Watery diarrhea	Infants <1 y of age
Enteroaggregative (EAggEC)	Watery diarrhea, persistent diarrhea	Infants <6 mo of age, AIDS patients
Enteroinvasive (EIEC)	Bloody diarrhea	Uncommon, often foodborne
Enterohemorrhagic (EHEC)	Bloody diarrhea, hemorrhagic colitis, hemolytic–uremic syndrome, thrombotic thrombocytopenic purpura	Western nations

is to determine the antigenic reactivity of the **O antigen** of the outer membrane LPS (see Chapter 3). There are 173 different *E. coli* O antigens. These O antigens can associate with the 60 different H antigens, resulting in a vast number of combinations. In addition, some strains have a capsular polysaccharide antigen called K. Determining the combination of O and H antigens helps identify certain virulent clones (see Table 16-3). Similar tests are also used to distinguish the cholera vibrios and the many distinct *Salmonella* serotypes.

ENCOUNTER

Some enteric pathogens are well adapted to the external environment and only incidentally cause disease. *V. cholerae* is a normal inhabitant of coastal estuarine waters, where it lives in close association with phytoplankton. Humans are incidentally infected when they enter this ecosystem or when the organisms contaminate drinking water or food. Seasonal variation in the *Vibrio* population can also occur, most likely as a result of the action of vibriophages that live in the same water as the bacteria. High temperatures, algal blooms, or changes in the local phage population can lead to *Vibrio* blooms, thereby increasing the likelihood of transmission to humans. If the organisms reach the drinking water and food supplies, epidemic spread can occur. The diarrhea that is so characteristic of this disease can be viewed as an evolutionary mechanism facilitating dispersal of the organisms and their transfer to new hosts.

Certain enteric pathogens (e.g., *Salmonella* and *Campylobacter*) are seldom found in the environment but are usually associated with humans or animals. Although these organisms display considerable host specificity, species barriers are often crossed. The diseases caused in humans by animal-specific strains are called **zoonoses** (see Chapter 73).

The route for transmission of enteric pathogens is from feces to mouth; however, many intermediary vehicles intervene, characterized as the "seven Fs": feces, food, fluids, fingers, flies, fomites (inanimate objects), and fornication. The number of organisms required to cause

disease (**inoculum size**) is probably better known for enteric bacteria than for most other organisms. Experimental infections have been induced in human volunteers who agree to drink buffered solutions containing a known number of living bacteria. A few hundred *Shigella dysenteriae* type 1 are sufficient to cause disease in many volunteers. In contrast, 1,000 to 10,000 *Shigella flexneri* and more than 100 million enterotoxigenic *E. coli* are required to cause the same attack rate. A direct consequence of a small infective dose is that, under the same conditions, *Shigella* are generally transmitted from person to person, because small inocula are readily passed by fingers or objects after contact with stool or soiled diapers. Directly transferring an infectious dose of enterotoxigenic *E. coli* is more difficult because transmission requires a visible lump of feces. It is more likely that large numbers of *E. coli* enter humans when they ingest contaminated food or water in which the organisms have already multiplied.

Despite the high standards of modern hygiene, we are in constant contact with enteric bacteria. Feces are an approximate 20% suspension of bacteria in water. Each day we are in contact with and ingest fecal microorganisms to a greater or lesser extent, depending on our age (which determines behavior) and the state of environmental sanitation. Because potential pathogens are so common, why do we not get diarrhea every day? The answer to this question requires an understanding of the mechanisms of pathogenesis of these diseases and host defenses, both specific and nonspecific.

ENTRY

Having arrived at the mouth, microorganisms face a perilous journey along the alimentary canal to their final destination. The gastrointestinal tract is a tube lined with differentiated epithelial cells that keep bacteria "outside" the body and deliver them to the environment through the anus. The journey is perilous because the microorganisms face host defenses and hostile conditions. The pH of the stomach is highly acidic, a condition lethal to most microorganisms. In the duodenum near the **ampulla of Vater**, surviving organisms are bathed in bicarbonate-buffered pancreatic juice with a pH that can be as high as 9. In the small intestine, microorganisms are smothered in mucus; rolled up in sticky polysaccharide balls; and kneaded, squeezed, and swept distally toward the anus by **peristaltic motions** of the bowel, unless they find a way to hold on. Throughout the journey, they encounter soluble proteins such as lysozyme, proteases, lipases, and secretory IgA, as well as bile salts and phagocytic and lymphoid cells. If they pause in the large intestine, they meet the populous normal microbiota that resists implantation by new species, in part by previous occupancy of adhesion sites on the gut wall and in part by producing inhibitory substances (e.g., bacteriocins).

The efficiency of these host defenses is the reason why the infectious dose of most noninvasive enteric pathogens is high and disease is not common. Some conditions, however, may be advantageous to the pathogen. For example, pathogens mixed with food are protected from stomach acid, and the infectious dose is therefore diminished. In some patients, the ability to secrete gastric acid is seriously impaired by intrinsic disease (pernicious anemia), infections (e.g., *Helicobacter pylori* or gastritis; see Chapter 22), prior surgery (gastric resection, diversions, or transections of the vagus nerve), or antiulcer drugs that inhibit or buffer gastric acid. These patients are at greater risk for infection with acid-sensitive bacteria like *V. cholerae* or *Salmonella*.

Mr. D. was at risk of developing clinical cholera on exposure to the organism for two reasons: he was an ulcer patient receiving H_2 blockers to reduce gastric acid secretion, and he was blood group O positive. For unknown reasons, O-positive persons are predisposed to develop more severe cholera, presumably because certain oligosaccharides on cells or in secretions enhance binding of the organism or cholera toxin production, or cause other altered responses of the mucosa.

SPREAD AND MULTIPLICATION

Cholera vibrios have several features that may help them reach the epithelial surface of the small intestine. Their flagella make them actively mobile, and they produce a protease that hydrolyses mucus. They colonize the intestine by adhering to the epithelial surface. **Adherence** is not a simple feat because the surfaces of both microbe and host are negatively charged (for optimal adherence, the surfaces should not be mutually repulsive). Cholera vibrios and other enteric pathogens have specific **pili** (**singular: pilus**) or **fimbriae** (see Chapter 4) that serve in part to increase the distance between the host cell surface and the bacterium and diminish the electrostatic repulsion. The mechanisms by which these adherence structure are assembled on the surface of the bacteria varies from one microbe to another, but the process is always complex and involves many proteins with specific roles in synthesis, transport, or assembly of the subunits that make up the structure.

Virtually all Gram-negative bacteria possess type 1 or **common pili**, which are protein rods that help the

bacteria stick to the mucosal surfaces of the gastrointestinal tract. Common pili have a special affinity for mannose-containing proteins and lipids in mucosal membranes. Despite their frequency, common pili are rarely involved in adherence of pathogenic microorganisms, which are endowed with more specialized adhesins. For example, cholera bacilli stick to one another using a specific pilus called the **toxin-coregulated pilus (TCP)**, so named because its synthesis is regulated by the same system that controls the production of cholera toxin (Fig. 16-2). This ability to stick to one another through the TCP is an important component of the

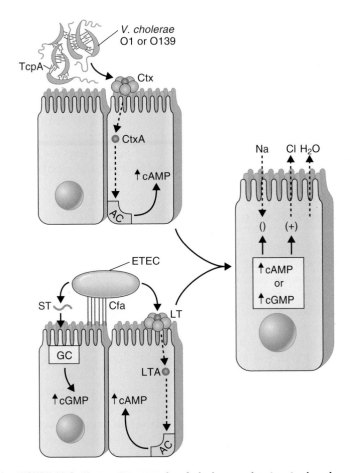

FIGURE 16-2. The pathogenesis of cholera and enterotoxigenic *Escherichia coli* (ETEC) infections. The organisms colonize the mucosal surface via microbial adhesins—for example, colonization factor antigen (Cfa) of enterotoxigenic *E. coli*. The factor that binds *V. cholerae* to cells is not clearly defined, but a toxin-coregulated pilus (TCP) causes the organisms to adhere to one another and form microcolonies on the epithelial surface. Once colonization has occurred, cholera toxin (Ctx) or labile toxin (LT) binds to a receptor, is taken up in vesicles, and an active subunit of each (CtxA or LTA) is transported to the basolateral membrane to the adenylate cyclase (AC) complex. The toxins transfer ADP ribose to the guanosine 5′-triphosphate (GTP)–binding protein of AC, elevating cAMP. ETEC also produces a heat-stable (ST) toxin that binds to the membrane guanylate cyclase (GC) and increases cyclic guanosine 5′-monophosphate (cGMP) levels. Both cAMP and cGMP reduce sodium absorption in villus cells and increase chlorine secretion in crypt cells, leading to watery diarrhea.

mechanism used by *V. cholerae* to colonize the small intestine.

After colonizing the intestinal brush border through the action of their pili, neither the cholera vibrios of Mr. D. or the *E. coli* of the baby were able to invade the mucosa. These pathogens can readily multiply because the resident microbiota at the level of the jejunum and upper ileum is scanty and thus pose no significant competition.

DAMAGE

V. cholerae and Enterotoxigenic *E. coli*

Mr. D.'s diarrhea was caused by colonization of the small bowel by organisms that survived their passage across the stomach. If the small bowel mucosa had been examined, no visible damage would have been noted. Instead, the pathology occurs at the biochemical level, that is, the increase in **adenylate cyclase** activity is caused by cholera toxin. In the small intestine, cholera bacilli make **cholera toxin**, the TCP, and several accessory virulence genes. Proving that nature is both parsimonious and creative, the genes for cholera toxin are encoded on the genome of a bacteriophage that is integrated into the chromosome and uses TCP as its receptor on the surface of the organism.

How do cholera bacilli "know" that they are in the small intestine? A number of their virulence genes, including the one for cholera toxin and TCP, are regulated by the activity of a complex but logical regulatory cascade that responds to cues within the human host. By switching on the virulence genes only when they are in a host, these pathogens do not waste energy making products not required in their natural aquatic environment. The switching occurs rapidly within the intestine and results in an ordered expression of the adherence organelle TCP followed by expression of cholera toxin. **Sensory mechanisms** of this sort that coordinate regulation of virulence are a common theme in bacterial pathogens (see Chapter 19 paradigm).

Once it is made, cholera toxin binds to a cell surface receptor (the **GM1 ganglioside**) and is internalized within a vesicle. The active subunit A of the toxin is routed to the basolateral membrane of the intestinal epithelial cell where the specific target of the cholera toxin, the **G_s regulatory protein** of the **adenylate cyclase complex**, is located. Cholera toxin can modify G_s by **adenosine diphosphate (ADP)-ribosylation** (the transfer of the ADP-ribosyl moiety of nicotinamide adenine dinucleotide to substrate proteins; see Chapter 9). The modification of G_s protein results in permanent activation of adenylate cyclase and an increase in intracellular **cyclic adenosine monophosphate (CAMP)**. Increased concentrations of cAMP inhibit sodium absorption by small bowel villous cells and increase chloride secretion by crypt cells. Because the amount of sodium chloride in the gut lumen increases, passive secretion of water occurs by osmotic force and generates watery, diarrheal stool. In a case of cholera like Mr. D.'s, the volume of water lost can be so prodigious that the patient is rapidly dehydrated, may go into shock, and, if not quickly treated, may die.

In endemic regions of Asia, Africa, and Latin America, cholera occurs primarily in children less than 10 years old, because older adolescents and adults are usually protected by adaptive immunity. During epidemics in previously cholera-free areas, all age groups are susceptible. This age-specific pattern is typical of endemic infections, not epidemic infections. Mortality is caused by electrolyte and water losses; therefore, with proper fluid replacement, no patient should die of cholera. Without therapy, as many as 50% of patients may die.

Related to cholera are infections caused by **enterotoxigenic *E. coli* (ETEC)**. These strains produce one or both **enterotoxins**, called **LT** and **ST**, for heat-Labile Toxin and heat-Stable Toxin, respectively. These toxins act by changing the net fluid transport in the gut from absorption to secretion. LT is structurally identical to cholera toxin and activates the adenylate cyclase–cAMP system in the same manner (Chapter 9).

Cholera is usually more serious than disease caused by ETEC, as the former leads to the secretion of much greater amounts of liquid stools. Unlike ETEC, *V. cholerae* has a very efficient mechanism for secreting toxin into its milieu, which may account for the different severities of two diseases caused by very similar toxins. In neither case is the intestinal mucosa visibly damaged; the watery stool does not contain white or red blood cells, and no inflammatory process occurs in the gut wall.

ST interacts with and activates the **guanylate cyclase (GC)** of intestinal cells. This interaction leads to an increase in the cyclic **guanosine monophosphate (GMP)** and altered sodium and chloride transport, much like LT and cholera toxin. Toxins related to cholera or ST toxins in activity or structure have also been found in other diarrheal pathogens such as *Salmonella* and *Yersinia*.

Enteropathogenic *E. coli*

Baby D. was infected with an EPEC, one of a small group of specific serotypes originally recognized because they cause outbreaks of diarrhea in the newborn nursery (see Table 16-3). This kind of diarrhea is caused by complex mechanisms that result in disruption of the microvillus surface and alteration of host cellular signaling processes by the action of a specialized mechanism, called a type III secretion system, that is elaborated by EPEC (for more on type III secretion, see Chapter 17 paradigm). Multiple steps in this pathogenesis have been uncovered. In the earliest stage, organisms adhere to target epithelial cells in a relatively distant ("nonintimate") manner. Binding occurs by means of a so-called **bundle-forming pilus** (Fig. 16-3), which is structurally similar to the TCP of *V. cholerae*. Subsequently, the type III secretion system is assembled and delivers some of its effector molecules into the host cells. One of these molecules, **Tir**, plays a critical role in the next step of the pathogenesis, which is characterized by intimate attachment and damage of the host enterocytes.

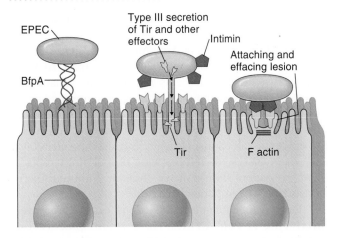

FIGURE 16-3. The pathogenesis of enteropathogenic *Escherichia coli* (EPEC). First, the organism attaches to the small bowel epithelial cell via a bundle-forming pilus (BfpA). Subsequently, a type III secretion system injects a membrane receptor protein, Tir, and other effectors to the host cell. In a third stage, intimin on the bacterial surface mediates intimate adherence to the cell by binding to the newly deployed Tir receptors. Polymerization of actin to filamentous actin (F actin) and other host cytoskeletal proteins is induced, and rearrangements of the cytoskeletal structure occur. Together these processes result in the characteristic EPEC pedestal with the intimately adherent organism (the attaching and effacing lesion).

Serving as the receptor for the bacteria, Tir enables the close attachment and subsequent enterocyte effacement. In essence, EPEC sends over its own receptor, which assembles in the host cell membrane. The microbes also produce a protein called **intimin** on their surfaces, and interaction between intimin and Tir serves to establish the intimate adherence of the microbes. Once this has occurred, Tir-mediated reorganization of the host actin cytoskeleton follows, and the surface of the enterocyte rearranges to form an actin-based "**pedestal**" underneath the EPEC. These pedestals and the disruption they cause to the host enterocyte surface represent the characteristic **attaching and effacing** EPEC lesion. How does this lesion cause diarrhea? The mechanism of this is an active area of investigation, but it likely includes malabsorption from the villus rearrangement and disruption of epithelial tight junctions that results in intestinal permeability. The production of a classic enterotoxin like LT or cholera toxin does not appear to be involved.

Other Infections Caused by Vibrios and *E. coli*

In late 1992 an unprecedented event occurred. Epidemic cholera caused by a non-O1 *V. cholerae* strain was detected in South India, rapidly spreading to Bangladesh and neighboring countries in Asia and displacing the resident O1 strain. Individuals immune to *V. cholerae* O1 were not immune to the new strain, *V. cholerae* O139. Thus, a new epidemic began that involved all ages in the endemic countries of Asia. This event is an example of the continuing emergence of new disease pathogens with extended virulence.

The appearance of the new strain was traced to exchange of the O-antigen synthesizing genes from another *V. cholerae* serogroup into an O1 El Tor strain. The precise source of the new DNA is not clear, but the outcome of the exchange was expression of a previously unknown LPS somatic antigen, O139. In addition, the organism acquired at least one new gene involved in making a capsule, an unusual feature in *V. cholerae* O1. The new organism traveled to Europe and the United States, although early concerns about a new pandemic, which would have been the eighth recorded cholera pandemic, were not borne out as *V. cholerae* O1 displaced O139 as the dominant cholera organism in cholera-endemic areas.

Other marine vibrios armed with virulence attributes different than those of *V. cholerae* can cause debilitating infections. One of these is *V. parahaemolyticus*, which causes bloody diarrhea associated with ingestion of sushi or raw shellfish, especially in Japan. Others, such as *V. vulnificus* and *V. alginolyticus*, may be acquired through an injury or a break in the skin and can cause severe subcutaneous and invasive illnesses.

EPEC and ETEC strains of *E. coli* represent only the earliest described diarrhea-causing *E. coli* species (see Table 16-3). The repertoire is already large and consists of a veritable alphabet soup of pathogenic groups—EPEC, ETEC, EIEC (enteroinvasive), EHEC (enterohemorrhagic), and EAggEC (enteroaggregative)—and more may be waiting in the wings. Each group is associated with identifiable genetic traits and characteristic epidemiology and causes distinctive conditions. EIEC and EHEC are discussed in Chapter 17. EAggEC autoagglutinate (aggregate) in tissue culture and are associated with diarrhea in children under 6 months old, often persisting for weeks with marked nutritional consequences. EAggEC may also be the agent of persistent diarrhea in some adults with HIV infection.

Other strains of *E. coli* involved in invasive disease in infants and young children and which cause bacteremia and systemic diseases such as meningitis or urinary tract infections in children and adults are discussed in Chapters 62 and 64, respectively. In every case, specific virulence factors are critical in determining the nature of the resulting disease. Many of these factors are known and are being investigated and, undoubtedly, still others remain to be discovered.

DIAGNOSIS

Mr. D. was diagnosed with cholera because his physician knew about the ongoing epidemic in the country Mr. D. visited and alerted the laboratory to use special media not routinely employed. On the usual media for bacterial diarrhea, *V. cholerae* is similar to commensals in its sugar fermentation patterns and is therefore not recognized for further diagnostic studies. On special media, however, the distinctive *V. cholerae* colonies are easily identified. Further analysis of the isolate from Mr. D. at the Centers for Disease Control and Prevention in Atlanta, Georgia, revealed it to be genetically identical to the Latin American epidemic and not to the Gulf Coast endemic strain. This information indicated that Mr. D.'s was an imported case and constituted no threat to the local population. The case was not attributed to contaminated seafood that could cause a local outbreak, nor was excretion of viable organisms a problem because of the effective water sanitation in Mr. D.'s hometown.

The stool from Baby D. was grown on cholera-selective media (because of the father's diagnosis) as well as on other media designed for both selection and differentiation of possible pathogens. By incubating the culture in air, the numerically dominant strict anaerobes in normal feces were eliminated. The media used permit the growth of enteric bacteria and not others by inclusion of inhibitors, such as dyes (e.g., eosin and methylene blue, as in the so-called EMB agar) or bile salts (as in MacConkey lactose agar), which selectively inhibit growth of Gram-positives. Because these media are not especially rich, they also exclude fastidious Gram-negatives (such as *Haemophilus influenzae*).

The diagnosis of Baby D. was not as simple as that of Mr. D. All the pathogenic groups of *E. coli* described look alike on agar plates and under the microscope, as do most other enteric Gram-negative rods. They must be further classified on the basis of their biochemical and nutritional properties, such as which sugars they ferment and other biochemical reactions. Some of the classical intestinal pathogens, notably *Salmonella* and *Shigella*, do not ferment lactose. Inclusion of lactose in the medium, together with a colored pH indicator, allows rapid selection of possible non–lactose-fermenting pathogens; the lactose-fermenting colonies (lactose-positives) turn a distinctive color because they produce acid. The lactose-negatives are picked for further determinative work. Other pathogens cannot be differentiated by this method and must be sought by different techniques. Probes and PCR primers against the components of the adherence system are the gold standard for diagnosis. However, these are virtually never used in clinical practice because the tests are not available in most laboratories and because the diagnosis rarely affects management. In the case of the remaining member of the D. family, Mrs. D., it is likely that she had an ETEC infection, but no lab studies were carried out.

TREATMENT

The therapeutic needs of Mr. D. and his son were to replace electrolyte and fluid losses and correct metabolic imbalances. Fortunately, secretory diarrheas are usually self-limiting and terminate without specific antibiotics, as long as the patient is well hydrated and prevented from going into shock. Mr. D. was so severely dehydrated that he required intravenous fluids. Baby D. did well with only an **oral electrolyte–glucose solution** designed to enhance a physiological sodium and glucose cotransport system in the small bowel epithelial cell. Mrs. D. had such a mild and self-limited disease that no specific therapy was needed.

Oral rehydration is a simple form of therapy that, if universally applied, could save the lives of millions of children every year throughout the developing world. Effective solutions can be made in the community by mixing salt, table sugar, and water. Unfortunately, it is not easy to ensure that such a simple solution is available in every country and household. Experience has shown that practical problems occur in ensuring that the solution is made correctly and that adequate amounts are given at the right times. The key is education of mothers, caretakers, and medical practitioners. Much effort is being devoted to determining how to teach the methodology. Given access to isotonic replacement fluids, no one should succumb to cholera. Mortality rates in cholera epidemics exceeding 1% point to a lack of public health resources and/or inappropriate case management by inexperienced clinical personnel.

PREVENTION

For most enteric diseases, the best preventive measures are those that interrupt the fecal–oral route of transmission. These may take the form of basic public sanitation efforts, water purification, or attention to proper food preparation (see Chapter 76). Nevertheless, infectious diarrhea continues to occur in societies where these efforts are maximized. Thus, other methods of personal protection, such as immunization, have also been considered.

Considerable efforts have been devoted to **vaccine** development for cholera as a prototype enteric infection. The challenge has been twofold: identify and prepare protective antigens, and find a way to present those in a way that leads to a local immune response in the intestine. Partial success has been achieved using live oral vaccines with attenuated genetically engineered strains or killed cholera vibrios given by mouth. The attenuated live vaccines have the most promise because they most closely mimic natural infection, which can confer long-lasting immunity. Vaccines for secretory diarrhea pathogens such as cholera are not widely recommended for use to control infection in endemic areas; they may sometimes be used in a highly targeted way to protect specific populations such as children or pregnant women. Cholera vaccines are approved and used for travelers, and these are killed, whole-cell preparations. However, improved live vaccine strains for cholera are on the horizon and may eventually be available for use in endemic areas.

CONCLUSION

Diarrhea is not simply a trivial bother that troubles everyone at some point. It is a major cause of infant death in the developing world. Symptomatic treatment by fluid replacement requires widespread educational efforts.

In every instance, local defenses of the gastrointestinal tract must be overcome for disease to occur. The efficacy of these defense mechanisms is best demonstrated by the relative rarity of intestinal infections in developed countries, even though the gut is a tube open to the exterior. Disease is seen when the load of pathogens in the environment and their opportunity for transmittal are high and when predisposing causes like malnutrition, which impair host defenses, are also present.

Suggested Readings

Bishop AL, Camilli A. *Vibrio cholerae*: lessons for mucosal vaccine design. *Expert Rev Vaccines*. 2011;10:79.

Chin CS, Sorenson J, Harris JB, et al. The origin of the Haitian cholera outbreak strain. *N Engl J Med*. 2011;364:33.

Croxen MA, Finlay, BB. Molecular mechanisms of *Escherichia coli* pathogenicity. *Nat Rev Microbiol*. 2010;8:26.

DiRita VJ. Molecular basis of infection by *Vibrio cholerae*. In: Groisman E, ed. *Principles of Bacterial Pathogenesis*. New York, NY: Academic Press; 2000.

Drazen JM, Klempner MS. Disaster, water, cholera, vaccines, and hope. *N Engl J Med*. 2005;352:827.

Faruque SM, Islam MJ, Ahmad QS, et al. Self-limiting nature of seasonal cholera epidemics: role of host-mediated amplification of phage. *Proc Natl Acad Sci USA*. 2005;102:6119–6124.

Faruque SM, Naser IB, Islam MJ, et al. Seasonal epidemics of cholera inversely correlate with the prevalence of environmental cholera phages. *Proc Natl Acad Sci USA*. 2005;102:1702–1707.

Gruenheid S, DeVinney R, Bladt F, et al. Enteropathogenic *E. coli* Tir binds Nck to initiate actin pedestal formation in host cells. *Nat Cell Biol*. 2001;3:856–859.

Mooi FR, Bik EM. The evolution of epidemic *Vibrio cholerae* strains. *Trends Microbiol*. 1997;5:161–165.

Nougayrede JP, Fernandes PJ, Donnenberg MS. Adhesion of enteropathogenic *Escherichia coli* to host cells. *Cell Microbiol*. 2003;5:359–372.

Sack DA, Sack RB, Nair GB, et al. Lysogenic conversion by a filamentous phage encoding cholera toxin. *Science*. 1996;272:1910–1914.

Chapter 17

Invasive and Tissue-Damaging Enteric Bacterial Pathogens: Bloody Diarrhea and Dysentery

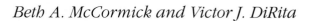

Beth A. McCormick and Victor J. DiRita

KEY CONCEPTS

Pathogens: *Shigella*, which causes dysentery and bloody diarrhea. *Shigella* is closely related to enteroinvasive *Escherichia coli* (EIEC).

Enterohemorrhagic *E. coli* (EHEC), which causes hemorrhagic colitis. The most common serotype is O157:H7.

Salmonella can cause nontyphoidal gastroenteritis and typhoid fever.

Encounter: All are acquired via the fecal–oral route of transmission. The mode of transmission depends on the infectious inoculum, for example, *Shigella* is the most infectious and can be transmitted by person-to-person contact. EHEC and *Salmonella* require larger inocula and are therefore usually transmitted in contaminated food or water.

Entry: Oral. Sensitivity to killing by gastric acid determines the infectious inoculum.

Spread and Multiplication: *Shigella* and *Salmonella* invade intestinal cells and enter the lamina propria. *Shigella* can spread directly from cell to cell. EHEC colonizes the surface of the mucosa.

Damage: *Shigella* and *Salmonella* produce damage by direct infection of cells and stimulation of a vigorous cytokine response. Hemorrhagic colitis is mediated by shigalike toxin production from EHEC.

Diagnosis: All three pathogens can be detected in stool cultures on selective indicator media. EHEC infection can also be diagnosed by assays of stool for shigalike toxin.

Treatment and Prevention: *Salmonella* gastroenteritis and EHEC are usually not treated with antibiotics. *Shigella* is treated when diagnosed, and typhoid is always treated, often on suspicion. Relapse of typhoid is common, and some individuals develop a carrier state associated with bacterial survival in the gallbladder.

THIS CHAPTER describes a group of intestinal pathogens that cause structural damage to the distal portions of the intestine, most commonly the large bowel. These organisms invade and damage the mucosa, leading to **bloody diarrhea** or **dysentery**. Dysentery is characterized by the frequent passage of stools (often more than 30 per day) that typically contain small volumes of blood, mucus, and pus. Other symptoms include cramps and pain caused by straining to pass stool (Table 17-1).

These serious, sometimes life-threatening, infections frequently require antibiotics. The use of antibiotics causes problems in some developing countries where antibiotic resistance is common and effective new drugs are either unavailable or too expensive. Rehydration therapies so useful in treating secretory diarrhea have little impact on dysentery.

The chapter focuses on *Shigella*, the prototypic invasive enteric pathogen and the closely related **enteroinvasive *Escherichia coli*** (EIEC). These organisms are contrasted with other tissue-damaging pathogens, including *Salmonella* and **enterohemorrhagic *E. coli*** (EHEC). Also discussed in the chapter is the agent of typhoid fever, *Salmonella typhi*, because that too enters the host by crossing the intestinal mucosa. However, typhoid fever, a systemic infection of mononuclear phagocytes, is a unique syndrome.

TABLE 17-1 Definitions of Clinical Types of Intestinal Infection

Infection	Stools	Site	Examples
Secretory or watery diarrhea	Copious, watery, no blood, no pus Tissue invasion: absent	Small intestine	*Vibrio cholerae*, ETEC strains
Dysentery	Scant volume, blood, mucus, pus Tissue invasion: present	Large intestine	Shigellae, *Entamoeba histolytica* (leukocytes absent in stool)
Hemorrhagic colitis	Copious, liquidlike, bloody, no leukocytes Tissue invasion: absent	Large intestine	EHEC strains
Bloody, watery diarrhea	Copious, liquidlike, bloody or blood-tinged, pus (sometimes) Tissue invasion: present	Ileum, colon	Salmonellae, *Campylobacter jejuni*, *Yersinia enterocolitica*

Enterohemorrhagic *Escherichia coli* (EHEC); enterotoxigenic *E. coli* (ETEC).

SHIGELLAE

The classic causes of **dysentery** are bacteria of the genus *Shigella* but also include the **ameba** *Entamoeba histolytica* (see Chapter 52). Approximately 15,000 to 20,000 cases of **shigellosis** are reported to the U.S. Centers for Disease Control and Prevention (CDC) each year. Because fecal cultures are infrequently obtained, it is estimated that the real number of cases is at least 10 times greater. Children less than 5 years old are 10 times more likely to contract this disease than the rest of the population. Severe and fatal cases are uncommon in industrialized countries.

The genus *Shigella* consists of **four species**, which are distinguished serologically by the **O antigen** of their lipopolysaccharide (LPS). The species are named **S. dysenteriae** (serogroup A), **S. flexneri** (group B),

S. boydii (group C), and **S. sonnei** (group D). Each group is further divided into subgroups. *S. dysenteriae* type 1 (which is now encountered primarily in developing countries) causes the most serious illness (dysentery), and *S. sonnei*, the predominant isolate in industrialized countries, causes the mildest one (watery diarrhea). *Shigella* species cannot be readily distinguished from *E. coli* by DNA hybridization and are actually differentiated pathogenic clones of *E. coli*.

ENCOUNTER

Shigellae are highly host specific, causing natural infections in humans and only occasionally in other higher primates. Encounter is most commonly by direct person-to-person

---

CASE • Infant T., a 22-month-old girl living in a low-income section of a Texas city near the Mexican border, became febrile, lost her appetite, and developed watery diarrhea. By the next day, her diarrhea had abated, but her parents noticed that her stools contained mucus and were blood tinged. The number of stools and the bloody appearance increased, and the baby began to vomit. The parents brought T. to a hospital emergency department. Her temperature was found to be 40°C. Shortly after arrival, she had a generalized seizure. Physical examination revealed an ill-appearing, somnolent infant with mild dehydration and hyperactive bowel sounds. Laboratory results showed leukocytosis and a mild decrease in serum sodium and glucose. T. was given fluids and an antibiotic. Several days later, *Shigella flexneri* grew from her stool culture. No further seizures occurred, and over the next few days, the dysentery subsided. The child had lost 2 pounds in weight but caught up to her growth curve 2 months later.

This case raises several questions:

1. What is the likely source of the shigellae?
2. How did these organisms enter into T.'s intestinal tract?
3. What bacterial properties were involved in producing the bloody diarrhea?
4. How should this disease have been treated?

See Appendix for answers.

contact, although transmission through food or water contaminated with feces also occurs. In contrast to cholera, enterotoxigenic *Escherichia coli* (ETEC), and enteropathogenic *E. coli* (EPEC) strains (see Chapter 16), the inoculum needed for *Shigella* infection is very small—a few hundred to a few thousand organisms. The small size of the effective inoculum allows the organisms to be easily transmitted from one person to another.

ENTRY, SPREAD, AND MULTIPLICATION

How do shigellae survive in the low pH environment of the stomach? These organisms are relatively acid resistant during certain phases of their growth, significantly more so than many other enteropathogenic bacteria. They sense the acid environment and adapt to it because they possess a global regulatory system of genes whose expression requires a **sigma factor** of **RNA polymerase (RpoS)** that is made only in the stationary phase of growth. When exposed to acid, the organisms survive but are less able to invade cells, at least in cell culture. Once they reach the small bowel (an alkaline or neutral environment) and begin to grow again, their acid resistance is repressed, and the invasive phenotype is restored. **Acid resistance** is also enhanced by anaerobiosis, the condition the organisms later encounter in the colon. It is likely, therefore, that when shigellae are excreted in the stool, they express the acid resistance phenotype. This phenotype is useful because the bacteria are already prepared to survive passage through the stomach when a new host ingests them. Thus, acid resistance may well contribute to the shigellae's success as pathogens.

After passing the stomach, the organisms go through the small bowel and enter the colon. Bacterial multiplication occurs mainly in the intracellular environment of the intestinal epithelial cell. Invasion and survival of shigellae within gut cells is a complex process that involves multiple genes present on both a large virulence plasmid and the chromosome. This is an interesting story and makes a good model for understanding the invasive properties of other enteric bacteria. Several steps are involved:

1. The shigellae approach the mucosal surface by an unknown mechanism (they are nonmotile). Intestinal epithelial cells are resistant to invasion by *Shigella* at their luminal surface, although they are susceptible at their basal surface.

2. How do the shigellae reach the lower portion of the intestinal cells? By stealth, first entering specialized **M cells**, which are antigen-sampling cells that overlie the lymphoid follicles (Fig. 17-1). Shigellae can also alter the intestinal barrier function facilitating paracellular passage through the intestinal epithelial barrier. Thus, the ability of shigellae to regulate the tight junction complex leads to direct entry of the organism at the basolateral epithelial surface. Invasion of both M cells and epithelial cells is effected by plasmid-encoded proteins (**invasion plasmid antigens** or Ipa proteins) delivered by a type III secretion system, which is also plasmid encoded (see paradigm).

3. If the shigellae invade the M cells, the bacteria are released into the **lamina propria**, where they are ingested by macrophages that may undergo apoptosis as a result. Macrophages release interleukin 1 (IL-1), causing a marked inflammatory response with recruitment of neutrophils (the process can be inhibited by IL-1 antagonists or by an antibody to CD18, a surface determinant that mediates migration of neutrophils in inflammation). This initial inflammatory response to small numbers of invading shigellae markedly increases the subsequent invasion—which itself leads to further release of proinflammatory cytokines and eicosanoids (i.e., hepoxilin A_3)—and is essential to causing clinical illness. The host leukocytic response is thus a key part of pathogenesis. At this stage the invading organisms are near the susceptible basal surface of the epithelial cells.

4. Like many other pathogens, shigellae can stimulate their uptake into epithelial cells. Unlike M cells, typical mucosal epithelial cells are not "professional phagocytes" and usually do not ingest large particles. *Shigella*-induced entry requires major reorganization of actin and cytoskeletal elements, just as occurs in typical phagocytosis. These changes are elicited by the action of *Shigella* type III secretion effectors to stimulate signaling pathways regulating actin dynamics.

5. Once inside the epithelial cells, the organisms escape the **phagosomal vesicle**, assisted by two Ipa proteins that disrupt the phagosome membrane. They then enter the cytoplasm where they multiply.

6. Having successfully invaded an epithelial cell, how do the organisms infect other epithelial cells? Rather than starting over from the intestinal lumen, they invoke a particular example of **molecular parasitism** that involves appropriating elements of the host cell's cytoskeleton. As they multiply, the shigellae make a protein called **IcsA** (*Ics* stands for "intracellular spread") at one pole of the rod-shaped organisms. IcsA induces polymerization of host cell **actin** (see Fig. 8-2). The rapid polymerization and depolymerization of actin filaments at one end of the bacterium (the "rear") propels the organisms forward. The force exerted is strong enough to push the organism and the overlying cell membrane into a fingerlike projection that pokes into the adjacent cell (see Figs. 8-2 and 17-1). The bacterium is now surrounded by two cell membranes: one from the old (previously invaded) cell and one from the new cell. When these membranes lyse, the organism is released in the cytoplasm of the new host cell, and the process can begin again. In this manner, **cell-to-cell spread** occurs without the need to reenter the extracellular milieu. The mechanism

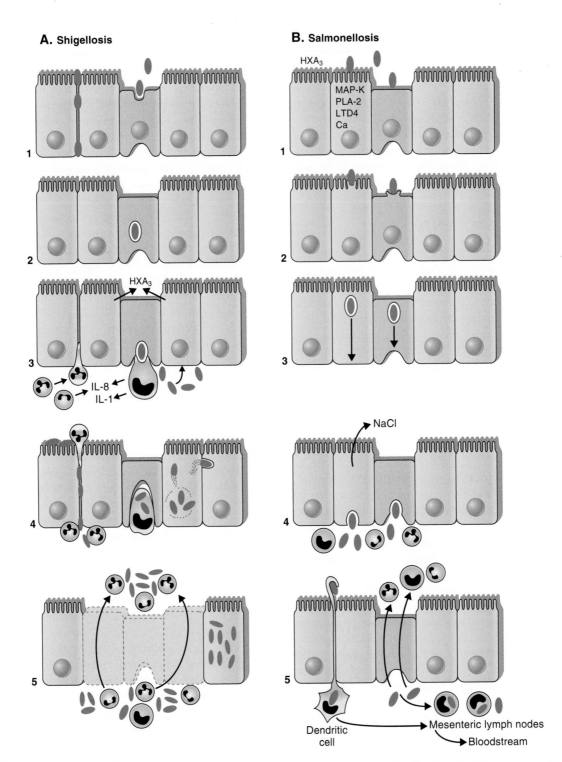

FIGURE 17-1. Invasion strategies of *Shigella* compared with *Salmonella* in the intestinal epithelium. A. Shigellae cannot invade intact epithelial cells from the luminal surface. Instead, they initially enter the mucosa overlaying intestinal lymphoid follicles through specialized M cells or alter tight junctional proteins for paracellular passage (*1*). Having transited through the M cells (*2*), some bacteria enter underlying macrophages (*3*). There cytokines IL-1 and IL-8 are induced by the action of proteins secreted by the *Shigella* type III system (see paradigm). A cascade of additional cytokines or eicosanoids (hepoxilin A$_3$ [HXA$_3$]) generates an influx of polymorphonuclear leukocytes (*3*), which migrate through the mucosa and cause separation of tight junctions between columnar epithelial cells (*4*). This separation subsequently permits the organisms to penetrate the disturbed epithelium. Once in the lamina propria, shigellae can invade the basal surface of epithelial cells (*3*). Internalized bacteria escape from phagosomes and travel from an infected cell to adjacent ones, using a mechanism that depends on actin and other host cytoskeletal proteins (*4*). Cell death results in a focal ulcer and exudation of inflammatory cells into the lumen, along with red blood cells to produce the dysentery stool (*5*). **B.** In *Salmonella* infection, organisms approach the mucosal surface (*1*), where they induce MAP-kinase (MAP-K), PLA-2 activity, production of leukotriene LTD4 and hepoxilin A$_3$ (HXA$_3$), and mobilization of intracellular Ca^{++} (*2*). These events induce surface ruffles (*3*, and see Fig. 17-3), leading to uptake of organisms within host cell membrane–bounded vesicles (*4*). These mediators result in electrolyte accumulation in the lumen (*4*) and an inflammatory exudate (*5*) to produce the diarrhea of *Salmonella* gastroenteritis. Bacteria are captured from the lumen by dendritic cells and transported to mesenteric lymph nodes. Some bacteria transit to the lymph nodes and are taken up by macrophages. Some escape to the bloodstream, resulting in transient bacteremia (*5*).

CHANGING NATURE OF INFECTIONS BY SHIGELLAE

The known history of shigellosis has followed an interesting course. Originally described in 1898, *Shigella dysenteriae* was the major isolate until it was replaced by *S. flexneri* after World War I, which was in turn supplanted by *S. sonnei* in industrialized countries following World War II. Beginning in 1969, however, epidemic *S. dysenteriae* reappeared in Latin America, Asia, and Africa. The reasons for these changes in prevalence over time are not known. *S. flexneri* increased again in the United States among young adult males, apparently related to homosexual practices, but not in the rest of the population.

used by *Shigella* for cell-to-cell spread is remarkably similar to the mechanism for cell-to-cell spread used by the Gram-positive pathogen *Listeria monocytogenes*, a foodborne pathogen that causes abortions, septicemia, and meningitis (see Chapter 21 paradigm).

DAMAGE

When a sufficient number of contiguous invaded cells die and slough off, the result is surface erosion in the gut wall, or an **ulcer.** Neutrophils that accumulate in large numbers in the mucosa are shed in the stool, where they are easily detected by light microscopy.

Bloody and pus-containing stools and pain associated with bowel movements (**tenesmus**) are characteristic of *Shigella* dysentery. Despite the ulcers and the inflammatory response, bacteremia is uncommon, except for *S. dysenteriae* type 1 infection. Bacteremia is most often encountered in poorly nourished infants in developing countries and is promoted by defects in host defenses associated with malnutrition, such as depressed complement activity.

One species, *S. dysenteriae* type 1, produces **Shiga toxin**, a cytotoxin that kills intestinal epithelial and endothelial cells. Shiga toxin cleaves the mammalian 60S ribosomal subunit, thereby stopping protein synthesis. Shiga toxin also causes cells to undergo apoptosis. The action of Shiga toxin has two effects: First, by targeting the sodium-absorptive villus cell and decreasing sodium absorption, it leads to an excess of fluid in the lumen. Second, effects of the toxin on mucosal endothelial cells contribute to the bloody diarrhea that follows.

Experimental infections in monkeys have shown that strains with inactivated Shiga toxin gene still cause disease but with much less damage to the mucosa and less bleeding. Thus, both invasion and toxin production are important in pathogenesis, which may explain why the highly toxigenic *S. dysenteriae* type 1 causes the most severe clinical illness of all *Shigella* species. *S. flexneri* also causes severe illness, dysentery, and bloody diarrhea despite its lack of the genes for shiga toxin.

It is curious that *S. sonnei* uses the same mechanisms of invasion as *S. dysenteriae* type 1 and *S. flexneri* but only rarely causes the dysentery syndrome; most commonly, it leads to a self-limited watery diarrhea. The basis for these differences is not understood but is probably related to the fact that these organisms do not induce as intense an inflammatory response and do not make shiga toxin.

DIAGNOSIS

When patients develop bloody diarrhea or dysentery, *Shigella* must obviously be included in the list of possible causes. In some parts of the world, up to 50% of patients with bloody diarrhea or dysentery are culture positive for *Shigella*. In contrast, this diagnosis may escape consideration in the mild watery diarrhea caused by *S. sonnei*, which grossly resembles that of other pathogens such as ETEC, EPEC, or even rotavirus. The presence of leukocytes in diarrheal stool is a simple indicator of an invasive pathogen, and their detection provides immediately useful diagnostic information.

The specific diagnosis of shigellosis relies on culturing the organisms. Because shigellae die off rapidly when excreted in stool, isolation rates depend on rapid processing of the stool sample, by either streaking directly onto isolation agar or, in field studies, into a transport medium to maintain viability until the sample can be processed. As with other enteric bacteria, media have been designed to detect the lactose-negative phenotype characteristic of *Shigella*. A rapid presumptive diagnosis can be made by suspending suspicious colonies in saline and carrying out **agglutination reactions** with antisera to group antigens of *Shigella*. Testing for biochemical and fermentation patterns allows genus and species identification.

In the era where so many bacterial genomes have been sequenced, it has become possible to identify *Shigella* and EIEC strains more rapidly by looking for specific genes using **DNA probes** or **amplification methods** such as polymerase chain reaction (PCR; see Chapter 58). These methods can be used on stool samples or environmental

PARADIGM BOX

BACTERIAL–HOST COMMUNICATION USING SPECIALIZED SECRETION MECHANISMS

Microbes have evolved a variety of mechanisms for secreting proteins into the environment. Often this ability allows microbes to survive within a host because the secreted molecules aid in microbial survival or dissemination. The challenge for microbes is how to transmit water-soluble proteins across their own membranes and the host's lipid membranes. Complex and incompletely understood mechanisms operate in these processes. In Gram-negative cells, toxins are typically delivered extracellularly in a two-step process. The toxin is first secreted into the periplasmic space—through the standard secretory pathway also used by many other (non–toxin-related) molecules—where it assembles into its final quaternary structure. In a second step, the toxin is transferred across the outer membrane, apparently without unfolding. Translocation across the outer membrane may require a dedicated protein pore through which the toxin, but not other proteins, can pass. Once extracellular, the secreted toxins gain access to the host cell by first binding to host surface molecules. This process of extracellular secretion is sometimes termed **type II secretion** and is the subject of intense study. The cholera toxin is secreted from *Vibrio cholerae* by this mechanism.

Another mechanism for transmitting proteins from the microbe to the host cell that has received a great deal is called **type III secretion** (formerly termed **contact-dependent secretion**). In contrast to the process described in the previous paragraph, there is no detectable periplasmic form of the protein secreted in this system. In some examples of type III secretion, there is no detectable extracellular form. Rather, the secreted protein is delivered directly from the microbe into the host cell by a process that has been likened to injection with a syringe. The complex of proteins required for this mechanism is collectively called the **injectisome**.

Type III secretion systems (T3SS) have been studied in a wide range of pathogens that cause disease in both animals and plants. Examples are *Yersinia* (responsible for mild diseases such as food poisoning as well as the more notorious and life-threatening plague), *Shigella*, and EPEC. The type of molecule delivered into the host cell differs in each case. *Yersinia* species us a T3SS to translocate toxin molecules that disrupt monocyte signaling pathways, thereby eliminating a major arm of the immune system. For *Shigella* the system is used to transfer proteins that cause the host cell to take up the microbe. Host cell invasion by shigellae is the first step in its eventual intracellular survival and cell-to-cell spread. EPEC transfers its own receptor, called Tir, which assembles into the host membrane and binds another EPEC protein, intimin.

How type III systems function is the focus of much current research. Each type III system that has been studied consists of several proteins that are genetically conserved, that is, they share sequence similarity and therefore are likely to have similar functions. Many proteins of the T3SS from one organism can functionally replace those of another. Some of the conserved proteins appear to form a pore within the host cell membrane, through which other proteins can pass into the cytosol of the host. In addition, in the *Yersinia* type III system, an outer membrane protein has biochemical and sequence similarity to the proposed outer membrane pore of the type II system described earlier. This suggests that the protein of the two systems may share common functions. Type III systems are structurally and evolutionarily related to the apparatus that some Gram-negatives use for assembling their flagella proteins. In fact, some pathogens use the flagellar pore to secrete virulence proteins, instead of a dedicated type III system. Once the flagellum is finished being assembled, secretion of the other proteins then ceases.

In these days of rapidly diminishing antibiotic choices, the possibility that type III secretion systems may prove useful targets for antimicrobial drug design has captured the imaginations of investigators, and small molecules that inhibit various features of T3SS have been identified as potential lead compounds. Another possibility for exploiting type III secretion lies in the notion of using suitably engineered microbes to deliver therapeutic molecules into eukaryotic cells with the same efficiency that they currently deliver toxins and invasion proteins.

samples such as food or water for quick diagnosis or to trace transmission routes.

TREATMENT AND PREVENTION

Shigellosis does not usually cause severely dehydrating diarrhea; therefore, intravenous fluids are rarely needed to treat the infection. Oral fluids usually suffice to correct the mild-to-moderate degree of dehydration and electrolyte abnormality. In more severe cases that involve bloody diarrhea or dysentery and high fever, the use of effective antibiotics reduces the duration of illness and the period of infectivity to others. Reducing the infective period is particularly important because the small inoculum needed for infection with *Shigella* frequently results in transmission to other household members.

The use of antibiotics is complicated by the ease with which the organisms acquire **antibiotic resistance**; it is not pure chance that transferable antibiotic resistance was first discovered in *Shigella*. The problem is greatest in developing countries where multiresistant *S. dysenteriae* type 1 is most commonly found and where cost and availability of the newest antimicrobials are limiting factors. The most reliably effective drugs at present are the **fluoroquinolones**. However, fluoroquinolone resistance is emerging. Some β-lactam and cephalosporin antibiotics are also effective. To make educated empiric decisions on which drug to use, clinicians should be aware of the drug susceptibility pattern of pathogens encountered in their communities and institutions.

No vaccine for shigellosis has been licensed, but many studies are under way using a number of strategies. In some approaches, virulence antigens, the Ipas, are being altered and packaged in various ways; other strategies depend on delivering the O antigen of *Shigella* in the vaccine preparation. A major goal is to produce live, attenuated vaccines that can be administered by mouth and will immunize the gut itself. Subunit vaccines for parenteral administration are also under investigation. Ultimately, however, these vaccines must be tested in humans because no animal model truly mimics human shigellosis.

ENTEROHEMORRHAGIC *E. COLI*

The EHEC strains include a number of *E. coli* serotypes that can cause a characteristic nonfebrile bloody diarrhea known as **hemorrhagic colitis**. The most commonly identified serotype in the United States is **O157:H7**. It is estimated that EHEC strains cause at least 20,000 to 40,000 infections annually in the United States. Approximately 250 to 500 deaths are caused by the **hemolytic–uremic syndrome (HUS)**, a complication of hemorrhagic colitis consisting of a particular form of hemolytic anemia, thrombocytopenia, and renal failure. Death from HUS occurs most commonly in young children, and the disease is the most frequent cause of acute renal failure in children in the United States. EHEC produces one or two related but antigenically distinguishable toxins that share the same enzymatic specificity and binding site as Shiga toxin of *S. dysenteriae* type 1. These constitute a family of protein toxins; the *E. coli* versions are known as Shiga toxins 1 and 2 (also called shigalike or vero toxins). Less often in the United States, bloody watery diarrhea is caused by other pathogens, including *Shigella*, *Salmonella*, *Campylobacter jejuni*, or, more uncommonly, *Yersinia enterocolitica*.

CASE • Mr. R., an 85-year-old resident of a nursing home, was awakened by the onset of severe abdominal cramps, primarily in the right lower quadrant of the abdomen. Later that morning, he had a watery diarrhea every 15 to 30 minutes, initially with small amounts of visible blood. Later that day, bright red stools consisting of what seemed to be pure blood appeared. He was nauseated but did not vomit. When seen the next morning by the physician on call, he did not have a fever. However, clinical examination of the abdomen revealed tenderness over the colon.

Because of the clinical findings, Mr. R. was hospitalized. Frankly bloody stools continued. A barium enema revealed edema of the ascending and transverse colon with areas of spasm. Routine stool cultures were negative for *Salmonella* and *Shigella*. However, **sorbitol nonfermenting** *E. coli* were subsequently identified by the state public health laboratory as serotype O157:H7, an EHEC strain. The patient was treated with intravenous fluids and gradually recovered over the next 7 days. By the time he was discharged and returned to the nursing home, his stool was negative for that particular *E. coli* strain.

The day before he became ill, Mr. R. was visited by E., his 3-year-old granddaughter. The two shared a fast-food hamburger for lunch. Two days after Mr. R. fell ill, E.

developed watery diarrhea. The diarrhea increased over the next 2 days and then became tinged with blood. When E. began to vomit and her urine output appeared to diminish, her parents took her to the pediatrician. E. was somewhat pale and lethargic, with a fluctuating level of consciousness. The laboratory reported a significant decrease in platelets and red blood cells, many of which looked abnormal. A diagnosis of diarrhea-associated hemolytic–uremic syndrome (HUS) was made, and the child was hospitalized. A stool culture was negative. E. was treated conservatively, and no antibiotics were given. No hypertension developed, the renal failure and hemolytic anemia did not progress, and dialysis was not performed. She was discharged 1 week later with no further diarrhea and improvement in the blood count.

This case raises several questions:

1. What is the likely source of the organisms that caused these diseases?

2. Why do only certain strains of *E. coli* cause the clinical manifestations seen in these cases?

3. By what mechanism does the responsible etiological agent cause these diseases?

4. What are the principal therapeutic concerns in such cases?

See Appendix for answers.

ENCOUNTER

We know the most about *E. coli* O157:H7 because the organism can be easily identified in the clinical laboratory. These strains have a convenient distinguishing characteristic: the inability to ferment sorbitol. However, their real prevalence compared with other EHEC serotypes has not been determined. O157:H7 clearly causes both outbreaks and sporadic disease, primarily as a **zoonosis** transmitted from animals to humans. Undercooked hamburger is the principal vehicle, but other food vehicles have been described. Groundwater contaminated in the vicinity of cattle farms can transmit infection as well. The organism appears to be acid resistant, and the estimated infectious dose is very low, approximately 50 organisms per gram of hamburger. As in *Shigella* infections, person-to-person transmission of *E. coli* O157:H7 in day-care centers has been documented.

ENTRY, MULTIPLICATION, AND DAMAGE

Once past the stomach, EHEC colonize the terminal regions of the bowel where they remain confined to the surface of the gut mucosa and multiply locally. They do not invade the bloodstream. EHEC possess a homologue of the EPEC genes (see Chapter 16) that mediate the same dramatic rearrangements of actin and cytoskeletal elements leading to characteristic **attaching and effacing** lesion of the brush border (see Fig. 17-2A). Production of shigalike toxins by EHEC may be responsible for a local cytokine response in the colonic mucosa. It is currently believed that profuse bleeding is caused by the interaction of inflammatory cytokines and shigalike toxins, which damages blood vessels in the lamina propria.

The major complication of EHEC, which occurs in approximately 5% of severe clinical cases, is damage to small blood vessels. When this occurs, predominantly in renal glomeruli and usually in small children, HUS results. When the target is the brain, commonly in older adults, the syndrome is called **thrombotic thrombocytopenic purpura**. It is quite clear from various studies that the toxin causes these clinical pictures. HUS resulting from EHEC is the most common cause of acute renal failure in children in the United States. It is estimated that as many as 5 to 10% of HUS-affected children will die promptly, and an unknown number may require dialysis or, eventually, kidney transplants. Shiga toxin is cytotoxic, suggesting that direct damage to glomerular endothelial cells may be the initiating factor of these diseases. Endothelial cell products (including von Willebrand factor, plasminogen activator inhibitor, prostacyclin, nitric oxide, and others) can mediate local pathophysiology leading to **platelet thrombi**, the characteristic feature of the disease.

EHEC species are lysogens, carrying on their chromosomes a temperate bacteriophage that encodes shigalike toxin (see Chapter 4 for a discussion of bacteriophage biology and other examples of phage-encoded virulence factors). In the lysogenic state, the phage genes—including the toxin gene—are repressed so their levels are very low or nonexistent. The phage is induced to undergo **lytic growth** when the DNA of the EHEC lysogen is damaged. During lytic growth, toxin is expressed at high levels from the phage, and its release is the result of phage-mediated lysis of the host bacteria that occurs after induction. Spontaneous lysis occurs at a very low frequency, thereby maintaining a low rate of toxin expression and release in

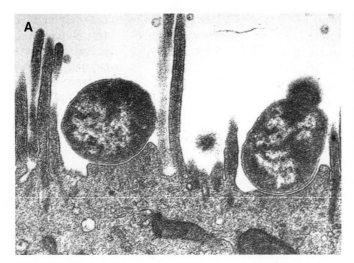
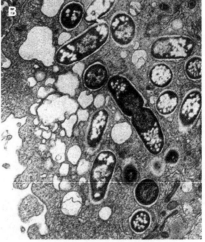

FIGURE 17-2. *Escherichia coli* **with distinctive interactions with host cells. A.** Electron micrograph of colon infected with the EHEC strain O157:H7. Notice the attaching bacteria and the altered epithelial cell membrane beneath them showing intimate attachment and "pedestal" formation. This attaching and effacing lesion is associated with EHEC and EPEC expressing the *eae* gene complex. (Original magnification, ×28,526.) **B.** Enteroinvasive *E. coli* within host cells.

infected people. However, phage-mediated toxin liberation can be dramatically increased when DNA-damaging antibiotics are used against the bacteria, because these can cause phage induction.

DIAGNOSIS

The classic syndrome of hemorrhagic colitis is sufficiently characteristic to be recognized clinically (as in the cases of Mr. R. and his granddaughter). Less severe bloody diarrhea is not so revealing, and diagnosis depends on detecting the organism in stool. Culture methods using MacConkey lactose agar identify just O157:H7 but miss the occasional sorbitol-positive O157:H7 and other EHEC strains, which, like most *E. coli*, ferment sorbitol. An enzyme immunoassay to detect Shiga toxins 1 and 2 is commercially available to detect toxin or any toxin-producing organisms in stool and is both highly sensitive and specific. Methods using PCR to detect specific DNA are also useful for detection.

TREATMENT

Treating EHEC infections is controversial. Some clinicians have suggested that antibiotic therapy may increase the likelihood of the HUS, and epidemiological data bear this out. This may not be strictly related to antibiotic-induced lytic growth of toxin-encoding phage in EHEC, because even antibiotics not known to significantly damage DNA appear to be associated with HUS. One explanation for this association may be that patients with more severe diarrheal disease are more likely to be treated with antibiotics and will thus fare worse than patients with less severe disease, with or without the drugs. Fluid therapy is relatively

simple because EHEC strains do not typically cause large volume losses and severe dehydration. The major challenge is to treat complications of EHEC by supportive measures, including dialysis for renal failure if needed. Thrombotic thrombocytopenic purpura usually responds rapidly to exchange transfusion, for unknown reasons.

NONTYPHOIDAL *SALMONELLA* AND TYPHOID FEVER: INTRODUCTION TO THE AGENTS

Four clinical syndromes, plus the carrier state, are associated with the genus *Salmonella*:

- Gastroenteritis: nausea, vomiting, and diarrhea, caused mainly by *S. enterica* subspecies *enterica*. This disease resembles some of those described in Chapter 16.
- **Focal infection of vascular endothelium**: caused by serovars Choleraesuis and Typhimurium.
- **Infections of particular organ systems**: osteomyelitis in patients with sickle cell disease, most commonly caused by *S. typhimurium*.
- **Typhoid fever**: caused mainly by serovars *S. typhi* and *S. paratyphi* A and B.

Some salmonellae are specific to animals and do not cause human disease; some, such as *S. typhi* and *S. paratyphi* subspecies A or B, are human specific and cause typhoid fever. A large number can cross host species. These are the most common causes of *Salmonella* diarrhea.

The genus *Salmonella* is vast, comprising more than 2,300 serological varieties (**serovars**), and the number is growing. The main antigens of *Salmonella* that

---

CASE • Ms. J., an Asian exchange student in the United States, returned home for a 3-month visit. Near the end of her visit, she cared for her aunt, who had high fevers and some diarrhea. Three weeks later, when she returned to the United States, Ms. J. had a shaking chill and fever to 38.5°C, with headache, muscle pain, and loss of appetite. The fever continued and progressively increased over the next several days. When seen at the student health service, she appeared ill and confused. Her abdomen was diffusely tender, and her liver and spleen were enlarged, although she did not have jaundice. In spite of the high fever, her pulse was relatively low at 90 beats per minute. Her white blood cell count was low, only 3,000/mm³, with a moderate monocytosis. An astute clinician made the presumptive diagnosis of typhoid fever, and therapy with ceftriaxone was initiated and continued for 14 days.

Admission blood cultures subsequently grew *Salmonella typhi*, thus confirming the diagnosis. The

fever gradually abated over the next 3 days, and Ms. J. made an uneventful recovery. However, 6 weeks later all her symptoms recurred, including a maximum fever of 38.5°C. *S. typhi* was again isolated from blood culture and was found to still be sensitive to trimethoprim–sulfamethoxazole. She was treated again for 2 weeks with the same drug with a rapid response. She experienced no further recurrence.

This case raises several questions:

1. Do the same salmonellae cause diarrhea, dysentery, and typhoid fever?
2. Can the epidemiology of typhoid fever be distinguished from that of other salmonelloses?
3. Why were organs other than those of the digestive system involved in Ms. J.'s disease?
4. Why is it particularly important to treat cases of typhoid fever with antibiotics?

See Appendix for answers.

distinguish its serovars are **somatic (O)**, **flagellar (H)**, and **capsular (K)**. Individual isolates express more than one O and H antigen at a time, and each strain is defined by a particular combination. The tremendous diversity of the genus stems from the ability of *Salmonella* to undergo **antigenic variation**, the ability to create mosaics of genes for their antigens through recombination, alterations in length, gene duplications, and point mutations. Only two species of *Salmonella* are now recognized: *S. enterica* and *S. bongori*. *S. enterica* consists of six subspecies, each of which contains multiple serovars (Table 17-2). Most human pathogens are grouped within a subdivision of *S. enterica* called subspecies *enterica* (subsp. I). However, it is still clinically useful to sort serovars into groups designated by the letters *A*, *B*, *C*, and so on. Serogrouping is usually the first information available from the clinical laboratory regarding a *Salmonella* isolate and provides a tentative clue to identification of the organisms likely to be involved.

ENCOUNTER

Salmonellae are common members of the normal flora of many animals, including chickens, cattle, and reptiles (e.g., pet turtles). The strains that cause **gastroenteritis** are usually transmitted by chicken meat, eggs, and dairy products. Unless care is taken in poultry farms, chicken eggs often become contaminated, both on their surface and within. Outbreaks are most frequent in summer months and are often related to contaminated egg or chicken salads. **Typhoid fever**, on the other hand, is traceable to

a human carrier (such as the infamous Typhoid Mary), although the routes of transmission often involve contaminated water or food. It is interesting that, because its host range is strictly limited to humans, *S. typhi* could potentially be eradicated, whereas organisms that colonize many other species cannot.

Like other enteric pathogens, salmonellae must travel from feces, whether human or animal, to the mouth. Significant changes and adaptations in the organisms are required for survival of this trip. The organism must use its genetic potential for attachment, replication, and survival. In addition, it must be able to disperse in the environment and infect new hosts.

ENTRY

Salmonellae are more acid sensitive than shigellae; therefore, susceptible individuals are often those who produce little or no stomach acid (a condition called **hypochlorhydria** or **achlorhydria**). In human volunteer experiments, a relatively large inoculum (10 to 100 million organisms) is required to infect those with normal gastric acid secretion, but the inoculum size is reduced 10 to 100 times when bicarbonate, which buffers the acidic pH of the stomach, is given along with the inoculum. Salmonellae also respond to the acidic environment of the stomach to express proteins of possible importance to its pathogenicity.

Organisms that successfully escape being killed in the stomach pass through the small bowel to the distal ileum and colon. There, like shigellae, they penetrate the mucosal barrier (see Fig. 17-1). Bacteria can enter M cells and the apical membrane of the gut epithelial cells. Contact of salmonellae with cells in culture induces a dramatic "**ruffling**" of the plasma membrane, a visual harbinger of cytoskeletal rearrangements that lead to uptake of the organisms within phagocytic vesicles (Fig. 17-3). Thus, the entry of salmonellae into cells is an example of **bacterial-mediated endocytosis (BME)**.

The process of BME in *Salmonella* is directed by a type III secretion system encoded on a large (more than 40 kbp) region of the genome called ***Salmonella* pathogenicity island 1 (SPI1).** Pathogenicity islands are found in many microbes and, as the name implies, typically encode features required for virulence. They often have a G + C content distinct from the overall G + C content of the genome and, curiously, are frequently inserted into genes that encode transfer RNA molecules. Pathogenicity islands are thought to be evidence of horizontally acquired genetic information that converts an otherwise nonpathogenic strain into a pathogen through acquisition of virulence genes en bloc. Within 30 minutes of contact with host epithelial cells in vitro, ruffles form on the host cell, and the microbe is taken up (see Fig. 17-3). Some experiments demonstrated the presence of nonpilus appendages on the surface of the bacteria before host cell ruffling, and these appendages were shown to require

TABLE 17-2 Classification and Serogroup of Some Human Pathogenic Salmonellae

Species	Group	Serovar
Salmonella enterica	A	Paratyphi A
	B	Typhimurium
		Derby
		Heidelberg
	C1	Choleraesuis
		Infantis
		Virchow
	C2	Muenchen
		Newport
	D1	Dublin
		Enteritidis
		Typhi
S. bongori		

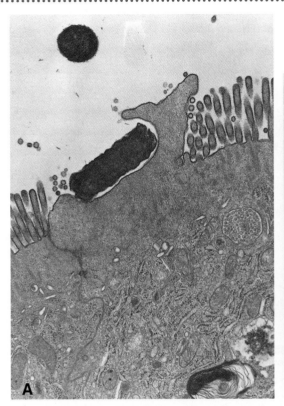
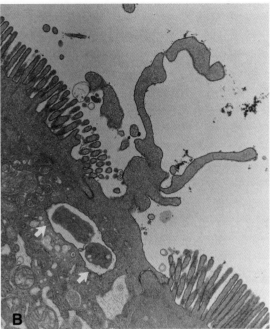

FIGURE 17-3. Ruffling of host cell membranes during intracellular *Salmonella* infection.
A mouse pathogenic *Salmonella* (var. *typhimurium*) was inoculated into ligated loops of mouse
ileum, and samples for electron microscopy taken after 30 minutes. At that time, the bacteria
were associated exclusively with M cells. **A.** A bacterium in contact with an M cell and the initial
phase of a ruffle response on the M-cell surface. **B.** Pronounced ruffling. The *arrows* point to two
bacteria seen in a vesicle inside the M cell. (Original magnification, ×12,000.)

genes of the type III system called *inv* genes, although the relevance of those structures is unclear.

In contrast to the shigellae, which escape to the cytoplasm and multiply intracellularly, salmonellae remain within vesicles. Salmonellae are unusually resistant to the lysosomal contents of cells and to the antibacterial peptides made by intestinal epithelial cells called **cryptins**. The bacteria-containing vesicles eventually travel to the basal membrane, and the organisms are released into the lamina propria. Thus, gut epithelial cells are not the main habitat for multiplication of salmonellae but rather are barriers to be crossed. After the alterations in the brush border are reversed, the gut cells are apparently not harmed.

The mechanisms determining whether *Salmonella* causes gastroenteritis or typhoid fever are not clear. The former is associated with production of inflammatory mediators and influx of neutrophils into the intestinal lumen, and bacteria are generally contained within the follicle-associated epithelium. The microbe appears to benefit to some degree from inflammation as reactive oxygen species arising during inflammation provide a respiratory electron acceptor that *Salmonella* preferentially uses to compete for growth with the normal microbiota. In contrast, typhoid fever is marked by little intestinal inflammation and dissemination of the bacteria from the intestine

to the reticuloendothelial system (Fig. 17-4). Experimental evidence suggests that expression of an antiphagocytic capsule termed the **Vi antigen** by typhoid fever–inducing salmonellae enables them to evade the intestinal inflammatory response and infect deeper tissue. Genes for synthesis and export of the Vi antigen are encoded on a region of the chromosome from typhoid strains that is missing from those strains associated with gastroenteritis only.

After salmonellae reach the lamina propria, they often enter the bloodstream and may be recovered in blood cultures early in the course of the disease. They normally do not cause sustained **bacteremia** because they are rapidly taken up by the phagocytic cell system and are effectively killed. Exceptions to this rule include some serovars (Typhimurium, Enteritidis, and Dublin) that spread systemically more often than the others and frequently cause focal systemic infections. Clinical conditions that impair mononuclear cells enhance susceptibility to *Salmonella* bacteremia. For example, patients with sickle cell anemia have a tenfold higher incidence of invasive salmonellosis. A marked increase in incidence and severity of infection is also observed in patients with AIDS, leukemia, diabetes, lymphoma, and chronic granulomatous disease.

Macrophage survival is associated with a second type III secretion system encoded on a pathogenicity

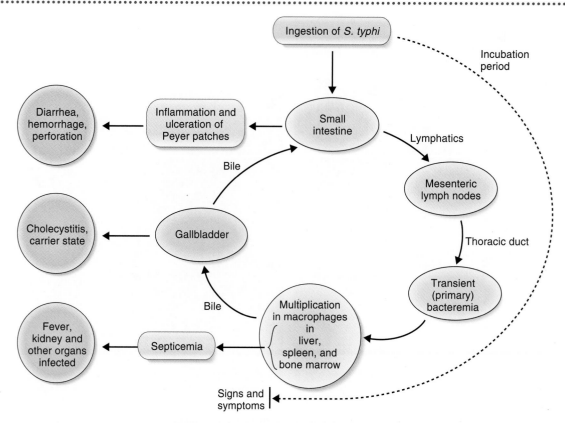

FIGURE 17-4. Pathogenesis of typhoid fever.

island called **SPI2**. Systemic spread of bacteria in typhoid fever is clinically silent and brief (see Fig. 17-4). As the organisms multiply in macrophages of liver, spleen, and mesenteric lymph nodes, patients are also clinically asymptomatic. When the number of intracellular organisms reaches a threshold, they are released into the bloodstream, initiating the continuous bacteremia characteristic of typhoid fever. This event signals the start of clinical illness, manifested by daily high fevers that continue for 4 to 8 weeks in untreated cases. This **second bacteremia** leads to invasion of the **gallbladder** and **kidney** and reinvasion of the **gut mucosa**, especially at the Peyer patches. At that stage the organism can be isolated not only from blood but also from stool and urine (Fig. 17-5). Uptake of organisms by monocytes or macrophages in bone marrow makes this site a useful source of culture material when other sites are negative, because the organisms can actually be enriched at this site.

That *Salmonella* enter through M cells likely facilitates uptake by underlying macrophages, which leads to dissemination. However, *Salmonella* can also disseminate into deeper tissue beyond the intestine by virtue of **intestinal dendritic cells**. These phagocytic cells of the innate immune system (see Chapter 6) can directly sample luminal contents by extending dendrites through the epithelial

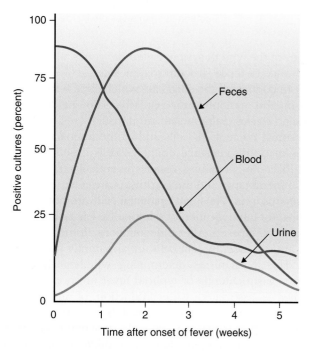

FIGURE 17-5. The isolation of typhoid bacilli from various sources in the course of untreated typhoid fever. The late rise in positive stool cultures is caused by secondary invasion of the gut by organisms from the gallbladder.

layer in such a way as not to disrupt the tight junctions between the enterocytes. Once ingested this way, the *Salmonella* can be disseminated by the bloodstream to deeper tissue. This pathway of dendritic cell-dependent dissemination does not require the SPI1 invasion genes required for epithelial cell invasion.

DAMAGE

Interaction of gastroenteritis-producing salmonellae with epithelial cells activates the inflammatory response and results in damage to the intestinal mucosa. Many biochemical events are activated by signals during invasion. Activation of the **mitogen-activated protein kinase (MAP kinase)** may be the first signal. MAP kinase is linked to a receptor on the cell surface. Binding of the organisms leads to activation of phospholipase A$_2$; release of arachidonic acid; production of prostaglandins, leukotrienes, and hepoxilins; and a sharp increase in intracellular calcium concentration. As yet, the mechanism by which fluid secretion is induced by *Salmonella* remains uncertain. Invasion induces production of inflammatory cytokines and lipids, such as IL-8 and hepoxilin A$_3$, leading to local leukocyte infiltration, particularly migration of neutrophils across the intestinal epithelium. This ability to invade and cause inflammation is necessary but not sufficient to cause diarrhea in experimental animals. Thus, additional traits need to be expressed. Disease is dependent on **transepithelial signals**, probably cytokines, elicited by the organism to recruit neutrophils.

The microbial contribution to macrophage survival has been extensively studied in *S. typhimurium* infection of mice. This organism typically causes a typhoid-like syndrome in mice and diarrhea in humans, whereas the human typhoid bacillus is not a mouse pathogen. Virulence of *S. typhimurium* is regulated by **two-component regulator or signal system** (see Chapter 19 paradigm), consisting of two genes, **PhoP** and **PhoQ**. These genes regulate a number of genes in *Salmonella*, most notably those whose products act to modify the bacterial LPS. The result of PhoP–PhoQ-regulated modification is microbial resistance to innate killing mechanisms of the host immune system, particularly killing by cationic peptides. This type of surface remodeling is seen in both Gram-negative and Gram-positive pathogens.

Invasive nontyphoidal salmonellae (such as serovar Dublin) possess a virulence plasmid that shares a conserved 8–kbp region of DNA containing *spv* (for *Salmonella* plasmid virulence) genes. This region encodes genes that are turned on when salmonellae enter eukaryotic cells. Other plasmid genes encode resistance to complement by blocking assembly of the terminal attack complex on the cell surface, thus enabling the organisms to resist that host defense mechanism.

Host proteins also contribute to survival of salmonellae within macrophages. For example, the susceptibility of some inbred strains of mice to several intracellular pathogens, including *Salmonella*, the protozoan *Leishmania*, and the attenuated tuberculosis vaccine strain BCG, is due to mutation in a gene called *NRAMP1*. Susceptibility to all three microbes is a result of a mutation at amino acid 169 of this gene, which eliminates its activity and enables intraphagosomal survival. In normal phagocytes, NRAMP1, which is a transporter, localizes to the membranes of phagosomes and is critical for phagosome maturation required to defend against pathogens. NRAMP regulates availability of iron or other cations to phagosomes and thus serves as a **metal withdrawal** defense against pathogens. A human homologue of this gene has been identified and is part of a family of at least three genes that control a natural macrophage-specific membrane transport protein.

Invasion of the gallbladder by typhoid bacilli may be temporary or may result in the long-term colonization that characterizes the **typhoid carrier state**, especially in the presence of gallstones. Occasionally, acute necrotizing cholecystitis may result. Typhoid bacilli survive well in gallstones and can be recovered from the center of a stone; viable organisms may still be obtained after dipping stones in antibiotics. Gallstones are a source of prolonged asymptomatic carriage and excretion of the organism in stool.

The source of secondary gut invasion may be bacteria from the bloodstream during the prolonged secondary bacteremia or bacteria shed in the bile that penetrate M cells. Such secondary reinvasion leads to severe bleeding and/or perforation attributable to the marked inflammatory response induced in the **Peyer patches**. We do not know why the invasion of the gut at this stage results in more extensive damage to the intestinal mucosa than the primary invasion, but severity could be immunologically mediated. Invasion of the liver, spleen, or kidney can result in hepatitis, splenitis that makes the spleen prone to rupture, or glomerulonephritis. The clinical prognosis is much worse when those events occur.

Endocarditis and **vascular infection** are caused by specific *Salmonella* serovars capable of adhering to endovascular surfaces. *S. choleraesuis* and *S. typhimurium* adhere well to endothelial cells and may cause aortitis or endocarditis. These conditions are difficult to treat and often require surgical intervention. *S. typhimurium* also causes osteomyelitis in individuals with hemoglobinopathies (e.g., sickle cell anemia), trauma, and underlying bony abnormalities. Despite its predilection to cause continuous bacteremia, *S. typhi* only rarely adheres to vascular epithelia and is an uncommon cause of endocarditis.

DIAGNOSIS

Salmonellosis is generally diagnosed in the laboratory by culture on selective media and a combination of serological and biochemical tests to identify individual serovars. The salmonellae are lactose nonfermenters, and the same media used for shigellae allow them to be selected for further testing as well. Most clinical laboratories can identify *S. typhi*, determine the O serogroup for other isolates (A through E for human *Salmonella*), and deduce the most likely serovars, but they are not usually equipped for more detailed diagnoses. Further identification is most useful for epidemiological purposes and usually requires the assistance of a state public health laboratory or the CDC.

Typhoid fever is not recognized in the asymptomatic incubation period. The specific diagnosis is usually made by blood culture, which becomes positive early in the course of clinical illness (see Fig. 17-5). Isolation of *S. typhi* is helped by their resistance to bile salts (the organisms survive in bile itself within the gallbladder). *S. typhi* also produces the capsular antigen **Vi**, the antiphagocytic virulence factor that may reduce intestinal inflammation and enable invasion into deeper tissue.

Typhoid fever can also be diagnosed by **serology**. A rising titer or a single very high anti-O-antigen titer is suggestive. The Vi antigen also elicits an antibody response; however, because other organisms produce that antigen as well, the response is suggestive but not definitive for *S. typhi*. These tests rely on **agglutination** of the organisms by antibodies present in patient sera. In a positive test, the bacteria make clumps visible to the naked eye. The highest dilution of serum that results in agglutination is the antibody titer.

TREATMENT AND PREVENTION

In the past, *Salmonella* **gastroenteritis** was not usually treated with antibiotics, because the drugs did not shorten the duration of the disease but rather prolonged carriage of the organisms in the stool. This is not the case with newer fluoroquinolones, which both eradicate the organism and decrease the period of illness. Resistance to these drugs has arisen, however, and they may therefore be less effective in the future.

Systemic nontyphoidal *Salmonella* infections require antimicrobial therapy. A number of drugs may be used, depending on antibiotic resistance patterns. Prevention of salmonellosis relies on avoiding potentially contaminated water or foods that contain raw eggs or unpasteurized milk or milk products, or cooking these foods enough to kill the organisms. Preventive measures are especially important for people with diminished gastric acid or an immunodeficiency disease, such as HIV infection. However, it is neither easy nor foolproof. Considerable work is currently under way to develop attenuated vaccine strains for immunization.

The morbidity and mortality from typhoid fever have been significantly reduced by antibiotic therapy. Most cases in the United States are now imported. It must be remembered that therapy does not eradicate the organism. Oddly, the relapse rate is higher in treated individuals, possibly because early therapy aborts the immune responses necessary for preventing relapse. Without effective cell-mediated immunity, surviving bacteria can

multiply to the point where they again cause clinical symptoms.

Progress has been made in developing a **typhoid vaccine**. Live, attenuated vaccines are under investigation, and one, Ty21a, is approved and used for travelers, with the standard exception of those who are immunocompromised. Other live, attenuated strains are being investigated for possible use, including those with mutations in the *galE* gene required for LPS synthesis, or in genes for aromatic amino acid biosynthesis, or in the *PhoP* and *PhoQ* regulatory genes. Each class of mutant is immunogenic but sufficiently growth-impaired in vivo to render them unable to cause systemic infection. Thus, natural immunity can develop while the organism self-destructs. A cell-free Vi polysaccharide vaccine is available that induces protection in older children and adults, and a Vi–protein conjugate vaccine is being developed to immunize infants too young to respond to the polysaccharide alone, and this has shown early promise.

Typhoid carriers are a public health concern because they are often asymptomatic shedders; they not only carry the organism but constantly spread them through their feces. Treatment of typhoid carriers has been difficult but also represents a social imperative. Because no successful treatment was available in her day, Typhoid Mary was jailed. Today the recommended course of action is prolonged antibiotic therapy (a new fluoroquinolone may be the most effective form) with removal of the gallbladder if gallstones are present.

CONCLUSION

Bacterial pathogens may damage the intestinal mucosa and lead to bloody and/or inflammatory enteritis. Damage results from the invasion or intimate interaction with the surface of the intestinal mucosa, the elicitation of an inflammatory response alone or in concert with the production of cytotoxins that alter gut epithelial cells or endothelial cells, or production of bacterial protein toxins. Multiple chromosomal, plasmid, or phage genes are required for virulence. The inflammatory response may not only be a response to injury but also, as in the example of *Shigella*, be required for pathogenesis.

Watery diarrhea appears the same, on the clinical level, whether it is caused by nontyphoidal *Salmonella*, ETEC strains, certain *Shigella* species, or rotavirus. Shigellae and occasionally certain salmonellae may produce frankly bloody diarrhea or dysentery. The noninvasive EHEC typically cause nonfebrile grossly bloody diarrhea known as hemorrhagic colitis, with the potentially fatal sequela of HUS. These organisms share virulence traits with EPEC and *Shigella*. The differences in clinical manifestations can be ascribed to the specific virulence factors these organisms express, but this extrapolation is less than perfect.

Typhoid bacilli are highly human-specific organisms that enter the host through the fecal–oral route and invade the intestinal mucosa. However, unlike nontyphoidal

Salmonella, they produce typhoid fever, a fundamentally different infection in which the organism behaves as an intracellular pathogen of mononuclear phagocytes. Both microbial and host genes affect this interaction. The identification of these genes has yielded new information about the basic pathogenic mechanisms involved.

Suggested Readings

Mrsny RJ, Gewirtz AT, Siccardi D, et al. Identification of hepoxilin A₃ in inflammatory events: a required role in neutrophil migration across the intestinal epithelia. *Proc Natl Acad Sci USA*. 2004;101:7421–7426.

Mumy KL, Bien JD, Pazos M, et al. Distinct isoforms of phospholipase A2 mediate the ability of *Salmonella enterica* serotype Typhimurium and *Shigella flexneri* to induce the transepithelial migration of neutrophils. *Infect Immun*. 2008;76:3360–3373.

Niedergang F, Didierlaurent A, Kraehenbuhl JP, et al. Dendritic cells: the host Achille's heel for mucosal pathogens? *Trends Microbiol*. 2004;12:79–88.

Pazos M, Siccardi D, Mumy KL, et al. Multi-drug resistance transporter 2 regulates mucosal inflammation by facilitating the synthesis of hepoxilin A3. *J Immunol*. 2008;181:8044–8052.

Raffatellu M, Chessa D, Wilson RP, et al. Capsule mediated immune evasion: a new hypothesis explaining aspects of typhoid fever pathogenesis *Infect Immun*. 2006;74:19–27.

Sansonetti PJ, Egile C, Wenneras C. Shigellosis: from disease symptoms to molecular and cellular pathogenesis. In: Groisman EA, ed. *Principles of Bacterial Pathogenesis*. San Diego, CA: Academic Press; 2001.

Takanori S, Köhler H, Gu X, et al. *Shigella flexneri* regulates tight junction associated proteins in human intestinal epithelial cells. *Cell Microbiol*. 2002;4:367–381.

Vazquez-Torres A, Fang FC. Cellular routes of invasion by enteropathogens. *Curr Opin Microbiol*. 2000;3:54–59.

Valdez Y, Ferreira RB, Molecular mechanisms of Salmonella virulence and host resistance. Finlay BB. *Curr Top Microbiol Immunol*. 2009;337:93–127.

Winter SE, Thiennimitr P, Winter MG, et al. Gut inflammation provides a respiratory electron acceptor for Salmonella. *Nature*. 2010;467:426–429.

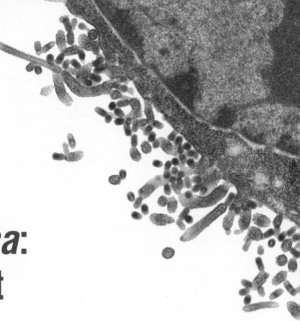

Chapter **18**

Pseudomonas aeruginosa: A Ubiquitous Opportunist

Joanna B. Goldberg

KEY CONCEPTS

Pathogen: *Pseudomonas aeruginosa* is a nonfermenting, aerobic, motile Gram-negative bacillus that is ubiquitous in the natural environment, for example, soil and water.

Encounter: *Pseudomonas*

- has minimal nutritional requirements and can easily contaminate wet surfaces in the hospital, as well as equipment, devices, and solutions.

- rarely colonizes healthy humans but frequently colonizes hospitalized patients

Entry: *Pseudomonas* may enter

- through abrasions or breaks in the skin

- by contaminating devices that bypass the normal barriers that protect the lungs (e.g., endotracheal tubes)

- by invasion of the intestinal tract (in neutropenic patients). Patients with neutropenia, cancer, burns, and cystic fibrosis are at special risk.

Spread and Multiplication: The bacteria secrete a biofilm that protects them and allows them to adhere to tissues. Infection is limited by neutrophils, so systemic spread typically occurs only in neutropenic or immunocompromised individuals.

Damage: *P. aeruginosa* secrete exotoxin A (with diphtheria toxin–like activity) several proteases that degrade specific host macromolecules. A type III secretion delivers virulence factors directly to host cells.

Diagnosis: The bacteria are easily cultured and identified in the laboratory. Antibiotic resistance testing of each isolate is critically important.

Treatment: Pseudomonads are naturally resistant to many antibiotics. Extended-spectrum β-lactams, carbapenems, aminoglycosides, and fluoroquinolones are often effective.

Prevention: Adherence to infection control measures may prevent the spread of drug-resistant *Pseudomonas* in the hospital.

PSEUDOMONADS are Gram-negative bacteria that inhabit soil and water; contact with healthy humans is widespread but usually insignificant. As a group, pseudomonads have flexible nutritional requirements and are capable of using a wide variety of carbon and nitrogen sources to grow in diverse environments. Among this group, *Pseudomonas aeruginosa* is the most prevalent **opportunistic pathogen** that causes a variety of infections in immunocompromised patients, such as burn victims and cancer patients, and persons with cystic fibrosis.

Because of its adaptability and intrinsic and acquired resistance to many common antibiotics, *P. aeruginosa* finds the hospital environment accommodating. Equipment that requires a wet, body-temperature environment, such as dialysis tubing and respiratory therapy equipment, is particularly susceptible to contamination by this organism. In the hospital, *P. aeruginosa* can be cultured from hand-washing sinks, hand creams, and even certain cleaning solutions. Although few healthy humans are colonized with *P. aeruginosa*, colonization rates can be high in hospitalized patients.

P. aeruginosa generally causes disease in humans only when a local or systemic breach occurs in the immune system (Table 18-1). Local lesions are often seen in people with corneal abrasions, burns, and surgical wounds. Puncture wounds of the foot, such as those caused by stepping on a nail while wearing tennis shoes, can give rise to *P. aeruginosa* **osteomyelitis** and **cellulitis**. *P. aeruginosa* infects chronic cutaneous

TABLE 18-1 Relationship Between Various *Pseudomonas aeruginosa* Infection and Predisposing Factors

Site of Infection	Predisposing Factors
Respiratory tract	Immunocompromised status, including neutropenia and AIDS
	Chemotherapy, ventilator associated
	Chronic lung disease, congestive heart failure
	Cystic fibrosis
Cardiac system	Prosthetic heart valves
	Intravenous drug abuse
Central nervous system	Trauma, surgery
Ear	Diabetes and age
	Injury, maceration, inflammation
	Wet or moist conditions
Cornea and eye	Injury
	Extended wear contact lenses
Bone and joint	Puncture, trauma
	Intravenous drug abuse
Bacteremia and septicemia	Immunocompromised status including diabetes mellitus, immunodeficiency, neutropenia, and burns
	Catheterization
Urinary tract	Obstruction, catheterization, surgery
Gastrointestinal	Immunocompromised status, portal for bacteremia
Skin and soft tissue	Burns, puncture, trauma
	Associated with contaminated pools or hot tubs

ulcers in persons with impaired local circulation, such as diabetics. Once the organism has gained entry, dissemination through the bloodstream and sepsis are possible. Patients with severe defects in immunity, such as those induced by malignancies or chemotherapeutic or other immunosuppressive agents, are at greatest risk from systemic pseudomonal infections. As such, acquisition of *P. aeruginosa* and other Gram-negatives in the hospital is an important problem. Infections in hospital patients are most often caused by the bacteria with which they are colonized.

CASE

Infection of an Immunocompromised Patient

H., a 4-year-old white boy on maintenance chemotherapy for acute lymphocytic leukemia (in remission), was brought by his parents to the emergency room because of fevers as high as 41°C over the preceding 24 hours. In the emergency room, he was alert but appeared ill and preferred to sit on his mother's lap. His skin was pale, his breath and pulse were rapid, and he was in mild respiratory distress with clear lung fields. Despite his fever, his extremities were cool and clammy. A central venous catheter had been surgically implanted because of the many intravenous medications he required. The site where the catheter entered the skin was intact and dry without any redness.

Blood analysis revealed that he had a white blood count of 2,000/mm³, of which 30% were neutrophils (an absolute neutrophil count of 600, normal being >1,000). A third-generation cephalosporin (ceftazidime) and an aminoglycoside (tobramycin) were started intravenously. Within the next few hours, H.'s status deteriorated, with worsening respiratory distress requiring intubation and mechanical ventilation and circulatory failure requiring fluid therapy

continued on page 222

and drugs to increase his blood pressure. He was tentatively diagnosed with shock probably caused by sepsis, due to the host response to the bacterial infection of the bloodstream.

The initial blood cultures were positive for *Pseudomonas aeruginosa,* but those obtained during fevers the second and third days of hospitalization were negative. H. gradually improved, and he was slowly weaned from the drugs used to increase his blood pressure and from ventilatory support. His next course of cancer chemotherapy was delayed because his blood counts remained low, but eventually, they did improve and his therapy was continued.

This case raises several questions:

1. What was the main predisposing factor for H.'s illness?
2. Where did *P. aeruginosa* come from? How did it gain entry into H.'s bloodstream?
3. What caused the symptoms of the infection?
4. What other sites could become infected in such a patient?

See Appendix for answers.

H.'s impaired host defenses, a consequence of his cancer and treatment, put him at increased risk for infection. Although not a factor in this case, an endotracheal tube or an indwelling catheter in the bladder or a vein increases risk by serving as a portal for infection.

CASE

Infection of a Cystic Fibrosis Patient

The parents of Z., a 2-year-old girl with a chronic cough, became alarmed because her cough worsened over a week's time and her color "became poor." Her parents told the pediatrician that they could not remember when she was last cough-free and that she would sometimes spit yellow–green mucus after forceful coughing, most often on arising in the morning.

On examination, Z. was an alert but pasty and pale-looking child with increased respiratory effort and rapid breathing. On inspiration, crackles were heard throughout the lung fields. Her extremities showed moderate clubbing with mild cyanosis. A chest radiograph showed increased (abnormal)

interstitial and peribronchial markings (Fig. 18-1A). By gagging the child with a sterile swab, a specimen of the green mucus was obtained and sent for Gram stain and culture.

Based on the history, physical examination, and radiograph, a tentative diagnosis of cystic fibrosis was made. Intravenous ceftazidime and tobramycin were administered while awaiting the results of a sweat chloride test (diagnostic of cystic fibrosis) and sputum culture. The sputum Gram stain showed many Gram-negative bacilli. In culture, the bacteria were initially described as non–lactose-fermenting Gram-negative rods and then identified as *Pseudomonas aeruginosa.* Z. gradually improved, and after 2 weeks of therapy, her radiograph showed improvement (Fig. 18-1B).

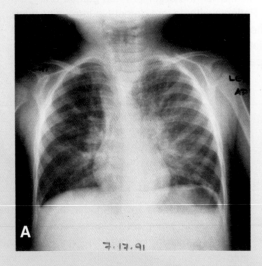
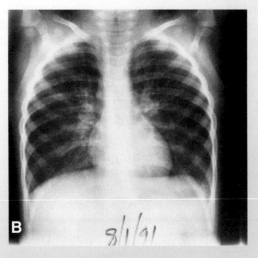

FIGURE 18-1. Chest radiograph of a patient before and after antibiotic treatment. A. X-ray shows interstitial and peribronchial markings. **B.** X-ray of the same patient after 2 weeks of intravenously administered ceftazidime and tobramycin.

This case raises several questions:

1. How does the *P. aeruginosa* infection in Z.'s case differ from that of H.?
2. Is the strain of *Pseudomonas* that infects patients with cystic fibrosis the same that infects other people?
3. What was the route of entry of the organism in Z.'s case?
4. Would antibiotics help in Z.'s case?

See Appendix for answers.

This case illustrates an early episode in the course of *P. aeruginosa* infection in **cystic fibrosis**. Cystic fibrosis is an autosomal recessive disease affecting many organs, including the gastrointestinal and respiratory tracts and the pancreas. Patients can be identified by their failure to gain weight and high concentrations of sweat electrolytes. Many of the clinical manifestations can be treated with pancreatic enzymes. However, the lung is the primary site of infection; chronic respiratory infections, particularly with *P. aeruginosa*, are the major cause of morbidity and mortality in cystic fibrosis patients. Bronchopulmonary *P. aeruginosa* infection in this disease is characterized by exacerbations and remissions. Although the organism is probably never completely eradicated, antipseudomonal antibiotic therapy leads to a decrease in the number of organisms in the sputum and improved pulmonary function.

Interestingly, some antibiotics with little in vitro antipseudomonal activity often appear to improve the clinical status of patients with cystic fibrosis. It is possible that these antibiotics downregulate the production of virulence factors by *P. aeruginosa* in the cystic fibrosis lung. In fact, laboratory studies with subinhibitory concentrations of antibiotics have shown this effect.

In chronic infections in the cystic fibrosis lung, *P. aeruginosa* strains have a mucoid appearance that is not found among environmental isolates or those causing other infections; mucoid strains are associated almost exclusively with this disease. Overproduction of polysaccharide alginate, responsible for the mucoid phenotype, does not by itself cause tissue destruction, but it can enable the organism to evade host defenses and persist in the lung.

P. aeruginosa infection in cystic fibrosis is unique because of its exceptionally chronic course. Individuals can become infected in childhood and, despite continued infection, live into the fourth or fifth decade of life with ongoing therapy. Although the infection is never cleared and lung function progressively declines, *P. aeruginosa* bacteremia virtually never occurs in cystic fibrosis.

THE PATHOGEN: *PSEUDOMONAS AERUGINOSA*

The members of the genus *Pseudomonas*, colloquially called the pseudomonads, belong to a large group of aerobic nonfermenting, actively motile Gram-negative rods. Pseudomonads generally appear positive in an oxidase test, frequently used in diagnostic microbiology to distinguish them from other Gram-negative bacteria, such as *Escherichia coli*. Pseudomonads often produce water-soluble pigments, giving them distinctive colors on solid media. They are motile bacteria owing to the presence of one or several polar flagella. Rapidly growing, robust organisms, pseudomonads can persist in marginal environments. Consequently, they are difficult to eradicate from contaminated areas, such as hospital rooms, clinics, operating rooms, and medical equipment, including respiratory support devices. They may even survive in some antiseptic solutions used to disinfect instruments and endoscopes.

These organisms do not carry out fermentations; rather, they obtain energy from the oxidation of sugars. Many strains can grow anaerobically using nitrate as a terminal electron acceptor. Pseudomonads have minimal nutritional requirements, needing only acetate and ammonia as sources of carbon and nitrogen, respectively. In addition, these simple needs are met by a large number of organic compounds, so they grow well on relatively simple minimal media in addition to common complex laboratory media. However, pseudomonads generally cannot break down polymers into monomers and thus cannot use lactose or sucrose as their sole source of carbon.

Medically, the most important species of this genus is *P. aeruginosa*, but others also cause disease, albeit infrequently. Colonies of *P. aeruginosa* are distinguished from other bacteria of this genus by the production of the water-soluble pigments **pyocyanin** and **pyoverdin**, giving them a characteristic blue-green and yellow-green color on agar media, respectively (Fig. 18-2). On agar plates, colonies of the organism have a characteristic fruity, grapelike, or corn tortilla–like odor, which is sometimes noticed near wounds or other sites that are heavily colonized. *P. aeruginosa* can grow between 20°C and 43°C; growth at the higher temperature can distinguish it from other pseudomonads.

A large number of cell-associated and secreted molecules participate in the pathogenesis of *P. aeruginosa* infections (Table 18-2). As discussed in the case of Z., some strains associated with lung infections in cystic fibrosis patients make a capsule composed of the polysaccharide **alginate** that gives colonies a distinctive mucoid phenotype.

To analyze the importance of potential virulence factors as well as to test new therapeutic strategies to

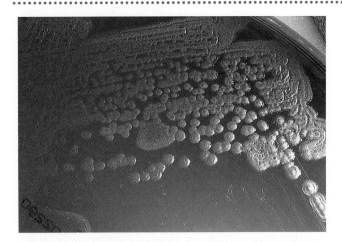

FIGURE 18-2. Appearance of *Pseudomonas aeruginosa* growing on a colorless media. Notice the staining of the media with pyoverdin, the green pigment produced by this organism.

combat *P. aeruginosa*, animal models of infection have been developed. Models that involve injury of epithelium or immune suppression before exposure to the organism have proven particularly informative. These models are attractive because they take into account the clinical observation that *P. aeruginosa* infections occur when the immune system—local or systemic—is breached.

Although appropriate animal models have been developed to study the pathogenesis of acute *P. aeruginosa* infections such as those occurring after corneal injury, burns, or administration of cytotoxins as chemotherapeutic agents, developing an animal model of the chronic, persistent lung infection seen in cystic fibrosis is more difficult. When *P. aeruginosa* is instilled intratracheally in an animal, the bacteria are either cleared or the animal dies of acute pneumonia. To overcome this problem and establish experimental chronic infection, bacteria are embedded in agar beads or alginate before instillation. Histological changes resembling those seen in cystic fibrosis lung infection then occur. These acute and chronic infection models are useful for studying therapeutic interventions or, by studying mutant strains constructed in the laboratory, it is possible to study the role of specific bacterial gene products during infection. Epidemiological and animal studies demonstrate the importance of various virulence factors (see Table 18-2).

TABLE 18-2 Notable Virulence Factors of *Pseudomonas aeruginosa*

Product	Location	Mechanism of Action	Possible Contribution to Virulence
Pili	Polar	Adherence, twitching motility	Biofilm formation, colonization
Flagellum	Polar	Motility, adherence	Dissemination and initiation of the innate immune response
Siderophores (pyoverdin and pyochelin)	Secreted	Scavenge iron	Acquisition of iron
Pyocyanin	Secreted	Generates reactive oxygen species	Tissue damage
Exotoxin A	Secreted	ADP-ribosylation of EF-2	Inhibits host cell protein synthesis
Exoenzymes: ExoS, ExoU, ExoT, ExoY	Secreted via type III secretion system	Interaction with components of the host cell cytoskeleton	Cytotoxicity, tissue damage, antiphagocytosi
Elastase	Secreted	Proteolysis of proteins such as elastin, collagen, immunoglobulins, complement components	Tissue damage
Proteases	Secreted	Proteolysis	Tissue damage
Phospholipases	Secreted	Hydrolysis of phospholipids, especially in eukaryotic membranes	Tissue damage, obtaining phosphate
Rhamnolipid	Secreted	Biosurfactant	Hemolysin, dispersion of biofilms
Alginate	Cell associated	Adherence, protection from dehydration, and immune evasion	Antiphagocytic, biofilm formation
Other polysaccharides	Cell associated	Adherence	Biofilm formation
Lipopolysaccharide	Outer membrane	Lipid A is endotoxic; core interacts CFTR; O antigen protects from complement-mediated killing	Sepsis, internalization, serum resistance

ENCOUNTER AND ENTRY

Because *P. aeruginosa* lives in the water and soil, it can be found on vegetables and living plants as well as in water taps, drains, and other wet surfaces. Humans can ingest the *P. aeruginosa* from such sources. Splashed water from a contaminated sink or shower, or droplets suctioned from a colonized endotracheal tube can spread the organism. This is generally not a cause for worry because, for the most part, *P. aeruginosa* relies on a breakdown of normal human defenses before it can cause infection. In fact, while it can be found in normal intestinal microbiota and on the skin, *P. aeruginosa* does not adhere well to normal intact epithelium. However, if present in large enough numbers, *P. aeruginosa* can enter the skin, possibly through insignificant abrasions. Infections involving the hair follicles (**folliculitis**) can occur as a result of bathing in contaminated hot tubs. The temperature in hot tubs favors *Pseudomonas* reproduction: a hot tub can contain up to 100 million organisms per milliliter. Such large inocula can overwhelm normal defenses and result in infections, even in immunocompetent people. In swimmers, *P. aeruginosa* can cause **otitis externa** that may be benign or serious and is often recurrent. In the case of immunosuppressed or otherwise compromised people, *P. aeruginosa* can cause infections that initiate at the site of compromise. Particularly in hospitalized patients, these localized infections can lead to more severe disease. For example, aspiration of *P. aeruginosa* into the respiratory tract can lead to serious **pneumonia**. Similarly, **gastrointestinal colonization** or **catheter-related infections** can lead to bacteremia. Importantly, the gastrointestinal tract can be the portal when neutropenic patients get *P. aeruginosa*, as chemotherapy can be distributive to the gastrointestinal mucosa.

SPREAD

To cause disease, *P. aeruginosa* must get to and establish itself at the site of infection. *P. aeruginosa* has at least three distinct modes of motility. It has the typical **flagella-mediated motility**, whereby the bacteria swim, and a second system of **twitching motility**. This latter form of motility results from the extension and retraction of the organism's polar pili. *P. aeruginosa* also has **swarming motility** that is dependent on both flagella and pili.

Adherence and Colonization

Aside from their functions in motility, both these factors have other roles with respect to virulence. Flagella and pili mediate adherence to epithelial cells. This capability may result from their interactions with the glycolipid **asialo GM1** on the host cell surface. In addition, flagella interact with one of the components of the innate immune system, the **toll-like receptor** (TLR) TLR5, to initiate an inflammatory response. **Type IV pili** are important for the initiation of the formation of structures called **biofilms**. These complex structures house bacteria held together by polysaccharides and other polymers and proteins and are responsible for adherence to surfaces, protection from dehydration, and increased antibiotic resistance. The so-called biofilm mode of growth is distinct from how bacteria grow in culture and in blood infections and may aid in attachment to cells and avoidance of immune cell recognition. The polysaccharide **alginate** can also act as an adhesin that offers protection. Alginate is one of the major components of the biofilm in isolates from the lungs of cystic fibrosis patients.

Lipopolysaccharide (LPS; endotoxin) can act as an adhesin. LPS is composed of three parts. The first is the lipid A portion, which is the biologically active component of LPS that interacts with the host cell receptor TLR4 to initiate the inflammatory response. This interaction is responsible for inducing many inflammatory effectors that lead to the production of acute-phase proteins, fever, hypotension, and other effects generally known as Gram-negative sepsis. In the case of *P. aeruginosa*, lipid A is generally less inflammatory than that of other typical Gram-negative bacteria, such as *E. coli* and *Salmonella typhimurium*. However, in susceptible patients like H., *P. aeruginosa* can cause hypotension and shock. The second part of LPS is the core oligosaccharide that interacts with the cystic fibrosis transmembrane conductance regulator (**CFTR**) on epithelial cells. This interaction leads to bacterial internalization and initiation of innate immune resistance to the pathogen. The third part of LPS is the O-antigen side chain; expression of long O-antigen side chains is responsible for resistance to normal human serum, detergents, and some antibiotics (see Chapter 3); strains without O antigen can be killed by normal human serum. Strains of *P. aeruginosa* isolated from chronic lung infections in cystic fibrosis patients often have an O-antigen defect and thus are serum sensitive, which explains in part why bacteremia is so rare in cystic fibrosis.

MULTIPLICATION

P. aeruginosa are typical extracellular pathogens. Their growth in tissue depends largely on their ability to resist ingestion by neutrophils. The low frequency of *P. aeruginosa* infections in healthy persons shows that the phagocytes and epithelial cells usually have the upper hand. Patients with reduced numbers of circulating neutrophils, like H. in the case presented earlier, are at high risk for *P. aeruginosa* infection.

What determines whether colonization, local infection, or systemic infection occurs after contact with *P. aeruginosa*? Examining mutant strains of *P. aeruginosa* in animal models has allowed the role of specific gene products to be studied. In these experiments, animals can be infected with strains differing only in one gene, and thus, any pathogenic differences can be attributed to the product of this gene. In a burned mouse model, strains deficient in any of a number of products (exotoxin A, elastase, or ExoS; see Table 18-2) persist in the wound but do not disseminate. Strains lacking flagella are also less virulent than wild-type strains. In an experimental model of ulcerative keratitis, ExoU and ExoT are virulence factors and pili and flagella act as adhesins. In this model, LPS–CFTR-mediated internalization leads to survival within buried epithelial cells and increased corneal injury.

P. aeruginosa employs several strategies to obtain scarce nutrients during infection. Obtaining iron is vital and difficult; virtually all the iron in human serum is tightly bound to transferrin. *P. aeruginosa* produces iron-binding **siderophores** (see Chapter 3), which compete with transferrin for iron. Iron limitation increases the production of secreted products of *P. aeruginosa*, including siderophores, exotoxin A, proteases, and the biosurfactant **rhamnolipid**. In turn, these molecules may damage tissues, making iron more accessible to the organism. When another necessary nutrient, phosphate, is limited, *P. aeruginosa* increases production of **phospholipase C**. This enzyme can hydrolyze phospholipids from host cell membranes to release phosphate in an available form.

P. aeruginosa elaborates a wide variety of exotoxins that can cause local inflammation and tissue destruction. This damage can degrade tissues and enable *P. aeruginosa* to obtain the nutrients it needs to persist. Damage may also be necessary for dissemination; as mentioned previously, strains lacking exotoxins and elastase persist locally in burn wounds but fail to disseminate.

To survive in the host, *Pseudomonas* must not only obtain nutrition but also be able to evade host defenses. In the bloodstream, the organisms do not usually survive and only cause bacteremia and sepsis in immunocompromised patients, as in the case of H. **Neutrophils** are clearly involved in curbing the proliferation of the organism, as seen by the increased incidence of *P. aeruginosa* sepsis in persons with severe neutropenia.

P. aeruginosa specifically colonizes the lungs of patients with cystic fibrosis, like Z., even though these individuals have an apparently functional immune system. Several independent, although not completely mutually exclusive, theories explain the hypersusceptibility of cystic fibrosis patients to chronic *P. aeruginosa* lung infections. In this disease, ion transport across the respiratory epithelium is abnormal because of a defect in CFTR. Persistence of the organism may be attributable, in part, to dehydration of respiratory secretions resulting in impairment of the mucociliary system, which normally rids the lungs of inhaled particles and bacteria. A controversial theory holds that the cystic fibrosis lung environment inhibits the effectiveness of antimicrobial peptides. One finding suggests that *P. aeruginosa* binds to asialo GM1, and the expression of this glycolipid is increased on epithelial cells from cystic fibrosis patients. On the other hand, *P. aeruginosa* can activate and be internalized into CFTR-expressing cells; internalization, which may be responsible for clearance, is defective in cystic fibrosis. Moreover, although high levels of antibodies to *P. aeruginosa* antigens have been found in serum from cystic fibrosis patients, they

appear to be ineffective at clearing the infection. This may be a result of specificity of the antibodies, particularly in their ability to opsonize *P. aeruginosa*.

P. aeruginosa also changes in character during the chronic lung infections in cystic fibrosis patients. As mentioned earlier, the production of alginate is increased, resulting in a mucoid appearance. In addition, strains express an altered LPS that has a modified lipid A structure and are defective for O-antigen production. These cystic fibrosis isolates also express fewer proteases and toxins and become nonmotile, all of which may serve to hide the organism from the immune system. The switch to a "chronic" phenotype is under complex regulation. Chronically infecting strains are generally not transferred between cystic fibrosis patients; however, epidemic lineages have now emerged. The determination of complete genome sequences of *P. aeruginosa* strains from various types of infections has enabled investigations into the regulation of virulence factor production and the similarities and differences between clinical and environmental isolates of this ubiquitous opportunist.

DAMAGE

For a generally innocuous bacterium, *P. aeruginosa* produces a wide variety of damage-causing factors. It secretes a toxin, **exotoxin A**, whose activity is identical to that of the diphtheria toxin, ADP-ribosylating host elongation factor 2, which is required for protein synthesis. *P. aeruginosa* also secretes a number of extracellular proteases of varying specificities. **Elastase**, as its name suggests, can degrade elastin in host cells. However, it is actually a zinc metalloprotease that degrades a myriad of other proteins as well. Another protease, **LasA**, is a serine protease that acts synergistically with elastase to degrade elastin. Other proteases, including alkaline protease and protease IV, have activities on components of host cells. Phospholipases hydrolyze phospholipids and cause membrane perturbation. While mutant strains lacking genes encoding these enzymes are often defective in animal models of infection, they often have overlapping specificities, making it difficult to identify the exact functions of any of these in a natural infectious process. Injury of host cells and tissues by these bacterial factors may also lead to increased attachment and colonization. In fact, *P. aeruginosa* appears to bind much more avidly to damaged epithelium.

P. aeruginosa also injects a number of virulence factors directly into host cells. These proteins are delivered using a **type III secretion system (T3SS)**. With its structure similar to flagella, the T3SS targets specific proteins from the cytosol of the bacteria into the cytoplasm of the host cell, thereby avoiding diffusion of the transferred proteins and their recognition by the immune system. Secretion is induced by host cell contact or environmental signals such as low calcium that apparently mimic this situation. In the case of *P. aeruginosa*, secretion of the effectors **ExoS**, **ExoT**, **ExoU**, and **ExoY** is controlled by the transcription activator ExsA. ExoS and ExoT have similar activities: both can ADP-ribosylate target proteins. However, each also has unique functions: ExoS causes rounding of cells, and ExoT interferes with internalization of *P. aeruginosa* by epithelial cells and macrophages. ExoY has adenyl cyclase activity. ExoU is a phospholipase that readily causes lysis of host cells. The production of this latter cytotoxin is associated with more severe disease; strains isolated from lung infections in cystic fibrosis patients rarely produce ExoU. More recently, a newly identified secretion system, called **type VI secretion**, has been described in *P. aeruginosa*; however, the effects of factors secreted by this system and its role in pathogenicity—if any—have not been fully elucidated.

In addition to the detection of and response to host cells, *P. aeruginosa* can sense and react to the presence of other bacteria in their environment. This **quorum-sensing** activity results from the production of **autoinducers**, of which *P. aeruginosa* can synthesize at least three: two that are derivatives of the molecule **homoserine lactone** and one that is similar to **quinolones**. These molecules readily diffuse out of the bacteria. With increasing cell density, the autoinducers can accumulate inside the bacteria and, once they reach a threshold level, can bind to a regulatory protein and together activate transcription of a number of genes. Up to 10% of *P. aeruginosa* genes may be regulated by quorum sensing, and many of these genes encode known or potential virulence factors. In fact, biofilm formation is regulated by one of the autoinducers. The use of quorum sensing to control expression of these factors may allow *P. aeruginosa* to accumulate in the host before inducing the expression of immunoactivating factors. *P. aeruginosa* quorum-sensing mutants are less virulent in many animal models of infection. In addition, *P. aeruginosa* can likely sense and respond to molecules released by other species of bacteria in their environment. Aside from its role in regulation, one of these *P. aeruginosa* autoinducers itself can induce a potent immune response.

The antimicrobial resistance of *P. aeruginosa* is a predisposing factor in treatment failure. This resistance of *P. aeruginosa* is the result of the limited permeability of the outer membrane as well as the presence of numerous multidrug resistance efflux pumps. As is typical for all bacteria, *P. aeruginosa* can also readily acquire antibiotic resistance genes from other bacteria by transformation, conjugation, and transduction. In addition, the biofilm mode of growth provides protection from antibiotics.

DIAGNOSIS

P. aeruginosa is easily cultured and identified by the clinical microbiology laboratory. Culture of the organism is essential because *P. aeruginosa* is resistant to many commonly used antibiotics, including first- and second-generation penicillins and cephalosporins, tetracyclines, chloramphenicol, and vancomycin. Because the resistance pattern among *P. aeruginosa* isolates varies from hospital to hospital and changes from year to year, knowledge of prevailing patterns of susceptibility and resistance in a given hospital allows for empiric therapy while awaiting culture and sensitivity results.

TREATMENT AND PREVENTION

The outcome of *P. aeruginosa* infection depends on the nature and severity of the infection, the state of host defenses, and the promptness and efficacy of treatment. A high-grade bacteremia in a neutropenic patient carries a 50 to 70% mortality rate. Because *P. aeruginosa* is relatively resistant to most antimicrobials, serious infections are sometimes treated with two antibiotics in combination to achieve an additive or synergistic effect. The extended-spectrum β-lactams, carbapenems, aminoglycosides, and fluoroquinolones are often effective. Clearly, the ability to develop and acquire antibiotic resistance contributes to the success of *P. aeruginosa* in the hospital environment, as does the resistance of the organism to many commonly used disinfecting agents. In some hospitals, *Pseudomonas* isolates resistant to all available antibiotics have been encountered, portending a potentially frightening future unless novel means of controlling these bacteria are discovered. In the absence of better antibacterial agents, careful attention to infection control measures may prevent the spread of *P. aeruginosa*—particularly the highly resistant isolates—among hospitalized patients.

CONCLUSION

P. aeruginosa is a model opportunistic environmental bacterium. It is abundant in our environment but causes diseases mainly in individuals who have impaired defenses. Occasionally, if the inoculum size is very large, it overcomes the defenses of healthy persons. Preventing and treating *P. aeruginosa* infection in patients debilitated by major underlying diseases, by developing either new antimicrobials or vaccines, is an important goal in modern medicine.

Suggested Readings

Gómez MI, Prince A. Opportunistic infections in lung disease: *Pseudomonas* infections in cystic fibrosis. *Curr Opin Pharmacol.* 2007;7:244–251.

Harmsen M, Yang L, Pamp SJ, et al. An update on *Pseudomonas aeruginosa* biofilm formation, tolerance, and dispersal. *FEMS Immunol Med Microbiol.* 2010;59:253–268.

Hauser AR. The type III secretion system of *Pseudomonas aeruginosa*: infection by injection. *Nat Rev Microbiol.* 2009;7:654–665.

Nordmann P, Naas T, Fortineau N, et al. Superbugs in the coming new decade; multidrug resistance and prospect for treatment of *Staphylococcus aureus, Enterococcus* spp. and *Pseudomonas aeruginosa* in 2010. *Curr Opin Microbiol.* 2007;10:436–440.

Wolfgang MC, Kulasekara BR, Liang XY, et al. Conservation of genome content and virulence determinants among clinical and environmental isolates of *Pseudomonas aeruginosa*. *Proc Natl Acad Sci USA.* 2003;100:8484–8489.

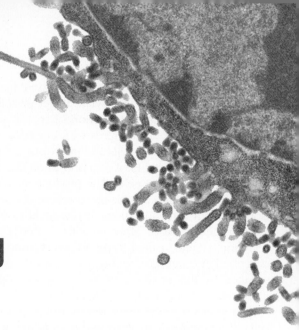

Chapter 19

Bordetella and Whooping Cough

Victor J. DiRita and Peggy A. Cotter

KEY CONCEPTS

Pathogens: *Bordetella pertussis* and *Bordetella parapertussis*

Encounter: These agents infect only the human respiratory tract. Therefore, infected humans are the source of all transmission, and older adolescents and adults are frequently the source of infection for susceptible infants.

Entry: Pertussis is extremely contagious and is acquired by direct contact or inhalation of respiratory droplets.

Spread and Multiplication: The organisms colonize upper and lower respiratory airways, but they do not disseminate or invade deeper tissues.

Damage: Pertussis (aka whooping cough) is a disease that causes characteristic paroxysmal cough in infants and prolonged hacking cough in adults.

Disease depends on several virulence factors, including microbial adhesins and toxins.

Diagnosis: Can be cultured from nasopharyngeal swabs on Bordet-Gengou media, but culture becomes less sensitive as the disease progresses. A rapid diagnosis is usually made with a direct fluorescent antibody test or molecular techniques.

Treatment: Macrolides and tetracyclines are active against *B. pertussis* but yield a significant improvement and reduction of bacterial shedding only when given early in the course of illness to infected patients.

Prevention: Infection can be prevented by immunizing with DPT or DTaP vaccines containing *B. pertussis* antigens, along with diphtheria and tetanus antigens.

PERTUSSIS, or whooping cough, is caused by *Bordetella pertussis* and *Bordetella parapertussis*, two extremely closely related bacteria that specifically colonize ciliated epithelial cells in the nasopharynx, trachea, bronchi, and bronchioles of humans. These **Gram-negative coccobacilli** produce powerful toxins that penetrate tissues, kill cells, immobilize the ciliary escalator, and cause the accumulation of thick mucus in the airway. The characteristic paroxysmal coughing spasms followed by a long, inspiratory "whoop" are thought to be caused by sensitization of cough receptors in the trachea and by the patient's effort to expectorate the accumulated mucus and cell debris. Killed whole *B. pertussis* cells added to diphtheria and tetanus toxoids yields the **DPT vaccine**, which has been given to infants for many years. Rare but unpleasant adverse effects of the DPT vaccine compelled the development of a widely used **acellular** vaccine consisting of inactivated toxins and adhesins. Along with the diphtheria and tetanus toxoids, the triple vaccine is called **DTaP**.

Whooping cough, or **pertussis**, is a respiratory disease that is especially severe in infants and young children. It is one of the most contagious infectious diseases known with transmission rates among household contacts nearing 90%. Before the advent of pertussis vaccines, incidence of pertussis was high, peaking at 260,000 cases in the United States in 1938. The original pertussis vaccine (the "P" in DPT) contained killed *B. pertussis* cells and was effective in preventing the disease. A steady decline in pertussis cases followed its introduction in 1949 from an average of 150 cases per 100,000 persons to 0.5 cases per 100,000 in 1976. However, the vaccine was responsible for rare episodes of fever with convulsions. As a result, reduced compliance with vaccine regimens in the 1970s reversed the downward trend and spurred the development of new acellular pertussis vaccines (the "aP" in DTaP). DTaP contains two to four *B. pertussis* proteins rather than whole, killed bacteria.

Although the availability of DTaP vaccines has increased compliance rates and hence decreased incidence, the number of pertussis cases in the United States and other countries with universal vaccine programs has been on the rise in recent decades and was 8.6 per 100,000 persons in the United States in 2005. The recent increase has been attributed to waning immunity in older adolescents and young adults, as well as increased awareness of the disease and improved diagnostics. In countries without widespread vaccination programs, pertussis continues to be a highly prevalent disease. Worldwide, there are currently nearly 50 million cases annually with about 300,000 deaths, mostly in infants.

Whooping cough is an important disease for four reasons:

1. Adults with mild disease, indistinguishable from a cold, are the reservoir.
2. It is highly communicable among susceptible infants less than 1 year old.
3. It is life threatening in infants with underlying cardiac or pulmonary disease.
4. It can lead to neurological sequelae.

Local manifestations of whooping cough are **tracheitis** and **bronchitis**, with accumulation of mucus, inflammatory cells, bacteria, and dead epithelial cells in the airway lumen. The **mucociliary escalator** is impaired by damage to ciliated epithelial cells, and the cough is easily triggered because cough receptors are sensitized. Intense straining against closed vocal cords (known as a **Valsalva maneuver**) in an effort to expel mucus and debris in the lower airway can lead to hemorrhages in the brain, conjunctiva, and beneath the tongue. The result is the violent cough with gasping for air that gives the disease its name. Systemic manifestations include low-grade fever, malaise, and lymphocytosis. Swallowing can precipitate a coughing attack and therefore infants and young children may resist feeding, leading to dehydration.

THE PATHOGENS: *BORDETELLA PERTUSSIS* AND *BORDETELLA PARAPERTUSSIS*

Bordetella species are small, Gram-negative, aerobic coccobacilli belonging to a group of nutritionally fastidious organisms that includes the genus *Haemophilus*.

They grow on complex media containing blood, which fulfills nutritional requirements, plus other additives to neutralize fatty acids and other inhibitory compounds. *B. pertussis* and *B. parapertussis*, the causative agents of whooping cough, belong to an extremely closely related group of bacteria known as the *Bordetella bronchiseptica* cluster. *B. pertussis* and *B. parapertussis* diverged recently and independently from a *B. bronchiseptica*–like ancestor, infect only humans, and do not survive outside the body for appreciable amounts of time. *B. bronchiseptica*, by contrast, has a broad host range and can survive in the environment indefinitely. Although typically considered a veterinary pathogen, *B. bronchiseptica* can infect humans and has been associated with serious disease in immunocompromised patients.

Bordetellae have specific proteins (adhesins) on their surface that allow them to attach to ciliated epithelial cells of the respiratory tract. They also secrete toxins that penetrate host cells and ultimately cause the signs and symptoms of the disease. Like other Gram-negative bacteria, *Bordetella* contain **endotoxin** (lipopolysaccharide [LPS]), which likely initiates induction of the innate inflammatory response and consequent disease symptoms, including fever.

CASE • Eight weeks after her birth, L. was taken to her family doctor for a checkup and her first baby shot. The immunization was postponed for a month because she had a slight cold and a runny nose. The baby may have acquired her cold from one of her three siblings or a grandfather living with the family, who all had colds recently. Subsequently, L. began sneezing and coughing. Any loud noise would bring on a coughing spell. L.'s mother became concerned when the baby turned blue after a series of coughing spells that ended with vomiting. Later, during an examination of the infant by a physician, L. had a series of "barky" coughs, after which she vomited and could not catch her breath. L.'s mother was told that her baby had whooping cough and needed to be hospitalized.

The laboratory report showed an elevated white blood cell count, due specifically to an increased number of lymphocytes. A nasopharyngeal specimen, evaluated using an immunofluorescent assay, contained *Bordetella pertussis*, the causative agent of whooping cough.

This case raises several questions:

1. How dangerous is whooping cough?
2. Why was the physician sure of the diagnosis?
3. Where did L. catch the "bug"?
4. Will antibiotics make L. better?
5. When can L. start getting her vaccinations?

See Appendix for answers.

ENCOUNTER

B. pertussis and *B. parapertussis* appear to be exclusively human-specific pathogens; there are no known environmental or animal reservoirs. Their persistence in the human population is thought to be due to infection of older adolescents and adults with fading immunity. The basis of the exceptional contagiousness of pertussis is unknown and puzzling, since the ability to recover *B. pertussis* or *B. parapertussis* from patients with whooping cough is low and decreases as the disease progresses. The bacteria are rarely recovered from the nasopharynx of healthy persons.

Not all people will recognize that they have been infected by *B. pertussis* or *B. parapertussis* because symptoms are dependent on several factors, including age and the state of immunity. Infants and young children typically will have "classic whooping cough," characterized by three stages. The **catarrhal stage** is often indistinguishable from initial stages of the common cold with signs including rhinorrhea, lacrimation, and mild cough. The **paroxysmal stage** initiates over a 7- to 14-day period, as symptoms worsen and the characteristic paroxysmal coughing spasms develop. Paroxysms are characterized by 10 or more forceful coughs during a single expiration followed by a massive inspiratory effort against a closed glottis, which produces the classic "whoop." During the paroxysm, cyanosis, bulging eyes, protrusion of the tongue, salivation, lacrimation, and distension of the neck veins may occur. At the end of a paroxysm, the patient frequently vomits. Paroxysms usually occur in groups, and there may be several groups per hour, round the clock, at the height of the disease. The paroxysmal stage lasts 2 to 8 weeks. The **convalescent stage**, during which paroxysms decrease in frequency and intensity, can last up to 6 months. Older adolescents and adults are more likely to experience mild disease or be asymptomatically infected, and therefore, the incidence of pertussis is probably vastly underestimated. It is becoming increasingly clear that neither immunization nor previous infection provides lifelong immunity. It is important, therefore, that physicians treating babies like L. take a complete history of all family members and alert them of the possibility that they may contract or already have whooping cough.

ENTRY

B. pertussis and *B. parapertussis* most likely enter the trachea and bronchi by inhalation. The organisms attach specifically to the cilia of epithelial cells in the nasopharynx and the large airways and are seldom found elsewhere (Fig. 19-1). Although there is some evidence to the contrary, whooping cough is believed to be an entirely superficial infection, that is, the organisms remain on the mucosal surface and do not invade tissues. Other important bacterial diseases with this characteristic include diphtheria and cholera. All of these bacteria secrete toxins

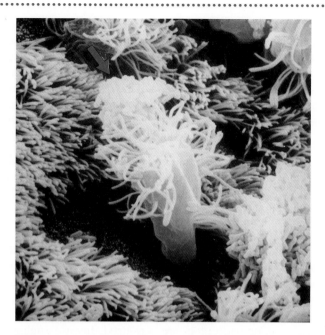

FIGURE 19-1. *Bordetella pertussis* **adhering to ciliated respiratory epithelial cells seen by scanning electron microscopy.** The *arrow* points to the clump of bacteria attached to the partially extruded epithelial cell.

that have dramatic effects on host cells and that appear to be responsible for a majority of disease manifestations.

The molecular basis of the tropism of *Bordetella* for cilia is not understood but is likely the result of specific interactions between bacterial adhesins and host receptor proteins that are present exclusively on cilia. Several surface-localized proteins produced by *B. pertussis* and *B. parapertussis* have been proposed to function as adhesins. These include **fimbriae** (**Fim**) (also called pili), **filamentous hemagglutinin** (**FHA**), and **pertactin** (**Prn**), all of which are included in acellular pertussis vaccines, the rationale being that antibodies against these proteins may block bacteria from adhering to their receptors and therefore prevent the establishment of infection. Host cell receptors to which these proteins bind are not known, but several proteins of the integrin family have been implicated.

SPREAD AND MULTIPLICATION

Experiments with animal models indicate that *Bordetella* multiply dramatically during the first few weeks of infection and can spread quickly from the nasopharynx to the trachea, bronchi, and bronchioles. Masses of bacteria become entrapped in the cilia and thick mucus. It has been suggested that the bacteria may contribute to the process by producing an exopolysaccharide matrix and forming a biofilm. Although the epithelium may remain predominantly intact, sloughing of ciliated epithelial cells occurs, possibly as a host defense mechanism. The submucosa beneath the bacteria becomes increasingly inflamed, and peribronchial lymph nodes enlarge. Reactive hyperplasia in the lymph nodes indicates that bacteria, their toxins, or

PARADIGM BOX

REGULATION OF VIRULENCE PROPERTIES

Like all organisms, bacteria must adapt to changing environmental conditions. Pathogenic bacteria likely encounter a variety of different environments as they travel within and between their eukaryotic hosts. Production of factors that are advantageous in one environment may offer no advantage or even be detrimental in other environments. Consequently, microbes have evolved sophisticated regulatory systems to control production of environment-specific molecules, such as virulence factors.

The signal transduction mechanism used most commonly by bacteria to sense and respond to changing environmental conditions is the two-component regulatory system (TCS). In these systems, a sensor histidine kinase, which usually resides in the cytoplasmic membrane with its signal recognition domain facing outward, phosphorylates itself on a histidine residue (a process called autophosphorylation) in response to "activating" conditions. The phosphoryl group is then transferred to an aspartic acid residue on a response regulator protein, which is usually located in the cytoplasm (Fig. 19-2A). Phosphorylation of the response regulator renders it competent to activate or repress transcription of genes encoding proteins that are needed or not, respectively, in that specific environment. A more complex variant of the TCS is the phosphorelay, which incorporates two additional phosphotransfer steps, presumably to afford the system additional levels of control.

In *Bordetella*, expression of genes encoding all known protein virulence factors is regulated by a phosphorelay system called BvgAS (for *Bordetella* virulence genes). BvgS is a hybrid sensor kinase that undergoes autophosphorylation on a histidine residue in the kinase domain. The phosphoryl group is then transferred to an aspartic acid in the receiver domain, then to a histidine in the C-terminal histidine phosphotransfer domain, and then finally to an aspartic acid residue on the response regulator protein BvgA (Fig. 19-2B). Phosphorylated BvgA activates transcription of genes encoding virulence factors, such as FHA, Fim, adenylate cyclase toxin (ACT), and pertussis toxin (PT), and represses transcription of genes that are not required for virulence.

The basic functions performed by TCS and phosphorelay proteins (autophosphorylation, phosphotransfer, and DNA binding) are similar among the various systems, and hence, the amino acid sequences of the functional domains are highly conserved. It is therefore possible to identify genes encoding potential TCS and phosphorelay systems by sequence analysis tools that can recognize the conserved domains. A single microbe may have several TCS and phosphorelay systems, each

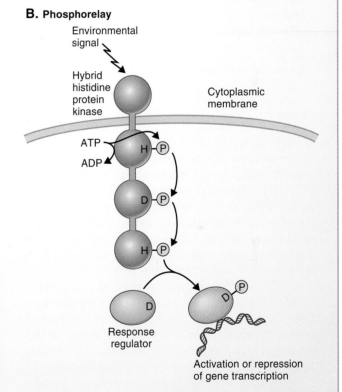

A. Two Component Regulatory System

Environmental signal

Histidine protein kinase

Cytoplasmic membrane

ATP
ADP

H–P

D

D–P

Response regulator

Activation or repression of gene transcription

B. Phosphorelay

Environmental signal

Hybrid histidine protein kinase

Cytoplasmic membrane

ATP
ADP

H–P

D–P

H–P

D

D–P

Response regulator

Activation or repression of gene transcription

FIGURE 19-2. Two-component regulatory systems (TCS) and phosphorelays. A. The histidine protein kinase of a TCS autophosphorylates on a conserved histidine residue in response to activating environmental cues. The phosphoryl group is transferred to an aspartic acid residue on the response regulator. The phosphorylated response regulator protein binds DNA to either allow or prevent the expression of a specific set of genes. **B.** Hybrid histidine kinases also autophosphorylate in response to activating environmental cues. The phosphoryl group is transferred to an aspartic acid residue in the adjacent "receiver" domain, then to a histidine in the C-terminal "histidine phosphotransfer" domain, then to an aspartic acid on the response regulator, which then activates and/or represses transcription of specific genes.

continued on page 232

TABLE 19-1 Examples of Two-Component Regulatory Systems in Pathogenic Bacteria

Organism and Manifestation	Sensor/Regulator	Signals	Regulated Virulence Properties
Bordetella pertussis Whooping cough	BvgS/BvgA	SO_4^{-2}, nicotinic acid, temperature	Pertussis toxin, adenylate cyclase Toxin, fimbriae, filamentous hemagglutinin, and many others
Pseudomonas aeruginosa Lung infections in cystic fibrosis patients	PilS/PilR ?/A1gR	? ?	Pilus colonization factor Alginate biosynthesis, mucoidy
Salmonella Gastroenteritis, typhoid fever, bacteremia	PhoQ/PhoP	Mg^{+2}, cationic antimicrobial peptides	Macrophage survival, invasion of epithelial cells, resistance to innate immune mechanisms
Staphylococcus aureus Abscesses	AgrC/AgrA	Peptide pheromone	Exoprotein production, including activation of hemolysins, proteases, and toxins; repression of coagulase and protein A
Enterococcus faecalis Urinary, biliary, cardiovascular infections	VanS/VanR	Vancomycin	Enzymes for vancomycin resistance
Streptococcus pyogenes Invasive skin infection, necrotizing fasciitis	CsrS/CsrR (CovR/CovS)	Mg^{+2}	Repression of hyaluronic acid capsule and other virulence factors; activation of some genes associated with pathogenicity

controlling a specific set of genes. The genome sequence of *Escherichia coli*, for example, contains 62 genes that are predicted to encode proteins that are components of TCS and phosphorelay systems. The number of TCS and phosphorelay systems produced by a particular bacterial system likely reflects the diversity of environments it encounters. *Helicobacter pylori*, which is thought to live only in the human stomach, produces only a very small number of TCS and phosphorelay proteins.

TCS and phosphorelay systems that regulate a variety of phenotypes in pathogenic microbes have been identified (Table 19-1). Because these systems are unique to bacteria, their exploitation as targets for new classes of broad-spectrum antimicrobials has been proposed and investigated with some limited success.

The possibility that strains of pathogenic bacteria with mutations in specific TCS and phosphorelay systems may be good candidates for vaccine use has also been tested. The rationale for this approach is that some of these regulatory systems may control gene expression only during certain stages of the interaction between the microbe and its human host. Mutants deficient for such systems might survive within the host long enough to elicit an immune response before becoming growth-limited because of the mutation. *Salmonella typhi*, the agent of typhoid fever, was mutated by deletion of the *phoP–phoQ* two-component system that regulates survival of this organism within macrophages. When tested in human volunteers, a single dose of the resulting strain, Ty800, induced greater intestinal and humoral immune responses than did four doses of the approved oral typhoid vaccine strain, Ty21a. This work established a precedent for studying the use of regulatory mutants as vaccines against other important pathogens.

other products have moved to those sites from their origin in the bronchial lumen. The ability to culture *B. pertussis* or *B. parapertussis* from the nasopharynx or from cough specimens of pertussis patients decreases dramatically after the catarrhal stage. Whether the bacteria have actually been eliminated at this point (despite the fact that symptoms are most severe for several weeks afterward) or have moved to deeper, less accessible sites within the respiratory tract is unknown.

DAMAGE

B. pertussis and *B. parapertussis* produce an impressive array of virulence factors (Table 19-2). These can affect a number of cell types, including immune cells, thereby enabling the microbe to significantly modulate the host response. PT, which is produced only by *B. pertussis* and is associated with lymphocytosis, resembles many other bacterial toxins (e.g., cholera toxin, diphtheria toxin, and

TABLE 19-2 Major Toxins and Virulence Factors of *B. pertussis* and *B. parapertussis*

Name	Chemical Nature	Site of Action	Biochemical Activities	Physiological Effects
Pertussis toxin (*B. pertussis* only)	Protein	Local and systemic	ADP-ribosylates G protein	Impairs neutrophil chemotaxis, phagocytosis, and bactericidal activity; lymphocytosis
Adenylate cyclase toxin	Protein	Local	Converts ATP to cAMP Membrane insertion	Histamine sensitization mimics pertussis toxin activity on neutrophils; increases capillary permeability leading to edema Hemolytic activity
Tracheal cytotoxin	Murein	Local	Stimulates nitric oxide production	Cytopathological damage to tracheal epithelia Kills ciliated respiratory epithelial cells; adjuvant
Endotoxin	Lipopolysaccharide	Systemic	Binds CD14 and TLR4 to stimulate pro-inflammatory response	Fever; adjuvant
Fimbriae (pili)	Protein	Local	?	Facilitating adherence to respiratory epithelium
Filamentous hemagglutinin	Protein	Local	Heparin binding; agglutinates red blood cells	Adherence and modulation of innate immunity
Pertactin	Protein	Local	?	Possibly adherence

ADP, adenosine diphosphate; ATP, adenosine triphosphate; cAMP, cyclic adenosine monophosphate.

Pseudomonas exotoxin A) by affecting **cyclic adenosine monophosphate (cAMP) metabolism**. Also like the toxins produced by these other bacteria, PT is an A-B toxin, consisting of an A (active) subunit and a B (binding) domain composed of five nonidentical subunits (see Chapter 9). The toxin attaches to host cells via the B domain allowing the A fragment to enter and act in the cytoplasm. Toxins like PT are **ADP-ribosyltransferases**; they split the nicotinamide portion from nicotinamide adenine dinucleotide (NAD) and attach the remaining ADP-ribose to specific host cell proteins. One of the target proteins is a **G protein** involved in regulation of adenylate cyclase. PT ADP-ribosylates an inhibitory G protein, resulting in constitutive activity of the cellular adenylate cyclase enzyme, and hence, high levels of cAMP are produced inside intoxicated cells, which inhibits important microbicidal activities of phagocytic cells, such as chemotaxis and the oxidative burst. Why PT results in lymphocytosis is not understood. Given that *B. parapertussis* does not produce PT but causes a disease nearly indistinguishable from that caused by *B. pertussis*, lymphocytosis is not a definitively defining feature of pertussis.

Both *B. pertussis* and *B. parapertussis* produce and secrete a protein that can enter eukaryotic cells and function directly, upon activation by calmodulin, as an adenylate cyclase enzyme. Similar to PT, this protein, called **adenylate cyclase toxin** (**ACT**), results in very high cAMP levels in intoxicated cells, inhibiting the microbicidal functions of phagocytic cells. ACT is actually a **bifunctional molecule**; its amino terminus contains the adenylate cyclase catalytic activity, and its carboxyl terminus, in addition to mediating entry of the catalytic domain into the cell, can form cation-selective channels in membranes and has weak hemolytic activity.

Local damage to respiratory epithelium is due, in large part, to another toxin called **tracheal cytotoxin** (**TCT**), which kills ciliated cells specifically and causes their

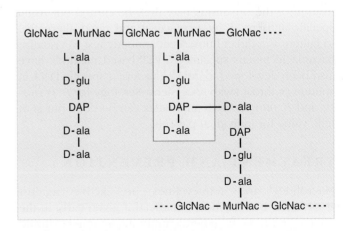

FIGURE 19-3. Portion of cell wall murein that corresponds to the structure of tracheal cytotoxin. ala, alanine; GlcNac, *N*-acetylglucosamine; DAP, diaminopimelic acid; glu, glutamic acid; MurNac, *N*-acetylmuramic acid.

extrusion from the epithelium (see Fig. 19-1). Curiously, this exotoxin is not a protein but consists of a **peptidoglycan fragment** called 1,6-anhydromuramic acid–N-acetylglucosamine tetrapeptide (Fig. 19-3). A similar compound is produced by gonococci and acts in an analogous fashion by killing ciliated epithelial cells in fallopian tubes (see Chapter 14). It is likely that additional factors that have yet to be identified and characterized also contribute to the ability of B. pertussis and B. parapertussis to cause local damage in the nasopharynx and trachea.

Given the nature of the local damage, is it likely that antibodies will have a significant effect on the cause of the disease? Preexisting antibodies produced by previous infections or by vaccination prevent the disease, especially if they are of the IgA type. However, once the disease is established, antibodies may play a lesser role because once exotoxins enter their target host cells, they become inaccessible to antibodies.

DIAGNOSIS

Whooping cough is uncommon in countries where the vaccine is widely used. Although the clinical signs and symptoms (particularly the characteristic "whoop") are usually quite distinctive, neither clinicians nor the laboratory are always alert to this particular diagnosis. It is also important to remember that laboratory diagnosis of B. pertussis is difficult because the number of organisms decreases as the severity of symptoms increases. Thus, B. pertussis and B. parapertussis can be cultured from only a small number of infected patients.

To culture B. pertussis, a small swab is placed on the posterior wall of the pharynx, which usually makes the patient cough. The swab is often treated with a drop of penicillin solution to kill other normally occurring bacteria that are sensitive to the drug (to which B. pertussis is intrinsically resistant). The swab is then applied to the surface of a plate containing a medium called **Bordet-Gengou** then incubated for 2 to 4 days. Positive identification of the organisms may then be carried out using specific antisera. A more practical and rapid alternative to culture is a direct fluorescent antibody test to visualize bacteria in mucus specimens. PCR-based methods have also been developed to detect Bordetella-specific DNA in sputum or throat swab specimens. Serology for B. pertussis and B. parapertussis antibodies can be done but is of little value for individual patients.

TREATMENT AND PREVENTION

Macrolides and tetracyclines are active against B. pertussis but are most beneficial if given early in the course of illness. In general, antibiotic treatment should reduce the shedding of bacteria, and it may shorten the course of disease and lessen symptoms, but the beneficial effects of treatment are not as dramatic as they are with other infections, such as pneumococcal pneumonia.

It is well established that vaccination should be widespread. Countries that suspended pertussis vaccination requirements in response to public concern about adverse effects, or because sufficient high-quality vaccine was unavailable or undeliverable, have seen dramatic increases in whooping cough cases. All states in the United States require children to be immunized against pertussis prior to enrollment in schools and, in some areas, day care centers. Because it is now apparent that neither immunization nor infection induce lifelong immunity and that adults appear to form the reservoir from which infants become infected, booster vaccinations every 10 years or so are recommended. Time will tell whether this strategy will be effective at reducing the burden of disease in the population and especially young children and infants, who are at greatest risk of severe disease.

CONCLUSION

The study of B. pertussis pathogenicity has revealed basic mechanisms general to many bacterial pathogens. As a superficial pathogen, B. pertussis does not penetrate into deep tissues. It produces a number of powerful toxins, most of which function to counteract the defense mechanisms of the lower respiratory tract. The disease it produces, whooping cough, can be virtually eliminated by vaccination. Another consequence of this basic research has been development of effective acellular vaccines, which are given in combination with vaccines for diphtheria and tetanus.

Suggested Readings

Bijlsma JJ, Groisman EA. Making informed decisions: regulatory interactions between two-component systems. *Trends Microbiol.* 2003;11:359–366.

Carbonetti NH, Artamonova GV, Mays RM, et al. Pertussis toxin plays an early role in respiratory tract colonization by *Bordetella pertussis. Infect Immun.* 2003;71:6358–6366.

Cotter PA, Jones AM. Phosphorelay control of virulence gene expression in *Bordetella. Trends Microbiol.* 2003;11:367–373.

de Gouw D, Diavatopoulos DA, Bootsma HJ, et al. Pertussis: a matter of immune modulation. *FEMS Microbiol Rev.* 2011;35:441–474

Hewlett EL, Edwards KM. Pertussis—not just for kids. *N Engl J Med.* 2005;352:1215–1222.

Robbins JB, Schneerson R, Trollfors B, et al. The diphtheria and pertussis components of diphtheria-tetanus toxoids-pertussis vaccine should be genetically inactivated mutant toxins. *J Infect Dis.* 2005;191:81–88.

Chapter **20**

Clostridia: Diarrheal Disease, Tissue Infection, Botulism, and Tetanus

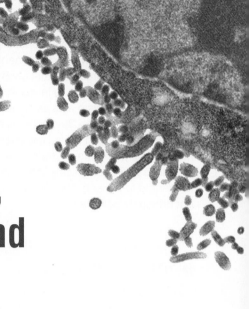

Stephen Melville

KEY CONCEPTS

Pathogens: Clostridia are Gram-positive, anaerobic, spore-forming rods. They include pathogens such as *Clostridium difficile*, a cause of antibiotic-associated diarrhea and pseudomembranous colitis; *C. perfringens*, the cause of gas gangrene; *C. botulinum*, the cause of botulism; and *C. tetani*, the cause of tetanus.

Encounter: Most pathogenic clostridia are acquired from the environment. Some colonize the mammalian colon and are returned to the environment as spores from the feces.

Entry: Antibiotic-associated colitis is acquired by ingestion of clostridial spores in the context of antibiotic therapy and disruption of the normal intestinal microbiota. Clostridial wound infections occur after contamination of wounds with soil. Botulism can occur after ingestion of preformed clostridial neurotoxin in contaminated food.

Spread and Multiplication: Clostridia can grow in the anaerobic environment of the gastrointestinal tract or in the devitalized, anaerobic tissue of a necrotic wound.

Damage: Expression of disease depends on the production of clostridial cytotoxins or neurotoxins.

Diagnosis: Clostridia in wounds can be detected with Gram stains and cultured under anaerobic conditions. *C. difficile* infection is usually diagnosed by detecting the characteristic toxins in feces. Neurotoxic clostridial infections (tetanus and botulism) are usually recognized by their characteristic clinical presentations.

Treatment: Surgical debridement of all devitalized tissues is critical to the management of clostridial wound infections. *C. difficile* infection is treated with oral metronidazole or vancomycin. Tetanus and botulism may be improved with the administration of antitoxins.

Prevention: Proper wound management to prevent wound infection and judicious use of antibiotics to avoid *C. difficile*. Attention to sterility in canning foods to prevent contamination with *C. botulinum* spores. A "toxoid" vaccine prevents the neurotoxic features of tetanus.

THE MANY species of clostridium are strictly anaerobic Gram-positive rods responsible for several unrelated diseases with various clinical manifestations. These include **pseudomembranous colitis** (PMC) (an inflammatory disease of the colon); soft tissue infections, including muscle invasion (**gas gangrene**) and **cellulitis** (an infection of subcutaneous connective tissue); **tetanus**; **botulism**; and food poisoning. Many of the clostridial diseases are serious and life threatening. All are caused by exotoxins secreted by the clostridia. In the case of botulism, the disease is acquired by eating toxin-contaminated food; the clinical symptoms are produced by the toxin without colonization or invasion by the organism.

Production of protein toxins by at least 14 clostridial species is associated with a range of diseases, including botulism, tetanus, gas gangrene, food poisoning, diarrhea, and PMC. The toxins responsible for botulism and tetanus are **neurotoxins**, whereas those causing gas gangrene and intestinal infections are **cytotoxins**; that is, they cause direct damage to cells. **Botulism** is caused by preformed botulinum toxin in contaminated food; thus, the *Clostridium botulinum* organism itself need not be present in the victim. In tetanus and PMC, the organisms are ensconced in the host, either in a wound (in the case of tetanus) or in the bowel lumen (in PMC). However, the organism itself does not invade the tissues; it merely produces toxins that cause the disease. The organism that causes gas gangrene, *Clostridium perfringens*, produces multiple virulence factors and is highly tissue invasive. Clostridia can also produce **suppurative wounds** and **tissue abscesses**, in which the organism acts as a simple invader, without systemic signs of toxin production (Table 20-1).

In addition to the 30 clostridial species encountered in human infections, another 50 or more species are found in the environment, particularly in soil and in animal wastes. Clostridia are highly active metabolically, and many strains have important industrial uses. Clostridial fermentation of crude substrates produces useful chemicals like alcohols and acetone, and some species are used in the production of fermented foods and cheese. The clostridia used for these purposes, like most members of the genus, are not ordinarily pathogenic.

CLOSTRIDIUM DIFFICILE AND DIARRHEAL DISEASE

An anaerobic, Gram-positive, spore-forming rod, *C. difficile*, was first identified in 1935. As the name implies, it has fastidious growth requirements. Although isolated occasionally in blood cultures and in wounds, it went unrecognized as a cause of diarrheal disease until 1977, when it was identified as the organism responsible for a severe ulcerating disease of the large bowel known as **pseudomembranous colitis** (**PMC**; *pseudomembranous* refers to the yellowish plaques composed of fibrin with cellular debris that overlay the ulcerations in the colonic mucosa). Since then, the organism has been linked to a spectrum of intestinal disorders associated with antibiotic treatment, ranging from an asymptomatic carrier state, to mild or moderate diarrhea, to fulminating, life-threatening PMC.

ENCOUNTER, ENTRY, SPREAD, AND MULTIPLICATION

C. difficile is harbored in the large intestine of a small percentage of healthy humans, where it tends to remain in low numbers. It can also be found in environmental sources, particularly hospitals in its highly resistant spore form. The spores can be cultured from the floor, bedpan, and toilet in a hospital room occupied by a patient with *C. difficile*, as well as from the hands and clothing of medical and nursing personnel. The mode of transmission is via the spore form, which is extremely difficult to eradicate from the environment and is often carried on the hands of health care personnel who are caring for multiple patients. *C. difficile* is currently the major cause of diarrhea acquired in a hospital. In nursing homes, where patients tend to stay for prolonged periods, 20 to 30% of the residents are asymptomatic carriers of *C. difficile*. In 2000, a new hypervirulent strain, called NAP1/BI/027, began to appear. It produces significantly higher levels of toxin A and toxin B, secretes a binary toxin related to the iota toxin of *C. perfringens*, and is resistant to fluoroquinolones, which are widely used in clinical settings. This epidemic strain resulted in a significant increase in the frequency and severity of *C. difficile* infections and also increased the development of toxic megacolon, which was rarely seen before this strain became widespread.

CASE • Mrs. T., a 79-year-old diabetic resident of a nursing home, developed a persistent leg ulcer. The ulcer was cleaned by debridement, and she was treated with cephalosporins and ampicillin for 2 weeks to prevent the ulcer from spreading. Two weeks after the antibiotic treatment was completed, Mrs. T. began suffering from fever, along with bouts of watery diarrhea and lower abdominal pain, whereupon she was sent to a local hospital.

A stool specimen was sent to the laboratory, which within 24 hours yielded a positive result for toxin A and toxin B of *Clostridium difficile*. Specific treatment for antibiotic-associated diarrhea caused by *C. difficile* was begun with oral metronidazole. Mrs. T. became afebrile within 36 hours, the diarrhea and abdominal pain gradually subsided, and she was returned to the nursing home. Three weeks after her return to the nursing home, she again developed fever, watery diarrhea, and abdominal pain, and her stool was positive for toxin A and toxin B. This time, she was treated with oral vancomycin and her symptoms abated within the next few days.

This case raises several questions:

1. What was the most likely source of the *C. difficile* that infected Mrs. T?

2. Is the history of previous treatment with cephalosporins and ampicillin pertinent to *C. difficile* infection?

3. Why was vancomycin not given at the initial occurrence of *C. difficile* infection?

4. What was the likely source of bacteria for the relapse that occurred in the *C. difficile* infection?

TABLE 20-1 Major Clostridial Diseases

Disease	Toxin Production	Tissue Invasiveness
Botulism		
Botulinum food poisoning	+	–
Infant botulism	+	–
Wound botulism	+	±
Tetanus	+	±
Pseudomembranous colitis	+	±
Gas gangrene	+	+
Suppurative wounds and abscesses	–	+

A remarkable feature of *C. difficile* diarrhea is its association with antimicrobial drugs. Most symptomatic patients have received an antimicrobial agent in the recent past. Virtually all antimicrobial drugs have been implicated; however, the most common antimicrobial drugs associated with *C. difficile* diarrhea are cephalosporins, ampicillin, and clindamycin. (This order reflects the frequency with which these drugs are used in clinical practice; in fact, clindamycin is associated with a higher incidence of disease per administration.)

The risk associated with use of a particular antimicrobial drug is not necessarily related to its in vitro activity against *C. difficile* but rather to the relative resistance of the spore form of *C. difficile* to almost all antimicrobial drugs. The sequence of events in antibiotic-associated *C. difficile* diarrhea begins with suppression of normal microbiota by the antimicrobial drug, with persistence of the spore form of *C. difficile*. Clindamycin suppresses anaerobic bacteria, the most common type of bacteria in the microbiota; this suppression may explain the strong association of its use with *C. difficile* diarrhea. *C. difficile* is either present already in the microbiota or is acquired from the hospital environment during antibiotic treatment.

At some time during or after antibiotic administration, the spores germinate and the vegetative form of *C. difficile* grows in large numbers, producing its toxins. When toxin production achieves a critical level in the large bowel, diarrhea begins. As the disease progresses, PMC may develop. Sigmoidoscopy of the patient's colon is the most reliable way to diagnose PMC, since the lesions are readily visible in the sigmoidoscope. Because 10 to 20% of patients will suffer a relapse of the disease, they should be closely monitored for symptoms.

DAMAGE

Like other toxin-related gastrointestinal infections (notably, diarrhea caused by *Vibrio cholerae* and toxigenic *Escherichia coli*), bacterial invasion of the bowel wall is not a feature of *C. difficile* diarrhea. Instead, the organism produces its toxins in the intestinal lumen, and the toxins cause damage to the epithelial lining of the bowel wall. The major toxins are designated A and B. **Toxin A** (also called TcdA) causes both fluid production and damage to the mucosa of the large bowel. **Toxin B** is a cytotoxin that causes rounding up of tissue-culture cells. Toxin B (also called TcdB) is thought to work in conjunction with toxin A to cause the symptoms associated with the clinical disease. Toxins A and B are enzymes, which act in the cytoplasm of the host cell to glucosylate **Rho-GTPases** such as **Rho**, **Rac**, and **Cdc42**, using UDP-glucose as the substrate. Glucosylation inactivates these regulatory proteins, and the cell loses its cytoskeletal structure and can die as a result. The standard laboratory diagnosis of the disease detects toxin A or toxin B or both in the feces of patients using an immunological test called an **enzyme-linked immunosorbent assay** (**ELISA**; see Chapter 58).

TREATMENT AND PREVENTION

In some cases, cessation of the original antibiotic treatment that led to the development of *C. difficile* diarrhea will limit the duration of the infection and associated symptoms. The antibiotics metronidazole and vancomycin can be used to successfully treat the overgrowth of *C. difficile* in the intestine (see case study). Vancomycin should be used judiciously, in order to prevent the development of vancomycin-resistant strains of intestinal pathogens (e.g., *Enterococcus* species).

Preventing *C. difficile* diarrhea and PMC can be achieved using a variety of strategies. The antibiotics most commonly associated with the disease (cephalosporins, ampicillin, and clindamycin) should not be used on susceptible populations of patients (e.g., those in nursing homes) if other antibiotics are available. The transmission of the disease most often occurs via the hands and instruments of health care personnel who carry the heat-resistant spores from patient to patient. Proper education in the methods of transmission of the disease and frequent changes of gloves and outer clothing can reduce the spread of the spores. Extensive disinfection of the rooms of patients with the disease can lower the number of spores in the environment, and in some cases, isolation of infected patients may be called for.

CLOSTRIDIUM PERFRINGENS AND TISSUE INFECTIONS

Traumatic wounds are commonly contaminated with clostridial spores other than those of *C. botulinum* and *C. tetani*. These other clostridial spores are widespread in soil. In contrast to *C. tetani* and *C. botulinum*, which have little or no invasive properties, the other clostridia in wound infections cause local damage in addition to systemic effects. The major pathogen of wound infections, *C. perfringens*, produces a variety of toxins that act both locally and systemically. The more common form of clostridial wound infections is a localized cellulitis that can usually be cured with surgical management and antibiotics. More severe trauma can be associated with gas gangrene, a necrotizing, gas-forming infection of muscle associated with systemic signs of shock. Cessation of the original antibiotic treatment that led to the development of *C. difficile* diarrhea can limit the duration of the infection and associated symptoms. The antibiotics metronidazole and vancomycin can be used to successfully treat the overgrowth of *C. difficile* in the intestine (see case study).

Preventing *C. difficile* diarrhea and PMC can be achieved using a variety of strategies. Antibiotics most commonly associated with the disease (cephalosporins, ampicillin, and clindamycin) should not be used on susceptible populations of patients if other antibiotics are available. Transmission of the disease most often occurs when health care personnel carry the heat-resistant spores from patient to patient. Proper education about disease transmission and frequent changes of gloves and outer clothing can reduce the spread of the spores. Extensive disinfection of the rooms of patients with the disease can lower the number of spores in the environment. In some cases, isolation of infected patients may be called for.

ENCOUNTER, ENTRY, SPREAD, AND MULTIPLICATION

C. perfringens and a variety of other clostridia are found in soil and in the intestinal tract of many animals. In wartime, 20 to 30% of wounds are contaminated by these organisms. The physiological condition of the wound site is critical in allowing the organism to germinate and to produce its toxins. The proper conditions are a low oxidation reduction potential (anaerobic conditions), compromised blood supply, calcium ions, and the availability of various peptides and amino acids. All these conditions are characteristic of damaged tissue.

DAMAGE

C. perfringens produces 12 toxins, but the α-toxin, a **lecithinase** that damages cell membranes, is the toxin most responsible for the symptoms of gas gangrene. A phospholipase type C, it interacts with eukaryotic cell membranes and **hydrolyzes phosphatidylcholine and sphingomyelin**, leading to cell death. Because the muscle tissue is destroyed (myonecrosis), it no longer reacts to stimuli. The muscle tissue appears reddish-blue to black. Large Gram-positive bacteria can be readily detected in the infected area (Fig. 20-1), and there is nearly a complete absence of leukocytes in the infected region. Abundant gas is produced by the organism, resulting in crepitus, which can be palpated as small gas bubbles under the

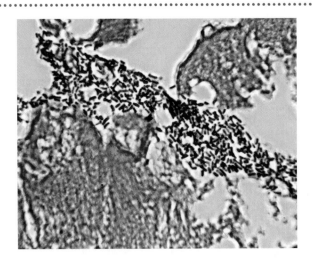

FIGURE 20-1. Hematoxylin and eosin stain of *Clostridium perfringens* in muscle tissue from gas gangrene. The bacteria (*purple rods*) are interspersed with muscle fibers (*red areas*). Note the hallmarks of gas gangrene: the absence of neutrophils and the nearly complete degradation of muscle fibers in the infected tissue.

skin. Systemically, the patient develops fever, sweating, low blood pressure, and decreased urinary output. The mortality rate for untreated gas gangrene approaches 100%; the patient generally succumbs to shock and renal failure within a few days of onset.

TREATMENT AND PREVENTION

Treatment of gas gangrene should be administered promptly because the organism can spread rapidly through healthy tissue. Treatment involves surgical removal of the involved muscle, which may necessitate extensive resection and even amputation of the affected limb. Antibiotics such as penicillin are administered to control the wound infection, but they are ineffective without adequate surgical debridement and drainage. Antitoxin, which is produced in horses, has had a negligible effect in this disease and is not recommended for treatment. Oxygen administered under high pressure (hyperbaric) is used in centers with appropriate chambers but appears to work in only a subset of cases. Milder forms of clostridial wound infection, without evidence of myonecrosis or systemic effects, can be managed with more conservative surgical intervention and appropriate antibiotics.

Prevention of gas gangrene and other clostridial wound infections involves prompt and appropriate attention to traumatic injuries. Under war conditions, frontline hospitals and evacuation facilities have ameliorated the damage caused by gunshot and shrapnel. Trauma units, now available in most US cities, have reduced the incidence of clostridial soft tissue infections by initiating prompt attention to wounds. Restoration of the arterial blood supply to the affected area is the most effective means of preventing gangrene from developing in traumatic wounds.

CLOSTRIDIUM PERFRINGENS AND FOOD POISONING

Food poisoning is unrelated to gas gangrene but is caused by sporulating *C. perfringens* cells that produce an **enterotoxin** in the intestines of people who have consumed contaminated food, usually a substance containing meat. The enterotoxin causes diarrhea about 12 to 24 hours after the contaminated food is eaten. The disease is self-limiting, and the symptoms disappear after 1 to 3 days. *C. perfringens* food poisoning is one of the most common types of bacterial food poisoning in the United States, with 10,000 cases per year estimated by the Centers for Disease Control.

CLOSTRIDIUM BOTULINUM AND BOTULISM

Although rarely seen in the United States, botulism is one of the most feared diseases because of the incredible potency of the botulinum toxin. The toxin has frequently been identified as a potential weapon of bioterrorism because of its potency and means of ingestion by contaminated food or water. Methods to detect the bacterium and the toxin in the food supply are becoming a high priority to prevent both the natural form of the disease and the use of the toxin as a biological weapon.

ENCOUNTER, ENTRY, SPREAD, AND MULTIPLICATION

C. botulinum spores found in soil or marine sediments contaminate meats, vegetables, and fish. Because the spores are relatively heat resistant, they survive food processing and canning when the temperatures are insufficiently high. Under anaerobic conditions, as found in canned foods, the spores germinate and release potent toxins. Proteolytic enzymes produced by some strains of the organism cause spoilage of the food; however, in many cases, the food has a normal appearance and taste. Even an experimental nibble of such food can contain enough toxin to cause lethal disease.

DAMAGE

C. botulinum produces eight immunologically distinct neurotoxins (types A, B, Cα, Cβ, D, E, F, and G). Human cases are associated mostly with types A and B and occasionally with type E, which is formed in fish products. As the interest in home canning and prepared foods has increased, cases of foodborne botulism have risen concomitantly. Among the most potent poisons known, botulinum toxins are protein **neurotoxins**. One microgram is sufficient to kill a large family, and 0.4 kg could kill all the people on Earth.

Botulism is an intoxication caused by the ingestion of a preformed toxin. The toxin prevents release of the neurotransmitter acetylcholine, thereby interfering with neurotransmission at **peripheral cholinergic synapses**. The toxin is a zinc metalloprotease that cleaves proteins involved in the docking of neurotransmitter-filled vesicles with the cytoplasmic membrane of neurons, thereby preventing transmission of the neurological signal to muscles to contract. This accounts for the symptoms of the clinical disease, **flaccid paralysis** of muscle, which occurs within 12 to 36 hours after ingestion of the toxin. Cranial nerves are affected first, particularly those involving the eyes, producing diplopia (double vision) and blurred vision. Difficulty swallowing is an early sign. The paralysis descends, and striated muscle groups weaken, especially those in the neck and extremities, with subsequent involvement of respiratory muscles. The toxin does not produce systemic signs of fever or sepsis. Patients generally succumb to paralysis and respiratory failure.

Infant botulism is a paralytic disease occurring in infants between 3 and 20 weeks of age. It produces a generalized hypotonic ("floppy") state. The infant's cry becomes feeble and the suck reflex weakens. In this disease, *C. botulinum* colonizes the large intestine, where it produces toxin. Infant botulism differs from the classic botulinum food poisoning in three ways: (1) The toxin is not found in food but rather is produced in the infant's intestinal tract; (2) the condition has a slow onset, probably because the toxin is absorbed more slowly from the large intestine; and (3) the disease has a favorable outcome in most cases, without specific treatment.

Wound botulism is a very rare form of the disease in which a traumatic wound is contaminated by spores of *C. botulinum*, which can multiply in the wound if the tissue is anaerobic. Toxins are produced at the wound site and absorbed into the tissues, causing a severe neurological disease similar to that of foodborne botulism.

TREATMENT AND PREVENTION

A heptavalent **antitoxin** is available for treatment against noninfant intoxication by the major toxin types A to G. This should be administered as soon as possible to bind any circulating toxin. Because this antitoxin is acquired from horses, a high incidence of hypersensitivity reactions is associated with its use. (Antitoxin antibodies derived from humans is available for infant cases.) The most important aspect of treatment for botulism is supportive care, including placement on a respirator, which is necessary to maintain breathing and other vital functions. Patients should be given parenteral nutrition. The illness may last for many weeks, and individual muscles may be paralyzed for months or even permanently. With good supportive care, the mortality from botulism is currently 25%.

Botulism can be prevented by proper canning methods. Although the spores are heat resistant, the toxins are heat labile, and terminal heating of contaminated food can kill *C. botulinum* spores. As a result of improvements in the canning industry, outbreaks associated with commercial foods are quite rare, and most cases of botulism are now associated with home canning.

CLOSTRIDIUM TETANI AND TETANUS

Tetanus, which is caused by *C. tetani*, is a tragic disease not only because of its severity but also because it can be completely prevented by appropriate immunization. Indeed, prevention of tetanus by active immunization has been one of the triumphs of modern bacteriology. Experience with tetanus in the two world wars of the past century demonstrated beyond doubt the benefits of the tetanus toxoid vaccine. Universal immunization of the American forces in World War II virtually eliminated the disease as a complication of traumatic injuries in soldiers. In developing countries where immunization is not widely practiced, tetanus remains a serious public health problem.

ENCOUNTER, ENTRY, SPREAD, AND MULTIPLICATION

C. tetani is ubiquitous in the gastrointestinal tract of humans and animals and in soil samples. Because of their resistance to environmental conditions, tetanus spores contaminate wounds of trauma victims.

Most cases of tetanus are associated with a **traumatic wound**. Tissue necrosis, anoxia, and other bacterial contaminants in the wound provide an optimal environment for germination of tetanus spores and production of toxin. Neonatal tetanus results from contamination of the umbilical cord at the time of delivery, either through unsanitary procedures or local customs of wrapping the cord in dung or mud.

DAMAGE

The major toxin, known as **tetanospasmin**, accounts for all the symptoms of tetanus. Tetanospasmin is a 150-kDa protein molecule composed of a heavy chain and a light chain held together by a disulfide bridge. Like other A-B two-chain toxins, the individual heavy and light chains are nontoxic (see Chapter 9). The complete toxin attaches to peripheral nerves in the region of the wound, where it is transmitted to **cranial nerve nuclei** either through intraspinal transmission among involved motor neurons or bloodstream delivery of toxin to other neuromuscular junctions. The major action of tetanus toxin is **inhibition of neurotransmitter release** and **normal inhibitory input**, thereby causing the lower motor neuron to increase resting tone and producing the characteristic **reflex spasms** (see Chapter 9). Several types of neurotransmitters are blocked, including γ-aminobutyric acid (GABA). Clinically, the disease presents as a **spastic paralysis**. Despite causing symptoms exactly opposite that of botulinum toxin, tetanus toxin works in the same manner as botulinum toxin by cleaving proteins involved

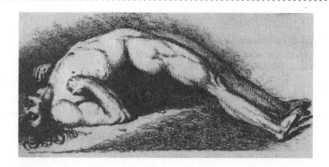

FIGURE 20-2. Advanced tetanus may lead to opisthotonos, the bending backward of the body caused by spastic paralysis of the strong extensors of the back. This classic painting of a British soldier wounded in 1809 in the Napoleonic Wars portrays this condition, as well as the "sardonic smile" and lockjaw caused by spasms of facial muscles.

in neurotransmitter-filled vesicular secretion. Like botulinum toxin, it is also a zinc metalloprotease but it acts on a different set of neurons (as described earlier), resulting in a spastic paralysis, unlike botulism, which is characterized by a flaccid paralysis.

Generalized tetanus, responsible for about 80% of cases, usually begins with trismus, or "lockjaw." Trismus is caused by tetanic spasm of the masseter muscles and prevents opening of the mouth. The disease typically descends, initially involving the neck and back muscles, progressing to produce boardlike rigidity of the abdominal musculature, eventually causing stiffness of the extremities. Individual muscle groups spasm, leading to a generalized spasm that is characterized by a tonic seizure, adduction of the arms, arching of the neck and back, extension of the legs, and clenching of the fists (Fig. 20-2). Death usually results from respiratory failure caused by paralysis of chest muscles.

TREATMENT AND PREVENTION

The treatment of tetanus is mainly a physiological exercise in preventing complications. Antitoxins (human and equine) are available and should be given at the earliest possible moment, but it is often a futile gesture because any toxin that has been produced is already irreversibly fixed to the nerve cells. Antibiotic treatment, particularly penicillin G, is directed at the organism because it may continue to produce toxin in the wound. In addition, surgical debridement of the involved wound should be performed to eliminate the environmental niche of the organism.

Prevention of tetanus is achieved through immunization. Active immunization should be carried out in all infants and children and in pregnant women who have not been previously immunized. The vaccine consists of **tetanus toxoid**, a form of the toxin that has been inactivated in formalin but retains its antigenicity. Tetanus toxoid is the *T* of the DPT vaccine given to infants and children. Passive immunization in the form of human globulin is administered to people with a "tetanus-prone wound." Because the disease itself does not produce sufficient antibody reaction for subsequent protection, it is necessary to immunize tetanus patients with the toxoid as well. Antibodies are insufficiently produced during the disease state because the amount of toxin present in the patient is too small to be immunogenic. It is a testament to the enormous potency of tetanus toxin that such a small amount is still sufficient to produce severe symptoms.

CONCLUSION

The pathogenic clostridia have a broad spectrum of colonization and invasiveness features. In botulism, the organisms do not invade the body at all; in tetanus, they barely set up housekeeping in tissues; and in clostridial gangrene, they show considerable invasiveness. The production of a wide range of toxins is a key feature of clostridial infections.

Suggested Readings

Johnson EA. *Clostridium botulinum* and *Clostridium tetani*. In: Borrelio SP, Murray PR, Funke G, eds. *Topley and Wilson's Microbiology and Microbial Infections*. London, UK: Arnold; 2005:1035–1088.

Mallozzi M, Viswanathan VK, Vedantam G. Spore forming *Bacilli* and *Clostridia* in human disease. *Future Microbiol*. 2010;5:1109

Popoff MR, Bouvet P. Clostridial toxins. *Future Microbiol*. 2009;4:1021–1064.

Rupnik M, Wilcox MH, Gerding DN. *Clostridium difficile* infection: new developments in epidemiology and pathogenesis. *Nat Rev Microbiol*. 2007;(7):526–536.

Stevens DL. Necrotizing Clostridial soft tissue infections. In: Rood JI, McClane BA, Songer JG, et al., eds. *The Clostridia: Molecular Biology and Pathogenesis*. San Diego, CA: Academic Press; 1997:141–152.

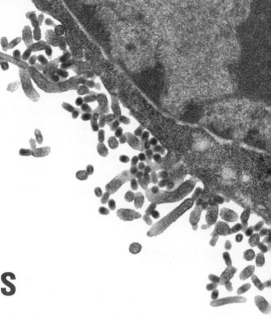

Chapter **21**

Legionella: Parasite of Amoebae and Macrophages

Michele Swanson and Cary Engleberg

KEY CONCEPTS

Pathogen: There are numerous *Legionella* species, but *Legionella pneumophila* is the most prevalent opportunistic pathogen of humans.

Encounter: Fresh water or soil reservoir, where bacteria multiply within free-living amoebae

Entry: Inhalation of aerosols or aspiration of contaminated water

Spread: Point-sources outbreaks occur from contaminated environmental sources, but there is no human-to-human transmission.

Multiplication: A specialized bacterial secretion system establishes a protected intracellular replication vacuole. Then, exhaustion of nutrients

or starvation within the infected cell triggers expression of a transmissive (virulent) phenotype.

Damage: Damage is due to the host inflammatory response. *Legionellae* express no classical toxins.

Diagnosis: Antibody-based tests or culture on specialized medium, which is slow and insensitive

Treatment and Prevention: Only antibiotics that can penetrate macrophage membranes (where the bacteria replicate) are effective for treatment. Risk is reduced by case surveillance and by monitoring and decontaminating institutional plumbing systems.

THE LEGIONELLAE are a diverse genus of aerobic Gram-negative bacilli that includes opportunistic pathogens of macrophages in humans. These bacteria parasitize amoebae and protozoa that reside in aquatic and soil habitats and occasionally colonize man-made water distribution systems. Humans acquire infection by inhalation. In the patients with impaired host defenses, you may see a severe form of pneumonia called Legionnaires disease. Because this infection is often associated with contaminated water systems, you may also encounter institutional outbreaks of Legionnaires disease in hospitals, hotels, and other large buildings.

EPIDEMIOLOGY

Legionella was first recognized as a bacterial species when researchers from the Centers for Disease Control investigated a highly publicized outbreak of pneumonia at an American Legion convention in Philadelphia in 1976. In all, 182 attendees became ill, and 29 died. Once the bacterium (*Legionella pneumophila*) was isolated, culture and serological methods were developed to facilitate the clinical diagnosis of Legionnaires disease. We now know that many species of *Legionella* are ubiquitous in aquatic environments or soil, and a few are a significant cause of

pneumonia. Although outbreaks of legionellosis continue to attract the most attention from the general public, by far the more typical form of infection is sporadic, community-acquired pneumonia. However, hospital-acquired legionellosis in vulnerable in-patients tends to be especially severe.

CHARACTERISTICS OF LEGIONELLAE

Legionella species do not grow on routine bacteriological media. Instead, the microbes form colonies visible after incubation for 3 to 5 days on special medium that

CASE • Mrs. R., a 59-year-old female schoolteacher was admitted to the hospital with high fever and altered mental status. Eight days earlier, she developed a "flu-like" illness with fever, anorexia, malaise, headache, and muscle aches. These symptoms were followed by a cough that became progressively worse but was productive of only scanty, clear sputum. Five days before admission, she saw a local physician who ordered a chest x-ray. The x-ray showed a small left upper lobe infiltrate, consistent with pneumonia. She was treated with an oral cephalosporin. In spite of the antibiotic treatment, her fever and chills increased steadily, she developed watery diarrhea, and she became confused and lethargic. Mrs. R.'s past medical history was unremarkable, but she had smoked one pack of cigarettes a day for 40 years. Two weeks earlier, Mrs. R had returned from a 2-week holiday at a resort in Southern Florida. None of Mrs. R's family members, coworkers, or students had a similar illness.

On admission, her temperature was 40°C, her heart rate was 88 beats per minute. The patient was severely hypoxic, and her white cell count was 13,700/mm³. A Gram stain of the sputum showed numerous neutrophils but no bacteria. A chest x-ray showed extension of her left upper lobe infiltrate and a new right middle lobe infiltrate.

High-dose erythromycin was added to the patient's antibiotic regimen on suspicion of Legionnaires disease. She was intubated and placed on mechanical ventilation in the intensive care unit (ICU). After a stormy ICU course, the patient began to improve slowly and eventually recovered. A culture of respiratory secretions obtained by aspiration through the endotracheal tube grew *Legionella pneumophila* after 4 days of incubation.

The case of Mrs. R. raises several questions for you to consider:

1. How did Mrs. R. acquire *L. pneumophila*, and why was not anyone in her family or workplace also infected?

2. Why was the diagnosis of Legionnaires disease initially overlooked in this case?

3. Why did Mrs. R.'s pneumonia worsen during treatment with an antibiotic that kills *L. pneumophila* growing in bacteriological media?

See Appendix for answers.

---

contains a source of amino acids to supply carbon and energy, inorganic iron, high levels of cysteine, charcoal to absorb inhibitory substances in the agar, and low sodium to avoid inhibiting virulent forms. Some species do not grow even on this special media and can only be cultured in amoebae. These species are known as *Legionella*-like amoebal pathogens.

More than 50 species of *Legionella* have been identified, but the majority have not been linked to human disease. In nature, the Legionellaceae inhabit ponds, lakes, and hot springs, where they are found in complex, adherent microbial communities. Amoebae and protozoa prey upon these biofilms, but *Legionella* actually profit from ingestion. Instead of being killed and digested like other bacteria, they replicate to large numbers inside these unicellular organisms. Once nutrients inside the eukaryotic host are depleted, the intracellular bacteria differentiate to a motile, resilient, and infectious form suited for transmission to another host cell.

ENCOUNTER

Numerous outbreaks have established a link between the occurrence of Legionnaires disease and the **colonization of plumbing systems** with *L. pneumophila*. In hospitals or hotels where epidemics have occurred, the *L. pneumophila* strain isolated from respiratory cultures of patients can usually be found in tap water or in sediments from hot water tanks. Nonpathogenic amoebae and protozoans are also common inhabitants of potable water supplies, and they may serve to amplify the population of infectious microbes and perhaps to promote *L. pneumophila* infection of human lungs when inhaled with bacteria. In some aquatic hosts, the bacteria differentiate into a small, thick-walled "mature intracellular form" that is highly resistant to biocides and antibiotics. In certain respects, *Legionella* is particularly well adapted to warm water supply systems of buildings. The bacterium grows at temperatures up to 46°C and tolerates much higher temperatures. It is **relatively chlorine resistant** compared with enteric bacteria. In addition, bacterial biofilm communities are notoriously resistant to biocides.

Legionnaires disease is nearly always a **primary pulmonary infection**. The pathogen is never transmitted from person to person; instead, humans acquire the infection from an **environmental source**, usually a water distribution system colonized with the microorganism (Fig. 21-1). Showers, humidifiers, water fountains, respiratory therapy equipment, or evaporative cooling towers associated with institutional central air conditioning systems produce **infectious aerosols** that can transmit *Legionella*. An alternative mode of entry is by microaspiration of bacteria from the oropharynx or mouth into the lower respiratory airways, during or after the ingestion of contaminated water or ice. The circumstances of Mrs. R.'s exposure are unknown, but if water was the likely source, she may have acquired the infection at home, at work, or at any place where tap water is available.

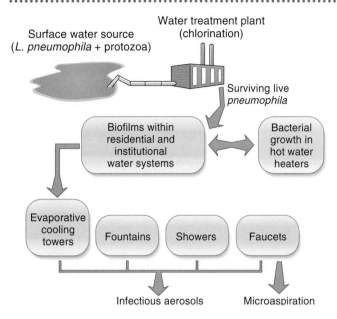

FIGURE 21-1. Sources of legionellae for human disease.

In outbreak situations, the risk of infection depends not only on the size of the inhaled inoculum but also on the susceptibility of the individual host. Several **host factors** are known to predispose individuals to infection. These include cigarette smoking, advanced age, chronic pulmonary disease, and immunosuppression (e.g., transplant patients, patients on corticosteroid therapy). Mrs. R. may have been particularly susceptible to infection because of her age and significant smoking history. Although the source of her infection is unknown, it is possible that other less susceptible individuals were exposed to the same source as Mrs. R. but did not become infected. Because she was vacationing at the time of her likely exposure, the water system at the Florida resort became suspect and was investigated.

ENTRY

In the air spaces of the lung, *Legionella* are ingested by **resident alveolar macrophages**. These phagocytic cells, which are normally regarded as a front line of defense against contaminants, fail to kill or even inhibit the growth of *L. pneumophila* in the lung. In the laboratory, the microbe grows faster in human macrophages than in artificial media. In the lung, inhaled *L. pneumophila* must be able to grow in phagocytic cells; bacterial strains that lack this capacity cannot cause pneumonia.

MULTIPLICATION AND SPREAD

After ingestion by phagocytes, most other bacteria are killed after their **phagosome acidifies and fuses with lysosomes**. In contrast, the *L. pneumophila* phagosome is enveloped by **endoplasmic reticulum** (Fig. 21-2). This process resembles **autophagy**, a stress response pathway by which eukaryotic cells sequester and digest their own cytoplasmic material, including organelles. If nutrients are available within this compartment, *L. pneumophila* differentiates into a **replicative form**. Eventually, the host cell becomes literally packed with bacteria, and nutrients are depleted. At this point, the organisms stop replicating and switch to the **transmissible form**. Their differentiation is coordinated by the same stress response mechanism that mediates the transition of most bacterial species into stationary phase, known as the **stringent response** (see Paradigm Box).

In the transmissible form, *L. pneumophila* express factors that lyse eukaryotic membranes, thus releasing

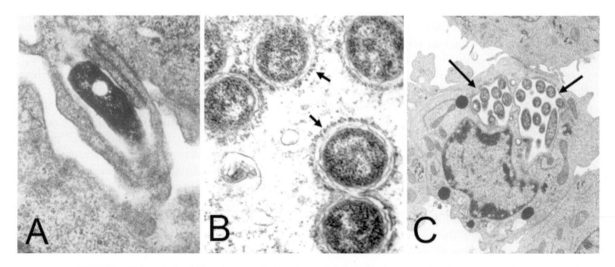

FIGURE 21-2. Electron micrographs. A. Uptake of *Legionella pneumophila* by a macrophage. **B.** At 4 hours after infection, a single organism in cross section is seen within an endosome that has associated with rough endoplasmic reticulum. Note the studding of the membrane with ribosomes. **C.** *L. pneumophila* begin to multiply to large numbers within membrane-bound vesicles.

the progeny from the infected host cell. The transmissible form also expresses **flagella** to facilitate spread in the aquatic environment and **resistance to osmotic shock** and other environmental stresses to ensure extracellular survival. Also critical to transmission are factors that **block phagosome–lysosome fusion** after ingestion by the next host cell. To establish an intracellular replication niche, transmissible *L. pneumophila* delivers numerous proteins directly into eukaryotic cells through a specialized secretion apparatus that evolved from a plasmid conjugation system. For example, *L. pneumophila* relies on its **type IV secretion system** to deliver several proteins that target **Rab1**, a small GTPase that regulates vesicle traffic in the secretory pathway of eukaryotic cells. Therefore, type IV secretion systems perform a similar role as the type III secretion systems of other pathogens, described in Chapter 17.

L. pneumophila virulence is almost certainly a product of its coevolution with amoebae and protozoa. Many of the same phenomena that occur when *L. pneumophila* infect macrophages have also been observed within amoebae. *L. pneumophila* is naturally competent to take up exogenous DNA, and its genome includes numerous

eukaryotic-like domains with protozoan origins. Several other pathogens that successfully replicate in human macrophages also parasitize amoebae and protozoa; these include species of *Mycobacteria, Listeria*, and *Cryptococcus*. We hypothesize that microbes that are pathogenic for human cells can emerge from the environment as a consequence of the selective pressures exerted by amoebae and other protozoa, which routinely eat and digest microorganisms as food.

The host may be able to inhibit the intracellular growth of *L. pneumophila* by innate immune mechanisms. Upon contact with *L. pneumophila*, macrophages secrete **tumor necrosis factor-alpha** (TNF-α), which inhibits intracellular growth of the bacteria. Thus, healthy hosts may be able to avoid *L. pneumophila* infection without ever inducing a specific immune response. Perhaps this explains why most healthy humans are resistant to Legionnaires disease.

Once infection is established, its outcome depends on the specific immune response. Experience with animal models suggests that antibodies play a minor role in containing infection by intracellular *L. pneumophila*. Instead, a **cell-mediated immune response** is required

PARADIGM BOX

STARVATION AND VIRULENCE

Like all microbes, the goal of every pathogenic organism is to survive and replicate. However, to overcome the formidable defenses of their hosts, pathogens are endowed with virulence traits, such as cell surface attachment, cell or tissue invasion, and transmission. A wide variety of pathogens couple the expression of their specific virulence mechanisms with more general adaptations, like stress resistance. Many of nature's most dreaded bacteria rely on small molecules known as **alarmones** that appear in response to metabolic disturbances and then coordinate survival and virulence programs.

ppGpp (guanosine 5′-diphosphate-3′-diphosphate) is an example of an alarmone that is critical to the expression of virulence in *L. pneumophila*. This molecule was discovered over 40 years ago when Cashel and Gallant visualized it as a "magic spot" on thin layer chromatography that appeared when well-nourished *Escherichia coli* were abruptly starved of amino acids. The appearance of this spot correlates with arrest of ribosomal RNA synthesis, a process referred to as the **stringent response**. The ppGpp alarmone mediates this and other physiological effects by selective control of gene transcription. These controls result in a transition of the organism from what we observe as the log phase of growth in cultures to the stationary phase when essential nutrients are exhausted.

The levels of ppGpp in the cell increase when two classes of synthetic enzymes, **RelA** and **SpoT**, become active. The synthetase activity of RelA is elicited at the ribosome by uncharged tRNAs that accumulate during amino acid starvation. In contrast, the SpoT responds to a variety of stimuli, including phosphate, carbon, and iron starvation, as well as perturbations in fatty acid metabolism.

Although new roles for ppGpp continue to be discovered, the alarmone generally functions to promote adaptation and resilience of bacterial cells faced with adversity. For many pathogenic bacteria, ppGpp also equips the cell to respond to metabolic stress by expressing necessary virulence factors. In *L. pneumophila*, ppGpp mediates the transition from the replicative to the transmissive phase when intracellular bacteria run out of nutrients (Fig. 21-3). Thus, by turning on the genes responsible for the *L. pneumophila* transmission, the ppGpp alarmone converts the bacteria from a nonvirulent, rapidly growing, intracellular form to a virulent one that will be released from the exhausted cell and be capable of establishing infection in new host cell.

When you consider the reasons for this level of control, the use of the stringent response to trigger expression of bacterial virulence makes sense from a teleological point of view. When a pathogen is starved, the expression of virulence may serve to improve its access to essential nutrients. So, it is not surprising that numerous other

continued on page 246

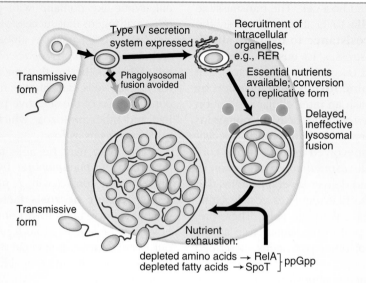

FIGURE 21-3. Key events in the life cycle of _L. pneumophila._ _L. pneumophila_ in the flagellate, transmissive form survives in the cell. Survival depends on the transfer of bacterial proteins to the host cell via a type IV secretion system. These proteins alter the trafficking of the phagosome within the cell. Instead of being delivered to lysosomes, the phagosome associates with intracellular organelles (e.g., ER) in a process akin to autophagy (see text). In the presence of abundant nutrients, the bacteria convert to the nonvirulent, replicative form and grow to large numbers in an ever-enlarging membrane-bound vesicle. Eventually, the depletion of amino acids and/or fatty acids in the cell results in the expression of the RelA and SpoT enzymes, which generate ppGpp. The ppGpp alarmone triggers the transcription of the transmissive phase genes that mediate release from the cell, motility (flagellation), and infectivity (altered trafficking) in the next host cell.

pathogens have been shown to rely on the elements of the stringent response (ppGpp, RelA, and SpoT) to regulate their virulence programs. There are numerous examples of this mode of gene regulation summarized in Table 21-1, and there are several others that are being investigated in such diverse genera as _Helicobacter, Listeria, Borrelia_, and _Streptococcus_. If the assumption that virulence serves in part to acquire nutrients for pathogens, then one might expect evolution to converge on the stringent response as a signal to express virulence in unrelated species.

TABLE 21-1 Some Bacterial Pathogens that Use the Stringent Response as a Regulator of Virulence Mechanisms

Pathogen	Environment Triggering the Stringent Response	Virulence Mechanisms Regulated	Chapter Reference
Enterohemorrhagic _Escherichia coli_	Colon	Locus of enterocyte effacement	16, 17
Uropathogenic _E. coli_	Bladder	Type 1 fimbriae and internalization into epithelial cells	63
Pseudomonas aeruginosa	Cystic fibrosis (CF) lung and others	Quorum-sensing systems that control virulence programs	18
Salmonella enterica	Small intestine	Type 3 secretion systems 1 and 2; cellular invasion	17
Yersinia pestis	Lymph node	Mortality in a mouse model of bubonic plague	57
Mycobacterium tuberculosis	Lung	Establishment of dormancy and persistence	23

for recovery from infection. By cellular immune processes described in Chapter 7, *Legionella*-immune lymphocytes proliferate and secrete **cytokines** after contact with cells presenting *Legionella* antigens with Class II histocompatibility molecules. One of the most important of these lymphokines, **γ-interferon**, can suppress the growth of *L. pneumophila* in macrophages, in part by inducing cells to sequester **iron** from the intracellular bacteria. Limiting access to this essential nutrient may be the critical function of the immune system in controlling *L. pneumophila* infection.

DAMAGE

Macrophages infected with *L. pneumophila* release **cytokines** that contribute to the influx of blood monocytes and neutrophils into the air spaces of the lung. As nodular areas of infection enlarge, they become visible as infiltrates on the chest x-ray. These areas typically evolve into microabscesses and may coalesce to form cavities. The bronchi and bronchioles are not affected. Rarely, *L. pneumophila* can be isolated from the blood or from organ tissues.

Most of the local damage produced by the infection is attributable to the vigor of the host inflammatory response. The *L. pneumophila* lipopolysaccharide is weaker than most other Gram-negative endotoxins. However, when macrophages detect *L. pneumophila* flagellin within their cytoplasm, they secrete the proinflammatory cytokines interleukin (IL)-1β and IL-18.

Legionnaires disease usually begins with "flulike" complaints, as in the case of Mrs. R. Virtually all patients have **fever** and develop clinical features of pneumonia: **cough, shortness of breath**, and possibly **chest pain**. Patients rarely have the grossly purulent (thick yellow or green) sputum associated with bacterial bronchopneumonias. **Watery diarrhea**, nausea, vomiting, or abdominal pain may also be present. Blood oxygen levels may be low, which may contribute to confusion and lethargy seen in Mrs. R.'s case. Typically, blood counts show only moderate elevation of total leukocytes, without a preponderance of neutrophils. In many patients, other laboratory tests may suggest dysfunction of the kidneys or liver. However, none of these clinical features is sufficiently specific to establish the diagnosis of Legionnaires disease, because any of them can occur in association with other pneumonias.

DIAGNOSIS

The laboratory diagnosis of Legionnaires disease may be difficult. The bacteria are not present in large numbers in the sputum and stain poorly. The Gram stain usually shows abundant neutrophils but no distinguishable bacteria. Several **rapid identification techniques** can be used to make a prompt diagnosis. They include examination of sputum by direct **fluorescent antibody** (DFA) staining or detection of *L. pneumophila* serogroup 1 antigen in the urine by an **enzyme immunoassay**. Although these tests may be useful in guiding the initial therapy of the patient, none of them is sufficiently sensitive or specific to be relied upon as the sole method of diagnosis. For example, diagnostic tests for serogroup 1 antigen in urine may miss as many as half of all *Legionella* infections: those caused by other *Legionella* species or other *L. pneumophila* serogroups. Culture is the most specific way to diagnose the infection, but it is not sensitive on sputum samples, and it has the drawback of requiring 3 to 5 days of incubation before *Legionella* colonies can be detected.

TREATMENT AND PREVENTION

Legionella grown in culture are sensitive to most antibiotics. However, successful antibiotic therapy requires drugs that can **penetrate** into infected cells where the bacteria grow. These include macrolides/ketolides, fluoroquinolones, and tetracyclines. As in Mrs. R.'s case, it is not unusual for patients to become worse while on treatment with a penicillin or cephalosporin antibiotic, because these antibiotics penetrate eukaryotic cells poorly.

Because the laboratory diagnosis of Legionnaires disease is imperfect and occasionally untimely, it is usually necessary to treat patients for this potentially fatal disease on suspicion alone. As a case in point, Mrs. R. was recognized as having a severe, atypical pneumonia that progressed in spite of treatment with an oral cephalosporin antibiotic. In the absence of an alternative etiological diagnosis, she was treated with an antibiotic that is known to be effective in Legionnaires disease, pending the results of the culture. This clinical decision may have saved her life.

Prevention of Legionnaires disease is presently practiced at an institutional level by monitoring water systems and by clinical surveillance for sentinel cases of legionellosis. In hospitals, hotels, and other large buildings where cases have occurred, **water systems are checked regularly for *Legionella***. When found, the systems are flushed and decontaminated by superheating of the water to 60°C, ultraviolet irradiation, or treatment with copper and silver ions or monochloramine. Because a single case of legionellosis may reflect a larger outbreak, clinical diagnosis is often the critical first step in prevention. Following Mrs. R's case, *L. pneumophila* serogroup 1 was cultured from the water system of the Florida resort where she vacationed. Decontamination of this system may have prevented numerous subsequent cases.

OTHER *LEGIONELLA* AND *LEGIONELLA*-ASSOCIATED DISEASES

In addition to *L. pneumophila*, several other species of *Legionella* cause human disease. In general, these are also water-related infections, and they produce clinical features comparable to Legionnaires disease, for example, *Legionella micdadei*. In Australia and New Zealand, a significant cause of legionellosis is *Legionella longbeachae*, which is typically acquired by inhalation of contaminated potting soil, rather than water aerosols.

Certain *Legionella* have also been associated with an illness called Pontiac fever. The illness was first recognized during a 1968 outbreak at the county health department building in Pontiac, Michigan. In this outbreak, 95% of the departmental employees became ill with fever, muscle aches, headache, and dizziness that resolved spontaneously in 2 to 5 days. The cause of this flulike illness was not identified at the time, but serum samples from patients and lung tissue from guinea pigs exposed to the building air were kept frozen for future reference. After the identification of *L. pneumophila* 9 years later, the frozen specimens were retested. The Pontiac patients were found to have had a rise in specific *Legionella* antibodies, and the guinea pig lungs yielded growth of *L. pneumophila* in culture.

Like Legionnaires disease, Pontiac fever is an airborne disease; but there the similarity ends. Unlike Legionnaires disease, Pontiac fever typically affects a high proportion of exposed individuals, and it affects healthy, as well as high-risk, individuals. It does not produce pneumonia and is never fatal. It may not involve bacterial infection, as the microbe has not been cultured from these patients. How the same bacteria can produce two such different clinical syndromes is still a mystery.

CONCLUSION

L. pneumophila is an opportunistic pathogen that can produce an airborne infection of the lungs that may develop into a life-threatening pneumonia. Infection depends upon the capacity of the bacterium to grow within phagocytic macrophages of the host. Treatment and immune mechanisms are beneficial insofar as they can affect the bacteria that occupy this intracellular niche.

Suggested Readings

Dalebroux ZD, Svensson SL, Gaynor EC, et al. ppGpp conjures bacterial virulence. *Microbiol Mol Biol Rev.* 2010;74:171–199.

Ensminger AW, Isberg RR. *Legionella pneumophila* Dot/Icm translocated substrates: a sum of parts. *Curr Opin Microbiol.* 2009;12:67–73.

Fraser DW, Tsai TR, Orenstein W, et al. Legionnaires' disease: description of an epidemic of pneumonia. *N Engl J Med.* 1977;297:1189–1197.

Lamoth F, Greub G. Amoebal pathogens as emerging causal agents of pneumonia. *FEMS Microbiol Rev.* 2009;34:260–280.

Molofsky AB, Swanson MS. Differentiate to thrive: Lessons from the *Legionella pneumophila* life cycle. *Mol Microbiol.* 2004;53:29–40.

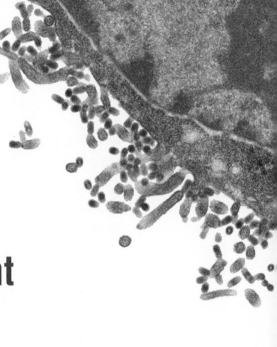

Chapter **22**

Helicobacter pylori: Pathogenesis of a Persistent Bacterial Infection

Jennifer M. Noto and Richard M. Peek Jr

KEY CONCEPTS

Pathogen: Gram-negative, helical-shaped microbe with high degree of genetic diversity

Encounter: *Helicobacter* infects half of the world's population. It is acquired in childhood likely through fecal–oral or oral–oral routes.

Entry: It is notable for its ability to survive and to thrive in the highly acidic stomach. It produces a urease that can buffer the local environment by production of ammonium from urea.

Spread and Multiplication: It colonizes the mucus layer and the epithelial surface of the stomach and adheres to the epithelium through multiple outer membrane proteins. It evades host immunity through a variety of mechanisms including a vacuolating toxin (VacA) that suppresses T-cell responses.

Damage: VacA can cause cell death of the gastric epithelium; another virulence factor CagA disrupts tight junctions between cells.

Low-level inflammation within the gastric mucosa leads to persistent superficial gastritis. Most colonized persons have asymptomatic, chronic gastritis, but approximately 10% develop gastric or duodenal ulcers. It may cause atrophic gastritis, a well-established risk factor for gastric adenocarcinoma. Gastric cancer and—more rarely—gastric MALT lymphoma may occur.

Diagnosis: Rapid urease test, histology, and microbial culture on endoscopic biopsy. Urea breath test does not require endoscopy and is easy to perform. Biochemical confirmation includes tests for urease, catalase, and oxidase. Other tests are based on *H. pylori*–specific serology and stool antigens by immunoassay. Testing stool for antigen is highly accurate.

Treatment: Triple therapy—two antibiotics with a proton pump inhibitor—is common.

Prevention: Vaccinology against *H. pylori* targeting its multiple virulence factors is an active area of research, but a human vaccine has yet to be developed.

CASE • A 45-year-old African American male was evaluated for recurrent burning epigastric discomfort. Seven years earlier, he had noted abdominal pain that often woke him from sleep, was associated with nausea, and improved with meals. He was initially treated with a proton pump inhibitor (PPI) for 8 weeks to reduce the production of gastric acid, and his symptoms resolved. However, 4 months later, his symptoms recurred. At endoscopy, a 1-cm ulcer was seen in the duodenal bulb. The patient was once again given PPI therapy. However, four times in the ensuing 6 years, his burning epigastric pain recurred. The patient's mother and one of his two siblings also had a history of peptic ulcer disease. Another endoscopy showed that a duodenal ulcer was still present. Biopsies from two sites in the stomach were taken for histologic examination and culture. These specimens showed chronic active gastritis

continued on page 250

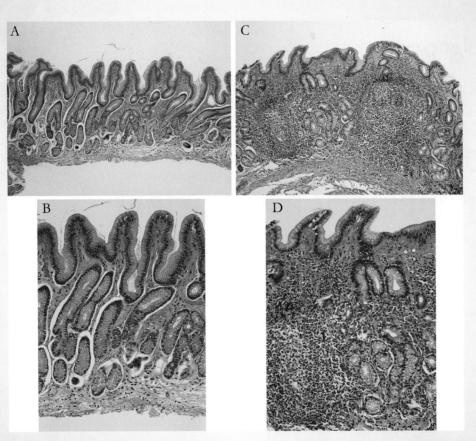

FIGURE 22-1. hematoxylin and eosin stain of *helicobacter pylori*–**associated gastritis.**
A. Normal gastric epithelium (10×) **B.** Normal gastric epithelium shown at higher magnification (20×). **C.** Active gastritis showing immune cell infiltration into the lamina propria as well as lymphoid follicle formation (10×). **D.** Active gastritis shown at higher magnification (20×).

with elevated numbers of neutrophils and mononuclear cells in the lamina propria and the glandular epithelium in addition to **lymphoid follicle** formation (Fig. 22-1). Curved, Gram-negative, rod-shaped bacteria were identified on the gastric mucosal surfaces of all samples, and cultures grew *Helicobacter pylori*.

In addition to acid reduction therapy with a PPI, the patient began a 10-day course of amoxicillin and clarithromycin. A repeat endoscopy 6 weeks after completion of therapy showed healing of his ulcer, and biopsies of his stomach showed resolution of gastritis. No *H. pylori* was found on histologic examination or culture. The patient remained symptom free after 6 months and required no further therapy.

This case raises a number of questions:

1. Was *H. pylori* the cause of the patient's 7-year bout of recurrent duodenal ulceration?
2. What features permit *H. pylori* to colonize the stomach when other bacteria cannot survive in this harsh environment?
3. What bacterial and/or host factors allow an infection with such high specificity for gastric epithelium to cause disease at an anatomically distinct site such as the duodenum?
4. How can *H. pylori* infection be detected in patients with disease?
5. How can *H. pylori* be eliminated from the stomach?

See Appendix for answers.

THE PATHOGEN: *HELICOBACTER PYLORI*

Helicobacter pylori is a Gram-negative bacterium that selectively colonizes the human stomach. In 1983, Barry Marshall and Robin Warren first identified *H. pylori* within the gastric epithelium of patients with chronic gastritis. They were subsequently awarded the Nobel Prize of Medicine in 2005 for their discovery of this pathogenic bacterium and its role in peptic ulcer disease. Since that discovery, a strong link has been established between *H. pylori* and a diverse spectrum of gastrointestinal diseases, including **gastric and duodenal ulceration**, **gastric adenocarcinoma**, **mucosa-associated lymphoid tissue (MALT) lymphoma**, and

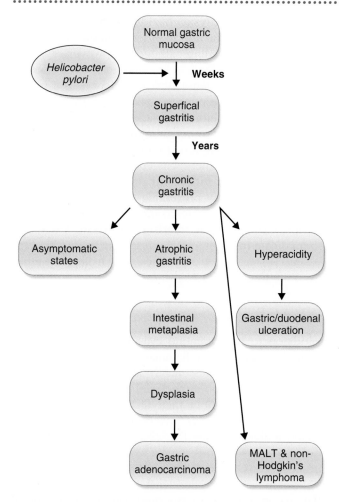

FIGURE 22-2. Diversity of clinical outcomes following *H. pylori* infection. *H. pylori* colonizes the human gastric mucosa and causes superficial gastritis within weeks. Over the years, *H. pylori*–induced gastritis can either remain clinically asymptomatic or lead to different disease outcomes, including duodenal ulcer, gastric adenocarcinoma, or, rarely, MALT or non-Hodgkin lymphoma.

non-Hodgkin lymphoma of the stomach (Fig. 22-2). As a result, the World Health Organization classified *H. pylori* as a class I carcinogen for gastric cancer in 1994.

H. pylori inhabits the human stomach for decades, not days or weeks as is usually the case for bacterial pathogens. The longevity of colonization and chronic, low-grade gastric inflammation with gradual progression to disease suggest that *H. pylori* is a prototypic persistent bacterium. In that sense, *H. pylori* resembles *Treponema pallidum*, *Borrelia burgdorferi*, and *Mycobacterium leprae*, which cause chronic, low-grade host inflammatory responses that ultimately lead to chronic disease, such as syphilis, Lyme disease, and leprosy, respectively. Recent insights into *H. pylori* pathophysiology are beginning to answer perplexing questions raised by its unique ecological niche, including why an organism that colonizes approximately half of the world's population leads to overt clinical disease in only 10 to 15% of infected individuals, and how *H. pylori* infection can cause such divergent clinical sequelae.

EPIDEMIOLOGY

Present in approximately half of the world's population, *H. pylori* remains one of the most common bacterial infections in humans. The precise mechanism by which *H. pylori* is transmitted remains undefined, in part because of its long-term persistence within the stomach as well as the nonspecific nature of symptoms associated with acute infection. Risk factors for infection include poor socio-economic status, familial overcrowding, ethnicity, and infection rates endemic to the country of origin. Though *H. pylori* can be found in all regions of the world, the prevalence of infection is significantly higher in developing countries. Most infections are thought to be acquired during childhood through fecal–oral or oral–oral modes of transmission. Eradication of *H. pylori* has been shown to significantly decrease the risk of gastric adenocarcinoma in persons who do not possess premalignant lesions, such as **intestinal metaplasia**, providing evidence that *H. pylori* influences the early stages of gastric carcinogenesis. The variable outcomes of *H. pylori* infection likely depend on strain-specific virulence determinants, responses governed by the genetic diversity of the host, or environmental factors, which ultimately influence the outcome of host–pathogen interactions. Thus, it is important to understand the pathogenesis of this persistent bacterial infection and how *H. pylori* colonizes the gastric niche, persists, and induces gastric damage and disease.

ENCOUNTER AND ADHERENCE

One of the initial obstacles encountered by *H. pylori* is the harsh, acidic (pH 1 to 2) environment of the stomach. To circumvent this deterrent, *H. pylori* is a robust producer of **urease**, which catalyzes the hydrolysis of urea into ammonia and carbon dioxide to neutralize the surrounding acidic environment (Fig. 22-3). Another fundamental barrier to successful *H. pylori* colonization of the stomach is gastric peristalsis. *H. pylori* uses several mechanisms to overcome this host defense, including efficient motility, chemotaxis, and adherence to the gastric epithelium (see Fig. 22-3). *H. pylori* have multiple **polar flagella** to penetrate and colonize the gastric mucus layer and its spiral shape confers efficient hydrodynamic movement within the mucus gel layer. In addition to flagella-mediated motility, **chemotaxis** plays a role in the ability of *H. pylori* to colonize and persist in the gastric niche.

Though most *H. pylori* are free living within the mucus layer of the gastric epithelium, approximately 20% adhere to gastric epithelial cells. Adherence of *H. pylori* to gastric epithelial cells is a critical step in establishing chronic infection, and a number of bacterial adhesins and host cell receptors have been identified that facilitate *H. pylori* colonization of the gastric epithelium. *H. pylori* express numerous outer membrane proteins that are important for adherence to and persistent colonization of the gastric epithelium. Some of the most well studied

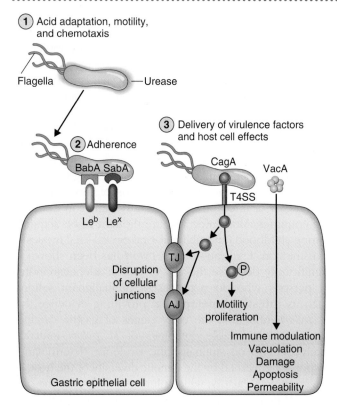

1 Acid adaptation, motility, and chemotaxis

Flagella — Urease

2 Adherence

3 Delivery of virulence factors and host cell effects

BabA SabA

CagA

VacA

T4SS

Le^b Le^x

Disruption of cellular junctions

TJ

P

AJ

Motility proliferation

Immune modulation
Vacuolation
Damage
Apoptosis
Permeability

Gastric epithelial cell

FIGURE 22-3. *H. pylori* virulence factors associated with adherence, persistence, and damage. Initial steps of *H. pylori* pathogenesis include acid adaptation, motility, and chemotaxis to the mucus layer and gastric epithelium. Next, a subpopulation of *H. pylori* colonizes the gastric epithelium via adhesin-mediated adherence to epithelial cell receptors. Following adherence, *H. pylori* can then initiate epithelial damage through release and delivery of effector proteins that induce an array of pathologic effects on the gastric epithelium. (BabA, blood-group antigen-binding adhesin; Le^b, Lewis^b blood-group antigen; SabA, sialic acid–binding adhesin; Le^x, Lewis^x blood-group antigen; CagA, cytotoxin-associated gene A; T4SS, type 4 secretion system; VacA, vacuolating cytotoxin A; TJ, tight junction; AJ, adherens junction; P, phosphorylated.)

are **blood-group antigen-binding adhesin, BabA,** and **sialic acid–binding adhesin, SabA** (see Fig. 22-3). BabA binds Lewis^b (Le^b) blood-group antigens, while SabA binds sialyl Lewis^x (Le^x) antigens that are expressed on gastric epithelial cells. The expression of both *H. pylori* BabA and SabA adhesins is associated with increased gastric cancer risk, indicating the importance of bacterial colonization on disease progression and carcinogenesis.

MULTIPLICATION, SURVIVAL, AND PERSISTENCE

The host immune system is a formidable obstacle that *H. pylori* must also overcome to establish residence within the stomach and cause disease. *H. pylori* possess numerous mechanisms to evade and manipulate the host immune response. Bacterial components, such as

flagella and **lipopolysaccharide (LPS)**, are usually readily detected by the host in order to mount an immune response against invading pathogens; however, *H. pylori* flagella and LPS are far less immunogenic than those of other invading pathogens. Typically, LPS elicits a robust host inflammatory response; however, *H. pylori* LPS is relatively anergic, exhibiting as little as 10^3 less endotoxin activity than LPS from other Gram-negative bacteria. Furthermore, *H. pylori* express a repertoire of human Lewis antigens on LPS, and these antigens undergo **phase variation** as a means of **molecular mimicry** to evade host immune responses by preventing the formation of antibodies against shared bacterial and host epitopes. Another *H. pylori* factor, the **vacuolating cytotoxin, VacA,** can also modulate the host immune response by directly suppressing T lymphocyte responses, which likely contributes to the longevity of *H. pylori* infection.

DAMAGE

In addition to host immune evasion, *H. pylori* induces low-grade, persistent inflammation within the gastric mucosa. As a result, essentially all individuals infected with *H. pylori* develop **superficial gastritis**, which typically persists throughout their lifetime. Long-term consequences of chronic *H. pylori* infection vary among infected individuals (see Fig. 22-2). Although the majority of colonized persons remain asymptomatic with only chronic gastritis, approximately 10% of infected individuals develop gastric or duodenal ulcers. For others, the inflammatory process is associated with loss of epithelial glands, termed **atrophic gastritis**, which occurs over the course of decades and is a well-established risk factor for the development of **gastric adenocarcinoma**. Gastric cancer develops in approximately 1 to 3% of infected individuals, and gastric **MALT lymphoma** occurs in less than 0.1% of infected individuals. Despite these low frequencies, gastric cancer remains the second leading cause of cancer-related death worldwide and *H. pylori* remains the strongest known risk factor for this disease.

H. pylori pathogenesis is complex, in keeping with the ability of this pathogen to cause a variety of diverse clinical manifestations. Although most *H. pylori*–infected individuals never develop clinical sequelae, colonization can lead to the development of peptic or duodenal ulceration and gastric carcinoma. *H. pylori* isolates exhibit substantial genetic diversity, and several virulence factors have been associated with peptic ulceration and carcinogenesis (see Fig. 22-3). One such factor is encoded by the **cytotoxin-associated gene**, *cagA*. This gene is a member of a 40-kilobase genomic element known as the ***cag* pathogenicity island** (PAI). Genes within the *cag*-PAI possess homology to components of a bacterial **type IV secretion system** that delivers bacterial effector proteins into host cells. The *H. pylori* effector protein, **CagA**, is translocated into host epithelial cells following *H. pylori* attachment, where it can be modified by phosphorylation of tyrosine residues. CagA activates several host signaling pathways through either phosphorylation-dependent or phosphorylation-independent mechanisms, ultimately leading to cell morphological changes, including disruption of junctional complexes (tight [TJ] and adherens junctions [AJ]) and increases in cell motility and proliferation (see Fig. 22-3).

CagA is present in approximately 70% of US *H. pylori* strains. Serum and mucosal antibodies to CagA are present in approximately 90% of patients with duodenal ulceration, and expression of CagA in vivo is highly correlated with peptic and duodenal inflammation and ulcer disease. *H. pylori* isolates that encode CagA (*cagA*+ strains) induce higher degrees of inflammation and damage in the gastric mucosa than do *cagA*− strains. In addition, mucosal levels of **interleukin 8** (**IL-8**), a potent proinflammatory cytokine, are significantly higher in persons harboring *cagA*+ strains compared to *cagA*− strains, which may explain the link between *cagA*+ strains and peptic ulcer disease.

Another *H. pylori* constituent that is associated with disease is the vacuolating cytotoxin, **VacA**. Present in virtually all strains of *H. pylori*, the gene *vacA* exists as different alleles which produce VacA proteins with different levels of vacuolating activity. *H. pylori* clinical isolates that produce a functional and potent VacA cytotoxin are more frequently associated with peptic ulcer disease and increased inflammatory infiltrates within the gastric antrum. In addition to vacuolation, VacA exerts other effects that may influence clinical outcome. Inoculation of mice with VacA leads to epithelial cell damage, and VacA causes gastric epithelial cells in vitro to undergo a specific form of cell death termed **apoptosis** (see Fig. 22-3). Although *H. pylori* can induce apoptosis, there is also evidence that very locally near the bacterium, the effects of its CagA protein are to inhibit the apoptosis caused by VacA. Thus, the microbe fine-tunes its effects on the host. VacA also functions as a transmembrane pore, permeabilizing host epithelial cells to urea, which in turn may allow *H. pylori* to manipulate the pH of its environment by generating ammonia with its urease. VacA also increases the paracellular permeability to important nutrients. Collectively, these findings indicate that VacA can induce multiple physiologic consequences that may contribute to gastric epithelial damage and disease pathogenesis.

It is likely that the complex interplay among bacterial and host factors contribute to different disease manifestations. However, the mechanism of ulcer development resulting from *H. pylori* infection is not completely understood. Continuous inflammation within the gastric mucosa may be sufficient to lead to mucosal breakdown, erosive gastritis, and ultimately gastric ulceration. *H. pylori* infection results in downregulation of somatostatin-producing D cells in the gastric mucosa, which in turn leads to inappropriately elevated gastrin levels and enhanced gastric acid secretion, all of which heighten the risk for duodenal ulceration (Fig. 22-4). In addition, duodenal intestinal-type tissue is often replaced by gastric tissue in patients

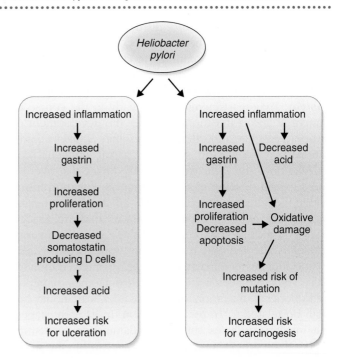

FIGURE 22-4. Potential mechanisms of ulceration and carcinogenesis following *H. pylori* infection. *H. pylori* increases the risk for gastric ulceration and carcinogenesis. The development of these disease states is complex, but a number of *H. pylori*–induced alterations have been shown to predispose the gastric epithelium to these different disease outcomes.

with hyperacidity. *H. pylori* can then populate regions of gastric metaplasia in the duodenum, establish infection, cause inflammation, and, in concert with elevated gastric acid levels, ultimately lead to ulceration at this distal site.

H. pylori infection is also associated with the development of adenocarcinoma of the stomach. The sequential progression of the most common form of this malignancy, intestinal-type gastric cancer, is lengthy, from chronic superficial gastritis to chronic atrophic gastritis, through intestinal metaplasia to dysplasia, and finally to invasive adenocarcinoma (see Fig. 22-2). After the onset of superficial gastritis, the entire process can take decades. *H. pylori* infection has also been shown to increase cellular proliferation while concomitantly decreasing the rate of apoptosis within colonized tissue, leading to increased cellular survival within an environment rich in inflammatory mediators (see Fig. 22-4). Increased gastric inflammation followed by increased cellular proliferation, both of which develop secondary to chronic *H. pylori* infection, may increase the likelihood of oxidative DNA damage in response to inflammation-induced oxygen or nitrogen free radicals. Cumulatively increased proliferation in combination with increased DNA damage heightens the risk for retention of genetic mutations and therefore increased carcinogenic potential. The risk of gastric cancer is also related to certain strain-specific factors. Infection with *cagA*+ toxigenic *H. pylori* strains is associated with a significantly increased risk for gastric adenocarcinoma, perhaps caused by the heightened inflammatory response and/or disruption of normal gastric epithelial turnover and homeostasis.

Host factors also contribute to carcinogenesis within *H. pylori*–infected gastric mucosa. One host determinant that may influence the development of gastric cancer is **gastrin**. Hypergastrinemia occurs early in the course of human *H. pylori* infection, precedes the development of atrophic gastritis, and often resolves after *H. pylori* eradication. In vitro, gastrin stimulates gastric epithelial cell proliferation, and *Helicobacter*-infected mice that overexpress gastrin develop gastric carcinomas. Polymorphisms within the human interleukin-1β (*IL-1β*) and tumor necrosis factor-α gene promoter sequences that are associated with increased expression of these proinflammatory cytokines also increase the risk for atrophic gastritis and gastric adenocarcinoma among *H. pylori*–infected individuals. Thus, the seemingly divergent outcomes of peptic and duodenal ulceration and gastric adenocarcinoma can both be related to *H. pylori* infection. In its early stages, the infection induces sufficient inflammation to disrupt mucosal integrity, alter acid homeostasis within the stomach, and potentially lead to ulcers, while in its later stage, it may promote the development of atrophic gastritis and subsequent neoplastic transformation.

In addition to ulcer disease and gastric adenocarcinoma, individuals infected with *H. pylori* have an increased risk of developing MALT lymphoma and non-Hodgkin lymphoma of the stomach. T cells that participate in the chronic inflammatory process can react with *H. pylori* antigens to produce inflammatory cytokines driving the uncontrolled growth and proliferation of B lymphocytes, leading to malignant lymphomatous degeneration. Although MALT lymphomas are rare in the United States, elimination of *H. pylori* leads to complete regression of these tumors in more than 80% of cases, a remarkable demonstration that removal of *H. pylori* can affect a clonal lesion.

DIAGNOSIS

Several techniques are currently available to diagnose *H. pylori* and can be classified as either invasive or noninvasive (Table 22-1). All the tests are quite sensitive and specific, and the choice of which test to use depends on the laboratory resources available and the clinical situation. Invasive methods involve obtaining gastric tissue biopsies by endoscopy and include **rapid urease tests**, **histology**, and **microbial culture**. Most pathologists initially use the Giemsa stain because it is sensitive and inexpensive; the **Steiner stain** (Fig. 22-5) and Warthin-Starry stain are more sensitive but also more expensive. Detection of *H. pylori* by culture is less reliable than other available methods because of the fastidious growth characteristics of the organism. Biochemical confirmation of *H. pylori* includes utilization of tests to assess production of **urease**, **catalase**, and **oxidase**. A rapid urease test detects urease activity within a gastric biopsy sample. When a biopsy containing *H. pylori* is placed into a

TABLE 22-1 Diagnosis of *Helicobacter pylori* Infection

Method	Specimen	Sensitivity
Invasive Tests		
Urease test	Mucosal gastric biopsy	High
Histology	Mucosal gastric biopsy	Very high
Culture	Mucosal gastric biopsy	Very high
Noninvasive Tests		
Serologic test	Serum	High
Urea breath test	Breath sample	Very high
Stool antigen test	Stool	Very high
Tests Used in Research		
Polymerase chain reaction	Stool sample, gastric juice, gastric biopsy	High

urea-containing indicator medium, ammonia is produced from urea, the pH increases, and the indicator turns red. The rapid urease test is less expensive than either histology or culture and is often the method of choice when endoscopy is used.

Noninvasive diagnostic tests include serology, the **urea breath tests**, and stool antigen tests. Serologic tests measure levels of circulating IgG antibodies directed against a variety of *H. pylori* antigens by enzyme-linked immunosorbent assay (ELISA) and are very sensitive and specific for primary diagnosis of *H. pylori* infection. However, serological methods have limited utility in assessing posttreatment *H. pylori* status because serologic titers fall

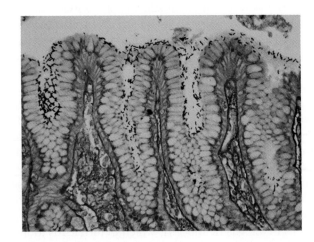

FIGURE 22-5. Steiner stain of *H. pylori*. *H. pylori* stain black because they are impregnated with silver and are therefore easily detectable in biopsy specimens. Numerous bacteria can be seen in the mucous layer and adherent to gastric epithelial cells.

gradually, and 6 months may be required before a sufficient decrease is observed. Urea breath tests involve ingestion of radioactive carbon-labeled urea, and if *H. pylori* is present, urea is metabolized to ammonia and carbon dioxide, and radioactive carbon dioxide is detected in breath samples. The urea breath test is a convenient method to document *H. pylori* eradication because it does not require endoscopy and is easy to perform.

An enzymatic immunoassay, HpSA, detects the presence of bacterial antigens in feces and is available as an alternative noninvasive *H. pylori* diagnostic technique. The *H. pylori* stool antigen test is both sensitive and specific, and the Food and Drug Administration (FDA) has approved HpSA for initial diagnosis of *H. pylori* and for monitoring posttherapy responses. Following successful treatment of *H. pylori,* stool antigen levels rapidly decline and, in the majority of patients, are undetectable by 5 days after treatment. Stool samples can be stored for prolonged periods and multiple samples can be assayed at once. Testing stool for *H. pylori* antigens is a highly accurate technique that is cost-effective compared with both serologic testing before therapy and urea breath testing after therapy.

TREATMENT

Physicians should only attempt to diagnose *H. pylori* if they are unequivocally committed to treating the infection. Currently, it is recommended that individuals with a present or past history of peptic ulcer disease or gastric MALT lymphoma or nonulcer dyspepsia be tested for *H. pylori* and treated if positive. Less clear indications exist for close family relatives of patients with gastric cancer or persons who have migrated from regions where the background prevalence of gastric cancer is high. An ideal treatment for *H. pylori* would be inexpensive, safe with minimal side effects, simple, effective, and short in duration. In addition, treatment should not induce significant antibiotic resistance. All regimens used to date fall short of these parameters. Several factors that limit the effectiveness of therapy for *H. pylori* include (1) rapidly developing bacterial resistance to metronidazole, quinolones, and macrolides; (2) reduced efficacy of certain drugs, such as clarithromycin and amoxicillin, under acidic conditions; and (3) patient noncompliance owing to side effects or the burden of ingesting multiple medications for 7 to 14 days.

The goal of *H. pylori* therapy is to eliminate the organism from the stomach, and successful eradication is defined as a negative test for the bacterium 4 or more weeks after completion of therapy. In general, antisecretory agents such as PPIs relieve ulcer symptoms and promote ulcer healing. In addition, the gastric pH is raised by these agents, which in turn increases the efficacy of antibiotics such as amoxicillin and clarithromycin. Initially, several large multicenter eradication trials documented that eradication rates of more than 85% could be achieved with triple therapies lasting 7 to 10 days and consisting of a PPI and two antibiotics (usually **clarithromycin** and either **amoxicillin** or **metronidazole**; Table 22-2). There

TABLE 22-2 Optimal Treatment Regimens for *Helicobacter pylori* Infection

Regimen	Drug	Dose	Duration
Triple therapy			
	Proton pump inhibitor (PPI)	Twice daily	7–10 d
	and amoxicillin	1 g twice daily	7–10 d
	and clarithromycin	500 mg twice daily	7–10 d
Quadruple therapy			
	PPI	Twice daily	14 d
	and bismuth subsalicylate	120 mg four times daily	14 d
	and tetracycline	500 mg four times daily	14 d
	and metronidazole	250 mg four times daily	14 d
Sequential therapy			
	PPI	Twice daily	1–10 d
	and amoxicillin	1 g twice daily	1–5 d
	then clarithromycin	500 mg twice daily	6–10 d
	and metronidazole	250 mg twice daily	6–10 d

are no consistent advantages to using a particular PPI for *H. pylori* eradication; therefore, any agent in this class can be used as a component of triple therapy.

However, the prevalence of antimicrobial resistance in *H. pylori* is increasing, particularly to metronidazole and clarithromycin, thus requiring the development of effective second-line therapies. Because the most effective second-line regimens contain metronidazole, it is advisable to use clarithromycin and amoxicillin instead of clarithromycin and metronidazole in first-line regimens to optimize treatment efficacy should subsequent therapy be required. Other therapies exist if first-line regimens fail to eliminate *H. pylori*. One effective regimen is quadruple therapy combining a PPI, bismuth subsalicylate, metronidazole, and tetracycline for 14 days (see Table 22-2). Another more novel, innovative strategy for the treatment of *H. pylori* is sequential therapy. This 10-day treatment regimen consists of a PPI and amoxicillin twice daily for the first 5 days followed by triple therapy of PPI, clarithromycin, and metronidazole twice daily for the remaining 5 days (see Table 22-2). This new regimen has achieved high eradication rates and is often effective in patients infected with clarithromycin-resistant *H. pylori* strains.

Although eradication rates in controlled trials often exceed 90%, efficacy in clinical practice is usually lower, primarily because of differences in patient populations, differences in infecting *H. pylori* isolates, and/or antibiotic resistance patterns of strains in a particular geographic area. As a result of the current availability and accuracy of noninvasive diagnostic tests for *H. pylori,* it is recommended that urea breath or stool antigen tests be performed following intervention to confirm successful eradication.

PREVENTION

The potential to prevent *H. pylori*–associated diseases with a vaccine is exciting. However, this strategy is likely to be most appropriately applied in areas where childhood infection is endemic. To develop an effective vaccine against *H. pylori*, factors important for its virulence must be identified, characterized, produced on a large scale, and then administered in an immunologically relevant way. In mice, an oral vaccine consisting of *H. pylori* urease prevented chronic infection by the related, murine-specific species *H. felis*. Interestingly, infected mice that received an oral treatment with recombinant urease were able to eliminate a chronic *H. felis* infection and developed protection against subsequent *H. felis* challenge. Thus, therapeutic vaccination may be possible, and there are many appealing *H. pylori* antigenic targets worth pursuing.

CONCLUSION

H. pylori infects approximately one-half of the world's population, but in most individuals, the infection is clinically asymptomatic. Transmission occurs likely via fecal–oral and/or oral–oral routes. *H. pylori*–induced gastritis is a necessary condition for the development of peptic ulceration. The infection is also linked with gastric adenocarcinoma, MALT lymphoma, and non-Hodgkin lymphoma of the stomach. Several excellent diagnostic tests are currently available, and effective therapeutic regimens now exist. The overwhelming evidence linking peptic ulcer disease to *H. pylori* infection indicates that ulcer patients infected with the organism should receive antimicrobial therapy directed toward *H. pylori* to decrease ulcer recurrence. However, antibiotic resistance is an increasing concern for *H. pylori* treatment and eradication; thus, discovery of new *H. pylori* therapies and vaccines will likely continue to be important areas of research. In the future, vaccines may not only provide a means to prevent *H. pylori* infection but also offer a therapeutic intervention.

Suggested Readings

Amieva MR, El-Omar EM. Host-bacterial interactions in *Helicobacter pylori* infection. *Gastroenterology*. 2008;134(1):306–323.

Atherton JC, Blaser MJ. Coadaptation of *Helicobacter pylori* and humans: ancient history, modern implications. *J Clin Invest*. 2009;119(9):2475–2487.

Graham DY, Shiotani A. New concepts of resistance in the treatment of *Helicobacter pylori* infections. *Nat Clin Pract Gastroenterol Hepatol*. 2008;5(6):321–331.

Israel DA, Peek RM. Surreptitious manipulation of the human host by *Helicobacter pylori*. *Gut Microbes*. 2010;1(2):119–127.

McColl KEL. *Helicobacter pylori* Infection. *N Engl J Med*. 2010;362(17):1597–1604.

Polk DB, Peek RM. *Helicobacter pylori*: gastric cancer and beyond. *Nat Rev Cancer*. 2010;10:403–414.

Vakil N, Megraud F. Eradication Therapy for *Helicobacter pylori*. *Gastroenterology*. 2007;133:985–1001.

Chapter 23

Mycobacteria: Tuberculosis and Leprosy

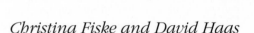

Christina Fiske and David Haas

KEY CONCEPTS

Mycobacterium tuberculosis

- Is a slow-growing, obligate aerobe.

- The acid-fast staining characteristic of *Mycobacteria* spp. results from the mycolic acid linked to the cell wall.

Encounter: This agent infects one-third of the world's population, but only 10% of those infected develop clinical disease.

Entry: The bacterium is usually acquired by inhaling aerosolized droplet nuclei.

Spread and Multiplication: *M. tuberculosis* can cause illness that begins soon after initial infection (primary disease) or can remain latent for years before reactivating and causing illness (endogenous reactivation).

Damage: Infection may elicit a cellular immune response that controls infection, with the only sequelae being a positive tuberculin skin test.

Or, infection may elicit a host immune response responsible for the pathologic features of the disease.

Active tuberculosis (TB) most often causes pulmonary disease associated with fever, weight loss, and drenching night sweats.

Diagnosis: TB is usually diagnosed by microscopy and culture of sputum.

Treatment and Prevention: TB is treated with combination antimicrobial therapy.

Mycobacterium leprae

- Is a slow-growing, acid-fast bacillus that is the causative agent of leprosy.

- Causes illness that ranges between two polar forms: tuberculoid (strong immune response with few organisms) and lepromatous (minimal immune response with immense numbers of organisms).

TUBERCULOSIS (TB) is the illness caused by *Mycobacterium tuberculosis* (also called the **tubercle bacillus**). Worldwide, the disease is **second only to HIV** as the most common cause of death from a single infectious agent. In 1993, TB was declared a global public health emergency by the World Health Organization. TB can affect any organ, but the lungs are the most important site. The outcome of infection depends on the timing of exposure to *M. tuberculosis*, age of the individual, and overall immunocompetence. At least 90% of healthy persons who become infected with *M. tuberculosis* never become ill. However, the organism can survive within macrophages and persist in tissues for many years. In some individuals, previously dormant (**latent**) bacteria can cause illness months or years later, with tissue damage caused mostly by hypersensitivity of the sensitized host to bacterial products. In contrast, almost all persons with AIDS who are coinfected with *M. tuberculosis* eventually develop active TB. Already one of the most important infectious diseases in the world, TB has become even more significant with the rise of the **AIDS pandemic** and the spread of **multidrug-resistant** strains.

This chapter discusses the pathogenesis and selected clinical aspects of TB. Leprosy, a relatively common mycobacterial disease in some resource-limited countries, is also discussed. For clarification, the term *infection* describes entry, multiplication, and survival of an organism within the host, regardless of whether symptoms develop; the term *disease* indicates illness resulting from infection.

CASE • Ms. A., a 35-year-old child care worker, had been in good health until she began experiencing chronic cough and weight loss. Over 2 months, she developed gradually worsening cough productive of yellow sputum. She also noted decreased appetite, a 15-lb weight loss, daily fever, and drenching night sweats. She did not improve despite being prescribed a routine antibiotic for 1 week. A chest radiograph revealed infiltrates in the apices of both lungs (Fig. 23-1). On further questioning, she described visiting South Africa several years earlier, where she worked briefly on an AIDS ward. She also recalled that her mother had a positive tuberculin skin test about 20 years ago, but her mother was never ill.

Ms. A. had a tuberculin skin test placed (intradermal injection of tuberculin on the volar aspect of the forearm), but it showed no induration (thickening) when examined 48 hours later. She was referred to a local health department, where acid-fast staining and microscopy of her sputum showed acid-fast bacilli. She was placed on respiratory isolation at home and prescribed four antituberculous drugs. Within 1 week she felt much better, after 2 weeks was taken off respiratory isolation, and after 1 month was allowed to return to work. She was cured after receiving 6 months of therapy, with every dose administered under direct observation by a health department nurse, as required by local public health authorities.

This case raises several questions:

1. How and when did Ms. A. most likely become infected with *Mycobacterium tuberculosis*?

2. Why did it take so long for Ms. A. to develop active tuberculosis (TB)?

3. By what route did the tubercle bacilli most likely arrive at the apices of her lungs?

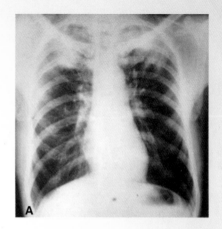

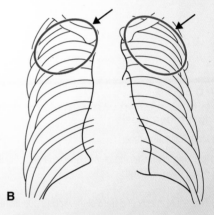

FIGURE 23-1. Pulmonary tuberculosis (TB). A. Chest radiograph from a young adult with TB involving the apices of both lungs. **B.** The areas most affected are *circled*.

4. Which individuals are most likely to develop active TB from contact with Ms. A.?

5. How would her illness have differed if she had had AIDS?

See Appendix for answers.

MYCOBACTERIUM TUBERCULOSIS

THE PATHOGEN

The genus *Mycobacterium* includes closely related species of **obligate aerobes** (Table 23-1). Species other than *M. tuberculosis* are often called atypical mycobacteria. These organisms are usually acquired from the environment rather than from person-to-person spread and tend to cause diseases distinct from TB. This genus also includes the agent of leprosy, *M. leprae* (discussed later in the chapter). Many mycobacteria are harmless, and some live on the human body without causing disease (e.g., *M. smegmatis*), while others are found in soil and other niches in the environment. Mycobacteria are **acid fast**, are unusually **resistant to drying**, and **grow slowly** compared with most other bacteria.

Acid Fastness: A Hallmark of Mycobacteria

Mycobacteria have the unusual property of retaining basic dyes when treated with acidic solutions. This property is a consequence of the mycobacterial envelope, which contains waxes composed of long-chain branched hydrocarbons. The most abundant wax, **mycolic acid**, is an α-alkyl-hydroxy fatty acid covalently linked to the cell wall. The name *Mycobacteria* reflects the presence of mycolic acid in the organisms. The waxy barrier greatly reduces permeability to many molecules, including Gram stain, and

TABLE 23-1 Characteristics of Clinically Important Species of Mycobacteria[a]

Species	Reservoir	Virulence for Humans	Main Disease Caused	Case-to-Case Transmission	In Vitro Growth Rate	Optimum Growth Temperature (°C)
Mycobacterium tuberculosis	Human	+ + +	TB	Yes	S	37
Mycobacterium bovis	Animals	+ + +	TB	Rare	S	37
Bacillus Calmette-Guérin (BCG)	Artificial culture	±	Local lesion	Very rare	S	37
Mycobacterium kansasii	Environment	+ +	TB-like	No	S	37
Mycobacterium scrofulaceum	Environment	+	Lymphadenitis	No	S	37
Mycobacterium avium-intracellulare	Environment; birds	+	TB-like *or* disseminated disease in AIDS	No	S	37
Mycobacterium fortuitum	Environment	±	Skin abscesses	No	F	37
Mycobacterium marinum	Water, fish	±	Skin granuloma	No	S	30
Mycobacterium ulcerans	Probably environment; tropical	+	Skin ulcerations	No	S	30
Mycobacterium leprae	Human	+ + +	Leprosy	Yes	None	Not applicable

[a]This table omits many essentially saprophytic mycobacteria.
S, slow; F, fast; BCG, Bacillus Calmette-Guérin; TB, tuberculosis.

mycobacteria are neither Gram-positive nor Gram-negative. However, they can be stained with special techniques such as briefly heating in the presence of a basic red dye called fuchsin. In some cases, detergent is added to the stain. The specimen is then treated with 3% hydrochloric acid in ethanol, which removes the stain from nearly all organisms except mycobacteria (thus, they are **acid fast**). The smear is then counterstained with a blue dye to provide a contrasting background. Mycobacteria appear as slender red rods. **Fluorochrome dyes** are now commonly used instead of fuchsin because they are more easily detected by fluorescence microscopy. The principle of staining with fluorochrome is otherwise similar to staining with fuchsin.

The waxy coat makes *M. tuberculosis* **resistant to drying** and to chemicals, which helps them survive both inside and outside the body. They are unusually resistant to killing by phagocytes. The resistance of mycobacteria to drying also facilitates airborne transmission. Their waxy coat does not, however, help them withstand heat. For example, in milk, the bacteria are killed by **pasteurization** (heating to 60°C for 30 minutes).

Slow Growth

Mycobacteria grow much more slowly than most other bacterial pathogens. The generation time of *M. tuberculosis* is 15 to 20 hours compared with less than 1 hour for most bacterial pathogens. Because of this long generation time, visible growth on solid media may take up to 6 weeks. Some mycobacteria grow faster than *M. tuberculosis* but still more slowly than other bacteria. Slow growth may delay diagnosis by culture methods alone. Even using specialized liquid broth media, detection can take 2 weeks or longer. Testing for drug susceptibility requires additional time after the organism

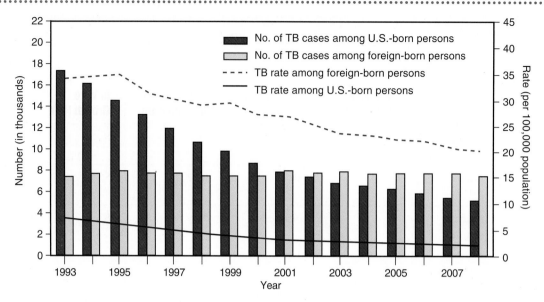

FIGURE 23-2. Number and rate of TB cases in the United States among US-born and foreign-born persons, by year reported—1993 to 2008. Data are updated as of February 18, 2009. Data for 2008 are provisional.

is recovered in culture. Thus, the patient who appropriately initiates therapy based on a positive sputum smear showing acid-fast organisms may wait many weeks before knowing whether the organism is susceptible to the prescribed antimicrobials.

ENCOUNTER

TB is an ancient disease. Evidence of TB has been found in the bones of Neolithic, pre-Colombian, and early Egyptian remains. It became a major public health problem during the Industrial Revolution, when crowded living conditions favored its airborne spread. In the eighteenth century, TB killed one-fourth of all adults in Europe. Major improvements began in the 1940s with effective antituberculous drugs. In the United States, TB case rates have declined ever since accurate statistics became available, even before the use of effective drugs. However, in the late 1980s, rates in the United States increased sharply because of infections in individuals with AIDS and transmission from them to others. Inadequately funded TB control programs in some major cities could not manage this problem, and large outbreaks resulted. Because of incomplete adherence with therapy, there were epidemics of multidrug-resistant TB, especially in Miami and New York City. Fortunately, TB case rates in the United States have declined since 1992, and in 2002, the rates were the lowest in history (<10 cases per 100,000 population). Foreign-born persons now comprise more than one-half of all TB cases in the United States (Fig. 23-2).

M. tuberculosis infects one-third of the world's population. Its rapid spread requires crowded living conditions and a population with little native resistance. Certain risk factors such as illicit drug use, excess alcohol use, homelessness, and HIV infection are interrelated

and lead to an increased risk of both TB reactivation and transmission. In Europe, case rates began declining before the turn of the century as those with less native resistance succumbed to the disease and living condi-

TABLE 23-2 Estimated Incidence of TB Among Countries that Account for 70% of Reported Cases Worldwide, 2007

Country	Cases	Rate per 100,000 Population
India	1,962,000	168
China	1,306,000	98
Indonesia	528,000	228
Nigeria	460,000	311
South Africa	461,000	948
Bangladesh	353,000	223
Ethiopia	314,000	378
Pakistan	297,000	181
Philippines	255,000	290
DR Congo	245,000	392
Russian Federation	157,000	110
Vietnam	150,000	171

Data from Global tuberculosis control: epidemiology, strategy, financing. *WHO report 2009*. Geneva, World Health Organization, 2009 (WHO/HTM/TB/2009.411). (http://www.who.int/tb/publications/global_report/2009/pdf/full_report.pdf).

MYCOBACTERIA AND AIDS

The interaction between *M. tuberculosis* and HIV is causing global devastation. Nearly all persons coinfected with HIV and *M. tuberculosis* will eventually develop active tuberculosis (TB) unless the HIV or the tuberculous infection is effectively treated. Persons with AIDS are predisposed to reactivation of remote infection and to rapid progression of recently acquired infection. TB is somewhat unique among opportunistic infections in persons with AIDS because of its person-to-person airborne spread. AIDS patients with TB are likely to develop widespread **extrapulmonary disease** as depletion of CD4+ T cells impairs cell-mediated immunity. Fortunately, persons with AIDS respond well to antituberculous therapy.

Patients with advanced AIDS are also very susceptible to disease caused by *Mycobacterium avium* complex (MAC). This organism is often found in water and soil and is generally harmless to immunocompetent individuals. Before the AIDS epidemic, MAC occasionally caused chronic pneumonia in patients with underlying lung disease, but disseminated infections were rare. In contrast, MAC frequently colonizes the gastrointestinal tract of patients with advanced AIDS before invading deeper tissues and causing disseminated disease. Patients with disseminated MAC may experience a nonspecific chronic illness with fever, malaise, and wasting, or such patients may have local manifestations, including diarrhea with involvement of the intestine or abdominal pain from involvement of the liver, spleen, and retroperitoneal lymph nodes. As with *M. tuberculosis*, effective therapy for MAC requires prolonged administration of multiple drugs.

tions improved. The rate of decline doubled after chemotherapy became widespread, and epidemiologists once thought TB would eventually disappear. Currently, TB has its greatest impact in resource-limited countries where HIV rates are often high (Table 23-2). With more than 30 million persons now living with HIV, the potential for interaction between AIDS and TB is immense (see the box titled "Mycobacteria and AIDS"). The situation is worst in Africa, where half of all HIV-infected adults also are infected with *M. tuberculosis* and 30 to 40% of all deaths due to AIDS are from TB.

ENTRY

Almost all tuberculous infections result from inhaling infectious particles that were aerosolized by coughing, sneezing, or talking. The initial source of infection is the lung in almost all cases. These so-called **droplet nuclei** dry while airborne, can remain suspended for hours, and when inhaled can reach the terminal air passages (Fig. 23-3). A cough or sneeze can produce thousands of droplet nuclei, as can talking for several minutes. Accordingly, the **air in a room occupied by a person with pulmonary TB may remain infectious even after the person has left the room**. Fortunately, prolonged exposure and multiple aerosol inocula are generally required to establish infection. Brief contact carries little risk, and infection rarely occurs outdoors because ultraviolet light kills *M. tuberculosis*. Large drops of respiratory secretions or contaminated inanimate objects infrequently result in transmission. In the past, TB of the intestine or the tonsils was common from ingestion of contaminated milk. This form of TB was caused by *M. bovis*, an organism that is

genetically similar to *M. tuberculosis* and causes infection in cattle.

Airborne spread of TB is efficient for several reasons. In source cases, the host inflammatory response to TB creates open lung lesions (**pulmonary cavities**) that contain huge numbers of organisms. Coughing spreads

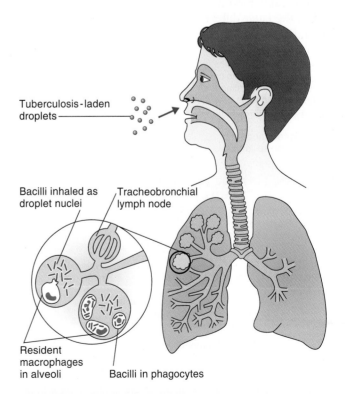

Tuberculosis-laden droplets

Bacilli inhaled as droplet nuclei

Tracheobronchial lymph node

Resident macrophages in alveoli

Bacilli in phagocytes

FIGURE 23-3. *Mycobacterium tuberculosis* **transmission by inhalation of droplet nuclei.**

the organisms from such lesions into the air. Contagiousness roughly correlates with the number of acid-fast bacilli visible by microscopy of sputum. Patients who are acid-fast smear positive are more contagious than those who are acid-fast smear negative but culture positive. However, many new infections are acquired from smear-negative but culture-positive patients, reflecting the limited sensitivity of acid-fast staining. The small size of droplet nuclei is also ideal for bypassing the mucociliary lining of large airways to reach the alveoli.

SPREAD, MULTIPLICATION, AND DAMAGE

Tubercle bacilli do not produce exotoxins or endotoxin. Instead, the clinical manifestations of TB result largely from the host immune response. Damage is caused by chronic inflammation and survival of organisms within macrophages.

Primary Tuberculosis

In **primary infection**, airborne droplet nuclei reach the alveoli where multiplication begins. This primary infection usually involves the middle lung zone, where airflow is greatest. There, the bacteria are ingested by alveolar macrophages, which may eliminate small numbers of bacilli. However, *M. tuberculosis* multiplies mostly unimpeded, destroying the macrophage (Fig. 23-4). Its capacity to multiply both inside and outside cells makes *M. tuberculosis* a **facultative intracellular pathogen**. Lymphocytes and monocytes are attracted from the bloodstream, the latter differentiating into macrophages, which ingest bacilli released from dying cells. Infected mac-

rophages are carried by lymphatics to regional lymph nodes. Some individuals develop the so-called **Ghon complex**, in which an area of lung inflammation is associated with enlarged hilar lymph nodes draining the area. In the nonimmune host, organisms may spread hematogenously throughout the body. During this early **lymphohematogenous dissemination**, the organisms preferentially localize in certain tissues, including lymph nodes, vertebral bodies, and meninges but most importantly the apices (upper parts) of the lungs. During the days and weeks before an effective cellular immune response develops, the organisms grow uninhibited in the initial pulmonary focus and the additional sites.

Primary infection can have various outcomes (Fig. 23-5). Cellular immunity and tissue hypersensitivity usually appear 3 to 8 weeks after infection and are marked by a positive tuberculin skin test (discussed later in the chapter). In most affected individuals, this response controls infection (although viable organisms may persist in the tissues), no symptoms develop, and the only evidence of infection is a positive tuberculin skin test. However, in some cases, the immune response does not control the primary infection, and progressive primary TB develops. This manifestation usually affects the very young, the elderly, and persons with advanced AIDS. In such individuals, the primary focus directly progresses to worsening pneumonia, and the very young may develop tuberculous meningitis. The most important consequence of lymphohematogenous dissemination is seeding of the lung apices, where either progressive primary or secondary disease can occur.

In persons with immunity from previous exposure to *M. tuberculosis*, organisms in newly inhaled droplet nuclei are destroyed before significant multiplication occurs. Nearly all TB in previously infected patients is the result of endogenous reactivation. However, when the airborne inoculum is large, or when host defenses are compromised, exogenous reinfection can occur.

Age influences the course of infection. Infants and children younger than 5 years of age who become infected are at high risk for developing progressive primary disease. In contrast, from age 5 to puberty is a period of relative resistance to progressive disease, although not to infection. From puberty until young adulthood, formation of apical cavities soon after primary infection is common. Most disease in this age group is caused by relatively recent infection rather than reactivation of childhood infection. Infection in mid-adulthood has a much better immediate and probably long-term prognosis, presumably because of a reduced tendency to develop tissue necrosis. In the elderly, infection acquired years earlier can progress as age compromises immunity, leading to production of apical pulmonary cavities. In elderly persons who lack preexisting immunity to TB, new infection can cause progressive primary disease resembling primary infection in children, with involvement of lower or middle lobes and often without cavities.

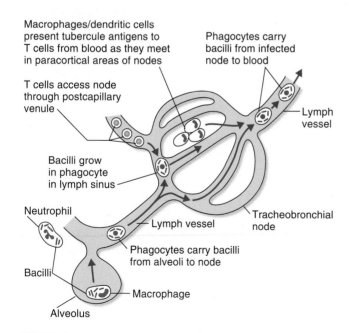

FIGURE 23-4. *Mycobacterium tuberculosis* **multiplication in alveolar macrophages and spread to lymph nodes and beyond.**

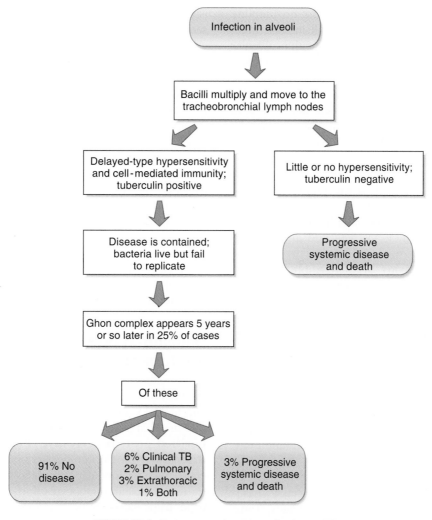

FIGURE 23-5. Outcomes of untreated primary TB.

Endogenous Reactivation (Secondary Tuberculosis)

Endogenous reactivation usually occurs within 2 years after initial infection but can occur at any time thereafter (see Fig. 23-5). Clearly, any impairment of the cellular immune system can render a person vulnerable to reactivation of latent mycobacteria. Subtle depression of the immune system resulting from stress or hormonal factors may go undetected. Other factors include malnutrition, therapy with corticosteroids or other immunosuppressive drugs, malignancy, and end-stage renal disease. Worldwide, the most important cause of reactivation is coinfection with HIV. The higher frequency of certain histocompatibility types (i.e., human leukocyte antigen or HLA) in persons who develop active TB suggests a genetic predisposition. The disease may reactivate in the elderly because of a poorly understood loss of immune competence that can occur with aging. In addition, local physical disturbances at the site of a latent focus can alter the balance between host and pathogen. For example, lung surgery can disturb quiescent pulmonary foci and cause active TB at that site.

The most common site of reactivation is **the apex of the lung** (see Fig. 23-1). Lesions slowly become necrotic, undergo **caseous necrosis** (named for its cheesy appearance), and eventually merge into larger lesions. With time, the caseous lesions liquefy and discharge their contents into bronchi. This event has several major consequences. It creates a well-aerated cavity in which the organisms proliferate. The discharge of caseous material also distributes the organisms to other sites in the lung, which can lead to a rapidly progressive **tuberculous pneumonia**. In addition, the bacteria-laden contents of caseous lesions are coughed up and become infectious droplet nuclei. Although the reason for the apical pulmonary localization is not known with certainty, it is likely that deficient lymphatic flow at the apices, where the pumping effect of respiratory motion is minimal, favors retention of organisms. When hypersensitivity develops, tissue damage creates apical cavities characteristic of pulmonary TB in adults.

Immune Response

TB requires a cellular immune response for control, with antibodies playing no apparent role. In the first few weeks after exposure, the host has almost no immune defense against *M. tuberculosis*, and small inhaled inocula multiply freely in alveolar spaces or within alveolar macrophages. Once inside the cell, mycobacteria increase their chance of survival by preventing acidification of the phagolysosome. Unrestrained replication proceeds for weeks, both in the initial focus and in metastatic foci, until tissue hypersensitivity and cellular immunity supervene. This tissue hypersensitivity is florid compared with other intracellular infections.

All persons have CD4+ T lymphocytes that can recognize mycobacterial antigens if processed and presented by macrophages in the context of major histocompatibility complex class II proteins. When lymphocytes encounter antigen in this manner, they are activated and proliferate, producing clones of similarly reactive lymphocytes. These in turn produce many distinct lymphokines that attract, retain, and activate macrophages at the site of antigen exposure. Activated macrophages accumulate lytic enzymes and reactive metabolites that increase their capacity to kill mycobacteria, but if released into surrounding tissues, these macrophage products can cause necrosis.

When the population of activated lymphocytes reaches a certain size, cutaneous delayed-type hypersensitivity to tuberculin becomes manifest. This response generally takes 3 to 8 weeks. At the same time, enhanced macrophage microbicidal activity, or cellular immunity, appears.

The pathologic features of TB are the result of hypersensitivity to mycobacterial antigens. The classic tissue response involves organization of macrophages, Langhans giant cells, and lymphocytes resulting in formation of **granulomas** (sometimes called tubercles). This pattern constitutes a successful tissue reaction with containment of infection, healing with eventual fibrosis, encapsulation, and scar formation. However, with time, the centers of the tubercles may become necrotic. Necrosis in TB tends to be incomplete, resulting in semisolid caseous material. Caseous necrosis is unstable, especially in the lungs, where it tends to liquefy and discharge through the bronchial tree, producing a cavity and providing conditions in which bacteria multiply to very high numbers.

Sustained immunity to new infection that follows natural infection is likely the result of persistent viable tubercle bacilli in the tissues with in vivo boosting. Although activated macrophages usually kill intracellular bacteria, intracellular mycobacteria may persist. An uneasy equilibrium is reached; some macrophages kill the organisms, others are themselves killed and release their bacterial contents, and still others harbor dormant bacteria for long periods. Proteolytic processing of killed bacteria leads to continued immunological stimulation.

Immunocompromised persons may not contain the primary infection, and organisms may invade the bloodstream and disseminate to cause a life-threatening infection known as **miliary tuberculosis**. The term *miliary*

is derived from the resemblance of the tubercles to millet seeds (bird seed). Characteristic of the disease are tubercles found in many organs, including the liver, spleen, kidneys, brain, and meninges. Caseation and cavitation are less frequent than in secondary TB.

The involvement of macrophages in the containment of *M. tuberculosis* comes at a price. Two cytokines produced by these cells, **IL-1** and **TNF-α** (see Chapter 6), contribute to symptoms of the disease. Among their various activities, these cytokines mediate **fever, weight loss, and night sweats**. In response to the carbohydrates, lipids, and proteins of the tubercle bacilli, macrophages also produce many other cytokines that modulate the immune response. In particular, increased production of IL-10 may suppress the immune response and promote disease progression. The net effects of these complex events are the local pathological manifestations of TB, including caseous necrosis and fibrosis with **calcification**.

Delayed-Type Hypersensitivity and the Tuberculin Skin Test

Immunological reactivity to TB can be demonstrated by tuberculin skin testing. This test involves the intradermal injection of proteins, or **tuberculin**, from tubercle bacilli. The material used is a poorly defined mixture known as **purified protein derivative** (**PPD**). A positive reaction is indicated by thickening (induration) of the skin several days after inoculation, which results from infiltration by mononuclear phagocytes and T cells. This **delayed-type hypersensitivity** reaction recapitulates the local events that take place in the lung and other infected tissue. Depending on the site of the reaction, delayed-type hypersensitivity may account for diverse manifestations, such as pleurisy with effusion (the sometimes massive accumulation of exudate in the pleural cavities) or sudden inflammation of the meninges. Surprisingly few tubercle bacilli are present in the pleural fluid or cerebrospinal fluid during these infections, but they are able to cause considerable inflammation.

The tuberculin skin test is most useful for diagnosing latent tuberculous infection. It is especially useful in places like the United States, where TB is relatively uncommon. The test is much less useful in countries where most of the population is tuberculin positive or has received the bacille Calmette-Guérin (BCG) vaccine (discussed later in the chapter). A newly positive test after a previous negative test (**tuberculin conversion**) indicates recent tuberculous infection and is an indication for chemoprophylaxis. Medical personnel who may have contact with infected patients are at increased risk of becoming infected and are regularly tested for skin test conversion.

There are caveats regarding the tuberculin test. About 15% of individuals with active TB have negative tuberculin tests. In some cases, this tuberculin negativity appears to be specific for *M. tuberculosis* because reactivity to other skin test antigens (e.g., *Candida*, mumps, or tetanus) is preserved. Soon after effective antituberculous therapy is initiated, the tuberculin test usually becomes positive as general overall health improves. Importantly, many immunocompromised persons with tuberculous infection (especially those with AIDS) have negative tuberculin tests. These individuals often lack skin test reactivity to other antigens. Thus, a negative tuberculin skin test does not exclude active TB. Conversely, a false-positive tuberculin test may be caused by exposure to atypical mycobacteria, although in such cases the diameter of induration is usually small.

Interferon Gamma Release Assays

Given the limitations of the tuberculin skin test in diagnosing latent *M. tuberculosis* infection, newer assays that quantify the immune response to *M. tuberculosis* have been developed. Interferon-γ plays a critical role in regulating the cellular immune response to *M. tuberculosis*. There are now FDA-approved assays that measure the in vitro production of interferon-γ in response to antigens specific for *M. tuberculosis*. These tests have increased specificity for diagnosing latent TB infection because the antigens used are not present in nontuberculous mycobacteria or BCG vaccine strains. Interferon-γ release assays are approved for every circumstance in which a tuberculin skin test would be used. These assays may be particularly appropriate for screening individuals who have been previously vaccinated with BCG.

DAMAGE: CLINICAL MANIFESTATIONS

TB is insidious. Most people are unaware of their initial encounter with the organism. However, some persons, particularly the very young, the elderly, and those who are immunocompromised, may not develop sufficient cellular immunity to contain the organisms and develop disseminated TB (see Fig. 23-5). This rampant infection differs from endogenous reactivation (although it sometimes occurs in patients with secondary TB).

Endogenous reactivation can affect virtually any organ in the body. However, the most common manifestation of TB in adults is a chronic pneumonia that characteristically forms cavities in the apices of the lung. Persistent fever, weight loss, and drenching night sweats are common during TB. *M. tuberculosis* also can affect vertebral bodies (**Pott disease**), in which patients present with chronic back pain. Failure to diagnose and treat Pott disease can result in destruction of vertebrae and permanent disability. Painless enlargement of lymph nodes resulting from infection by *M. tuberculosis* can affect virtually any region of the body. Less common manifestations include chronic inflammation of the meninges, pericardium, peritoneal cavity, or adrenal glands.

Considering that tissue damage is caused by the immune response to *M. tuberculosis*, one might ask which is worse: a robust cell-mediated immune response or no immune response at all. Effective immunologic control of TB is a matter of balance. Without cellular immunity and delayed-type hypersensitivity, caseous necrosis would not develop, but the tubercle bacilli would proliferate unchecked. The result could be miliary TB, a disease that can kill much more rapidly than chronic pulmonary TB. For example, the loss of CD4+ T cells as a result of HIV infection leads to rapid progression of TB and death. In addition, persons with AIDS may not develop the lesions typical of reactivation TB. Thus, the immune response contains the disease, even if it eventually causes damage. In fact, the body relies on two defensive strategies: the first involves the antimicrobial action of activated macrophages, and the second consists of walling off and containing the lesion by fibrosis and calcification. In short, defense mechanisms provide lifelong control of infection in most individuals.

DIAGNOSIS

The diagnosis of asymptomatic tuberculous infection is usually based on tuberculin skin test results. In contrast, active disease is usually diagnosed by acid-fast staining and culture of sputum or affected tissues.

The initial diagnostic approach includes a careful history, direct examination of sputum or exudates, and a chest radiograph (see Fig. 23-1). Direct examination of sputum can yield a rapid presumptive diagnosis. Importantly, contagiousness correlates with sputum smear positivity. Acid-fast stains are rapid and relatively sensitive, especially with cavitary pulmonary TB (Fig. 23-6). The yield increases by examining sputa collected on three separate days. Early morning sputa have the best yields because pulmonary secretions accumulate during sleep.

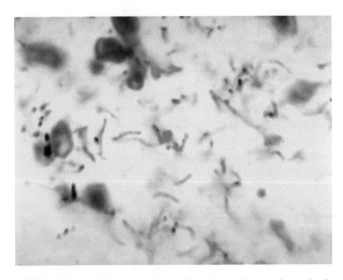

FIGURE 23-6. Acid-fast stain of *Mycobacterium tuberculosis* from a pulmonary cavity.

The **gold standard** for diagnosis of TB is **culture**. Sputum from some patients with active TB but too few organisms to detect microscopically may have positive cultures. Detection of colonies on solid media usually takes 3 to 6 weeks. **Radiometric culture techniques** accelerate the diagnosis by early detection of radioactive CO_2 released by organisms metabolizing ^{14}C-labeled palmitic acid, providing results within 7 to 14 days. If growth of tubercle bacilli occurs, it is important to test for antibiotic susceptibility. Overall, the process may take 6 or more weeks. More sensitive nucleic acid amplification methods for rapid diagnosis are occasionally used in practice but have not replaced smear and culture.

What other infections can resemble TB? There are many, as shown in Table 23-2. They include those caused by atypical mycobacteria such as *Mycobacterium avium complex (MAC)* and *M. kansasii*. Disease caused by these organisms tends to be less severe and more indolent. MAC causes disseminated illness during advanced AIDS. Other diseases in the differential diagnosis of TB are those caused by actinomycetes, nocardia, and systemic fungi.

TREATMENT

Excellent drugs are available for treating TB. These include **isoniazid (INH)**, **rifampin, pyrazinamide (PZA)**, and **ethambutol**. Persons with pulmonary TB usually become noncontagious within 2 weeks of therapy if the organisms are sensitive to the drugs administered. Unlike most bacterial infections that can be cured with a single drug, **active TB requires multiple drugs for cure** because of the remarkable propensity of the organism to **develop resistance**. In any population of tubercle bacilli, chromosomal mutations associated with resistance to any single drug are already present in about one of every 10^6 to 10^7 bacteria, even though the organisms have never been exposed to the drug. Because tuberculous cavities can contain in excess of 10^{11} organisms, many of the bacteria present will be resistant to any single drug, even before treatment is begun. In fact, some organisms will be resistant to drugs that are yet to be developed.

Fortunately, the chance that one organism will become resistant to two drugs simultaneously is small. Therefore, prescribing multiple drugs in combination prevents resistance. Unfortunately, adherence with complex and prolonged treatment regimens is difficult. If treatment is sporadic, **multidrug-resistant strains** can emerge, making treatment more difficult or impossible. Spread of such strains to other individuals can be catastrophic. For this reason, directly observed therapy for TB has become the standard of care, with every dose directly administered by a health care provider, usually a public health worker.

Prescribing multiple drugs also allows for a shorter duration of therapy. In cases of drug-sensitive TB, 18 months of INH plus ethambutol was once required for cure. In the 1970s, it was discovered that including rifampin in the regimen allowed therapy to be shortened to 9 months. Later, it was discovered that adding PZA allowed cure in 6 months. In the United States, individuals at risk for exposure to TB (e.g., health care professionals as well as medical students and residents) are routinely screened for tuberculin conversion. INH is administered to persons who convert to a positive reaction, which indicates recent infection. Such treatment of latent infection is called **chemoprophylaxis**. Unlike treating active TB, chemoprophylaxis requires only a single drug (e.g., INH) because there are so few organisms that it is highly unlikely that resistant organisms will be present.

Drug-Resistant Tuberculosis

Drug-resistant TB is a major challenge to TB control worldwide. Resistance can be either **primary**, as is the case when a person becomes infected with a drug-resistant strain, or **secondary**, which arises in a person who has received TB therapy and is often associated with treatment nonadherence. Mycobacterial strains that are resistant to INH and rifampin are designated multidrug resistant, or MDR TB. Strains resistant to INH, rifampin, and second-line agents such as fluoroquinolones and aminoglycosides are designated extensively drug resistant, or XDR TB. Approximately 7% of TB cases worldwide are multidrug resistant. Drug-resistant TB is associated with decreased cure, increased morbidity and mortality, and can be disseminated to susceptible persons.

PREVENTION

The history of TB suggests that improving the standard of living decreases rates of disease. In many resource-limited countries, that is unfortunately not a reality. Currently, an effective vaccine made from killed *M. tuberculosis* does not exist. The immunology of TB tells us why: killed vaccines may generate antibodies, but humoral immunity does not protect against TB. Cell-mediated immune responses are best elicited when antigens are presented by live organisms.

The **bacille Calmette-Guérin (BCG) vaccine** is a strain of *M. bovis* made relatively avirulent (attenuated) by multiple passages in culture. It is routinely given to newborns and young children in many countries, including those with limited resources. Administering BCG vaccine causes tuberculin skin test positivity, a criterion for a successful "take" of the immunization. Long-term persistence of tuberculin positivity varies depending on the patient's age at BCG vaccination; the earlier the vaccination, the less durable the skin test positivity. Because BCG-induced tuberculin positivity would decrease the value of tuberculin skin testing to diagnose new infections, BCG is not used in the United States. The safety and immunogenicity of BCG also make it a potential vector to deliver protective antigens from other pathogenic organisms. Genes encoding such antigens have been introduced into BCG to generate "multivaccines" that might protect against multiple pathogens.

MYCOBACTERIUM LEPRAE

Leprosy is the disease caused by *M. leprae*. It shares some pathobiological features with TB, but it differs in its clinical manifestations. Leprosy has historically been more feared and resulted in more social stigmatization than other infectious diseases. Because the skin lesions of leprosy are often obvious, persons with this disease were once vehemently shunned, even though leprosy is much less contagious than TB. Although rare in the United States, leprosy is still important worldwide. An estimated 6 million people have leprosy, mainly in tropical, resource-limited countries, where the disease causes economic loss and human suffering.

The mode of transmission of *M. leprae* is not certain. Leprosy is clearly communicable, and acquisition requires prolonged contact with infectious cases. With skin involvement as a major feature, leprosy was once thought to be transmitted by contact with skin lesions. However, persons with leprosy shed *M. leprae* in their nasal secretions, and it is now thought that the disease is transmitted by the airborne route. Because leprosy is primarily a rural and not an urban disease, transmission by soil also has been suggested.

Studies of *M. leprae* are difficult because **the organism cannot be continuously grown in vitro**. *M. leprae* was one of the first microbes to be linked to a human disease. In 1873, G. A. Hansen discovered *M. leprae* in lesions of leprosy patients. In recognition of this discovery, leprosy is often called **Hansen disease**. It was not until 1960 that researchers discovered that *M. leprae* can grow in the footpads of mice. Even there, it grows very slowly (doubling once every 14 days), and yields of the organisms are low. In 1970, *M. leprae* was found to naturally infect the nine-banded armadillo, where it grows to more than 10^{10} bacilli per gram of tissue. In fact, 15% of wild armadillos in Louisiana and Texas are infected with *M. leprae*. This finding revolutionized leprosy research because it provided sufficient quantities of the organism for basic studies. Many genes encoding important *M. leprae* antigens have since been identified and expressed in *Escherichia coli* and other organisms, providing novel reagents to study the host immune response.

M. leprae, like *M. tuberculosis* and MAC, survives and multiplies within macrophages. This mycobacterium has an arsenal of defenses to escape killing by phagocytes. For example, **phenolic glycolipid**, a surface lipid of *M. leprae*, may provide a defense against oxidative killing. To exert their maximal killing potential, macrophages must be activated by cytokines produced by CD4+ T cells.

Leprosy bacilli grow best at low temperatures. Accordingly, they multiply most rapidly in the skin, nose, and other superficial tissues. Clinical leprosy ranges between two polar forms, tuberculoid and lepromatous. The prognosis of leprosy has dramatically improved with the introduction of effective drugs like **dapsone**, **rifampin**, and **clofazimine**.

Tuberculoid Leprosy

Tuberculoid leprosy is often characterized by red blotchy lesions with localized anesthesia (loss of sensation) on the face, trunk, and extremities. The organisms grow and cause thickening in nerve sheaths. These thickened nerves can be felt through the skin, a characteristic of leprosy. Such patients usually demonstrate delayed-type hypersensitivity to **lepromin** (the *M. leprae* equivalent of tuberculin) prepared from infected tissues. Patients with tuberculoid leprosy have a vigorous cell-mediated immune response to *M. leprae*, which mediates the nerve damage, but few acid-fast bacilli can be found in the tuberculoid lesion.

Tuberculoid leprosy is analogous to secondary TB in that it invokes a robust cell-mediated immune response and tissue hypersensitivity. The prognosis with tuberculoid leprosy is better than that with lepromatous leprosy and, in some cases, tuberculoid leprosy is a self-limited disease.

Lepromatous Leprosy

M. leprae can reduce or suppress specific T cells produced by the host that activate infected macrophages and provide cell-mediated immunity. **In lepromatous leprosy, there is little or no delayed-type hypersensitivity to lepromin**. This lack of cellular immunity is associated with enormous numbers of *M. leprae* in the skin and superficial nerves. The number of bacilli harbored by a lepromatous patient (10^{15}) is far greater than in any other human disease. Both **skin and nerves may be involved**. With time, the loss of local sensation leads to inadvertent, traumatic lesions of the face and extremities. These may become secondarily infected, resulting in additional disfigurement.

Lepromatous leprosy is the more debilitating form of the disease. Pathogenically, it is analogous to systemic, progressive (miliary) TB, in which the organisms grow profusely. In both diseases, the cell-mediated immune response is weak. It is not clear why cell-mediated immunity is decreased in persons with leprosy. The infecting organisms may play a role in this immunosuppression, and host genetic factors also may be involved.

CONCLUSION

TB is one of the most important diseases in the world. Tissue damage occurs primarily because of exuberant hypersensitivity to the organism. The tubercle bacillus has a waxy coat, grows very slowly, and is a highly successful intracellular pathogen. Clinical manifestations differ between the initial and subsequent encounters with the organism. *M. tuberculosis* may not cause illness in the infected individual for many years, if at all. In the absence of HIV infection or other immunocompromising illness, a pivotal event in the pathogenesis of TB is the formation of a pulmonary cavity, where organisms grow to huge numbers, ensuring airborne spread and increasing the chance of transmission. Although the availability of effective antituberculous drugs once raised hope of eliminating TB, the AIDS pandemic and increasing drug resistance has made this plan unrealistic in the foreseeable future.

Leprosy is rare in the United States but still a significant problem in many countries. Studying *M. leprae* is particularly difficult because it cannot be cultivated in vitro. The two polar forms of leprosy are tuberculoid and lepromatous. Tuberculoid leprosy is characterized by a vigorous cell-mediated immune response with few organisms present. In contrast, lepromatous leprosy is associated with diminished delayed-type hypersensitivity to *M. leprae* and enormous numbers of organisms. Fortunately, there are now effective drugs for treating leprosy.

Suggested Readings

Barker LF, Brennan MJ, Rosenstein PK, et al. Tuberculosis vaccine research: the impact of immunology. *Curr Opin Immunol.* 2009;21:331–338.

Edlin BR, Tokars JI, Grieco MH, et al. An outbreak of multidrug-resistant tuberculosis among hospitalized patients with the acquired immunodeficiency syndrome. *N Engl J Med.* 1992;326:1514–1521.

Hale YM, Pfyffer GE, Salfinger M. Laboratory diagnosis of mycobacterial infections: new tools and lessons learned. *Clin Infect Dis.* 2001;33:834–846.

Havlir DV, Barnes PF. Tuberculosis in patients with human immunodeficiency virus infection. *N Engl J Med.* 1999;340:367–373.

Murray JF. Cursed duet: HIV infection and tuberculosis. *Respiration.* 1990;57:210–220.

Nash DR, Douglass JE. Anergy in active pulmonary tuberculosis: a comparison between positive and negative reactors and an evaluation of 5 TU and 250 TU skin test doses. *Chest.* 1980;77:32–37.

Selwyn PA, Hartel D, Lewis VA, et al. A prospective study of the risk of tuberculosis among intravenous drug users with human immunodeficiency virus infection. *N Engl J Med.* 1989;320:545–555.

Snider DE Jr. The tuberculin skin test. *Am Rev Respir Dis.* 1982;125:108–118.

Swaminathan S, Padmapriyadarsini C, Narendran G. HIV-associated tuberculosis: clinical update. *Clin Infect Dis.* 2010;50:1377–1386.

Pai M, Minion J, Sohn H, et al. Novel and improved technologies for tuberculosis diagnosis: progress and challenges. *Clin Chest Med.* 2009;30:701–716, viii.

Trends in tuberculosis—United States, 2008. *MMWR Morb Mortal Wkly Rep.* 2009;58:249–253.

Updated guidelines for using interferon gamma release assays to detect *Mycobacterium tuberculosis* infection—United States, 2010. *MMWR Morb Mortal Wkly Rep.* 2010;59:1–25.

World Health Organization. Global tuberculosis control: a short update to the 2009 report. 2009. Available from: http://www.who.int/tb/en

World Health Organization. Multidrug and extensively drug-resistant TB (M/XDR-TB): 2010 global report on surveillance and response. 2010. Available from: http://www.who.int/tb/en

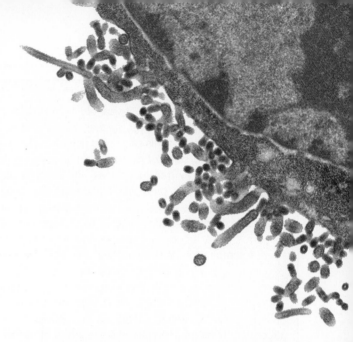

Chapter **24**

Syphilis: A Disease with a History

John R. Ebright and Jack D. Sobel

KEY CONCEPTS

Pathogen: Syphilis is caused by the noncultivable spirochete *Treponema pallidum*.

Encounter: Most commonly acquired by sexual contact

Entry: The bacterium usually enters through genital mucosa or skin. However, it can also be transmitted from mother to fetus (congenital syphilis).

Spread and Multiplication: Disease is characterized by three stages: primary syphilis, in which the organism is localized to a chancre, or skin lesion; secondary syphilis, in which the organism disseminates to distant sites; and tertiary syphilis, in which the immune response to the organisms leads to the destruction of tissue.

Damage: Mechanisms of disease are not understood.

Diagnosis: Syphilis is initially diagnosed by tests such as Venereal Disease Reference Laboratory test; positive results should be confirmed with more specific tests.

Treatment and Prevention: Syphilis is readily treated with penicillin. There is currently no vaccine.

THE AGENT OF SYPHILIS, **Treponema pallidum**, although most commonly acquired by sexual contact, can be transmitted from an infected mother to her fetus and may cause congenital syphilis; it has often occupied center stage in the history of medicine. A recent resurgence of syphilis in select populations within the United States has once again focused attention on this ancient infectious disease. Syphilis is a multistage disease, and each stage has a dramatically different clinical presentation. The first two stages (**primary and secondary**) manifest as acute and subacute disease, respectively, whereas **tertiary syphilis** is a chronic disease that lasts many years.

   T. pallidum, a spirochete, cannot be cultured in artificial media. It does not produce toxins. In fact, it is not known how *T. pallidum* causes disease. Nevertheless, scientific observations are beginning to elucidate why the organism is able to escape the immune system and how it induces disease. Fortunately, *T. pallidum* remains sensitive to penicillin, which is why the disease is easily treatable today.

CASE

CASE • Mr. B., a 24-year-old homosexual man, came to the clinic with fever, swollen lymph nodes, and spotty discolorations of his skin, most notably on the palms of his hands and soles of his feet. He had recently noted a penny-sized, gray, translucent lesion on the inner aspect of his lower lip. The physician recognized the "macular rash" on the palms and soles and the lesion on his lip as characteristic of secondary syphilis. Mr. B. reported that he engages in oral sex as well as anal-receptive intercourse.

A scraping of Mr. B.'s lip lesion was examined under a dark-field microscope; it revealed the presence of large numbers of corkscrew-shaped spirochetes. The laboratory reported "positive serology," indicating the presence of the characteristic serum antibodies to *T. pallidum*. These laboratory findings confirmed the diagnosis of secondary syphilis. Because his sexual behavior put him at high risk of other sexually transmitted diseases, Mr. B. consented to a serum test for the presence of antibodies to the human immunodeficiency virus (HIV). He was serologically negative for HIV at that time. Mr. B. was treated with a course of penicillin, and his lesions and symptoms abated. He was considered cured, as his syphilis serologic titers (the level of antibodies in serum) declined over months.

This case raises several questions:

1. Is it possible that this patient was not aware of having had a chancre before presenting with secondary syphilis?

2. How did the spirochetes travel from the chancre to the patient's skin, lower lip, and lymph nodes?

3. Are the clinical features of secondary syphilis (rash, swollen lymph nodes, mucous membrane lesions) fully explained by spirochetes invading skin, lymph nodes, and lower lip? What host factors may be contributing to the disease process?

4. Are the skin lesions and mouth lesions infective? Could another person acquire syphilis by touching them?

5. What will happen to this person's skin rash, lip lesion, and swollen lymph nodes if he is not promptly treated with antibiotics?

See Appendix for answers.

The agent of syphilis belongs to the genus *Treponema* and is a **spirochete**, a type of bacteria with a highly characteristic appearance. Spirochetes are helical, slender, and relatively long cells (Fig. 24-1). They are widespread in nature but only a few cause disease in humans and animals. The principal human spirochetoses are syphilis, Lyme disease (Chapter 25), relapsing fever (caused by members of the genus *Borrelia*), and leptospirosis (caused by members of the genus *Leptospira*). Other organisms of the genus *Treponema* cause rare diseases such as yaws, pinta, and bejel that are found mostly in tropical countries. These exotic diseases pose no medical problem in the United States, but patients who may have acquired one of these infections in a tropical country may develop positive serologic tests for syphilis that may remain positive for life.

T. pallidum is so narrow (0.1 to 0.2 mm) that it cannot be seen by standard microscopic techniques. It can be visualized by special stains (silver impregnation or immunofluorescence) or with special lighting (*dark-field microscopy*). When observed in a freshly prepared wet mount using a dark-field microscope, it exhibits a characteristic *corkscrew-like movement and flexion*. Its cell structure is similar to Gram-negative bacteria with an inner cytoplasmic membrane, a thin peptidoglycan cell wall and an outer membrane. However, the outer membrane differs from most Gram-negative bacteria in that it lacks lipopolysaccharide and

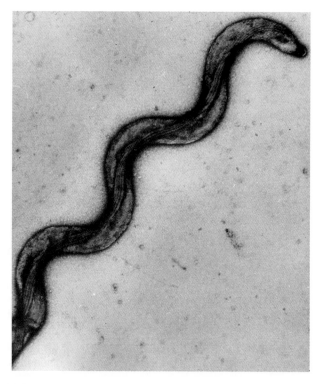

FIGURE 24-1. Electron photomicrograph of *Treponema pallidum*, negatively stained. At the dark end of the organism are the insertion points of the periplasmic flagella (ropelike contractile structures), which enable the organisms to engage in their typical corkscrew-like motility.

appears to have a relatively small number of surface antigens. Unlike the flagella of other bacteria, which protrude freely into the medium, those of spirochetes are contained within the periplasm. This location probably accounts for the characteristic movement of the organism.

Understanding of the mechanisms by which *T. pallidum* causes disease has been limited both by the inability to cultivate the organisms serially in artificial media and by the lack of a suitable animal model. In artificial media, these bacteria can be kept alive for only short periods of time (a few divisions at most). To bypass these constraints, research efforts have focused on producing and characterizing specific proteins of *T. pallidum* using genes cloned into *Escherichia coli*.

ENCOUNTER, ENTRY, SPREAD, AND MULTIPLICATION

T. pallidum is sensitive to drying, disinfectants, and heat (as low as 42°C). Therefore, they are unlikely to be acquired by means other than personal contact. The two major routes of transmission are **sexual** and **transplacental**. Sexual exposure to a person who has an active syphilitic chancre carries a high probability of acquiring syphilis.

The organisms enter a susceptible host through the mucous membranes or the minute abrasions in the skin surface that occur during sexual intercourse. Once in the subepithelial tissues, the organisms replicate locally in an extracellular location (Fig. 24-2). In culture, they adhere

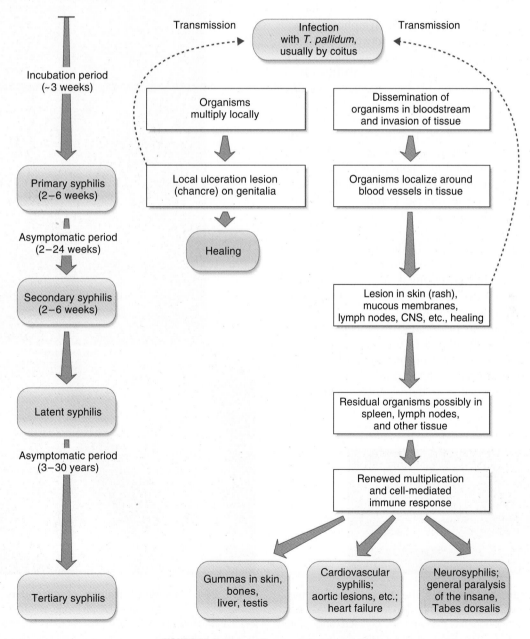

FIGURE 24-2. The pathogenesis of syphilis.

to cells by their tapered ends and probably stick to cells in tissue by the same means. Not all of them stick, and many are soon carried through lymphatic channels to the systemic circulation. Thus, even if the initial manifestation of the disease consists of an isolated skin lesion, syphilis is a systemic disease almost from the outset.

Treponemes can cross the placental barrier from the bloodstream of an infected mother and cause disease in the fetus. It is not known how the organisms cross this barrier. (Chapter 72 provides a general discussion of this issue.)

DAMAGE

Primary Syphilis

Initially, neutrophils migrate to the area of inoculation and are later replaced by plasma cells, lymphocytes, and macrophages. The result of the battle between the locally replicating treponemes and the cellular defenses of the host is the lesion of primary syphilis, the **syphilitic chancre** (Fig. 24-3). The chancre usually is painless. The time between the initial introduction of the organisms and the appearance of the ulcer depends on the size of the inoculum. The larger the size of the inoculum, the earlier the chancre appears. This lesion heals spontaneously within 26 weeks, but by this time, the spirochetes have spread through the bloodstream and may cause lesions in other parts of the body. These diverse lesions comprise the cluster of findings that characterize "secondary syphilis," such as that manifested in Mr. B.

The syphilitic chancre and other genital ulcer diseases are associated with increased risk of HIV transmission. Patients who have genital ulcers are estimated to have a three- to fivefold increased risk of acquiring HIV infection. Furthermore, recent studies have demonstrated that HIV can be isolated from genital ulcers, which increases the likelihood of transmitting the virus. The possible role of genital ulcers in facilitating the transmission of HIV underscores the importance of recognizing and promptly treating primary syphilis, chancroid, or herpes.

Three to six weeks after the ulcer heals, the secondary form of the disease occurs in about 50% of infected individuals. **Secondary syphilis** results from the systemic spread of the infection when treponemes replicate in the lymph nodes, the liver, joints, muscles, skin, and mucous membranes distant from the site of the primary chancre (Fig 24-4). The signs and symptoms of secondary syphilis may be so varied and involve such different tissues and organs that the disease has been called "the Great Imitator." The rash and other manifestations of secondary syphilis resolve within weeks to months, but one-fourth of affected individuals experience a recurrence of the secondary stage (relapse) within approximately 1 year or so (Fig. 24-2).

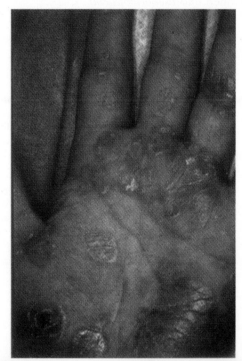

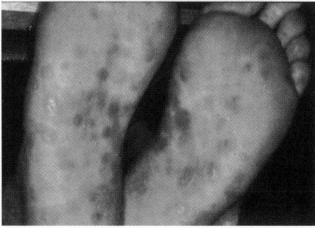

FIGURE 24-4. Cutaneous lesions of secondary syphilis. In addition to fever, headache, lymph node enlargement, and oral lesions, a scaly papular eruption involving the trunk and extremities including palms and soles is characteristic of secondary syphilis.

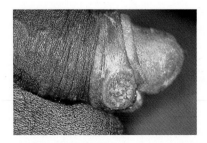

FIGURE 24-3. Chancre of the penis. The chancre is the first manifestation of syphilis in some patients. The lesion is painless and, on dark-field examination, has many motile "corkscrewing" spirochetes, thus confirming the diagnosis of syphilis.

This biphasic course of the disease is puzzling for several reasons. We do not understand how spirochetes kill so many epidermal cells to create a chancre or how the ulcer heals. Why do the defense mechanisms that are so successful in resolving the primary chancre fail to function systemically during secondary syphilis? How does the organism survive in the body for long periods of time? Where are the organisms located, intracellularly or extracellularly? What is the role of the specific immune response in the disease process? We do not have answers to these questions or to others regarding other aspects of syphilis. It remains one of the more fascinating and puzzling of infectious diseases. However, there are a few clues. Recently, it has been demonstrated that *T. pallidum* contains 100-fold fewer membrane-spanning proteins than the outer membrane of typical Gram-negative bacteria. This finding suggests that, in the case of *T. pallidum*, antibodies against surface proteins may not play their usual protective antimicrobial role. In addition, when the organism is isolated from tissues, it has been found to be coated with plasma proteins, which may play a protective role against human host defense mechanisms.

Tertiary Syphilis

The mystery deepens with the resolution of the secondary stage. In about one-third of individuals, the organisms disappear and the person is spontaneously cured. In the remaining two-thirds of individuals, the treponemes persist without causing signs or symptoms for years (**latent syphilis**, Fig. 24-2). In about one-half of this group, the manifestations of tertiary syphilis eventually develop, sometimes years or even decades after the primary infection.

In adults, **tertiary syphilis** is responsible for a majority of the morbidity and mortality associated with the disease. Fortunately, tertiary syphilis is uncommon in the United States, where routine serological screening identifies most cases before this stage develops. The hallmark of tertiary syphilis is the destruction of tissue caused by a response to the presence of treponemal antigens. This change manifests as **vasculitis** and **chronic inflammation**. Soft masses, or **gummas**, composed of few treponemes and inflammatory cells, are lesions that may destroy bone and soft tissue ("**late benign syphilis**"). However, they may also involve vital organs, such as the liver. In cardiovascular syphilis, vasculitis involves the arteries (vasa vasorum) supplying the thoracic aorta. Destruction of the elastic tissue in the aorta media leads to dilatation of the wall and **aortic valve insufficiency** or to the formation of **aortic aneurysms** with resultant **rupture of the aorta**.

The central nervous system may also be involved, either by direct invasion of the parenchyma by treponemes or by brain infarction caused by vasculitis.

The clinical findings of **neurosyphilis** can be subtle. The severity of signs and symptoms depends on the location of the lesions. Involvement of the dorsal columns of the spinal cord results in loss of position sensation, a classic condition known as **tabes dorsalis**. It often manifests as a staggering, or **ataxic gait**. In turn, the loss of position sensation causes trauma in the knee and occasionally the ankle joints, which results in bone overgrowth and instability known as "**Charcot joint**." A generalized involvement of the brain leads to impaired motor function (paresis) as well as to gradual loss of higher integrative functions and personality changes. This clinical picture is known as **general paresis** or paralysis of the insane. A physical sign of neurosyphilis is the **Argyll Robertson pupil**: the pupil does not react to light but does contract when an object is moved from far to near the eye. If untreated, neurosyphilis may be fatal.

The lesions of tertiary syphilis usually contain few or no treponemes. What then accounts for the presence of lesions in the tissues? Researchers have demonstrated that the immune system likely plays a deleterious role in the development of the syphilitic lesions. Human cells exposed to treponemes in culture elaborate intercellular adhesion molecules, which facilitate the chemotaxis and attachment of inflammatory cells. Does this mobilization of inflammatory cells contribute to the disease? Further elucidation of this complex process awaits more research.

Congenital Syphilis

Despite serological tests that are easily available to detect syphilis, and antibiotics available to treat the disease, thousands of babies are born with congenital syphilis in the United States each year (the exact figures are hard to come by). This number actually underrepresents the problem, as the majority of infected fetuses likely die in utero. The manifestations of congenital syphilis are varied and include life-threatening organ damage, silent infections, congenital malformations, and developmental abnormalities. Congenital anomalies include **premature birth**, **intrauterine growth retardation**, and **multiple organ failure** (e.g., central nervous system infection, pneumonia, and enlargement of the liver and spleen). The most common manifestations of syphilis become evident at about 2 years of age and include **facial and tooth deformities** (the so-called **Hutchinson incisors** and "**mulberry**" molars). Other less common manifestations include **deafness**, **arthritis**, and "**saber shins**." Congenital syphilis is especially tragic because it is completely preventable by penicillin therapy of women with a positive serological test for syphilis early in pregnancy. Prevention of congenital syphilis is one reason why prenatal care is essential.

HISTORY OF SYPHILIS: "FOR ONE SMALL PLEASURE I SUFFER A THOUSAND MISFORTUNES"

The route of the global spread of syphilis is a controversial subject that is not likely to be resolved. One view is that Christopher Columbus brought the syphilis agent back to Spain from the New World, since the first documented outbreaks of syphilis occurred in Europe shortly after Columbus's return. Whether or not Columbus' crew was the source of the outbreak, the spread of the disease through Europe was rapid and, initially, was accompanied by a high mortality rate. In 1494, King Charles VIII of France invaded Italy with an army of mercenaries from many countries, including Spain. Because the mercenaries initially saw little fighting, much of the campaign was spent consorting with female camp followers. In returning to their home countries, the mercenaries carried syphilis to all of Europe. Understandably, no country wanted to claim syphilis as its own:

"The Italians called it the Spanish or the French disease; the French called it the Italian or Neapolitan disease; the English called it the French disease; the Russians called it the Polish disease. And… the first Spaniards who recognized the disease called it the disease of Espaniola, which meant, at that time, the disease of Haiti."

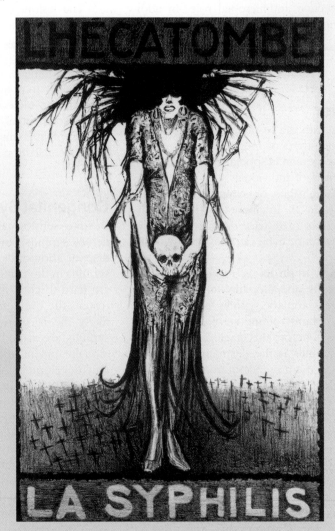

FIGURE 24-5. In previous years, syphilis stirred the imagination to extremes of gloom and hysteria. This French illustration ascribes to syphilis a degree of mortality that has not been seen since the advent of serological testing and penicillin therapy in this century.

(continued)

Interestingly, it was the poet Fracastorius who gave the disease the name by which we know it today. Fracastorius' poem, *Syphilis Sive Morbus Gallicus*, published in 1530, assigned a nonpolitical name to the "venereal pox" that of the shepherd Syphilos. Ambroise Paré, in 1575, referred to it as "Lues Venerea," the lover's plague.

During the 16th and 17th centuries, many clinical manifestations of syphilis were observed and catalogued. One of the most puzzling aspects of the disease is that within a few years of its emergence, it ceased to be a rapid killer and acquired the complex clinical manifestations that today characterize the disease (Fig. 24-5). The change in the organism's virulence, from high to moderate, supports the notion that the most successful pathogens do not kill their host. In fact, the less severe the symptoms, the less likely the pathogen will be eliminated. The epitome of this principle is the organism that causes asymptomatic disease, since the host is neither diagnosed nor treated. An organism that goes undetected is able to reproduce, and it is this ability and not the ability to cause disease that is the main selective force in nature. *T. pallidum* is particularly successful as a human parasite because it possesses, among others, the following traits: spread by sexual transmission, efficient transmission from one adult to another (horizontal transmission), a long infectious period, transmission from mother to child (vertical transmission), long persistence in the host, and, usually, lethality only after decades of infection.

In general, sexually transmitted diseases do not "travel alone." Thus, early physicians found it difficult to separate the manifestations of one disease—for instance, gonorrhea—from another (syphilis) because one person might have both diseases simultaneously. Many physicians who studied these diseases thought that they were separate entities. Unfortunately, however, John Hunter confused the issue for six decades. In 1767, Hunter, in a courageous but ill-conceived experiment, placed onto his skin pus taken from the urethra of a man with gonorrhea. A chancre developed. Undoubtedly, Hunter had taken pus from a man coinfected with both *Neisseria gonorrhoeae* and *T. pallidum*. It was not until 60 years later that Philippe Ricord correctly distinguished the two diseases. Ricord also recognized the **stages of syphilis** (**primary**, **secondary**, and **tertiary**).

The incidence of syphilis has changed in recent decades. Between 1947 and 1965, a dramatic decline in the cases of syphilis was reported in the United States. However, from 1986 through 1990, the nation experienced a syphilis epidemic. Although the incidence fell during the following decade, the rate of primary and secondary syphilis has again increased in 2001 and 2002, especially among men. This suggests the increase results primarily among men who have sex with men.

DIAGNOSIS

In the past, physicians relied on the clinical signs and symptoms of the disease to make a diagnosis of syphilis. Therefore, only individuals with obvious skin or mucosal lesions were considered to have syphilis and, thus, received therapy. Patients with asymptomatic or latent syphilis were undiagnosed and, therefore, untreated. Early in the 20th century, Wassermann, Neisser, and Bruck discovered that the sera of patients with syphilis have antibodies that react with normal human tissue. The tissue component was found to be a lipid present in the membranes of mitochondria, called **cardiolipin**. Why patients with syphilis form these curious antibodies is not known. In fact, these antibodies are produced in patients with other diseases as well; **biological "false-positive" tests** for syphilis occur in patients with hemolytic anemia, systemic lupus erythematosus, leprosy, narcotics abuse, and aging.

The original test of Wassermann and colleagues led to the development of more rapid and reproducible tests. Several variations exist and are known by their eponyms (e.g., the Venereal Diseases Reference Laboratory test, **VDRL**, or the rapid plasma reagin, **RPR**). Although nonspecific, these tests are cheap and easy to perform, which makes them suitable for initial screening of large numbers of serum samples, as in premarital "blood tests." However, their relative lack of specificity makes it necessary to test all positive samples by more specific, technically demanding, and expensive tests directed against treponemal antigens. One such **treponeme-specific test** is the fluorescent treponemal antibody (**FTA**) test, an indirect fluorescent antibody test (see Chapter 58).

The diagnosis of syphilis can be established by one of two methods: (1) obtaining a positive specific serologic treponemal test (usually following a positive nonspecific screening test such as the RPR or VDRL) or (2) directly visualizing the organisms scraped from mucocutaneous lesions by dark-field or immunofluorescence microscopy (in primary, secondary, or early congenital syphilis only).

TREATMENT—"ONE NIGHT WITH VENUS, THE REST OF LIFE WITH MERCURY"

Two major advances in the diagnosis and management of syphilis have occurred during the 20th century: the development of serological tests for diagnosing syphilis and the use of penicillin for treating the disease. Fortunately for Mr. B. and for the rest of the world, the organisms are still exquisitely sensitive to penicillin.

Before penicillin, treatment depended on an arsenic-containing compound synthesized by Ehrlich early in the 20th century (it was the first effective synthetic chemotherapeutic agent). This compound was called "606," in recognition of 605 previous failures in that laboratory. Before the introduction of penicillin, therapy consisted of the tedious, expensive, and dangerous administration of arsenic and **mercury or bismuth** for a minimum of 2 months and as long as 2 or 3 years. An alternative therapy was the induction of high fevers in individuals with neurosyphilis. The basis of the therapeutic use of fever was the known heat sensitivity of *T. pallidum*. Fever first was induced by the production of erysipelas (streptococcal skin infections). However, when the streptococcal infections spread to and killed others who did not have syphilis, this method was abandoned. Subsequent efforts focused on malaria as the fever-inducing agent. Deaths were not unexpected, especially when the extremely virulent and deadly *Plasmodium falciparum* was inadvertently used instead of the more innocuous *Plasmodium vivax*.

Currently, the treatment of all stages of syphilis relies on the continued sensitivity of *T. pallidum* to **penicillin**. The optimal strengths and types of penicillin (aqueous, procaine, or benzathine penicillin) and duration of therapy for each stage are still not known with certainty. In general, however, patients with primary and secondary syphilis are treated with an injection of penicillin (benzathine type) that provides effective tissue levels for at least 1 week; whereas patients with late latent or tertiary syphilis are treated with repeated injections in order to provide effective tissue levels for approximately 3 weeks. Reports of treatment failures following accepted and standard regimens of penicillin have surfaced with increasing frequency. Treatment failure is believed to be due to lack of penetration of penicillin into the central nervous system harboring treponemes. Known infection of the central nervous system (neurosyphilis) should be treated with high-dose intravenous penicillin for 10 days. Similarly, the lack of immunity in patients infected with HIV has also contributed to treatment failure. These failures have caused tremendous uncertainty. Accordingly, some experts recommend intensified treatment of patients with later stages of syphilis and of individuals coinfected with HIV. Although cases of treatment failure are dramatic, they are difficult to interpret without knowing how many individuals are successfully managed by the same regimen. Without further evidence to justify major changes in the approach to syphilis treatment, current recommendations by the Centers for Disease Control and Prevention have remained conservative.

CONCLUSION

From the mid-1980s to the mid-1990s, the largest single-year increase in infectious syphilis in more than a quarter of a century was reported in the United States. During this period, the incidence of congenital syphilis also increased. In addition, genital ulcer diseases, such as syphilis, increase the risk of HIV transmission, contributing to the epidemic of AIDS.

Several factors are fueling the syphilis epidemic: drug use, high-risk sexual activity, a decline in socioeconomic and educational levels among groups at risk, and limited access to health care, due in part to the overburdening of health care facilities by the AIDS epidemic.

Among all the sexually transmitted diseases, syphilis is one of the easiest to control for the following reasons:

- The cases are clustered. Most of the current increase is occurring in low-income, minority heterosexuals and their children.
- Good diagnostic tests are available. These tests are inexpensive and give accurate, fairly rapid results.
- Treatment is available. An inexpensive antibiotic, penicillin, is effective for primary and secondary syphilis in single doses. Furthermore, antibiotic resistance is not a problem.

Suggested Readings

Centers for Disease Control and Prevention. Sexually transmitted diseases treatment guidelines 2006. *Morb Mortal Wkly Rep.* 2006;55(RR 11):1–94.

Erbelding E, Rompalo A. Changing epidemiology of syphilis and its persistent relationship with HIV. *Curr Infect Dis Rep.* 2004;6(2):135–140.

Lukehart SA. Biology of treponemes. In: Holmes KK, et al., eds. *Sexually Transmitted Diseases.* 4th ed. New York: McGraw Hill; 2008:647–659.

Sorgel F. The return of Ehrlich's "Therapia magna sterilisans" and other Ehrlich concepts?. Series of papers honoring Paul Ehrlich on the occasion of his 150th birthday. *Chemotherapy.* 2004;50(1):6–10.

Sparling PF, Swartz MN, Musher DM, et al. Clinical manifestations of syphilis. In: Holmes KK, et al., eds. *Sexually Transmitted Diseases.* 4th ed. New York: McGraw Hill; 2008:661–684.

Tramont EC. The impact of syphilis on humankind. *Infect Dis Clin North Am.* 2004;18(1):101–110.

Chapter 25

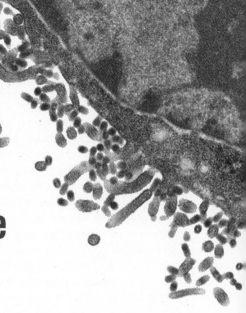

Borrelia burgdorferi and Lyme Disease

Mollie W. Jewett, Jenifer Coburn, and John Leong

KEY CONCEPTS

Pathogen: Lyme disease is caused by the spiral-shaped bacterium (spirochete) *Borrelia burgdorferi*.

Encounter: The infection is acquired by the bite of an infected deer tick.

Entry: Initial infection is characterized by the hallmark erythema migrans or bull's-eye rash that expands out from the tick bite site.

Spread and Multiplication: Lyme disease is a multistage disease that spreads from the tick bite site to infect the skin, joints, heart, central nervous system, and other tissues.

Damage: The host immune response to the *B. burgdorferi* infection causes injury to the host tissues.

Diagnosis: Diagnosis is based on the presence of an erythema migrans and antibodies against *B. burgdorferi*, along with a history that suggests exposure to infected ticks.

Treatment: Lyme disease is effectively treated with antibiotic therapy if detected early.

Prevention: The disease is not preventable by any currently available vaccine.

LYME DISEASE, or **Lyme borreliosis**, is the leading vectorborne bacterial disease of humans in the world. Lyme disease is caused by the spirochete ***Borrelia burgdorferi***. The infectious cycle of *B. burgdorferi* involves passage between the tick vector (*Ixodes sp.*) and mammalian host. Humans do not serve as natural reservoirs for *B. burgdorferi*, but the spirochete can be transmitted to humans by the bite of an infected tick, resulting in Lyme disease. Lyme disease diagnosis and treatment is complicated by its multisystem involvement, occurrence in stages (Fig. 25-1), and mimicry of other diseases. Lyme disease typically begins with a localized infection of the skin, resulting in a characteristic expanding skin lesion called **erythema migrans** (Fig. 25-2) emanating from the site of the tick bite (stage 1). Within several days to weeks, the spirochete may transiently enter the blood to spread to other tissues (stage 2), particularly to other skin sites, the nervous system, joints, heart, and/or eyes. Signs and symptoms change and are typically intermittent during this stage of the illness. After months to years, sometimes following long periods of latent infection, the spirochete may cause late stage disease manifestations (stage 3), most commonly of the joints, nervous system, or skin, depending on the tissue(s) in which the spirochetes reside.

CASE • Mr. G., a 48-year-old resident of a suburb of Boston, Massachusetts, spent a weekend on Nantucket Island in June. Activities during the weekend included hiking through scrubby, grassy, and lightly wooded areas. When he returned home he felt well, but over the next few days his wife noticed a slowly expanding red rash on one shoulder blade. As the rash expanded, the outer margins stayed red but the center started clearing, giving a bull's-eye appearance. Approximately 2 weeks later, while visiting Arizona, he developed a severe headache, fever, myalgia, and malaise. Mr. G. sought medical attention and was told that he probably had a viral infection. The symptoms gradually abated, but he later developed a somewhat droopy eyelid on one side and transient aches in multiple joints, which also spontaneously resolved with time. However, several months later at home in Boston, he again sought medical attention because he had developed considerable pain and swelling in one knee. At that time, based on his medical history and current symptoms, he was tested for *Borrelia burgdorferi* infection (Lyme disease). Serological tests revealed a high IgG titer to *B. burgdorferi* antigens by enzyme-linked immunosorbent assay (ELISA) and an IgG response to more than 10 different spirochetal proteins in an immunoblot. A polymerase chain reaction of joint fluid aspirated from the affected knee revealed the presence of *B. burgdorferi* DNA. He was treated with a 1-month course of oral doxycycline and made a slow but complete recovery.

The case of Mr. G. raises several questions:

1. How did Mr. G. acquire the infection? What is the likely significance of his vacationing in Nantucket in June? Is he likely to transmit the infection to anyone else?

2. What early clinical feature did Mr. G. exhibit that might have provided his physician with the best diagnostic hint that he had Lyme disease? Why was the diagnosis of Lyme disease overlooked when he saw a doctor while visiting Arizona?

3. What feature(s) of the spirochete are responsible for Mr. G. suffering such diverse signs and symptoms, including headache, myalgia, facial droop, arthralgia, and arthritis?

4. Why was an immunoblot performed in addition to ELISA?

See Appendix for answers.

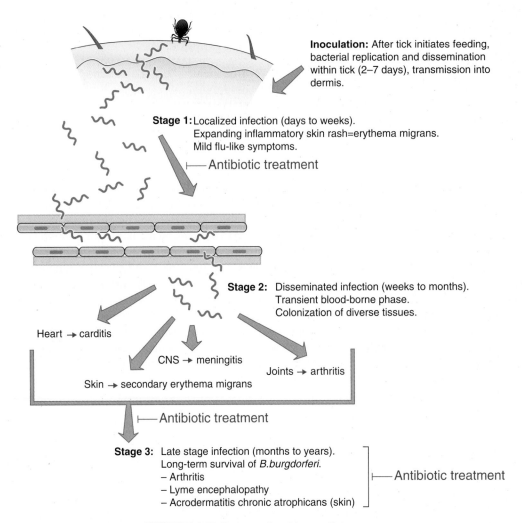

Inoculation: After tick initiates feeding, bacterial replication and dissemination within tick (2–7 days), transmission into dermis.

Stage 1: Localized infection (days to weeks). Expanding inflammatory skin rash=erythema migrans. Mild flu-like symptoms.

├── Antibiotic treatment

Stage 2: Disseminated infection (weeks to months). Transient blood-borne phase. Colonization of diverse tissues.

Heart → carditis

CNS → meningitis

Joints → arthritis

Skin → secondary erythema migrans

├── Antibiotic treatment

Stage 3: Late stage infection (months to years). Long-term survival of *B.burgdorferi*.
– Arthritis
– Lyme encephalopathy
– Acrodermatitis chronic atrophicans (skin)

├── Antibiotic treatment

FIGURE 25-1. Pathogenesis of Lyme disease.

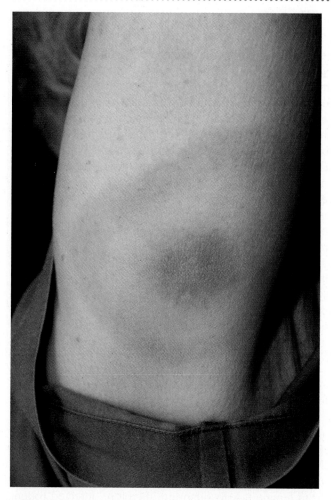

FIGURE 25-2. Erythema migrans, the characteristic rash of Lyme disease. This photograph depicts the "bull's-eye" pattern rash at the site of a tick bite on a woman's upper arm who subsequently contracted Lyme disease.

THE PATHOGEN: *BORRELIA BURGDORFERI*

Borrelia species, along with the leptospires and treponemes, are **spirochetes**. Like all spirochetes, *Borrelia* structure consists of a long, thin corkscrew-shaped cell (Fig. 25-3) surrounded first by an inner (cytoplasmic) membrane, then by a thin peptidoglycan layer, and finally by an outer membrane that is only loosely associated with the underlying structures. Flagella, which provide spirochetes with the ability to swim rapidly through viscous environments, such as host tissues, are contained between the two membranes and determine the corkscrew shape of the cell. The *Borrelia* species are fastidious, lacking the ability to synthesize amino acids, fatty acids, nucleotides, and enzyme cofactors, and need to scavenge numerous metabolic components from the host. In the laboratory, *B. burgdorferi* can be cultivated in a complex, chemically undefined liquid medium at 35°C with a generation time of approximately 8 hours. Until recently, only three *Borrelia* species were known to cause human Lyme disease: *B. burgdorferi*, *B. garinii*, and *B. afzelii*. Newly discovered *Borrelia* species found to cause disease in humans include *B. valaisiana*, *B. lusitaniae*, *B. bissettii*, and *B. spielmanii*. Infection in North America is caused solely by *B. burgdorferi*, but all species are a significant source of Lyme disease in Europe and Asia. All species cause similar but not identical clinical patterns and will generally be referred to as *B. burgdorferi* throughout this chapter.

The genome of *B. burgdorferi* is remarkably complex, consisting of a small linear chromosome and about 22 linear and circular plasmids, depending on the particular strain. More than half of the open reading frames present on the *B. burgdorferi* plasmids encode proteins of unknown function and unique to *Borrelia*. The *B. burgdorferi* outer membrane lacks lipopolysaccharide; rather, the outer membrane is decorated with a large array of lipoproteins. The repertoire of proteins expressed on the surface of the spirochete undergoes rapid changes in response to the diverse environments *B. burgdorferi* encounters throughout its infectious cycle.

HISTORY OF LYME DISEASE

Lyme disease was first described in 1975 as a distinct entity associated with a geographic cluster in Lyme, Connecticut, of children who received the diagnosis of juvenile rheumatoid arthritis. The rural setting of the case clusters and the identification of the characteristic erythema migrans as a feature of the illness suggested that the disorder was transmitted by an arthropod. Epidemiologic studies implicated certain *Ixodes* ticks as vectors of the disease (see Chapter 56). It soon became apparent that Lyme disease was a multisystemic illness that affected primarily the skin, nervous system, heart, and joints.

In addition to providing clues about the cause of the disease, erythema migrans helped link Lyme disease in the United States to certain syndromes in Europe. Early in the 20th century, several European investigators described the characteristic expanding skin lesion of erythema migrans, which they attributed to *Ixodes* tick bites. Many years later it was recognized that erythema migrans was often followed by a chronic skin disease (acrodermatitis chronica atrophicans), which had already

continued on page 280

(continued)

been described as a separate entity. In the 1940s, a neurologic syndrome was described in Europe (called Bannwarth syndrome, meningopolyneuritis, or meningoradiculitis). That syndrome was sometimes preceded by an **erythematous rash**. The various syndromes were linked conclusively in 1982 when the causative agent, a previously unrecognized spirochete now called *Borrelia burgdorferi*, was isolated from *Ixodes* (deer) ticks. The spirochete was then recovered from patients with Lyme disease in the United States, as well as from individuals in Europe with erythema migrans, Bannwarth syndrome, or acrodermatitis. Moreover, serological analysis demonstrated that all of these patients produced *B. burgdorferi*–specific antibodies. Although regional variations exist, the basic outlines of the disease are similar worldwide, and its most common name is Lyme disease or Lyme borreliosis.

Lyme disease is categorized as an emerging disease by the National Institute of Allergy and Infectious Diseases as the number of reported cases has more than doubled over the past 15 years. In 2008, there were approximately 29,000 confirmed cases of Lyme disease in the United States. Why has Lyme disease become a major concern in certain parts of the world? The most obvious reason is the recent recognition of a disease that has escaped definition in the past. Since 1982, diagnosis and reporting of Lyme disease have undergone vast improvements. Furthermore, Lyme disease is now causing **focal epidemics** as it spreads in the Northeastern and Upper Midwestern United States (see Fig. 25-6). These epidemics are thought to be the result of a large increase in the number of deer in those parts of the country, and, by extension, the deer ticks that transmit this disorder. At the same time, rural areas where deer and the deer ticks live have become increasingly populated by susceptible suburbanites who have never been exposed to the spirochete.

ENCOUNTER

Humans are "accidental" hosts for *B. burgdorferi* because spirochetes from infected people are not transmitted to other hosts. In most cases, small vertebrates, such as the **white-footed mouse**, participate with the *Ixodes sp.*

(**deer**) **tick** (Fig. 25-4) to maintain the reservoir of *B. burgdorferi* in nature. Additional potential reservoir hosts include voles, rats, squirrels, chipmunks, and even birds. There is no vertical transmission of the spirochete from female tick to offspring; therefore, infected rodents provide the critical means for the indirect transmission of spirochetes from one generation of deer tick to the next (Fig. 25-5). After being fed upon for several days by nymphal-stage deer ticks, these rodents become chronically infected with *B. burgdorferi*, particularly in the skin, enabling them to months later efficiently pass the spirochete back to uninfected larval ticks of a new generation. Therefore, while deer are the most common hosts for adult stage ticks, it is the transmission of spirochetes between small vertebrates, larval ticks, and nymphal ticks that is essential for the maintenance of *B. burgdorferi* in nature, and the nymphal tick is the major vector of transmission to humans (Fig. 25-5).

The infectious cycle of *B. burgdorferi* has significant implications for human disease. First, the geographic regions endemic for Lyme disease are restricted to those where all the essential elements of the natural cycle coexist, including populations of *Ixodes* ticks, populations of small vertebrates, appropriate vegetation, and optimal climatic conditions. Lyme disease in the United States is concentrated in the Northeastern and mid-Atlantic coastal states and the Great Lakes region with more sporadic cases occurring elsewhere (Fig. 25-6). Second, the ability of the spirochete to establish a chronic infection of rodents, with efficient colonization of the skin in particular, presents a challenge to eradication. Third,

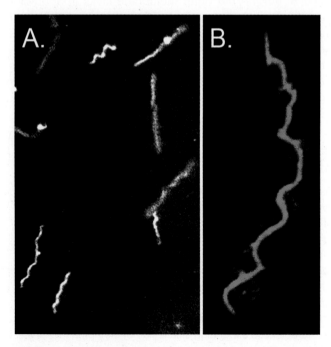

FIGURE 2-3. Micrographs of *Borrelia burgdorferi.* **A.** Dark-field micrograph of wet mount live *B. burgdorferi.* **B.** Confocal fluorescent micrograph of ALEXA 488–labeled *B. burgdorferi.*

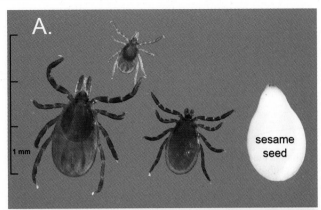

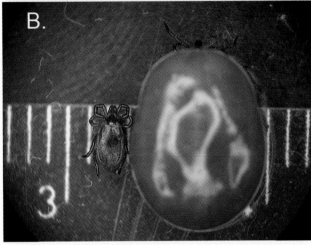

FIGURE 25-4. *Ixodes scapularis*: **black-legged deer ticks**. *Ixodes scapularis* ticks are the arthropod vectors that transmit the spirochete *Borrelia burgdorferi* to humans causing Lyme disease. **A.** From **left** to **right**, an unfed *I. scapularis* adult female, nymph, and adult male. The sesame seed demonstrates relative size. **B.** An unfed *I. scapularis* adult female (**left**) and a fully engorged *I. scapularis* adult female (**right**).

most human infections occur in the spring and summer months, when outdoor activities bring people into contact with feeding nymphal ticks. Moreover, one of the factors that have contributed to a dramatic increase in the incidence of Lyme disease over the past 10 years is the movement of people out of cities to rural, undeveloped areas resulting in a greater likelihood of coming in to contact with infected ticks.

ENTRY

Deer ticks are extremely small (~1 to 2 mm in length; see Fig. 25-4) and in many instances are not discovered by the individuals that they feed on, a feature that allows the tick to remain attached for several days. If left undetected, deer ticks feed continuously for 3 to 5 days and undergo a dramatic increase in body size due to the ingested blood meal (see Fig. 25-4). Spirochete transmission to the host typically does not occur until day 3 of tick feeding. Thus, if an individual removes a tick from his/her skin prior to the third day of feeding, it is likely that the person has not become infected with *B. burgdorferi* and will not contract Lyme disease.

While in the midgut of the *Ixodes* tick between feeding periods, the spirochetes of *B. burgdorferi* are in a dormant, nonreplicating state attached to epithelial cells. There they express a plasmid-encoded, major outer surface protein (**OspA**) that, although not required for persistence in the tick vector, plays a critical role in protection of *B. burgdorferi* from antibodies present in the blood meal from immune hosts and may also promote tick midgut colonization by binding to tick midgut cell receptors. When the tick feeds on a mammalian host, the spirochetes are exposed to a higher temperature and to the contents of mammalian blood. In response, the spirochete undergoes a number of phenotypic changes over the next 2 or 3 days. Most notably, expression of OspA decreases, and expression of **OspC**, a second outer surface protein encoded on a different plasmid, increases. Although the precise function of OspC is not entirely characterized, it is required for successful mammalian infection.

During the blood meal, the spirochetes replicate and invade the gut wall to spread throughout the tick, including to the salivary glands. Interestingly, the host protease plasmin, present in ingested blood, binds to and becomes activated on the bacterial surface and is required for efficient tick dissemination. From the salivary glands, the spirochetes are injected into the skin of the mammalian host. The change in the gene expression profile of the spirochetes in response to tick feeding, typified by the switch from OspA to OspC, is essential, because if feeding ticks are removed within the first 2 days of feeding, before the spirochete can complete these events, transmission of the spirochete to the mammalian host is abrogated. In addition, *B. burgdorferi* transmission from the tick to the mammal during the blood meal is facilitated by an increase in the expression of certain tick genes that encode proteins with immunosuppressive properties.

SPREAD AND MULTIPLICATION

The ability of *B. burgdorferi* to multiply and establish infection in the skin of the mammalian host is reflected in one of the characteristic signs of **localized infection** or **stage 1** Lyme disease in humans, the erythema migrans rash (Fig. 25-2 and see Fig. 25-1). The spirochetes are highly motile and probably still coated with the host protease plasmin; thus, over a period of days, they are able to spread through the skin, resulting in expansion of the rash, leaving a blanched central area, and a bull's-eye appearance. Some but not all strains of *B. burgdorferi* are capable of further multiplication and dissemination in humans in the following days to weeks, spreading to multiple tissues, including the nervous system, musculoskeletal tissues, and the heart. This stage is known as **early**

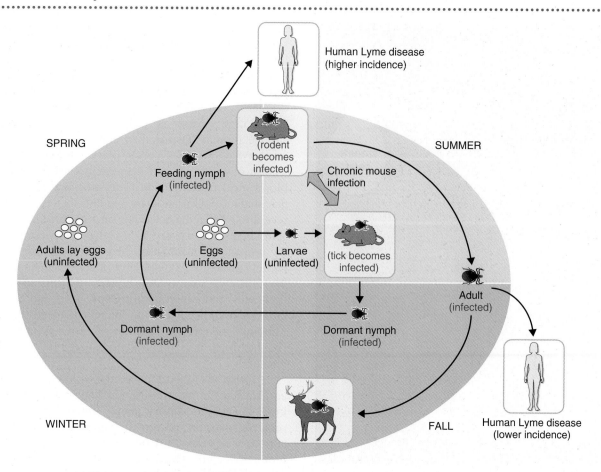

FIGURE 25-5. The natural cycle of Lyme disease. Deer ticks undergo a 2-year cycle that encompasses four stages: eggs, larvae, nymphs, and adults. In the summer, larvae hatch in an uninfected state and then acquire *B. burgdorferi* by feeding on infected rodents. *B. burgdorferi* survives in the midgut as the larvae molt into nymphs in the fall and are dormant through the winter. Infected nymphs feed on rodents in the late spring and early summer, resulting in the chronic infection of this natural reservoir of *B. burgdorferi*. The population of chronically infected rodents transmits *B. burgdorferi* to a new generation of larval-stage ticks. Nymphal ticks can also feed on humans, giving rise to the peak of human Lyme disease in the late spring and summer. The ticks molt into adults in the fall, and while their preferred host is deer, they can occasionally feed on humans, giving rise to a smaller peak of human Lyme disease in the fall.

disseminated infection or **stage 2** Lyme disease. Later, in **late stage** or **stage 3** Lyme disease, the rate of bacterial multiplication appears to be significantly reduced or is kept in check by the host defenses, resulting in the very low number of bacteria present in tissues. These bacteria, however, are not eradicated by the host immune response.

Although the bacterial properties that allow the spirochete to cause infection in a variety of tissues are still being defined, adherence of the spirochete to host cells and extracellular matrix (ECM) is likely one critical factor in colonization of diverse tissues. In vitro studies have demonstrated that *B. burgdorferi* utilizes several binding pathways to attach to diverse cell types and to ECM. Spirochetal binding to cells and ECM can be mediated by recognition of **glycosaminoglycans**, such as heparan sulfate and dermatan sulfate, which are long, linear

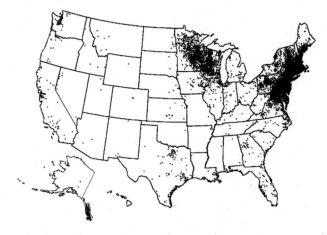

FIGURE 25-6. Risk areas for Lyme disease within the United States. Reported cases of Lyme disease in the United States in 2008. One dot represents a reported case of Lyme disease.

polymers of repeating disaccharides, as well as to **proteoglycans**, such as decorin, which contain glycosaminoglycans linked to a protein core. Other components of ECM that *B. burgdorferi* is able to bind to are the glycoproteins **fibronectin**, **laminin**, and **collagen**, the major protein of connective tissue ECM. In addition, *B. burgdorferi* attaches to receptors that belong to the **integrin** family, which normally mediate adherence of mammalian cells to ECM proteins (including fibronectin). Moreover, in vivo experimental models for infection have demonstrated roles for decorin-binding and fibronectin-binding proteins in the pathogenesis of *B. burgdorferi*. Studies are on going to further elucidate the contribution each of these interactions has on the ability of *B. burgdorferi* to colonize a specific tissue and the mechanisms by which these interactions likely cooperate to promote colonization of multiple tissues.

The ability to chronically infect the natural mammalian host, a characteristic that is essential for the ability of *B. burgdorferi* to complete its infectious cycle, is reflected in human Lyme disease. Once human infection is established, the spirochete can survive for years, despite the development of a vigorous host immune response. Several mechanisms that promote long-term survival of the organism have been identified to date. First, *B. burgdorferi* is able to bind mammalian complement regulatory factors, which may provide resistance to complement-mediated lysis and opsonization during persistent infection of host tissues. Second, the pathogen appears to be quite adept at turning on and off the expression of many genes encoding surface proteins, or altering their structure, thus presenting a "moving target" to the immune system.

An important example of the downregulation strategy is the seroreactive major outer surface protein OspC, which is expressed on the *B. burgdorferi* surface in feeding ticks and is required for the spirochete to initiate infection in the mammal. The protein is no longer required after day 8 of infection, and expression of the *ospC* gene is rapidly downregulated. Experiments have shown that spirochetes expressing a constitutive allele of *ospC*, resulting in continued production of the OspC protein, elicit an antibody response that clears the infection. Therefore, downregulation of *ospC* expression is essential for *B. burgdorferi* to persist in the mammalian host.

The spirochete can also alter the antigenic nature of at least one surface protein. Production of the outer surface protein **VlsE** is increased concomitant with the decrease in OspC production, and VlsE shares some general structural features with OspC. Unlike OspC, however, VlsE is subject to continual antigenic variation during an active infection, providing a mechanism for immune evasion while allowing sustained production of the protein. Adjacent to the *vlsE* gene are highly variant "cassettes" of nonexpressed DNA homologous to *vlsE*, and portions of the expressed *vlsE* gene are continually replaced with corresponding fragments of the nonexpressed cassettes by recombination. The *vls* locus can, in theory, generate on the order of 10^{30}

variants of the protein. The *vlsE* gene itself and recently identified factors required for VlsE switching are essential for *B. burgdorferi* immune evasion and persistence in mice. In sum, not only is *B. burgdorferi* required to sense and adapt to the disparate environments of the tick vector and mammalian host, but success of the pathogen depends on important changes in gene expression and sequence that occur at each stage of mammalian infection.

DAMAGE

Stages 1 and 2: Early Localized and Disseminated Infection

Evidence of damage is present at each stage of Lyme disease. Local skin infection at the tick bite site results in erythema migrans, which reflects infiltration of lymphocytes and macrophages (stage 1; see Fig. 25-1). Disseminated infection (stage 2) includes transient colonization of the bloodstream. At this stage some degree of vascular damage, including mild vasculitis or hypercellular vascular occlusion, may be seen in multiple sites, suggesting that the spirochetes colonize the vessel wall. In fact, microscopic analysis of mice infected with fluorescently labeled *B. burgdorferi* has demonstrated that the spirochete attaches to the vessel wall in stages, first transiently binding, then stably binding, followed by penetration of the endothelium and localization in the underlying tissue. Stage 2 of disease is often heralded by signs and symptoms reflecting colonization of the skin, nervous system, heart, and musculoskeletal sites, such as secondary erythema migrans lesions, excruciating headache, mild neck stiffness, and migratory pain in joints, bursae, tendons, muscle, or bone. Neurologic abnormalities can include meningitis and neuritis. Inflammatory manifestations of ocular infection can include conjunctivitis, iritis, choroiditis, or panophthalmitis. Cardiac involvement may result in fluctuating degrees of atrioventricular block or myopericarditis. These clinical manifestations are likely to be a result of direct infection of the affected tissue, because spirochetes have been detected in or recovered from most of these sites during this stage of the illness.

B. burgdorferi is not known to produce toxins that directly damage any tissue. Rather, the spirochete persists in infected tissues and thereby elicits an immune response that causes "bystander" injury to the host. The spirochete does not produce lipopolysaccharide (LPS, also called endotoxin), but as mentioned earlier, its genome encodes an unusually large number of **lipoproteins**, which are potent stimulators of proinflammatory cytokine production via toll-like receptors. Moreover, it has recently been demonstrated that the intracellular pattern recognition receptor **NOD2**, which recognizes **muramyl dipeptide** (**MDP**), a component of the cell wall of Gram-negative and Gram-positive bacteria, is important for recognition of *B. burgdorferi* and induction of cytokine production by human peripheral blood mononuclear cells following exposure to the spirochete. Consistent with this, infected tissues show an infiltration of lymphocytes and macrophages, and sometimes plasma cells and/or neutrophils.

Stage 3: Late Stage Infection

In untreated patients, diverse objective manifestations of late stage Lyme disease (stage 3; Fig 25-1) can occur months to years after disease onset, reflecting the ability of the spirochete to establish a chronic infection in many tissue sites. Patients, particularly those in the United States, may suffer from repeated episodes of pauciarticular arthritis (i.e., arthritis involving a few joints), the most common presentation of late Lyme disease due to chronic infection of the joints.

Neurologic involvement, affecting either the peripheral or central nervous system, may also occur in late stage Lyme disease, sometimes following years of latent infection. *B. burgdorferi* DNA has been detected in cerebrospinal fluid in patients with **Lyme encephalopathy** many years after disease onset. In Lyme disease, the most common form of chronic central nervous system involvement affects memory, mood, or sleep, sometimes with subtle language disturbance.

Another example of prolonged latency followed by appearance of clinical signs of persistent infection in Lyme disease is a late skin manifestation called **acrodermatitis chronica atrophicans**, which has been observed primarily in Europe after infection with *B. afzelii*. This skin lesion usually begins with bluish-red discoloration and swollen skin on an extremity. The lesion's inflammatory phase may persist for many years or decades, and it gradually leads to atrophy of the skin. *Borrelia* has been cultured from such lesions as much as 10 years after their onset.

It is well documented that Lyme disease is successfully treated with antibiotics. In rare cases, however, patients who have been diagnosed with Lyme disease and who have received the recommended course of antibiotics continue to suffer from symptoms such as fatigue, musculoskeletal pain, and loss of cognitive functions. These patients are classified as having **post–Lyme disease syndrome**. The causes of post–Lyme disease syndrome are not known. Post–Lyme disease syndrome appears to correlate with greater severity of disease at the onset and delayed antibiotic treatment, but NOT with a lack of appropriate initial antibiotic treatment. In many patients, these manifestations represent a slow response to the antibiotic therapy, as patients report a gradual decrease in symptoms over time following treatment. The symptoms of post–Lyme disease syndrome may also be attributed to autoimmunity triggered by the initial *B. burgdorferi* infection. This appears to be the case in patients with specific HLA-DR alleles that are also associated with susceptibility to rheumatoid arthritis. It has been postulated that in genetically susceptible people, *B. burgdorferi* triggers a self-damaging immune response that continues even after apparent eradication of the spirochetes from the joint,

perhaps owing to the presence of bacterial antigens that are cross-reactive with human proteins. Although the mechanisms underlying post–Lyme disease syndrome are not completely understood, there is no evidence that the associated symptoms are due to a persistent *B. burgdorferi* infection. Thus, prolonged antibiotic therapy is believed to be medically unjustified and in fact may expose patients to risks associated with any extended antibiotic treatment.

DIAGNOSIS

The ability to culture the organism from infected sites is often the gold standard for diagnosis of bacterial infections. Rare case studies demonstrated isolation of *B. burgdorferi* from the erythema migrans skin lesions and/or blood samples from Lyme disease patients, and even then sophisticated culturing techniques and long incubation times were required. It is usually difficult to visualize spirochetes in histologic sections due to the low number of spirochetes present even during an active infection. Although it is possible to detect *B. burgdorferi* DNA in tissue biopsies from some of the affected sites, such as joints, technical challenges that limit the sensitivity and specificity of DNA-based tests have hindered the development of a widely available, routine, definitive diagnostic test for Lyme disease. Furthermore, detection of spirochete DNA in tissues still falls short of the definitive diagnosis of an active *B. burgdorferi* infection with replicating, viable spirochetes. Instead, the diagnosis of Lyme disease is first and foremost a process of identifying clinical features, particularly erythema migrans, suggestive of Lyme disease coupled with a history that is compatible with exposure to infected deer ticks.

In cases in which the clinical assessment leads to the suspicion of Lyme disease, but not its definitive diagnosis, serologic testing, such as enzyme-linked immunosorbent assay (**ELISA**) and **immunoblot**, to detect anti–*B. burgdorferi* antibodies can be employed to confirm the diagnosis. After the first several weeks of infection, particularly if the spirochete disseminates, most patients become seropositive. However, even these serologic tests have their limitations, and interpretation requires some experience and skill. As early diagnosis of Lyme disease is critical to successful treatment, development of new antibody-based assays with enhanced sensitivity and reliability is an active area of Lyme disease research.

The fact that the manifestations of Lyme disease are quite varied and not entirely specific has given rise to considerable dispute surrounding the diagnosis of Lyme disease. For example, the term "chronic Lyme disease" has been used by some to describe patients with persistent pain, neurocognitive symptoms, and fatigue but with no objective clinical or serological evidence of the patient ever having been infected with *B. burgdorferi*. Equating such syndromes with chronic *B. burgdorferi* infection is a misnomer. In addition, once a person has

TABLE 25-1 Clinical Presentation and Recommended Therapy for Patients with Lyme Disease

Disease Stage	Clinical Presentation	Treatment	Duration (d)
Stage 1, early localized	Erythema migrans	Oral	14–21
Stage 2, early disseminated	Multiple erythema migrans	Oral	14–21
	Cranial nerve palsy	Oral	14–21
	Meningitis	Intravenous followed by oral	14–21
	Cardiac disease		
	Ambulatory	Oral	14–21
	Hospitalized	Intravenous followed by oral	14–21
	Borrelia lymphocytoma	Oral	14–21
Stage 3, late stage	Arthritis	Oral	28
	Encephalitis	Oral or intravenous	28

received the diagnosis of chronic Lyme disease (typically due to subjective clinical criteria followed by the use of unproven and/or unvalidated laboratory tests), the patient is often subjected to treatment over the course of months to years with multiple antibiotics, some of which have no demonstrated antimicrobial activity against *B. burgdorferi*. As with post–Lyme disease syndrome, antibiotic treatment of patients with so-called chronic Lyme disease poses substantial risk with little to no demonstrable benefit. Thus, physicians have a responsibility to appropriately diagnose their patients using validated laboratory tests and clinical criteria and follow up with a suitable treatment regime.

TREATMENT

Lyme disease patients typically respond well to appropriate antibiotic treatment, which is guided by the stage and manifestation of the disease (Table 25-1). For stage 1 or 2, the duration of therapy is generally 2 to 4 weeks and is guided by the clinical presentation of illness. *B. burgdorferi* is only moderately sensitive to penicillin; consequently, doxycycline is the most commonly prescribed antibiotic for adults, and amoxicillin is the primary choice for children. Patients with late stage Lyme disease, manifesting as arthritis, typically respond well to oral therapy with doxycycline or amoxicillin over a 4-week period. Two

COMPARISON OF VARIOUS SPIROCHETOSES

The spirochetoses that affect humans in the United States in addition to Lyme disease include **syphilis**, **relapsing fever**, and **leptospirosis** (Table 25-2). Except for syphilis, these are animal diseases that only incidentally affect humans when they are bitten by *Borrelia*-infected ticks or when they come in contact with animal urine contaminated with leptospires. All these spirochetes are highly motile, and all are capable of spreading from the initial site of infection. The initial phases of these infections have many similarities to Lyme disease, including the possible presence of fever, headache, muscle pain, meningitis, photophobia, malaise, or fatigue. However, each disease also has unique clinical features. Relapsing fever is associated with intermittent episodes of high fever, which are thought to occur because of variation of the major antigen, a surface protein of the spirochete. Leptospirosis often affects the kidney, but infection of many tissues is seen and can result in hemorrhage. Both Lyme disease and syphilis occur in stages over a period of years and typically cause neurologic abnormalities late in the illness. However, the neurologic syndromes of the two diseases are different. For syphilis and Lyme disease, diagnosis is usually made by recognition of a characteristic clinical picture with serologic confirmation. All the spirochetes are susceptible to a wide range of antibiotics.

TABLE 25-2 Main Features of the Spirochetoses

Name of Disease	Causative Agent	Mode of Transmission	Characteristic Clinical Aspects
Lyme disease	*Borrelia burgdorferi*	Ticks of the *Ixodes ricinus* complex	Erythema migrans, recurrent arthritis
Relapsing fever	*B. hermsii, B. recurrentis,* others	*Ornithodoros* ticks, human body louse	Recurrent high fever
Syphilis	*Treponema pallidum*	Sexual contact	Chancre, tabes dorsalis, aortitis
Leptospirosis	*Leptospira* spp.	Contact with infected animals or their urine	Jaundice, renal involvement

to four weeks of intravenous therapy is generally necessary for patients with objective neurologic involvement, such as Lyme meningitis, and the third-generation cephalosporin drugs (e.g., ceftriaxone or cefotaxime) are used most often for this purpose. Ceftriaxone is also used for treatment of patients presenting with myocarditis. Once symptoms begin to improve, these patients can complete their treatment regime with oral antibiotics.

PREVENTION

Given the potential difficulties in early diagnosis of Lyme disease, the prevention of infection has been emphasized. Currently, the best advice for prevention is behavioral: people should be warned to minimize the chances of tick bites by wearing long pants tucked into socks, spraying clothing with insect repellent, and performing careful checks for feeding ticks daily when engaging in outdoor activities in Lyme-endemic areas, particularly in the spring and summer. As described above, removal of an *Ixodes* tick within the first 2 days of feeding is likely to prevent transmission of the spirochete.

A Lyme vaccine based on OspA was available in the United States for several years. It has since been withdrawn from the market for various reasons, but provides interesting insight into *B. burgdorferi* biology. As discussed earlier, OspA is expressed while the spirochete is in the tick midgut but is not usually expressed while the spirochete is in the mammalian host. Thus, anti-OspA antibody does not promote clearance of bacteria in the mammalian host. Instead, the anti-OspA antibody present in blood is ingested by the feeding tick and leads to killing of spirochetes in the tick midgut, thereby interrupting the activation and migration of spirochetes from the tick midgut to the salivary glands, a process required for mammalian infection. Although not all vectorborne pathogens require growth and/or development in the gut of

the vector for transmission, the OspA vaccine highlights the potential efficacy of transmission-blocking vaccines. In the Lyme disease field, researchers are actively examining a variety of novel vaccine approaches, including utilizing alternative *B. burgdorferi* surface antigens as well as targeting molecules produced by the tick vector that the spirochete requires for infection of the mammalian host.

CONCLUSION

Lyme disease is an insidious disease that can be readily treated if diagnosed at an early stage. Untreated, the spirochete can cause a long-term, multisystemic illness that can be divided into three stages based on the site(s) and duration of infection. Because diagnosis is still largely dependent on clinical suspicion and evaluation of the patient rather than on laboratory tests, physicians and other health personnel must be alert to the possibility of this disease among people living in affected areas, especially those who are frequently outdoors.

Suggested Readings

Edlow JA, ed. Tick-borne diseases, part I: Lyme disease. *Infect Dis Clin N Am.* 2008;22(2):195–380.

Olson D, Heys J, Czark G. Lyme Disease Guidelines Review. Available from: http://www.idsociety.org/Content.aspx?id=16501. Last accessed April 22, 2010.

Samuels DS, Radolf JD, eds. *Borrelia: Molecular Biology, Host Interaction and Pathogenesis.* Caister Academic Press: Norfolk, UK; 2010.

Wormser GP, Dattwyler RJ, Shapiro ED, et al. The clinical assessment, treatment, and prevention of Lyme disease, human granulocytic anaplasmosis, and babesiosis: clinical practice guidelines by the Infectious Diseases Society of America. *Clin Infect Dis.* 2006;43(9):1089–1134.

Wormser GP, Schwartz I. Antibiotic treatment of animals infected with *Borrelia burgdorferi. Clin Microbiol Rev.* 2009;22(3):387–395.

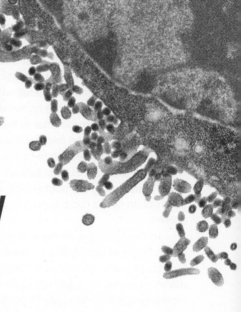

Chapter 26

Cat Scratch Disease, Bacillary Angiomatosis, and Other Bartonelloses

Christoph Dehio

KEY CONCEPTS

Pathogens: *Bartonella* species are slow-growing Gram-negative bacteria. They include *Bartonella henselae*, the cause of cat scratch disease (in immunocompetent persons), peliosis hepatis, and bacillary angiomatosis (in immunocompromised persons); *B. quintana*, which causes trench fever and bacteremia (in immunocompetent persons) and bacillary angiomatosis (in immunocompromised persons); *B. bacilliformis*, the agent of Oroya fever and verruga peruana; six additional zoonotic species listed in Table 26-1 that can cause endocarditis and other rare manifestations in humans

Encounter and Entry: Transmitted by a cat scratch or bite (*B. henselae*), the feces of the body louse (*B. quintana*), and the bite of a South American sandfly (*B. bacilliformis*) or unknown routes (other human-pathogenic *Bartonella* species)

Spread, Multiplication, and Damage: The extent of *B. henselae* and *B. quintana* infections in humans is determined by the adequacy of the immune response. In immunocompetent hosts, the infection tends to be limited or localized. In immunocompromised hosts, the growth of the organisms is uncontrolled.

Diagnosis: Requires prolonged cultivation to isolate organisms, microscopic examination of biopsies using special stains, detection of specific antibodies in blood, or PCR.

Treatment: *B. henselae* is susceptible to macrolide antibiotics, but treatment in immunocompetent hosts may not be necessary.

BARTONELLA species can cause serious infections of both immunocompetent and immunocompromised persons, with markedly different consequences depending on the state of host defenses. *B. henselae* is the major cause of two diseases: **cat scratch disease**, a prevalent, self-limited infectious lymphadenitis transmitted by the scratch or bite of a healthy-appearing infected cat, and **bacillary angiomatosis**, cutaneous and visceral tumorlike proliferations of blood vessels principally in people with AIDS. *B. quintana* causes also two diseases: **trench fever**, a 5-day relapsing fever transmitted by the body louse, and **bacillary angiomatosis**. In South America, an endemic bartonellosis, caused by *B. bacilliformis*, is transmitted by sandflies and results in **Oroya fever**, a febrile illness with severe hemolytic anemia, and/or subsequent vasoproliferative skin lesions.

Cat scratch disease is a significant infection in the United States, with more than 20,000 cases reported annually. M. developed the typical clinical features and a self-limited course of cat scratch disease, whereas J. developed a more indolent and relapsing disease in the context of AIDS. In addition to *B. henselae* causing cat scratch disease and bacillary angiomatosis, there are two other medically important *Bartonella* infections, as well as a steadily growing number of species causing zoonotic infections at rather low incidence (Table 26-1).

In parts of Peru, Ecuador, and Colombia, a skin disorder called **verruga peruana** ("Peruvian wart") has been recognized since pre-Columbian times. The indolent angioma-like lesions of this condition resemble those seen in the case of J. In late 19th century Peru, an epidemic of fever and anemia (**Oroya fever**) occurred among railroad construction workers. At that time, a Peruvian medical student named Daniel Carrión demonstrated that the lesions of verruga peruana contain the same infectious agent responsible for Oroya fever. He injected himself with material from a skin lesion and unfortunately died of the acute febrile illness. His legacy was the important discovery that the two seemingly disparate diseases have a common etiology. It is now known that in the natural course of infection, the febrile illness occurs first and may resolve to be followed months later by the skin lesions. In honor of the medical student whose autoexperiment permitted this connection to be recognized, the disorder was renamed **Carrión disease**. The etiologic agent of Carrión disease, *B. bacilliformis*, was observed in 1913 by its discoverer, Alberto Barton, to infect red blood cells during the acute stage of infection. Blood infection leads to extreme anemia because of massive destruction of the red blood cells by the mononuclear phagocytes in lymphoreticular organs such as the spleen.

In the Northern Hemisphere, **trench fever** caused by *B. quintana* was one of the major causes of morbidity in World War I. The disease has appeared again in new forms in people with AIDS and in homeless persons. Immunocompromised persons are particularly susceptible to this infection, which may manifest as febrile bacteremia or tumorlike proliferations in blood vessels of the skin and visceral organs, indistinguishable clinically or pathologically from *B. henselae* bacillary angiomatosis. Homeless persons in Europe and North America have been found to have *B. quintana* infections of the bloodstream and cardiac valves. The chronic bacteremia of this infection can extend for months beyond clinical recovery. Originally, the trench fever bacterium was believed to be a species of *Rickettsia*. In 1961, cell-free cultivation of this etiologic agent on blood agar demonstrated that it was not an obligate intracellular bacterium. For many years, the trench fever agent was called *Rickettsia quintana* and later *Rochalimaea quintana* in honor of the Brazilian microbiologist da Rocha-Lima. However, contemporary molecular tools revealed that the bacterium, now known as *B. quintana*, is a close relative of *B. bacilliformis* and *B. henselae* (see Paradigm Box).

In addition to these three major human pathogens, at least six other *Bartonella* species were reported to cause human disease at low incidence, most prominently endocarditis (Table 26-1). However, the real incidence of infection by these species is likely underestimated due to the lack of appropriate diagnostic tools and the broad spectrum of disease manifestations. Due to our lack of knowledge on the epidemiology and virulence properties of these emerging pathogens, they are not further discussed in this chapter.

CASE • Two brothers, M. and J., became ill after having been scratched by a new kitten given to them by an aunt. M. is 5 years old and has been healthy all his life. He developed a 6-mm cutaneous papule on the right hand where the kitten had scratched him 1 week before. After another week, he developed numerous enlarged lymph nodes in the right axilla. Acute and convalescent sera collected by M.'s pediatrician showed an eightfold rise in titer of antibodies to Bartonella henselae. M.'s lymph nodes returned to normal size and consistency over a 3-month period without antimicrobial treatment.

J. is 3 years old. Unlike M., he acquired infection with HIV-1 congenitally from his mother and has AIDS. J. developed three painless, red protuberant skin lesions that resembled tumors. Biopsy of the largest of the lesions revealed proliferation of small blood vessels and numerous colonies of small bacteria. A diagnosis of bacillary angiomatosis was made. The lesions resolved after a month of continuous treatment with oral erythromycin. However, another crop of similar lesions developed 3 weeks after discontinuing the antibiotic. With the recurrence, J. also developed fever and chills. Blood cultures for *Bartonella* organisms were obtained, and J. was treated with intravenous erythromycin until his fever resolved. Oral erythromycin was continued thereafter. His skin lesions disappeared on treatment, but he died of other complications of AIDS 4 months later. After 2 weeks of incubation, his blood culture grew *B. henselae*.

This case raises several questions:

1. Why did J. develop a different disease than M. when both were infected with the same organism, *B. henselae*?

2. Why did M. get well without treatment, while J. suffered a relapse despite treatment with an appropriate antibiotic?

3. What was the source of the infection?

4. By what route(s) did the organisms travel to the skin papule, the lymph nodes, and the pseudoneoplastic skin lesions?

See Appendix for answers.

PARADIGM BOX

NEW METHODS AND THE DISCOVERY OF NEW ETIOLOGIC AGENTS

Ever since microscopy, microbial cultivation, and animal inoculation led to the concept that living things invisible to the naked eye could cause diseases, advances in technology have led to the discovery of new infectious agents. Cell culture has enabled the discovery of viruses and other etiologic agents that cannot be cultivated on agar or in broth. Electron microscopy allowed visualization of viruses and bacteria for which effective methods of growth had not been developed.

Recently, the application of molecular methods, particularly polymerase chain reaction (PCR) and amplification and sequencing of DNA derived from the infectious agent, has fostered the discovery of previously undetermined or undiscovered etiologic agents of infectious diseases. The major causative agent of bacillary angiomatosis, *Bartonella henselae*, was initially identified using this approach. Classic serologic, epidemiologic, and ecological investigations later revealed that it also causes cat scratch disease.

Other pathogens that had yet to be cultivated, including the agents that cause **human granulocytic anaplasmosis** and **Whipple disease**, have been identified by DNA analysis. Human granulocytic anaplasmosis is a life-threatening disease that was recognized as a veterinary pathogen in Great Britain in 1932 but was just recently discovered to pose a threat to humans. Whipple disease, on the other hand, has been known as a human disease since 1907. In both instances, scientists obtained affected tissues from patients and used PCR to amplify a structural RNA gene known to be present in all bacteria—namely, **16S ribosomal RNA** (**16S rRNA**). The amplified RNA was sequenced and compared with the 16S rRNA sequences of other known bacteria stored in computerized data banks. Because certain variations in the 16S rRNA sequence are known to occur during the evolution of bacterial species, scientists can identify the closest relatives of the unknown pathogen even when an exact match is not available from the data bank. Subsequently, both *Anaplasma phagocytophilum* and *Tropheryma whippelii* have been propagated in cell culture.

Similarly, to identify the culprit causing the deadly, acute respiratory disease outbreak of 1993 in the Four Corners area of New Mexico, Arizona, Colorado, and Utah, researchers used a variation of this method. Based on serology, investigators suspected a Hantavirus-like agent. Consequently, researchers added a reverse transcription step to convert viral RNA in patient samples into DNA. Then primers for conserved Hantavirus sequences were used for PCR. These studies revealed that the etiologic agent was indeed a novel strain of Hantavirus. Many of the riddles of newly emerging and poorly understood infectious diseases will surely yield to the study of genomic sequences by ever-improving methods.

TABLE 26-1 Etiology and Epidemiology of Bartonella Infections

Organisms	Diseases	Reservoir in Nature	Transmission
B. henselae	Cat scratch disease, bacillary angiomatosis	Cats	Cat scratch or bite (cat to human), cat flea (cat to cat)
B. quintana	Trench fever, bacillary angiomatosis	Humans	Louse feces, possibly other arthropods, and contaminated drug paraphernalia
B. bacilliformis	Oroya fever (or Carrión disease), verruga peruana	Humans	Sandfly bite
B. alsatica	Endocarditis, lymphadenitis	Rabbit	Not known
B. elizabethae	Endocarditis	Rat	Not known
B. koehlerae	Endocarditis	Cat	Not known
B. grahamii	Neuroretinitis	Mouse	Not known
B. rochalimaea	Bacteremia with fever	Fox	Not known
B. vinsonii subsp. *arupensis*	Endocarditis Bacteremia with fever	Mouse	Not known
B. vinsonii subsp. *berkhoffii*	Endocarditis	Dog/coyote	Not known

ENCOUNTER AND ENTRY

Bartonella henselae is introduced into human skin by a scratch or bite from an infected cat, likely by inoculation with the feces from cat fleas that contain infectious bacteria. Transmission from cat to cat occurs through fleas. In contrast, *B. quintana* infections during World War I were transmitted among humans by the human body louse. Many affected individuals in modern times have not shown any signs of having lice. Other possible, but unproven, modes of transmission of *B. quintana* include contaminated intravenous drug paraphernalia or other arthropods. The third *Bartonella* species, *B. bacilliformis*, is transmitted through the bite of a phlebotomine **sandfly**, which takes a blood meal from an infected host, possibly amplifies the quantity of organisms, and then transmits the organisms by feeding on a new susceptible host. Humans may be the only reservoir for *B. bacilliformis*, but other species of *Bartonella* infect a variety of mammals (e.g., rodents, felines, and canines) in endemic areas and throughout the world.

SPREAD, MULTIPLICATION, AND DAMAGE

In cat scratch disease, *B. henselae* causes a small papule at the site of inoculation. The organism then spreads via the lymphatic vessels to the draining regional lymph nodes where bacterial proliferation and a vigorous mixed **granulomatous** and **suppurative** host response occur. This response typically limits the infection, and very few bacteria are found in infected lymph nodes (Fig. 26-1). In some patients, however, particularly people with AIDS, the host response is insufficient to control the infection. The organisms multiply freely and disseminate in large numbers through the bloodstream, often manifesting clinically as sepsis or as localized infection of the skin, liver, and other viscera. In infections of skin and other organs, the bacteria secrete substances and trigger cytokine production that stimulate proliferation of small blood vessels, resulting in the lesions of **bacillary angiomatosis** (Fig. 26-2).

B. quintana has been found to cause an indistinguishable angioproliferative lesion in people with AIDS, although the source of infection and mode of entry are not always clear. Both *B. quintana* and *B. henselae* are

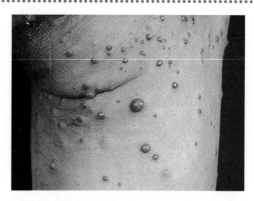

FIGURE 26-2. Multiple violaceous papules and nodules in a case of bacillary angiomatosis.

also frequent causes of culture-negative endocarditis, so called because routine cultures do not recover the organisms. In the course of trench fever, *B. quintana* enters human erythrocytes and replicates. This may explain the characteristic relapsing fever, but intraerythrocytic growth typically does not lead to anemia or any other life-threatening condition.

B. bacilliformis attaches to the erythrocyte, deforms the cell membrane as it enters the cell, and then multiplies within the erythrocyte cytoplasm. **Massive anemia** can then ensue from greatly enhanced erythrophagocytosis. This process can also alter host defenses. The pathogenesis of the ensuing chronic nodular skin lesions is similar to that of bacillary angiomatosis.

DIAGNOSIS

Bartonella infections can be diagnosed by cultivation of the organisms from blood or skin lesions; however, growth is slow, and routine cultures are often discarded before organisms are detected. Alternatively, diagnosis of *B. henselae* or *B. quintana* infection can be made by detecting specific antibodies in patients with suspicious clinical signs and symptoms. *Bartonella* species can also be detected in biopsies with the use of special silver-staining methods. In people with AIDS, biopsies of lesions are often performed to rule out the similar-appearing, malignant angiomatous lesion of Kaposi sarcoma. Likewise, *B. bacilliformis* can be visualized diagnostically in Romanowsky-stained smears of peripheral blood of patients with Oroya fever. *Bartonella* infection in blood or tissues can also be diagnosed by PCR. PCR with primers to amplify members of the genus *Bartonella* in combination with DNA sequence analysis has also facilitated the identification of previously unrecognized *Bartonella* species as causes of human disease (see Table 26-1).

TREATMENT

In cat scratch disease, the course of illness is only marginally affected by antibiotic treatment. Although various

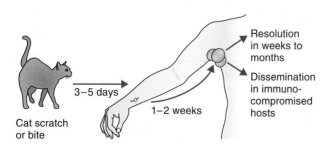

Cat scratch or bite → 3–5 days → 1–2 weeks → Resolution in weeks to months / Dissemination in immunocompromised hosts

FIGURE 26-1. Acquisition and courses of infection with *Bartonella henselae*.

antibiotics (rifampin, ciprofloxacin, trimethoprim/sulfamethoxazole, and gentamicin) have been used, there is no established, effective antimicrobial therapy. The drug of choice for bacillary angiomatosis or bacteremia caused by either *B. henselae* or *B. quintana* is **erythromycin**; doxycycline and azithromycin also produce good results. Unfortunately, relapses requiring repeated or long-term maintenance treatment occur in patients with inadequate host defenses. For *B. bacilliformis* infection, chloramphenicol was traditionally given in the acute febrile stage (Oroya fever) because of the frequency of complications resulting from *Salmonella* superinfection. Currently, **ciprofloxacin** is a drug of choice but a combination with another antimicrobial is often used to prevent resistance. **Rifampin** is used for the much less serious verrucous stage.

CONCLUSION

Organisms of the genus *Bartonella* belong to a large and heterogeneous group of fastidious Gram-negative bacilli that infect a variety of mammals. Decades of confusion passed before they were assigned a logical taxonomic home based on nucleic acid homology of evolutionarily conserved genes. The three species that cause most cases of human disease, *B. henselae*, *B. quintana*, and *B. bacilliformis*, produce angiomatous skin lesions, sepsis, or visceral organ infection (e.g., peliosis hepatis and endocarditis), depending on the circumstances of infection and the immune status of the host. When the organisms proliferate in tissues or blood, treatment with an antibiotic is effective and warranted. In lymphadenopathic cat scratch disease, a vigorous host response limits bacterial growth but also produces lymphadenitis, which is a hallmark of the disease. Antimicrobial therapy is of minimal, if any, value in such situations.

Suggested Readings

Bass JW, Vincent JM, Person DA. The expanding spectrum of *Bartonella* infections: I. Bartonellosis and trench fever. *Pediatr Infect Dis J.* 1997;16:2–10.

Bass JW, Vincent JM, Person DA. The expanding spectrum of *Bartonella* infections: II. Cat-scratch disease. *Pediatr Infect Dis J.* 1997;16:163–179.

Florin TA, Zaoutis TE, Zaoutis LB. Beyond cat scratch disease: widening spectrum of *Bartonella henselae* infection. *Pediatrics.* 2008;121:e1413–e1425.

Maguina C, Guerra H, Ventosilla P. Bartonellosis. *Clin Dermatol.* 2009;27:271–280.

Relman DA, Loutit JS, Schmidt TM, et al. The agent of bacillary angiomatosis: an approach to the identification of uncultured pathogens. *N Engl J Med.* 1990;323:1573–1580.

Schultz MG. Daniel Carrión's experiment. *N Engl J Med.* 1968;278:1323–1326.

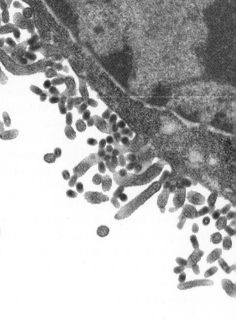

Chapter 27

Chlamydiae: Genital, Ocular, and Respiratory Pathogens

Toni Darville

KEY CONCEPTS

Pathogen: Chlamydiae are obligate intracellular Gram-negative bacteria.

Encounter: Chlamydiae cause a wide variety of genital, ocular, and respiratory infections in humans; certain animal and avian isolates cause disease.

Entry: Depending on the species, infection may be sexually transmitted, acquired from human-to-human droplet spread, or acquired from contact with infected animals.

Spread: Chlamydiae undergo a unique developmental cycle within eukaryotic host cells.

Multiplication: There are two distinct morphological forms termed elementary bodies (EBs) and reticulate bodies (RBs). EBs are small (0.25-μm)

extracellular infectious particles that attach to and enter into host cells but are metabolically inert; that is, they do not grow or divide. RBs are derived from EBs after uptake by cells; they are larger (0.6- to 0.8-μm), intracellular, noninfectious but metabolically active forms that divide by binary fission within a membrane-bound inclusion in eukaryotic host cells.

Damage: Most tissue damage is related to a host hypersensitivity reaction.

Diagnosis: Genital infection can be diagnosed by polymerase chain reaction; other infections generally depend on serologic diagnosis.

Treatment and Prevention: Chlamydiae are sensitive to macrolides, tetracyclines, and fluoroquinolones.

THE CHLAMYDIA genus includes species of Gram-negative bacteria that have an obligatory requirement to grow and to propagate within eukaryotic cells. They cannot be cultured in nutrient broth media or on agar plates. One evolutionary result of their restricted growth within eukaryotic cells is that chlamydiae are extremely isolated within their own phylogenetic grouping and are genetically distant from other eubacteria. Interestingly, these organisms have acquired several genes from eukaryotes that have never been found in other bacteria. *Chlamydiae* are widespread in humans, animals, and birds, and they have achieved a remarkably balanced relationship with their hosts. Thus, they are often referred to as "stealth pathogens." Although they cause many serious diseases with apparently immune-mediated complications, the organisms themselves have an extraordinary ability to evade host immune responses.

CLASSIFICATION AND BASIC BIOLOGY

Current, ongoing molecular analyses of a variety of chlamydial isolates confirm that the order Chlamydiales encompasses a wide range of pathogenic bacteria that share a unique biphasic developmental cycle within eukaryotic host cells. Presently, the taxonomical terms for human chlamydial pathogens that have been used since the early 1970s are most commonly used in the literature. In this nomenclature, the order Chlamydiales contains one family, Chlamydiaceae; one genus, *Chlamydia*; and two species, *C. trachomatis* and *C. pneumoniae*. Organisms are also subdivided according to specific biological traits (i.e., biovariants, or biovars) as well as serology (i.e., serovariants, or serovars). Molecular studies do indicate that *C. pneumoniae* could be recategorized into a separate genus (*Chlamydophila*). Although this designation has been

CASE • Mr. C., who is 24 years old, saw a physician because of a purulent discharge from his penis. A diagnosis of gonorrhea was made (see Chapter 14), and he was given a cephalosporin, ceftriaxone, by intramuscular injection and two capsules of a second oral antibiotic. Mr. C. improved but felt guilty when confessing the situation to his latest sexual partner, Ms. N. He urged her to make an appointment to be tested for infection.

Ms. N. had no complaints of pain, vaginal irritation, or discharge. However, on physical examination, she was found to have a mucopurulent discharge emanating from her cervix. Her cervix was inflamed and bled easily when a swab was used to remove adherent secretions. Gram stain of the secretions revealed numerous neutrophils but no Gram-negative diplococci. Ms. N. was told she probably had a chlamydial infection, chlamydial cervicitis. An endocervical swab was collected for nucleic amplification assays for both chlamydiae and gonococci. Ms. N. was also given an intramuscular injection of ceftriaxone, as an added precaution against *Neisseria gonorrhoeae*, and two capsules of an oral antibiotic, which she took in the presence of the physician. The physician then questioned Ms. N. about other sexual partners before releasing her.

These cases raise several questions:

1. What was the second antibiotic taken by Mr. C. and Ms. N., and why was it given?

2. Why were nucleic acid amplification assays performed instead of culture on Ms. N.'s endocervical specimen?

3. If Ms. N. had not heeded Mr. C.'s advice and sought medical attention, what might have been the consequences for her? What are the pathophysiological mechanisms of such sequelae?

See Appendix for answers.

adopted by taxonomists, many investigators have been slow to adopt this new genus name. You may find either designation used in different learning resources. Analysis of 16S rRNA for the purpose of taxonomy has been particularly beneficial for speciation of chlamydiae associated with animal diseases. These animal pathogens are important in human medicine because accidental transmission to humans can produce acute, life-threatening illnesses. Table 27-1 briefly describes the chlamydial agents and associated illnesses.

Chlamydiae are small in size (0.25 to 0.8 μm in diameter) compared with typical bacteria such as *Escherichia coli* (1.0 μm) and have small chromosomes ranging from 1.0 to 1.2 megabases in size. They are **Gram-negative** in architecture and composition, with an outer membrane containing lipopolysaccharide (truncated and not very endotoxic) and a cytoplasmic membrane. While the classic bacterial cell wall component peptidoglycan (murein) has not been confirmed by isolation and identification, chlamydiae are susceptible to β-lactam antibiotics and possess all the genes for murein synthesis and penicillin-binding proteins. A distinct layer located just beneath the outer membrane can be seen by freeze-fracture electron microscopy, suggesting a structure analogous to peptidoglycan. Chlamydiae also contain a plasmid, which confers the virulence properties of enhanced attachment/uptake and activation of innate immune receptors. Bacteriophages have been identified in *C. pneumoniae* and *C. psittaci*, but the roles and consequences of the viral agents are unknown at this time.

These **obligate intracellular bacteria** parasitize their host epithelial cell for nutrients and are **auxotrophic** for several amino acids and three of the four nucleoside triphosphates; the demand for host cell adenosine triphosphate (ATP) has led to their designation as an "energy parasite." Although whole genome sequencing revealed that chlamydiae can produce limited ATP by glycolysis, their genomes contain two separate loci for the production of ATP/ADP (adenosine diphosphate) translocases that would function in taking ATP from the host to ensure sufficient quantities to drive their synthetic and metabolic needs.

ENCOUNTER

C. trachomatis and *C. pneumoniae* are among the most common bacterial disease agents observed in the human population in both developed and developing countries. The estimated annual incidence for genital infections by *C. trachomatis* serovars D through K is 4 million in the United States and 90 million worldwide. *C. trachomatis* is the leading bacterial agent of **sexually transmitted disease (STD)**, and overall infections are perhaps second only to human papillomavirus as the most common STDs overall. In 2007, 1,108,374 chlamydial infections were reported to the U.S. Centers for Disease Control and Prevention (CDC) from 50 states and the District of Columbia, the highest rate ever reported. The reported number of cases of chlamydial infection was over three times greater than the reported cases of gonorrhea (355,991 gonorrhea cases were reported in 2007). From 1988 through 2007, the reported rate of chlamydial infection in women increased approximately fivefold. Possible reasons for the increase are increased screening, increased use of nucleic acid amplification tests (NAATS), and improved reporting, as well as continuing high burden of disease. Chlamydia case rates continue to remain high in all races and ethnicities. However, the rate of chlamydia among blacks was over eight times higher than that of whites in 2007 (1,398.7 and 162.3 cases per 100,000 population,

TABLE 27-1 Chlamydial Agents and Diseases

Agent	Disease Manifestation
Agents of Human Chlamydial Infections	
Chlamydia trachomatis biovar trachoma serovars A–C	Trachoma
C. trachomatis biovar trachoma serovars D–K	Sexually transmitted infections (urethritis, cervicitis, endometritis, salpingitis, pelvic inflammatory disease, epididymitis, prostatitis, proctitis, reactive arthritis, conjunctivitis, pneumonitis)
C. trachomatis biovar lymphogranuloma venereum (LGV) serovars L1–L3	Invasive sexually transmitted infections (proctitis, lymphadenopathy, buboes)
C. pneumonia	Pneumonia, bronchitis, pharyngitis, association with asthma and atherosclerosis
Agents of Animal Chlamydial Infections	
C. muridarum	Pneumonitis in mice
C. suis	Sexually transmitted infections in pigs
C. pneumoniae biovar Koala	Pneumonitis in koala bears
C. pneumoniae biovar equine	Pneumonitis in horses
C. psittaci serovars A–F[a]	Respiratory and gastrointestinal illnesses in wild and domesticated birds
	Acute respiratory disease (psittacosis) in humans
C. abortus[a]	Abortion in sheep, lambs
	Abortion in humans
C. felis[a]	Conjunctivitis in cats
	Conjunctivitis in humans
C. caviae	Guinea pig inclusion conjunctivitis
C. pecorum	Polyarthritis, encephalomyelitis, and pneumonia in sheep and cattle

[a]Agents for which zoonotic transmission to humans has been confirmed.

respectively). The highest age-specific rates are among 15- to 19-year-old women (2007: 3,004.7 cases per 100,000 females) and 20- to 24-year-old men (2007: 932.9 cases per 100,000 males). It is estimated that *C. trachomatis* is responsible for approximately one-half of all cases of **pelvic inflammatory disease (PID)**.

Lymphogranuloma venereum (LGV, serovars L1 through L3), a genetically related biovariant of *C. trachomatis* serovars D through K, also causes STDs but with different clinical manifestations. LGV causes an invasive disease primarily of the lymph nodes and is more common in Africa, Asia, India, and South America. The disease was reported only sporadically in North America and Europe until 2004 when an outbreak of LGV was reported among men who have sex with men (MSM) in the Netherlands. Soon after, cases were identified in MSM in several US border cities. Diagnosis was hindered

by the fact that symptoms usually associated with LGV (i.e., inguinal adenopathy) were rare. The majority of patients presented with anorectal symptoms (e.g., bloody proctitis with a purulent or mucous anal discharge and constipation). Almost all LGV cases reported in the United States have occurred among MSM and most reported unprotected receptive anal intercourse within 6 months. Additionally, the majority were coinfected with HIV, and nearly half had a prior syphilis diagnosis.

Trachoma, caused by *C. trachomatis* serovars A through C, is an ocular disease that is the leading cause of preventable visual impairment globally. Distribution is worldwide, and the disease occurs chiefly in poor communities in the tropics. Sub-Saharan Africa and Asia, parts of the Middle East, the Americas, and the Pacific Islands are most affected. Areas without clean water sources, with poor hygiene, and with crowded living conditions are at highest risk. More than 50 million people are infected, and between 3 and 10 million are blind as a result of the infection.

Chlamydophila pneumoniae was identified in 1989 as an agent of "walking pneumonia" of endemic proportions. Numerous serological studies indicate that 70 to 90% of all adults either have been or are infected with *C. pneumoniae*. The proportion of community-acquired pneumonia in children and adults associated with *C. pneumoniae* infection has ranged from 0 to over 44%, varying with geographic location, the age group examined, and the diagnostic methods used. Early studies that relied on serology suggested that infection in children younger than 5 years old was rare; however, subsequent studies using culture and/or polymerase chain reaction (PCR) have found the prevalence of infection in children beyond early infancy to be similar to that found in adults. In addition to **respiratory illness** and contributory roles in **asthma**, viable *C. pneumoniae* have also been directly isolated from human monocytes, foam cells, and smooth muscle cells in atherosclerotic lesions and likely participate in exacerbating the chronic inflammatory process of **atherogenesis** and **coronary artery disease**.

The most common **chlamydial zoonoses** involve accidental transmission of **Chlamydophila psittaci** to humans. **Psittacosis** was recognized as early as 1879 and is primarily associated with ownership or care of exotic psittacine birds such as parrots, parakeets, cockatoos, cockatiels, and macaws. The term *ornithosis* is interchangeable with *psittacosis* in reference to the illness observed in humans but is indicative of infections originating from nonpsittacine birds such as turkeys and pigeons. Psittacosis is an occupational disease of zoo and pet shop employees, poultry farmers, and ranchers. Human-to-human transmission is rare but possible. These cases may cause more severe disease than avian-acquired psittacosis. Reports show up to 200 cases of psittacosis annually in the United States, which is probably an underestimate of the actual number of cases because psittacosis is difficult to diagnose, is covered by macrolide antimicrobials (which may be used empirically for therapy of community-acquired pneumonia), and often goes unreported.

C. abortus infections represent a major economic burden for farmers of domestic sheep and lambs; although human infections are extremely rare, there are reports of human abortion among pregnant female farmers assisting with lambing. In recent years, *C. felis*, which is a common cause of conjunctivitis in cats, particularly kittens, has been recognized as a cause of conjunctivitis and atypical pneumonia in humans who have frequent and close contact with cats.

ENTRY

The two proposed genera of Chlamydiaceae are acquired by different routes. *Chlamydia* spp. are acquired by direct contact with mucous membranes or abraded skin, that is, by sexual contact or by direct inoculation into the eye in the case of trachoma or neonatal conjunctivitis. The major species that have been reclassified as *Chlamydophila* spp. (*C. pneumoniae* and *C. psittaci*) are typically acquired via the respiratory route (e.g., by respiratory droplets or aerosols).

SPREAD AND MULTIPLICATION

Growth of chlamydiae in their target columnar epithelial cells is characterized by a unique developmental cycle (Fig. 27-1). Two forms of the organism are needed (or required) for infection and disease to occur: the infectious, extracellular form called an **elementary body** (**EB**) and the noninfectious but metabolically active intracellular form called a **reticulate body** (**RB**). Infection is initiated by attachment of EBs to the apical surfaces of epithelial cells of the conjunctiva, respiratory, gastrointestinal, or urogenital tracts, followed by entry by **receptor-mediated endocytosis** (Fig. 27-2A). The EBs quickly modify their early endosomal membrane to exit the endosomal pathway, thereby avoiding fusion with lysosomes and traffic on microtubules to the peri-Golgi/nuclear hof region. The EB-containing endosomes of *C. trachomatis* then fuse homotypically with one another to form their one nascent microcolony called an **inclusion** (Fig. 27-3A); the EB-containing endosomes of *C. pneumoniae* and *C. psittaci* (Fig. 27-3B) develop independently and form multiple inclusions in each infected cell.

The EBs then transform into RBs, the chromosome becomes relaxed and transcriptionally active, and metabolic growth and binary fission ensue to generate progeny (Fig. 27-2B). Chlamydiae-directed modification of their inclusion membrane permits interception of trans-Golgi vesicles for transfer of sphingomyelin and glycerolphospholipids to the inclusion membrane, which can expand to accommodate some 200 to 1,000 progeny; this strategy of acquiring host cell markers for the inclusion also provides some degree of camouflage for the chlamydiae within.

It is speculated that RBs obtain their nutrients from the epithelial cytoplasm using at least two strategies: (1) insertion of chlamydial proteins (Incs) into the inclusion membrane, some of which likely have autotransporter functions and (2) insertion of a unique appendage through the inclusion membrane. On the surface of chlamydiae are 18 to 23 projections arranged in a hexagonal array (Fig. 27-2C); they span the envelope and can be seen passing through the inclusion membrane into the host cytoplasm (Fig. 27-2D). As the projections are hollow, they are thought to act as "drinking straws," allowing the prokaryotic chlamydiae to feed from their eukaryotic host without having to leave the confines of their protective inclusion vacuole. Isolated projections have a nail-like morphology remarkably similar to that of flagella. Even though the chlamydiae are not motile, the *C. trachomatis* D genome sequence revealed the existence of some flagella gene

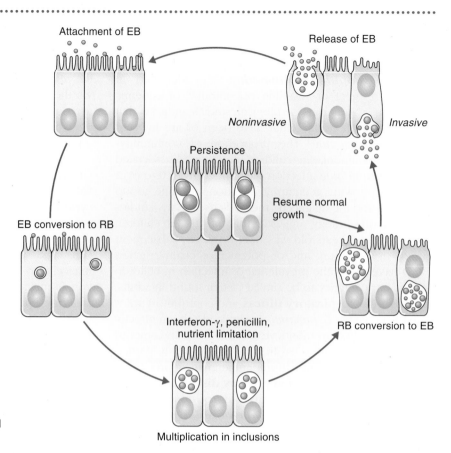

FIGURE 27-1. The *Chlamydia* developmental cycle.

orthologues, including some basal body structural and flagella-associated transport functional equivalents, suggesting a possible common evolutionary origin of flagella and the hollow "drinking straws" we see in chlamydiae.

More recently, some type III secretion homologues have been identified in chlamydiae, causing speculation that the chlamydial projections might serve an alternative function as a type III secretion system. As with other Gram-negative bacteria, the projections might function during contact-dependent attachment to prime the epithelial cell signal transduction and trafficking pathways for EB entry (from outside to inside; see Fig. 27-2A). A new, alternative concept is that they might function later in chlamydial development to deliver RB-secreted

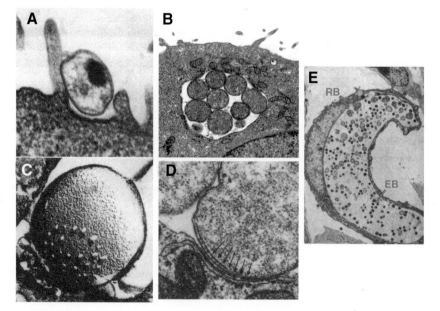

FIGURE 27-2. The *C. trachomatis* infectious process. A. Infection is initiated by attachment of elementary bodies (EBs) to epithelial cells; notice projections facing down into the coated pit. **B.** Metabolically active reticulate bodies (RBs) in an early inclusion. **C,D.** Projections on an EB and RB penetrating through the inclusion membrane into epithelial cytoplasm. **E.** A single mature inclusion containing RBs and EBs.

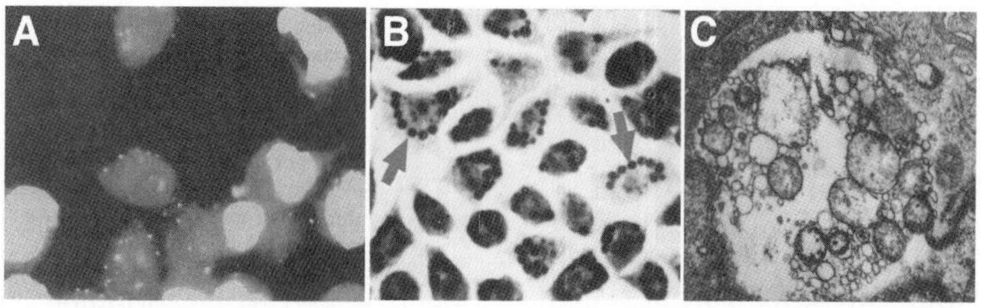

FIGURE 27-3. Chlamydial inclusions and effect of antibiotic exposure. A. Fluorescence photograph of *Chlamydia trachomatis* inclusions (*white patches*), one per infected epithelial cell (*light gray*); note few residual EBs (*tiny white dots*) attached to the host cells. **B.** Giemsa stain of multiple *Chlamydia psittaci* inclusions (*arrows*) per infected host cell. **C.** Disruption of chlamydial protein synthesis by azithromycin on growing RBs damages RBs.

effector molecules into the host cytoplasm to further modulate host–pathogen interactions (from inside to outside). Potential type III secretion functions include blocking acidification of the nascent chlamydial endosome and its fusion with lysosomes, perturbation of host cell signaling events and membrane recycling, and the modulation of apoptosis.

RBs are osmotically fragile and do not survive outside their inclusion nor can they bind to epithelial cells. Thus, to perpetuate the infectious process, RBs must mature back into infectious EBs before escaping from infected cells (Fig. 27-2E). The signal for this conversion may be detachment from the inclusion membrane of the now replete RB. Numerous disulfide bonds are formed, cross-linking three major outer membrane proteins and helping to provide the rigidity and stability EBs need for their sojourn into the extracellular environment to find a fresh susceptible epithelial cell to infect. The inclusion membrane may then fuse with the host plasma membrane to release chlamydiae, or the host cell, depleted of nutrients and energy, may lyse. Luminal *C. trachomatis* progeny are released at the apical surfaces of polarized columnar epithelial cells to spread canalicularly to the upper genital tract, whereas the invasive LGV serovars are released at the basal domain into the submucosa en route to the regional lymph nodes. This developmental cycle takes 2 to 3 days to complete, depending on the species.

Exposure of chlamydiae-infected cells in vitro to **interferon**-γ induces an altered state in RB known as **persistence** (see Fig. 27-1). Chlamydiae are auxotrophic for tryptophan, and interferon-γ activates a mammalian enzyme that catabolizes L-tryptophan. The persistent state is characterized by morphologically enlarged, aberrant RBs that are transcriptionally active but have lowered metabolic rates. The chromosome can be replicated and segregated, but some cell division gene transcription is halted, resulting in the lack of production of infectious EBs and a culture-negative scenario. Activated CD4+ and CD8+ T cells may secrete interferon-γ in response to chlamydial antigen-activated macrophages that may inhibit chlamydial replication and drive the bacteria into a persistent state. Such "persistent" forms have not been visualized in infected tissues from animals or

humans, and it is possible that the culture-negative scenario simply represents a low level of replicating organisms that may be difficult to detect by relatively insensitive culture methods. Whether present in a "persistent" nonreplicating state that intermittently reactivates or at constant low level of replication, either of these states would promote low-grade chronic inflammation that may cause long-term sequelae.

DAMAGE

C. trachomatis serovars A through K initially infect and grow within epithelial cells of the ocular and genital mucosae; resident macrophages and dendritic cells are also exposed to released EBs but do not sufficiently support bacterial development. Inflammatory mediators and chemokines produced in infected epithelial cells serve as initial triggers for an influx of leukocytes including neutrophils, natural killer cells, dendritic cells, monocytes, and lymphocytes. Infected epithelial cells and early infiltrating natural killer cells activate antigen-presenting cells into programming the cell-mediated immune response. As the host immune response develops, active sites of infection show an infiltration of lymphocytes, plasma cells, and macrophages. Lymphoid follicles containing macrophages, T cells, and B cells subsequently develop. The chronic inflammatory process leads to epithelial cell necrosis, fibroblast proliferation, and eventual scar tissue formation. Thus, the serious sequelae of *C. trachomatis* infections are mediated by the **host immune response**.

Clinically, the early stages of *C. trachomatis* serovars D through K genital infections are either extremely subtle or completely asymptomatic. Thus, most patients do not seek treatment, leading to the high prevalence of infection. In women, the endocervix is sometimes reddened and friable with a mucoid exudate that is less purulent than that observed for *N. gonorrhoeae*. In men, there may be a scant amount of a mucoid urethral exudate. Depending on sexual practices and hygiene, the rectal and ocular mucosae of both men and women can become infected. Importantly, isolates of *C. trachomatis* serovars D through K are not invasive and do not penetrate or invade the submucosa but remain at the luminal surface of the epithelium and spread in an ascending manner in the genitourinary tract. Infections in women progress from the cervix (**cervicitis**) to the endometrium (**endometritis**), then to the fallopian tubes (**salpingitis**), and eventually into the peritoneum. In men with **urethritis**, the organisms can eventually colonize the epididymis (**epididymitis**) and the prostate (**prostatitis**) but rarely the testicles. Approximately 1% of men with chlamydial urethritis develop acute aseptic arthritis of presumed immune-mediated etiology. One-third of patients have the full complex of Reiter syndrome (arthritis, urethritis, and conjunctivitis); most such patients carry the histocompatibility antigen HLA-B27.

Chronic infections, as well as repeated reinfections, lead to more serious disease sequelae, such as **tubal factor infertility** and PID. When these later complications occur, patients can be treated for eradication of the organisms, but the tissue damage is generally irreversible, and women are at risk for life-threatening **ectopic pregnancy**.

Infants born vaginally to infected mothers acquire EBs in their eyes, ears, nose, and mouth and may develop **conjunctivitis** and **pneumonia** that is characterized by a chronic, repetitive cough without wheezing. Symptoms of pneumonia characteristically develop between 4 and 11 weeks of age. Most infants are only moderately ill and are afebrile. Physical findings include tachypnea and rales but not wheezing. About 50% of the affected infants have a history or evidence of conjunctivitis. Follow-up evaluation of a small cohort of children who had *C. trachomatis* pneumonia in infancy has shown an increased prevalence of chronic cough and abnormal lung function compared with age-matched controls.

The invasive LGV serovars of *C. trachomatis* can enter small breaks in the skin and initiate an inconspicuous genital papule or herpetic-like ulcer. Patients with these infrequent primary lesions are usually asymptomatic. LGV may also produce rectal ulcers, bleeding, pain, and discharge, especially among those who practice receptive anal intercourse. Genital lesions caused by LGV can be mistaken for other ulcerative STDs such as syphilis, genital herpes, and chancroid. Complications of untreated LGV may include enlargement and ulcerations of the external genitalia and **lymphatic obstruction**, which may lead to elephantiasis of the genitalia.

Similar to *C. trachomatis* infections, those with *C. pneumoniae*, a common agent of **atypical pneumonia**, can evolve into chronic inflammatory events mediated by the host immune response. *C. pneumoniae* EBs are spread by respiratory secretions. Respiratory infections are generally mild or asymptomatic in healthy individuals, and in adults, symptoms are often clinically indistinguishable from those caused by *Mycoplasma pneumoniae*. Patients may present with pharyngitis, laryngitis, bronchitis, sinusitis, otitis media, or

pneumonia that evolves over an extended number of weeks. Prolonged respiratory infection, documented by culture, lasting from several weeks to several years has been reported. Reliable diagnosis of respiratory infection due to *C. pneumoniae* remains difficult due to the absence of well-standardized and commercially available diagnostic tests. Infection with *C. pneumoniae* has been linked to development of asthma and to asthma exacerbations by a large number of epidemiologic and clinical studies. It has been hypothesized that an inadequate or delayed clearance of the pathogen may fuel a low-grade chronic immune response that increases asthmatic disease.

C. pneumoniae infects and multiplies within a wide range of host cells, including epithelial cells, endothelial cells, monocytes, macrophages, lymphocytes, and cells that participate in atherogenesis. Indeed, the ability to grow in various cells represents the likely vehicle in which *C. pneumoniae* is distributed from the lungs into the circulation. The hypothesis that *C. pneumoniae* contributes to **coronary artery disease** is supported by several lines of evidence: adults with coronary artery disease have high titers of *C. pneumoniae*–specific antibodies, the organisms have been directly cultured from **atherosclerotic lesions**, and the organisms stimulate inflammatory events consistent with atherosclerosis and can promote the development of coronary lesions in animal model studies.

C. trachomatis serovars A through K and *C. pneumoniae* are similar in that initial infections are often mild or asymptomatic, and the organisms can produce long-term chronic infections within host tissues culminating in chronic inflammatory pathology. Conversely, the **invasive and lymphotropic** sexually transmitted LGV biovariant of *C. trachomatis* and the zoonotic chlamydial animal pathogens generally cause acute, sometimes life-threatening, illnesses.

Inhalation of *C. psittaci*, present in fecal aerosols excreted by stressed or sick birds, initially causes an abrupt flulike illness in humans but can rapidly progress to severe pneumonia. Rarely, it may lead to hepatitis, endocarditis, and/or encephalitis. Pregnant female farmers that assist in the birthing of lambs are at risk of infection with *C. abortus*, which can cause abortion, renal failure, disseminated intravascular coagulation, or death. Because these illnesses are not common, a detailed patient history, including travel, pet ownership, and profession, is essential to prompt diagnostic consideration and testing.

DIAGNOSIS

Until recently, diagnosis of chlamydial infections was made following growth and culture of the organisms from patient specimens. This task was performed only by a limited number of experienced laboratories. Subsequently, antigen detection methods, either **direct fluorescence assay** or **enzyme immunoassay**, became popular and are still used in certain clinical studies. Currently, **nucleic acid amplification tests** (**NAATs**), such as PCR, ligase chain reaction, or transcription-mediated amplification, represent the most common and sensitive methods used for *C. trachomatis* detection and screening. One prominent advantage of NAAT is that specimens may be obtained by noninvasive procedures such as first-void urine.

Because these organisms reside within epithelial cells, obtaining an appropriate specimen requires rotating a fibrous swab on affected mucosal epithelium. For suspected cases of genital *C. trachomatis* infection in women, any cervical exudate should be collected on a swab of the endocervix at the squamocolumnar junction and assayed for both chlamydiae and *N. gonorrhoeae*. Likewise, in men, excess discharge can be collected on a swab or samples can be obtained by inserting a swab 3 to 4 cm into the urethra with rotation. Because the latter procedure is uncomfortable, this invasive procedure is rarely performed and is one reason why our knowledge of chlamydial genital infections in men is incomplete. The adaptation of NAAT for first void urine samples, which contain infected epithelial cells, and self-collected vaginal swab material has been a major advance in diagnosing chlamydial genital infections.

DNA amplification methods will hopefully be available in the near future for diagnosis of infections by *C. pneumoniae*. Culture and immunofluorescence microscopy are presently used by some laboratories, but commercially available *C. pneumoniae*–specific antibody reagents are limited. A confirmatory diagnosis requires an experienced laboratory to differentiate between *C. pneumoniae* and *C. trachomatis* or *C. psittaci*, all of which can cause respiratory illness. The optimal sample for the laboratory is obtained using a wire-shafted swab to obtain epithelial cells from the nasopharynx; throat swabs and sputum samples may not yield sufficient numbers of organisms. Because the clinical presentation of *C. pneumoniae* infections resemble those caused by *M. pneumoniae*, the cold hemagglutinin reaction may be helpful to distinguish them (see Chapter 29). *M. pneumoniae* infection may induce cold agglutinins; *C. pneumoniae* does not.

TREATMENT AND PREVENTION

Antimicrobial therapy regimens for chlamydial infections require agents that have excellent tissue penetration properties; moreover, bactericidal concentrations should be maintained for an extended period because of the slow-growing and persistent nature of chlamydiae. Patients diagnosed with infections by *C. trachomatis* serovars A through K are prescribed azithromycin (Fig. 27-3C) or multiple doses of doxycycline over 7 days; erythromycin is an alternative for pregnant women and children where doxycycline is contraindicated. Azithromycin's half-life allows a large single dose to be administered and yet maintain bacteriostatic levels in the infected tissue for several days. Currently, recommended treatment for LGV is doxycycline for 21 days or erythromycin base for 21 days. Sex

partners should be evaluated, tested, and treated if they had sexual contact with the patient during the 60 days preceding either diagnosis of *Chlamydia* or onset of symptoms in the patient. The most recent sex partner should be treated even if the time of the last sexual contact was greater than 60 days before diagnosis of the index case.

For patients with pneumonia suspected to be due to *C. pneumoniae*, doxycycline is the treatment of choice except in children younger than 9 years and in pregnant women. Treatment should be continued for at least 10 to 14 days after defervescence. If symptoms persist, a second course with a different class of antibiotics is usually effective. Alternatives include azithromycin or clarithromycin for 7 to 10 days. Studies have suggested that antibiotics with activity against *C. pneumoniae* are beneficial for asthmatics with proven or presumed *C. pneumoniae* infection. However, many of the studies were not randomized, or contained small numbers of patients with documented *C. pneumoniae* infection, and data supporting or refuting the use of macrolides in asthmatics are inconclusive.

The development of a vaccine against human chlamydial infections represents a long-term objective requiring continual investigation. Numerous studies indicate that a Th1 cell–mediated immune response favors resolution of infection and protective immunity. In female patients with genital tract infection and in patients with trachoma, a decreased Th1-related response is associated with increased risk of infection and disease, whereas an increased Th1-related response is associated with protection. Since the host immune response to infection is what causes tissue damage, prevention of tissue damage likely requires an optimal Th1 response, that is, one that is sufficient to resolve infection but that does not promote ongoing cellular influx and production of potentially tissue-damaging mediators of inflammation. Chlamydiae-infected patients also produce a wide array of specific antibodies, and certain antibodies may limit spread of infectious EB. However, limited data indicate that protective humoral immune responses are strain-specific and of short duration. High serum antibody titers reflect increased exposure and are associated with complications of chlamydial disease. The programming of T lymphocytes toward the most effective response for pathogen clearance is a central issue for vaccination, and it is crucial to delineate chlamydial antigens that can promote protective immunity.

CONCLUSION

Chlamydiae sequester themselves inside host cells in vacuoles that protect them from the array of hostile armaments the host cell reserves for invading pathogens. Infections due to *C. trachomatis* and *C. pneumoniae* are frequently asymptomatic and chronic in nature. *Chlamydia trachomatis* infects mucosal epithelial surfaces of the eye and the genital tract. The host's inflammatory response leads to epithelial cell necrosis, and as part of the healing process, scarring occurs that leads to the sequelae of blindness (trachoma) or infertility. *Chlamydophila pneumoniae* infects the respiratory epithelium where it can cause acute bronchitis and pneumonia, but chronic respiratory infection is linked to enhanced asthmatic disease. It also chronically infects endothelial cells and inflammatory cells and is linked to acceleration of atherosclerosis. Zoonotic infections due to *C. psittaci* and *C. pecorum* are more acutely inflammatory in nature, and may result in life-threatening disease. Current research is focused on how chlamydiae behave inside eukaryotic cells and what the host response strategies are: What receptors do chlamydiae activate in infected cells to induce innate responses, and how can we harness the innate responses to induce protective adaptive immunity?

ACKNOWLEDGMENT

The author thanks Priscilla B. Wyrick and Jane E. Raulston for their valuable contributions to this chapter in previous editions of the text.

Suggested Readings

Belland RJ, Ouellette SP, Gieffers J, et al. *Chlamydia pneumoniae* and atherosclerosis. *Cell Microbiol.* 2004;6:117–127.

Grayston JT. Background and current knowledge of *Chlamydia pneumoniae* and atherosclerosis. *J Infect Dis.* 2000;181(suppl 3):S402–S410.

Hammerschlag MR. Pneumonia due to *Chlamydia pneumoniae* in children: epidemiology, diagnosis and treatment. *Ped Pulmonol.* 2003;36:384–390.

Hogan RJ, Mathews SA, Mukhopadhyay S, et al. Chlamydial persistence: beyond the biphasic paradigm. *Infect Immun.* 2004;72:1843–1855.

Johnson S, Johnson FN. *Chlamydia trachomatis* and azithromycin. *Rev Contem Pharmacother.* 2000;11:139–256.

Longbottom D, Coulter LJ. Animal chlamydioses and zoonotic implications. *J Compar Pathol.* 2003;128:217–244.

Maybey DC, Solomon AW, Foster A. Trachoma. *Lancet.* 2003;362:223–229.

Stephens RS, ed. *Chlamydia: Intracellular Biology, Pathogenesis, and Immunity.* Washington, DC: ASM Press; 1999.

Wyrick PB. Intracellular survival by *Chlamydia. Cell Microbiol.* 2000;2:275–282.

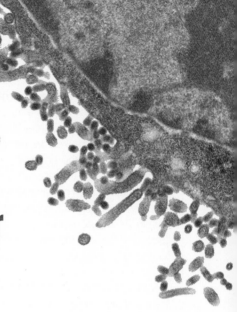

Chapter 28

Rocky Mountain Spotted Fever and Other Rickettsioses

David H. Walker

KEY CONCEPTS

Pathogens: Rickettsiae are obligate intracellular bacteria (i.e., cannot be grown on artificial media) and are not resolved by light microscopy.

Encounter: The distribution of various rickettsiae tends to be geographically limited and dependent on the distribution of suitable arthropod vectors or animal reservoirs.

Entry: Humans usually acquire infection by arthropod bites (exception: *Coxiella burnetii* may be acquired by inhalation and other routes).

Spread and Multiplication: The organisms have a predilection for vascular endothelial cells, causing blood vessel damage and bleeding in various organs. In the skin, vascular damage results in rashes.

Damage: Rickettsiae can cause several severe diseases: Rocky Mountain spotted fever (*Rickettsia rickettsii*), typhus (*R. prowazekii*), murine typhus (*R. typhi*), scrub typhus (*Orientia tsutsugamushi*), and others.

Diagnosis: Depends on clinical suspicion and acumen, since laboratory studies are seldom helpful in establishing a diagnosis during the acute stage

Treatment and Prevention: Rickettsial infections can be treated with antibiotics that penetrate into host cells.

THE RICKETTSIA genus comprises a large number of bacteria that can only grow inside eukaryotic cells. With the chlamydiae, the rickettsiae are the principal medically important **obligate intracellular bacteria**. The other defining characteristic of these organisms is their epidemiology. Most rickettsioses are **zoonoses**, infections that are transmitted from animals to humans and are spread mainly through arthropod vectors (ticks, mites, fleas, lice, and chiggers). Table 28-1 outlines the etiology and epidemiology of the most common diseases caused by the *Rickettsia* bacteria.

The most important rickettsiosis in the United States, **Rocky Mountain spotted fever**, is a serious, life-threatening disease. Like many other species of rickettsiae, the causative agent invades vascular endothelial cells, resulting in generalized vascular damage. Other important rickettsioses are **Q fever** (which often manifests as pneumonia), **human monocytotropic ehrlichiosis**, and **human granulocytotropic anaplasmosis** (both of which infect leukocytes and cause thrombocytopenia). Some rickettsioses have played important roles in history, and some have appeared to emerge as previously unknown infectious diseases.

The classic rickettsiosis, epidemic **typhus**, has been one of the most significant infectious diseases in history because of its devastating effects on humanity, particularly in its influence on the outcome of most European wars between 1500 and 1900. During and immediately after World War I and the Russian Revolution, 30 million people suffered from epidemic typhus, and 3 million of them died. The human body louse transmits *Rickettsia prowazekii* by depositing its feces on the skin. With the discovery of effective insecticides, delousing interrupted the transmission of epidemic typhus in World War II and greatly reduced its incidence.

CASE • S., a 9-year-old girl, was taken to her pediatrician on May 31, 2 days after the onset of fever reaching 40.5°C, severe headache, and muscle pains. The next day, she developed nausea, vomiting, and abdominal pain and was admitted to the hospital for observation for possible appendicitis. On the second day following admission, an erythematous rash consisting of 2- to 4-mm macules (areas of pink discoloration) appeared on her wrists and ankles. Within 24 hours of its onset, the rash involved the arms, legs, and trunk, and many of the lesions had become maculopapular (discolored and raised) with petechiae (dark red spots caused by bleeding in the skin). A serological test for Rocky Mountain spotted fever and cultures of the blood, cerebrospinal fluid, and urine were negative. S. became stuporous and had edema in her face and extremities.

Treatment with intravenous doxycycline was begun for the suspected diagnosis of Rocky Mountain spotted fever. Within 72 hours, S. was alert and afebrile. She was sent home after 4 days in the hospital with instructions to take oral doxycycline for three more days. By the time of her discharge from the hospital, the rash had faded remarkably.

S. lived in a mobile home on the outskirts of Burlington, North Carolina, and played after school in the nearby high grass and weeds. Her mother had removed several ticks from her body nearly every day during the month of May before she became sick. When S. returned to her pediatrician at the end of June, she was completely recovered. A serum sample was collected and sent, along with one collected during the acute phase of her hospitalization, to the state public health laboratory. A dramatic rise in titer of antibody to *Rickettsia rickettsii* was detected in the convalescent sample.

This case raises several questions:

1. What caused the rash, stupor, and gastrointestinal symptoms?

2. Why was the serological test for Rocky Mountain spotted fever negative in the hospital?

3. Assuming that rickettsiae were circulating in the blood, why were the blood cultures negative?

4. How did a girl from an eastern state get "Rocky Mountain" spotted fever?

See Appendix for answers.

The most common rickettsiosis in the United States is Rocky Mountain spotted fever. It affects approximately 2,000 people annually, mostly in the eastern and southern states rather than in the Rocky Mountains where it was first described. This disease can be extremely serious and, if untreated, has a mortality rate of about 20%. Because the disease responds well to certain antibiotics, especially in the early stages, a speedy diagnosis is essential. The

TABLE 28-1 Etiology and Epidemiology of Principal Rickettsioses

Rickettsial Agent	Diseases	Reservoir in Nature	Transmission	Geographic Distribution
Rickettsia rickettsii	Rocky Mountain spotted fever	Ticks (transovarian transmission)	Tick bite	North and South America
Rickettsia conorii	Boutonneuse fever	Tick (transovarian transmission)	Tick bite	Southern Europe, Africa, and Asia
Rickettsia prowazekii	Epidemic typhus	Humans, flying squirrels	Louse feces	Potentially worldwide
	Recrudescent typhus	Humans	None	Potentially worldwide
Rickettsia typhi	Murine typhus	Fleas and rats	Flea feces	Worldwide, especially tropics and subtropics
Orientia tsutsugamushi	Scrub typhus	Chiggers (transovarian transmission)	Chigger bite	Asia, Oceania, and northern Australia
Ehrlichia chaffeensis	Human monocytotropic ehrlichiosis	Deer, goats, dogs	Tick bite	North America, Africa, Asia
Anaplasma phagocytophilum	Human granulocytotropic anaplasmosis	Deer, elk, wild rodents	Tick bite	North America and Eurasia
Coxiella burnetii	Q fever	Cattle, sheep, goats, other livestock; cats	Aerosol from infected birth products; ticks	Worldwide

spotted fever group of rickettsioses and the typhus group are characterized by disseminated vascular infection. Injury in the lungs, central nervous system, and other systemic microcirculation may cause neurological signs, seizures, coma, acute respiratory failure, shock, and acute renal failure. Other spotted fever group rickettsiae which are less pathogenic (e.g., *R. parkeri*) and of undetermined pathogenicity (e.g., *R. amblyommii*) are also prevalent in the United States.

Q fever differs significantly from the typhus and spotted fever infections in that it has an acute form, manifested mainly as pneumonia, and a chronic form, in which the heart valves are usually affected. The causative agent, *Coxiella burnetii*, grows in the macrophages in the lung, liver, bone marrow, and spleen, where it stimulates granuloma formation. A method to cultivate *Coxiella* in cell-free medium has been devised, removing its obligate intracellular status. In another kind of rickettsiosis, called ehrlichiosis, the organisms grow in white blood cells. Ehrlichioses are tick-transmitted infections of monocytes and macrophages or neutrophils with systemic manifestations caused by the host response.

THE PATHOGENS: RICKETTSIAE

Rickettsiae are small Gram-negative rods that have an outer membrane and a thin murein layer (Fig. 28-1). However, they are not readily stainable by the Gram method. DNA homology studies reveal that spotted fever and typhus rickettsiae are relatively closely related to other strict intracellular parasites, the *Ehrlichia* and *Ana-*

plasma, as well as facultatively intracellular *Bartonella*. In contrast, *C. burnetii* is more closely related to *Legionella* and only distantly related to the other rickettsiae. Spotted fever and typhus rickettsiae have lipopolysaccharides that are antigenically distinct for each group. *Ehrlichia* and *Orientia* lack both lipopolysaccharides and peptidoglycan.

Rickettsiae are highly adapted to the intracellular niche, where they propagate by binary fission with a generation time of 8 to 10 hours. They have reduced their genome size by elimination of genes which served functions that the host cell provides. Rickettsiae thrive in the eukaryotic cytosol and have specific membrane transport systems for acquiring adenosine triphosphate (ATP), amino acids, and other metabolites from the host cell. These small bacteria can grow more efficiently because their genomes are smaller and they require fewer building blocks and less energy. Unlike chlamydiae, rickettsiae are not strict energy parasites; they are also able to synthesize at least some of their required ATP. In addition, rickettsiae are capable of **independent metabolism** (e.g., tricarboxylic acid cycle and electron transport system) and use their own biosynthetic machinery to make proteins and other complex components. However, they cannot be cultivated on artificial medium, and in the laboratory, they must be grown in animals, embryonated eggs, or cell cultures.

RICKETTSIA RICKETTSII: ROCKY MOUNTAIN SPOTTED FEVER

ENCOUNTER

The geographic distribution of cases of the disease occurring in the United States from 1994 to 1998 is shown in Figure 28-2. *R. rickettsii* organisms are transmitted from tick to tick by the transovarian route and usually cause little harm to that host. The ticks involved in Rocky Mountain spotted fever (*Dermacentor* species) are different from the *Ixodes* involved in Lyme disease (see Chapter 25). When some wild animals are bitten by *Dermacentor* ticks, they become transiently infected and a transient reservoir of the rickettsiae. Thus, the disease cannot be eradicated by public health measures.

ENTRY

Signs and symptoms of Rocky Mountain spotted fever begin an average of 1 week after an infected adult tick inoculates *R. rickettsii* into the skin while taking a blood meal. The risk of transmission can be reduced by the use of tick repellents and protective clothing. Individuals can prevent this illness by removing ticks from the skin before the bacteria are inoculated, usually between 6 and 24 hours after attachment (for a discussion of insectborne diseases, see Chapter 33 paradigm).

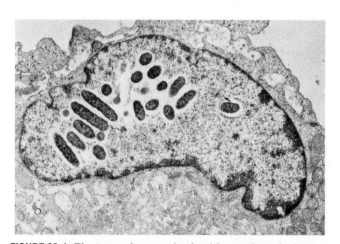

FIGURE 28-1. Electron micrograph of a thin section of a human endothelial cell infected with *Rickettsia rickettsii,* the etiological agent of Rocky Mountain spotted fever. The rickettsiae are the dark, rod-shaped bacteria in the nucleus, about the same size as the mitochondria and smaller than most other bacteria. These rickettsiae have invaded the nucleus. Although *R. rickettsii* organisms usually occupy the cytoplasm and few enter the nucleus, their presence in this location is characteristic of spotted fever rickettsiae and would be most unusual for other rickettsiae as well as *Mycobacteria, Salmonella,* and *Legionella* organisms.

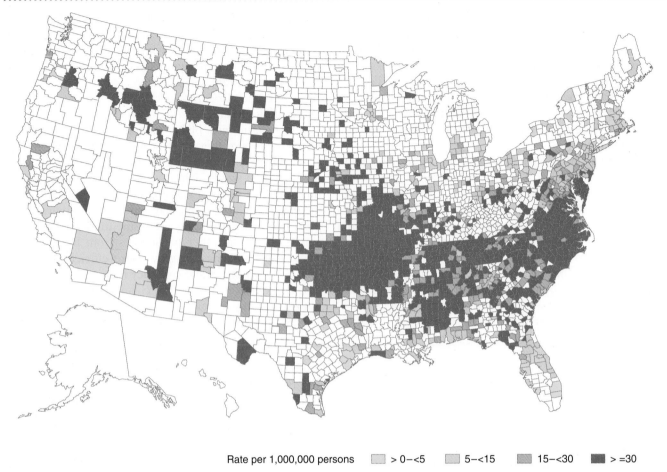

Rate per 1,000,000 persons ☐ > 0–<5 ☐ 5–<15 ☒ 15–<30 ■ > =30

FIGURE 28-2. National Rocky Mountain spotted fever incidence by county, 2000 to 2007.

SPREAD AND MULTIPLICATION

After inoculation, rickettsiae spread throughout the body via the bloodstream. On encountering vascular endothelial cells, rickettsiae attach to the cell membrane and induce the cells to engulf them (Fig. 28-3 and Table 28-2). Once inside the cells, rickettsiae rapidly escape from the phagosome into the cytosol, apparently by lysis of the phagosomal membrane by a phospholipase.

Ensconced in the cytosol, *R. rickettsii* multiply and are propelled through the cytoplasm by polymerization of the host cell actin at one pole. The organisms then spread to other endothelial cells through long cellular projections of the cell membrane (see Chapter 17).

DAMAGE

Injury to the host cell correlates with the quantity of bacteria accumulated intracellularly. The subcellular target of injury appears to be the cell membrane, and the mechanism of damage to that structure appears to be the result of the action of free radical–induced membrane lipid peroxidation.

The effects of damage to foci of contiguous endothelial cells are visible in the skin, where dilation of the blood vessels first produces a pink rash. Later, leakage of red blood cells results in hemorrhagic spots (or **petechiae**), from which the name of the disease is derived (Fig. 28-4). Within the blood vessels of the brain, lung, heart, liver, and other visceral organs, these pinpoint hemorrhages lead to encephalitis, pneumonitis, cardiac arrhythmia, nausea, vomiting, and abdominal pain.

Even before the introduction of the effective antimicrobial treatment, 75% of patients with Rocky Mountain spotted fever survived. Clearance of intracellular rickettsiae from the endothelium is achieved through the strong effects of the immune system with important contributions by cell-mediated immunity, particularly T lymphocytes and their cytokines, such as interferon-γ and tumor necrosis factor. Older individuals are more likely to die from the disease.

Similar diseases are caused by antigenically related organisms. The geographic distribution of these diseases coincides with a population of infected ticks (e.g., in Southern Europe, Asia, and Africa, boutonneuse fever and **African tick bite fever**; in Australia, **Queensland tick typhus** and Flinders Island spotted fever; in northern Asia, Siberian tick typhus) or mites (in North America, Europe, and Asia, **rickettsialpox**). A substantial number of people become infected while traveling in Africa, where their activities expose them to ticks. On returning to North America or Europe, they seek medical attention

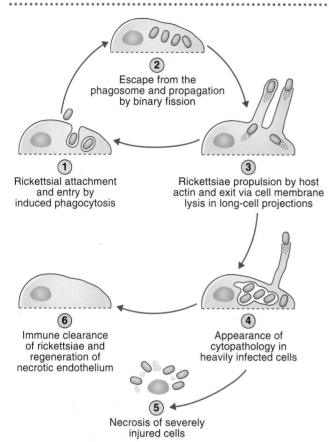

FIGURE 28-3. Sequence of rickettsia–host cell interactions in Rocky Mountain spotted fever.

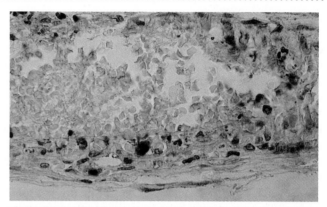

FIGURE 28-4. Cross section of a blood vessel from the dermis of a patient with Rocky Mountain spotted fever. The rickettsiae are visualized within endothelial cells and vascular smooth muscle cells as tiny *purple-red dots* in clusters. Notice the infiltration of the vessel with lymphocytes and histiocytes.

for what is recognized by astute physicians as African tick bite fever. The prevalence of antibodies to spotted fever group rickettsiae among healthy subjects in the affected countries suggests that many infections are not diagnosed.

OTHER RICKETTSIAE AND RICKETTSIA-LIKE INFECTIONS
Rickettsia prowazekii and *R. typhi*: Typhus Group Fevers

The classic epidemic disease, **typhus fever**, is spread among humans by the body **louse** and is associated with high mortality and dramatic epidemics. Epidemics begin

with a single case of **recrudescent typhus (Brill-Zinsser disease)**, which is caused by reactivation of the agent, *R. prowazekii*. This agent can remain latent in the body for years or even decades after recovery from epidemic louseborne typhus or zoonotic typhus transmitted by fleas from flying squirrels. Recrudescent typhus was described in the late 1800s in New York City among immigrants from eastern Europe, where epidemics of typhus were notorious. It is presumed that typhus epidemics can be ignited from a patient with recrudescent typhus and body lice, which spread the infection to other persons. Absence of epidemic typhus in developed countries today is an effect of the socioeconomic conditions and low prevalence of human body lice. Where war, natural disasters, and famine occur, epidemic typhus has often followed; thus, the disease is associated with crowding, poverty, and "lousy" sanitary conditions. It is foolish to believe that epidemic typhus could never return.

The reservoir of the epidemic typhus rickettsiae is not only human beings but also flying squirrels and their fleas and lice. The infection has been transmitted from this source to humans in the eastern United States. Could an epidemic of typhus arise from one of these cases if it occurred among a louse-infested population? Possibly.

A more prevalent and widely dispersed rickettsiosis is **murine typhus**. This endemic disease is caused by *R. typhi*, which is transmitted in a natural cycle between rats and rat fleas. Humans become infected by the deposition of infected flea feces on their skin. Murine typhus occurs throughout the tropics and subtropics and was an important problem in the southern United States until the development of insecticides and intense rat control efforts.

Orientia tsutsugamushi: Scrub Typhus
Scrub typhus is a disease of major importance with one million cases annually in parts of the world distant from the everyday lives of Americans and Europeans.

TABLE 28-2 Cellular and Subcellular Locations

Rickettsial Agent	Host Target Cell	Cellular Location
Rickettsia	Endothelium	Cytosol
Coxiella	Macrophages	Phagolysosome
Ehrlichia	Leukocytes	Cytoplasmic endosomal vacuole

However, during World War II and the Vietnam War, Americans and Europeans came into contact with the ecological conditions in the South Pacific, Burma, and China. As a result, *Orientia tsutsugamushi* infected 18,000 soldiers in World War II and was one of the major causes of undiagnosed febrile illness among soldiers in Vietnam. The indigenous populations of endemic areas in many countries of Asia are continuously exposed to the agent of this infection. In a study in rural Malaysia, scrub typhus was the most frequent reason for febrile hospitalization.

Several factors exacerbate the problem of scrub typhus. The organisms exist in various antigenic types, and immunity to one strain wanes over a period of a few years and to other strains after a few months. Subsequently, the patient becomes fully susceptible to reinfection. To make matters worse, clinical diagnosis is difficult because rash and eschar (a dry scab), considered the textbook hallmarks of the disease, are absent in most cases. In many endemic areas, medical care is suboptimal and laboratory diagnosis is virtually nonexistent. Scrub typhus is a life-threatening neglected disease that, from time to time, rivets the attention of missionaries, the military, and medical examination committees.

Coxiella burnetii: Q fever

Q fever is short for "Query fever," referring to its unknown etiology when it was first described. The etiologic agent, *C. burnetii*, stands apart from other rickettsiae, and the disease differs from other rickettsioses in its clinical manifestations, pathological lesions, and epidemiology. Extracellularly, the organisms are much more resistant than the other rickettsiae to the many deleterious effects of the environment. Resistance may result from the formation of a sporelike structure that has been observed by electron microscopy. Consequently, this agent does not require the protection afforded by a living vector but may also be transmitted through aerosols. Q fever is distinctly zoonotic, and the main reservoirs are infected sheep, cattle, cats, rabbits, and other animals. The organisms are present in large amounts in the placenta and fetal membranes and are spread in copious numbers when ewes give birth. The disease is most often seen among sheep farmers, veterinarians, and workers in laboratories that use sheep for experimentation.

The kind of disease produced by *C. burnetii* varies from acute pneumonia to chronic endocarditis. Acute infection may be asymptomatic or associated with nonspecific flulike febrile illness, atypical pneumonia, or granulomatous hepatitis. Chronic infection is usually diagnosed in patients with a long course, cardiac valvular infection, and negative routine blood cultures for bacteria. The pathogenic mechanisms appear to be largely immunopathological with T lymphocyte–mediated granulomas in self-limited disease and an immune complex–mediated component in some cases of chronic illness.

Ehrlichiae: Ehrlichioses and Anaplasmosis

Previously unrecognized infectious diseases continue to be described; two human diseases caused by *Ehrlichia* species are among the newest to be discovered. *E. chaffeensis* and *E. ewingii* are transmitted by the Lone Star tick. They infect mainly monocytes and macrophages or neutrophils, respectively. Another intracellular pathogen of neutrophils, *Anaplasma phagocytophilum*, also infects rodents, ruminants, and deer and is transmitted by the same *Ixodes* ticks as Lyme disease. These obligate intracellular pathogens replicate intracellularly in membrane-bound vesicles. Occasionally, these vesicles can be seen by light microscopy of stained blood smears as round inclusions in either monocytes or neutrophils, depending on the bacterial species.

Most cases of ehrlichiosis and anaplasmosis are clinically similar to Rocky Mountain spotted fever and are characterized by fever, headache, and often severe multisystem involvement but with a lower incidence of rash. The spectrum of severity is quite broad and ranges from mild to fatal. Many patients with these infections have reduced numbers of circulating leukocytes as well as low platelet counts. Human granulocytic anaplasmosis is diagnosed much more readily than human monocytic ehrlichiosis because the organisms are visible more often in circulating leukocytes.

DIAGNOSIS

The clinical diagnosis of rickettsioses is difficult, particularly when the patient first visits a physician and treatment is most effective. At the time of presentation during the first 3 days of illness, only 3% of patients with Rocky Mountain spotted fever have the classic triad of fever, rash, and history of tick bite. In contrast to most infectious diseases, laboratory studies are seldom helpful in establishing a diagnosis of rickettsial disease in the acute stage of the illness. Very few laboratories attempt to isolate rickettsiae because of the technical requirements for inoculation of antibiotic-free cell culture. In addition, the handling of these agents is notoriously hazardous.

For these reasons, the diagnosis of most rickettsioses requires considerable diagnostic acumen by physicians. Laboratory confirmation of rickettsioses is usually achieved in the convalescent stage by demonstrating a fourfold or greater rise in the titer of antibodies to rickettsial antigens. The only rickettsial disease that can be expected to have diagnostic levels of antibodies at the time the patient seeks medical attention is chronic Q fever. The serological methods usually employed are indirect fluorescent antibody assay or enzyme immunoassay (see Chapter 58); newer methods are currently being developed. The **Weil-Felix test**, an archaic test still in use in few laboratories, relies on the agglutination of certain strains of the enteric bacterium *Proteus vulgaris*, which shares cross-reactive antigens with certain rickettsiae. The

A FRAUDULENT EPIDEMIC SAVES LIVES

Although it is now antiquated, it is worth recounting how the Weil-Felix test was put to a humanitarian use by two Polish physicians in World War II. These physicians were aware that the occupying Germans did not send people suspected of having epidemic typhus to labor camps. Ingeniously, these doctors inoculated the population of several villages with an innocuous vaccine consisting of killed P. vulgaris. The high Weil-Felix titer of these people's sera was taken by the German medical staff to indicate that these villages were hotbeds of epidemic typhus. The inhabitants were thus spared, thanks to the microbiological stratagem of the two physicians.

Serologic tests are not useful for making an early diagnosis of rickettsioses but are used to confirm the diagnosis in convalescing patients. An early diagnosis is sometimes possible, however, by taking a biopsy of a skin lesion and treating it with antirickettsial antibodies. Localization of these antibodies to endothelial cells by immunochemical staining is diagnostic of acute Rocky Mountain spotted fever (see Fig. 28-4).

---

results of the Weil-Felix test are nonspecific and insensitive, yet some hospitals persist in using it despite the availability of better methods.

TREATMENT

Rickettsial diseases generally respond well to antimicrobial agents that enter host cells and are active in the intracellular environment. Most of these diseases respond to oral or intravenous therapy with doxycycline (the drug of choice), tetracycline, or chloramphenicol, each of which has its advantages and disadvantages under particular circumstances. Ketolide and fluoroquinolone antimicrobial drugs are becoming a popular treatment for some of the milder rickettsioses. Penicillins, aminoglycosides, and other antimicrobials do not affect the course of rickettsial diseases. Sulfa drugs actually seem to exacerbate both spotted and typhus fevers.

CONCLUSION

Although rickettsial infections are not common in the United States, some can be life threatening. The diseases must be diagnosed promptly, and antibiotic therapy must be instituted quickly. The most devastating disease caused by these organisms, epidemic typhus, has receded in importance as a result of louse control but could emerge among the homeless in the United States; an epidemic occurred in Burundi during its civil war, and outbreaks have been identified in Russia and the Andes.

Rickettsiae are delicate organisms (except that which causes Q fever) but are well adapted to intracellular life and to passage from reservoir to host via arthropods. Their localization in blood vessels causes vascular injury with increased permeability and hemorrhages, sometimes with severe consequences.

Suggested Readings

Bechah Y, Capo C, Mege JL, et al. Epidemic typhus. *Lancet Infect Dis.* 2008;8:417–426.

Chapman AS, Bakken JS, Folk SM, et al. Diagnosis and management of tickborne rickettsial diseases: Rocky Mountain spotted fever, ehrlichioses, and anaplasmosis—United States. *MMWR Recomm Rep.* 2006;55:1–27.

Harden VA. *Rocky Mountain Spotted Fever: History of a Twentieth Century Disease.* Baltimore, MD: Johns Hopkins University Press; 1990.

Holman RC, Paddock CD, Curns AT, et al. Analysis of risk factors for fatal Rocky Mountain spotted fever: evidence for superiority of tetracyclines for therapy. *J Infect Dis.* 2001;184:1437–1444.

Marrie TJ, Raoult D. Update on Q fever, including Q fever endocarditis. *Curr Clin Top Infect Dis.* 2002;22:97–124.

Olano JP, Walker DH. Human ehrlichioses. *Med Clin North Am.* 2002;86:375–392.

Paddock CD, Childs JE. *Ehrlichia chaffeensis*: a prototypical emerging pathogen. *Clin Microbiol Rev.* 2003;16:37–64.

Raoult D, Fournier P-E, Fenollar F, et al. *Rickettsia africae*, a tick-borne pathogen in travelers to sub-Saharan Africa. *N Engl J Med.* 2001;344(20):1504–1510.

Walker DH. Rickettsiae and rickettsial infections: The current state of knowledge. *Clin Infect Dis.* 2007;45(suppl 1):539–544.

Chapter **29**

Mycoplasma: Curiosity and Pathogen

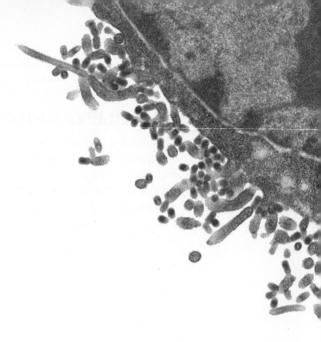

Joel B. Baseman and Ken B. Waites

KEY CONCEPTS

Pathogen: Mycoplasmas:

- are the smallest organisms capable of growth on cell-free media
- lack a rigid cell wall
- require sterols for growth
- include at least five species that are proven causes of significant human disease: Mycoplasma pneumoniae, M. genitalium, M. hominis, Ureaplasma urealyticum, and U. parvum

Encounter: *M. pneumoniae* is a common cause of tracheobronchitis and atypical pneumonia.

Entry: *M. pneumoniae* are acquired by respiratory droplet spread. The other species mentioned are transmitted by sexual contact.

Spread and Multiplication: *M. pneumoniae* are extracellular pathogens that attach to and grow on the respiratory tract mucosa.

Damage: *M. pneumonia* may cause a range of other acute and chronic airway diseases and extrapulmonary manifestations, including neurologic conditions and hemolytic anemia mediated by cold hemagglutinin IgM antibody.

Diagnosis: *Mycoplasma* infections are usually diagnosed by clinical features, measurement of serological response, and/or polymerase chain reaction testing.

Treatment and Prevention: *Mycoplasma* infections are treated with macrolides, tetracyclines, or quinolones.

Genital Mycoplasmas and Ureaplasmas:

- *M. genitalium* causes urethritis, cervicitis, and endometritis.
- *M. hominis* causes pelvic inflammatory disease, pyelonephritis, chorioamnionitis, postpartum endometritis, arthritis, and wound infections. It has also been isolated from the central nervous systems of newborns with meningitis.
- *U. urealyticum* and *U. parvum* cause urethritis, arthritis, chorioamnionitis, postpartum endometritis, and preterm labor. They are also associated with congenital pneumonia and chronic lung disease in premature infants with very low birth weights and have been isolated from the central nervous systems of newborns with meningitis.

MYCOPLASMAS and Ureaplasmas belong to the class Mollicutes and are a highly distinct group of bacteria that **lack a cell wall**, are bounded by a plasma membrane, and **require sterols for growth**. Most human-associated species are innocuous members of the normal flora. One species, however, is a common cause of **tracheobronchitis** and **pneumonia**, and others cause infections in the genitourinary tracts of adults and in the respiratory tracts and central nervous systems of newborn infants. These infecting organisms are usually susceptible to broad-spectrum antibiotics that inhibit functions other than cell wall synthesis. However, mycoplasma persistence following antibiotic treatment has been observed, and acquired antimicrobial resistance is now becoming more common.

CASE • B., a 7-year-old girl, who previously had been in good health, developed fever, headache, and a dry cough. Her 12-year-old brother had had similar symptoms 2 weeks earlier. Over the next 2 days, her temperature increased and the cough worsened, producing small amounts of clear sputum. Her physician noted that she appeared slightly pale and had a temperature of 39.3°C and a respiratory rate of 40 breaths per minute. Scattered rales (abnormal respiratory sounds) were heard through the stethoscope over the left posterior lung.

Her white blood cell count was in the normal range, 8,600 per μL, with a normal differential count. She was slightly anemic (hematocrit of 29%) and had an increased number of reticulocytes. A Gram stain of her sputum revealed only a few neutrophils and no bacteria. A chest radiograph showed an infiltrate of the left midlung field (Fig. 29-1). A rapid test for IgM antibody to *Mycoplasma pneumoniae* was positive. This finding and the clinical picture allowed the tentative diagnosis of **primary atypical pneumonia** caused by *M. pneumoniae*. B. was treated with azithromycin and made an uneventful recovery.

This case raises several questions:

1. How did B. acquire the organism?
2. What are distinguishing features of the organism and the treatment process?

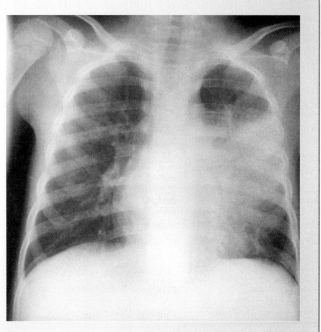

FIGURE 29-1. Chest radiograph reveals an infiltrate in left midlung field.

3. How can a definitive diagnosis of mycoplasmal infection be made?

See Appendix for answers.

Mycoplasma pneumoniae is a common cause of pneumonia in children and young adults. As in B.'s case, the illness usually has a less abrupt onset and a milder course than pneumococcal pneumonia. A rather imprecise term, "walking pneumonia," has been used to describe mycoplasmal infections. Occasionally, cases are quite severe in healthy and immunocompromised individuals and children with sickle cell disease. Headache and cough are prominent clinical features. Before the etiology of this disease became known, it was referred to as primary atypical pneumonia to distinguish it from "typical" cases of lobar pneumonia (usually caused by pneumococci). Clinicians knew that patients with typical pneumonia responded to penicillin but those with atypical pneumonia did not.

PATHOGEN: MYCOPLASMAS AND UREAPLASMAS (CLASS MOLLICUTES)

The mycoplasmas have a number of unusual features:

- They are the smallest prokaryotes capable of growth on cell-free media, although the highly fastidious nature and very slow growth of some pathogenic species, especially *Mycoplasma genitalium* and *M. pneumoniae*, make culture less useful than other methods of laboratory detection, such as serological and polymerase chain reaction (PCR) assays.

- Unlike any other bacteria, mycoplasmas lack a rigid cell wall (no murein) and can assume a variety of shapes. This characteristic has important implications for antibiotic therapy because many commonly used antibiotics (especially the β-lactams) act by inhibiting cell wall murein synthesis and thus are ineffective against mycoplasmas.

- Their cell membrane contains **sterols**, which must be supplied in culture medium by the addition of serum to support their growth.

Mycoplasma and *Ureaplasma* species are capable of causing disease in a wide range of animals, plants, and insects. Among the species for whom humans are the primary host, five are known to cause significant human disease; several others have been implicated in a range of pathologies, while other species exist mainly as harmless commensals in the respiratory or genitourinary tracts. A summary of the human Mollicute flora is provided in Table 29-1. *M. pneumoniae* is a common cause of respiratory infections; *M. genitalium* is a frequent cause of genitourinary tract infections; and *M. hominis* causes a variety of infections of the genitourinary tract and joints as well as meningitis in newborns. *Ureaplasma urealyticum* and *U. parvum* can also infect the genitourinary tract and have been implicated in preterm labor as well as infections of the respiratory tract and central nervous system in newborns. *M. fermentans* has been linked to a wide range of

TABLE 29-1 Human Mycoplasmas and Diseases They Cause

Organism	Disease	Primary Habitat
Mycoplasma pneumoniae	Primary atypical pneumonia, pharyngitis, tracheobronchitis, reactive airway disease, and extrapulmonary pathologies	Respiratory tract
Mycoplasma genitalium	Male urethritis, cervicitis, pelvic inflammatory disease	Genitourinary tract
Mycoplasma hominis	Pelvic inflammatory disease; postpartum endometritis; pyelonephritis; neonatal infections involving the bloodstream, lungs, and central nervous system; extragenital infections in immunocompromised hosts including arthritis	Genitourinary tract
Mycoplasma fermentans	Arthritis, pneumonia	Respiratory tract, genitourinary tract
Ureaplasma urealyticum and *Ureaplasma parvum*	Male urethritis; urinary calculi; abscesses; chorioamnionitis; postpartum endometritis; prematurity/low birth weight; neonatal infections involving the bloodstream, lungs, and central nervous system; extragenital infections in immunocompromised hosts including arthritis	Genitourinary tract
Mycoplasma penetrans	Possibly HIV cofactor	Genitourinary tract
Others[a]	None	Genitourinary tract or oropharynx

[a]Other species for which humans are the primary host that normally do not cause disease in immunocompetent persons include *Acholeplasma laidlawii*, *M. buccale, M. faucium, M. lipophilum, M. orale, M. salivarium, M. pirum, M. spermatophilum, M. primatum,* and *M. penetrans*. A newly described species, *M. amphoriforme,* has been isolated from the lower respiratory tracts in a small number of immunocompromised persons suffering from bronchitis.

disease processes, including secondary complications in immunocompromised individuals, although its direct relationship to disease etiologies is not fully understood. It has been speculated that *M. fermentans* and *M. penetrans* may contribute to various conditions such as the progression of AIDS, chronic fatigue syndrome, and malignant transformation, but conclusive evidence for these associations is lacking. While most human mycoplasmal or ureaplasmal infections in individuals beyond the neonatal period are limited to the respiratory or genitourinary tract mucosae, persons with congenital antibody deficiencies or other immunological impairments are at risk for invasive systemic infections due to a variety of human mycoplasmal species and occasionally mycoplasmal species of nonhuman origin. Other *Mycoplasma* species commonly

found as part of the normal human flora have not been linked to disease.

Many *Mycoplasma* and *Ureaplasma* species can be readily cultivated in the laboratory, providing special media containing sterols and other growth factors are supplied. *M. pneumoniae* grows slowly, and several weeks may be required for colonies to become evident. The colonies are much smaller than those of common bacteria and require a dissecting microscope to visualize them. Some species such as *M. hominis* grow within 2 to 3 days and have a dense center that gives them a "fried egg" appearance (Fig. 29-2). *M. hominis* can sometimes be grown on the blood agar plates used in clinical microbiology laboratories. However, this organism often goes undetected, probably because of its relatively small

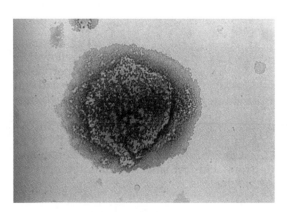 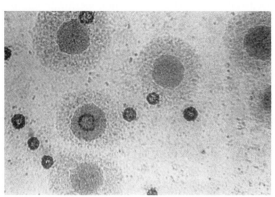

FIGURE 29-2. Photomicrograph of colonies of *Mycoplasma hominis* and *Ureaplasma* species colonies grown on agar. Note the "fried egg" appearance of the larger *M. hominis* colonies and the smaller dark granular ureaplasma colonies.

colonies and overgrowth by rapidly growing bacteria. Ureaplasmas grow readily within 1 to 2 days in specialized broth or agar containing urea as a metabolic substrate (Fig. 29-2), but they are not cultivable on growth media normally used to detect conventional bacteria.

MYCOPLASMA PNEUMONIAE
ENCOUNTER AND ENTRY

Infected humans constitute the only known reservoir of *M. pneumoniae*. Patients become ill following exposure to the respiratory secretions of persons harboring the organism. As with the pneumococcus, prolonged asymptomatic colonization with *M. pneumoniae* can occur even after proper antibiotic therapy. In some cases, the source of the infection is not recognized because the typical *M. pneumoniae* infection is mild. However, *M. pneumoniae* infections are fairly contagious. Cases of spread within households and residential institutions have been reported, some with intervals of 2 to 3 weeks between cases. Persons of all ages, including infants and the elderly, may develop respiratory infections due to *M. pneumoniae*.

  M. pneumoniae infection begins with the binding of organisms to the respiratory epithelium. Microscopic studies of *M. pneumoniae* have revealed a unique terminal attachment structure. Specialized adhesin and adherence accessory proteins are part of this tip-mediated attachment organelle that helps the organisms bind to carbohydrate-containing receptors on the respiratory epithelium. Monoclonal antibodies to adhesin proteins inhibit the attachment of *M. pneumoniae,* and mutants lacking the proteins exhibit marked reduction in cytadherence and virulence in experimentally infected hamsters. Also, alternate adherence pathways that target fibronectin and surfactant protein A provide additional mechanisms for mycoplasma parasitism. Although *M. pneumoniae* is usually considered a respiratory mucosal surface pathogen, evidence obtained in cultured mammalian cells suggests it may also invade and replicate in host cells. Intracellular localization may facilitate establishment of chronic infections and evasion of the host immune response as sometimes occurs with other facultative intracellular microorganisms.

SPREAD, MULTIPLICATION, AND DAMAGE

The pathogenesis of *M. pneumoniae* infection differs markedly from other forms of pneumonia, such as that caused by the pneumococcus or *Legionella pneumophila,* mainly because its involvement is largely limited to the respiratory mucosa that lines the airways.

  In experimentally infected tracheal organ cultures, the organisms line up along the mucosa, with the terminal attachment structure in contact with the epithelium (Fig. 29-3). In this model, ciliary function is impaired

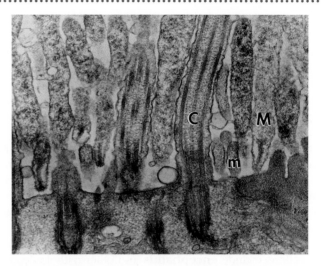

FIGURE 29-3. Transmission electron photomicrograph of a hamster tracheal ring infected with *M. pneumoniae*. Notice the orientation of the mycoplasma (M) through its specialized tip-mediated attachment organelle, which permits close association with the respiratory epithelium (original magnification ×50,000). m, microvillus; c, cilia.

and tissue cytopathology observed, probably as a result of local elaboration of tissue-toxic substances. Recently, a protein known as the community-acquired respiratory distress syndrome (CARDS) toxin has been identified, which exhibits similarities to pertussis toxin. This protein functions as an ADP-ribosylating and vacuolating toxin and appears to play a role in damaging the respiratory epithelium and disrupting ciliary activity as CARDS toxin alone elicits vacuolization and cytotoxicity of the bronchiolar epithelium in animal models. The CARDS toxin and other mycoplasmal components may also elicit cellular toxicity by induction of cytokines and other inflammatory mediators. The main inflammatory response is characterized by perivascular and peribronchial infiltration of mononuclear leukocytes with few neutrophils. These infections can cause chronic lung damage and reduced lung function, leading to wheezing, asthma, and other reactive airway diseases. Some immunocompromised patients with mycoplasmal infection do not have visible pulmonary infiltrates, suggesting that the immune response may play a role in causing disease pathogenesis.

  The clinical manifestations of *M. pneumoniae* infections are generally limited to the respiratory tract, but other organs are occasionally involved. B. had a mild **hemolytic anemia**, which was caused by an antibody stimulated by mycoplasmal infection. An IgM antibody, it binds to red blood cells and, at reduced temperatures, causes them to agglutinate. The antibody is called a **cold hemagglutinin**, which is detectable in about 50% of severe *Mycoplasma* infections. Only a small number of patients with cold hemagglutinins actually experience clinically significant hemolysis. The reason *M. pneumoniae* infection stimulates the production of cold hemagglutinins is likely linked to a combination of molecular mimicry and shared antigens between *Mycoplasma* and mammalian proteins and autoimmunity. The most characteristic clinical features of mycoplasmal infection are a sore scratchy throat and persistent cough that occurs as a result of the damage that the organisms cause on the respiratory tract epithelium. Most of the time, the illness is limited to tracheobronchitis, an inflammation of the large airways of the lung, but some persons progress to pneumonia. An infiltrate of mononuclear cells surrounds infected bronchi and bronchioles, but there is no evidence of involvement of the lung alveoli. The pattern of involvement is that of a **bronchopneumonia** rather than a lobar process typically seen with pneumococcal infection.

Extrapulmonary complications of *M. pneumoniae* infections include **encephalitis** and other pathologies of the central nervous system. Some patients develop a rash known as erythema multiforme, renal and cardiac disorders, or arthritis. These manifestations that sometimes occur in *M. pneumoniae* infections may result from direct spread of the organisms and the CARDS toxin from the respiratory tract to other parts of the body, or systemic host inflammatory and immune reactions that occur in response to the infectious process. Interestingly, the discovery of the CARDS toxin provides a possible pathogenic mediator of metabolic pathway abnormalities, cytopathologies, and tissue injury distal to the airway.

DIAGNOSIS

Culturing *M. pneumoniae* from clinical specimens can take several weeks, requires special media and experienced personnel, and frequently fails. Consequently, the diagnosis of mycoplasmal pneumonia is usually suspected from clinical features and reinforced by serologic tests and/or PCR assays. Comparisons of *M. pneumoniae* IgM and IgG antibody titers between acute and convalescent phase sera can be diagnostic. However, such results become available long after therapeutic decisions about the patient must be made. Elevation of specific IgM antibodies may occur after about 1 week of illness suggesting the diagnosis of *M. pneumoniae* infection in children and young adults, but older persons may not mount an IgM response as a consequence of repeated past infections. However, IgM may persist in some persons for prolonged periods after initial infection, making it somewhat unreliable when used alone for diagnostic purposes. PCR assays can detect the presence of *M. pneumoniae* DNA in single specimen and will be positive earlier in the course of illness than serological tests. However, PCR is expensive and is currently available only in reference laboratories. Recent observations suggest that PCR for the CARDS toxin gene, serological, and direct toxin detection assays may provide improved diagnostic options.

In contrast to pneumococcal pneumonia, sputum production in *M. pneumoniae* infections is scanty and the sputum may be nonpurulent. The peripheral blood usually does not show the leukocytosis and marked increase in young leukocyte forms characteristic of pneumococcal infection. The chest radiography in mycoplasmal pneumonia is highly variable but usually reveals a patchy infiltrate suggestive of bronchopneumonia.

TREATMENT AND PREVENTION

Treatment with a macrolide, tetracycline, or quinolone is usually effective, although persistence of mycoplasmas following completion of antibiotic therapy has been reported. While macrolide antibiotics have been considered first-line treatments, within the past decade, there have been reports from Asian countries as well as Europe and the United States of *M. pneumoniae* infections that are highly resistant to erythromycin and other drugs in the macrolide class. This resistance can be clinically significant, although fluoroquinolones and tetracyclines are not affected by this resistance. No vaccine is currently available to prevent *Mycoplasma* infections.

GENITAL MYCOPLASMAS

In epidemiology and pathogenesis, *M. genitalium* is among the newest emerging pathogenic bacteria for humans. It is an important cause of chlamydia-negative, nongonococcal urethritis in men and has been directly linked to cervicitis, endometritis, and pelvic inflammatory disease in women. Also, this mycoplasma has been isolated, along with *M. pneumoniae*, from the synovial and respiratory fluids of diseased individuals. As such, both *M. pneumoniae* and *M. genitalium* share common biological features, including tip-mediated attachment organelles and amino acid sequence–related adhesin and adherence-accessory protein homologues. Also, *M. genitalium* can be readily visualized extracellularly and intracellularly in vaginal cells of women, indicating that mycoplasmas are capable of invading cells and persisting and replicating for extended periods with high likelihood of transmission through sexual contact.

U. urealyticum, U. parvum, and *M. hominis* are common flora of the genitourinary tract, especially of sexually active people and may occur in many persons in the absence of any clinical disease. They are almost certainly transmitted through sexual contact among adults and are transmitted vertically, from mother to newborn infant, during pregnancy and birth. Ureaplasma species have been clearly established as a cause of male urethritis, and *M. hominis* is a proven cause of pelvic inflammatory disease. Both organisms can cause chorioamnionitis (inflammation of the fetal membranes) and postpartum endometritis. Intrauterine infection with ureaplasmas has been associated with onset of preterm labor. Several studies have demonstrated that ureaplasmas can cause congenital pneumonia and are associated with chronic lung disease in premature infants with very low birth weights. *M. hominis* and *Ureaplasma* species have also been isolated from the cerebrospinal fluid of newborn infants with meningitis. Some evidence suggests that *U. urealyticum* may be of more pathogenic significance in some conditions than the more common species, *U. parvum*. However, definitive proof for this concept has not yet been demonstrated.

While culture using special media is useful for the rapidly growing *M. hominis* and *Ureaplasma* species, PCR is required for detection of the very slow growing and fastidious *M. genitalium*. Antibiotic treatment options for the genital mycoplasmas are generally similar to those for *M. pneumoniae* and are limited mainly to macrolides, lincosamides, tetracyclines, and quinolones. However, uniform susceptibility of the genital mycoplasmas to all agents in these classes can no longer be assumed. Tetracycline resistance may occur in up to 50% of clinical isolates of *M. hominis* and *Ureaplasma* species. *M. hominis* is resistant to many drugs in the macrolide class, including erythromycin and azithromycin, but is susceptible to clindamycin. The reverse is true for *Ureaplasma* species. *M. genitalium* is usually susceptible to macrolides and tetracyclines, but treatment failures have been reported. Quinolones are generally active against all of the genital mycoplasma species, but resistance has been documented occasionally.

CONCLUSION

Mycoplasmas are unique among the prokaryotes in that they lack a cell wall, require sterols for growth, and make characteristically small colonies on agar. These organisms show a marked tropism for mucous membranes and can cause varied clinical manifestations.

M. pneumoniae is unequivocally responsible for a common form of pneumonia in humans, and *M. genitalium* is clearly emerging as a significant cause of genitourinary tract infections in men and women. *M. hominis* and *Ureaplasma* species are commonly found in the genitourinary tracts of adults and can cause infections of the respiratory tracts and central nervous systems of newborn infants.

Our knowledge about the mycoplasmas and their role in disease is accumulating at a rapid pace with the advent of new detection and diagnostic assays and genetic and molecular biological strategies in pathogenesis. However, only limited data exist concerning long-term antibiotic treatment and eradication of mycoplasmal infections. The association of mycoplasmas with a variety of clinical symptoms in humans suggests the need to clarify virulence determinants, host immune responsiveness, and effective therapies so that mycoplasmal disease transmission and progression can be controlled and prevented.

Suggested Readings

Baseman JB, Tully JG. Mycoplasmas: sophisticated, reemerging and burdened by their notoriety. *Emerg Infect Dis*. 1997;3:21–32.

Kannan TR, Baseman JB. ADP-ribosylating and vacuolating cytotoxin of *Mycoplasma pneumoniae* represents unique virulence determinant among bacterial pathogens. *PNAS*. 2006;103(17):6724–6729.

Stein MA, Baseman JB. The Evolving saga of *Mycoplasma genitalium*. *Clin Micro Newsletter*. 2006;28(6):41–48.

Waites KB, Balish MF, Atkinson TP. New insights into the pathogenesis and detection of *Mycoplasma pneumoniae* infections. *Future Microbiol*. 2008;3(6):635–648.

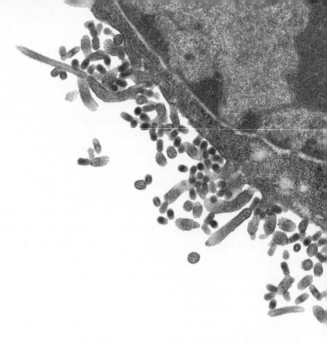

Chapter **30**

Strategies to Combat Bacterial Infections

Cary Engleberg

OVER THE LAST two centuries, the health and longevity of people living in developed countries have taken a quantum jump forward. We take for granted that we, our relatives, and our acquaintances have survived infancy and will reach old age. Disease is an exceptional event for most people, and premature death is relatively uncommon. Two interrelated factors have contributed to this increased life expectancy: improvement in nutrition and control of infectious diseases. Initially, the most important factors in reducing the incidence of infectious disease were preventive measures, largely purification of the water supply and control of human wastes and disease vectors. Later, in the last 100 years, these measures were supplemented with effective medical interventions: vaccination and antimicrobial therapy. Clearly, preventive measures, not therapy, have played the greatest role in the control of infectious diseases.

This chapter discusses strategies that have been developed for prevention and therapy of infectious diseases. The emphasis here is on bacteria, but the basic principles apply to other infectious agents. Related topics also addressed in this text include the biological basis of antimicrobial activity and resistance (see Chapter 5), antiviral strategies (see Chapter 44), and immunization (see Chapter 45).

ANTIMICROBIAL THERAPY

Despite the great advances in preventive medicine in the last century, little could be done to treat patients with infectious diseases until relatively recently. Medical literature from the early decades of the 20th century is full of vivid descriptions of gruesome infections caused by streptococci, staphylococci, and clostridia. At the dawning of the age of antimicrobial therapy, with the introduction of the sulfonamides in the 1930s, physicians could finally cure many of those once-fatal infections. Here is a description of the first time penicillin that was used clinically:

The time had now come to find a suitable patient for the first test of the therapeutic power of penicillin in man..... In the septic ward at the Radcliffe Infirmary (Oxford, England), there was an unfortunate policeman aged 43 who had a sore on his lip four months previously, from which he developed a combined staphylococcal and streptococcal septicaemia. He had multiple abscesses on his face and orbits: he also had osteomyelitis of his right humerus with discharging sinuses, and abscesses in his

lungs. He was in great pain and was desperately ill. There was all to gain for him in a trial of penicillin and nothing to lose. Penicillin treatment was started on 12 February 1941, with 200 mg (10,000 units) intravenously initially and then 300 mg every three hours.... Four days later there was striking improvement, and after 5 days the patient was vastly better, afebrile and eating well, and there was obvious resolution of the abscesses on his face and scalp and in his right orbit.

Unfortunately, this first clinical trial of a β-lactam antibiotic ended abruptly because the total supply of the drug was exhausted by the 5-day course of treatment. Despite efforts to recover the drug from the patient's urine, he died 4 weeks later.

Although the experiment ended tragically, it served to demonstrate the efficacy and superiority of the new therapy over any that was available until that time. Today, it has become increasingly difficult to prove the superiority of new antibiotics over those already in use. In assessing new drugs, pharmaceutical companies must carry out complex and expensive trials that include laboratory work, experimental animals, and lengthy clinical studies. The practicing physician may often find it difficult to evaluate such intricate studies.

The selection of the most appropriate drug to treat a particular infection is also not a simple matter. For example, when the first carbapenem antibiotic, imipenem, was introduced in the 1980s, it was treated as a true "wonder drug." It had the widest antibacterial spectrum of activity of any antibiotic available at the time, and it was resistant to all of the contemporary β-**lactamase** enzymes. So, how could penicillin, which has neither of these desirable properties, ever have a therapeutic role after the introduction of such an advanced antimicrobial agent? In fact, penicillin remains the drug of choice for several infectious diseases; even the most advanced antimicrobial drugs come with some excess baggage, and imipenem is no exception. Because of its broad spectrum, imipenem can wipe out much of the normal bacterial microbiota and lead to colonization by resistant species. Imipenem is more likely than penicillin to cause seizures if the drug accumulates. Imipenem is substantially more expensive than penicillin. And finally, like all antimicrobials that find a place in medical practice, resistance eventually emerges. In recent years, we have seen the emergence of **carbapenemase** enzymes that render imipenem and other drugs in this class useless against bacteria that were sensitive in earlier times. Thus, the pharmacological properties of the drugs, their adverse effects, their cost, their propensity to allow resistance to emerge, and many other factors must be considered in making an appropriate therapeutic choice. When deciding which antibiotic to use for a patient, the clinician must consider the following questions:

- Which pathogens are causing the infection? If their identity cannot be determined at this time, what are the likely possibilities?
- What antibiotics are active against the suspected pathogen or pathogens?
- Will the drug penetrate the site of infection, and will it work under the conditions at that site?
- What is the toxicity of the drug to the patient?
- What is the effect of the drug on the microbial ecology? Will its use lead to the emergence of broadly based antibiotic resistance, thereby posing a threat to the patient being treated and to other infected patients in the community?
- Are other host factors relevant to the proposed therapy?

In some cases, the proper conclusion will be that the patient should not be treated with antimicrobial drugs at all because the benefits of such treatment are not likely to outweigh the drawbacks.

Infecting Organisms

Choosing the proper antimicrobial drug depends on the identification of the infecting organisms. Consider, for example, patients with recurrent urinary tract infections.

Often, the infections are caused by *Escherichia coli*, but they can also be caused by *Enterococcus, Pseudomonas aeruginosa*, or one of the other Enterobacteriaceae, such as *Klebsiella, Enterobacter*, or *Serratia*. Each organism has a unique set of susceptibilities, and the determination of its antimicrobial susceptibility is mandatory.

Physicians treating first-time, uncomplicated urinary tract infections usually do not wait for the results of laboratory cultures and drug susceptibility testing. These infections are known to be almost always caused by *E. coli*. Other situations that require empiric therapy are those in which an adequate sample of infected material for direct analysis or culture cannot be obtained. In such cases, **empiric treatment** is based on the clinician's knowledge of the usual causative agents in a particular clinical situation: factors pertinent to the individual patient and the local environment, large studies of similar cases in the medical literature, recent local experience with similar cases, and antibiotic susceptibility patterns in the local hospital or community. Failure to analyze the best empiric therapy invariably results in an attempt to treat all possible bacteria with one or several antibiotics. This "shotgun" approach to antibiotic therapy has several drawbacks:

- Failure to "cover" the pathogen
- Synergistic toxicity of multiple drugs
- Possible antagonism between drugs
- Increased likelihood of superinfection by resistant bacteria or fungi
- Increased cost of therapy

Obviously, these disadvantages are minimized when the identity of the infectious agent can be determined. In general, the more rapid the diagnosis, the sooner proper therapy can be instituted. Much effort is directed toward the development of rapid diagnostic methods, but most still require one or several days (see Chapter 58).

Antibiotic Susceptibility

Susceptibility to antibiotics varies among the many kinds of bacteria. Gram-positive bacteria, possibly because they lack an outer membrane, are potentially more susceptible than Gram-negative bacteria. For example, streptococci are generally about a 1,000-fold more susceptible to penicillin G than is *E. coli*. However, the exceptions are too numerous to make these generalizations very useful (mechanisms of bacterial resistance are outlined in Chapter 5). Much depends on the presence of antibiotic-resistant strains in a particular environment. Monitoring resistant strains nationwide and locally is helpful in providing general guidelines, but basically, each isolate should be tested for susceptibility.

Two fundamental shifts occurred in the 1990s in the spectrum of antibiotic resistance among clinically important pathogens. First, antibacterial resistance, which first appeared among Gram-negative bacteria, has become widespread in medically important Gram-positive bacteria. These include methicillin-resistant *Staphylococcus aureus*,

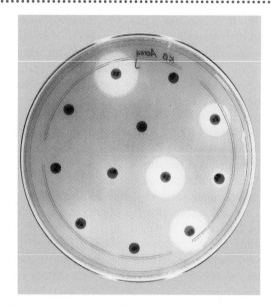

FIGURE 30-1. The disk-diffusion method for determining antibiotic susceptibility. Bacteria were uniformly seeded on the surface of a nutrient agar plate, and filter paper disks containing various antibiotics were placed at intervals over the surface. After incubation, susceptibility to some of the antibiotics becomes apparent as clear areas around the disks. The diameter of the clear area depends on the extent of diffusion of the drug throughout the agar. Resistance to other antibiotics is indicated by growth (turbidity) up to the edge of the disks.

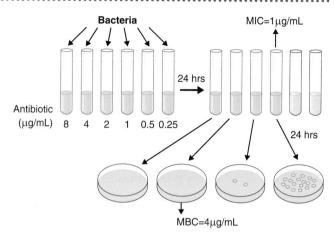

FIGURE 30-2. Antimicrobial susceptibility testing by measurement of the minimal inhibitory concentration (MIC) and minimal bactericidal concentration (MBC). A series of tubes containing liquid media and decreasing concentrations of the antibiotic to be tested are inoculated with equal amounts of the bacterial isolate of interest. After incubation overnight, growth occurs in all tubes that have noninhibitory levels of the antibiotic. The first tube in the series in which no growth occurs contains the MIC of the antibiotic. To determine the MBC, 1 per 1,000 of the volume from each of the inhibited cultures is plated on agar media. The last tube from which no bacteria are isolated reflects a 99.9% kill of the bacteria, which defines the MBC of the antibiotic.

vancomycin-resistant enterococci, and penicillin-resistant *Streptococcus pneumoniae*. Organisms such as *S. aureus* and *S. pneumoniae*, which were among the most frequent killers in the preantibiotic era, have become increasingly serious therapeutic problems once again. Second, antimicrobial-resistant organisms have spread from hospitals into the community and now affect children in day-care centers and elders in nursing homes.

It is extremely important that drug resistance be monitored both across the nation and on a local basis and that the information be readily available to medical personnel. The simplest and most widely used assay for microbial susceptibility, the **disk-diffusion method**, involves placing a paper disk infused with an antibiotic on an agar plate that has been inoculated with the organism of interest (Fig. 30-1). As the antibiotic diffuses into the agar, it inhibits bacterial growth up to the limit of the effective concentration. This test is not a truly quantitative technique, because many factors influence the diffusion of the drug. Quantitative techniques require the use of dilutions of the drug in liquid media. These techniques provide an estimate of the **minimum inhibitory concentration** (**MIC**), a parameter that is used to ascertain whether an effective antibiotic concentration is attainable in body fluids (Fig. 30-2).

Static versus Cidal Drugs

The MIC indicates the **bacteriostatic** concentration of a drug but not the **bactericidal** one. The two concentrations

are not usually the same: most agents that are bactericidal are bacteriostatic at lower concentrations. The **minimum bactericidal concentration** (**MBC**) is determined by subculturing the tubes or microtiter plates that have no visible growth into antibiotic-free media. This subculturing allows the bacteria that were inhibited from growing in the first culture, but are still alive, to replicate (see Fig. 30-2). Although this technique is time consuming and has some technical problems, it can yield important information because bactericidal and bacteriostatic drugs are not equally effective in all situations. A bacteriostatic therapy requires that the host clears the inhibited bacteria. However, if host immune response is inadequate to this task, either because the effector cells are absent (as in neutropenia) or because the site of infection is inaccessible to effective immune clearance (as in endocarditis or meningitis), then bactericidal antibiotics are required.

Multiple-Drug Therapy

The use of combinations of antibiotics (usually two drugs) is clearly needed in a number of clinical situations. As discussed in Chapter 5, when drugs are combined, three results are possible:

1. **Indifference**: The actions of neither drug are affected by the presence of the other.
2. **Antagonism**: One drug prevents the full effect of the other (e.g., bacteriostatic drugs and penicillin).
3. **Synergism**: Two drugs work better together than the sum of their individual activities because their

mechanisms of action complement and enhance one another (e.g., penicillin and gentamicin against enterococci).

In some situations, combined antibiotic therapy is desirable:

- **Treating severe infections when no single agent is sufficiently effective**: Synergistic combinations of antibiotics could create a bactericidal effect at nontoxic concentrations (e.g., enterococcal endocarditis).
- **Preventing the emergence of resistant organisms**: In active tuberculosis, for example, combination therapy is essential.
- **Treating polymicrobial infections, such as intra-abdominal abscesses**: Each organism causing the infection could be susceptible to different drugs.
- **Initiating empiric therapy to "cover" multiple potential pathogens**.

PHARMACOKINETICS AND PHARMACODYNAMICS

The pharmacokinetic factors that should be considered in the choice of drugs include absorption, distribution in tissues, and excretion. The **absorption** profile of a drug dictates its route of administration. The proportion of an administered dose of a drug that reaches the systemic circulation is referred to as its **bioavailability**. The most convenient route is usually by mouth, and this route is used with highly absorbable (or highly bioavailable) antibiotics like the fluoroquinolones, trimethoprim/sulfamethoxazole, linezolid, metronidazole, and rifampin. Of course, these medications cannot be given orally if the patient is vomiting, has impaired gastrointestinal absorption, or is in shock. Many antibiotics, such as vancomycin, the aminoglycosides, and the newer β-lactams, are not absorbed in a normal gastrointestinal tract and must be given by parenteral injection for systemic infection. However, nonabsorbable antibiotics can be used to treat infections limited to the lumen of the gastrointestinal tract. An example is the use of oral vancomycin to treat diarrhea or colitis induced by *Clostridium difficile* (see Chapter 20).

Distribution of drugs takes place through the circulation and is followed by entry into tissues by passive diffusion. The diffusion and polarity properties of antibiotics are relevant in this process, as they are with all drugs. Some antibiotics bind to plasma proteins; this has a good and a bad side. On one hand, protein binding limits the amount of unbound drug available for diffusion. On the other hand, the drug remains available in the bloodstream for a much longer time.

Consideration must be given to the speed of **excretion** of the drug. Most drugs are excreted by the kidney, but some drugs (e.g., nafcillin, ceftriaxone) are excreted primarily by the liver through the biliary tree and still others use both pathways. Patterns of excretion can be

used to advantage in infections of the urinary tract or the biliary tree. However, the level of renal or hepatic function must also be taken into account because the excretion mechanisms must be working properly to achieve effective drug concentrations. If they are not, the drug could accumulate in the bloodstream with toxic consequences.

Antibiotics with similar activities against a particular bacterial pathogen and similar pharmacokinetics can nevertheless differ in their ability to clear an infection, depending on how they are administered. The **pharmacodynamic** profiles of the antibiotics—that is, their ability to clear infection—may differ because of their respective mechanisms of action. Antibiotics that kill bacteria slowly, such as the β-lactams, are most effective when given frequently or continuously. Larger doses to obtain higher levels of the antibiotic are not necessarily helpful, and the pharmacodynamic parameter that correlates best with therapeutic success is the time that the drug level exceeds the MIC (Fig. 30-3). In contrast, antibiotics that kill bacteria rapidly, such as fluoroquinolones and aminoglycosides, are most effective when administered at high doses at extended intervals. The pharmacodynamic parameters that best predict their effectiveness are the ratio of the maximum drug concentration to the MIC (**C_{max}/MIC**) and the area under the drug-level curve that is above the MIC (**area under the inhibitory curve [AUIC]**).

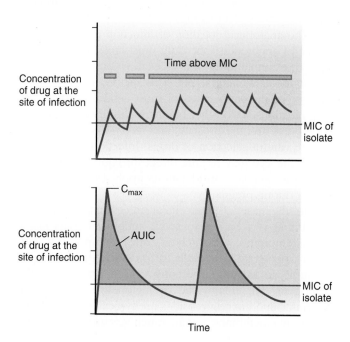

FIGURE 30-3. Pharmacodynamic properties of antibiotics. A slowly bactericidal antibiotic is best administered to maximize the time that drug levels remain above the minimal inhibitory concentration (MIC) of the organism being treated. In contrast, rapidly bactericidal antibiotics are best administered so that the maximum drug concentration (C_{max}) is many multiples of the MIC, that is, high C_{max}/MIC ratio, or the area under the inhibitory curve (AUIC) is maximized.

TABLE 30-1 Physiochemical Conditions that Affect the Activity of Antimicrobial Agents

Condition	Decrease	Increase
Low pH	Aminoglycosides Some β-lactams (porin changes) Erythromycin	Tetracycline Chloramphenicol
Low redox potential	Aminoglycosides	Metronidazole
High divalent cation concentration	Aminoglycosides Tetracyclines (Ca^{2+}) Fluoroquinolones	

LOCAL FACTORS

Tissue inflammation, which occurs early in many infections, changes the environment in which an antibiotic is to work. If infection is not controlled, local tissue necrosis can alter conditions even further. In an abscess caused by staphylococci or a mixed anaerobic–aerobic flora, the environment becomes anaerobic and the pH may drop as low as 5.5. Antibiotics must be selected for their ability to function under those conditions. As shown in Table 30-1, the efficacy of aminoglycosides is diminished at low pH, at low redox potential, or in the presence of a high concentration of divalent cations.

The anatomical location of infection can dictate the choice of antibiotics if the drug must cross a natural barrier. For example, drugs that cross the blood–brain barrier are nonpolar at neutral pH. This factor may be critical because of the seriousness of most central nervous system infections. Two other organs with important barriers are the eye and the prostate, and infections at these sites require careful selection of drugs. Infections of the interior of the eye may require direct injection of drugs into the tissue. Similar considerations apply to the placental barrier during pregnancy.

In the case of intracellular infections, the plasma membrane is a barrier to some antibiotics. Macrolides, fluoroquinolones, tetracyclines, and rifampin can efficiently penetrate host cells, a property that is highly desirable in treating infections caused by intracellular pathogens like chlamydiae or legionellae. In contrast, β-lactams and aminoglycosides are typically excluded by the plasma membrane and are much less useful in treating intracellular infections.

ANTIBIOTIC TOXICITY

Like any drug, an antibiotic can have both toxic and beneficial effects. Sometimes toxicity is so severe that it limits the drug's efficacy. For example, chloramphenicol, an antibiotic commonly prescribed in past decades, has virtually disappeared from clinical practice because of a rare and fatal aplastic anemia associated with its use. The following sections present a brief overview of the main categories of adverse reactions associated with antibiotics. Practicing physicians need more detailed information and must constantly update it.

Allergy

Antimicrobial agents may be recognized as foreign substances by the immune system, resulting in sensitization of some individuals. The most common antibacterial drugs associated with severe allergic reactions are the penicillins, cephalosporins, and sulfonamides. A likely reason why penicillins lead this list is that they readily bind to proteins and function as haptens to elicit IgE antibody responses. The most severe reactions result in immediate hypersensitive responses—**hives**, **angioneurotic edema**, and **anaphylactic shock**—and can be fatal. Mild to fairly severe allergic reactions include rash, urticaria (hives), lymphadenopathy, asthma, and fever. In some cases, fever confuses the clinical picture because it is attributed to the infection and not to the drug. Previous history of drug sensitivity often dictates the choice of other agents.

Other Systemic Reactions

All major organs of the body can be affected by toxicity from antimicrobial drugs. The most frequent reactions involve the **gastrointestinal tract**. Gastrointestinal distress and diarrhea are the most common reactions and often require discontinuation of the drug. These manifestations are often caused by a direct stimulatory effect of the drug on the sympathetic nervous system. However, diarrhea can also result from changes in the intestinal flora. This form of toxicity usually occurs late in the course of treatment and may manifest only after treatment is stopped. About one-third of the cases of antibiotic-associated diarrhea have been associated with the toxin produced by *C. difficile* (see Chapter 20). The spectrum of diseases caused by this organism ranges from a trivial and self-limiting diarrhea to a severe and life-threatening pseudomembranous colitis.

The **liver** is the major site of drug metabolism and is frequently affected. Many drugs induce mild alterations of function of the hepatic parenchyma, usually manifested by an increase in the serum level of certain transaminases. Some drugs affect biliary excretion. Most of these manifestations are mild and reversible, although cases of liver failure have been reported in pregnant women treated with tetracycline.

The **kidney** is also a frequent site of adverse reactions, resulting in decreased renal function. These reactions are caused by three general mechanisms: immunological damage to the glomeruli, which blocks filtration; damage to the tubules; and obstruction of the collecting system by crystals of the drug. Reactions in the kidney are an important problem because many drugs are excreted through the urinary tract. An unrecognized decrease in renal function could result not only in ineffective levels in the urine but also in toxic serum levels of the drug. The aminoglycosides are the most important class of drugs that cause these side effects. They also cause inner ear toxicity (hearing loss and imbalance). The frequency of toxic reactions in the kidney is so high that frequent monitoring of renal function and blood levels of the drug is required during aminoglycoside therapy.

The **skin** can also be affected by antimicrobial agents and is often the site of an allergic reaction. More serious skin reactions include **exfoliative dermatitis** and a disease known as **Stevens-Johnson syndrome**, which leads to the formation of bullae, large vesicles on the skin, and inflammation of the eyes and mucous membranes.

The **hematopoietic system** can be adversely affected, leading to decreased production of red and white blood cells in the bone marrow. Further, peripheral red and white blood cells can become immunologically sensitized, resulting in their hemolysis or sequestration by fixed macrophages. Antibiotics can also affect the circulatory system, central nervous system, musculoskeletal system, and respiratory tract. Most reactions at these sites are specific to individual drugs. Information about the reactions caused by antibiotics is made available to physicians in reference manuals published periodically; physicians should consult this information before prescribing any medication.

Interactions with Nonantimicrobial Drugs

Antimicrobial drugs sometimes interact with other medications a patient is taking. The drugs can interact directly or by affecting enzymes that influence their pharmacology. The drugs most commonly involved are anticoagulants and anticonvulsants. The following case is an example.

PROPHYLACTIC USE OF ANTIMICROBIAL DRUGS

Soon after the introduction of effective antibacterial agents in the 1930s, it became clear that they could be used not only to treat infections but to prevent them as well. However, prophylaxis is a complex and controversial subject because the use of antibiotics to prevent infections carries risks as well as benefits. Antimicrobial drugs can be used prophylactically for two purposes:

- **To prevent disease caused by exogenous pathogens**: An example is the administration of antibiotics to persons exposed to patients with meningococcal infections. The meningococcus spreads rapidly among susceptible individuals, but antibiotics such as rifampin can usually forestall its clinical manifestations. Likewise, the antituberculous drug isoniazid is given to persons who are at high risk of acquiring tuberculosis, such as children living in the same quarters as a patient with pulmonary tuberculosis (see Chapter 23).
- **To prevent commensal organisms from spreading from their usual residence to normally sterile sites of the body**: The use of antibiotics to prevent postoperative infections after certain high-risk surgical procedures also falls in this category. Another example is the administration of antibiotics to patients with certain valvular heart conditions, including prosthetic heart valves. The drugs are used to prevent bacteremia and infection of the abnormal valves when patients undergo medical procedures that carry a risk of bacteremia (see Chapter 12).

The risks involved in antibiotic prophylaxis must be clearly understood. They include allergy or other toxic reactions to the drugs, selection of resistant mutants, and masking or delaying the diagnosis of the infection. The following criteria should be met for the prophylactic use of antibiotics:

- A surgical or medical intervention carries a significant risk of microbial contamination. When a surgeon

CASE • Mrs. O., a 67-year-old woman with recurrent thrombophlebitis and pulmonary embolism had been asymptomatic on an oral anticoagulant (warfarin), which maintained her prothrombin (clotting) time at 24 seconds, twice the normal value. Recently diagnosed with pulmonary tuberculosis, Mrs. O. began taking a four-drug regimen her physician prescribed. Several days later, she required hospitalization for recurrence of her thrombophlebitis. Laboratory evaluation revealed that her prothrombin time was only 2 seconds above normal, despite taking the same amount of warfarin. Her physician then learned that rifampin, one of the four antituberculous drugs she was taking, induces the liver to accelerate the clearance of warfarin. Rifampin was

stopped, and Mrs. O. was treated with intravenous heparin to raise her clotting time.

This case illustrates one of the numerous interactions that can occur between drugs. The potential consequences can be catastrophic for the patient, particularly if the therapy affected is life saving, as in this case. Imagine if Mrs. O. had required anticoagulation therapy to prevent clotting on an artificial heart valve. An opposite effect, prolongation of clotting time, could also occur with sulfonamides and metronidazole and lead to massive gastrointestinal bleeding. The severity of such complications cannot be overestimated, and the message must not be lost on the practitioner.

crosses a tissue plane that contains a rich microbial flora, such as the colon or the oral cavity, the risk of infection is unacceptably high, and the administration of prophylactic antibiotics is necessary. Antibiotic prophylaxis should also be used when infection is not extremely likely but could have disastrous effects—for instance, in surgery to implant a heart valve or hip prostheses. Antibiotic prophylaxis is not indicated when the risk of infection is low and the outcome trivial, such as in a hernia operation.

- The antibiotics used prophylactically should be directed against the most likely pathogens. Previous studies should suggest which infectious agents are likely to be involved and what drugs are likely to be effective. In operations involving the colon, antibiotics should cover the microbiota of the intestine. When surgery crosses the oral mucosa, a prophylactic antibiotic with a narrow spectrum is indicated because most of the bacteria in the oral cavity are susceptible to penicillin.
- A suitable concentration of the drug must be achievable at the right time in the relevant tissues. Studies in experimental animals (which have also been confirmed in randomized human studies) have shown that prophylactic antibiotics are of no value when given after surgery is completed. However, their effectiveness is readily apparent when they are given just before surgery and adequate tissue levels are sustained during the operation. It makes sense that a drug should be present in the body when the wound is likely to be contaminated; once the wound is closed, it rapidly becomes impermeable to exogenous bacteria.
- Antimicrobial drugs should be used for a short time to minimize the emergence of drug resistance. Indications for the prophylactic use of antibiotics are expanding with the occurrence of new diseases, new drugs, and new therapeutic methods. The guidelines presented here should be applicable in the development of new indications.

CONCLUSION

Bacterial infections are no longer the inevitable threat to life they often were in the preantibiotic era. Today, the clinician can choose from a vast array of antimicrobial agents with various kinetics, mechanisms, and spectra of activity against microbes. However, the wise clinician uses these agents judiciously, knowing that they pose risks of toxicity, allergy, drug interactions, and selection of resistant flora. Antibiotics can also be used to prevent infections, but the occasions when prophylaxis is appropriate are strictly limited.

Suggested Readings

Bratzler DW, Houck PM, et al. Antimicrobial prophylaxis for surgery: an advisory statement from the National Surgical Infection Prevention Project. *Clin Infect Dis*. 2004;38:1706–1715.

Craig WA. Basic pharmacodynamics of antibacterials with clinical applications to the use of beta-lactams, glycopeptides, and linezolid. *Infect Dis Clin North Am*. 2003;17:479–501.

Fishman N. Antimicrobial stewardship. *Am J Med*. 2006;119(6 suppl 1):S53–S61.

Gandhi TN, DePestel DD, Collins CD, et al. Managing antimicrobial resistance in intensive care units. *Crit Care Med*. 2010;38(8 suppl):S315–S323.

Gold HS, Moellering RC. Antimicrobial-drug resistance. *N Engl J Med*. 1996;335:1445–1454.

Handbook of Antimicrobial Therapy. Medical Letter. Published yearly.

Jacoby GA, Munoz-Price LS. The new beta-lactamases. *N Engl J Med*. 2005;352:380–391.

Pillai SK, Eliopoulis GM, Moellering RC. Principles of anti-infective therapy. In: Mandel GL, Bennett JE, Dolin R, eds. *Principles and Practice of Infectious Diseases*. 7th ed. New York, NY: Churchill Livingstone, 2009.

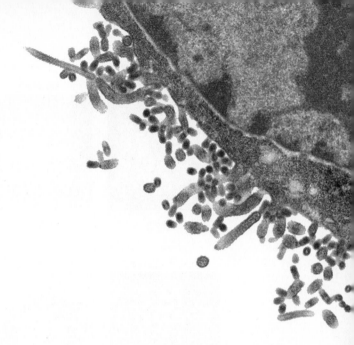

Chapter **31**

Biology of Viruses

Terence S. Dermody and Jeffrey M. Bergelson

KEY CONCEPTS

Pathogens: Viruses are obligate intracellular parasites that use the machinery of the host cell to replicate. They consist of a nucleic acid core surrounded by a protein capsid; the capsid of some viruses is surrounded by an envelope.

Encounter: Infection can be acquired from other humans or from the environment. Direct contact routes include sexual contact and vertical transmission, and environmental routes include respiratory (aerosols), gastrointestinal (fecal–oral contamination), and transcutaneous (inoculation) transmission.

Entry: The viral capsid permits delivery of the genome into the cell; the genome encodes proteins that permit the virus to control the cell and replicate.

Spread: Viral infection can spread through nerves to the central nervous system or through the blood to many organs. Some viruses use multiple pathways to spread.

Replication: Viral infection is often characterized by an incubation period, during which the virus replicates within the host before disease symptoms become evident.

Damage: Viral infection can be acute, latent, or chronic. Damage may be due to direct effects of viral replication on host cells or to the host response to the infection. Infections are controlled primarily by cell-mediated immunity. Humoral immunity prevents reinfection. Innate immunity and intrinsic cellular defenses must be evaded for infection to occur.

Diagnosis: Diagnosis depends on virus isolation in tissue culture or identification of viral antigens or nucleic acids. Some viral infections are diagnosed by the detection of antiviral antibodies.

Treatment: Some viral infections can be attenuated by specific antiviral medications.

Prevention: Many infections can be prevented with vaccines that induce cell-mediated immunity, neutralizing antibodies, or both.

THE FUNDAMENTAL difference between viruses and other infectious agents is in their mechanism of reproduction. Unlike bacteria, viruses do not simply divide. Virus replication is carried out by the host cell machinery, which synthesizes multiple copies of the viral genome and viral proteins. These viral components assemble spontaneously within the host cell to form progeny virus particles. Viruses have no means to produce energy and contain a few enzymes at most. Thus, totally dependent on host cells, viruses are **obligate intracellular parasites**. They are important pathogens of virtually all forms of life, including humans and other animals, plants, and fungi. One type of virus, called bacteriophage, infects bacteria (see Chapter 4). Because they are relatively amenable to study, viruses serve as important models for examination of basic cellular processes.

Viruses are small, although the largest ones (e.g., smallpox virus and the giant mimivirus that infects amoebas) are barely visible with the light microscope. Viruses vary in volume over a 1000-fold range and in structure from relatively simple to very complex (Fig. 31-1). The genomic nucleic acid of a virus is either DNA or RNA.

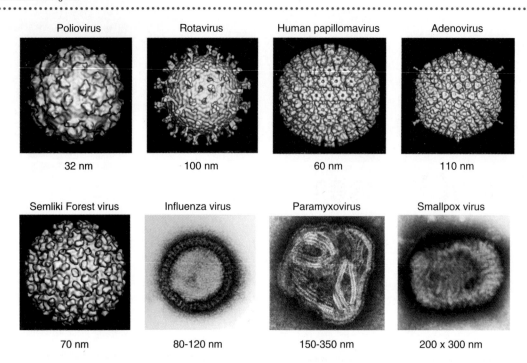

Poliovirus   Rotavirus   Human papillomavirus   Adenovirus

32 nm   100 nm   60 nm   110 nm

Semliki Forest virus   Influenza virus   Paramyxovirus   Smallpox virus

70 nm   80-120 nm   150-350 nm   200 x 300 nm

FIGURE 31-1. Examples of virus morphology. These images of selected viruses were obtained using either cryoelectron microscopy and three-dimensional computer processing or transmission electron microscopy. Poliovirus, rotavirus, HPV, and adenovirus are nonenveloped viruses with icosahedral capsids. Semliki Forest virus, influenza virus, paramyxovirus, and smallpox virus are enveloped viruses. The envelope of Semliki Forest virus is hidden by a dense outer shell formed by the major envelope glycoproteins. The envelope glycoproteins of influenza virus, paramyxovirus, and smallpox virus are less densely arrayed, and their envelopes have less defined structure. Note the characteristic wiggly helical nucleocapsid of the paramyxovirus and the complex structure of smallpox virus.

STRUCTURE AND CLASSIFICATION OF VIRUSES

A virus particle, called a **virion**, can be thought of as a delivery system that surrounds a payload (Fig. 31-2). The delivery system consists of structural components used by the virus to survive in the environment and bind to host cells. The payload contains the viral genome and often includes enzymes required for the initial steps in

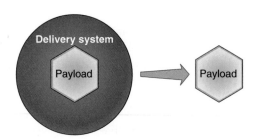

FIGURE 31-2. Schematic diagram of a virus particle. Viruses are simple structures consisting of a delivery system and a payload. The delivery system of a virus protects it against degradation in the environment and contains structures used to bind to target cells in the host. The payload of a virus contains the genome and enzymes necessary to initiate the first steps in virus replication.

virus replication. An eminent scientist once characterized a virus as "a piece of bad news wrapped in a protein coat."

Viral genomes are incredibly diverse. The smallest viral genomes encode three or four proteins, and the largest encode more than 100 structural proteins and enzymes. The number of proteins encoded may be greater than predicted from the size of the nucleic acid. For some viral genomes, the same stretch of nucleic acid may contain multiple open reading frames or overlapping regions that can be transcribed into several distinct messenger RNAs (mRNAs). The viral nucleic acid is surrounded by a **capsid**, a single- or double-layer protein shell. Together, the nucleic acid and the capsid are often referred to as the **nucleocapsid**. Capsids are composed of subunits (sometimes called "capsomers") arranged in symmetric patterns. Each capsid subunit has the capacity to bind to other subunits in specific ways; these physical interactions between subunits permit the subunits to self-assemble to form the virus capsid.

Viral capsid proteins are arranged in two basic structural patterns, **icosahedral** and **helical**. Viruses with icosahedral symmetry contain a defined number of structural subunits (20 triangular faces and 12 vertices), whereas the number of subunits varies in viruses with

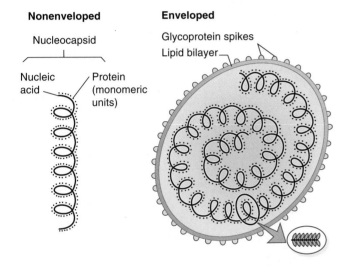

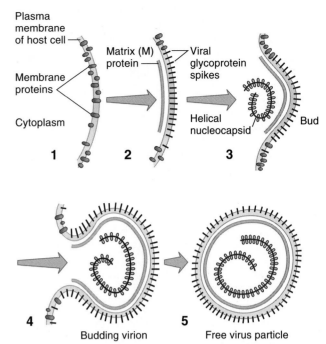

FIGURE 31-4. Virus budding through the cytoplasmic membrane. The host cell plasma membrane seen early in infection (1). Virus-encoded matrix (M) proteins become associated with the plasma membrane (2). Viral glycoprotein spikes are incorporated into the membrane, the viral nucleocapsid is assembled near the membrane, and budding begins (3). Budding continues with further insertion of viral spikes in the membrane (4). Budding is completed, releasing a free virion (5).

FIGURE 31-3. Basic viral forms. The inset depicts the nucleic acid–protein complex, often called the nucleocapsid. The arrow indicates proteins aligned at regular intervals in the helical nucleocapsid.

helical symmetry. Viruses with icosahedral symmetry usually have a spherical shape, like a soccer ball (Fig. 31-3). In those viruses, the nucleic acid is packed inside the spherical core and often tightly associated with specific viral capsid proteins. A general feature of viruses with helical symmetry is that the protein subunits of the capsid are bound in a regular, periodic fashion along the nucleic acid. Some of the largest viruses, such as the poxviruses, have complex structural arrangements.

Many viruses possess an **envelope** that surrounds the nucleocapsid (see Fig. 31-3). Those viruses are called **enveloped viruses**; viruses without an envelope are called **nonenveloped viruses**. The viral envelope is composed of virus-specific proteins plus lipids and carbohydrates derived from host cell membranes (e.g., the nuclear membrane, endoplasmic reticulum, Golgi apparatus, or plasma membrane). In some cases, virus-specific envelope proteins include a **matrix (M) protein** that lines the inner surface of the envelope and is in contact with the nucleocapsid (Fig. 31-4). M proteins may stabilize the interaction between viral glycoproteins and the lipid envelope, direct the viral genome to intracellular

sites of virus assembly, or help in virus budding. Virus-specific envelope glycoproteins protrude from the outer surface of the envelope.

The principal viruses that cause disease in humans belong to about a dozen families containing hundreds of species (Table 31-1, Fig. 31-5). Each species may contain many individual strains that differ in virulence and antigenic properties (serotypes). Viruses are classified according to a number of factors, including their structure, the nature of their genome, and their replication strategy, as well as their immunologic properties and the diseases they cause.

VIRUS REPLICATION

The steps in virus replication include infection of a susceptible cell, reproduction of the viral nucleic acid and proteins, and assembly and release of infectious progeny. The structural and genetic diversity of viruses is reflected in the variety of replicative strategies that they employ (Fig. 31-6). Every event in the virus life cycle makes some use of the host cell's own machinery, and, not surprisingly, viruses have evolved many ways to use and manipulate the host cell for their own ends. Viruses can regulate cellular enzymes, modify cellular structures, and perturb metabolic and signaling pathways. Understanding

TABLE 31-1 Classification of Viruses

Family	Example	Nucleic Acid Polarity or Structure	Genome Size (kb or kbP)	Envelope
RNA Viruses				
Single Stranded				
Picornaviridae	Poliovirus	(+) RNA	7–9	No
Caliciviridae	Norwalk virus	(+) RNA	7–8	No
Togaviridae	Rubella virus	(+) RNA	10–12	Yes
Flaviviridae	Yellow fever virus	(+) RNA	10–12	Yes
Coronaviridae	SARS-CoV	(+) RNA	28–31	Yes
Rhabdoviridae	Rabies virus	(−) RNA	11–15	Yes
Paramyxoviridae	Measles virus	(−) RNA	13–18	Yes
Arenaviridae	Lassa fever virus	Two ambisense RNA segments	11	Yes
Bunyaviridae	Hantavirus	Three (−) RNA segments	11–19	Yes
Orthomyxoviridae	Influenza virus	Eight (−) RNA segments[a]	10–15	Yes
Double Stranded				
Reoviridae	Rotavirus	10–12 dsRNA segments[b]	19–32	No
RNA and DNA Reverse-Transcribing Viruses				
Retroviridae	HIV	Two identical molecules (+) RNA	7–13	Yes
Hepadnaviridae	Hepatitis B virus	Circular dsDNA with ss portions	3–4	Yes
DNA Viruses				
Single Stranded				
Parvoviridae	Human parvovirus B-19	(+) or (−)	4–6	No
Double Stranded				
Polyomaviridae	JC virus	Circular	5	No
Papillomaviridae	Human papillomavirus	Circular	7–8	No
Adenoviridae	Human adenoviruses	Linear	26–45	No
Herpesviridae	Herpes simplex virus	Linear	125–240	Yes
Poxviridae	Vaccinia virus	Linear with covalently closed ends	130–375	Yes

[a]Influenza C has 7 segments.
[b]Reoviruses and orbiviruses have 10 segments; rotavirus has 11 segments; Colorado tick fever has 12 segments.
(+) positive sense; (−) negative sense; ds, double-stranded; SARS, severe acute respiratory syndrome; ss, single-stranded.
Adapted from Condit RC. Principles of virology. In: Knipe DM, Howley PM, eds. *Fields Virology*. 5th ed. Philadelphia, PA: Lippincott-Raven Press; 2007:24–57.

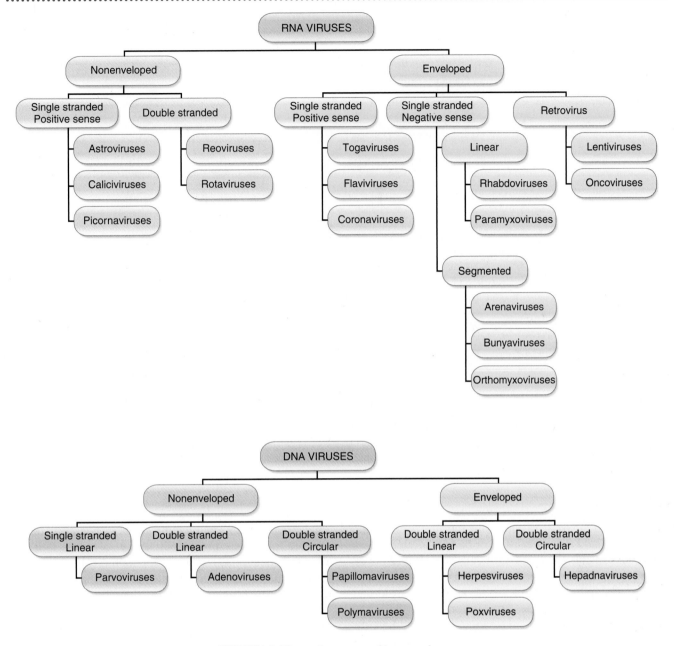

FIGURE 31-5. The main groups of human viruses.

the details of the virus life cycle is important for designing specific antiviral drugs.

Attachment and Penetration

The first step in viral infection of target cells is the attachment of the virus to the host cell surface. That step, which is also called **adsorption**, is initially reversible and results from random collisions between virions and target cells. For enveloped viruses, the attachment protein is usually one of the spikes exposed on the outer surface of the viral envelope, such as the hemagglutinin of influenza virus. Some enveloped viruses, such as the herpesviruses and poxviruses, have more than one type of attachment protein. For nonenveloped viruses, surface-exposed regions of capsid proteins function to mediate virus attachment.

Viruses have adapted to attach to a variety of molecules (receptors) on the cell surface. Viral receptors can be highly specialized proteins with limited tissue distribution, such as CD4 on T cells or neurotransmitter receptors in the brain, or they can be more ubiquitous components of cellular membranes including adhesion molecules, complement regulatory proteins, phospholipids, or carbohydrates. Some viruses use multiple receptors, which may allow them to invade a variety of cell types as infection in the host progresses. Many viruses use distinct molecules for attachment and internalization. For example, HIV binds to both CD4 and one of several chemokine receptors. Utilization of multiple receptors may be important to ensure precise targeting of the virus to particular host cells.

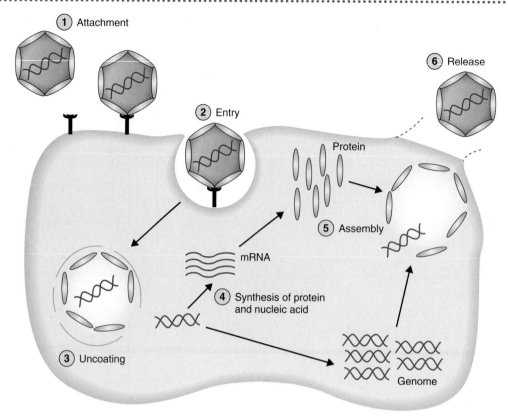

FIGURE 31-6. A prototypical viral life cycle. The process of viral infection begins with attachment to a receptor *(1)* and entry of the virion into the cell *(2)*. The viral capsid (delivery system) is uncoated to release the genome (payload) *(3)*. New viral proteins and genomes are synthesized *(4)*, and progeny virions are assembled *(5)* and released from the cell *(6)*.

Once adsorption has occurred, the entire virion or a component of the payload containing the viral genome and virion-associated polymerases must be translocated across the plasma membrane of the host cell. The entry of enveloped viruses involves fusion of the viral envelope with cell membranes, followed by release of the nucleocapsid into the cell (Fig. 31-7). In some cases, fusion occurs directly at the plasma membrane (measles virus). In others, the virus is taken inside the cell by endocytosis, and fusion occurs with an endosomal membrane inside the cell. Viruses are internalized by a number of endocytic routes. Influenza virus and many others bind receptors that aggregate at distinct sites on the plasma membrane (**clathrin-coated pits**) and then are endocytosed within clathrin-coated vesicles before delivery to endosomes. Nonenveloped viruses cannot fuse with cellular membranes; in many cases, these viruses are endocytosed and escape into the cell by disrupting the endosomal membrane.

The next step in virus replication is **uncoating**, the process in which the capsid is removed to make the viral genome accessible to the cellular transcription and translation machinery. For many viruses, penetration and uncoating occur simultaneously. For certain viruses, contact with the receptor induces conformational changes in the capsid that facilitate release of the viral nucleic acid into the cytoplasm.

Some nonenveloped viruses require host cell enzymes for removal of their capsids. For certain reoviruses, proteases present in late endosomes and lysosomes sequentially remove the outer capsid proteins to produce a "subvirion particle." Those particles penetrate endosomal membranes, leading to activation of virus transcription in the cytoplasm. SV40 needs to pass through the endoplasmic reticulum, where specific

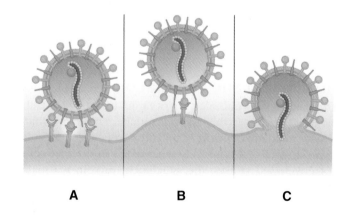

A   **B**   **C**

FIGURE 31-7. Fusion and cell entry of an enveloped virus. **A.** Attachment to cell-surface receptors. **B.** Penetration of the host-cell membrane by a fusion protein. **C.** Merging of the viral envelope and cell membrane.

enzymes reduce disulfide bonds that hold the capsid subunits to each other.

Macromolecular Synthesis

The synthesis of all viral macromolecules first requires the translation of viral mRNA into virus-specific proteins. How is viral mRNA made? Viruses that contain double-stranded DNA synthesize mRNA just as the host cell does, using a DNA-dependent RNA polymerase. RNA viruses, however, must make their mRNA from RNA, which involves a different mechanism. Viruses use several strategies to synthesize viral mRNA and translate it into protein (Fig. 31-8). The variations are described in more detail in the chapters covering the individual virus groups (see Chapters 32 to 43).

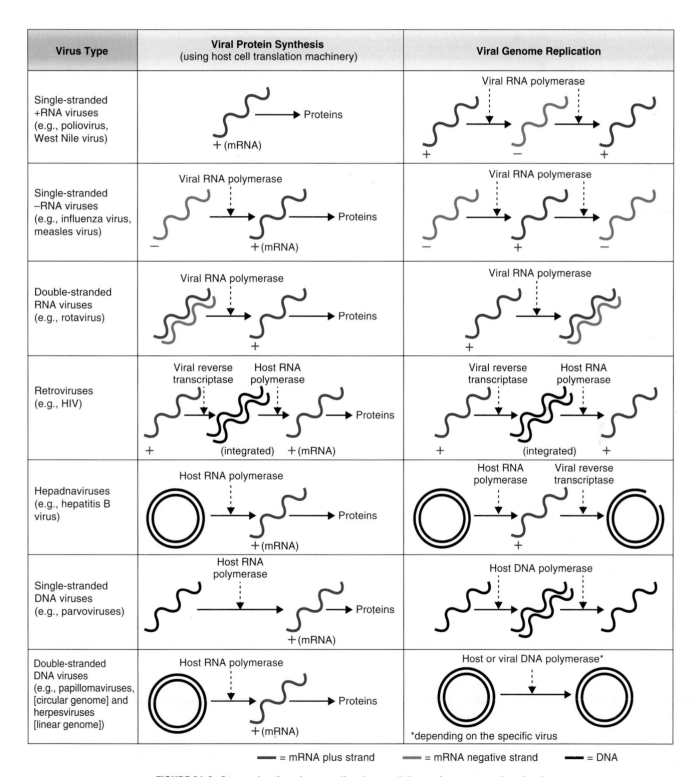

FIGURE 31-8. **Strategies for virus replication and the main enzymes involved.**

Single-Stranded Positive-Sense RNA Viruses

The simplest translation strategy is for the nucleic acid of the virion to function directly as mRNA. Examples of viruses that use that approach are the picornaviruses (e.g., poliovirus) and flaviviruses (e.g., West Nile virus). By convention, the genomes of those viruses are said to have **positive-sense polarity**. Following entry into the host cell, the viral genomic RNA acts as mRNA and is translated by cellular ribosomes to produce the various viral proteins. For certain viruses, such as poliovirus, mRNA is translated into a single large polyprotein that is sequentially cleaved by virus-encoded proteases to release the individual viral proteins; this process leads to expression of viral proteins in equimolar amounts.

For positive-sense RNA viruses, how is the viral RNA synthesized? A **virus-encoded RNA-dependent RNA polymerase** synthesizes a complementary **negative-sense** RNA using genomic RNA as a template. In turn, the newly synthesized negative-sense RNA serves as a template for the synthesis of additional copies of genomic positive-sense RNA. The newly produced genomic RNA may serve as mRNA or may be packaged into progeny virions.

Single-Stranded Negative-Sense RNA Viruses

The RNA of negative-sense viruses does not carry instructions for synthesis of viral proteins; only its complementary strand does. These viruses must therefore use a different strategy to make mRNA. The genomic negative-sense RNA is used as a template to produce mRNA transcripts corresponding to each viral gene. The transcripts differ in abundance, which allows the synthesis of each viral protein to be regulated independently. The genome is replicated by production of a full-length single-stranded positive-sense RNA intermediate, which then serves as a template to synthesize new copies of single-stranded negative-sense genomic RNA. Mammalian cells do not possess enzymes that use RNA as template for making RNA. Therefore, viruses using that strategy must contain an RNA-dependent RNA polymerase in the virion (i.e., part of the payload), which is introduced into host cells during infection.

Some single-stranded negative-sense RNA viruses (e.g., influenza virus) have **segmented genomes**, which consist of more than one RNA molecule. As with the nonsegmented negative-sense RNA viruses, transcription results in unique mRNAs for each viral protein rather than a single large polycistronic mRNA molecule.

Double-Stranded RNA Viruses

The information encoded in double-stranded RNA (like that encoded in DNA) first must be copied into a positive-sense single strand of RNA to act as mRNA. Because of its double-stranded character, the virion RNA cannot function directly as mRNA (even though it contains a positive-sense strand). Viruses with double-stranded RNA genomes, such as the reoviruses and rotaviruses, contain a virus-encoded RNA-dependent RNA polymerase that transcribes single-stranded positive-sense RNAs using the negative-sense strands of the double-stranded RNA segments as templates. The double-stranded RNA genome is always found as segments, each of which is transcribed to produce a unique mRNA.

RNA Viruses That Replicate through a DNA Intermediate

The retroviruses, such as HIV, contain single-stranded positive-sense RNA but employ a unique replicative strategy using a DNA intermediate. Viral positive-sense RNA serves as a template for a virion-associated RNA-dependent DNA polymerase (reverse transcriptase). The DNA is then integrated into host chromosomal DNA, where it resides for the life of the cell. Transcription of the integrated viral DNA, like transcription of host cell genes, is carried out by host cell DNA-dependent RNA polymerases.

DNA Viruses

In general, DNA-containing viruses make mRNA using strategies similar to those of host cells. In cells infected with adenoviruses, herpesviruses, papillomaviruses, and polyomaviruses, transcription of viral DNA into mRNA occurs in the host cell nucleus and depends on host cell enzymes. Transcription of most DNA-containing viruses is tightly regulated and results in synthesis of early and then late mRNA transcripts (Fig. 31-9). The early transcripts encode regulatory proteins and the proteins required for DNA replication, while the late transcripts encode mainly structural proteins of the virion. Several DNA-containing viruses, such as adenovirus and human papillomavirus (HPV), induce cells to express host proteins required for viral DNA replication by stimulating cell cycle progression. For example, the HPV E7 protein binds the retinoblastoma gene product pRB and liberates the transcription factor E2F, which drives the cell to progress through the cell cycle. To prevent programmed cell death in response to E7-mediated unscheduled cell cycle progression, the HPV E6 protein induces the ubiquitylation and degradation of tumor suppressor protein p53.

The individual mRNAs for both early and late viral proteins often correspond to sequences of viral DNA called **exons**, separated by spacer sequences called **introns**. The products of transcription are RNA molecules with sequences identical to those of the DNA. The immature mRNA molecules are cut and then spliced back together to remove the intervening introns. For many viruses, mRNAs are synthesized from overlapping regions of the viral DNA. This redundancy reduces the amount of viral DNA required to encode some viral proteins and is another example of the genetic economy among viruses.

Poxviruses are the most structurally intricate of the animal viruses, and their replicative cycle is correspondingly complex. The initial steps of transcription and translation occur in the host cell cytoplasm. Therefore, poxviruses viruses cannot use host RNA polymerases,

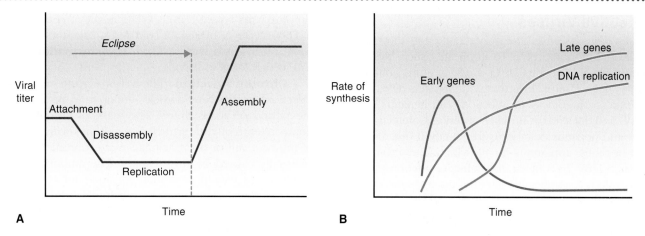

FIGURE 31-9. Virus replication events during a single infectious cycle. A. Viral titer. A single cycle of virus replication can be studied by determining the titer of infectious virus (e.g., by plaque assay) over time. Cells are adsorbed with virus, and at various intervals after adsorption, the cells are lysed, and viral titer is determined. Viral titer is stable during the brief period of virus attachment, indicating that removal of the virus after attachment but before internalization does not diminish infectivity. Following attachment, viral titer declines precipitously as the virus undergoes disassembly, transcription, translation, and genome replication. That interval is termed the eclipse. Viral titer begins to increase as progeny virions, which are fully infectious, are assembled. **B. DNA virus transcription.** Transcription of most DNA viruses results in synthesis of early and late mRNA transcripts. The early transcripts encode regulatory proteins and enzymes required for DNA replication. The late transcripts encode mainly structural proteins of the virion. Initiation of DNA synthesis precedes transcription of the late genes.

which are located in the nucleus. Consequently, poxviruses carry their own DNA-dependent RNA polymerase to initiate transcription. One of the virus-encoded early proteins is responsible for a second stage of uncoating in which the viral DNA is made fully accessible for transcription and replication. Replication, transcription, and virus assembly all occur within virus-initiated organelles, known as "factories," located in the host cell cytoplasm. Early proteins include a number of enzymes (e.g., DNA polymerase and thymidine kinase) and some structural proteins. As infection progresses, DNA replication begins, the synthesis of the early nonstructural proteins ceases, and the synthesis of late proteins takes place. Many of the late proteins are structural proteins, but other late proteins include enzymes and proteins that function in virus assembly.

Assembly of Progeny Virions and Release from the Host Cell

Once new viral genomes and proteins have been synthesized, intact virions are assembled and released from host cells. Assembly of the nonenveloped viruses and the nucleocapsids of enveloped viruses often occurs spontaneously, resulting in crystalline arrays of viral capsids. Once the capsid is formed, it becomes filled with viral nucleic acid, resulting in the production of viable virions (Fig. 31-9).

Nonenveloped viruses are usually released when the cell lyses. Events leading to cell disruption include inhibition of the synthesis of host cell macromolecules,

disorganization of the host cell cytoskeleton, and alteration of host cell membrane structure. Membrane disruption may result in increased cell permeability and the release of proteolytic enzymes from lysosomes. Failure of the host cell to replenish energy-rich substrate molecules inhibits the function of ion transport pumps and disturbs transport of essential nutrients and cellular waste products.

Enveloped viruses are usually released from infected cells by budding. This process may or may not be lethal to the cell. In all cases, virus-encoded proteins inserted into host cell membranes displace some of the normal protein components, which results in restructuring of the membrane. Viral capsids may then bind to virus-encoded M (matrix) proteins lining the cytoplasmic surface of the altered patches of membrane (see Fig. 31-4). Many viruses are capable of inducing the genetically programmed mechanism of cell death that leads to **apoptosis** of host cells. Apoptotic cell death is characterized by cell shrinkage, membrane blebbing, condensation of nuclear chromatin, and cleavage of cellular DNA. These changes occur according to predetermined developmental programs or in response to certain environmental stimuli. In some cases, apoptosis serves as an antiviral defense mechanism to limit virus replication by either the destruction of virus-infected cells or the reduction of potentially harmful inflammatory responses elicited by infection. In other cases, apoptosis results from viral induction of cellular factors required for efficient virus replication and may aid in virus release.

Defective Viruses

Certain viruses cause disease even though they cannot replicate autonomously. To replicate, such **defective viruses** (e.g., hepatitis delta virus) require coinfection with a "helper" virus. Infection with hepatitis delta virus is dependent on coincident infection with hepatitis B virus (HBV) and does not occur in its absence. Coinfection with HBV and hepatitis delta virus frequently results in fulminant hepatitis, apparently by allowing increased multiplication of HBV. In contrast, the defective adeno-associated viruses do not significantly alter the disease caused by the helper adenovirus. Defective viruses can be detected by searching for their antigens or nucleic acids or by culture in the presence of helper viruses.

VIRAL DISEASES
PATHOBIOLOGY

The signs and symptoms of viral disease are the culmination of a series of interactions between the virus and the host. After encountering a host cell, a virus must be able to enter it, undergo primary replication, and then spread to a final target tissue. Once a virus reaches its target organs, it must infect and successfully replicate in a susceptible population of host cells.

One of three possible outcomes follows infection of a host organism by a virus: acute infection, latent infection, or chronic infection (Fig. 31-10). In an **acute infection**, the virus undergoes multiple rounds of replication. Replication results in the death of the host cell, which is used as a factory for virus production. Examples of acute infections are those caused by poliovirus or influenza virus.

At the opposite end of the spectrum is **latent infection**, which does not result in the production of progeny virus. Latent infections, which are caused by DNA viruses or retroviruses, reflect the persistence of viral DNA either as an extrachromosomal element (herpesviruses) or as an integrated sequence within the host genome (retroviruses). During cell growth, the genome of the virus is replicated along with the chromosomes of the host cell. An example of latent infection is that produced by herpes simplex virus type 1 (HSV-1). The result of **reactivation** of HSV-1 is fever blisters or cold sores. Latent infection by some retroviruses may result in **transformation** of the cell, which leads to cancer.

Chronic infection differs from acute and latent infections in that virus particles continue to be shed after the period of acute illness. The mark of chronic infection is release of virus particles, sometimes without death of the host cell or overt cellular injury. Chronic infection is usually caused by RNA viruses. The amount of virus produced is usually less than in acute infections, and the viruses are often altered ("mutated") from the original ones. Chronic infections are associated with defective host immune responses that are insufficient to clear the infection. Some chronic infections do not result in overt disease, although they can produce disease after a prolonged interval. For example, hepatitis C virus can cause a chronic infection in the liver that eventually leads to chronic hepatitis and even liver cancer.

ENCOUNTER AND ENTRY

Transmission of a virus from an infected host to a susceptible individual can occur in various ways (Table 31-2). The sources of human-to-human transmission of viruses are acutely ill individuals or chronic carriers; pregnant women also can transmit viruses to their fetuses. Transmission is accomplished by direct contact, such as sexual contact (as in HIV infection) or through the environment. Environmental spread may involve fecal–oral contamination (as in the diarrhea caused by rotaviruses), aerosols (as in chickenpox), or direct inoculation from infected needles or blood products (as in hepatitis B or C). Animal-to-human transmission usually occurs from the bite of a diseased animal (as in rabies) or the bite of an insect vector (as in many types of viral encephalitis).

For most viruses, it is not known how many particles are required to initiate an infection. For adenovirus, coxsackie A21 virus, and influenza A virus, as few as 10 particles may suffice. In other cases, the number is likely to be considerably larger.

Respiratory Route

Respiratory infection takes place by means of aerosol droplets, nasal secretions, or saliva. Respiratory aerosolization usually occurs from coughing or sneezing. A cough can generate up to 90,000 aerosol particles, and a sneeze up to 2 million! The fate of those particles depends on both ambient environmental conditions (e.g., humidity and wind currents) and particle size. Small particles remain airborne longer and may escape the filtering action of the nose, which traps particles larger than 6 μm in diameter; viruses transmitted in small droplets (e.g., varicella-zoster virus [VZV]) are highly contagious. Aerosolization is not the only possible route of respiratory transmission. Epstein-Barr virus (EBV) is usually spread by saliva, and some respiratory viruses can spread in

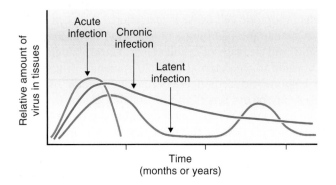

FIGURE 31-10. The three types of viral infections.

TABLE 31-2 Routes of Virus Transmission

Route	Virus
Respiratory	
Airborne small droplet	Influenza virus
	Measles virus
	Smallpox virus (?)
	Varicella-zoster virus
Airborne large droplet	Adenovirus
	Parainfluenza virus
	Parvovirus
	Smallpox virus
Direct contact with respiratory secretions	Respiratory syncytial virus
	Rhinovirus
Gastrointestinal	
Fecal–oral	Enteric adenovirus
	Hepatitis A virus
	Norwalk virus
	Poliovirus and other enteroviruses
	Rotavirus
Contact with lesions	Herpes simplex virus
	Smallpox virus
	Varicella-zoster virus
Blood and body fluids	Cytomegalovirus
	Epstein-Barr virus
	Hepatitis B virus
	Hepatitis C virus
	HIV
Insect bites	Chikungunya virus
	Dengue virus
	Eastern, western equine encephalitis virus
	La Crosse virus
	West Nile virus
	Yellow fever virus

child-care facilities by persisting on contaminated toys. Rhinoviruses, which cause the common cold, are most efficiently spread not by aerosols but from contaminated hands to eyes, nose, or mouth—a cycle that can be interrupted by hand washing.

Entry via the respiratory route requires that the virus overcome a formidable series of host defenses. Respiratory epithelial cells are covered by a thick glycocalyx and tracheobronchial mucus that can trap virus particles. Ciliated respiratory epithelial cells continually sweep mucus up from the lower respiratory tract into the upper respiratory tract, where it is usually swallowed. In the lung, immunologic defenses include secretory IgA, natural killer (NK) cells, and macrophages.

Gastrointestinal Route

Gastrointestinal transmission occurs when viruses shed in feces contaminate food or water subsequently ingested by a susceptible individual (fecal–oral spread). Stool-tainted hands, resulting from poor personal hygiene, provide another vehicle of spread for enteric viruses. The high incidence of enteric virus infections in child-care centers reflects the difficulty of maintaining hygiene in those settings.

Gastrointestinal transmission is limited to viruses that can withstand the harsh environment of the gastrointestinal tract. The acidity of the stomach inactivates acid-labile viruses such as rhinoviruses. Bile salts, present in the lumen of the small intestine, can destroy the lipid envelopes of many viruses and may explain why entry via the gastrointestinal route is limited largely to nonenveloped viruses. Proteolytic enzymes and secretory IgA also contribute to host antiviral defenses in the gastrointestinal tract. However, certain proteolysis-resistant viral capsid proteins allow some viruses to withstand digestion in the gut.

For some enteric viruses, passage across the mucosal barrier of the gut is mediated by **microfold (M) cells** overlying mucosal lymphoid tissues known as Peyer patches. M cells, and perhaps their analogs in bronchial lymphoid tissue, appear to facilitate transport of some viruses across the mucosal epithelium.

Transcutaneous Route

The stratum corneum of the skin provides both a physical and biological barrier against the entry of viruses. Some viruses overcome the skin barrier by direct inoculation from insect or animal bites or from mechanical devices such as needles.

In viral diseases in which the vector is an insect or an infected animal, the disease cycle may be complex. For example, transmission of dengue virus is characterized by a continuous cycle between humans and infected mosquitoes. Dengue viruses multiply in the gut of a mosquito, spread to its salivary glands, and are injected into a human as the mosquito takes a blood meal. Virus replication within the host leads to a high titer of virus in the bloodstream (**viremia**), which is sufficient to allow the virus to be picked up by an uninfected mosquito during biting. In other arthropodborne virus infections, humans are "dead-end" hosts because the degree of viremia in infected individuals is insufficient to transmit the infection to a new group of insect vectors. Examples of that type of cycle are found in the togaviruses, such as the various equine encephalitis viruses. The normal animal reservoirs for togaviruses include small birds and mammals. Horses, like humans, are also usually dead-end hosts, although in Venezuelan equine encephalitis, horses may be a reservoir of virus.

Some arthropodborne viruses do not require a viremic vertebrate intermediate host to maintain a transmission cycle in nature. These viruses are passed in transovarian fashion to the progeny of infected insects or by sexual transmission between males and females. Transovarian transmission may allow survival of arthropodborne viruses through the winter months.

Iatrogenic inoculation (caused by diagnostic or therapeutic procedures) sometimes allows the entry of viruses. Cytomegalovirus (CMV), HBV, and HIV may be present in contaminated blood products used for transfusion, although various screening procedures have diminished the risk of that means of transmission. Iatrogenic inoculation can be purposeful and benevolent, as in the case of vaccination using live, attenuated viruses (e.g., the measles virus or Sabin poliovirus vaccines).

Sexual Route

Sexual transmission with entry across the genitourinary or rectal mucosa is important for HBV, HSV, HIV, and some types of HPV. The virus can spread to other organs, but with some viruses, such as HSV, lesions are often found near the site of entry.

Endogenous and Exogenous Viruses

Most viral diseases result from exposure to **exogenous** virus. However, some viral diseases result from the reactivation of an **endogenous** virus that has been latent within specific host cells. Examples of infections caused by reactivated endogenous viruses include shingles (VZV), progressive multifocal leukoencephalopathy (caused by JC or BK polyomaviruses), recurrent oral and genital herpes (HSV), and some types of CMV infections. Many latent viruses are held in check by the cellular immune system, and aging or immunosuppressive therapies can lead to virus reactivation.

For the majority of viral diseases, transmission of viruses occurs between members of a susceptible host population (**horizontal spread**). **Vertical spread** of infection occurs when the fetus becomes infected in utero through virus carried in the germ cell line, virus infecting the placenta, or virus in the maternal birth canal. CMV, HBV, HIV, HSV, rubella virus, and VZV can produce vertically transmitted congenital infections.

SPREAD AND REPLICATION

For some viruses, the processes of entry, primary replication, and tissue tropism all occur at the same anatomic site. Examples of that type of viral infection include the upper and lower respiratory infections caused by the orthomyxoviruses, paramyxoviruses, and rhinoviruses, the enteritis caused by rotaviruses, and the dermatologic lesions induced by HPV (warts). Other viruses enter at one site and, to produce disease, subsequently spread to a distant area, such as the central nervous system (CNS). In these diseases, it is useful to distinguish between primary virus replication near the entry site and secondary replication at the eventual target organ or tissue. Enteroviruses enter via the gastrointestinal tract and spread to the CNS to produce meningitis, encephalitis, or poliomyelitis. Measles virus and VZV enter the body through the respiratory tract but then spread to produce skin disease (resulting in a rash or **exanthem**) and often generalized organ involvement. Neural, hematogenous, and lymphatic pathways can be used by viruses to spread to target tissues.

A great deal of virus replication can occur before any signs or symptoms of clinical illness are evident. The **incubation period** varies from a few days (influenza) to weeks (measles and varicella) or months (hepatitis and rabies). Viral infection does not always lead to overt clinical disease. The percentage of infected people who develop overt disease ranges from 100% (measles and rabies) to nearly zero (BK and JC polyomaviruses). For many viral infections, symptomatic disease is less common in children than in adults (e.g., EBV mononucleosis, hepatitis A, and paralytic poliomyelitis).

Neural Spread

Examples of viruses that spread through nerves include HSV, rabies virus, and VZV. HSV is thought to enter nerves through receptors located primarily near synaptic endings rather than on the nerve cell body. Rabies virus accumulates at the motor end plate of the neuromuscular junction and may use the acetylcholine receptor or a closely related structure to enter the distal axons of motor neurons. Rabies virus also infects muscle and spreads through motor and sensory nerves to the spinal cord.

The kinetics of neural spread for HSV, poliovirus, and rabies virus suggest that these agents use intraneuronal mechanisms involved in fast axonal transport. Infection of Schwann cells may provide another pathway of dissemination to the CNS. Neural spread is important not only for entry into the CNS but also for spread within the CNS and from the CNS to the periphery (as in reactivation of latent HSV infections).

The olfactory system presents a special pathway for neural spread. The rod processes of olfactory receptor cells lie exposed in the olfactory mucosa and are the only place in the body where the nervous system is in direct contact with the environment. Experimental intranasal or aerosol inoculations of HSV, poliovirus, rabies virus, and some togaviruses have led to CNS infection via the olfactory route. That route may provide a pathway to the CNS in humans for rabies virus and possibly other viruses in circumstances where high-titer aerosols are present, such as in caves occupied by large numbers of rabid bats or in accidental laboratory-acquired infections. The olfactory route of spread might explain the localization of HSV in the orbitofrontal and medial temporal cortex in cases of HSV encephalitis.

Hematogenous Spread

Hematogenous spread is an important mechanism of dissemination for many viruses. A period of primary replication usually precedes the initial viremia and may be asymptomatic or result in prodromal symptoms. For enteric viruses, primary replication often occurs in Peyer patches and peritonsillar lymphatic tissue. For respiratory viruses, primary replication is thought to take place in epithelial or alveolar cells. In some cases, virus travels through lymphatics from the site of primary replication to regional lymph nodes before entering the bloodstream. The initial (primary) viremia often disseminates the virus to tissues like the spleen and liver, where continued replication in parenchymal cells leads to an amplified secondary viremia. Growth in endothelial cells may help sustain the viremic phase in some togavirus infections. Sustained secondary amplification of the viremia is required if the virus is to overcome clearance by lymphoreticular cells.

Bloodborne virus particles may travel free in the plasma or in association with cells. Enteroviruses, HBV, and togaviruses all travel free within plasma; Colorado tick fever virus and Rift Valley fever virus are associated with red blood cells; CMV, EBV, HIV, and rubella virus are associated with lymphocytes or monocytes.

Multiple Pathways for Spread

Some viruses use different pathways of spread at different stages in the infectious cycle. VZV disseminates to the skin by the hematogenous route to produce "chickenpox" (varicella) and then spreads centripetally along nerves from the skin to neurons in the dorsal root ganglion, where it becomes latent. Reactivation results in centrifugal spread of virus along sensory nerves to their skin dermatome, which produces "shingles" (zoster). Neural spread of virus accounts for recurrent episodes of oral and genital infections caused by HSV. Poliovirus is an example of a virus capable of spreading by both hematogenous and neural routes. The hematogenous route is generally accepted as the primary pathway to the CNS, although the virus may spread to the CNS from the gut through autonomic nerves or from infected muscle through peripheral nerves.

HOST FACTORS IN DEFENSE AND DAMAGE

A large number of innate and adaptive host defense mechanisms are involved in protection against viruses. The age and genetic makeup of the host have a strong influence on the outcome of certain viral infections. For example, newborns are particularly susceptible to severe disseminated HSV infections. In contrast, many of the exanthematous illnesses, EBV infections, and poliovirus infections are usually more severe in older individuals than in children. Specific host genes may help determine susceptibility to certain viral infections by influencing immune responsiveness or altering viral receptors. Inadequate host nutrition may increase susceptibility to some viruses such as measles virus, perhaps by depressing cell-mediated immunity; malnutrition accounts for the high mortality associated with measles in some developing countries. The host may influence viral infections in other ways that are still poorly understood. For example, stress can trigger recurrent fever blisters (herpes labialis), but how that occurs is unknown.

The most important adaptive defense mechanism against viral infections is cell-mediated immunity. Persons with defective cell-mediated immunity but normal capacity to make antibodies often have prolonged viral infections. This situation is most evident in persons with AIDS or in stem cell transplant recipients, who may suffer fatal infections with herpesviruses and respiratory viruses that normally cause self-limited illnesses in immunocompetent persons. Antibody deficiency by itself usually does not change the outcome of viral infections (although antibody-deficient persons can suffer from severe and chronic infections caused by enteroviruses). However, the protective effects of viral vaccines depend largely on antiviral antibodies that neutralize viruses and prevent them from establishing infection. Phagocytosis by neutrophils does not play an important role in defense against viral infections. Macrophages, on the other hand, are often involved in virus containment and can limit the spread of viruses in the body.

Intrinsic Protective Mechanisms

Beyond the extrinsic protective mechanisms (anatomic barriers and innate and adaptive immune responses) discussed in Chapters 6 and 7, mammalian cells have evolved a number of intrinsic mechanisms that act to limit viral infections. Cells respond to many virus infections by activating a cell death program (apoptosis) that prevents completion of the viral life cycle. Virus infection can induce a cellular stress response (**autophagy**) that results in viral sequestration and degradation in cytoplasmic organelles called autophagosomes. There exist several host proteins that restrict infection by certain viruses. For example, a cytidine deaminase called APOBEC induces multiple mutations in the HIV genome. Other restriction factors inhibit uncoating (TRIM5) or trap newly budded virus on the cell surface (tetherin) preventing release and spread. Successful viruses have evolved specific mechanisms to counteract apoptosis, autophagy, or cellular restriction factors.

Innate Immune Responses

The innate immune system (discussed in more detail in Chapter 6) recognizes macromolecules likely to be expressed by microbial pathogens but not by host cells (pathogen-associated molecular patterns). Tolllike receptors (TLRs) and intracytosolic sensors (e.g., RIG-I) are activated by viral components such as viral glycoproteins and double-stranded RNA, respectively, triggering inflammatory responses, cytokine and interferon secretion, and activation of the adaptive immune system. Virtually all viruses deploy countermeasures to evade recognition by the innate immune system and block its functions. Patients with defects in innate immunity—for example, those with defects in specific TLRs or interferon production or signaling—may suffer from devastating viral infections.

Cell-Mediated Immunity

Cell-mediated immunity is a major factor in both the termination of viral infections and the pathogenesis of viral diseases. Because of the viral intracellular habitat, infected cells are susceptible to the action of lymphocytes that recognize viral antigens bound to major histocompatibility complex (MHC) proteins on their surface (see Chapter 7). Virus-infected cells can be lysed by several types of lymphoid cells through antibody-independent and antibody-dependent pathways.

Cytotoxicity by **NK cells** provides one of the earliest host defenses against viral infection (peak activity at 2 to 3 days) and precedes the appearance of cytotoxic T lymphocytes (CTLs) and virus-specific antibody responses. NK cells are large granular lymphocytes that recognize and kill some virus-infected cells. Activation of NK cells is regulated by signals from a variety of cell-surface receptors that recognize the presence or absence of ligands, such as MHC antigens, on target cells. Viruses, by modulating expression of these ligands, may render cells susceptible to NK-mediated lysis. NK cells appear to be particularly important for the control of CMV and other herpesvirus infections.

CTLs constitute a **specific** virus-induced defense mechanism because they must be activated by antigen presented by macrophages or other antigen-presenting cells. Lysis of infected cells mediated by CTLs is restricted to cells that express MHC class I proteins, although examples of MHC class II-restricted CTLs have been described (see Chapter 7). In contrast to neutralizing antibodies, which usually recognize epitopes on intact viral surface proteins, CTLs recognize protein fragments derived from both viral surface and internal proteins.

Antibody Response

Most viruses are sufficiently antigenic to stimulate a specific immune response. Viruses contain many foreign proteins, each of which may contain multiple antigenic sites. Although the amount of viral antigenic material may be initially quite small, it is amplified during virus replication.

Antibodies do not usually play a primary role in terminating acute viral infections. Instead, antibodies are important in preventing reinfection. In some cases, antibodies may themselves be implicated in the pathogenesis of disease (e.g., in dengue hemorrhagic fever).

Antibodies that protect the host by destroying the infectivity of the virus are called **neutralizing antibodies**. They are usually directed against epitopes present on viral proteins located on the surface of the virus particle. Neutralizing antibodies are thought to reduce viral infectivity by inhibiting early steps of the replication cycle such as attachment, penetration, or uncoating of the virus. In addition, such antibodies may produce aggregation of virions or enhance viral opsonization and subsequent phagocytosis. If two isolates of a virus are neutralized by the same specific antibody, they are said to belong to a single **serotype** (or "type"). Neutralizing antibodies directed against one member of a serotype will protect against reinfection by other members of the same serotype but not against viruses belonging to a different serotype. There are nearly 100 serotypes of rhinovirus; therefore, after recovering from an upper respiratory infection caused by a rhinovirus, a person remains susceptible to many other types. Although polioviruses, like rhinoviruses, belong to the picornavirus family, there are only three poliovirus serotypes. Poliovirus vaccines include each of the three serotypes to provide protection against poliomyelitis.

Antibodies also can participate in lysis of virus-infected cells via **antibody-dependent cell-mediated cytotoxicity** (ADCC; see Chapter 7). In ADCC immune responses, virus-specific antibodies bound to antigens on the surface of infected cells interact with receptors for the Fc portion of IgG on the surface of NK cells. Binding of IgG to Fc receptors activates the NK cells and results in target cell killing. Macrophages, lymphocytes, and neutrophils also have Fc receptors and may participate in ADCC.

Interferons

In addition to adaptive humoral and cellular defense mechanisms, viral infections elicit an inducible defense mechanism, the **interferons**. These are proteins synthesized by host cells in response to viruses and other proinflammatory agents. Interferons inhibit virus replication indirectly by inducing the expression of cellular proteins that inhibit the protein synthesis machinery. The discovery and practical applications of interferons are discussed in Chapter 44.

There are three main kinds of interferons: interferon-α is produced by leukocytes, interferon-β is produced by fibroblasts and epithelial cells, and interferon-γ is usually produced by T cells activated by specific antigens.

Interferon-α and interferon-β are induced by viable and inactivated viruses, double-stranded RNA, and a number of other compounds. Newly produced interferon is released into the extracellular fluid and binds to specific interferon receptors on adjacent cells. Consequently, interferon tends to act locally rather than systemically. Binding of interferon to its receptor leads to a series of intracellular signaling events. These events in turn lead to the expression of a large number of cellular genes that act in concert to create an "antiviral state." For example, interferon induces the expression of a protein kinase called **PKR** that phosphorylates a protein synthesis initiation factor. In the phosphorylated form, this factor cannot participate in the formation of the protein synthesis–initiation complex, thus leading to inhibition of viral protein synthesis. Other interferon-induced factors degrade viral RNA (RNase L), interfere with trafficking of nucleocapsids, inhibit viral budding, and stimulate production of nitric oxide. Interferons also increase the activity of NK cells, CTLs, and cells involved in ADCC.

Virus-Induced Immunopathology

Immunological injury results from cell lysis elicited by one or more of the antiviral host defense mechanisms. Such damage was seen in children immunized with an inactivated measles virus vaccine who experienced severe disease when later infected with measles virus. The role of cell-mediated immunity is dramatically illustrated in mice infected with the virus that causes lymphocytic choriomeningitis. When inoculated intracerebrally with the virus, normal mice die within about a week. However, mice with defective cell-mediated immunity survive inoculation even though virus multiplication is unaffected. In humans, lymphocytic infiltrates are responsible for much of the myocardial damage that follows viral infections of the heart.

Virus-induced immunopathology also can result from antibody production. Viruses may combine with virus-specific antibodies to form circulating immune complexes to cause a variety of diseases. Immune complexes become trapped in basement membranes at various sites, including the skin, kidney, choroid plexus, and walls of blood vessels. Accumulation of immune complexes results in tissue injury by attracting and activating a variety of inflammatory mediators. In addition, virus stimulation of B lymphocytes can induce cross-reacting antibodies to normal host structures that contain antigenic regions similar to those of the virus (**molecular mimicry**).

Virus Evasion of the Immune System

Viruses have evolved several mechanisms to evade the immune response. Perhaps the best adapted is HIV, which replicates and spreads within macrophages and T lymphocytes of the immune system itself. Other viruses avoid CTL responses by blocking antigen processing (CMV and HSV) or by inhibiting MHC expression (adenovirus and CMV). To prevent NK cell recognition of MHC-deficient cells, CMV encodes an MHC-like protein that engages inhibitory receptors on NK cells. HSV and some poxviruses express glycoproteins that interfere with complement activation, and a number of viruses encode cytokine homologs that interfere with normal immunologic functions. Other viruses express molecules that inhibit interferon responses or block effectors of apoptosis.

DIAGNOSIS

A reasonably accurate diagnosis of some viral illnesses, such as measles or varicella, can be made on clinical grounds alone. In other cases, the best that can be done clinically is to identify the group of viruses that are the likely pathogens. More definitive diagnosis is often necessary because many of the available antiviral agents have activities that are limited to certain types of viruses. To make a definitive diagnosis, the clinician must isolate the virus in tissue culture, identify the virus or detect virus-specific antigens or viral nucleic acids in tissues or body fluids, or demonstrate specific serologic responses (Table 31-3).

Isolation of virus from clinical specimens usually involves inoculation of cultured cells. The cultures are then examined for distinctive patterns of **cytopathic effect**. Viruses such as HSV and many enteroviruses produce cytopathic effect within a few days, whereas cytopathic effect due to CMV, rubella virus, and some adenoviruses may take weeks to appear. The identity of the virus can be confirmed by staining infected cells with antibodies to

TABLE 31-3 Diagnostic Methods for Common Human Viruses

Virus	Method
Adenovirus (gastrointestinal)	ELISA
Adenovirus (respiratory)	Antigen, PCR, culture
Cytomegalovirus	Antigen, PCR, culture
Enteroviruses (echovirus, coxsackievirus, poliovirus)	PCR, culture
Epstein-Barr virus	PCR, serology
Hepatitis A virus	Serology
Hepatitis B virus	Antigen, PCR, serology
Hepatitis C virus	PCR, serology
Herpes simplex virus	Antigen, PCR, culture
HIV	PCR, serology
Influenza virus	ELISA, antigen, culture, PCR
Parainfluenza virus	Antigen, PCR, culture
Respiratory syncytial virus	ELISA, antigen, PCR, culture
Rotavirus	ELISA
Varicella-zoster virus	Antigen, PCR

ELISA, enzyme-linked immunosorbent assay; PCR, polymerase chain reaction.

detect specific viral antigens. Different viruses may grow in different cells, and some clinically important viruses cannot be detected in routine cultures.

A specific diagnosis also can be made serologically by detecting IgM antibodies to a specific agent or measuring antibodies in both the acute and convalescent stages of illness (a period of 3 to 4 weeks) and showing a significant (greater than or equal to fourfold) rise in titer. The timing of antiviral antibody responses and their sensitivity and specificity differ greatly.

Virus culture and serologic tests are quite slow, and most viral diagnosis now depends on direct detection of viral antigens or nucleic acids in clinical specimens. Rapid antigen tests are available for influenza and other respiratory viruses, and many clinical laboratories provide a variety of polymerase chain reaction (PCR) tests for common viruses. In special cases, less common viruses can be identified by nucleic acid hybridization using "virochips," which include thousands of probes to detect virtually all identified viruses. Another new approach involves high-throughput nucleic acid sequencing of clinical samples and comparison with sequence databases. Of course, as diagnostic tests become broader and more sensitive, it may become harder to know whether the identified virus is a true pathogen or just an innocent bystander.

EMERGING VIRUSES

New viruses continue to be identified, and new viral diseases continue to appear. During our careers, the authors of this chapter have experienced the identification of human herpesvirus 6 (HHV-6) as the cause of roseola (1986), the isolation of hepatitis C as the agent for non-A, non-B hepatitis (1988), and the identification of human metapneumovirus as a common agent of pneumonia in young children (2002). More dramatically, the emergence of new illnesses—such as the AIDS epidemic first noted in 1981, the outbreak of hantavirus pulmonary syndrome in 1993, and the severe acute respiratory syndrome (SARS) epidemic of 2003—has led to the discovery of new viral agents. The ease of international travel and the threat of bioterrorism have caused concerns that relatively exotic pathogens (Ebola virus, Lassa fever virus, and West Nile virus) or viruses from the past (smallpox virus) may appear unexpectedly. The general principles discussed in this chapter may provide a framework for understanding the biology of these emerging pathogens, but each new virus is likely to have its own specific life cycle, evolutionary adaptations, and interactions with the immune system.

CONCLUSION

Viruses are simple structures that contain two components: a delivery system (the viral envelope and capsid) and a payload (the information contained in the viral genome). Viruses are obligate intracellular parasites that depend on the host cell for most essential enzymatic functions. Depending on the virus replication strategy, the virus may need to encode some enzymes or incorporate an essential replication enzyme in the virion. Viral pathogenesis depends on an ordered series of interactions between a virus and its host: entry, uncoating, and primary replication; many viruses then spread to other target tissues within the body. Many components of innate and adaptive immunity act to defend against viral infections. Cell-mediated immunity is responsible for termination of acute viral infections, and humoral immunity is responsible for protection against reinfection. New viruses likely will continue to emerge, posing unique challenges for the development of antiviral drugs and vaccines.

Suggested Readings

Baranowski ECM, Ruiz-Jarabo CM, Domingo E. Evolution of cell recognition by viruses. *Science.* 2001;292:1102–1105.

Condit RC. Principles of virology. In: Knipe DM, Howley PM, eds. *Fields Virology.* 5th ed. Philadelphia, PA: Lippincott Williams & Wilkins; 2007:24–57.

Chappell JD, Dermody TS. Introduction to viruses and viral diseases. In: Mandell GL, Bennett JE, Dolin R, eds. *Mandell, Douglas, and Bennett's Principles and Practices of Infectious Diseases.* 7th ed. New York: Churchill Livingstone; 2010: 1907–1921.

Collinge DB, Jørgensen HJ, Lund OS, et al. BST-2/tetherin: a new component of the innate immune response to enveloped viruses. *Trends Microbiol.* 2010;18:388–396.

den Boon JA, Diaz A, Ahlquist P. Cytoplasmic viral replication complexes. *Cell Host Microbe.* 2010;8:77–85

Feng H, Shuda M, Chang Y, Moore PS. Clonal integration of a polyomavirus in human Merkel cell carcinoma. *Science.* 2008;319:1096–1100.

Mercer J, Schelhaas M, Helenius A. Virus entry by endocytosis. *Annu Rev Biochem.* 2010;79:803–833.

Novel Swine-Origin Influenza A (H1N1) Virus Investigation Team. Emergence of a novel swine-origin influenza A (H1N1) virus in humans. *N Engl J Med.* 2009;360:2605–2615,

Sharp PM. Origins of human virus diversity. *Cell.* 2002; 108:305–312.

Virgin S. Pathogenesis of viral infections. In: Knipe DM, Howley PM. *Fields Virology.* 5th ed. Philadelphia, PA: Lippincott Williams & Wilkins; 2007:327–388.

Wilkins C, Gale M Jr. Recognition of viruses by cytoplasmic sensors. *Curr Opin Immunol.* 2010;22:41–47.

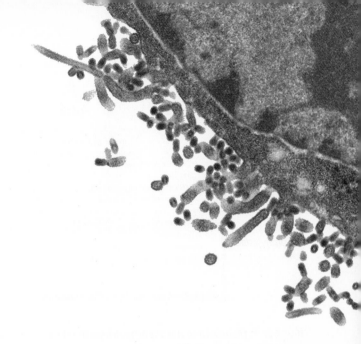

Chapter **32**

Picornaviruses and Coronaviruses

Vincent R. Racaniello and Mark R. Denison

KEY CONCEPTS

Pathogens: Picornaviruses are a family of small, positive-sense RNA viruses, including enteroviruses and hepatitis A virus. Enteroviruses include polioviruses, coxsackieviruses, echoviruses, rhinoviruses, and others.

Enteroviruses (except rhinoviruses)

Encounter: Wild-type polioviruses have been eradicated from the Western Hemisphere because of immunization programs, but they persist in some parts of Asia and Africa. Coxsackieviruses and echoviruses are common infections worldwide.

Entry: Originally named because they infect the gastrointestinal (GI) tract.

Replication: These viruses replicate in the intestine and can be shed in the stool weeks to months after infection.

Spread: Polioviruses can spread from the GI tract to the central nervous system. Other enteroviruses also enter from the GI tract but have tropisms for different organs.

Damage: Polioviruses can cause asymptomatic infection, aseptic meningitis, or flaccid paralysis. Other enteroviruses may cause aseptic meningitis, myocarditis (heart), pleuritis (lung), herpangina (pharynx), febrile rashes, or other manifestations.

Diagnosis: Suspected polio warrants viral detection with nucleic acid amplification and culture. Clinical features of most enterovirus infections are rarely specific. Moreover, detecting the virus in patients is not sufficient for diagnosis because of the high frequency of asymptomatic infection.

Treatment: There is no currently available antiviral treatment.

Prevention: Poliovirus infection can be prevented with either an inactivated vaccine (Salk) or an infectious, attenuated vaccine (Sabin).

Rhinoviruses

Encounter: Transmitted person-to-person through contamination or aerosols.

Entry: Viruses bind to specific receptors on respiratory epithelial cells.

Spread and Replication: Rhinoviruses infect the upper respiratory tract and cause mild infections (common cold) but also can produce severe lower respiratory tract disease.

Damage: Probably cause damage by mechanisms other than virus-induced cytopathology.

Diagnosis: Diagnostic testing is not routinely done.

Treatment: An acceptable antiviral treatment is not currently available.

Prevention: Rhinoviruses comprise more than 100 serotypes, making development of an effective vaccine difficult.

THE PICORNAVIRIDAE (*pico* means "small," and *rna* is the type of nucleic acid that makes up the viral genome) is a family of small RNA viruses divided into 12 genera, 4 of which include human pathogens: the **enteroviruses**, such as **poliovirus**, **coxsackievirus**, **echovirus**, **rhinovirus**, and others, the **parechoviruses**, the hepatovirus **hepatitis A virus**, and the **koboviruses**, which cause gastroenteritis (Fig. 32-1).

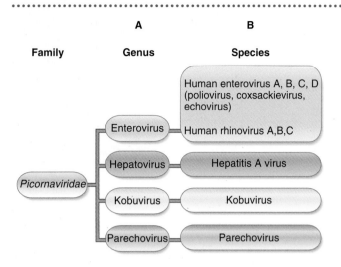

FIGURE 32-1. Members of the *Picornaviridae* family. A. Four genera of picornaviruses include viruses that cause human disease. **B.** The genus *Enterovirus* consists of 10 species, of which 7 contain human pathogens: human enterovirus A–D and human rhinovirus A–C. Examples of each species are shown.

THE PATHOGENS: ENTEROVIRUSES

Enteroviruses were originally named because of their capacity to replicate in the gastrointestinal tract. The best studied enteroviruses are the polioviruses, the etiologic agents of poliomyelitis (see Fig. 32-1). There are three antigenic types, or serotypes, of polioviruses; most epidemics were caused by **type 1**. Other enteroviruses include **coxsackieviruses**, first isolated during a polio outbreak in Coxsackie, New York, and echoviruses (for "enteric cytopathic human orphan viruses"). Echoviruses were so named because they were initially isolated from the feces of individuals who had no symptoms, and the viruses could not be linked to any human disease. More recently discovered enteroviruses are simply assigned a number, as in enterovirus 70. Rhinoviruses, which are respiratory pathogens, are now classified within the enterovirus genus based on sequence homology. These viruses are discussed in the section "Rhinoviruses." The genus enterovirus comprises 10 viral species, of which 7 are human pathogens (see Fig. 32-1).

Hepatitis A virus was originally classified as enterovirus type 72. Information about the biology and replication of this virus, and comparisons of the nucleotide and amino acid sequence of the viral genome with that of other picornaviruses, led to reclassification of hepatitis A virus into a separate genus, hepatovirus.

ENCOUNTER AND ENTRY

Like many of the enteroviruses, polioviruses are excreted in large amounts in feces. In some outbreaks of poliomyelitis,

CASE

Outbreak of Poliomyelitis

In October 1972, 11 of 130 students attending a private school in Greenwich, Connecticut, were diagnosed with paralytic poliomyelitis. Three weeks elapsed between the first and the last cases. Nine of the eleven cases were boys 12 to 17 years of age, and all nine were members either of the football or soccer team. The clinical histories of those patients were similar: They reported "flulike" symptoms, fever up to 39°C, sore throat, and muscle pains. Symptoms lasted on average 13 days. Two to three days later, they complained of a stiff neck, increased muscle pain, and fever up to 41°C. Those symptoms were followed by flaccid paralysis of the legs that varied in intensity from relatively minor to totally incapacitating. During the first 3 weeks of October, 17 other students were seen at the school infirmary with nonspecific complaints that suggested an acute viral syndrome.

Poliomyelitis was diagnosed by serological studies that demonstrated a rising titer of antibodies to type 1 poliovirus but not types 2 and 3. The diagnosis was confirmed by the isolation of type 1 virus from the feces and throat washings of patients with paralytic disease. More than 50% of the school's students had not received oral polio vaccine because of religious convictions. A small number of day students at the school lived at home, where they interacted with friends from surrounding towns in activities that included swimming classes at the local YMCA. Paralytic disease did not occur among youths who did not attend the private school.

An immunization survey of the public schools revealed that more than 95% of their students had been vaccinated.

This case raises several questions:

1. What was the origin of the virus, and how did it spread among the students?
2. What caused the illness among the 17 students who complained of nonspecific signs and symptoms?
3. Why did the disease not spread to all of the students or to the community outside the school?
4. How does poliovirus cause paralysis and other symptoms of disease?
5. What could have been done to halt further spread of poliovirus in the school?

Poliomyelitis has been eradicated from the United States and nearly eliminated from most countries. Paradoxically, its dreaded consequences, paralysis and death, are more common in unvaccinated individuals living in countries with a high standard of sanitation. Poliomyelitis remains an excellent model for understanding the epidemiology and pathogenesis of viral infections because of its well-understood and comparatively simple replication cycle and the relative ease with which it can be studied in the laboratory. Several related viruses (other enteroviruses) continue to cause important diseases in the United States.

See Appendix for answers.

a single individual who sheds high amounts of virus from the gastrointestinal tract can be the source of infection. In countries with temperate climates, outbreaks of enterovirus disease usually occur in the summer or early fall; in the tropics, the diseases caused by these viruses are endemic and occur throughout the year. The major portal of entry is the mouth, and transmission is primarily from person-to-person via the fecal–oral route, through contaminated surfaces or drinking water.

SPREAD AND REPLICATION

After ingestion, poliovirus replicates in the oropharyngeal and intestinal mucosa, most likely in epithelial and lymphoid cells. Virus particles then traverse the basement membrane, invade the subepithelial tissues, and enter the

bloodstream to establish a **viremia**. From the blood, the virus can spread throughout the body (Fig. 32-2). In most infections, virus replication does not progress beyond the mucosa or the initial stage of viremia. These infections may not be apparent (i.e., no symptoms are evident) or present as minor illnesses characterized by fever and headache. The incubation period for a minor illness is approximately 7 days. Poliovirus can continue to replicate in the intestine and be shed in the stool for weeks to months after the symptoms subside. In the Connecticut school outbreak, virus continued to circulate and infect new students for some time. The capacity to replicate weeks to months after infection explains the varying onsets of symptoms in students at the school over a 3-week period.

In about 1% of infections, poliovirus invades the brain and spinal cord. Virions can enter the central nervous

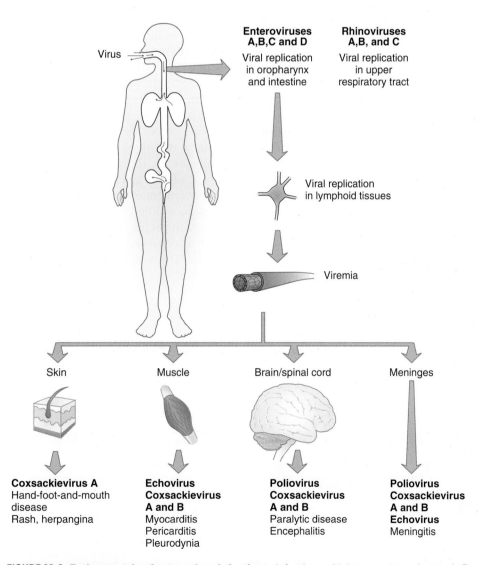

FIGURE 32-2. Pathogenesis of enterovirus infections. Infections with human enteroviruses A–D begin in the alimentary tract; spread of virus through the blood to target organs is shown. The various clinical syndromes caused by some enteroviruses are listed. Rhinovirus infection initiates in the mucosal epithelial cells of the respiratory tract. In the common cold, viral replication is limited to upper respiratory tract. Human rhinovirus C infections also involve the lower respiratory tract.

system directly from the blood or by retrograde axonal transport in peripheral or cranial nerves. Paralysis usually occurs 11 to 13 days after infection.

Although the viremia allows virus access to all sites in the body, the organs infected by poliovirus are limited. The basis for this restricted **tropism**, defined as the organs where the virus replicates, is thought to be determined by the early, innate immune response of the host. The poliovirus receptor, CD155, is necessary for replication but does not explain poliovirus tropism. The protein is expressed within a broad range of animal tissues, some of which do not serve as sites for poliovirus replication. These cells are protected from poliovirus infection by producing interferon, which induces an antiviral state. Why the brain and spinal cord are not similarly protected from infection is not understood.

The replication cycle of poliovirus has been studied in great detail, in part because the virus multiplies efficiently in cell culture and is experimentally highly manipulable. Polioviruses are a prototype of **positive-sense RNA viruses**, which means that the **genomic RNA** can be translated and is therefore a messenger RNA (mRNA). The first step in the poliovirus replication cycle is attachment of the virus to a cellular receptor, which is a glycosylated membrane protein called **poliovirus receptor (PVR)** or **CD155**. The receptor binds to a cleft, called the canyon, on the surface of the viral capsid. The virion is taken into the cell by endocytosis, and the viral genome is released into the cell cytoplasm. The CD155 protein is thought to trigger the release of viral RNA from the virion. Poliovirus RNA is single stranded and, like most eukaryotic mRNAs, has a **poly(A) tract** at the 3′ end. The 5′ end of the genomic RNA is unusual in that it lacks the 5′-terminal cap structure typical of many eukaryotic

mRNAs (Fig. 32-3). Instead, the 5′ end of the genomic RNA is covalently linked to a viral protein called **VPg**. The VPg protein is a primer for viral RNA synthesis catalyzed by the viral RNA-dependent RNA polymerase.

Studies of the synthesis of poliovirus proteins have revealed several unexpected findings. The genomic RNA is translated by internal ribosome binding mediated by an **internal ribosome entry site (IRES)** within the 5′ untranslated region. The viral genome is translated in the cytoplasm by the cellular translation apparatus to produce a single polypeptide called a **polyprotein** (see Fig. 32-3). The production of a polyprotein allows the synthesis of multiple proteins from a single mRNA, a process that does not usually occur in eukaryotic cells. The polyprotein precursor is processed by 2 virus-encoded **proteases** to produce 4 **structural proteins** and 10 **nonstructural proteins**. The structural proteins, VP1, VP2, VP3, and VP4, are the constituents of the viral capsid. The nonstructural proteins include the viral proteases, an **RNA-dependent RNA polymerase**, VPg, and the other proteins involved in viral RNA synthesis.

The poliovirus RNA-dependent RNA polymerase, the enzyme that replicates the viral RNA genome, is an unusual enzyme not found in eukaryotic cells. The viral enzyme copies the positive-sense RNA to form complementary negative-sense strands, which in turn serve as templates for the synthesis of additional positive-sense copies of the genome. The poliovirus RNA-dependent RNA polymerase uses the viral protein VPg linked to two U residues (VPg-U-U) as a primer for viral RNA synthesis. Late in the replication cycle, as the viral structural proteins accumulate, viral RNA is encapsidated into mature virions. The virus particles are released when the host cell lyses.

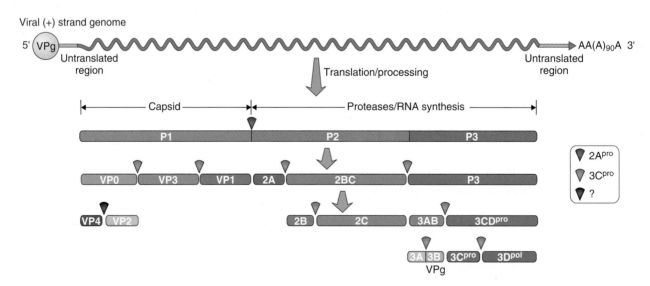

FIGURE 32-3. Picornavirus genome organization. A. The poliovirus RNA genome has a VPg protein covalently attached to the 5′ end. **B.** In the polyprotein precursor, viral polyprotein is cleaved by two virus-encoded proteases, 2A^{pro} and 3C^{pro}. Cleavage sites for each protease are indicated. The protease responsible for cleavage between VP4 and VP2 has not been identified.

Under optimal conditions of cell culture, approximately 1,000 infectious virus particles are released per cell. A complete cycle of replication, from virus attachment to the release of progeny virions, is completed within 6 to 8 hours. The replication cycles of other enteroviruses are likely to proceed in a similar manner.

DAMAGE

Poliovirus is called a **lytic** virus because replication leads to the destruction of infected host cells. The virus replicates in neurons of the gray matter of both the brain and spinal cord. The characteristic **flaccid paralysis** of limb muscles occurs when **anterior horn cells** of the spinal cord are destroyed. However, it is not known if those neurons are destroyed only by viral lysis or if the immune response of the host plays a role. The most severe form of disease is **bulbar poliomyelitis**, the paralysis of the respiratory muscles resulting from involvement of the **medulla oblongata**. That type of poliomyelitis led to the development of "iron lungs," cumbersome predecessors of modern ventilators that enabled patients to inhale and exhale by external changes in pressure. The mortality rate in paralytic cases of poliomyelitis is approximately 50%. Fortunately, bulbar poliomyelitis is rare, comprising less than 0.1% of all infections. Spinal paralytic poliomyelitis, which involves weakness and asymmetric flaccid lower limb paralysis, comprises less than 1% of all infections and is accompanied by an approximately 10% fatality rate.

In the outbreak of poliomyelitis at the Connecticut school, one strain of virus caused a spectrum of disease. Why are poliovirus infections so frequently mild or asymptomatic? The answer is not known, but many factors are likely responsible. The size of the viral inoculum, the concentration of virus in the blood, the virulence of individual virus strains, levels of circulating antibodies, and the efficiency of the innate immune response all are likely to determine whether an infection is symptomatic. Risk factors for poliomyelitis include physical exertion and trauma. Those factors may explain, in part, the observation that 9 of the 11 affected students were actively participating in football and soccer. Another predisposing factor for paralytic poliomyelitis is intramuscular injection. Skeletal muscle injury appears to increase axonal transport, thereby facilitating viral invasion of the central nervous system. Antibodies play an important role in controlling enteroviruses, as illustrated by the inability of patients with hypogammaglobulinemias to readily resolve enterovirus infections.

Diseases Caused by Other Enteroviruses

The most frequent diseases caused by enteroviruses in the United States are caused by the coxsackieviruses (Table 32-1). These viruses produce a variety of illnesses, with some differences among the members of group A and group B. Viruses of both groups cause **aseptic meningitis**, a term used to describe nonbacterial meningitis. Group A viruses cause **herpangina**, a fever of sudden onset with vesicles or ulcers on the tonsils and palate. Group B viruses also infect other organs, particularly the heart. In general, echoviruses produce similar diseases (see Table 32-1).

Most enterovirus infections are not sufficiently unique to allow diagnosis solely on clinical grounds. For example, the skin rashes (**exanthems**) caused by coxsackieviruses and echoviruses are indistinguishable. One important exception is **hand-foot-and-mouth disease**, a readily identifiable febrile illness that is associated with blisters on the palate, hands, and feet. This disease is usually caused by a specific type of coxsackievirus, **type A16**, and enterovirus 71 (see Table 32-1).

Most enterovirus infections are accompanied by viremia, allowing virus access to many organs. Nevertheless, the tropism of different enteroviruses is distinct (see Table 32-1). All enteroviruses replicate in the central nervous system, but some also replicate in the heart (**myocarditis**), the respiratory tract (**pleurodynia**), or the mucous membranes of the eye (**hemorrhagic conjunctivitis**). Infected newborns are at high risk for developing severe enterovirus disease unless they have acquired protective maternal antibodies. The neonatal immune system may not be sufficiently developed to curtail an enterovirus infection. Neonates can acquire coxsackievirus or echovirus by transplacental passage of the virus near term, from contact with maternal fecal material during birth, or from contact with an infected individual at or shortly after birth.

It has been suggested that **type 1 autoimmune diabetes mellitus** may be associated with enterovirus infection. Coxsackievirus B4 infection of certain strains of mice can lead to pancreatitis, and the virus has been isolated from rare cases of fatal human diabetes. In one hypothesis, an initial infection with coxsackievirus or echovirus of the pancreas may trigger autoimmune destruction of β cells in genetically susceptible individuals. Additional work is necessary to confirm or refute the role of enteroviruses as a possible cofactor in the etiology of diabetes.

DIAGNOSIS

Diagnosis of enterovirus disease is challenging because the symptoms of infection are generic. Furthermore, during endemic months when enteroviruses circulate in a community, they can be readily isolated from throat washings or fecal specimens from symptomatic as well as asymptomatic persons. Consequently, recovery of an enterovirus from the throat or feces of an ill person does not prove that the symptoms are the result of an enterovirus. However, certain epidemiological features of enterovirus infection may permit a presumptive diagnosis. For example, enterovirus infections are seasonal in temperate latitudes and tend to cause community outbreaks. Therefore, cases

TABLE 32-1 Disease Caused by Enteroviruses A–D

Disease	Poliovirus	Coxsackievirus Type A	Coxsackievirus Type B	Echovirus	Enterovirus 70	Enterovirus 71	Parechovirus
Asymptomatic infection	+	+	+	+	+	+	+
Paralytic disease	+	+	+	+	+	+	+
Encephalitis, meningitis	+	+	+	+		+	+
Myocarditis		+	+	+			
Pleurodynia			+				
Herpangina		+					
Hand-foot-and-mouth disease		+				+	
Acute hemorrhagic conjunctivitis		+			+		
Respiratory tract disease	+	+		+			+
Gastrointestinal disease				+			+
Diabetes, pancreatitis			+				
Orchitis			+				

of aseptic meningitis in the summer months are likely to be caused by an enterovirus.

Identification of enterovirus infection is done by inoculating a cell culture with a clinical sample, isolating the virus, and neutralizing by reference antisera. Typical specimens for isolating enteroviruses include stool samples, rectal swabs, throat swabs, and cerebrospinal fluid. Reverse transcription-polymerase chain reaction to detect viral genomic RNA is increasingly employed to diagnose enterovirus infections.

TREATMENT

No drug therapy for enterovirus infections exists, although several antiviral compounds have been studied extensively in clinical trials. The administration of pooled immunoglobulin is effective in preventing central nervous system disease in immunocompromised persons with severe coxsackievirus or echovirus infections.

PREVENTION

Two excellent vaccines are available for preventing poliomyelitis. Both were made possible by the seminal finding of Enders, Weller, and Robbins in 1949 that poliovirus could be propagated in cultured nonneural cells. The formalin-inactivated, noninfectious **Salk vaccine** was introduced in the United States in 1955 and led to a precipitous decline in the incidence of poliomyelitis (Fig. 32-4). In 1961, the orally administered **infectious, attenuated Sabin vaccine** was introduced in the United States, and it soon replaced the Salk vaccine for routine

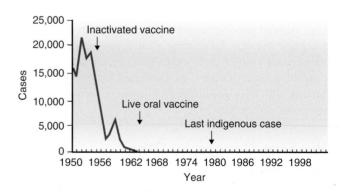

FIGURE 32-4. Effect of immunization on poliomyelitis cases in the United States, 1950 to 1998.

TABLE 32-2 Poliovirus Vaccines

	Sabin (Infectious, Attenuated)	Salk (Inactivated)
Advantages	• Easy to administer • Produces intestinal immunity • Spreads to contacts • Inexpensive	• When properly prepared does not cause disease • Safe for immunodeficient persons
Disadvantages	• May revert during intestinal replication (vaccine-associated poliomyelitis) • Not safe for immunodeficient persons	• Must be injected • Produces reduced intestinal immunity compared with natural infection • More costly than Sabin vaccine

use. Both vaccines have advantages and disadvantages (Table 32-2).

Both the Salk and Sabin vaccines induce serum antibody (Fig. 32-5). However, because the Sabin vaccine is administered orally, an infection of the intestine ensues that stimulates the formation of secretory antibodies. The immune response elicited by the infectious, attenuated vaccine therefore closely resembles the response brought about by natural poliovirus infection. In contrast, the Salk inactivated vaccine is administered by injection and produces immunity in the circulation but not in the intestine (see Fig. 32-5). A recipient of the inactivated vaccine is protected from symptomatic disease, but poliovirus can still replicate in the intestine and spread to others. The Sabin vaccine is therefore highly effective at halting outbreaks of poliomyelitis because it interrupts the chain of virus transmission. Another advantage of the Sabin vaccine is that it can spread from immunized to unimmunized persons. That property is desirable because immunization rates in most countries are less than 100%. Because the Sabin vaccine is administered orally, trained health care personnel are not required for its distribution.

Compared with the inactivated vaccine, the infectious, attenuated vaccine has an important disadvantage. During replication of the Sabin strains in the human intestine, the mutations that reduce the virulence of the vaccine strains can be lost. Consequently, vaccine recipients shed revertant viruses that can cause disease in either the recipients or their contacts. The risk of developing vaccine-associated poliomyelitis is one case of paralytic poliomyelitis per 1.4 million first doses of vaccine. From 1980 to 1998, 144 cases of vaccine-associated paralytic poliomyelitis were reported in the United States. Of those cases, 59 occurred in vaccine recipients, 44 in healthy contacts of vaccine recipients, 30 in individuals with immune defects, and 7 in hosts with no known contact with recipients. From 1979 to 1999, all cases of poliomyelitis in the United States occurred as a consequence of the Sabin vaccine. The Advisory Committee for Immunization Practices therefore recommended that the Salk

vaccine be used exclusively in the United States beginning in 2000.

Because only three serotypes of poliovirus exist and humans are the only known reservoir for the virus, the virus is a candidate for eradication. Smallpox is the only virus that has been eradicated; the last case of smallpox occurred in 1978, and the virus is known to exist only in secure freezers in the United States and Russia. In 1988, the World Health Organization declared that poliovirus would be eradicated from the globe by 2000. Although that goal was missed, the global incidence of poliomyelitis has been significantly reduced (1,294 cases in 2010). Paradoxically, the eradication campaign is threatened by the use of the Sabin vaccine, which has been instrumental in the reduction of poliomyelitis worldwide. Vaccine-derived poliovirus revertants now circulate freely in global sewage and aquifers and are capable of causing poliomyelitis in unimmunized recipients. That problem confounds the plan to cease poliovirus immunization, a step that would occur 5 to 10 years after eradication. Once vaccination against poliovirus stops, it is not known whether circulating revertant poliovirus vaccine strains will cause outbreaks of paralytic disease.

THE PATHOGENS: HUMAN RHINOVIRUSES

Human rhinoviruses are the viruses most frequently isolated from patients with mild upper respiratory infections (common cold) and are probably the most frequent causes of acute infectious human illness. Rhinoviruses are members of the *Picornaviridae* family, initially placed in a separate genus because they differ markedly from enteroviruses. They have now been classified with the enteroviruses based on comparative sequence analysis of viral genomes (see Fig. 32-1). Antigenic diversity is a striking characteristic of the rhinoviruses, with more than 100 serotypes recognized to date classified as human rhinovirus A (75 serotypes) and human rhinovirus B (60 serotypes) (any two rhinovirus isolates are considered to be of different serotypes if their infectivity is not neutralized by the

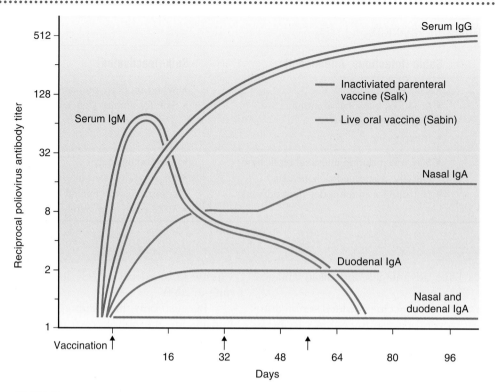

FIGURE 32-5. Antibody responses to poliovirus vaccines. Serum and secretory (IgA) antibody response at different times after immunization with Salk vaccine (*red line*) or Sabin vaccine (*blue line*). The *y*-axis is the reciprocal of the dilution of antiserum that causes 50% inhibition of poliovirus infectivity.

same antiserum). Incorporating such diversity into a rhinovirus vaccine is a seemingly impossible problem given current technology, but it may be solved in the future.

The use of molecular diagnostics (nucleic acid sequencing, polymerase chain reaction) led to the discovery of a new species of rhinovirus, called human rhinovirus C, for which 48 types have been designated. These rhinoviruses cannot yet be propagated in cell culture, explaining why they were not discovered previously. In contrast to rhinoviruses A and B, they appear to be associated with severe lower respiratory tract disease.

The differences in the physical properties of rhinoviruses and enteroviruses partly explain why the two agents cause very different diseases. Enterovirus particles are highly resistant to gastric acidity (pH 3.0) and to bile; therefore, enteroviruses can initiate infection in the alimentary tract. Rhinoviruses are acid labile and readily inactivated by gastric secretions. Rhinoviruses replicate best at 33°C, a temperature found within the upper respiratory tract. Those features of rhinoviruses may help explain why they infect the upper respiratory tract and not the gastrointestinal tract.

CASE

Common Cold

Ms. C., a 28-year-old woman, realized she was getting a cold when she noticed a scratchy feeling in her throat, sneezing, nasal discharge, low-grade fever, and malaise. The symptoms worsened, reaching a peak after 48 hours. Her nasal discharge thickened and was slightly yellowish. It slowly subsided over the next several days. All of her other symptoms resolved completely within about 7 days of onset. She thought that she had acquired the illness from her 7-year-old child, who had similar symptoms a few days earlier.

This case raises several questions:

1. What viruses can cause these symptoms?
2. How was the infection transmitted from the child to the mother?
3. Will this infection induce immune responses that protect against future infections of the same type?

See Appendix for answers.

ENCOUNTER

Rhinovirus infections are very common. The average person experiences approximately one rhinovirus infection per year, and school-age children and their contacts may experience many more. Rhinovirus infections occur most commonly in the fall and spring. Multiple serotypes circulate simultaneously, but the prevalent serotypes change from year to year.

Infected humans, particularly children, are the only known reservoir for rhinoviruses. The mode of transmission has been the subject of intense experimental study. One series of experiments demonstrated that transmission occurs if individuals touch their nose or eyes after their hands become contaminated with rhinovirus (either from contaminated nasal secretions or environmental objects). In other experiments, susceptible volunteers played cards with persons who had symptomatic rhinovirus infection, and the volunteers became infected even if they were restrained from touching their faces. The finding indicates that rhinovirus infection can be transmitted by **aerosols** as well as by direct contact. Sneezing effectively produces and disperses aerosol droplets. Results of experimental infections demonstrate that a small inoculum of rhinovirus is sufficient to initiate an infection.

ENTRY

Once rhinovirus has entered the respiratory tract, the first step in infection is the binding of the virus to specific receptors on respiratory epithelial cells. The cellular receptor for 91 rhinovirus serotypes, also known as the "major group," is **intercellular adhesion molecule 1 (ICAM-1)**, a cellular adhesion protein that plays a role in the recruitment of inflammatory cells. The remaining rhinovirus serotypes, the "minor group," bind to the **very-low-density lipoprotein (VLDL) receptor**. The results of structural studies have revealed that ICAM-1 binds within a canyon on the capsid surface of the major group rhinoviruses in a manner similar to the binding of CD155 by poliovirus. In contrast, the VLDL receptor binds to a flat dome at one end of the capsid of minor group viruses. The replication of rhinovirus within infected cells is similar to that described for poliovirus. The receptor for human rhinovirus C has not been identified.

SPREAD AND MULTIPLCATION

The primary site of rhinovirus infection is the epithelial surface of the nasal mucosa. The release of rhinovirus particles from infected cells is thought to facilitate spread through the respiratory epithelium. In experimental colds, the **posterior nasopharynx** is the site of the most intense infection. The incubation period, from infection to onset of virus shedding, is 1 to 4 days. Virus shedding decreases after 2 to 3 days but may be detectable for up to 3 weeks, long after symptoms have subsided. Such prolonged asymptomatic virus shedding likely facilitates transmission.

DAMAGE

The nose of a patient with a cold becomes swollen and red (**hyperemic**) as a consequence of blood vessel dilation. The thin nasal discharge contains large amounts of serum proteins. As the cold progresses, the discharge becomes **mucopurulent** and contains many cells, especially **neutrophils**. Respiratory epithelial cells are also present, some of which contain rhinovirus antigens, indicating that they are infected by the virus. Biopsy of the mucosa early in the course of a cold reveals edema of subepithelial connective tissue with relatively small numbers of inflammatory cells. In contrast to other viral respiratory infections, particularly influenza, a cold causes only minimal histopathological changes, even in areas where viral antigens are present.

What produces the symptoms of the common cold? A clear correlation exists between the severity of the cold and the amount of rhinovirus recovered from the respiratory tract. However, even when high levels of virus particles are produced, tissue destruction does not occur. The clinical symptoms of a rhinovirus infection are probably not caused by virus-induced cytopathology but are **immunopathological**, a consequence of the immune response to the virus. Supporting that hypothesis is the finding that nasal secretions of persons with colds contain large amounts of the vasoactive substance, **bradykinin**, and **proinflammatory cytokines** that recruit inflammatory cells into the infected area. In addition, rhinovirus infection of a cell leads to increased expression of ICAM-1 on the cell surface. Because ICAM-1 is an important mediator of inflammatory cell recruitment, its upregulation is likely to play a role in airway inflammation. Understanding the immunopathology of rhinovirus infection might allow development of therapies to treat the cold symptoms.

Many rhinovirus common colds are mild, although they may involve secondary complications such as **sinusitis** or **otitis media**, which are usually caused by bacterial infections that develop because the normal draining of the sinuses or the middle ear is blocked. Rhinoviruses also can cause **lower respiratory tract disease** and **asthma exacerbations**. Rhinoviruses are the second most frequently isolated virus from infants, children, older adults, and immunocompromised hosts with pneumonia and bronchiolitis. Infection with rhinovirus is associated with up to 50% of asthma attacks in children and adults, many of whom require hospitalization. Understanding the physiological basis of airway inflammation that occurs during rhinovirus infection is clearly essential for developing therapies for virus-induced asthma exacerbations. Thus, the medical consequences of rhinovirus infections are likely to be much greater than previously thought.

TREATMENT AND PREVENTION

Following most rhinovirus infections, neutralizing antibodies develop in serum and nasal secretions. Unfortunately, those antibodies are only effective in preventing infection by the same rhinovirus serotype. Therefore, reinfection with a different serotype can readily occur. A vaccine to prevent rhinovirus infection does not appear feasible because it would have to comprise more than 100 serotypes. Nevertheless, several novel approaches to prophylaxis have been explored. One is the use of **recombinant interferon-α** administered by nasal spray. When given for 5 days before viral infection, interferon was 80% effective in preventing illness. However, when given for longer than 5 days, interferon led to nasal symptoms as bothersome as those of a cold. Interferon treatment of rhinovirus infection is no longer being pursued because it is not effective in clearing an established viral infection. Antiviral drugs that inhibit various stages of the viral life cycle have been developed. They include compounds that bind the viral capsid and block uncoating of the viral RNA and inhibitors of the viral proteases. Although some of the compounds have proven safe and effective in clinical trials, their effectiveness is reduced by the emergence of resistant viral strains. Further compromising the effectiveness of antiviral drugs is the short duration of virus shedding and illness.

CORONAVIRUSES, SARS, AND EMERGING INFECTIONS: AN OLD FAMILY WITH NEW DISEASES

Coronaviruses are a family of enveloped, positive-sense RNA viruses known for more than 30 years to cause significant and economically important illnesses in many animal species including dogs, cats, cattle, pigs, and chickens. Studies of human coronaviruses in the 1960s and 1970s confirmed the capacity of these viruses to cause up to 30% of common colds. However, the limited frequency of severe human disease and the difficulty in growing human respiratory coronaviruses from clinical specimens were obstacles to identifying coronaviruses and understanding their potential to cause human illness.

Research studies using animal coronaviruses have demonstrated that coronaviruses can undergo rapid genetic change with alterations in clinical disease and "trans-species" movement to new animal hosts. These laboratory observations were dramatically confirmed in nature during the spring and summer of 2003 with the recognition that a new human coronavirus was the cause of **severe acute respiratory syndrome (SARS)**. Within several months of its emergence in the Guangdong province of southeastern China, the SARS coronavirus (SARS-CoV) demonstrated worldwide spread and the potential for high mortality with dramatic economic and societal consequences. The SARS epidemic raised important questions about coronaviruses and their biological potential to cause new diseases in humans and other animals. Where did SARS-CoV come from? Why was it able to cause such severe disease in humans? Why did it disappear, and will it reemerge to cause new outbreaks of disease?

Recent studies of coronavirus genomics and evolution give important clues to the answers to those and other questions. At least two additional human coronaviruses have been identified due to increased surveillance after the SARS epidemic, HKU1 and NL63. Genomic studies of "viromes" of other species have identified in many bat species a large number of coronaviruses related to SARS-CoV and more generally to all mammalian coronaviruses. Bat coronaviruses have not been cultured and do not appear to cause disease in bats, suggesting a long coevolution and possible reservoirs in bats for trans-species movement of SARS-like viruses to new hosts. The data so far suggest that SARS-CoV is a zoonotic virus derived from bats. In support of this hypothesis, a "synthetic" bat coronavirus RNA genome with a small portion from the SARS-CoV genome was engineered and used to recover replicating bat SARS-like coronaviruses in cultured primate and human cells. This approach will allow the study of new zoonotic viruses.

Advances in understanding the molecular biology of coronaviruses have defined several biological characteristics that may influence the capacity of these viruses to move from one species to another. The coronaviruses contain single-stranded, positive-sense RNA genomes, which in addition to replication of full-length genomic RNA, synthesize a set of subgenomic mRNAs that are used for translation of structural and other viral proteins. To accomplish these steps in RNA synthesis, coronaviruses use a viral RNA-dependent RNA-polymerase that can "jump" across an RNA template or between two different templates, resulting in RNA–RNA recombination. The coronavirus polymerase has a high intrinsic error rate with the potential to introduce multiple nucleotide changes during each genome replication. However, coronaviruses express a unique RNA exonuclease that may mediate RNA proofreading and regulate replication fidelity. This combination of RNA recombination, high polymerase error, and regulated replication fidelity appears to favor the generation of recombinant and highly diverse populations of viruses with the potential to cross species and subsequently adapt to new hosts. However, the experience with SARS also demonstrates that the biological potential for emergence of new human coronaviruses is limited by natural barriers, which make such emergences uncommon.

CONCLUSION

Human enteroviruses A–D commonly cause infections in humans. Although readily communicable, only rarely do they cause severe disease. Illnesses caused by enteroviruses may be highly tissue specific (poliovirus) or can affect many organs (coxsackievirus and echovirus). These diseases are often difficult to distinguish clinically, and their presumptive diagnoses are often based on epidemiological features. The success in eradicating poliovirus with vaccination is providential because no other way is known to control the disease.

Rhinoviruses cause half of all common colds. Although it is a benign illness, associated complications such as asthma and lower respiratory tract infection can be life threatening. Furthermore, newly discovered members of the rhinovirus C species are now known to cause severe, life-threatening lower respiratory tract infections. It is therefore essential to develop effective means of controlling rhinovirus infections. Because conventional vaccine approaches do not appear feasible, current efforts are directed toward identifying novel approaches to immunization and effective antiviral compounds against rhinoviruses.

Suggested Readings

Gern JE. The ABCs of rhinoviruses, wheezing, and asthma. *J Virol.* 2010;84(15):7418–7426.

Pallansch MA, Roos RP. Enteroviruses: polioviruses, coxsackieviruses, echoviruses, and newer enteroviruses. In: Knipe DM, Howley PM, eds. *Fields Virology.* 5th ed. Philadelphia, PA: Lippincott Williams & Wilkins, 2007:839–893.

Racaniello VR. Picornaviridae: the viruses and their replication. In: Knipe DM, Howley PM, eds. *Fields Virology.* 5th ed. Philadelphia, PA: Lippincott Williams & Wilkins, 2007:795–838.

Turner RB, Couch RB. Rhinoviruses. In: Knipe DM, Howley PM, eds. *Fields Virology.* 5th ed. Philadelphia, PA: Lippincott Williams & Wilkins, 2007:895–909.

World Health Organization. *Global Polio Eradication Initiative Strategic Plan 2010–2012.* Available at: http://www.polioeradication.org/Resourcelibrary/Strategyandwork/Strategicplan.aspx

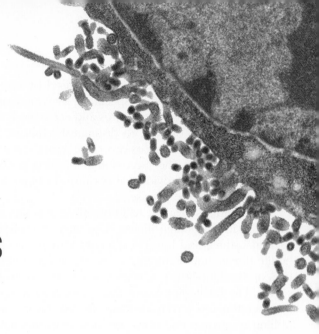

Chapter **33**

Arthropodborne Viruses

Diane E. Griffin

KEY CONCEPTS

Pathogen: Arthropodborne viruses belong primarily to the Togaviridae, Flaviviridae, and Bunyaviridae families of enveloped RNA viruses.

Encounter: Arthropodborne viruses are maintained in natural cycles between insects and birds, wild animals, or humans. They have seasonal transmission in restricted geographic regions.

Entry: Transmission to humans occurs by mosquito, tick, or sandfly bites.

Spread and Replication: Replication occurs in both invertebrate and vertebrate hosts.

Damage: Infection may cause fever, encephalitis, rash, arthritis, or hemorrhagic fever.

Diagnosis: Disease is usually diagnosed by serology or reverse transcription-polymerase chain reaction.

Treatment and Prevention: These infections cannot currently be treated, but vaccines exist for a few and are under development for others.

ARTHROPODBORNE viruses (**arboviruses**) are transmitted by insects, usually mosquitoes, ticks, or blood-feeding flies. More than 100 arboviruses are known to infect humans. These viruses belong to several different virus families, the most important of which are the Togaviridae, Flaviviridae, and Bunyaviridae. Human infection is often asymptomatic, but when disease occurs, it can be manifested by mild to severe febrile illness, rash, arthritis, meningitis, encephalitis, or hemorrhagic fever. Each virus causes a characteristic spectrum of illness, but the same virus can produce diseases of differing severity depending on the viral inoculum and host factors such as age, genetic background, and immunological status.

An arbovirus must replicate in its arthropod vector and spread to the arthropod's salivary glands before the virus can be transmitted to a vertebrate host. After an infected insect bites a human or reservoir host, the virus replicates locally, enters the blood, and then spreads to target cells and organs, such as the brain, liver, skin, or endothelium. Virus in the blood provides the means for infection of new susceptible insects that feed on the infected individual during that time. This transmission increases the number of infected mosquitoes, ticks, or flies and amplifies the infection in nature. The amount of virus in the blood determines the likelihood of the insect becoming infected during feeding. For many arboviruses, humans are "dead-end" hosts because the viremia is of short duration and levels of virus in blood are low. For these viruses, amplifying infections occur in birds or small mammals (Fig. 33-1). However, for yellow fever and dengue viruses, and occasionally for Chikungunya and Ross River viruses, humans are important vertebrate hosts for amplifying viral infection. The paradigm box provides a fundamental understanding of infection by arthropods.

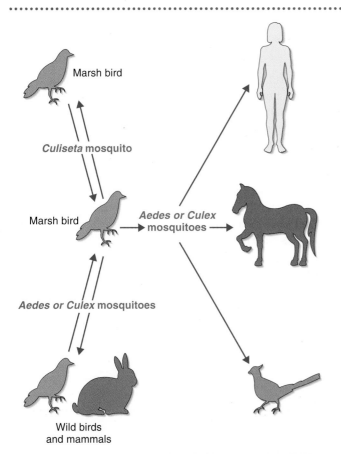

FIGURE 33-1. Life cycles of mosquitoborne arboviruses with nonhuman reservoirs. For eastern equine encephalitis virus, the natural cycle is maintained between birds in salt marshes and *Culiseta* mosquitoes. Transmission to other hosts requires infection of "bridge" mosquito species, such as *Aedes* and *Culex*, that feed on a variety of hosts, including humans. Other animals, such as humans and horses, are susceptible to these infections but are unimportant for maintaining these viruses in nature. Other arboviruses may use the same mosquito species for transmission to humans and other hosts.

Arboviruses are a large group of viruses that share three characteristics: transmission by arthropod vectors, enveloped virions, and an RNA genome (Table 33-1). Many cause encephalitis, while others produce fever, rash, arthritis, hepatitis, or hemorrhagic disease. Arboviruses are often named after the disease they cause or the place where they were first isolated (e.g., La Crosse, Rift Valley, Venezuelan equine encephalitis, Ross River, West Nile, etc.). Vectors include mosquitoes, ticks, and biting flies. The natural cycle for many arboviruses involves transmission between the insect vector and wild animals or birds. Humans are often only accidentally infected and unimportant for maintaining the virus in nature (see Fig. 33-1). However, for dengue and yellow fever viruses, humans are important hosts for the natural cycle and, in concert with the urban mosquito *Aedes aegypti* as a vector, can lead to explosive outbreaks of human disease.

PATHOGEN: ARTHROPODBORNE VIRUSES

Members of the Togaviridae and Flaviviridae families are enveloped viruses that contain a nonsegmented, single-stranded, positive-sense RNA genome. The RNA serves as messenger RNA and is translated directly into large polyproteins that are subsequently processed into the individual proteins necessary for replication and assembly of new virions. Members of the Bunyaviridae family are enveloped viruses that contain a segmented, single-stranded, negative-sense or ambisense RNA genome. The virion carries an RNA polymerase for production of messenger RNA. For all groups, the lipid-containing envelope, acquired during budding from host cell membranes, contains surface glycoprotein spikes that are important for attachment and entry of the virion into new cells. These viruses are inactivated by detergents that disrupt the lipid envelope.

Togaviruses that are important causes of human disease include the encephalitic eastern, western, and Venezuelan equine encephalitis viruses (**EEE**, **WEE**, and **VEE**) in the Americas and the rash- and arthritis-causing **Sindbis virus** in northern Europe and South Africa, **Ross River virus** in Australia, and **Chikungunya virus** in Africa, India, and Southeast Asia. Flaviviruses that are important causes of human encephalitis include the mosquitoborne **West Nile virus** (**WNV**), **St. Louis encephalitis** virus, and **Japanese encephalitis** virus and the tickborne encephalitis viruses. **Dengue** virus usually causes a febrile rash disease, but it also can cause a severe vascular leakage syndrome. **Yellow fever virus** (**YFV**) causes jaundice and hemorrhagic fever. Bunyaviruses are the most varied and numerous of the arboviruses and include the mosquito-transmitted **La Crosse virus** in North America and **Rift Valley fever** virus in Africa, a group of viruses that cause **sandfly fever** around the Mediterranean, and tickborne **Crimean-Congo hemorrhagic fever** virus in Africa and Europe (see Table 33-1).

Some diseases not transmitted by arthropod vectors are caused by viruses in the same families as arboviruses. For example, the virus that causes rubella belongs to the Togaviridae family, the virus that causes hepatitis C belongs to the Flaviviridae family, and the viruses that cause Hantavirus pulmonary syndrome and hemorrhagic fever with renal syndrome belong to the Bunyaviridae family.

ENCOUNTER

The natural life cycle of the viruses that cause West Nile and eastern equine encephalitis involves birds and mosquitoes, while the natural cycle of Venezuelan equine encephalitis involves small mammals and mosquitoes (see Fig. 33-1). Transmission of yellow fever can involve monkeys or humans and mosquitoes. Several viruses in the tickborne encephalitis group of flaviviruses are transmitted between animals by ticks. The arthropod becomes infected by taking a blood meal from an infected

CASE

West Nile Virus

Mrs. K., a 72-year-old, previously healthy woman, was admitted to a hospital in Illinois in early September with high fever and altered mental status. For several days, she had experienced fever, headache, cognitive decline, and difficulty walking. Mrs. K.'s past medical history was unremarkable. She was active outdoors (president of the local garden club), had not traveled out of the area, and her husband was not ill.

On admission, her temperature was 39.5°C, and her heart rate was 120 beats per minute. On physical exam, she was disoriented, and her left leg was weak. Her white blood cell count was 6,500/mm³, and cerebrospinal fluid (CSF) showed 150 cells/mm³, with 75% mononuclear cells, glucose of 100 mg/dL, and protein of 90 mg/dL. Mrs. K. was given antibiotics for the fever but did not respond and became increasingly obtunded. No bacteria were isolated from blood or CSF.

Five days after admission, Mrs. K. had two generalized seizures, became deeply comatose, and required mechanical ventilation. Muscle tone was flaccid, and deep tendon reflexes were absent. She showed no signs of improvement over the next 2 weeks, and life support was withdrawn on day 19 of hospitalization. CSF and serum samples were positive for IgM antibody to West Nile virus, and RNA of the virus was detected by reverse transcription-polymerase chain reaction (RT-PCR). Serum collected just prior to death was positive for IgG antibody to West Nile virus.

This case raises several questions:

1. How and where did Mrs. K. become infected with West Nile virus?
2. What was her most important risk factor for severe disease?
3. How could this infection have been prevented?

See Appendix for answers.

TABLE 33-1 Important Human Arboviruses

Genus and Example	Main Disease	Primary Vector	Distribution
Togaviridae Family			
Eastern equine encephalitis	Encephalitis	Mosquito	Eastern United States, Caribbean
Venezuelan equine encephalitis	Encephalitis	Mosquito	Central and South America
Ross River	Rash, arthritis	Mosquito	Australia
Many others (e.g., Sindbis, Chikungunya)	Fevers, arthritis, rash, encephalitis	Mosquito	Worldwide
Flaviviridae Family			
West Nile	Encephalitis	Mosquito	Americas, Africa, Middle East, Europe
St. Louis encephalitis	Encephalitis	Mosquito	North America
Japanese encephalitis	Encephalitis	Mosquito	Asia, India, Australia
Dengue	Rash, hemorrhagic fever	Mosquito	Caribbean, South and Central America, Asia
Yellow fever	Hemorrhagic fever	Mosquito	Africa, South America
Tickborne encephalitis	Encephalitis	Tick	Russia, eastern and central Europe
Many others	Fever, encephalitis	Mosquito, tick	Worldwide
Bunyaviridae Family			
California/La Crosse	Encephalitis	Mosquito	North America
Rift Valley	Fever	Mosquito	Africa, Middle East
Sandfly fever	Fever	Sandfly	Mediterranean
Crimean-Congo hemorrhagic fever	Hemorrhagic fever	Tick, culicoid fly	Europe, Afric, Asia
Many others	Fever	Mosquito	Worldwide

PARADIGM BOX

PRINCIPLES OF ARTHROPODBORNE INFECTION

Many of the infections described in this text are acquired by exposure to arthropods. Nearly any insect that feeds on humans can also be a vector for infection, including mosquitoes, ticks, sandflies, tsetse flies, black flies, reduviid bugs, fleas, and lice. Viruses, bacteria, rickettsia, protozoa, and helminths are among the infectious agents that can be transmitted by insects. A few general principles can be applied to arthropodborne infections.

In most instances, the infectious agent must develop and multiply within the vector before it can be transmitted. Agents that do not infect arthropods (e.g., HIV) are rarely, if ever, transmitted by passive contamination of a biting insect's mouth parts.

The geographical distribution of an arthropodborne infection is determined by the habitat requirements of the vector. The temperature, humidity, altitude, and vegetation determine whether vector and host will survive in a specific location.

The feeding behavior of the vector often influences the epidemiology of an arthropodborne infection. Human disease requires vectors that feed on humans. For example, despite the wide distribution of the virus, eastern equine encephalitis virus has a low incidence of disease because *Culiseta* mosquitoes prefer to feed on birds that maintain the natural cycle. Only when there is "spill over" into mosquito species that feed on mammals do equine and human cases occur (see Fig. 33-1).

Human behaviors influence the likelihood of contact with arthropods. Diseases transmitted by fleas and lice are commonly associated with impoverished conditions or war. Mosquitoborne diseases tend to occur in locations where humans do not have the means to protect themselves from exposure.

Arthropods expose humans to agents that are otherwise restricted to animals or birds. For instance, mice are the reservoir for Lyme disease, and ticks transmit the agent to humans, as well as to mice.

West Nile virus (WNV) is widespread throughout Africa, the Middle East, and southern Europe. It was not recognized as an important cause of neurologic disease in those regions until the mid-1990s, suggesting the recent emergence of a new, more virulent strain of the virus. In 1999, an outbreak of viral encephalomyelitis in Queens, a borough of New York City, was surprisingly found to be caused by WNV, which was not previously known to exist in the Western Hemisphere. Whether it came across the Atlantic with an infected mosquito, bird, or human is not known. However, appropriate mosquito vectors and avian hosts were available in the new environment, and the virus spread across North America within a few years. WNV is now endemic in the Americas and infects thousands of people in the United States each year. Most infections are mild and not diagnosed. Of those reported to the Centers for Disease Control, approximately half have neurologic disease. All ages are susceptible to infection, but disease is age dependent. The median age for those with any illness is 47 years and for those with neurologic disease is 77 years. Most deaths occur in patients over age 60 (Fig. 33-2).

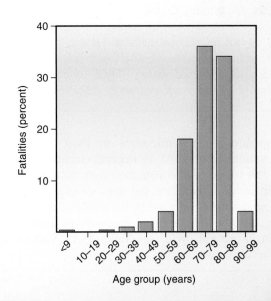

FIGURE 33-2. Age-dependent mortality caused by infection with West Nile virus in the United States. A graph of the percentage of all fatalities that occurred in each age group shows the largest proportion in patients older than 60 years.

vertebrate host with sufficient levels of virus in the blood to initiate infection or, for ticks, by cofeeding with an infected insect. Several days must pass before an insect that has acquired a virus can transmit it because the virus must first replicate in midgut cells and spread through the hemolymph to replicate in the salivary glands. Insect vectors survive infection with these viruses and remain infectious for life. For some virus–arthropod pairs, transmission occurs through germline cells to the next generation of insects constituting a true reservoir of infection.

Acquisition of arbovirus infection is seasonal because transmission depends on the presence of the insect vector.

CASE

Yellow Fever Virus

Mr. W., a 20-year-old college student, was admitted to the hospital with high fever, jaundice, and renal failure. Two days before admission, he had been seen in the emergency department for the abrupt onset of fever, chills, back pain, headache, nausea, and vomiting. At that time, his face was flushed, his temperature was 39°C, and his heart rate was 65 beats per minute. He was previously well and had recently returned from a 2-week trip to the Amazon basin where he collected plants for a summer research project. A malaria smear was negative. Gastroenteritis was considered the most likely diagnosis, and symptomatic treatment was prescribed. The next day, he felt better. However, the day of admission, his headache and back pain had returned, and he developed bloody diarrhea and was too weak to walk.

On admission, he was jaundiced but alert and had a temperature of 38°C, heart rate of 60 beats per minute, and blood pressure of 110/70 mm Hg. His white blood cell count was 4,100/mm³, creatinine 6.9 mg/dL, and bilirubin 3.5 mg/dL. He had albuminuria, and over the next 2 days, urine output declined to less than 100 mL in 24 hours. Hemodialysis was initiated. On the third day, his prothrombin time was very prolonged and he started to bleed from injection sites as well as mucosal surfaces. He was transfused but died from massive gastrointestinal bleeding and hypovolemic shock 4 days after admission. RT-PCR on plasma taken at the time of admission was positive for yellow fever virus RNA.

This case raises several questions:

1. How and where did Mr. W. become infected with yellow fever virus?
2. What was the reason for his bleeding disorder?
3. What could have been done to prevent this infection?

Yellow fever is historically important. It was first recognized as a clinical entity in the Yucatan region of Mexico in 1648, but the virus was probably introduced from Africa. Summertime epidemics occurred as far north as Boston and Halifax into the 20th century. Demonstration by Walter Reed and his colleagues that the disease was transmitted by the ***Aedes aegypti* mosquito** led to massive vector control programs (see the box entitled "Yellow Fever Board"), and in the 1930s, *Aedes aegypti* was eradicated from much of its range in the Americas. However, mosquito control was not sustained. *Aedes aegypti* has gradually repopulated its old habitats, and yellow fever is an emerging threat. Yellow fever virus can be maintained in a "jungle cycle" involving forest mosquitoes and monkeys. Humans that go into forested regions, as Mr. W. did for his summer project, can become infected. The disease typically has a biphasic course corresponding to the viremic and hepatic phases of infection and is fatal in 50% of cases. An effective live virus vaccine is available, which should be administered to individuals traveling to endemic regions.

See Appendix for answers.

In temperate climates, infections are most likely in the warm months (Fig. 33-3); in tropical climates, they can occur year-round or in conjunction with the rainy season. Arboviruses and, therefore, the diseases caused by them are geographically restricted by the availability of the vertebrate and invertebrate hosts necessary to maintain the virus in its natural cycle (see Table 33-1). Viruses with birds as natural hosts can be spread over wide ranges, while those with mammals as hosts are usually confined to smaller regions. Modern travel has provided ample opportunity for expansion of these historically confined ranges. That opportunity was dramatically demonstrated with the introduction of WNV into North America in 1999. This virus was previously found only in Africa and the

YELLOW FEVER BOARD

Large outbreaks of yellow fever affected the U.S. Army in Cuba during the Spanish American War and caused high mortality in workers attempting to build the Panama Canal. In 1881, a Cuban physician, Carlos Finlay, proposed that the disease was transmitted by mosquitoes, but he was unable to demonstrate this experimentally by feeding mosquitoes on an ill person and then on a healthy person. The Yellow Fever Board was established by the U.S. Army in 1900 and went to Cuba to help determine how the disease was spread. Walter Reed led the group.

The investigators demonstrated that a filterable agent in the blood of patients could transmit the disease. They also showed transmission by *Aedes aegypti* mosquitoes after an incubation period of several days. Jesse Lazear, one of the four members of the Yellow Fever Board, died from yellow fever during the investigations. Yellow fever was the first virus ("filterable agent") shown to cause a human disease and the first virus for which insect transmission was identified.

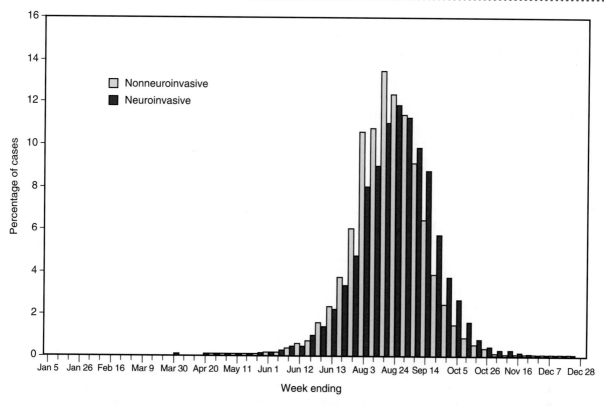

FIGURE 33-3. Seasonal incidence of West Nile virus infection in the United States. A graph of the week of illness onset for neuroinvasive and nonneuroinvasive disease caused by WNV from 1999 to 2008 shows that most cases occur during July to September with a peak in August.

Middle East. The virus can infect a wide variety of birds and mosquitoes, which aided its successful introduction into this new region. Interestingly, **corvid birds** in North America are very susceptible to infection, and the spread of the virus across North America was heralded by the deaths of large numbers of crows and blue jays.

With the resurgence of *Aedes aegypti* and the spread of Asian strains of dengue virus, the incidence of dengue and **dengue hemorrhagic fever** is increasing significantly. An estimated 50 to 100 million cases of dengue fever and 250,000 to 500,000 cases of dengue hemorrhagic fever occur annually worldwide. Multiple serotypes are now circulating in Latin America, the Caribbean, Africa, and Asia.

ENTRY, SPREAD, AND REPLICATION

Arboviruses gain access to humans through the bite of an infected arthropod. Saliva containing virus is introduced into the capillary bed, and the virus can initiate infection at that site or be carried by Langerhans cells from the skin to local lymphatic tissue, where replication occurs. As the virus replicates and is released into the blood from the primary site of infection, a viremia is established. In individuals without protective antibody, fever often appears at this time, and the virus can spread to new target organs such as the central nervous system, joints, liver, and skin. In many cases, infection does not progress past the stage of local replication. It is not known how encephalitic arboviruses cross the blood–brain barrier or why that only occurs in some infected individuals.

Other modes of infection are possible. Many arboviruses can cross the placenta to cause fetal infection that can result in abortion, stillbirth, or congenital disease. Tickborne viruses can be transmitted orally through the milk of infected animals, and Rift Valley fever can be contracted through contact with infected livestock. A number of cases of WNV have been acquired through transfusion of blood to a susceptible recipient from an asymptomatic viremic donor.

DISEASES CAUSED BY ARBOVIRUSES

Encephalitis

In addition to WNV, several other arboviruses can cause encephalitis. In the Americas, these viruses include two togaviruses: eastern and Venezuelan equine encephalitis viruses. EEE virus is endemic in a natural cycle involving marsh birds and *Culiseta* mosquitoes along the Atlantic and Gulf coasts and in the Great Lakes region of the United States. Eastern equine encephalitis has a high mortality, with the most severe disease occurring in children. Neurologic sequelae, such as mental retardation and motor deficits, are common in patients who survive. Fortunately, cases are few because the mosquito that transmits the virus between marsh birds does not usually feed on humans. People and horses are at risk only when mosquitoes that feed on mammals become infected (see Fig. 33-1). WEE virus has caused large outbreaks of equine and human encephalitis in the western United States. However, for reasons that are not known, very few cases have been recognized since 1994.

St. Louis encephalitis virus is a flavivirus related to WNV endemic in the United States. It causes periodic outbreaks of encephalitis and shares with WNV the capacity to cause more severe disease in the elderly. Japanese encephalitis virus is another flavivirus related to WNV and the most important cause of encephalitis worldwide. It is widely distributed throughout Asia and causes at least 10,000 deaths from encephalitis each year. Many of the fatalities are in children, probably because older individuals living in the region have already acquired infection and are immune. Adult travelers to endemic regions are susceptible to fatal disease.

La Crosse virus is a member of the California encephalitis group of bunyaviruses and one of the most common causes of central nervous system infection in the group. The spectrum of illness caused by the California serogroup viruses ranges from mild febrile illness to aseptic meningitis and encephalitis. Neurologic disease occurs primarily in children under the age of 10 years living in the central United States. The case fatality rate is less than 1%.

Rash and Arthritis

Sindbis (also known as Ockelbo, Pogosta, or Karelian fever) and Ross River viruses are togaviruses that cause summertime outbreaks of rash and arthritis in northern Europe and Australia, respectively. In addition, there have recently been large epidemics of rash and arthritis due to Chikungunya virus in the Indian Ocean region. These viruses can cause substantial morbidity, with prolonged and recurrent joint pain, but little if any mortality.

Hemorrhagic Fever

Yellow fever and dengue viruses are transmitted by the *Aedes aegypti* mosquito, and humans are the primary vertebrate host. The geographic ranges of these viruses overlap, and they are found in tropical and subtropical regions of much of the world. Dengue is the most common arbovirus-induced disease, and there are four dengue virus serotypes. An initial dengue virus infection is rarely fatal and provides solid protection against reinfection with that serotype. Clinical manifestations include the sudden onset of fever, headache, and lumbosacral pain ("**breakbone fever**"), often followed by the appearance of a generalized rash. This infection does not provide protection against

other serotypes. In fact, partially cross-reactive immunity can result in enhanced disease following infection with a second dengue virus serotype. The enhanced disease is associated with increased capillary permeability and can lead to dengue shock syndrome. Multiple serotypes are circulating in most regions of the world, including much of South and Central America and the Caribbean. Dengue is frequently imported into the United States by returning travelers but has not spread widely, perhaps because, in contrast to WNV, the natural cycle requires dengue virus to infect humans, who can avoid mosquito contact.

DAMAGE

The clinical symptoms in Mrs. K.'s case of West Nile encephalitis are consistent with damage to the brain and spinal cord, while Mr. W.'s symptoms from YFV are consistent with damage to the liver. For WNV and other arboviruses that cause encephalitis, neurons are the primary target cell for virus replication and can be irrevocably damaged by the virus. Particular subsets of neurons may be more vulnerable to infection than others. Infection of spinal cord motor neurons leads to flaccid paralysis observed with flavivirus-induced neurologic disease, as seen in Mrs. K. Infection of basal ganglia neurons leads to symptoms resembling Parkinson disease in many individuals with Japanese encephalitis. In cases of eastern equine encephalitis, vascular damage is also prominent with many small hemorrhages throughout the central nervous system.

In YFV infection, the liver is a major target organ, and hepatocellular damage is mediated directly by viral infection. Failure to metabolize bilirubin leads to jaundice (and the name yellow fever). Decreased hepatic synthesis of vitamin K–dependent coagulation factors is an important part of the hemorrhagic disorder. The virus also infects monocytes and macrophages with extensive cell death in lymphoid tissue.

For Sindbis, Ross River, and Chikungunya viruses, synovial tissues are targets for infection with infiltration and infection of infiltrating monocytes and macrophages. In dengue virus infection, mononuclear cells are also major targets for infection. These cells have Fc receptors on the surface, and infection can be increased by the presence of cross-reacting antibodies, as seen during infection with a second dengue virus serotype. Through mechanisms that may be related to increased virus replication and cytokine production, a second infection can lead to increased vascular permeability manifested by serous effusions, hypovolemia, and shock.

DIAGNOSIS

Diagnosis of diseases caused by any arbovirus on clinical grounds alone is difficult, except in outbreak situations, because of the paucity of specific findings on physical examination. A travel history can provide important clues to virus exposure. Definitive diagnosis is usually made by detection of virus-specific IgM by enzyme immunoassay, viral RNA by reverse transcription-polymerase chain reaction (RT-PCR), or seroconversion.

TREATMENT AND PREVENTION

There is no specific therapy for any of the arbovirus diseases. Community mosquito control programs and the use of insect repellents and window screens for personal protection against mosquitoes are important for prevention of infection. Widespread aerial spraying of insecticides can decrease adult populations of mosquitoes, and treatment of water to control larvae can inhibit emergence. Vaccines against yellow fever, Japanese encephalitis, and tickborne encephalitis are available and should be used by travelers going to regions where exposure to these viruses is likely. Vaccines against other arboviruses, particularly WNV and dengue, as well as new-generation Japanese encephalitis vaccines are in development.

CONCLUSION

The diverse group of arthropodborne viruses are transmitted by insects, most commonly mosquitoes, and can cause diseases that include fever, encephalitis, hemorrhagic fever, rash, and arthritis. No specific treatment for any of these diseases is available. Prevention of infection is key to inhibiting arbovirus-induced morbidity and mortality.

Suggested Readings

Barnett ED. Yellow fever: epidemiology and prevention. *Clin Infect Dis.* 2007;44:850–856.

Gould EA, Solomon T. Pathogenic flaviviruses. *Lancet.* 2008;371:500–509.

Halstead SB, Thomas SJ. Japanese encephalitis: new options for active immunization. *Clin Infect Dis.* 2010;50:1155–1164.

Lambrechts L, Scott TW, Gubler DJ. Consequences of the expanding global distribution of *Aedes albopictus* for dengue virus transmission. *PLoS Negl Trop Dis.* 2010;4:e646.

Mansfield KL, Johnson N, Phipps LP, et al. Tick-borne encephalitis virus—a review of an emerging zoonosis. *J Gen Virol.* 2009;90:1781–1794.

Nielsen DG. The relationship of interacting immunological components in dengue pathogenesis. *Virol J.* 2009;6:211.

Sejvar JJ. The long-term outcomes of human West Nile virus infection. *Clin Infect Dis.* 2007;44:1617–1624.

Staples JE, Breiman RF, Powers AM. Chikungunya fever: an epidemiological review of a re-emerging infectious disease. *Clin Infect Dis.* 2009;49:942–948.

Weaver SC, Reisen WK. Present and future arboviral threats. *Antiviral Res.* 2010;85:328–345.

Chapter 34

Paramyxoviruses: Measles Virus and Respiratory Syncytial Virus

John V. Williams and James E. Crowe Jr

KEY CONCEPTS

Pathogen: Paramyxoviruses:

- Have single-stranded, nonsegmented, negative-sense RNA genomes.
- Have a lipid envelope derived from the host cell membrane.
- Contain membrane glycoproteins that are important functional and immunologic determinants of virulence.

Encounter: Paramyxoviruses include causes of some of the oldest known viral diseases (measles and mumps) and several respiratory diseases (respiratory syncytial virus and parainfluenza virus).

Measles
Entry: Measles virus is spread by aerosolized droplets.

Spread and Replication: Measles virus replicates in the respiratory tract and then spreads in the bloodstream.

Damage: Damage is associated with viral cytotoxicity and formation of giant cells in the respiratory epithelium and is enhanced by the host immune response.

Diagnosis: Usually clinical: The "three *C*'s" are cough, coryza, and conjunctivitis.

Treatment and Prevention: A live, attenuated virus vaccine is protective.

Respiratory Syncytial Virus
Entry: Respiratory syncytial virus (RSV) is spread to the respiratory tract by airborne droplets and fomites.

Spread and Replication: RSV infection is confined to the respiratory tract.

Damage: Damage is due both to viral cytotoxicity and to immune-mediated pathology.

Treatment and Prevention: There is currently no licensed vaccine, but a monoclonal antibody, palivizumab, can protect at-risk, immunocompromised children through the seasonal occurrence of RSV.

THE PARAMYXOVIRIDAE family includes major causes of childhood disease that have been recognized for centuries, such as measles and mumps (Table 34-1 and see History Box on measles). This family also includes viruses that have recently emerged as causes of human disease, such as Hendra and Nipah viruses and human metapneumovirus (HMPV). Another member of the family, respiratory syncytial virus (RSV), is the most common cause of lower respiratory tract infection in infants and children worldwide and a significant cause of acute respiratory tract illness in the elderly. Parainfluenza viruses types 1, 2, and 3 are also major causes of acute respiratory diseases such as croup or laryngitis in children and adults. Thus, many of the paramyxoviruses are of major medical and socioeconomic importance, particularly for children. Paramyxoviruses infect a diverse range of nonhuman hosts including mammals, birds, reptiles, and fish. This chapter focuses on two human paramyxoviruses that exemplify the varied patterns of disease caused by members of this group of viruses: **measles virus** and **RSV**.

TABLE 34-1 Family *Paramyxoviridae*

Subfamily *Paramyxovirinae*	Subfamily *Pneumovirinae*
Genus Respirovirus	**Genus Pneumovirus**
Parainfluenza virus 1, 3	Respiratory syncytial virus
Genus Rubulavirus	**Genus Metapneumovirus**
Mumps virus	Human metapneumovirus
Parainfluenza virus 2, 4	
Genus Morbillivirus	
Measles virus	
Genus Henipavirus	
Hendra virus	
Nipah virus	

PATHOGEN: THE *PARAMYXOVIRIDAE*

Common morphologic and genetic characteristics define the *Paramyxoviridae*. These viruses possess single-stranded, negative-sense RNA genomes (Fig. 34-1). Because humans do not possess RNA-dependent RNA polymerases, the virus particle must contain a polymerase. The viral **RNA-dependent RNA polymerase (large** or **L protein**) is required to transcribe both mRNA and a positive-sense, full-length RNA copy of the genome (antigenome) used to make negative-sense RNA genomes (Fig. 34-2). The viral polymerase transcribes individual mRNAs directly from the virus genome; the mRNAs are then translated by the host cell protein synthesis machinery.

At some point during the viral life cycle, the polymerase switches to making mostly full-length, positive-sense antigenome. The antigenome serves as template for replication of new full-length, negative-sense genomes for incorporation into progeny virions, which bud from the host cell membrane. The outer surface of paramyxoviruses is composed of a **lipid envelope** derived from the host cell plasma membrane. The envelope contains several viral integral membrane glycoproteins that are determinants of virulence and host cell tropism; those proteins also serve as targets for protective neutralizing antibodies (see Fig. 34-1). The surface glycoproteins also define antigenic subgroups of some paramyxoviruses, a characteristic important for vaccine development. In general, paramyxoviruses are spread by the respiratory route and cause respiratory infections that are limited to the most superficial epithelial cells lining the airway, although the central nervous system is another target tissue for some paramyxoviruses, notably measles, mumps, Hendra, and Nipah viruses.

Unlike influenza virus in the *Orthomyxoviridae* family, viruses with single-stranded, nonsegmented genomes cannot acquire genetic changes by mixing gene segments (reassortment or antigenic shift). In addition, paramyxoviruses rarely undergo recombination. Therefore, genetic diversity of paramyxoviruses is achieved almost solely through the process of nonsynonymous nucleotide point mutations arising from errors made by the error-prone viral RNA polymerase during virus replication (antigenic drift).

MEASLES VIRUS

PATHOGEN: MEASLES VIRUS

Measles virus contains an **RNA genome** that encodes eight proteins. The genome is complexed in a helical

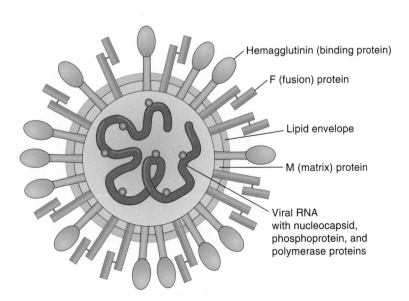

FIGURE 34-1. Schematic diagram of a paramyxovirus.

Hemagglutinin (binding protein)

F (fusion) protein

Lipid envelope

M (matrix) protein

Viral RNA with nucleocapsid, phosphoprotein, and polymerase proteins

CASE • B., an unvaccinated 7-year-old boy, visited Switzerland with his family in 2008. He developed fever and sore throat 1 week after returning to California, followed by cough, coryza, and conjunctivitis. He continued to attend school during this illness, and when symptoms persisted, he was evaluated by both his family physician and pediatrician. Scarlet fever was excluded on the basis of a negative rapid test for *Streptococcus pyogenes*.

This case raises several questions:

1. Why was the diagnosis of measles not considered by B.'s physicians?
2. Is there a concern that he might transmit the infection to others?
3. How could this illness be diagnosed as measles?

See Appendix for answers.

The boy remained ill and visited a children's hospital laboratory, where blood specimens were collected for measles antibody testing; later that day, he was taken to the same hospital's emergency department due to high fever 104°F (40°C) and generalized rash. No isolation precautions were insti- tuted at the doctors' offices or hospital facilities. The child's serum tested positive for measles virus IgM, and subsequently, 839 exposed individuals were identified. Eleven secondary cases of measles occurred, including three infants less than 12 months old (and thus too young to have received measles vaccine). One of these infants was hospitalized and had a prolonged convalescence; another infant traveled by plane to Hawaii during the contagious period, leading to further exposures. Nearly 10% of the patient's schoolmates also were unvaccinated. Forty-eight infants too young to be vaccinated following exposure were quarantined at home for the 21-day contagious period. Many exposed persons were vaccinated, and several high-risk patients were administered measles immune globulin as passive prophylaxis. The estimated cost was more than $176, 000.

This case highlights several points, including the extremely contagious nature of measles, the facile spread within a susceptible, unvaccinated population, and the lack of awareness of measles among both physicians and the public due to the success of vaccination against this disease.

nucleocapsid with the **nucleocapsid protein** and the **phosphoprotein**. Alternate open reading frames within the phosphoprotein gene encode two additional proteins designated **V** and **C**, which have roles in virus replication, pathogenesis, and host immune modulation. **Matrix (M) protein** localizes to the inner face of the viral envelope and is necessary for virion assembly. Measles virus has two important membrane glycoproteins embedded in the viral envelope and displayed on the outer surface of virions. **Hemagglutinin (H)** serves as the attachment protein and binds to host cell receptors, and the **F protein** mediates fusion of the viral envelope with the host cell

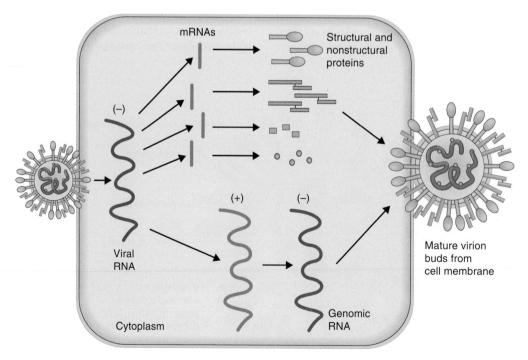

FIGURE 34-2. Schematic representation of the transcription, translation, and genome replication of paramyxoviruses in the host cell cytoplasm.

membrane to facilitate genome entry into the cell. The F protein also mediates cell-to-cell fusion of infected cells to adjacent uninfected cells, forming **giant cells** or **syncytia**, a hallmark of measles virus cytopathic effect in tissue culture and in vivo (Fig. 34-3, *arrows*). Although mutations do occur in measles viruses that circulate in humans, only one measles virus serotype exists. Therefore, a single vaccine strain is effective at preventing disease caused by naturally circulating viruses.

ENCOUNTER AND ENTRY

Persons infected with measles virus are most contagious 2 to 3 days before developing a rash, but they remain infectious until approximately 4 days after the rash appears. Thus, B. may have been infected by a contact who had not yet become symptomatic. The virus is easily spread by **aerosolized droplets**, which can transmit infection during a brief encounter on an elevator, plane, or other public space. Careful history for potential exposures to infected or susceptible persons or for recent travel to endemic areas is important for raising suspicion of this diagnosis. Knowing whether a patient has received a vaccination or not is essential in determining that person's susceptibility to infection.

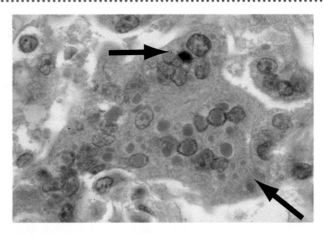

FIGURE 34-3. Formation of giant cells (syncytia) in measles pneumonia. Syncytia are indicated by *arrows*. Note the eosinophilic inclusions in both the cytoplasm and nuclei.

SPREAD AND REPLICATION

The route of infection is usually by inhalation or conjunctival inoculation, and virus initially replicates in respiratory epithelial tissues. Primary **viremia** spreads the virus to the lymph nodes, tonsils, lungs, gastrointestinal tract,

HISTORY OF MEASLES

Measles is one of the classical diseases of antiquity, first clearly described by the Baghdad physician Abu Bakr Muhammad ibn Zakariyya of Ray (latinized to Rhazes) in his AD 910 treatise on measles and smallpox. It is thought that measles virus became endemic within human populations when concentrated masses of people began living in urban areas. Humans are the only known host for measles virus, and infection leads to lifelong immunity. Therefore, the persistence of measles virus in a population requires a certain "size threshold" of susceptible humans being born or migrating into a population. That number has been estimated to be 250,000 at a minimum, and the first cities approaching that size developed in Sumer more than 5,000 years ago.

Measles has had a tremendous historical impact, perhaps surpassed only by smallpox and plague, because of its highly contagious nature and the significant morbidity and mortality associated with measles virus disease. The Italian physician Fracastorius appreciated the spread of measles from human to human in the 16th century, long before the development of the germ theory.

Measles virus is one of the most contagious viruses known. In an outbreak between April and October 1846 in the Faro Islands near Iceland, more than 6,000 of the 7,782 inhabitants were infected. Because no measles outbreaks had occurred in this insular population for 65 years, Faro natives were almost universally susceptible. Crowding facilitates measles epidemics; for example, epidemics were common in armies and decimated many regiments of both the North and South during the American Civil War. The introduction of measles to the Fiji islands in 1875 led to more than 40,000 deaths, one-fifth to one-quarter of the population.

In 1857, the Scottish physician Francis Home provided the first demonstration of virus in blood (viremia) before the actual discovery of viruses when he transmitted measles inadvertently by injecting blood from infected patients into volunteers in an attempt to immunize the recipients. Growth of measles virus in tissue cell culture by John Enders and Thomas Peebles in 1954 paved the way for the study of measles virus and the development of a live, attenuated vaccine. Although measles is no longer endemic in the United States because of high levels of vaccine coverage (more than 90% by age 3 years), deaths from the disease still exceed 150,000 annually worldwide, making measles a major vaccine-preventable disease.

and spleen. A few days later, a second wave of viremia coincides with the onset of major systemic symptoms and rash. This requirement for multiple cycles of replication and dissemination accounts for the 10- to 14-day incubation period for measles. Persons infected with measles virus are contagious prior to the onset of rash, which enhances the potential for spread to susceptible individuals prior to diagnosis.

DAMAGE

Many of the clinical manifestations of measles virus infection can be attributed to damage of host epithelial and endothelial cells caused by measles virus cytotoxicity. Infection of epithelial cells leads to the formation of giant cells, similar to those seen in tissue culture, while endothelial cell infection causes vascular dilation and increased vascular permeability. Although viral antigens are present in infected cells, histopathology of these lesions demonstrates intense inflammation and mononuclear cell infiltrates. Thus, the host immune response required to clear the infection also contributes to the disease. Epithelial giant cells are present in nasal secretions and conjunctivae, and the pathognomonic mucosal eruption (**enanthem**) of measles, **Koplik spots**, consists of epithelial giant cells with surrounding mononuclear cell infiltrates in the submucous glands. Measles virus infection is often accompanied by leukopenia. Organ-specific complications such as pneumonitis, diarrhea, and encephalitis can occur.

The host immune response is important for clearance of measles virus infection. The onset of rash coincides with the appearance of measles-specific antibodies in the normal host, initially of the IgM isotype. Over the next few weeks to months, IgG isotype antibodies appear and persist at low levels for life. Antibodies specific for measles virus mediate protection against disease and may play a role in clearance of acute infection. In a susceptible host exposed to measles, administration of measles virus–specific immune globulin ameliorates the course of disease. However, cellular immunity appears to be more important than humoral immunity for clearance of acute infection. Persons with primary antibody deficiencies (e.g., X-linked hypogammaglobulinemia) generally recover from measles virus infection, but patients with primary or acquired cellular immune deficiencies (e.g., severe combined immunodeficiency or AIDS) are prone to severe or fatal measles. Immunocompromised persons can develop giant cell pneumonia or chronic progressive encephalitis (measles inclusion body encephalitis), which is distinct from the encephalitis that can occur in normal hosts.

The most salient feature of the interaction of measles virus with the immune system is **immunosuppression** following infection. There is a high rate of secondary infections following measles, particularly bacterial and viral pneumonias and bacterial and protozoan intestinal infections. These infections are more frequent and associated with greater mortality in malnourished persons and those at the extremes of age. Measles-associated immunosuppression also leads to diminished responses to vaccines and tuberculin skin tests. Historically, secondary infections were the greatest cause of death in measles outbreaks, and the availability of antibiotics and other public health measures greatly decreased measles-associated mortality decades before the virus was identified or a vaccine developed. **Vitamin A deficiency** is particularly associated with poor outcome in measles virus infections in the developing world, and large studies have shown the benefit of vitamin A supplementation in that setting.

The exact mechanisms of immunosuppression following measles are not known, although several potential pathways exist. Receptors for measles virus have been identified, including **CD46** (membrane cofactor protein, expressed on epithelial cells), nectin-4 (expressed on epithelial cells), and **SLAM** (signaling lymphocyte activation molecule, expressed on B cells, T cells, and dendritic cells). Both molecules transduce powerful signals following engagement by their normal ligands, and interactions with measles virus might lead to attenuation of the immune response. In addition, measles virus nucleocapsid protein binds to an inhibitory immunoglobulin receptor on B cells (Fcγ receptor II) to diminish antibody production. It is likely that other mechanisms contribute to the immunosuppression observed following measles.

DIAGNOSIS

An experienced clinician can make the diagnosis of measles based on a patient's history and clinical presentation alone; almost all measles virus infections are symptomatic in susceptible persons. A 2- to 3-day prodrome of fever and the "**three Cs**" (**cough**, **coryza**, and **conjunctivitis**) followed by a rash are highly suggestive of the diagnosis. Koplik spots, which are small, bright-red spots with bluish centers that can be seen on the buccal mucosa during this period, are almost pathognomonic for measles (Fig. 34-4). The rash that follows the prodrome, with cephalocaudal progression and evolution from discrete maculopapules to confluence, is classic for the disease (Fig. 34-5). However, measles has become uncommon in many parts of the world, and many clinicians are no longer familiar with its presentation, as in the case of B. Furthermore, manifestations may be altered in persons who were previously immunized and thus partially protected or those who are immunocompromised.

Definitive diagnosis of measles is made by virus isolation in culture. Virus can be recovered from respiratory or conjunctival secretions, peripheral blood mononuclear cells, or urine. However, measles virus culture is difficult, time consuming, and not widely available. Serology is now the laboratory method employed to diagnose measles. Ideally, acute and convalescent sera are obtained to document a fourfold rise in measles-specific serum IgG levels, but in a potential outbreak, more rapid diagnosis is needed. Enzyme immunoassays to detect

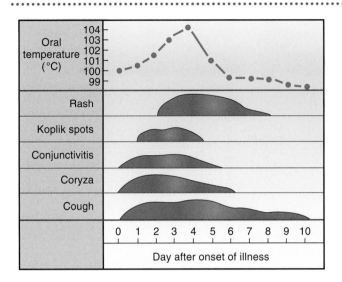

FIGURE 34-4. Signs and symptoms of measles infection.

measles-specific IgM antibodies are available and can establish the diagnosis of measles using a single blood sample. Other methods that use immunofluorescent antibodies to detect measles virus proteins or reverse transcription-polymerase chain reaction (RT-PCR) to detect measles virus genome are sensitive and specific but not widely available.

COMPLICATIONS

Immunologically normal, well-nourished individuals usually do not experience major complications or long-term consequences from measles, but even for those persons, acute measles is not a mild disease. Profound malaise and significant respiratory symptoms are common. Malnutrition

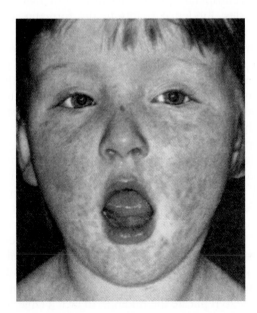

FIGURE 34-5. A child with measles showing classic rash and runny nose.

and other comorbid conditions are prevalent in most countries where measles still flourishes. The most frequent complications are respiratory superinfections such as pneumonia, otitis media, and laryngotracheobronchitis, usually caused by *Streptococcus pneumoniae, Staphylococcus aureus*, or *Haemophilus influenzae*. These infections can be devastating in the absence of appropriate antimicrobial therapy. Diarrhea also is common and, in the developing world, that complication is a major cause of morbidity and mortality in young children. Vitamin A provides clear benefit for respiratory complications and may improve gastrointestinal outcomes.

Eye disease can occur, particularly in vitamin A–deficient children, and is an important cause of blindness in measles-endemic areas of Africa and India. Cerebrospinal fluid pleocytosis is common in apparently uncomplicated measles and is usually asymptomatic. However, approximately 1 in 1,000 children with measles develop clinical signs of encephalitis, which appears to be caused by an inflammatory process known as **acute disseminated encephalomyelitis (ADEM)**. The disease usually has an abrupt onset of fever and altered mental status within 2 weeks following the rash. ADEM appears to be an autoimmune-mediated demyelinating disease and can follow a variety of other infections besides measles. Most survivors of measles encephalitis have profound neurological sequelae such as deafness or intellectual disability.

Although extremely rare (occurring in about 1 in 1,000,000 cases), a neurological complication of measles called **subacute sclerosing panencephalitis (SSPE)** can affect primarily immunocompetent children and young adults. The onset is insidious, 7 to 10 years after primary infection, with mental impairment, personality changes, or myoclonus. The disease course is marked by relentlessly progressive neurological deterioration, with death occurring months to years after onset. The pathophysiology of SSPE is not completely understood. Measles virus particles with defects in the envelope-associated proteins have been isolated from the brains of affected patients, and measles-specific antibodies are present in the cerebrospinal fluid. The incidence of SSPE declined dramatically with the introduction of measles vaccine (Fig. 34-6).

TREATMENT AND PREVENTION

The cornerstone of reducing morbidity and mortality from measles is prevention through vaccination. There is no effective antiviral therapy for established measles virus infection, although measles immune globulin given soon after exposure can ameliorate disease. The World Health Organization recommends administration of vitamin A to children with measles in high-risk regions. Vitamin A is inexpensive and widely used, while immune globulin is expensive and primarily directed toward preventing severe measles in immunocompromised individuals.

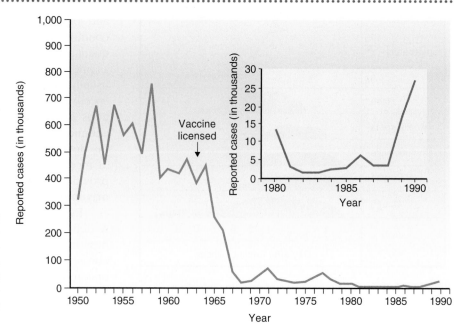

FIGURE 34-6. Reported cases of measles in the United States, 1950 to 1990. Immediately after the introduction of the vaccine, the incidence declined dramatically. A measles epidemic occurred between 1989 and 1991, with most cases affecting unvaccinated children younger than 5 years.

Live, attenuated measles vaccine has greatly diminished the incidence of measles in every country in which it has been used. The vaccine strains were generated by attenuation of the virus in the laboratory. Wild-type measles virus strains were passaged in chick embryo fibroblast cell culture until they sustained mutations and became avirulent for primates. However, these attenuated strains can still induce protective humoral and cellular immune responses. A number of such strains have been developed and used since the 1960s. In the United States, the current childhood vaccine employed for universal use is a combination measles–mumps–rubella (MMR) vaccine containing attenuated strains of all three viruses. A single dose, given intramuscularly at 12 to 15 months of age, induces measles-specific immunity in more than 95% of healthy children. The recommended second dose at 4 to 6 years of age serves principally to seroconvert children who missed or did not respond to the first dose.

The presence of passively acquired maternal antibodies inhibits the response to measles vaccine, which is a problem in measles-endemic areas where the risk of severe measles is greatest in infants and young children. If immunized at 12 months of age, most infants will seroconvert, but many infants with low maternal antibody levels will contract measles at ages younger than 12 months. Immunization at 6 months of age will protect some of these infants, but many others will fail to respond because of the presence of maternal antibodies and immunologic immaturity. These infants will require revaccination or will not be protected against exposure later in life.

Trials were conducted to evaluate the efficacy of a higher-titer, live, attenuated vaccine given to infants 4 to 6 months of age in an attempt to overcome the poor immunogenicity of the vaccine in young infants. The higher-titer vaccine induced higher rates of seroconversion, but female children at some trial sites had increased

mortality as a result of all causes over the next few years of follow-up. Although this observation has not been explained, the practice of immunizing 4- to 6-month-old infants with high-titer vaccine has been discontinued. Current recommendations are for immunization at 9 months of age in endemic areas and 12 to 15 months in areas where measles is rare.

A formalin-inactivated vaccine used in the mid-1960s proved surprisingly ineffective. In fact, recipients of the inactivated vaccine developed **atypical measles** when they were subsequently infected with wild-type measles virus. The clinical features of this altered illness were high fever, pneumonitis, and an unusual rash consisting of vasculitic, hemorrhagic, or vesicular lesions with a centripetal spread differing from that of typical measles. Evidence points to the formalin inactivation steps used in vaccine preparation possibly altering the conformation of the F protein, thus inducing low-affinity antibodies that did not inhibit virus or protect recipients against infection. Instead, these antibodies may have reacted with wild-type measles virus to form immune complexes with resultant immune dysregulation. This episode illustrates the complexity of vaccine development for paramyxoviruses.

The currently licensed vaccine is safe and well tolerated, with occasional mild side effects similar to natural measles virus infection, such as rash or fever. However, in 1998, a group of researchers in Great Britain published a study of 12 children with autism and "enterocolitis," which the authors claimed was associated with measles vaccine based on histological stains of intestinal biopsies from the affected individuals. This study was subsequently retracted, and no other investigators have been able to replicate the findings. In fact, a large number of subsequent epidemiologic studies involving hundreds of thousands of children in various countries, including studies that specifically included children with autism and gastrointestinal complaints, have refuted an association between measles vaccine and autism. Nonetheless, immunization rates fell in Great Britain following that initial report, and measles outbreaks occurred, resulting in the deaths of three children. The concern elicited by the original report has led to continued measles outbreaks in developed nations due to nonvaccinators, as in B.'s case. The United States experienced more than 131 cases of measles between January and July 2008, 75% of which were secondary spread from imported measles; ongoing outbreaks in Eastern and Southern Europe since 2008 have included thousands of cases.

Universal measles vaccination and the possible eradication of measles virus transmission face numerous obstacles. Sociopolitical upheaval and civil wars hamper the delivery of vaccine, and temperature instability of the live-virus vaccine requires a "**cold chain**" that is difficult and costly to maintain. Furthermore, many of the areas where measles virus persists have high birth rates and thus continue to introduce a susceptible population. Nonetheless, the World Health Organization, Pan American Health Organization, and Centers for Disease Control and Prevention have set an agenda for measles virus elimination from the Western Hemisphere, with the goal of measles eradication within the next 10 to 20 years. Remarkable progress has been made toward that goal. Measles remains a leading cause of death in Africa, India, and Southeast Asia with an estimated 40 million cases and 757,000 deaths in 2000; aggressive worldwide vaccination campaigns reduced this to an estimated 164,000 deaths in 2008. Reduction of this continued loss of life, despite a safe and effective vaccine, remains a challenging task.

RESPIRATORY SYNCYTIAL VIRUS

RSV is a ubiquitous cause of respiratory tract disease in children worldwide. In both developed and developing nations, approximately 75% of infants are seropositive for RSV by 1 year of age, and virtually all have been infected by age two. The classic illness associated with RSV is **bronchiolitis**, which is characterized by cough, wheezing, and dyspnea, although RSV also can cause laryngotracheobronchitis, or **croup**, and focal alveolar disease indistinguishable on chest radiographs from bacterial **pneumonia**. RSV is linked epidemiologically with asthma, although it is not clear whether infection with RSV increases a child's risk of developing asthma or whether RSV infection is more severe and thus more apparent in children who already have a genetic or physiologic predisposition for the illness.

PATHOGEN: RESPIRATORY SYNCYTIAL VIRUS

RSV has **nucleocapsid**, **matrix**, **phosphoprotein**, and **polymerase** proteins, similar to measles virus, which serve analogous functions. RSV does not encode additional proteins within the phosphoprotein gene, but it encodes the **nonstructural** (**NS**) proteins **NS1** and **NS2**, which are involved in replication and modulation of the host immune response. RSV has an additional membrane glycoprotein, the small hydrophobic or **SH protein**, the function of which is not known. The major RSV surface glycoproteins are the highly glycosylated **G protein** and the **fusion** (**F**) **protein**. G protein mediates virus attachment to host cells, although a definitive receptor has not been identified. Diversity within G protein defines the two antigenic subgroups of RSV. F protein mediates fusion of the viral envelope and the host cell membrane and release of the viral genome into the cytoplasm to begin the virus replication cycle. F protein also promotes cell-to-cell fusion, another mechanism by which virus spread may occur. F protein is conserved between the two virus subgroups, and neutralizing antibodies to F protein generally protect against lower respiratory tract disease caused by viruses of either subgroup.

CASE • In January, a mother brought her 2-month-old boy, N., to his pediatrician because the infant was coughing and breastfeeding poorly. The baby had rhinorrhea but no fever. His 2-year-old sibling was enrolled in a day-care facility. On examination, the physician noted that N. was tachypneic, with subcostal retractions and diffuse expiratory wheezes on auscultation. Pulse oximetry showed his oxygen saturation to be low, and he was administered oxygen and an aerosolized bronchodilator drug.

The treatment had little effect, and N. was admitted to the hospital for continuous oxygen therapy and intravenous hydration because he remained unable to nurse owing to tachypnea. A rapid antigen test performed on nasal secretions was positive for RSV, and a chest radiograph revealed hyperinflation with peribronchial thickening. He was hospitalized for 3 days, during which time he improved, began nursing again, and was weaned from supplemental oxygen. He was discharged home in good condition but continued to cough for 2 more weeks.

This case raises several questions:

1. What was the role of N.'s sibling in this case?
2. What is the significance of hyperinflation with peribronchial thickening on the chest radiograph?
3. Why did N.'s cough persist for 2 weeks after hospitalization?

See Appendix for answers.

ENCOUNTER AND ENTRY

Humans are the only known host for RSV, and respiratory droplets and fomites readily transmit the virus. Reinfection occurs throughout life, with repeat infections generally milder than those in early childhood. In one study, healthy adult volunteers were inoculated repeatedly with a single, wild-type strain of RSV and were reinfected successfully more than half the time. Many of these infections were symptomatic, causing rhinorrhea and cough. Thus, natural immunity to RSV protects against lower respiratory tract involvement but is not very effective at preventing disease of the upper respiratory tract. One of the features of RSV biology that has hindered successful vaccine development is the high rate of reinfection. An explanation for the lack of permanent immunity is not clear, but the likely contributing factors are antigenic variation of the virus, inhibition of host immune responses mediated by viral proteins, and rapidly waning mucosal IgA in the upper respiratory tract.

In temperate regions, RSV infection is seasonal, occurring most frequently in the winter months. In the tropics, infections occur throughout the year but peak in the rainy season. Almost all children are symptomatic with primary infection, and up to 40% of them have evidence of lower respiratory tract involvement. The risk of hospitalization is about 1 to 3% in otherwise healthy infants, but the hospitalization rate is higher in children with underlying problems such as prematurity, cardiopulmonary disease, or immune deficiency. In the United States, RSV is estimated to cause about 50,000 to 80,000 hospitalizations, at least 100 infant deaths, and 17,000 deaths in the elderly each year. Risk factors for acquisition of RSV include daycare attendance and the presence of school-age siblings in the home. Risk factors for more severe disease include prematurity, male sex, secondhand exposure to tobacco smoke, and lack of breastfeeding.

SPREAD AND REPLICATION

In contrast to measles virus infection, RSV infection is limited to respiratory epithelial cells and does not involve distant body sites. Signs of upper respiratory infection occur before lower respiratory tract signs, although it is not known if infection spreads by cell-to-cell fusion or aspiration of respiratory droplets. Peak virus replication in the host precedes the peak of clinical illness; therefore, children are infectious for a few days before they become sick. The mean duration of virus shedding in immunocompetent children is 12 days; virus shedding is shorter in adults and much longer in immunocompromised persons.

DAMAGE

RSV is cytotoxic to respiratory epithelial cells, with resultant damage to ciliary function. Necrosis of RSV-infected cells with sloughing into the bronchiolar lumen is seen in histological specimens from fatal cases. However, as with measles, the host immune response plays an important role in the pathogenesis of RSV disease. The amount of virus present in nasal secretions peaks just before the development of severe illness. Often when infants are hospitalized, the amount of virus being shed is declining even as the illness worsens. Histopathology of fatal cases shows an intense inflammatory infiltrate in a peribronchiolar distribution, with edema of the airway contributing to the obstruction. Narrowing of small airways leads to the classic manifestations of bronchiolitis: wheezing, dyspnea, and air trapping, with hyperexpansion of the lung and decreased ventilation.

Immunopathologic components of RSV infection are not well understood. RSV infection of epithelial cells induces the production of certain cytokines such as interleukin 6 (IL-6), IL-8, tumor necrosis factor-α, and RANTES (regulated on activation, normally expressed and secreted by T cells). Animal models suggest that a skewed CD4 T-cell response, marked by Th2 cytokines, may play a role in immunopathogenesis. Severely immunocompromised persons, such as hematopoietic stem cell transplant recipients, can develop fatal pneumonia with RSV that appears to be caused principally by cytotoxic viral damage.

TREATMENT AND PREVENTION

There is no highly effective antiviral therapy for RSV infection. The nucleoside analogue ribavirin has inhibitory activity in vitro, and it may have a role in severely immunocompromised patients. However, ribavirin does not benefit most children hospitalized with RSV. Supportive therapy with oxygen and intravenous fluids is of paramount importance. Bronchodilators have limited utility, underscoring the distinction between acute viral bronchiolitis and the reversible airway obstruction that occurs in asthma. Although the host immune response seems to be involved in disease production, immunomodulatory corticosteroids have shown no benefit in controlled trials. Currently, there is no licensed vaccine for RSV although several promising vaccine candidates are under study in clinical trials. The history of RSV vaccine development provides another illustration of the complexity of designing strategies to prevent paramyxovirus disease.

A formalin-inactivated RSV vaccine candidate was tested in the late 1960s, but vaccine recipients developed altered immune responses and experienced more severe disease when infected subsequently with wild-type RSV, and several deaths occurred. Those events slowed RSV vaccine development for decades. Subsequent studies have suggested that, like the inactivated measles vaccine, RSV antigens did not retain a fully native conformation following formalin inactivation and induced a Th2-biased cytokine response with low-affinity antibodies that did not protect against wild-type RSV infection. Later, live, attenuated virus strains were developed using the techniques of serial viral passage in cell culture and chemical mutagenesis to generate stably attenuated viruses. Several of these vaccine candidates have been tested in clinical trials, and some are promising for infant vaccination.

One challenge to the development of a safe and effective RSV vaccine is the need to vaccinate very early in life to protect those at highest risk. The immunological immaturity of young infants hinders effective antibody responses to attenuated vaccines, but more immunogenic and less attenuated viruses can cause unacceptable side effects of respiratory infection. Thus, a perfect balance between immunogenicity and suitable attenuation may be difficult to achieve in infants. Protein subunit vaccines are efficacious in older children, but in animal models, these vaccines induce a biased Th2 cytokine response similar to that induced by the formalin-inactivated RSV vaccine.

The most effective preventive strategy currently available for high-risk infants is passive immunoprophylaxis. **Palivizumab** is a humanized monoclonal antibody specific for the F protein that has high neutralizing activity against most RSV strains. This antibody product was developed by cloning sequences encoding the antigen-binding domain from a murine monoclonal antibody into the framework of a human antibody gene, thus producing a recombinant antibody that is mostly human derived. Palivizumab reduces RSV-related hospitalizations in high-risk infants by about 50%. The antibody is expensive and must be given intramuscularly once a month during the RSV season for the first year of life. Palivizumab is one of the most successful and widely used monoclonal antibodies licensed for use thus far. The high rates of hospitalization in the US and the high infant mortality in low-resource settings warrant continued efforts to develop prophylactic RSV vaccines.

RECENTLY DISCOVERED PARAMYXOVIRUSES

Hendra and Nipah Viruses

In 1994, an outbreak of severe respiratory disease in Australia killed 14 horses and affected 2 humans, 1 of whom died. The causative agent was determined to be a paramyxovirus based on virion morphology and genetic analysis. The virus was named **Hendra virus** after the location of the outbreak. Evidence for a latent reservoir of virus in horses or humans was not found, and sporadic cases continue to occur in horses and occasionally humans.

In September 1998, an outbreak of pneumonia and febrile encephalitis eventually resulted in 283 human cases and 109 deaths in Malaysia and Singapore. Most of the affected individuals had direct contact with pigs on farms or in slaughterhouses; the pigs were found to have a mild respiratory illness. More than 1 million pigs were destroyed in an effort to stop the outbreak, which subsided in May 1999. Another novel paramyxovirus was found to be the cause of this outbreak and was called **Nipah virus** after the village where it was recovered.

Extensive epidemiological and environmental investigations identified a **fruit bat** species as the asymptomatic natural host for both Hendra virus and Nipah virus. It appeared that deforestation had encroached on the fruit bat's natural habitat, thus bringing the animals into closer contact with domesticated pigs and allowing interspecies transmission. Subsequently, Nipah virus was shown to infect dogs, cats, horses, and goats, thus exhibiting a remarkable capacity to infect a variety of host species. Since 2004, ongoing outbreaks of Nipah virus in Bangladesh and India have caused more than 100 human cases, including dozens of fatalities; many of these infections have resulted from direct human-to-human transmission. The long-term relationship of these viruses with humans is not clear, but technological advances in modern molecular biology have allowed these new viruses to be identified and characterized rapidly.

Human Metapneumovirus

Investigators in the Netherlands in 2001 described a previously undetected paramyxovirus associated with severe acute respiratory tract infections in children and adults. Genetic analysis of the virus showed that it was similar to RSV but more closely related to an important bird pathogen called avian metapneumovirus. Thus, the new virus was designated human metapneumovirus (HMPV; see Table 34-1). The virus was difficult to grow and detect in culture, requiring special cells and conditions, likely accounting for the delay in its recognition. Further studies using molecular tests such as RT-PCR found evidence of HMPV infection worldwide. A large prospective study in the United States found HMPV to be one of the most common viruses associated with lower respiratory infection in children, causing bronchiolitis, croup, and pneumonia. Many subsequent epidemiologic investigations have identified HMPV as the second leading cause of lower respiratory infection in children after RSV. HMPV also is a common cause of upper respiratory infections, and reinfections can occur later in life, as with RSV. Furthermore, HMPV is an important cause of serious respiratory disease in older adults and persons with underlying conditions such as prematurity, asthma, chronic obstructive pulmonary disease, and immunodeficiency. Serological studies of archived sera indicate that HMPV has been infecting humans for at least 50 years, and thus, it is not truly a new pathogen but rather newly recognized. Live, attenuated vaccines using techniques developed for RSV vaccines are in development for HMPV.

CONCLUSION

Paramyxoviruses cause some of the most ancient as well as the newest diseases that plague humankind. Vaccines have dramatically diminished the incidence of diseases caused by some viruses in the *Paramyxoviridae* family, such as measles and mumps viruses. Others, like RSV and the parainfluenza viruses, are major causes of respiratory disease and so far have eluded the development of effective vaccines. Three paramyxoviruses—Hendra virus, Nipah virus, and HMPV—have emerged in the last two decades. All paramyxoviruses share common structural and genetic features and cause either respiratory or neurological infections or both. All are important human pathogens deserving of continued studies into mechanisms of pathogenesis and immunity.

Suggested Readings

Bellini WJ, Rota JS, Rota PA. Virology of measles virus. *J Inf Dis.* 1994;170(suppl):S15–S23.

Chua KB. Nipah virus outbreak in Malaysia. *J Clin Virol.* 2003;26:265–275.

Cliff, AD. Measles: an historical geography of a major human viral disease from global expansion to local retreat, 1840–1990. Cambridge, MA: Blackwell Reference; 1993.

Collins PL, Crowe JE Jr. Respiratory syncytial virus and human metapneumovirus. In: Knipe DM, Howley PM, Griffin DE, et al., eds. *Fields Virology.* 5th ed. Philadelphia, PA: Lippincott Williams & Wilkins; 2007:1601–1646.

Griffin DE. Immune responses during measles virus infection. *Curr Top Microbiol Immunol.* 1995;191:117–134.

Griffin DE. Measles virus. In: Knipe DM, Howley PM, Griffin DE, et al., eds. *Fields Virology.* 5th ed. Philadelphia, PA: Lippincott Williams & Wilkins; 2007:1551–1585.

Hall WR, Hall CB. Atypical measles in adolescents: evaluation of clinical and pulmonary function. *Ann Intern Med.* 1979;90:882–886.

Van den Hoogen BG, de Jong JC, Groen J, et al. A newly discovered human pneumovirus isolated from young children with respiratory tract disease. *Nat Med.* 2001;7:719–724.

Williams JV, Harris PA, Tollefson SJ, et al. Human metapneumovirus and lower respiratory tract disease in otherwise healthy infants and children. *N Engl J Med.* 2004;350:443–450.

Chapter 35

Rabies

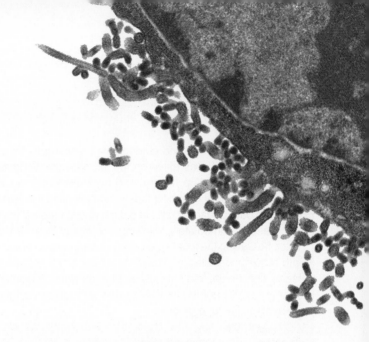

Charles E. Rupprecht and Brett W. Petersen

KEY CONCEPTS

Pathogen: Rabies virus is a zoonotic pathogen classified in the family Rhabdoviridae, genus *Lyssavirus*.

Encounter: Rabies is mainly a disease of dogs in developing countries; in developed countries, it is perpetuated by wildlife, such as bats and mammalian carnivores (foxes, skunks, raccoons, coyotes, mongooses, and jackals, among others).

Entry: Rabies virus is transmitted to humans by the bite of an infected wild or domesticated animal.

Spread: The virus spreads from the site of the bite via nerves in the peripheral nervous system to the central nervous system; the virus then travels back from the brain to peripheral sites.

Replication: The disease manifests after a variable incubation period of approximately 1 to 3 months, but the incubation period can range from a few weeks to more than 1 year.

Damage:
- Signs and symptoms include acute, progressive fever, headache, difficulty swallowing, paresthesia, increased muscle tone, hypersalivation, paralysis, and hydrophobia.
- Lesions are minimal and nonspecific in the brain, but microscopic pathology may include intracytoplasmic inclusions in neurons (known as Negri bodies).

Diagnosis: Rabies can be diagnosed postmortem by fluorescent antibody demonstration of viral antigen in the brain or antemortem by detection of viral antibody in patient serum or cerebrospinal fluid, viral antigen in a skin or brain biopsy, viral nucleic acid in saliva, skin biopsy, or brain biopsy, or infectious virus in saliva.

Treatment and Prevention:
- Rabies can be controlled by vaccination of domesticated and wild animals, stray animal management, and local leash laws.
- It has been prevented in humans by a combination of local wound treatment, passive administration of rabies immune globulin, and rabies vaccination.

RABIES is an acute, progressive encephalitis with no proven effective cure. It is a disease that has instilled terror in human society, and with good reason. Virtually all people who are bitten by a rabid animal and develop symptoms will die. Many of the symptoms are dramatic and frightening. In developed countries, the disease in dogs has been controlled with veterinary vaccines and, consequently, human rabies cases are rare. Surveillance in developed countries is still important, however, because the rabies virus is commonly found in a variety of wild animals (including bats, foxes, skunks, and raccoons). A limited number of places are considered "free" of the disease, mainly islands such as Hawaii and Japan and many of the small Caribbean islands. The disease is common in many developing countries, where canine rabies perpetuates, and millions of people are vaccinated after being bitten by potentially rabid animals, mainly dogs.

This chapter discusses the distribution of rabies in various parts of the world and the animals involved, replication and spread of the virus in those animals, diagnosis of the disease, and prevention of persons exposed to the virus (including the crucial question of whether or not to use postexposure prophylaxis).

CASE

A Bat Bite

Mr. B., a 55-year-old avid outdoorsman residing in Texas County, Missouri, was bitten on the left ear by a bat after allowing it to crawl up his arm and neck. He kept the bat unrestrained in his house for 2 days and released it outside after the bat appeared well. He did not obtain medical care for the bite immediately following the injury. Five weeks later, he went to the local emergency department complaining of numbness and pruritus of the left ear and face, headache, chest pain, and difficulty swallowing water. Based on his history of bat bite, he was treated with rabies vaccine and rabies immune globulin.

Over the next few days, Mr. B.'s symptoms progressed, and he showed steady neurological decline. He became febrile, confused, and disoriented. He received experimental treatment for rabies including coma induction and administration of amantadine. Despite these efforts, Mr. B.'s condition continued to deteriorate, and he died 7 days after admission.

Rabies virus RNA was detected by reverse transcription-polymerase chain reaction testing in saliva and a skin biopsy from Mr. B. Based on genetic sequencing, the rabies virus variant was identified as identical to those viruses found in silver-haired bats. Because of possible contacts Mr. B. had with people, including family and medical personnel while sick, rabies postexposure prophylaxis was provided to five persons.

This case raises several questions:

1. Is this a "typical" case of rabies in the United States?
2. What prophylaxis would Mr. B. have received had he gone to the emergency department immediately after he was bitten?
3. What would have been the chances of success if Mr. B. had been provided with the appropriate prophylaxis against rabies?
4. On average, how many cases of human rabies occur in the United States each year?
5. Approximately how many persons are vaccinated against rabies in the United States each year?
6. Were Mr. B.'s symptoms characteristic of human rabies cases?

See Appendix for answers.

RABIES VIRUS

THE PATHOGEN

Rabies virus can infect dozens of mammalian species, including humans. The reason for its unusually broad host range is not known. The agent that causes rabies belongs to the Rhabdoviridae family, genus *Lyssavirus*. The best known member of that genus is rabies virus, but rabies-related viruses from the Old World can also cause the disease. Rabies and rabies-related viruses are rod or bullet shaped and contain an envelope. These viruses are fairly large compared with most other viruses (~180 nm in length and 75 nm in width; Fig. 35-1). The rabies virus genome consists of only five genes that each encodes a single protein. The virus contains an **envelope glycoprotein (G protein)**, a **matrix (M) protein** underlying the envelope, and a **helical ribonucleoprotein (RNP) core**, or nucleocapsid, in which the **unsegmented**

CASE

A Dog Bite

As Mrs. X., a 38-year-old accountant, was jogging through her neighborhood in suburban Seattle, Washington, she was chased by an average-size black dog that bit her on the right ankle. The dog then ran away. Mrs. X. thought she recognized the animal as a Labrador mix from a few streets away, but she was not sure. Mr. X. cleaned his wife's puncture wounds when she got home. Both Mr. and Mrs. X. were concerned about rabies and called the local health department. An official told them that no cases of rabies in dogs had been reported in Washington for decades. Only bats had been reported rabid in the last few years. The couple was told not to worry about rabies in the dog. The county animal control department was dispatched to search for the dog, found a likely suspect, and placed the animal in quarantine, where it remained healthy for the next 10 days before being claimed by its owner.

This case raises several questions:

1. Should Mrs. X. still be concerned about rabies exposure?
2. If the dog had not been found, would the treatment have been different?
3. If this incident occurred outside the United States, would the protocol have been the same?

See Appendix for answers.

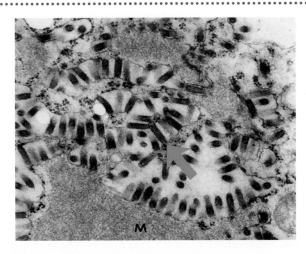

FIGURE 35-1. Neuron of a dog inoculated with rabies virus. This ultrathin section of a cell shows randomly spaced viral matrices (*M*) and virions (*arrow*) budding from endoplasmic reticulum membranes (original magnification, ×62,560).

single-stranded RNA is tightly encased with the **nucleoprotein (N protein)**. A **phosphoprotein (P protein)** also is found in the RNP core. Because the genome of rabies virus is of **negative polarity**, the virions contain an **RNA-dependent RNA polymerase (L) protein**. The replication cycle of rabies viruses takes place entirely in the cytoplasm of infected cells and results in the formation of numerous virus particles. Masses of nucleocapsids accumulate in the cytoplasm of neurons to form inclusions, called **Negri bodies**, which can be seen in specially stained preparations or by immunofluorescence (Fig. 35-2).

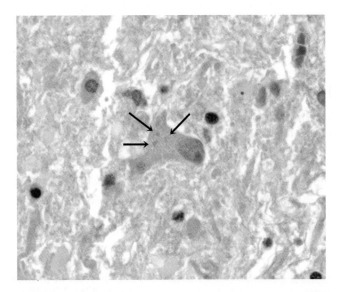

FIGURE 35-2. Negri bodies in a neuron of a human with rabies. Intracytoplasmic inclusions known as Negri bodies like those seen in this hematoxylin–eosin-stained section (*arrows*) of brainstem are highly pathognomonic for rabies (original magnification, ×158).

Resistance to rabies infection has long been correlated with the presence of neutralizing antiviral antibodies, and that relationship has been well established in a variety of experimental animal studies. Some of the viruses in this group may elicit the formation of antibodies that cross-react against other members of the group.

ENCOUNTER

In most years, only one to three human rabies cases are reported in the United States. Those cases are either imported or associated with exposures to wild or unidentified animals. Tens of thousands of cases of animal rabies occur annually worldwide, most of which are in domestic animals. Consequently, humans from regions of endemic rabies are vaccinated after exposure to dogs and cats that are known to be rabid or have escaped examination and observation. In contrast, most rabies cases in the United States are found in wild, not domestic, animals.

Rabies epidemiology varies greatly from country to country. In almost all of Africa and Asia, rabies continues to be a disease of dogs that accounts for more than 90% of human rabies deaths. Where canine rabies exists, human rabies remains common, and millions of persons are vaccinated annually for exposures to rabid animals, mostly dogs. Worldwide, an estimated 50,000 to 100,000 persons die of rabies every year, and most of those cases occur in developing countries. In much of the developed world, where rabies in dogs has been controlled, the disease primarily affects a variety of wild animals and the animals that they bite. In eastern Europe, for instance, the red fox is the primary transmitter of rabies, and most cases are found in that species. In the United States and Canada, rabies is maintained by skunks, raccoons, foxes, and insectivorous bats.

It is crucial to monitor the exact location of rabid animals within each state through state health departments or federal health agencies, because that information will assist in deciding whether to recommend prophylaxis for persons bitten by animals. If a given species has not been reported to be rabid in a certain area (e.g., terrestrial animals in the Pacific Northwest), prophylaxis of persons exposed to that species in that area is usually unnecessary. However, a person bitten by a bat in a geographic area where rabid bats have been found will require prophylaxis. Some animal species are almost never diagnosed as rabid, including rodents (mice, rats, hamsters) and lagomorphs (rabbits and hares). Approximately 25,000 to 40,000 persons are vaccinated against rabies each year in the United States. Only a small number of people who are vaccinated are known to have actually been bitten by rabid animals.

The bite of a rabid animal does not necessarily result in rabies. Contrary to popular beliefs, humans are somewhat refractory to the rabies virus. Historical records show that the average occurrence of disease after the bite of a known rabid dog is about 15%, although the percentage rises to more than 60% with severe bites on the face and head.

ENTRY

Rabies virus is transmitted most commonly through the bite of an infected animal. Nonbite exposures involving contact of saliva or other potentially infectious material (e.g., neural tissue) with mucous membranes or nonintact skin also can result in disease. In contrast, activities such as petting or handling an animal, saliva contact with intact skin, or contact with blood, urine, or feces do not constitute an exposure. Aerosol transmission of the virus has only been well documented in laboratory settings involving concentrated virus and is unlikely to pose a threat to nonlaboratory workers. Human-to-human rabies virus transmission has not been well documented except in cases of organ or tissue transplantation.

The problems associated with exposures to the rabies virus are very different from those with other viral diseases in which contact may be unknown, because the location and time of possible virus entry (by bite) are usually obvious in rabies. The following questions relate particularly to rabies:

- Did the bite result in a skin break?
- Has rabies been reported in the state or region where the bite occurred?
- Was the biting animal rabid? Is it available for laboratory diagnosis, or did it escape?
- Is the species known commonly to be infected with the virus?
- Is the biting animal a dog, cat, or ferret that can be observed? (If so, the period of shedding or potential virus transmission is usually concomitant with illness, or a few days before, up to a maximum of 10 days, which allows a generous safety margin. If a person has been bitten by a dog 11 days before the dog gets sick, no prophylaxis is needed.)

SPREAD AND REPLICATION

After rabies virus enters the body through a bite, the **incubation period** is usually between 1 and 3 months but can last up to 12 months and, in rare cases, years. The length of the incubation period depends in part on the size of the viral inoculum, the length of the neural path from the wound to the brain, and the type of virus. Thus, a severe bite on the face or head typically results in a shorter incubation period.

Studies using experimental animals have shown that during the incubation period, the rabies virus may move into the nervous system or remain at or close to the bite. It is not known exactly where the virus resides during that period or what factors stimulate the virus to advance to the peripheral and central nervous systems. When the virus eventually reaches the peripheral nerves, it quickly advances to the spinal ganglia, spinal cord, and brain (Fig. 35-3). The virus moves passively within the

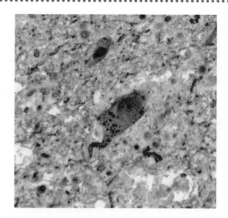

FIGURE 35-3. Rabies virus antigen in a neuron of a human with rabies. Advancement of rabies virus from peripheral nerves to the central nervous system results in infection of the brain as evidenced by the detection of rabies virus antigen, seen in *red* after immunohistochemical staining, in this section of human brainstem (original magnification, ×158).

axoplasm of peripheral nerves to the central nervous system in a retrograde fashion.

From the brain, the virus often returns to the periphery using the same axoplasmic route as used for centripetal movement. A favored peripheral site is the highly innervated **salivary glands**, but toward the end of the disease course, the virus may be found in many other tissues. In some cases, the virus never reaches the salivary glands or any exit route, and the host can die from acute encephalitis. The level of virus in the salivary gland tissue of rabid animals may be 1,000 or more times the level found in the brain, suggesting that the virus replicates at peripheral sites. The presence of virus in the salivary glands combined with altered and often aggressive behavior helps explain the transmission of virus from one animal to another through infectious saliva.

DAMAGE

A surprisingly limited amount of histopathological change occurs in the central nervous system of animals or humans dying of rabies. Neurons of infected animals and humans contain typical intracytoplasmic inclusions, the **Negri bodies** (Fig. 35-2). These inclusions are highly pathognomonic—that is, indicative of the specific disease. In the case of rabies, Negri bodies may be the only diagnostic feature, but they are not always detectable. In some cases, perivascular cuffing and limited neuronal necrosis also occur. These limited histopathological changes are in striking contrast to the marked symptoms seen in human rabies.

Symptoms usually start with fever, headache, **difficulty in swallowing**, and **increased muscle tone**. **Hydrophobia** (contractions of the muscles involved in swallowing) is sometimes elicited by the mere sight or sound of water or other liquids. Eventually, patients develop signs of extensive damage to the central nervous system, progress to coma, and die. Rabies virus can be detected in and isolated from almost all tissues in the body of the deceased host.

Two cases of rabies survivors have suggested that the disease may not be universally fatal and may in fact represent a spectrum of illness. In 2004, a 15-year-old girl in Wisconsin survived clinical rabies after undergoing intensive treatment including coma induction. In 2009, a presumptive abortive human rabies case occurred in a 17-year-old girl in Texas that required only supportive care. In both cases, the diagnosis of rabies was based on a compatible clinical syndrome, a history of bat exposure, and positive serology (rabies virus–specific antibodies detected in serum and cerebrospinal fluid). After recovery, both patients had minimal sequelae. Although reports of survival from rabies have been described, these patients were unique in that neither had received any form of postexposure prophylaxis before the onset of illness. Attempts to replicate the protocol used in Wisconsin have not demonstrated proven effectiveness, although research into treatment strategies is ongoing.

DIAGNOSIS

For the first half of the 20th century, rabies diagnosis in suspect animals was limited to the detection of Negri bodies in the Ammon horn and cerebellum (the inclusions were found in ~75% of positive cases) and intracerebral inoculation into mice of suspected brain specimens. Those tests resulted in immediate diagnosis of some positive cases but a delayed diagnosis of the remaining cases. Usually, a period of 24 days elapsed until the inoculated mice either died of rabies or survived.

In 1958, the **fluorescent antibody technique** was introduced. That test involves staining suspect brain impressions with a fluorescein-tagged antibody to rabies virus. Diagnosis also can be made in persons with encephalitis by fluorescent staining of skin biopsies of the nape of the neck where many hair follicles are found (the infected nerve network around hair follicles

HISTORY OF RABIES

Disease associated with the bite of many kinds of animals has been recognized for thousands of years. For example, in the Mesopotamian Eşhnunna Code, dating from about 2300 BC, it is written: "If a dog is mad, and if the authorities have made its owner aware of this fact; if... it bites a man and causes his death, the owner must pay two thirds of a mina." That amounted to about 40 shekels of silver. Whether this account was an early recognition of rabies or merely outright death from a vicious dog is uncertain. Nevertheless, in the glory that was Greece and the grandeur that was Rome lurked the horror that was recognized by the great thinkers of the time, including Democritus, Aristotle, Celsus, and Galen.

Evidence that saliva was infective came in the early 19th century when Georg Gottfried Zinke, a German scientist, demonstrated that saliva from a rabid dog placed in contact with the wounds on the leg of an uninfected dachshund caused the disease. In 1881, Louis Pasteur delineated the role of the central nervous system in rabies when he injected rabbits intracerebrally (rather than intramuscularly) with a suspension of brain taken from a rabid cow and thus reproduced the disease. Pasteur produced the first rabies vaccines by passing infectious spinal cord material (he did not know it was a virus at the time) through a series of rabbits. The then-infected spinal cords were partially inactivated by drying over potash for various periods. Pasteur's first rabies vaccination injection consisted of cords dried for 14 days. Subsequent injections used cords dried for shorter periods, until the last injection employed fully virulent cord suspensions.

Although Pasteur's early studies of vaccine were performed on dogs and other animals, the results from those studies led to the triumphant use of a spinal cord vaccine in a human in July 1885, when a 9-year-old boy, Joseph Meister, was successfully treated for severe wounds received from a rabid dog. Over the next few decades, the original vaccine underwent many changes, including chemical inactivation of the virus. Early vaccines were prepared from virus grown in nervous system tissue. Regrettably, those vaccines resulted in postvaccine demyelination and tissue destruction in approximately one-third of vaccinated individuals.

Today, safe and effective vaccines are produced from inactivated viruses grown in nonneural tissue culture. Recombinant rabies vaccines are also being tested and have been used to control rabies among wildlife in Europe and North America.

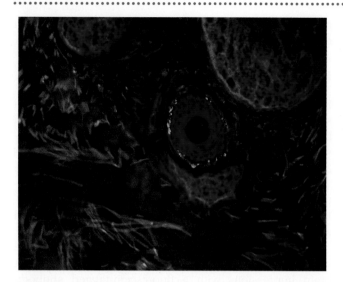

FIGURE 35-4. Rabies virus antigen in perifollicular nerves from a human skin biopsy of the nape of the neck. Viral antigens appear *apple green* after staining with fluorescein-tagged antibodies specific for rabies. Direct fluorescent antibody testing has become the procedure of choice for diagnosing rabies (original magnification, ×200).

fluoresces) during the encephalitic period (Fig. 35-4). The fluorescent antibody technique has become the diagnostic procedure of choice for use early in the disease. Neutralizing antibodies are found in the serum and cerebrospinal fluid later in infection, usually 8 to 10 days after the encephalitic symptoms appear. Virus can be isolated from saliva in cell culture, or viral nucleic acid can be amplified from saliva or infected tissues by a polymerase chain reaction test.

PREVENTION

Vaccination of Animals

Rabies is a zoonosis, a disease transmitted to humans by animals—in this case, by infected mammals. The best protection against the disease can be achieved by the elimination of rabies virus in dogs (and preventing exposure to cats) by requiring **vaccination of pets** by law, thereby creating a barrier to human exposure by the interruption of animal-to-animal transmission (either dog-to-dog or wild animal-to-dog). An additional approach is to vaccinate wild animals. Vaccination of red foxes has been performed successfully on a mass scale in Europe and Canada by dropping baited oral vaccines from airplanes. A similar strategy is being used to vaccinate raccoons, the major reservoir in the northeastern United States, and gray foxes and coyotes in Texas.

Prophylaxis of Humans

Because the incubation period of rabies is usually long, and because disease is preventable if neutralizing antibodies are present when the virus emerges in the central nervous system, rabies is one of the few infectious diseases for which there is highly effective prevention afforded by primary and secondary immunization after exposure to the infectious agent. A risk assessment should be performed after a potential exposure to determine the need for postexposure prophylaxis. For example, unnecessary postexposure prophylaxis can be avoided if the dog, cat, or ferret responsible for the exposure remains healthy after 10 days of observation. Once the decision to provide postexposure prophylaxis has been made, prophylaxis of humans consists of three steps: (1) **local wound treatment**, (2) **passive administration of antibody** (antiserum or rabies immunoglobulin), and (3) **vaccination** (Fig. 35-5). Superficial wounds can be washed with soap and water. The passive antibody administered in developed countries is **human rabies immune globulin** (**HRIG**) collected from immunized persons and administered as soon as possible after rabies exposure at a dose of 20 IU/kg; as much as possible is infiltrated at the bite site, and the remainder is administered intramuscularly.

Vaccination with modern tissue culture vaccines consists of a series of four doses, all administered intramuscularly in the deltoid region, 1 mL each, over a 2-week period (days 0, 3, 7, and 14). For persons with immunosuppression, the recommended postexposure prophylaxis series includes five doses of vaccine administered on days 0, 3, 7, 14, and 28. The most common vaccines are prepared with avian embryos or several kinds of human or monkey cells in culture from which the virus is purified and inactivated. All individuals given such vaccination have developed the expected level of antibodies. When the combination of globulin and vaccine has been properly applied promptly, no prophylaxis failures have been noted, and complications have been rare.

People in certain professions, such as veterinarians and animal handlers, are considered at higher risk of rabies virus exposure. These individuals may receive preexposure vaccination (usually three doses of vaccine on days 0, 7, and 21 or 28) and two booster vaccinations (on days 0 and 3) if they ever have a known exposure (such as an animal bite).

CONCLUSION

Rabies is a viral disease of mammals. The virus is neurotropic and shed in the saliva. Rabies is almost always caused by a bite. The disease may be prevented by avoiding exposure to animal bites. Rabies is almost always fatal after the onset of illness. A large part of disease control encompasses measures to prevent rabid animals from biting people. In the developing world, the prime offenders are dogs, and canine vaccination is essential in those areas. In many parts of the developed world, wildlife is the source of exposure. All mammals may be susceptible, but only certain hosts maintain the disease. Common animals include bats and carnivores such as foxes, raccoons, skunks, mongooses, and coyotes.

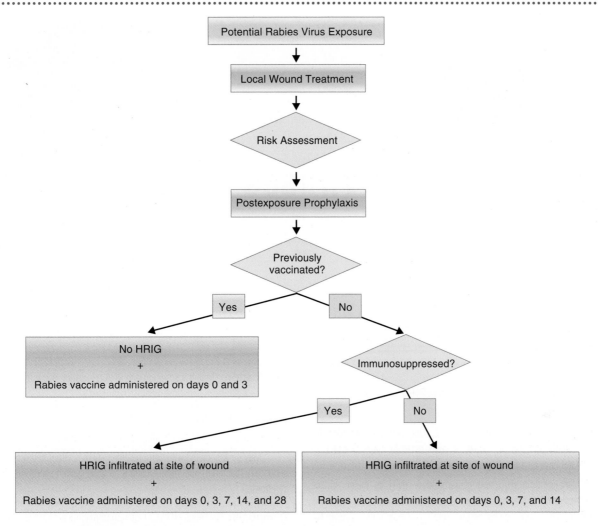

FIGURE 35-5. Algorithm for Postexposure Prophylaxis. All potential exposures to rabies virus should receive local wound treatment and a risk assessment. The recommended postexposure prophylaxis regimen varies based on history of previous rabies vaccination and immune status. (HRIG, human rabies immune globulin.)

Avoiding contact with strange-acting animals and wildlife can prevent exposure. Vaccinating pets and being a responsible owner by supervising pets are critical to avoiding rabies. Prompt first aid after a bite and proper prophylaxis by immune globulin and vaccine can prevent the disease. State and national public health officials can provide information about the current epidemiology of the disease and answer questions about the risk of acquisition from various exposure scenarios.

Suggested Readings

Centers for Disease Control and Prevention. Human rabies—Missouri, 2008. *MMWR Morb Mortal Wkly Rep.* 2009;58:1207–1209.

Centers for Disease Control and Prevention. Investigation of rabies infections in organ donor and transplant recipients—Alabama, Arkansas, Oklahoma, and Texas, 2004. *MMWR Morb Mortal Wkly Rep.* 2004;53:586–589.

Centers for Disease Control and Prevention. Presumptive Abortive Human Rabies—Texas, 2009. *MMWR Morb Mortal Wkly Rep.* 2010;59:185–190.

Compendium of Animal Rabies Prevention and Control, 2008: National Association of State Public Health Veterinarians, Inc. (NASPHV). *MMWR Recomm Rep.* 2008;57(RR-2);1–9.

Gibbons RV. Cryptogenic rabies, bats, and the question of aerosol transmission. *Ann Emerg Med.* 2002;39:528–536.

Human rabies prevention—United States, 2008. Recommendations of the Advisory Committee on Immunization Practices (ACIP). *MMWR Recomm Rep.* 2008;57(RR-3):1–26,28.

Jackson AC, Warrell MJ, Rupprecht CE, et al. Management of rabies in humans. *Clin Infect Dis.* 2003;36:60–63.

Messenger SL, Smith JS, Orciari LA, et al. Emerging pattern of rabies deaths and increased viral infectivity. *Emerg Infect Dis.* 2003;9:151–154.

Moran GJ, Talan DA, Mower W, et al. Appropriateness of rabies postexposure prophylaxis treatment for animal exposures. Emergency ID Net Study Group. *JAMA.* 2000;284:1001–1007.

Use of a reduced (4-dose) vaccine schedule for postexposure prophylaxis to prevent human rabies: recommendations of the Advisory Committee on Immunization Practices (ACIP). *MMWR Recomm Rep.* 2010;59(RR-2):1–9.

Willoughby RE Jr, Tieves KS, Hoffman GM, et al. Survival after treatment of rabies with induction of coma. *N Engl J Med.* 2005;352:2508–2514.

Chapter **36**

Influenza and Its Viruses

Peter Palese

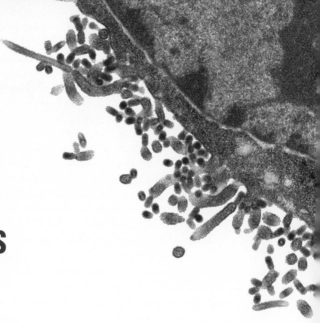

KEY CONCEPTS

Pathogen: Influenza viruses

- Contain a genome of segmented negative-sense RNAs.

- Belong to three types: A, B, and C.

- Can infect birds (including poultry), horses, pigs, and other animals, for example, ferrets, guinea pigs, minks, or seals (type A); types B and C in general do not have an animal reservoir.

- Possess hemagglutinin (HA) and neuraminidase (NA) as major surface antigens. Antigenic drift is caused by the yearly accumulation of mutations in the HA and NA; antigenic shift results from the acquisition of a novel HA and NA by the virus.

Encounter: Influenza occurs in epidemics and pandemics in the winter (seasonality).

Entry: Influenza viruses are acquired by person-to-person spread via respiratory droplets that infect the upper and lower respiratory tract.

Spread: Cell infection is initiated by attachment of the viral HA to sialic acid–containing glycoproteins or glycolipids and subsequent uptake into an endocytic vesicle.

Replication: Gene transcription and RNA replication occur in the nucleus, not in the cytoplasm like most other RNA viruses.

Damage: Causes clinical symptoms, including common cold, pharyngitis, tracheobronchitis, and bronchiolitis or croup in children.

May be associated with complications such as viral pneumonia, secondary (bacterial) pneumonia, central nervous system syndromes, or Reye syndrome.

Diagnosis: Still relies on virus isolation from clinical samples, including sputum and nose and throat washings or swabs, but rapid diagnostic tests are also available.

Treatment and Prevention: Antivirals active against influenza include rimantadine and amantadine (which inhibit viral uncoating after uptake) and NA inhibitors (which inhibit viral release from the infected cell and cause aggregation of viral particles).

Prevention is best achieved with either the inactivated vaccine or the live, attenuated, cold-adapted vaccine.

INFLUENZA can be a serious disease in humans and is characterized by repeated **epidemics** and **pandemics** (global epidemics). The cyclical nature of influenza reflects the characteristic of the virus to undergo **antigenic drift** (accumulating changes in the antigenic sites of the hemagglutinin [HA] and less importantly of the neuraminidase [NA]) or **antigenic shift** (capturing a novel HA and occasionally also an NA by exchange of genes with another virus in a process called **reassortment**). Despite the availability of vaccines and antiviral drugs, influenza ranks among the major public health threats in the United States, causing annually an average of about 20 million respiratory illnesses, 100,000 hospitalizations, and more than 20,000 deaths. Influenza virus types A and B (but not C) are mostly responsible for the disease in humans.

CASE • A woman brought her 2-year-old son, P., to the family physician in early January. The day before, her 6-year-old son, F., had developed high fever, sore throat, and muscle aches. When F. developed a runny nose, the boys' mother became concerned about P. He showed signs of crankiness, and his mother thought P. might have contracted the same disease as his older sibling.

The doctor did not order any laboratory work but wrote a prescription for an antipyretic and an antiviral drug active against influenza virus. In fact, he asked the mother to take that same drug as well. After the doctor discovered that the other members of the household, the father and another boy (15 years of age), did not show any signs of illness, he

suggested that they (but not the 6-year-old) also take that drug to prevent influenza.

This case raises several questions:

1. Why did the physician think P. would develop influenza even though no laboratory tests supported the assumption?

2. What was the most likely drug the physician prescribed to the patient and other family members? Why did he not give the medication to the 6-year-old sibling?

3. What should the physician have asked regarding all family members, and what should he have recommended the family do next year?

See Appendix for answers.

PATHOGEN: INFLUENZA VIRUSES

All influenza viruses possess a common structure (Fig. 36-1). Each RNA segment is encapsidated by the **viral nucleoprotein (NP)** and the three **virus-encoded polymerase proteins (PA, PB1, and PB2)**. The encapsidated RNAs are surrounded by the **matrix (M) protein**.

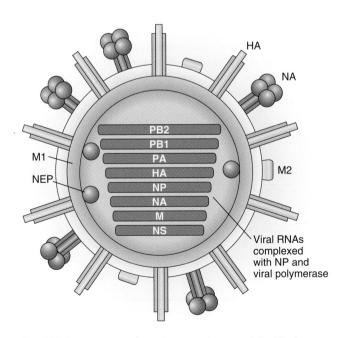

FIGURE 36-1. Diagram of an influenza virus particle. The hemagglutinin (HA) is a trimer, the neuraminidase (NA) is a tetramer, and the M2 ion channel is a tetramer. The matrix protein (M1) underlies the plasma membrane–derived lipid envelope. A nuclear export protein (NEP) is also associated with the virus. The eight viral RNA segments are coated with nucleoprotein (NP) and bound by the polymerase complex (PA, PB1, and PB2).

This complex in turn is surrounded by the host-derived lipid membrane, into which the surface glycoproteins, **HA** and **NA**, are embedded. The RNA genome of influenza A viruses consists of eight segments encoding up to 12 proteins (Fig. 36-2). Antibodies made against the internal proteins of a single strain of influenza A virus cross-react with the proteins of all other type A strains but not with those of an influenza virus type B or C. Influenza virus types B and C have diverged sufficiently from type A influenza viruses (and from each other) that no cross-reactivity with antisera can be detected. Possibly because they have an **animal reservoir**, only influenza A viruses (not influenza B or C virus) occur as **subtypes**; there are currently 16 HA subtypes and 9 NA subtypes.

Three instances of antigenic shift occurred in the 20th century. Figure 36-3 shows the circulation of influenza A viruses starting with the pandemic of 1918. During that well-documented event at the end of World War I, an estimated 50 million (or more) people died of what was called the **Spanish flu**, and countless millions had severe disease. Following the 1918 pandemic, influenza A viruses of the H1N1 subtype remained prevalent until 1957. During the next 11 years, from 1957 to 1968, H2N2 viruses (**Asian flu**) circulated, and since 1968, the **Hong Kong** subtype (H3N2) has predominated. Interestingly, H1N1 viruses reemerged in 1977 and have cocirculated with the H3N2 viruses since that time.

Predictions about the characteristics of novel pandemic strains cannot be made with certainty, but if the past is any guide to the future, we would expect reassortment between human and animal influenza viruses to result in new pandemic strains. For example, in 1968, a novel HA (H3) replaced the H2 HA, and the PB1 gene also changed. It is likely that the two genes were captured from an avian strain, and the remaining six genes were derived from the H2N2 virus circulating in humans during the previous

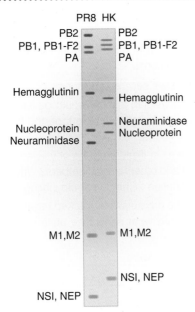

FIGURE 36-2. Eight RNA segments of influenza A/Puerto Rico/8/34 (PR8) and A/Hong Kong/8/68 (HK) viruses. The viral RNAs are separated on a polyacrylamide gel. The proteins encoded by the RNAs are indicated. The PB1 gene encodes the polymerase protein PB1 and the proapoptotic PB1-F2, which also has anti-interferon activity. The M gene encodes the matrix protein (M1) and the ion channel protein (M2). The NS gene encodes the nonstructural protein (NS1), which is an interferon antagonist, and the nuclear export protein (NEP, formerly called NS2).

subtype period (Fig. 36-4). In April 2009, a novel H1N1 virus appeared, which was designated a pandemic strain in June 2009 by the World Health Organization (WHO). This pandemic H1N1 virus also was derived by reassortment. Five genes were from swine viruses (including the HA and the NA), two genes were from an avian source, and a single gene came from a human influenza virus.

Antigenic drift occurs with both influenza A and B viruses. In general, drift over a period of 3 to 5 years is sufficient to allow a novel strain to cause disease. The antigenic sites in HA that undergo mutations (antigenic drift) have been defined (Fig. 36-5). Antigenic drift (as well as the occasional antigenic shift) requires that new vaccine formulations be used each year (see "Treatment and Prevention"). At the beginning of the 21st century, H3N2 and H1N1 influenza A viruses, as well as influenza B virus strains, were responsible for disease in humans. In 2010, the novel H1N1 pandemic virus appeared to replace the seasonal H1N1 strain. Thus, the 2010/2011 vaccine formulation contained three different strains (the seasonal H3N2, the novel H1N1, and a B virus component).

ENCOUNTER

Infections from influenza virus types A and B usually appear in the Northern hemisphere between October and April, with peaks between December and March. Influenza C virus infections are usually nonseasonal, and most occur in children between 1 and 4 years of age. In general, infections with influenza virus type C are less severe than those caused by influenza A and B viruses. However, most adults and children over 6 years of age are seropositive for influenza C viruses (Table 36-1).

ENTRY

Influenza viruses are transmitted from person to person by **airborne droplets** (most probably 1 to 5 μm in size) and possibly by direct contact. Coughing and sneezing

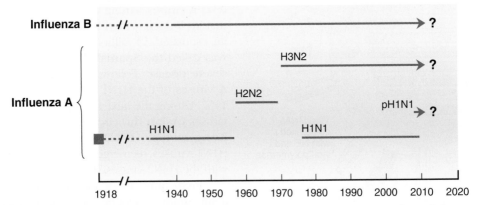

FIGURE 36-3. Epidemiology of influenza A and B viruses. The appearance of new influenza A virus subtypes in 1918, 1957, and 1968 resulted in pandemics. The broken lines indicate the probable prevailing strains before isolation of the first human influenza viruses. Sequence analysis of viral RNA obtained from formalin-fixed and frozen tissue samples indicates that the 1918 pandemic strain was an H1N1 virus (*solid square*). In 2009, yet another pandemic H1N1 (pH1N1) virus appeared. It is unpredictable whether these viruses will continue to circulate or whether new (pandemic) strains will emerge.

Antigenic shift

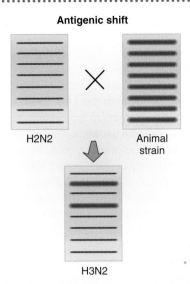

FIGURE 36-4. Antigenic shift: Reassortment of a human H2N2 and an animal (avian) influenza virus. The H3N2 virus responsible for the pandemic in 1968 is postulated to have derived its PB1 and HA genes (*red lines*) from an animal strain and its remaining six RNAs from an H2N2 parent virus (*blue lines*).

are obvious ways in which the virus becomes airborne. Although the precise mechanism of influenza transmission is unknown, the virus infects the mucosa of the upper and lower respiratory tract. The incubation period is usually 1 to 2 days, and virus shedding during uncomplicated influenza continues for 3 to 6 days. Influenza viremia or invasion of extrarespiratory tissues is very rare.

Influenza viruses infect the upper and lower respiratory tracts. The first cells to be infected are nonciliated epithelial cells. The preferred receptor for the virus on these cells is a terminal sialic acid in a (2-6) linkage to galactose. Whether the virus establishes infection depends mostly on the presence or absence of **neutralizing antibodies** in the host and the capacity of the virus to overcome the host **innate immune response (antiviral interferon response)**.

SPREAD AND REPLICATION

Infection of cells by influenza viruses is initiated by attachment of the HA to the viral receptor (sialic acid–containing glycoproteins or glycolipids on the cell surface) and subsequent uptake of the virus into an endocytic vesicle. Under the acidified conditions within the vesicle, the HA undergoes a structural change leading to fusion of the viral envelope with the membrane of the endocytic vesicle. At the same time, the M2 protein of the virus, which has **ion channel activity**, allows the influx of H+ ions from the vesicle into the interior of the virus, facilitating the uncoating of the virus and release of the viral gene segments (ribonucleoprotein) into the cytoplasm. The processes of viral uncoating and genome release are inhibited by the antiviral drugs **amantadine** and **rimantadine**. Subsequently, the viral ribonucleoprotein enters the nucleus, where

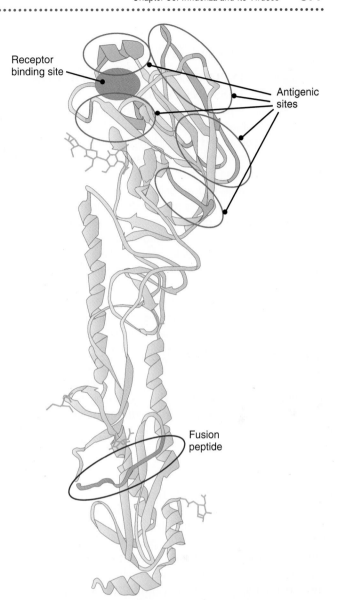

FIGURE 36-5. Ribbon representation of the HA monomer from the 1918 influenza virus based on X-ray diffraction analysis. The five predicted antigenic sites surround the sialic acid receptor–binding site. Viruses counter antibody reactivity by altering these sites or introducing new glycosylation sites (existing glycosylation sites are colored *orange*) through a process called antigenic drift. This fusion peptide is displayed toward the membrane proximal end (**bottom**).

TABLE 36-1 Characteristics of Influenza Virus Types A, B, and C

Characteristic	A	B	C
Frequency of isolation	+++	++	±
Severity of disease	+++	++	±
Animal reservoir	Yes	No	No
RNA segments	8	8	7

+++, high; ++, medium; ±, infrequent.

PARADIGM BOX

INFLUENZA PANDEMIC OF 1918: LESSONS LEARNED

A **pandemic** occurs when a highly virulent and transmissible virus emerges to which most people lack prior exposure and thus immunity. In the case of influenza, the virus can acquire a new surface antigen (e.g., HA) by exchanging its "old" HA for a "new" one. If a human influenza virus and an animal influenza virus happen to infect the same cell, a novel virus can form through **reassortment** of the genes of the two viruses (see Fig. 36-4). Influenza pandemics occurred in the 20th century in 1918, 1957, and 1968. In each case, it is likely that an antigenic shift occurred when the human strain acquired a new HA from an avian virus infecting the same cell. The estimated death toll from the 1918 pandemic exceeded 50 million people worldwide. Among the US military, approximately an equal number of men died from influenza as from direct military action in World War I.

Although no live 1918 virus is available, recent technological breakthroughs allow RNA sequences to be obtained from formaldehyde-treated lung samples (in paraffin blocks) by **reverse transcription polymerase chain reaction** (**RT-PCR**). Based on its sequence, a gene can be reconstructed by using synthetic oligonucleotides. Virus containing genes from the 1918 strain can then be rescued (in a high-containment facility) from the DNA by a technique called **reverse genetics**. The study of the resurrected **1918 virus** using animal models has revealed that the virus was unusually virulent. In fact, the reconstructed extinct 1918 virus can kill mice in as few as 3 days, faster than any other human virus tested thus far. The generation of reassortant viruses (i.e., replacing one of the genes of the 1918 virus with one from a low pathogenicity influenza virus strain) showed that the HA, NA, and PB1 genes are crucial for the extraordinary virulence of the 1918 virus. Nevertheless, currently available antivirals would be effective against the 1918 pandemic virus. Vaccines also have been shown (in mice) to be effective against the 1918 strain. In fact, vaccination with the current pandemic H1N1 influenza vaccine protects mice against a challenge with the 1918 virus. Thus, we have learned valuable lessons from the 1918 pandemic virus. We have gained an understanding of why the virus was so virulent, and we have developed effective countermeasures: antivirals and vaccines.

viral mRNA is synthesized. In this way, influenza virus is unlike most RNA viruses in that transcription and RNA replication occur in the nucleus and not in the cytoplasm. Viral protein synthesis and amplification of the viral RNA allows the formation of viral ribonucleoproteins and the assembly and budding of new particles from the cytoplasmic membrane. The function of the NA is to remove the sialic acid receptors from the virus particles and the cell surface. This process prevents new viruses from adhering to each other and the surface of the infected cell. **Neuraminidase inhibitors (oseltamivir, zanamivir, and peramivir)** effectively prevent the removal of cell-surface sialic acid, thereby inhibiting the spread of virus particles from infected cells to uninfected cells.

DAMAGE

In uncomplicated cases of influenza, respiratory epithelial cell function is affected by the infection- and inflammation-induced edema, and mononuclear cell infiltrates in the lamina propria are observed. In more severe disease, gross pathologic findings include hemorrhagic and airless lungs and necrotizing tracheobronchitis and bronchiolitis. Later in the infection, severe alveolar damage can occur, sometimes with extensive fibrosis. A direct cytopathic effect is most likely responsible for the pathologic changes observed following infection, and the direct involvement of the upper and lower respiratory tracts can account for most of the signs and symptoms of the disease (see the box entitled "Clinical Manifestations of Influenza"). Much of what we know about the pathogenicity of influenza viruses comes from experiments using animal models. The histopathological changes in the lungs of mice infected with even low-virulence influenza viruses are dramatic (Fig. 36-6).

Complications caused by infection with influenza virus have been described including **primary viral pneumonia, secondary bacterial pneumonia, and otitis media**. Reye syndrome in children is associated with infections by influenza virus type B (and occasionally type A), leading to brain swelling and a fatty degeneration of the liver. Interestingly, the incidence of Reye syndrome has been lowered dramatically as a result of the decreased use of aspirin (acetylsalicylate) in children, which had previously been identified as a cofactor in the disease.

DIAGNOSIS

The laboratory diagnosis of influenza in many cases still relies on virus isolation from clinical samples, including sputum and nose and throat washings or swabs. Embryonated chicken eggs or Madin-Darby canine kidney tissue-culture cells are the preferred substrates for isolation of the virus. Viral antigens can be detected in clinical samples by a variety of immunoassays, and RT-PCR can be used to detect viral RNA. Prior infections (as evidenced

A PBS

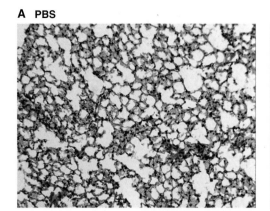

B Low virulence virus

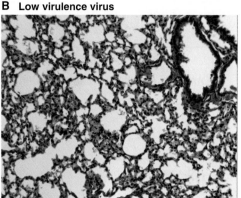

C High virulence virus

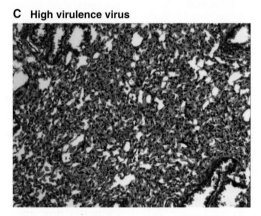

FIGURE 36-6. Lung histology of mice infected with influenza viruses of low and high virulence. Mice were inoculated with **(A)** phosphate-buffered saline (PBS) as a control or 10^4 infectious particles of either **(B)** low-virulence or **(C)** high-virulence influenza viruses. Lung sections (6 μm) were stained with hematoxylin and eosin and imaged using bright-field microscopy at 10× magnification. In mock-infected mice, the lung parenchyma demonstrates clear alveolar airspaces defined by thin septa of squamous epithelial cells and capillaries. In the lungs of mice infected with the low virulence virus, alveolar septa are widened with interstitial infiltration by inflammatory cells. Scattered alveoli demonstrate opacification by an inflammatory cell infiltrate and proteinaceous material. In the lungs of mice infected with the high virulence virus, diffuse airspace obliteration is seen, with a majority of alveoli filled by inflammatory cells and debris.

CLINICAL MANIFESTATIONS OF INFLUENZA

Symptoms and signs
- Malaise
- Myalgia
- Fever
- Chills
- Headache
- Respiratory symptoms
- Cough
- Substernal burning
- Gastrointestinal symptoms (rare)

Complications
- Pneumonia
- Secondary bacterial pneumonia
- Otitis media
- Reye syndrome
- Encephalitis (possibly Parkinson disease)

TABLE 36-2 Antiviral Drugs Active Against Influenza

Generic (Trade Name)	Antiviral Activity	Route of Administration
Amantadine	Influenza A	Oral
Rimantadine (Flumadine)	Influenza A	Oral
Oseltamivir (Tamiflu)	Influenza A and B	Oral
Zanamivir (Relenza)	Influenza A and B	Inhalation
Peramivir	Influenza A and B	Intravenous (emergency use against pandemic H1N1 only)

by the presence of anti-influenza virus antibodies) can be demonstrated by the classical **hemagglutination-inhibition test**. Sera from patients are used to measure the inhibition of agglutination of chicken or human red blood cells by known influenza viruses. However, the majority of clinical diagnoses do not involve the use of laboratory tests but are based on clinical symptoms, epidemiological evidence from the community, and knowledge concerning the seasonality of the virus. In the future, the use of rapid influenza virus tests will likely become much more widespread, because the reliability of these tests has been dramatically improved.

TREATMENT AND PREVENTION

Influenza is frequently treated only symptomatically. However, there are now specific antiviral therapeutics that arrest influenza virus replication (Table 36-2). Amantadine and rimantadine are effective only against influenza A viruses. That drawback—combined with known adverse reactions, including dizziness, central nervous system symptoms, and the emergence of drug resistance—makes those antiviral approaches less desirable. NA inhibitors such as oseltamivir and zanamivir are efficacious in the treatment of both influenza A and B viruses and also can be used prophylactically. Resistance to NA inhibitors has become a problem with some influenza virus strains (e.g., H3N2 viruses), but inhibitor-resistant mutants may be less pathogenic than the wild-type virus.

The most cost-effective treatment modality remains prophylactic vaccination (see the box entitled "Influenza Virus Vaccines"). Currently, **inactivated vaccines** and **live**, **attenuated**, **cold-adapted vaccines** are available. The inactivated vaccines are formaldehyde-treated preparations of whole virus or disrupted "split" virus. They are injected intramuscularly, and their level of efficacy is generally in the range of 60 to 90% in healthy children and adults. The injection may cause local reactions, but the killed inactivated vaccine cannot cause influenza-like symptoms in recipients. In contrast to the injectable killed virus vaccine, the live, attenuated, cold-adapted influenza virus vaccine induces a **local mucosal response** because it is given as a nasal spray, resulting in low-level replication in respiratory epithelial cells. Immunization with the live, attenuated virus vaccine also may induce a response that is more cross-reactive against different viral variants and thus may offer longer-lasting immunity than that resulting from vaccination with the inactivated preparation. Immunization against influenza is of paramount importance in curbing the disease and also reduces the risk of influenza-related complications, such as myocardial infarction in patients with coronary disease and otitis media in young children. Thus, the use of influenza virus vaccines is cost-effective and brings added benefits to certain risk groups. Efforts are ongoing to improve existing vaccines (through development of genetically engineered strains) and establish the safest and most effective regimens for special populations, such as very young children and the immunocompromised.

The current manufacturing process relies on the selection of antigenically appropriate strains by the Food and Drug Administration (FDA) in February of each year.

INFLUENZA VIRUS VACCINES

Killed (inactivated) virus
Split or whole (formaldehyde treated)
Live (attenuated) virus
Cold adapted
Genetically engineered viruses
In development

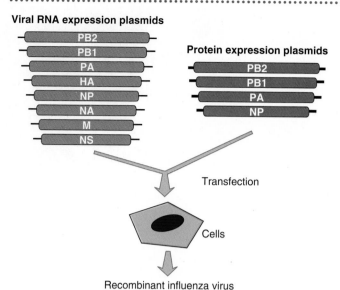

Viral RNA expression plasmids

PB2
PB1
PA
HA
NP
NA
M
NS

Protein expression plasmids

PB2
PB1
PA
NP

Transfection

Cells

Recombinant influenza virus

FIGURE 36-7. Reverse genetics: plasmid-based rescue of infectious influenza virus. Twelve plasmids are introduced into mammalian cells. Eight plasmids express precise copies of the eight viral RNA segments (PA, PB1, PB2, HA, NP, NA, M, and NS). Four plasmids lead to formation of the viral polymerase complex (formed by the PA, PB1, PB2, and NP proteins) required for replication of viral RNAs. The production of viral RNAs and proteins leads to the formation of infectious (recombinant) influenza viruses.

Selection is mostly based on the evaluation of strains that circulated in the previous season in the Northern and Southern hemispheres. Following the February decision, it takes several months to produce sufficient amounts of virus (at this point in embryonated eggs) to allow distribution of inactivated and live influenza virus vaccines in the fall. If this manufacturing process were accelerated, it would be possible to make the selection of strains in the summer, which might allow a better fit of vaccine strains with circulating strains. Other strategies involve the design of a universal influenza virus vaccine, which would use as antigen conserved parts of the virus. Such a vaccine could be effective against many different variants of influenza virus and may induce longer-lasting protective immunity against this ever-changing virus. A vaccine consisting of a "headless" HA, which lacks the highly variable head portion of the molecule but preserves the conserved stalk region, successfully protects mice against challenge with heterologous influenza viruses and offers hope that this approach might be successful in humans.

GENETIC ENGINEERING OF INFLUENZA VIRUSES: REVERSE GENETICS

Influenza viruses are negative-sense RNA viruses whose RNA is not intrinsically infectious. Thus, viral RNA transfected into cells does not produce infectious virus. To introduce specific changes into the genome of influenza viruses (**genetic engineering**), cells are transfected with plasmids expressing the eight viral RNAs as well as helper plasmids that express the viral polymerase proteins. This system, called **reverse genetics**, results in the rescue of infectious virus from DNA and thus can be used to study the effects of genetic changes in the virus (Fig. 36-7). Reverse genetics also allows the generation of **attenuated viruses** for possible use as vaccines. Similar techniques have been developed to generate from cDNA other infectious negative-sense RNA viruses, including bunyaviruses, filoviruses, and paramyxoviruses.

CONCLUSION

Three types of influenza virus (A, B, and C) occur in nature. Antigenic drift (A and B) and antigenic shift (A only) define the epidemiology of this family of negative-sense RNA viruses. Pandemics such as the one in 1918 are characterized by high morbidity and mortality in the human population. Recent developments have resulted in improved antivirals and vaccines against influenza.

Suggested Readings

Hayden FG, Palese P. Influenza virus. In: Richman DD, Whitley RJ, Hayden FG, eds. *Clinical Virology*. 3rd ed. Washington, DC: ASM Press; 2009:943–976.

Mendelman PM, Cordova J, Cho I. Safety, efficacy and effectiveness of the influenza virus vaccine, trivalent, types A and B, live, cold-adapted (CAIV-T) in healthy children and healthy adults. *Vaccine*. 2001;19:2221–2226.

Palese P, Shaw ML. Orthomyxoviridae: the viruses and their replication. In: Knipe DM, Howley PM, et al., eds. *Fields Virology*. 5th ed. Philadelphia, PA: Lippincott-Raven Press; 2007:1647–1689.

Steel J, Lowen AC, Wang T, et al. Influenza virus vaccine based on the conserved hemagglutinin stalk domain. *mBio*. 2010;1(1):e00018–10.

Treanor JJ, Hayden FG. Viral infections. In: Murray JF, Nadel JA, eds. *Textbook of Respiratory Medicine*. 3rd ed. Philadelphia, PA: WB Saunders; 2000:929–984.

Tumpey TM, Basler CF, Aguilar PV, et al. Characterization of the reconstructed 1918 Spanish influenza pandemic virus. *Science*. 2005;310:77–80.

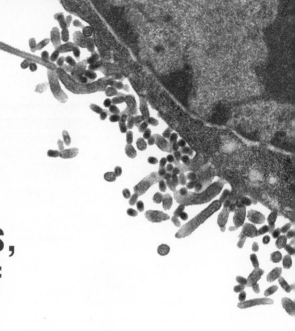

Chapter **37**

Rotaviruses, Noroviruses, and Other Viral Agents of Gastroenteritis

Robert L. Atmar and Mary K. Estes

KEY CONCEPTS

Pathogens:

Rotaviruses are wheel-shaped, double-stranded RNA viruses.

Noroviruses are small, single-stranded RNA viruses that currently cannot be cultivated.

Other viruses can also cause viral gastroenteritis (e.g., enteric adenoviruses, sapoviruses, astroviruses, and Aichi virus).

Encounter:
Rotaviruses

• Are the most common cause of viral gastroenteritis in young children. In the United States, they cause disease with peak incidence in the winter months.

Noroviruses

• Are the leading cause of viral gastroenteritis in adults and the second leading cause of severe disease in children.

• Are associated with disease in diverse settings, including schools and child-care centers, nursing homes, vacation settings (e.g., camps and cruise ships), military ships and maneuvers, restaurants and catered meals, and hospitals.

• Have a peak incidence in the winter months in the North America.

Entry: Rotaviruses, noroviruses, and others agents of viral gastroenteritis are all transmitted by the fecal–oral route, usually by person-to-person contact but also by ingestion of food or water.

Spread: These viruses usually do not invade the intestinal mucosa or spread to other organs.

Replication: Susceptibility to norovirus infection and disease is based on histoblood group antigen expression (e.g., blood type and secretor status).

Damage: Both of the principal viruses cause changes in the small intestinal mucosa that lead to diarrhea. Rotaviruses induce long-term immunity.

Diagnosis: Different viruses causing viral gastroenteritis cannot be distinguished based on the clinical presentation.

Treatment and Prevention: Viral gastroenteritis is not treatable by any specific therapy; rather, treatment is supportive to provide and maintain hydration.

Severe rotavirus-induced illness can be prevented or attenuated by vaccination with live virus vaccines.

ACUTE GASTROENTERITIS is one of the most common diseases in humans and continues to be a significant cause of morbidity and mortality. Worldwide, 2.5 million children die each year from the complications of **infectious gastroenteritis**. In the United States, fewer than 500 children per year die from infectious diarrhea, but more than 200,000 children under age 5 are hospitalized for diarrhea-induced dehydration. Before the 1970s, although viral agents were suspected to cause diarrhea, the only etiologic agents for diarrhea that could be diagnosed were bacteria or protozoa. Viral agents of diarrhea were difficult to identify because they do not grow well in cultured cells.

In the 1970s, electron microscopy allowed detection of viruses in stool specimens, and in 1972, Norwalk virus, a **norovirus** that is a type of **calicivirus**, was the first agent of viral diarrhea identified by electron microscopic analysis of stool. When a convalescent serum specimen was mixed with a diarrheal stool specimen, clumped virions were observed, suggesting an immune response had been elicited by a pathogenic virus. Noroviruses are now recognized as the most common cause of outbreaks of viral diarrhea in adults and the second most important cause of diarrhea in children. In 1973, **rotavirus** was identified by electron microscopic examination of stool specimens. Rotavirus is now known to be the most commonly recognized agent of gastroenteritis in children. Four additional viral agents of gastroenteritis have been identified: **enteric adenoviruses**, **sapoviruses**, **astroviruses**, and **Aichi virus** (Table 37-1). Since 40 to 50% of diarrhea cases are still of uncertain etiology, it is likely that additional viral agents will be discovered as causes of gastroenteritis.

ROTAVIRUS

ENCOUNTER

Almost every child in the United States becomes infected with rotavirus. The peak incidence of primary (or initial) rotavirus infection in the United States occurs between 6 months and 2 years of age. Most individuals have experienced infection and are immune to severe rotavirus disease by age 4. Seropositive older children or adults who are reexposed to a high inoculum of virus or who become immunocompromised may experience mild illness. Parents of young children experiencing a primary rotavirus infection may have mild symptoms. Certain individuals known to be at increased risk for complications of dehydration due to viral gastroenteritis include malnourished children and adults, particularly in developing countries, and the elderly, who may experience waning immunity with age.

Rotavirus-induced disease has a **seasonal distribution** in the United States, peaking in the winter and becoming rare in the warmer months. In tropical countries, endemic rotavirus infection occurs throughout the year. Other viruses, such as influenza virus and respiratory syncytial virus, also have characteristic seasonal appearances in temperate climates, but the reasons for the seasonality are not known. As with other viral illnesses, some children will develop rotavirus gastroenteritis without having had contact with symptomatic individuals. Acquisition may result from an encounter with an individual who is asymptomatically shedding virus. Such asymptomatic excretion of rotavirus can occur for weeks before the onset of diarrhea and for days following resolution of symptoms. Other children can shed rotavirus and never experience symptoms.

ENTRY

Endemic rotavirus disease is caused primarily by **person-to-person transmission**. The principal means of transmission is by the **fecal–oral route**. Rotavirus is excreted at levels that reach 10^{12} infectious particles per milliliter of stool. Transmission of as few as 10 infectious particles can result in infection. Outbreaks due to contamination of municipal water supplies and foodborne transmission have been reported but appear to be rare. Speculation exists that rotavirus may spread by the **respiratory route**

TABLE 37-1 Viral Causes of Gastroenteritis in Humans

Etiologic Agent	Virus Family	Genome	Seasonality	Medical Significance
Rotavirus	*Reoviridae*			
Group A		Segmented dsRNA	Predominantly winter	Major cause of diarrhea in children 6–24 mo
Groups B and C		Segmented dsRNA		Rare in United States
Norovirus	*Caliciviridae*	(+) ssRNA	Winter peak, year-round occurrence	Major cause of diarrhea outbreaks in children and adults
Sapovirus	*Caliciviridae*	(+) ssRNA	Year-round	Infects children and adults
Enteric adenovirus	*Adenoviridae*	Linear dsDNA	Year-round	Infects mainly children 2–10 y old
Astrovirus	*Astroviridae*	(+) ssRNA	Year-round	Infects mainly children
Aichi virus	*Picornaviridae*	(+) ssRNA	Not known	Infects children and adults

(+), positive-sense polarity; ds, double-stranded; ss, single-stranded.

CASE • M., a 7-month-old girl living in Washington, DC, was recently switched from breastfeeding to bottle feeding. Usually a satisfied and happy child, M. became irritable on March 29, began to vomit, and had a low-grade fever. She also had mild upper respiratory symptoms, with cough, nasal discharge, and pharyngitis. After 2 days, she was brought to the pediatrician, who diagnosed rotavirus gastroenteritis by detecting viral antigen in the stool with an enzyme-linked immunosorbent assay (see Chapter 58). Oral rehydration solution was given at home, and M. made an uneventful recovery by the sixth day.

This case raises several questions:

1. How did M. acquire the virus?
2. Is it significant that M.'s disease occurred in the spring?
3. Will M. ever have the same disease again?
4. Why did the pediatrician suspect this etiological agent?
5. Could this illness have been prevented?

See Appendix for answers.

via infectious aerosols. That possibility is based on well-described epidemics in which fecal–oral transmission cannot be documented and on the observation that respiratory symptoms may precede the development of gastroenteritis by a day or two.

STRUCTURE AND REPLICATION

Rotaviruses are among the few human viruses with a **double-stranded RNA genome**, which resembles double-stranded DNA in structure. Another distinguishing property (shared by the orthomyxoviruses) is that the genome of rotaviruses is **segmented**. In two-dimensional images, rotavirus particles appear wheel-shaped with short spokes and an outer rim (*rota* means "wheel" in Latin; Fig. 37-1). The particle possesses an icosahedral structure with inner and outer capsids. Infectivity requires an intact outer capsid layer that helps establish **acid stability**, a critical characteristic for viruses that gain entry through the gastrointestinal tract. Two outer-capsid

proteins, a hemagglutinin (VP4) and a glycoprotein (VP7), induce development of neutralizing antibodies.

The capsid contains 11 segments of double-stranded RNA as well as a viral **RNA-dependent RNA polymerase (transcriptase)** for transcription of individual RNA segments into messenger RNA (mRNA). The enzyme is absent in animal cells and must be introduced with the virion during infection. Most rotavirus strains require treatment with a protease to become infective. Virus penetration into cells is enhanced by proteolysis of the VP4 outer-capsid protein. Virus replication proceeds in the cytoplasm, resulting in the formation of both positive- and negative-sense RNA (Fig. 37-2). The positive-sense RNA functions as a template for both translation (like mRNA) and replication of negative-sense RNA. Production of negative-sense RNA using positive-sense RNA as a template results in the formation of progeny, double-stranded RNA gene segments. Virus particles are assembled in the cytoplasm and mature by budding through the endoplasmic reticulum. Mature virus particles are released into the extracellular environment with lysis of the infected cell.

Six groups of rotaviruses (A through F) have been identified based on antigenic characteristics. **Group A rotaviruses** share a common antigen and are the only rotaviruses recognized to cause frequent infections in the United States. **Group B rotaviruses** are best known as a cause of diarrhea in swine, but these viruses have caused outbreaks in children and adults in China. The other rotavirus groups are either infrequent human pathogens or their role in human disease is not clear.

DAMAGE

Rotaviruses produce a spectrum of disease ranging from asymptomatic infection to severe diarrhea with potentially fatal dehydration. Severe gastroenteritis generally occurs in children between 6 and 24 months of age, as in the case of M. Rotavirus infections typically have a 2-day incubation period. Vomiting often precedes the onset of diarrhea by

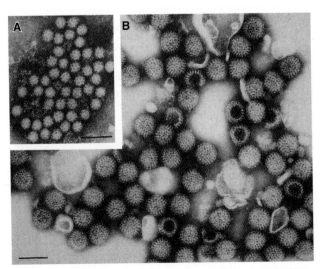

FIGURE 37-1. Electron micrograph of negatively stained virus particles. A. Norwalk virus. **B.** Rotavirus.

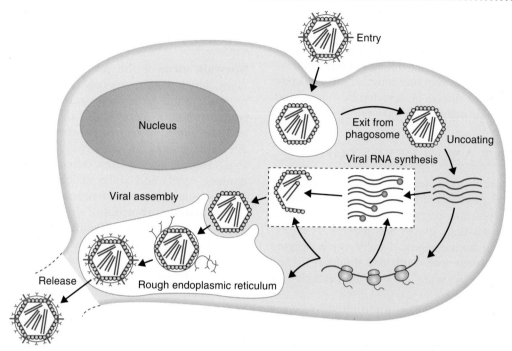

FIGURE 37-2. The rotavirus replication cycle. The virus binds to cell-surface receptors and is internalized into the cytoplasm. During that process, the outer shell of the virus is removed leaving behind the transcriptionally active viral core. Transcription of the viral genome within the core results in synthesis of viral mRNAs. The viral mRNAs serve as template for both translation and genome replication. Mature viral progeny are assembled in the endoplasmic reticulum and released when the cell lyses.

2 or 3 days. Watery diarrhea can last 3 to 8 days in infants who become symptomatic. Fever and abdominal cramps are common. Red blood cells or leukocytes are generally not found in the stool of patients with rotavirus gastroenteritis.

Morphological changes have been identified from biopsies of the mucosa of the proximal small intestine of infants and children with rotavirus gastroenteritis. Among the changes are shortening and atrophy of the villi, denuded villi, and mononuclear cell infiltration of the lamina propria. Virus invasion of the epithelial cells of the small intestine causes destruction of the mature absorptive cells that are then replaced with young, virus-free cells. That process results in diarrhea for at least four reasons: First, immature replacement cells have a reduced capacity to absorb salt and water. Second, immature cells have a reduced capacity to produce disaccharidases, which results in malabsorption of carbohydrates. Third, the virus produces a protein that functions as an enterotoxin, is released from virus-infected cells, and stimulates chloride and water secretion in the gut. Fourth, the enteric nervous system is activated. The severity of rotavirus-induced diarrhea may not be proportional to the extent of mucosal damage in the small intestine because the enterotoxin can cause diarrhea in the absence of histological changes.

In infants younger than 6 months of age, rotavirus diarrhea is less common, except for premature neonates who may acquire the infection during outbreaks in newborn nurseries. For reasons not well understood, normal full-term infants often become infected but remain asymptomatic even while shedding rotavirus in the stool. It may be that maternal antibodies transferred during the third trimester protect term infants, while premature infants born before they acquire maternal antirotavirus antibodies are susceptible. In children older than 6 months of age, rotavirus is a major nosocomial pathogen and a frequent cause of disease in child-care settings.

Adults generally experience a mild or even asymptomatic infection from rotavirus because long-term immunity generally follows a primary infection. Symptoms become apparent when the inoculum size is large enough to overcome preexisting immunity. In some instances, rotavirus causes travelers' diarrhea in children and adults, although it is a less common agent of that disease than are other pathogens.

Chronic diarrhea and prolonged shedding have been associated with rotavirus infection in children with **T-cell immunodeficiencies**. Patients undergoing immunosuppression for stem cell transplantation are also at increased risk.

DIAGNOSIS

Because most of the viral agents that cause gastroenteritis grow poorly in cell culture, assays that detect viral antigen in stool specimens have become the most commonly employed diagnostic tools. **Antigen detection** assays, as used in M.'s case, are widely available for rotavirus detection, but the commercially available assays detect only group A rotaviruses. Electron microscopy also is used, and group B and C rotavirus infections are often only suspected following use of that test. Electron microscopy allows the identification of other enteric viruses. However, this modality is not available in many clinical laboratories, and a relatively high viral titer must be present in the stool specimen for the virus to be detected by this method. Serologic diagnosis is possible but generally not useful.

TREATMENT AND PREVENTION

At present, no specific therapies are available for the management of viral gastroenteritis. Adherence to standard precautions for infection control, such as hand washing and barrier methods (e.g., gloves and gowns), is important for minimizing disease spread. Patient care is directed at supportive measures with particular attention to preventing dehydration by using intravenous hydration or oral rehydration therapy.

Oral immunization with a **live, attenuated rotavirus vaccine** is effective in preventing severe rotavirus disease. Live, attenuated vaccines induce a protective immune response without inducing illness. Rotaviruses of bovine, human, lamb, or rhesus origin have been evaluated as candidate vaccines. The first licensed rotavirus vaccine (derived from a rhesus rotavirus strain) was withdrawn from the market after 1 year owing to an unexpected, temporal association with **intussusception**, a telescoping of the intestine into itself. Since then, two other live, attenuated vaccines (of bovine and human origin, respectively) have been licensed, and vaccination should begin between 6 and 14 weeks of age. These vaccines are also associated with a low frequency of intussusception, but the benefit of vaccination outweighs the risk of intussusception. Since vaccine introduction in the United States, the prevalence of severe rotavirus gastroenteritis has declined dramatically. However, as live, attenuated virus vaccines, they should not be administered to severely immunocompromised children (such as those with severe T-cell immunodeficiency). The success of these vaccines now makes rotavirus-induced gastroenteritis a vaccine-preventable disease.

NOROVIRUS

ENCOUNTER

Norwalk virus is the prototype strain of the noroviruses, which were previously called Norwalk-like viruses or small, round, structured viruses (SRSVs; see Fig. 37-1). Noroviruses are members of the **Caliciviridae** family and the genus *Norovirus*. Norovirus strains are named after the geographic area where an outbreak occurs (e.g., Hawaii agent, Snow Mountain agent, and Montgomery agent) and are genetically very diverse. These viruses usually come to attention through the occurrence of **explosive outbreaks** of disease, with an incubation period of 1 to 2 days following a common source exposure. A seasonal peak of disease occurs in the winter, but infection can happen throughout the year. Noroviruses are highly stable in the environment and can be transmitted by contaminated **food** or **water** and by person-to-person contact. Fecal–oral transmission is the usual route, but transmission by aerosol also can occur following vomiting.

Noroviruses can infect persons of any age, but they are most frequently diagnosed in adults and school-aged children who are involved in outbreaks. However, noroviruses also cause disease in preschool children and are second to rotaviruses as a cause of diarrhea in children, including children hospitalized with gastroenteritis. With a decline in the incidence of severe rotavirus illness due to vaccination, noroviruses may soon become the most common cause of gastroenteritis in this age group. Noroviruses cause outbreaks in nursing homes, on cruise ships, and in essentially any setting where individuals are confined in close contact. International common source outbreaks related to food and water also can occur. Asymptomatic infection is common, and virus shedding can occur for prolonged periods (3 to 6 weeks or longer) after an individual recovers from illness. Transmission of virus from persons asymptomatically shedding virus is likely to be the source of many infections.

CASE • Mr. S., a 25-year-old chef who had just returned from a vacation on a cruise ship, presented to his primary care physician with a 2-day history of diarrhea. He also had abdominal cramps, vomiting, and malaise but no fever. He was anxious to go back to his job at a restaurant. His wife had also been sick for 1 day, but she only had vomiting. Their two children, who did not go on the cruise, were in good health. Without ordering any diagnostic tests, Mr. S.'s physician sent him home with the recommendation to drink fluids and be careful to wash his hands and disinfect the bathroom to prevent spreading the illness to others. Although he was advised to return to work when his illness ended, Mr. S. was cautioned to continue using good hygiene practices and be sure to wear gloves when handling food.

This case raises several questions:

1. How did Mr. S. acquire the virus?
2. Why did the physician not perform any diagnostic tests?
3. Why did the physician tell Mr. S. to use good hygiene practices at home and at work?
4. Will Mr. S. ever have the same disease again?

See Appendix for answers.

Host Factors Affect Infection

There are two major mechanisms responsible for protection against norovirus infection: genetic resistance and acquired immunity. Early volunteer studies showed that some individuals are resistant to infection with noroviruses. Recent studies have found that genetic factors affecting histoblood group antigen expression, including secretor status and ABO blood group type, influence whether an individual becomes infected with Norwalk virus. Nonsecretors are resistant to infection, and individuals with a blood group type B are less likely to become infected or develop symptomatic infection. Resistance to other norovirus strains that are genetically distinct from Norwalk virus is not well understood. Norovirus infection induces short-term immunity (6 to 26 weeks) to reinfection and disease, but reinfection with the same strain 2 to 3 years later can again lead to gastroenteritis. The acquired immunity is associated with the presence of serum antibodies that block norovirus binding to histoblood group antigens.

REPLICATION AND DAMAGE

The human noroviruses cannot be cultured in the laboratory. Therefore, knowledge about the pathogenesis of disease caused by these viruses has primarily come from volunteer studies. Norovirus gastroenteritis is generally considered to be mild and self-limiting, although illness can last from 24 to 48 hours and is often incapacitating during that time. A spectrum of clinical manifestations has been observe in adults infected with the same virus, with some having significant vomiting and diarrhea and others having only diarrhea or vomiting. Common symptoms (seen in >50% of patients) include nausea, abdominal cramps, diarrhea, vomiting, and malaise. Chills and fever occur less frequently. Bloody diarrhea does not occur. Prolonged (for months to years) gastroenteritis can occur in severely immunocompromised patients, such as stem cell transplant recipients. Small bowel biopsies of infected volunteers show villous blunting in the ileum and proximal jejunum, with the intestinal mucosa remaining intact. Gastric emptying is delayed, and malabsorption of fat, D-xylose, and lactose has been observed.

DIAGNOSIS

Enzyme-linked immunosorbent assays are available for the diagnosis of norovirus outbreaks but not for individual cases because of low assay sensitivity. The usual method for diagnosis of norovirus infection is by identification of the viral RNA in stools by using RT-PCR assays. Electron microscopy, antigen detection in stool, and serologic diagnosis using paired sera also are used but are not available in most clinical laboratories.

TREATMENT AND PREVENTION

No specific treatments for norovirus-induced disease exist. Symptoms usually resolve without complications, and oral fluid and electrolyte replacement therapy is normally sufficient to manage fluid loss. If severe vomiting or diarrhea occurs, parenteral administration of fluids may be required. Vaccines to prevent norovirus disease are being evaluated, but for now, prevention relies on the same basic infection-control measures described for rotavirus infections.

OTHER ENTERIC VIRUSES

Whereas rotaviruses and noroviruses are the most widely recognized causes of viral enteric infections, other agents contribute to the spectrum of viral gastroenteritis. **Adenoviruses** are best known as a cause of upper respiratory tract disease (see Chapter 39). However, two serotypes (40 and 41) cause diarrhea, especially in children who are less than 2 years of age. Outbreaks due to **sapoviruses**, another type of **calicivirus**, have been described, mainly in institutions. Based on the prevalence of specific antibodies, most individuals have been infected with those viruses by 12 years of age, but infections in adults are being recognized more frequently. **Astroviruses** are another group of viruses that cause enteric disease, primarily in children less than 5 years of age. **Aichi virus** is a **picornavirus** that causes disease in children and adults. Diagnostic assays for the adenoviruses, sapoviruses, astroviruses, and Aichi virus are not routinely available. Treatment for infections by those agents is supportive, similar to that described for the rotaviruses and noroviruses.

CONCLUSION

Rotaviruses and noroviruses are the most common causes of viral gastroenteritis worldwide. Rotavirus infections are almost universal in children; norovirus infections are associated with explosive outbreaks of disease. Both viruses are spread by the fecal–oral route. Rotaviruses and noroviruses contain RNA genomes and replicate in the cytoplasm of host cells. Virus replication leads to secretory diarrhea. Treatment of rotavirus and norovirus disease relies on fluid replacement. Vaccines are now available for rotaviruses, and vaccine development for noroviruses is an active area of research.

Suggested Readings

Glass RI, Bresee J, Jiang B, et al. Gastroenteritis viruses: an overview. *Novartis Found Symp.* 2001;238:5–19.

Glass RI, Parashar UD, Estes MK. Norovirus gastroenteritis. *N Engl J Med.* 2009;361:1776–85.

Greenberg HB, Estes MK. Rotaviruses: from pathogenesis to vaccination. *Gastroenterology.* 2009;136:1939–1951.

Koopmans M, Duizer E. Foodborne viruses: an emerging problem. *Int J Food Microbiol.* 2004;90:23–41.

Reeck AR, Kavanagh O, Estes MK, et al. Serological correlate of protection against norovirus-induced gastroenteritis. *J Infect Dis.* 2010;202:1212–8.

Chapter 38

The Human Retroviruses: AIDS and Other Diseases

Robert T. Schooley

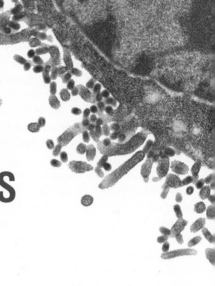

KEY CONCEPTS

Pathogens: Retroviruses are RNA viruses that contain the enzyme reverse transcriptase, which allows them to use RNA as a template to make DNA. They include human immunodeficiency virus (HIV), the virus that causes acquired immune deficiency syndrome (AIDS), human T-cell leukemia virus type I (HTLV-I), which is associated with leukemia and lymphoma, and HTLV-II.

Encounter: HIV infection has emerged as a worldwide pandemic since the first cases in the early 1980s. Other human retroviruses have limited geographic range and less tendency to result in serious disease.

Entry: HIV is transmitted through sexual contact, injection drug use, and vertically (mother to child).

Spread: HIV preferentially binds to the CD4 molecule found on helper T cells and monocytes, enters, and infects these cells.

Replication: Retroviruses may cause disease years after initial infection. HIV has a long latency period (average of 10 years).

Damage: HIV infection of CD4+ T lymphocytes results in the eventual destruction of these cells disabling the immune system and making the infected individual vulnerable to opportunistic infections. HIV displays antigenic variation.

Diagnosis: Screening is done by testing for antibodies specific to HIV (or other) retrovirus. Confirmation and quantification of infection can be done using nucleic acid amplification techniques.

Treatment: Treatment of HIV infection with antiviral drugs is now highly effective.

Prevention: Vaccine development has been slow, but recent advances in microbicides, the use of antiretroviral drugs as preventative agents, and the demonstration that male circumcision reduces HIV transmission have provided new approaches for reducing spread of the epidemic.

IN THE 30 YEARS since five previously healthy homosexual men were diagnosed with *Pneumocystis jiroveci* (formerly known as *Pneumocystis carinii*) pneumonia in May 1981, AIDS has grown from an epidemiologically isolated medical condition to a worldwide epidemic of mammoth proportions. During the initial phase of the epidemic, it became apparent that the disease was one likely caused by an infectious agent with a prolonged incubation period that could be transmitted sexually or by exposure to blood. By 1983, with the initial reports linking the presence of a retrovirus (subsequently designated human immunodeficiency virus type 1 or HIV-1) to the syndrome, the agent responsible for the illness had spread far beyond its initial epidemiological and geographic boundaries. The number of AIDS cases in the United States and Europe rose steadily through the mid-1990s and then plateaued as the combined effects of antiretroviral chemotherapy and increasingly effective prevention efforts synergized to delay the onset of new cases and reduce transmission of the etiologic retrovirus. By 2010, over 1 million Americans had received a diagnosis of AIDS, and over a half million had died. Although the yearly number of new cases peaked in 1999, the disease has continued to spread in resource-limited settings where it now exerts its most devastating medical and social effects. By

2010, it was estimated that approximately 33 million people were living with HIV-1 (Fig. 38-1). Most of these people are in sub-Saharan Africa, but the number of affected individuals in Asia has been rising steadily. Although antiretroviral therapy has not yet fully reached all of those in need, the increasing availability of treatment has resulted in a declining number of deaths since 2004. It is estimated that 1.6 to 2.1 million people died of AIDS in 2009. Two attributes make AIDS unique among infectious diseases: it is uniformly fatal, and most of its devastating effects are not caused directly by the causative agent. With suppression of the host immune response by HIV, opportunistic organisms cause a number of clinical syndromes. In fact, most symptoms in a person with AIDS result from secondary infections rather than the virus itself. The clinical manifestations of AIDS are described in detail in Chapter 71, "Acquired Immunodeficiency Syndrome."

THE PATHOGENS: RETROVIRUSES

Retroviruses have a small spherical virion surrounded by a lipid envelope (Fig. 38-2). The genome contains two identical RNA molecules. These molecules resemble eukaryotic mRNA because they contain a **cap structure** at the 5′ end and a **poly A sequence** at the 3′ end. Four viral genes are required for the replication of retroviruses (Fig. 38-3). The *gag* gene encodes several core (Gag) proteins. The *pol* gene encodes **reverse transcriptase** or **RNA-dependent DNA polymerase** (Pol), the enzyme responsible for replication of the genome, as well as **integrase**, the enzyme required for integration of viral DNA into the host cell genome. The *env* gene encodes the two **envelope glycoproteins**, **gp120** and **gp41**. Noncoding sequences include terminally redundant regions and unique regions near the ends of the genome. The *pro* gene encodes a **protease** necessary for cleaving the Gag and Pol proteins to their active forms.

In addition to the genes common to all retroviruses, *gag, pro, pol,* and *env,* the HIV genome contains at least six other genes. These genes encode proteins that are important in regulating the complex replication cycle of the virus, which may exist in a latent state in the infected cell and then undergo rapid replication at an appropriate time.

ENCOUNTER (HIV)

The distribution of HIV infection in the population is consistent with an agent that is extremely labile and cannot readily enter the host through intact body surfaces. In this respect, HIV resembles (but is much less contagious than) hepatitis B virus, which has a similar epidemiological pattern in the United States. HIV has been detected in a number of body fluids including peripheral blood, semen, cervical secretions, breast milk, urine, cerebrospinal fluid, saliva, and tears. The last four fluids do not represent important means of transmission. With few exceptions, HIV transmission occurs by one of three routes: sexual contact, injection drug use, and vertical passage from infected mothers to their offspring. In 1991, homosexual and bisexual men accounted for approximately 70% of AIDS cases in the United States (including 8% who were also injection drug users). Since that time, men who have sex with men have represented a progressively smaller proportion of the total cases, and heterosexual transmission and injecting drug use have become more important, especially among persons of color. Heterosexual transmission now accounts for nearly a third of new cases of HIV infection, and injecting drug use accounts for one in six new cases each year. In the past, injecting drug

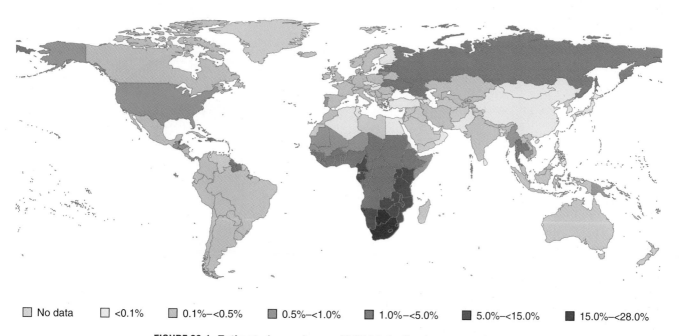

No data   <0.1%   0.1%–<0.5%   0.5%–<1.0%   1.0%–<5.0%   5.0%–<15.0%   15.0%–<28.0%

FIGURE 38-1. Estimated prevalence of HIV-1 infection by country in 2009.

CASE • A baby boy, G., was born by Cesarean section after a 36-week gestation to a 29-year-old commercial sex worker with AIDS. The mother had been diagnosed 4 years earlier when she developed *Pneumocystis jiroveci* pneumonia, but she had not had regular medical care since that time. She came to the hospital in labor. The delivery staff did not immediately inquire about her past medical history because her labor was quite advanced; thus, her prior history of *P. jiroveci* pneumonia was not known until after the delivery.

IgG antibodies to HIV were detected in the infant by both an enzyme-linked immunosorbent assay and immunoblot (Western blot) analysis (see Chapter 58). By 4 months of age, G. experienced poor weight gain, thrush (oral candidiasis), diffuse lymphadenopathy (enlargement of lymph nodes), and persistent diarrhea. HIV RNA and proviral DNA were detected in his peripheral blood, and a diagnosis of AIDS was made. Antiretroviral drugs were administered, and over several months, G.'s symptoms disappeared and weight gain resumed.

This case raises several questions:

1. Was the presence of HIV antibodies in G.'s blood diagnostic of HIV infection?
2. What was the basis of the initial diagnosis?
3. How was the diagnosis confirmed?

See Appendix for answers.

use–associated cases served as an important bridge to the heterosexual population. The heterosexual epidemic is now self-sustaining. Transmission among injection drug users occurs through sharing of contaminated needles and syringes that contain a residue of blood (including infected white blood cells) from previous users.

HIV transmission by blood transfusion has been very rare since March 1985 when routine screening of blood products was instituted. Persons with hemophilia are at risk for bloodborne viruses such as hepatitis B and C because they receive preparations of factor VIII and factor IX obtained from plasma pooled from thousands of donors. Since 1984, factor VIII concentrates have been unlikely to contain HIV because blood donors are screened for HIV antibodies. In addition, since 1984, plasma products have been treated with heat and chemicals to inactivate contaminating viruses. Approximately 80% of recipients of factor VIII prior to 1984 are now infected with HIV or deceased.

Vaginal intercourse can result in HIV transmission to partners of either gender. Heterosexual transmission is the most common form of spread of HIV in most countries other than the United States and northern Europe. For example, the overall ratio of male to female AIDS cases

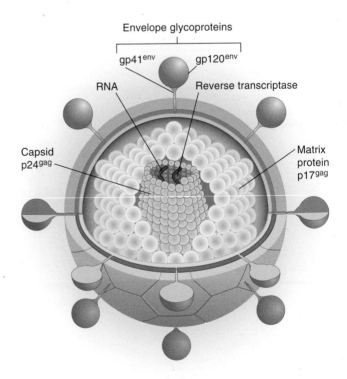

FIGURE 38-2. Retrovirus structure. A schematic drawing showing the virion proteins and other structures.

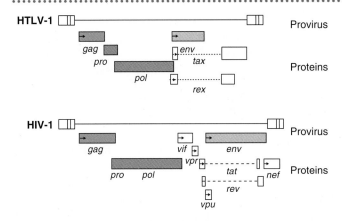

FIGURE 38-3. The genetic organization of human retroviruses. The top line in each case shows the provirus with control sequences shown as boxes at the termini. The boxes shown in color indicate locations of the viral structural genes, and the open boxes indicate locations of the viral accessory genes.

in sub-Saharan Africa is approximately 1:1 as opposed to 13:1 in the United States. In many areas of Africa, AIDS is now the leading cause of death among adults.

Transmission rates to long-term heterosexual partners of AIDS patients vary widely, from less than 10% to 70%. In some instances, transmission may occur after as few as one or two sexual contacts. The low transmission rate seen in spouses of HIV-positive hemophiliacs suggests that, in many instances, the virus is not easily transmitted even over periods of several years. Although there are differences among individuals in terms of both infectiousness and susceptibility, the average risk for each instance of heterosexual intercourse between infected and uninfected individuals has been estimated to be about 0.3%. Transmission rates are higher when the infected partner has a higher level of virus in the bloodstream (and presumably in the genital tract) such as during acute infection or in late stages of the illness. Uncircumcised men are more susceptible to infection following either vaginal or insertive anal intercourse. Sex that is associated with trauma also is associated with a higher rate of HIV transmission. Genetic factors are important determinants of susceptibility to infection. One such factor is the gene encoding CCR5, a chemokine receptor that serves as a coreceptor for HIV. The defective form of this gene is found in about 10% of individuals of European descent, but it occurs much less frequently in other populations. In the 1% of this group who are homozygous, it confers a very high (although not absolute) level of resistance to HIV infection. Heterozygous individuals are not protected from infection but seem to have a slower rate of progression to AIDS.

Congenital transmission, as in the case of baby G., is the most important route of transmission of pediatric AIDS. The Centers for Disease Control and Prevention estimates that between 1978 and 1993, 15,000 newborns in the United States acquired HIV infection by vertical transmission. Since the recognition that intervention with antiretroviral drugs can interrupt maternofetal transmission, new cases of pediatric AIDS have fallen sharply in the United States and Europe. In the absence of such intervention, between 25 and 33% of HIV-infected women transmit HIV to their children. When infection of the mother is recognized, and antiretroviral intervention is employed in the mother and child, the transmission rate falls to less than 1% of births. At this point in the epidemic, there are fewer than 50 perinatal transmissions in the United States each year. Although HIV transmission among health care workers is an area of particular concern, extensive studies have confirmed that HIV-transmission in a medical setting is rare. The risk of infection following an accidental stick with a needle used to draw blood from an HIV-infected patient is less than 0.3%. The risk from percutaneous transmission is greater if the sharp object is hollow, if the source patient is in a stage of illness with higher levels of virus, if the sharp object had been in a location where more virus is present (e.g., within a vein as opposed to within a muscle), or if the injury involves a laceration (rather than a simple puncture). The risk from exposure to mucous membranes or by contamination of apparently intact skin is considerably less. With the general adoption of "universal precautions," which assume that blood or other fluids from all patients is potentially infectious, and the increasing use of "smart" medical disposables that are designed to minimize risk to the user, HIV spread to health care workers should remain a rare event. The rate of HIV infection in the health care setting can be further reduced by immediate postexposure treatment with a combination of antiviral drugs. The spread of HIV from health care workers to patients is even less frequent. Spread of HIV among nonsexual household contacts or coworkers is exceedingly rare. More than 12 studies involving over 700 family members or boarding-school contacts of persons with AIDS failed to detect a single instance of transmission. Although arthropod vectors have been proposed as a route of transmission, there is no evidence to support this idea. If arthropods, such as mosquitoes or ticks, were important, children in developing countries would be frequently infected, as they are often victims of such bites. In fact, the occurrence of AIDS in children outside recognized risk groups is highly unusual, making arthropod vectors an unlikely mechanism of transmission.

ENTRY

The mechanism by which HIV establishes infection in the host is incompletely understood. HIV may enter the host contained within infected cells, for example, macrophages, lymphocytes, or spermatozoa, or as free virus. HIV also may enter the body through microabrasions on the surface of mucous membranes, through penetration of intact skin with a needle, or through grossly intact mucosal surfaces.

SPREAD

While HIV can infect a number of cell types, two major groups of cells in the body serve as preferred targets for infection by HIV: helper T lymphocytes and monocytes. These cells express CD4 and the appropriate coreceptors. They transport the virus to tissues in which these cells are abundant (e.g., lymph nodes, spleen, blood, and body fluids).

REPLICATION

The replication cycle of HIV (Fig. 38-4) includes the following steps:

* **Binding**. Once in close proximity to a **CD4+ T lymphocyte**, HIV binds to the **CD4 molecule** via envelope glycoprotein gp120. Antibodies to either gp120 or the cellular receptor block this interaction and prevent infection. The presence of CD4 on the cell surface, which plays an important role in immunological function (see Chapter 7, "Induced Defenses"), determines the primary target cells for infection. After binding to CD4, a secondary binding event occurs in which gp120 engages one of two coreceptor molecules (CCR5 or CXCR4). These molecules serve physiologically as receptors for chemokines, but in the case of HIV infection, they facilitate tight binding of the virus to the cell surface and induce a conformational change in gp41 that brings a hydrophobic domain of the protein into apposition with the cell membrane.

* **Fusion** of the viral envelope with the cell membrane is facilitated by a hydrophobic interaction between gp41 and the target cell membrane. Following fusion, the virion loses its integrity and characteristic morphology. The viral core, which contains the genomic RNA and molecules of reverse transcriptase, is released into the cytoplasm.

* **Synthesis of DNA**. Reverse transcriptase synthesizes a complementary DNA molecule corresponding to the viral RNA genome. The enzyme then synthesizes the second DNA strand (complementary to the first), generating a double-stranded DNA molecule. In the process of making the DNA, portions of the ends of the genomic RNA are copied twice, resulting in a structure at each end of the DNA called the **long terminal repeat (LTR)**.

* **Integration**. The double-stranded DNA molecule is transported to the nucleus and integrated into host cell chromosomes. The virus-encoded enzyme, **integrase**, is responsible for catalyzing this reaction, which involves joining the ends of each LTR to host cell DNA. The retrovirus integration process resembles the mechanism of action of some transposable elements of bacteria (see Chapter 4, "Genetic Approaches to Studying Bacterial Pathogenesis"). In the integrated state, the viral genetic material is called the **provirus**. The provirus is analogous to a cellular gene in that it is passed to daughter cells at division and contains signals that control its transcription into RNA.

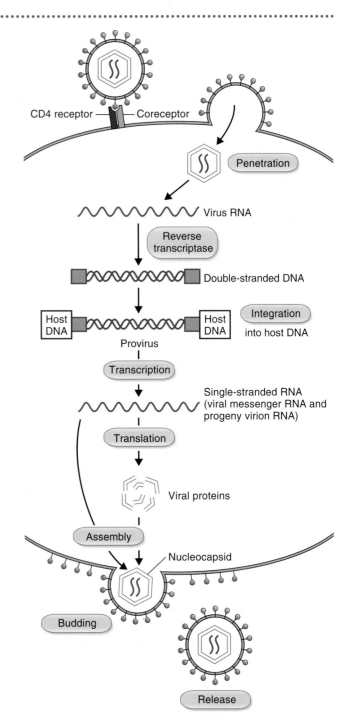

FIGURE 38-4. The retrovirus replication cycle.

* **Synthesis of progeny virus**. In the "productive phase," viral DNA is transcribed into mRNA by host cell DNA-dependent RNA polymerase. Signals that direct the RNA synthetic machinery of the cell are found in the LTR and resemble signals used by the cell for making its own RNAs. After transcription, some of these viral RNA molecules are used as mRNA for the synthesis of viral proteins. Others become incorporated as genomes into progeny viral particles. Assembly of virions takes place at the cell surface. The structural proteins coalesce with viral genomes and acquire their

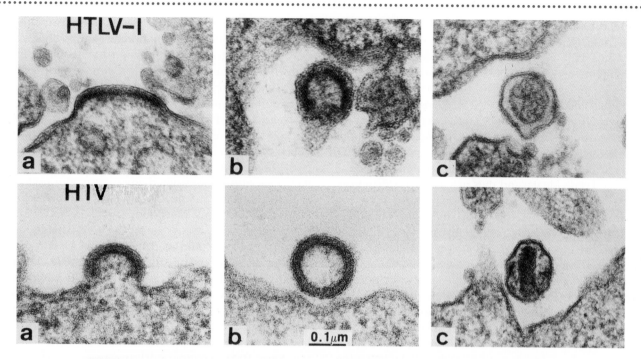

FIGURE 38-5. Electron micrographs showing successive stages in the assembly and budding of the human retroviruses HTLV-I (top row) and HIV (bottom row). Note the difference in structure of the core in the two types of mature virions (c).

envelope by passage through the host cell membrane (Fig. 38-5). Following budding through the membrane, the viral protease cleaves the viral protein precursors, and morphological changes in the virion are observed.

• **Latency and transactivation.** In general, the replication cycle described so far is common to all retroviruses. HIV and some related viruses have yet other features. First, infection also can involve a **latent** phase in which infected cells contain a provirus but do not express viral RNA or proteins. Second, expression of HIV macromolecules is subject to regulation by viral gene products that operate as soluble elements (in "trans"). This phenomenon is known as **transactivation.** At least two HIV genes (called *tat* and *rev*) encode **transactivating factors,** which greatly increase the expression of viral RNAs and proteins. The Tat protein accelerates the transcription of viral RNA by host RNA polymerase; the Rev protein enhances the transport of some viral RNAs from the nucleus to the cytoplasm. Third, HIV proviruses contain signals that induce expression when HIV-infected cells are stimulated by antigen or infected by some other viruses (such as a herpesvirus). These features appear to be related in an important way: after infection of lymphocytes and integration of the provirus, the infectious process may be halted, only to be reinitiated much later in an explosive way by unknown stimuli. The outcome is a high level of transactivation, resulting in a burst of virus production and rapid death of the cell. While only a small fraction of infected cells enter this latent state, these cells can defeat attempts to eradicate infection by antiviral therapy, even when administered for extended periods. Finally, in addition to the regulatory effects of Tat and Rev, HIV-1 has other gene products that interact with host cell proteins to facilitate evasion of virus-specific immune responses and intracellular protective mechanisms that can limit viral replication. For example, the **Nef** protein downregulates cell-surface expression of MHC class I molecules, which are responsible for presenting antigens to virus-specific cytotoxic T cells. Another viral protein, **Vif**, facilitates destruction of a cellular protein called **ABOBEC 3G**, which is capable of blocking reverse transcription when packaged within the viral particle. Finally, the **Vpu** protein downregulates an interferon-induced cellular protein called **tetherin**, which inhibits release of viral particles from the cell surface.

Antigenic Variation

A unique characteristic of infection by HIV is that the immune response of the host is unable to completely curtail viral replication (although it may be important in partially suppressing it during the latent phase of the disease). This characteristic is a paradox, since for most other viral infections, the presence of antibody indicates immunity, protection from infection, and a favorable prognosis. How does HIV persist in the host despite an antiviral immune response? Several mechanisms may be at work here: virus gene products may be relatively invisible to the immune response; the virus may mask or change its antigenic specificity; and the virus may replicate primarily in lymphoid follicles, locations within lymphoid tissues in which virus-directed immune cells do not migrate freely.

Which HIV gene products are important in directing the immune response of the host? A clue comes from studies of the genetic diversity of the virus genes. HIV genes that encode internal viral proteins (*gag* and *pol*) show relative stability from one isolate to the next, but the *env* gene displays many mutations that lead to variations in its products, the surface glycoproteins gp41 and gp120. Although antibodies to the Gag and Pol proteins are found in infected individuals, and thus are useful for diagnosis, these antibodies do not seem to be important in preventing viral replication. On the other hand, some antibodies to the envelope proteins can neutralize the virus, although their titers are low compared to those in other chronic viral infections. HIV envelope glycoproteins have two unusual features. First, they are extensively coated with polysaccharides, which are of only limited immunogenicity. Second, they contain **hypervariable regions** that permit the virus to present new antigenic configurations to the host. In contrast, sequences in the surface glycoprotein gp120 that are involved in interactions with cellular receptors must be genetically conserved. Conserved sequences may be hidden and thus protected from neutralizing antibodies by the carbohydrates and the hypervariable regions. As a result, HIV can constantly vary its surface antigenic composition, which may allow it to avoid neutralization. In this regard, HIV resembles influenza viruses and trypanosomes of sleeping sickness in its capacity to withstand the immune response by changing major surface antigens. Such a mechanism hinders the development of an effective vaccine containing the surface glycoproteins.

THE HISTORY OF RETROVIRUSES

Understanding the role of retroviruses as the etiologic agent of AIDS requires a historical detour through the puzzling connection between viruses and cancer. This history includes a challenge to a traditional tenet of molecular biology, which holds that genetic information flows from DNA through RNA intermediates to protein. In the late 1960s, researchers identified an unusual class of viruses that carried genetic information in molecules of RNA. While RNA-containing viruses were not a novelty, these viruses were unique because they contained the formerly unrecognized enzyme, reverse transcriptase. Using RNA as a template, this enzyme reverses the conventional flow of genetic information by synthesizing a copy of complementary DNA that ultimately integrates into the genome of the host cell. This DNA, called the provirus, serves as an intermediate stage in the replicative cycle.

Some of these viruses (now called retroviruses in recognition of their reverse or "retro" mode of replication) are capable of causing tumors. A virus of this type was first isolated in 1911, when Peyton Rous reported that tumors in chickens could be caused by a virus (later known as RSV, for Rous sarcoma virus) readily transmissible by filtered extracts. Since then, hundreds of retroviruses have been isolated from many groups of vertebrates. In the early 1960s, a cancer-inducing cat virus was discovered, now called the feline leukemia virus. This virus proved to be important in understanding the biology of retroviruses for two reasons. First, it facilitated the discovery in 1986 of a second feline retrovirus, feline immunodeficiency virus, which causes an immunodeficiency disease in cats similar to the one observed in humans with AIDS. Second, feline leukemia virus is transmitted among cats in a household setting, providing a valuable model for epidemiological analysis of retrovirus infection.

Until the late 1960s, there was considerable skepticism that a virus could mediate the transmission of cancer. Because cancer appeared to be a genetic alteration, it was difficult to conceive how an RNA-containing virus could interact with the DNA of the host cell to produce oncogenic changes. The discovery of reverse transcriptase suggested a mechanism for the induction of permanent genetic change.

Since 1980, two groups of retroviruses capable of causing disease in humans have been isolated and characterized (Table 38-1). For several years before 1980, researchers suspected that retroviruses might be agents of human disease, but the point could not be proved because these viruses did not grow in cultured cells. Several advances in cell-culture technology overcame this obstacle. One of the most important was the discovery of interleukin-2 (IL-2), which stimulates the growth of T lymphocytes in vitro. These lymphocytes could then be used for the isolation of human T-cell leukemia viruses (HTLVs).

The first of these viruses, HTLV-I, was isolated from the cells of two patients with adult T-cell lymphoma. Subsequent HTLV-I isolates from other patients with T-cell leukemia or lymphoma were shown to be closely related, as determined by serology and nucleic acid hybridization. Epidemiological studies suggested a causal relationship

TABLE 38.1 The Pathogenic Human Retroviruses

HTLV Group

HTLV-I	Causative agent of certain cutaneous T-cell leukemias and lymphomas as well as HTLV-I myelopathy (also called tropical spastic paraparesis)
HTLV-II	Not conclusively linked to a specific disease; found in cases of hairy cell leukemia

Lentiviruses

HIV-1	Causative agent of AIDS
HIV-2	Related to but distinct from HIV-1; described as a cause of AIDS, particularly in West Africa

between a childhood infection with HTLV-I and the development of leukemia or lymphoma in a few percent of infected individuals as many as 40 years later. A similar virus, HTLV-II, was later isolated from a patient with hairy cell leukemia, but its role in human disease is less clear. The malignant diseases caused by HTLV-I, adult T-cell leukemia and lymphoma, are uniformly fatal but relatively rare (even in infected individuals) and limited to certain specific populations. HTLV-I infection also is associated with certain progressive spinal cord diseases, such as tropical spastic paraparesis and HTLV-I-associated myelopathy.

As the first known human retrovirus, HTLV-I attracted considerable attention. Although uncommon in the United States, concern about the spread of this virus through the blood supply resulted in routine screening of donated blood for the presence of this virus. Fortuitously, studies of HTLV-I provided the technology required for the isolation of the AIDS agent several years later. Thus, AIDS was shown to be caused by a retrovirus within 3 years after the syndrome was first described in 1981. When first isolated, this virus had several names, but it is now known as human immunodeficiency virus type 1 (HIV-1). Years later, another member of this family, HIV-2, was discovered in West Africa. This virus shares many features of HIV-1, although it is generally less virulent. The remainder of this chapter focuses on HIV-1.

DAMAGE

The molecular events that modulate lymphocyte damage in HIV-infected persons are not fully understood. However, on the basis of known abnormalities of humoral and cellular immunity, it is possible to outline a sequence of events that follow HIV infection.

Infection and Depletion of Helper T Cells

During acute HIV infection, the virus infects CD4-expressing cells within local mucosal surfaces and then rapidly establishes infection in local lymphoid tissues. Studies using primate models suggest that in most cases of sexual transmission, a limited amount of virus is involved in the first cycles of replication in submucosal tissue. Over the next several days, local rounds of replication are restricted to cells that are already in place. With most exposures, the number of local susceptible cells declines and the infection "dies out" at the site of initial exposure. However, cytokines and chemokines are generated as part of the primary immune response. These signals recruit additional components of the immune system, and if these cells arrive after the first burst of infection is terminated, the infection is not productive and the exposed host is not infected. On the other hand, if local viral replication is still ongoing when these additional cells arrive, the virus is provided cellular fodder for additional rounds of replication, and the infection disseminates, becoming self-sustaining. This early window of vulnerability likely contributes to the relatively low level of infectivity of the virus with each sexual exposure and the capacity of relatively modest antiviral interventions to reduce transmission risk even further.

Following infection at the site of entry into the host, the virus quickly disseminates systemically, infecting remote lymphoid tissues and the central nervous system (CNS) in a brushfire of infection during which the virus exhibits some of its highest replication rates in the natural history of the disease. The virus appears in genital secretions, and as in many other infectious diseases, the propensity to transmit the virus may be highest during this initial phase of infection. Acutely infected persons are often asymptomatic or may manifest symptoms that can be confused with acute mononucleosis, such as fever, headache, malaise, and an evanescent rash. Within weeks of the initial infection, virus-specific cytotoxic T cells appear in the peripheral blood and lymphoid tissue, and shortly thereafter, neutralizing antibodies may be detected in the plasma. During this period of rapid viral replication, the lifelong process of viral diversification is initiated, and the host is confronted with the immunologic challenge of developing an immune response against a rapidly changing pathogen at the same time the virus is destroying the CD4+ T-cell pool—especially virus-specific CD4+ T cells—that are required for an effective immune response. Since HIV reverse transcriptase has an error rate of approximately 1 per 10,000 nucleotides copied, on average, a new nucleotide is introduced into the virus with each replicative cycle. Since there are up to a billion viral replication cycles in each HIV-infected person each day, the capacity for generation of viral diversity at both the individual and population level is enormous. For example, in the case of the viral envelope glycoproteins, viral diversity may occur at such a rate that 15 new amino acid changes become fixed within the host each year.

Cells infected with HIV-1 may be killed directly by viral replication or by virus-specific immune effector mechanisms (primarily HIV-specific cytotoxic T cells or antibody-dependent cellular cytotoxicity). After the first several months of infection, a balance among viral replication, immune effector mechanisms, and cells available for viral replication is established, and the infection enters its chronic phase during which the infected individual is generally asymptomatic. The so-called set point to which viral replication settles following acute infection is the prime determinant of the rate of disease progression. After the initial primary phase of HIV infection, virus replication is confined largely to the lymphoid organs where activated CD4+ T lymphocytes are the primary target in which approximately 99% of viral replication is thought to occur (Fig. 38-6). The remaining 1% of viral replication occurs in monocytes and resting CD4+ T cells, which are cell populations that serve as sites for viral latency. Loss of the CD4+ T-cell population results in progressive immunodeficiency

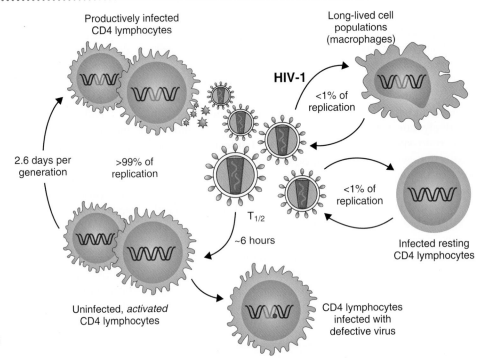

FIGURE 38-6. Pathogenesis of HIV-1 infection.

that ultimately leads to opportunistic infections and malignancies. Although substantial individual variation exists, the duration of the symptom-free period before the appearance of AIDS-defining infections is approximately 10 years. During this interval, CD4+ T-cell counts drop from the normal level of about 1,000 cells/mm³ to less than 500 cells/mm³. Persons with advanced HIV disease usually have CD4+ T-cell counts of less than 200 cells per mm³. The risk of opportunistic infections is greatest in the late-stage AIDS, when the CD4+ T-cell count drops to fewer than 50 cells/mm³. Serial measurements of CD4+ T-cell counts serve as indicators of the risk of such infections and guide management of antiretroviral therapy.

The rate of immunological and clinical progression is directly related to the extent of virus replication, which varies considerably from individual to individual. Viral replication rates within the host are highly correlated with the number of copies of HIV RNA in plasma. Individuals with high virus loads (10^5 copies/mL or more) are at greater risk for disease progression within a few years; infected individuals with lower loads (<10^4 copies/mL) may not progress to AIDS for 10 years or longer.

In addition to decreased numbers of T cells (**lymphopenia**), HIV induces abnormalities of T-cell function. Normally, T cells modulate the function of other cells in the immune system, including B cells, monocytes, and natural-killer cells. Although many persons with AIDS have elevated immunoglobulin levels in their serum, their ability to produce antibodies against specific antigens may be impaired. For example, children with HIV infection cannot make antibodies against the specific capsular polysaccharide antigens of *Haemophilus influenzae* type b and *Streptococcus pneumoniae*. This defect may be due to direct impairment of B lymphocytes in addition to the loss of helper T lymphocytes.

The specific CD4 marker characteristic of helper T lymphocytes is also found in membranes of other cell types, including circulating monocytes and macrophages, natural-killer cells, certain B lymphocytes, and cells of the CNS, such as glial cells. These cells also may become infected and damaged by viral replication or serve as reservoirs for latent virus. Defects in killing of ingested microorganisms may be attributes of HIV infection of macrophages and monocytes. Furthermore, macrophage-related cells called Langerhans cells, which form part of epithelial surfaces, have been found to be highly sensitive to HIV and may be an important entry point for sexually transmitted infection.

Clinical Consequences of HIV Infection

AIDS represents the terminal stage of infection by HIV. Clinical syndromes vary with different stages of infection.

Primary HIV infection may be associated with a mononucleosis-like syndrome that usually develops a few weeks after exposure. The infected individual then becomes asymptomatic, but HIV antibodies are detectable in serum, and viral replication continues during a period of clinical latency that is variable from patient to patient but averages 8 to 10 years.

As viral replication continues and CD4+ T cells are depleted, HIV-infected persons may remain completely asymptomatic or develop persistent generalized lymphadenopathy (Table 38-2). Lymphadenopathy may persist or resolve before progressing over months to years to pre-AIDS conditions, characterized by diarrhea, oral candidiasis, weight loss, and fever.

TABLE 38.2 Clinical Categories of HIV Infection in Persons More than 13 Years of Age

Category A (Excludes Patients with Conditions in Categories B and C):
- Asymptomatic
- Persistent generalized adenopathy
- Symptomatic, acute (primary) HIV infection

Category B (Excludes Patients with Conditions in Category C):

If the following conditions are attributable to HIV, follow a course complicated by HIV or require special management because of HIV:
- Bacillary angiomatosis (disseminated bartonellosis)
- Oropharyngeal candidiasis
- Persistent, recurrent, or poorly responsive vulvovaginal candidiasis
- Cervical dysplasia or cervical carcinoma in situ
- Constitutional symptoms, e.g., fever of >38.5°C or diarrhea for >1 mo
- Oral hairy leukoplakia
- Recurrent or multidermatomal herpes zoster
- Idiopathic thrombocytopenic purpura
- Listeriosis
- Pelvic inflammatory disease, particularly with tuboovarian abscess
- Peripheral neuropathy

Category C

If any of the following conditions are diagnosed:
- Candidiasis of the trachea, bronchi, or lungs
- Esophageal candidiasis
- Disseminated coccidioidomycosis
- Extrapulmonary cryptococcosis
- Chronic cryptosporidiosis, with diarrhea for >1 mo
- Cytomegalovirus infection (other than liver, spleen, or nodes)
- Cytomegalovirus retinitis (with vision loss)
- HIV encephalopathy
- Herpes simplex: chronic ulcers for >1 mo or bronchitis, pneumonia, or esophagitis
- Disseminated or extrapulmonary histoplasmosis
- Isosporiasis, with diarrhea for >1 mo
- Kaposi sarcoma
- Hodgkin lymphoma
- Non-Hodgkin lymphoma of B cell or unknown phenotype, including Burkitt lymphoma
- Primary lymphoma of the brain
- Disseminated *Mycobacterium avium* complex or *Mycobacterium kansasi*
- *Mycobacterium tuberculosis*, either pulmonary or extrapulmonary
- Other disseminated or extrapulmonary mycobacterial infections
- *Pneumocystis jiroveci* pneumonia
- Recurrent pneumonia
- Progressive multifocal leukoencephalopathy
- Recurrent *Salmonella* bacteremia
- Toxoplasmosis of the brain
- Wasting syndrome due to HIV
- Invasive cervical cancer

HIV-infected individuals will eventually progress to AIDS with opportunistic infections, Kaposi sarcoma, or B-cell lymphomas (Table 38-2, categories B and C). The specific distribution of AIDS-associated opportunistic infections in a given population is highly dependent on the background prevalence of these pathogens in the population of HIV-infected persons. For example, in the United States and Europe, *P. jiroveci* pneumonia is the most common presenting clinical manifestation in persons not receiving prophylaxis for this agent; in Zimbabwe, *Mycobacterium tuberculosis* is by far the most common clinical manifestation. A significant fraction of adult AIDS patients also may develop neurologic symptoms. Neurologic manifestations of AIDS may be due to viral replication in the CNS, secondary infection by opportunistic organisms such as the protozoan *Toxoplasma gondii* or the fungus *Cryptococcus neoformans*, or the development of CNS malignancies. It is not known if damage to brain cells is due to the release of toxic substances from infected monocytes or via direct damage to brain tissue by replicating virus.

The most important factor in the development of AIDS in HIV-infected individuals is time. In the absence of antiretroviral chemotherapy, most if not all HIV-infected individuals will ultimately develop AIDS. Over 95% of HIV-infected individuals progress to AIDS within 15 years of infection. The remaining small fraction of long-term nonprogressors has very low virus loads and may remain asymptomatic for prolonged periods. Several factors affect survival rates, including viral and host factors such as age, HLA haplotype, gender, and immune status. Effective antiretroviral chemotherapy (as assessed by the use of antiretroviral drugs that drive HIV RNA levels in the plasma to levels below the current limits of detection [20 to 50 copies/mL]) will reverse immunologic progression and may delay the onset of symptoms indefinitely.

DIAGNOSIS

Evidence of HIV infection is generally based on the presence of antiviral antibodies. The presence of virus in blood or tissues can be documented by growth of the virus in cell culture or by molecular methods, such as PCR-based assays that detect viral genetic material. Serologic tests for HIV infection detect specific anti-HIV antibodies in serum, which are present in close to 100% of HIV-infected individuals. The exceptions are a small group of individuals either in the earliest stages of the disease (before seroconversion) or even more rarely in the terminal stages (when B cells can no longer synthesize antibodies). On very rare occasions, certain individuals may "serorevert" (lose detectable antibodies while still carrying the virus). Thus, it is important to remember that in a very limited number of instances, the absence of antibodies does not completely exclude HIV infection.

Initial tests for HIV antibodies generally are performed using an ELISA (enzyme-linked immunosorbent assay). If

PARADIGM BOX

NEW EPIDEMICS OF INFECTIOUS DISEASES

How do new epidemics of infectious diseases arise? In some cases, such as influenza, the virus is already present in the human or animal population and undergoes antigenic change to produce new, more virulent strains. In other instances, the agent is present as a relatively innocuous commensal in animals, and by a genetic alteration, it becomes virulent in humans.

In the case of the AIDS epidemic, considerable genetic evidence suggests that viruses related to HIV have existed in nonhuman primates for a long time. The prevailing evidence is that retroviruses similar to HIV-1 were present in primate (simian) species and that the strain most like HIV-1, termed SIV_{cpz}, was carried by chimpanzees. In this host, the virus appears to be less virulent than in humans. Several transmissions of this virus from chimpanzees to humans are thought to have occurred in equatorial West Africa in the early part of the 20th century, probably in association with the butchering of these animals for food. The most important variable accounting for the rapid global spread of HIV-1 is increasing travel, which allowed the virus to become established and disseminate widely within the human population by sexual intercourse and maternofetal spread.

Will the AIDS epidemic ever come to an end? The AIDS epidemic of today has a vivid historical parallel.

At the end of the 15th century, syphilis, an apparently new disease, swept through Europe in epidemic proportions. For the first 60 years of its history, syphilis was a very different illness from the disease we know now: instead of progressing (if untreated) to the chronic manifestations of the tertiary stage, 15th- and 16th-century syphilis was an acute disease with a high mortality rate. We do not know what caused the abrupt change in the pathological picture of syphilis, but we can speculate as follows: For any disease that is spread directly among people, an agent that causes death of the host eliminates infected contacts. As a result, transmission of the agent is greatly reduced. Eventually, the deadly strain of the agent will be supplanted by a milder one that causes a chronic illness and thus has a greater chance of being transmitted to a new host. This scenario may in fact have occurred for HIV or HIV-like viruses in monkeys and apes. AIDS in humans, on the other hand, is unlikely to result in such a balanced situation any time in the near future. An HIV-infected person can be the source of transmission of the virus over a long period of time. Thus, the biological basis for the abatement of the AIDS epidemic is not obvious. Interrupting the AIDS epidemic cannot depend on evolutionary changes in either the host or the virus but will require effective antiviral vaccination or chemotherapy.

---

the serum is found to contain HIV antibodies, the test is usually repeated and confirmed by a secondary antibody test such as an immunoblot or "Western blot" assay.

The ELISA test has a false-positive rate of less than 0.1%. With confirmatory immunoblot tests, the joint false-positive rate approaches a remarkable 0.005%. Before the advent of effective antiretroviral therapy, it was necessary to carefully weigh whether low-risk individuals should be tested. The impact of a positive test result on a person's state of mind, social interactions, marriage, insurance eligibility, and employment opportunities is enormous. It is now recognized that the beneficial effects of initiating anti-HIV therapy prior to the onset of AIDS clearly justifies serologic testing of persons at risk for HIV infection.

TREATMENT

Over the past 25 years, major progress has been made in the development of antiretroviral therapy (see Chapter 44, "Antiviral Treatment Strategies"). The life cycle of retroviruses is intimately associated with the physiology of mammalian cells so that only a limited number of metabolic reactions can be singled out for targets of specific chemotherapy. Reverse transcriptase is an attractive target because inhibition of this enzyme should have no effect on the host cell. Several FDA-approved anti-HIV drugs inhibit this unique viral function. Zidovudine (azidothymidine or AZT) was the first of several dideoxynucleotides to be tested in clinical trials. Other approved drugs in this category include didanosine (ddI), zalcitabine (ddC), stavudine (d4T), lamivudine (3TC), emtricitabine (FTC), and tenofovir. These drugs inhibit reverse transcriptase after being phosphorylated intracellularly. Inhibition takes place by premature termination of growing strands of DNA into which the drugs have been incorporated. Mammalian DNA polymerases are more resistant to these drugs than is the viral reverse transcriptase.

A second class of reverse transcriptase inhibitors, the nonnucleoside inhibitors (or NNRTIs), act by binding to the enzyme at a site distant from the active site. This class includes the drugs nevirapine, efavirenz, and delavirdine. After reverse transcription produces a double-stranded DNA copy of the viral RNA, the viral integrase enzyme inserts the viral genetic information into host chromosomal DNA. A very potent and well-tolerated viral integrase inhibitor, raltegravir, has entered clinical practice and is providing additional treatment options in both treatment-naïve and treatment-experienced patients.

An additional group of antiviral drugs approved for use against HIV includes inhibitors of the viral protease, such as ritonavir, indinavir, saquinavir, amprenavir, nelfinavir, darunavir, and lopinavir. These drugs do not affect early stages of virus replication but rather prevent cleavage of the viral polyproteins into their mature, active forms. Finally, viral entry inhibitors that either prevent the virus from binding to its secondary receptor (CCR5) or block viral envelope fusion with the host cell membrane also have entered clinical practice. However, these agents currently have more limited use. CCR5 inhibitors are active only against virus that exclusively engages that receptor and thus require a complex susceptibility test before use. The only available fusion inhibitor is not orally bioavailable and must be given twice daily by subcutaneous injection.

The use of all antiviral agents is limited by the development of genetic resistance of the virus. Any of the antivirals individually is capable of rapidly and effectively halting most or all virus replication in the body. However, in virtually all cases of such monotherapy, virus replication rapidly rebounds and remains resistant to further treatment with the same or related compounds. Much more durable results, that is, strong suppression of virus replication combined with marked clinical improvement, can be achieved in most HIV-infected individuals by using combinations of three or four agents with diverse antiviral mechanisms. When such regimens achieve viral suppression to levels that are below the limit of detection of current commercial assays, antiretroviral therapy is effective for over 15 years with little evidence of failure in persons who are able to remain adherent to their treatment regimens. The impact of antiretroviral chemotherapy on HIV infection has been one of the most striking successes of modern medicine in that it has turned a disease that led inexorably to death in virtually all patients over a matter of years to a chronic infection that can be successfully managed for decades while patients resume the activities of daily life.

PREVENTION

Control of AIDS transmission has been difficult because a vaccine is not yet available. The most effective control of this disease requires a reduction in sexual activities associated with viral transmission or the cessation of using contaminated needles or syringes associated with injecting drug use. Education is the most important means of reducing the spread of AIDS at the present time. The most important measures include curtailing high-risk practices, such as multiple sexual contacts for both homosexual and heterosexual persons, the use of condoms, awareness of the danger of anal intercourse, and the use of uncontaminated needles for injection drug users. Circumcision makes men less likely to acquire the virus during insertive intercourse with either male or female partners. Evidence that education has an impact on sexual practices comes from experience in the gay community in San Francisco as well as in heterosexual populations in resource-limited countries where governments have openly advocated

for strategies to curtail the epidemic. Although not yet proven, effective integration of prevention and treatment programs likely will be even more successful in reducing spread of the virus. By providing medical care to those who need it, there is an incentive for individuals to submit to voluntary testing for HIV infection. Prevention messages targeted at the infected population can only be effective when such individuals are identified. For example, studies from Kenya have demonstrated that when an infected member of a serodiscordant steady sexual couple is placed on antiretroviral chemotherapy, the rate of new infections among uninfected partners falls sharply. Another study among high-risk men who have sex with men has demonstrated that daily administration of tenofovir and emtricitabine decreases the likelihood of becoming infected by over 50%. Thus, antiretroviral therapy is efficacious in reducing the likelihood of transmission whether it is given to the infected or the uninfected member of a sexually active couple. Indeed, it is possible that antiretroviral agents might reduce transmission when applied as a component of a gel prior to sexual intercourse.

What about an AIDS vaccine? Will it ever be possible? The capacity of HIV to change its antigenicity complicates conventional approaches to vaccine development and presents perhaps the most serious barrier to an effective HIV vaccine. Since the initial introductions of HIV-1 into the human population 70 to 80 years ago, the virus has diversified widely into multiple types, subtypes, and genome recombinants. Although immunization with viral envelope antigens failed to prevent viral transmission in humans, a study in which the viral envelope glycoprotein gp120 was used to boost a recombinant poxvirus vectorborne vaccine provided encouraging results. Although it is clear that vigorous virus-specific immune responses develop during the course of infection and that these immune responses are partially effective in controlling viral replication, it is not clear which (if any) of these immune responses are associated with reductions in acquisition of the virus. Furthermore, recent data indicating up to a 50% rate of superinfection with multiple strains of virus among highly exposed individuals, despite the presence of these immune responses, should provide a sobering reminder that it is possible that an effective AIDS vaccine may not be developed for several decades—if at all. Nonetheless, the challenge of AIDS vaccine development has been met with a variety of innovative approaches for antigen presentation and contributed immensely to the field of vaccinology. While these efforts must be vigorously supported, enthusiasm for an effective vaccine must not cloud the realization that such a vaccine may be far off, and in the meantime, prevention and treatment programs should be planned as if there will be no vaccine. If a vaccine is developed, it will be much easier to modify public health strategies to this reality than to face the long-term consequences of inadequate investments in conventional public health approaches.

CONCLUSION

AIDS is a uniquely devastating disease: it kills all those that exhibit symptoms. It is a chronic illness, often manifested years after the virus is acquired and after the infected individual has had the opportunity to transmit it. In the United States, the number of new AIDS cases has stabilized, and the number of AIDS deaths is declining due to the use of potent antiretroviral drug combinations.

By inactivating a central cellular component of the immune system, the CD4+ T lymphocyte, HIV produces severe impairment of both humoral and cellular immunity. The disease is lethal because defense mechanisms against opportunistic pathogens are eradicated. Diseases that were practically unseen before AIDS (e.g., encephalitis due to *T. gondii*), or under reasonable control (e.g., mycobacterial infections), have become common and highly dangerous among people with AIDS.

AIDS runs counter to the tenet that a successful parasite does not cause lethal injury to its host, suggesting that HIV may be a relative newcomer among human infectious agents. There is a great deal of knowledge about HIV and other retroviruses, but many features of the disease are unexplained. The virus is particularly elusive to vaccine development because of variability in its surface antigens and other features of its structure and replication program.

Antiretroviral therapy has made it possible to improve the quality and nearly indefinitely prolong the lives of those infected with the virus. In addition, as antiretroviral therapy has become more widely available, coupled with behaviorally based prevention efforts, it is likely that antiretroviral drugs also have contributed to reduced transmission rates in places where they have been made available.

Suggested Readings

Abdool Karim Q, Abdool Karim SS, Frohlich JA, et al. Effectiveness and safety of tenofovir gel, an antiretroviral microbicide, for the prevention of HIV infection in women. *Science.* 2010;329:1168–1174.

Chan M. Towards universal access: scaling up priority HIV/AIDS interventions in the health sector. Progress report. Geneva: World Health Organization; 2008. http://www.who.int/hiv/pub/2008progressreport/en/index.html

Chasela CS, Hudgens MG, Jamieson DJ, et al. Maternal or infant antiretroviral drugs to reduce HIV-1 transmission. *N Engl J Med.* 2010;362:2271–2281.

Gao F, Bailes E, Robertson DL, Chen Y, et al. Origin of HIV-1 in the chimpanzee Pan troglodytes troglodytes. *Nature.* 1999;397:436–441.

Grant RM, Lama JR, Anderson PL, et al. Preexposure chemoprophylaxis for HIV prevention in men who have sex with men. *N Engl J Med.* 2010;363:2587–2599.

Gray RH, Kigozi G, Servadda D, et al. Male circumcision for HIV prevention in men in Rakai, Uganda: a randomised trial. *Lancet.* 2007;369:657–666.

Johnston MI, Fauci AS. An HIV vaccine—evolving concepts. *N Engl J Med.* 2007;356:2073–2081.

Perelson AS, Neumann AU, Markowitz M, et al. HIV-1 dynamics in vivo: virion clearance rate, infected cell life-span, and viral generation time. *Science.* 1996;271:1582–1586.

Rerks-Ngarm S, Pitisuttithum P, Nitayaphan S, et al. Vaccination with ALVAC and AIDSVAX to prevent HIV-1 infection in Thailand. *N Engl J Med.* 2009;361:2209–2220.

Thompson MA (Panel Chair), Aberg JA, Cahn P, et al. Antiretroviral treatment of adult HIV infection: 2010 recommendations of the International AIDS Society-USA Panel. *JAMA.* 2010;304:321–333.

Wei X, Decker JM, Wang S, et al. Antibody neutralization and escape by HIV-1. *Nature.* 2003;422:307–312.

the viral genome, whereas herpesviruses (see Chapters 41 and 42) encode most of the enzymes involved in viral DNA replication. The adenoviruses fall between these extremes, employing both virus-encoded and host proteins in replication.

Adenovirus DNA possesses **inverted terminal repeats**: About 100 base pairs are repeated in an inverted orientation at each end of the genome. The two ends of the DNA molecule thus have identical sequences. DNA replication is initiated within these repeats at one or the other end of the adenovirus DNA molecule (Fig. 39-3). Initiation takes place at either end with about equal frequency. After initiation, DNA synthesis proceeds along the template DNA. One parental strand is copied, and the other is displaced. Completion of the synthesis of the first daughter strand produces a duplex molecule consisting of one parental strand and one daughter strand and leaves behind a displaced parental single strand. Because of the inverted terminal repeats, the displaced single strand assumes a "**panhandle**" configuration containing a short double-stranded region identical in sequence to the ends of the normal double-stranded genome. DNA synthesis is initiated on the panhandle, and the displaced single strand serves as template for the synthesis of the second daughter strand.

Synthesis of viral DNA differs from that of host DNA in three respects. First, a single DNA strand is copied at each virus replication fork, whereas in host cell replication, both strands are copied concurrently. Second, the synthesis of all new viral DNA is continuous; that is, it occurs by the uninterrupted elongation of the growing chain across the entire genome. In host cell DNA replication, one strand at each replication fork is produced continuously, but the other is synthesized discontinuously as short pieces (Okazaki fragments) that must be joined to produce the finished strand. Finally, host chromosomes replicate by a well-regulated process that occurs once in a division cycle, whereas virus replication is uncoordinated and takes place continuously over time. The latter strategy is a response to the need to produce as many viral DNA molecules as possible over the short course of a viral infectious cycle.

Studies carried out with purified proteins have led to a detailed biochemical understanding of the events in adenovirus DNA replication. Six proteins are required for optimal viral DNA replication in vitro. Three of the proteins are virally encoded—a **DNA polymerase (AdPol)**, a **DNA-binding protein (DBP)**, and the **preterminal protein (pTP)**, which is the precursor of the terminal protein found in virions. All three proteins are products of the E2 region. The remaining three replication proteins are cellular products. Two are transcription factors that normally function to regulate expression of cellular genes in uninfected cells; the third is a topoisomerase.

The initiation of DNA replication is carried out by a complex consisting of AdPol and pTP. The complex binds to a DNA sequence within the terminal repeat, a process **stimulated by the binding of the host transcription factors** to adjacent sequences. The end of the viral DNA molecule is unwound, exposing single-stranded DNA that serves as the template for the actual initiation event. That event is the formation of a phosphodiester link between the first nucleotide of the 5′ end of the new DNA strand (dC) and a serine residue in the pTP molecule. In that way, **pTP serves as the primer for adenovirus DNA replication** (see Fig. 39-3, Panel C). Protein priming of DNA replication is most unusual; in most cases, primers for DNA replication are short RNA molecules. After formation of the initial pTP–dC linkage, elongation of the new daughter strand proceeds conventionally, with AdPol sequentially adding nucleotides to the 3′ end of the pTP-bound growing chain. The viral DBP is essential for elongation and coats the displaced single strand, protecting it from nuclease attack. As DNA is packaged, proteolytic processing cleaves the pTP molecule bound to each DNA strand to generate the form found in mature virions. In principle, the unique features of adenovirus DNA replication present attractive targets for antiviral drug therapy. However, this opportunity has thus far not been exploited.

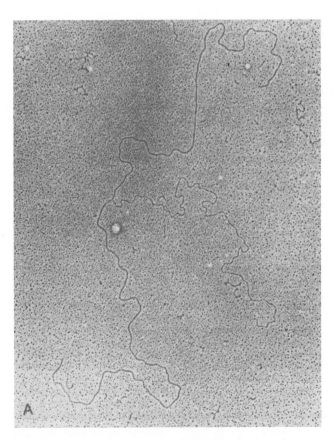

FIGURE 39-3. Adenovirus DNA replication. A. An electron micrograph of a DNA molecule of the type diagrammed in the second line of part B—that is, a duplex with one single-stranded branch.

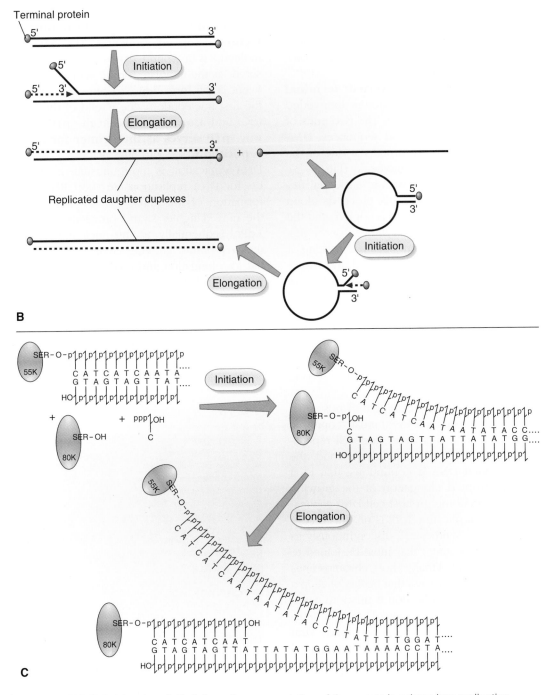

FIGURE 39-3. (*Continued*) **B.** Schematic representation of the events in adenovirus replication. **C.** Details of the initiation of adenovirus DNA replication showing the priming of DNA synthesis by the preterminal protein (pTP is labeled 80K; TP is labeled 55K).

Virion Assembly

Particle assembly begins when sufficient amounts of capsid proteins have accumulated. The first step is the assembly of individual capsid proteins into hexon and penton capsomeres. Pentons are assembled spontaneously, but hexon assembly requires the participation of a protein that does not appear in the mature particle. Such proteins that assist in assembly but do not appear in the virus are commonly referred to as **scaffold proteins**. Hexons and several minor virion components are next assembled into an empty particle that is later filled with DNA and core proteins. By analogy to bacteriophages, the DNA probably enters the empty virus particle through one of the open vertices. Finally, the pentons and fibers become associated with the capsid, and a series of proteolytic events converts precursor proteins within the virion into their mature forms. After assembly, adenovirus particles are slowly released as the dying cell lyses. A viral protease and the colorfully

PARADIGM BOX

DNA VIRUS REPLICATION AND CONTROL OF THE CELL CYCLE

The study of DNA viruses can teach us a great deal about the complicated workings of normal cells. Because DNA viruses either make use of host cell machinery (frequently modified by viral proteins) or employ general strategies similar to those of their host cells, understanding the events that occur in virus-infected cells often reveals much about the events that take place in uninfected cells. Adenoviruses have been particularly useful models for studies of DNA replication and gene expression. For example, **mRNA splicing** was first discovered in studies of the synthesis of adenovirus late mRNAs, and only later was the process found to occur in normal eukaryotic cells. Similarly, in vitro eukaryotic DNA replication systems first developed for adenovirus and polyomavirus DNAs have been extremely useful in understanding the biochemistry of cellular DNA replication. Of particular importance, studies of adenoviruses, papillomaviruses, and polyomaviruses have contributed to knowledge about mammalian cell cycle control that guarantees that cellular DNA replicates exactly once per cell division and that cells divide only on receipt of appropriate signals. Aberrations in cell cycle control are central to the growth abnormalities of cancer cells.

Most DNA viruses, including adenoviruses, exploit at least some elements of the cellular DNA replication machinery. This exploitation is economical for the virus, but it also creates a timing problem because the shared cellular factors are normally expressed only during the DNA synthesis (S) phase of the cell cycle. It is not advantageous for a virus to wait for the cell to begin its division cycle. Moreover, many of the cells targeted by

DNA viruses are differentiated and do not divide at all, never entering S phase (e.g., superficial epithelial cells). To overcome these obstacles and maintain a continuous large supply of the necessary host cell proteins, adenoviruses and most other DNA viruses encode proteins that force infected cells into the S phase of the cell cycle.

Viral proteins induce the S phase by interacting with key regulators of the normal cell cycle. In the case of adenoviruses, the products of the **E1A** region bind to and inactivate the cellular protein **pRb**, which normally maintains S-phase genes in a silent state. Inactivation of pRb is primarily responsible for continuous S-phase gene expression in adenovirus-infected cells. Additional adenovirus proteins, expressed from **E1B and E4**, inactivate the cellular protein **p53**, which cooperates with pRb in preventing a cell from advancing into S phase and also can induce **apoptosis** (programmed cell death) in cells that overexpress S-phase genes. Together, the viral proteins inactivate two key negative regulators of the S phase of the cell cycle and permit the infected cell to overexpress factors necessary for DNA replication and survive the cell death pathway that would be the normal consequence of this enforced overexpression.

Because of their effects on pRb and p53, adenoviruses possess **oncogenic potential**. Indeed, the cellular proteins are known as **tumor suppressors**, since mutations in their respective genes are associated with a wide range of nonviral human cancers. Adenoviruses are not alone in their effects on tumor suppressors: Papillomaviruses, polyomaviruses, and some herpesviruses encode proteins that subvert the functions of pRb and p53, resulting in the induction of tumors. Of note, both pRb and p53 were originally identified on the basis of their interactions with DNA virus proteins.

---

named adenovirus death protein (from E3) participate in the destruction of the host cell and virus release. Released virus can attach directly to adjacent cells or spread to cells in remote locations through the bloodstream.

DAMAGE

The usual symptoms of adenovirus respiratory infections resemble those of the **common cold**, including nasal congestion, inflammation of the upper respiratory tract, and cough. Systemic symptoms such as chills, headache, muscle aches, and fever are common, and **conjunctivitis** sometimes accompanies the other symptoms (**pharyngo-conjunctival fever**). In severe cases, **pneumonia** can develop. Different serotypes are associated with different disease manifestations (Table 39-1). Serotypes 1, 2, 5, and 6 are endemic in most populations, and 80% of all young adults have neutralizing antibodies to those types. Other serotypes (4 and 7) are associated with outbreaks of a

fairly severe febrile respiratory infection (**acute respiratory disease or ARD**).

Adenoviruses are also an important cause of acute gastrointestinal disease in children and may be responsible for up to 15% of childhood intestinal infections. Many serotypes of adenoviruses are present, not only in the stool of patients but in normal stool as well, in contrast to other serotypes that are only associated with disease. Adenovirus type 12 (Ad12) has been implicated in the development of celiac disease (gluten enteropathy). The development of that illness appears to depend on protein sequence homology between an Ad12 early protein and gliadin-α, a component of the cereal grains that activate the disease. It is possible that exposure to Ad12 induces an antibody response to gliadin-α, which predisposes to celiac disease in some persons.

Less common than respiratory and gastrointestinal disease is adenovirus-induced conjunctivitis without other symptoms. Mild "**swimming pool conjunctivitis**" is probably most often a result of adenovirus infection, as is the more serious, highly contagious **epidemic keratoconjunctivitis**.

Latent adenovirus infections are very common; adenoviruses can be recovered from as many as 80% of the tonsils or adenoids removed from children and young adults. The mechanism of persistence in those cases is not known. Viral DNA can persist in tonsillar tissue free of infectious virus, but it is also possible that persistence may be caused by a low-level active infection imperfectly controlled by the immune system. In fact, the majority of healthy adults examined have very small numbers of peripheral lymphocytes apparently undergoing a typical adenovirus lytic cycle. Early gene products that interfere with host defense mechanisms may play a role in persistence.

Adenoviruses frequently are recovered from immunocompromised individuals. Numerous isolations from patients with immunodeficiency resulting from HIV infection have been reported, and infection has been associated in some cases with mortality. Disseminated adenovirus infections also are a significant cause of mortality among stem cell transplant recipients. In these cases, reactivation of latent adenovirus infection is probably the source of the acute infection.

Interactions with Host Defense Systems

Adenoviruses carry several genes that function to evade or antagonize antiviral host defenses. The main immunological defense against viral infection, cell-mediated immunity, involves destruction of virus-infected cells by cytotoxic T lymphocytes (CTLs). CTLs have receptors for specific complexes of viral peptides bound to **major histocompatibility complex (MHC) class I** molecules on the surface of most cells. These receptors enable CTLs to recognize infected cells. Cells that do not express MHC class I molecules do not become targets for destruction by CTLs. Adenoviruses evade cell-mediated immune response using two independent mechanisms that interfere with expression of MHC class I molecules. First, an adenovirus early region protein **blocks the production of MHC class I mRNA** in infected cells. Second, an E3-encoded glycoprotein **prevents the transport of newly synthesized MHC class I proteins** to the cell surface. In cotton rats, infections of the lung with adenovirus mutants that do not express the E3 protein induce a striking pulmonary infiltration of neutrophils, suggesting that this protein influences the course of disease in vivo.

Another way in which adenoviruses escape cellular immunity is through resistance to signals from immune cells that would otherwise cause premature death of the infected cell. For example, both **tumor necrosis factor (TNF)**, produced by activated macrophages, and **Fas ligand**, found on the surface of many immune cells, can activate intracellular pathways that result in death of virus-infected cells. Adenoviruses produce proteins that block these death pathways and render cells relatively resistant to either death stimulus. In addition, adenovirus mediates the removal of a cell-surface receptor required for killing by Fas ligand.

A third line of defense against viral infection is the antiviral state induced in cells by **interferon-α** and **interferon-β**. Among other effects, the interferons prevent protein synthesis in virus-infected cells by initiating a chain of events that culminates in the inactivation of the cellular translation machinery. Central to inhibition of translation is a host cell protein (**PKR**) activated by double-stranded RNA produced in most viral infections, including adenovirus infection. Adenoviruses break the interferon chain and prevent the inhibition of protein synthesis through the action of small RNA molecules (**VA RNAs**) encoded by viral genes. The VA RNAs fold into partially double-stranded structures that bind to and prevent activation of PKR, preserving the cellular translational apparatus for use by the virus.

Adenoviruses also interfere with antiviral processes within individual cells. For example, many viral infections activate DNA repair pathways normally induced by DNA damage, and these pathways in turn reduce virus growth. Adenoviruses inactivate these pathways by destroying through proteolysis host cell proteins central to the DNA damage response, preventing their interference with viral replication.

Obviously, adenoviruses do not completely blunt antiviral responses, because most adenovirus infections eventually are cleared. However, it is likely that reductions or delays in these processes contribute to the success of adenoviruses as common human pathogens.

Oncogenicity and Cell Transformation

Adenovirus type 12 was the first DNA-containing virus shown to cause cancer in animals. That discovery sparked a massive search for evidence that adenoviruses (and other DNA viruses) cause cancer in humans. It is now clear that some DNA viruses, including papillomaviruses (see Chapter 40), are important causes of human cancer, but there is no convincing association between adenoviruses and cancer in people. Enormous efforts also have been made to determine mechanisms of tumorigenesis by animal DNA viruses. Those studies have contributed significantly to knowledge about the molecular basis of carcinogenesis.

While playing no apparent role in human cancer, adenoviruses induce phenotypic changes in cultured cells that resemble those that occur during natural carcinogenesis. This process is referred to as **transformation**. Transformation by adenoviruses requires the products of the E1A and E1B regions, which transform cells largely by interacting with the cellular tumor suppressor products **pRb** and **p53** (see the Paradigm Box). Importantly, transformation by adenoviruses is only an incidental consequence of the mechanisms that regulate viral gene expression.

ADENOVIRUSES AS VECTORS FOR GENE DELIVERY

Virus particles efficiently introduce foreign nucleic acid (the viral genome) into living cells. This property has been exploited to introduce nonviral genes into animals or animal cells. Because much is known about adenovirus biology and genetics, adenoviruses are considered to be particularly promising vectors for foreign gene delivery.

The development of safe and effective vaccines to combat ARD makes the use of recombinant adenoviruses to immunize against pathogens other than adenovirus itself an attractive idea. Several candidate **adenovirus-based vaccine strains** have been constructed. In these strains, a segment of DNA encoding an antigen derived from a pathogen, along with regulatory signals to direct expression of the antigen, replaces a segment of the adenovirus genome. Such genetically engineered adenoviruses direct the production of the foreign antigen in infected cells. Vaccines against pathogens including HIV, rabies virus, and the malaria parasite induce strong cellular and humoral immune responses and protect against the target pathogen in animal models.

A second potential application for adenovirus is as a vector for the introduction of an exogenous gene into an individual for therapeutic purposes. **Gene therapy** is usually envisioned as a therapeutic approach for an inherited disease. For example, the blood-clotting disorder hemophilia A results from the inheritance of nonfunctional alleles of a particular gene (the gene encoding factor VIII). Administration of purified factor VIII to affected persons corrects the defect. Therefore, delivery of the normal factor VIII gene to appropriate cells in a patient might restore enough factor VIII function to relieve symptoms of the disease. Accordingly, genetically engineered adenoviruses carrying the factor VIII gene in place of E1 (such viruses cannot conduct a lytic growth cycle in normal cells) have been constructed, and clinical improvement has been demonstrated in a mouse hemophilia A model after the administration of recombinant adenovirus. Significant technical problems, such as short-lived expression of the exogenous genes, need to be overcome before gene therapy of this sort becomes practical. The tragic death of a human volunteer in an adenovirus gene therapy trial in 1999 points out the social and ethical problems that also accompany the development of gene therapy.

A final promising application for adenovirus vectors is in cancer treatment. Numerous clinical trials with recombinant adenoviruses designed specifically to kill cancer cells are under way. Cell death is variously accomplished by delivery of toxic genes, by delivery of genes that stimulate antitumor immunity, or by use of adenovirus mutants that grow selectively in cells with genetic abnormalities frequently found in cancer cells. As with adenovirus vaccination and gene therapy, much work remains before adenovirus anticancer therapy becomes clinically useful.

PREVENTION AND TREATMENT

The public health impact of adenoviruses has not justified development of a vaccine for the general population. However, ARD presents a serious problem among military recruits during basic training. As many as 80% of some groups of recruits are affected, with one-fourth to one-half requiring hospitalization in some outbreaks. In response to ARD, a live oral adenovirus vaccine was developed by the US military in the 1960s. Given to newly inducted military personnel, it effectively eliminated ARD from the military for three decades. Recently, production of the vaccine was ended for economic reasons, and ARD has reappeared, resulting in at least one fatality. Vaccine manufacture is now being reestablished, and it is likely that the disease will again come under control. The military experience with ARD graphically illustrates the hazard to health created by eliminating costly vaccination programs when funds are short, and the problem seems to have disappeared (often through the use of vaccine).

Largely because of the risk of severe adenovirus disease in transplant recipients, significant efforts have been made to identify antiadenovirus drugs. Several established and developmental antiviral drugs show efficacy against adenovirus in tissue culture, but none has yet shown sufficient promise in animals to justify use in humans.

CONCLUSION

Adenoviruses are commonly found among healthy persons but also cause many types of infections that range in severity. The eye, the upper and lower respiratory tracts, and the gastrointestinal tract are often involved. Adenoviruses are capable of cellular transformation and oncogenesis in animals, but convincing evidence linking adenoviruses to cancer in humans is lacking. Adenoviruses are double-stranded DNA viruses whose life cycle has served as a model for the study of eukaryotic DNA replication and gene expression. The expression of adenovirus genes follows a defined program, some genes being expressed early, while others are expressed late. Modified adenoviruses may be suitable candidates for recombinant vaccines to be used in immunizing against a variety of antigens or for introducing genes into humans for correction of genetic diseases.

Suggested Readings

Berget SM, Moore C, Sharp PA. Spliced segments at the 5' terminus of adenovirus 2 late mRNA. *Proc Natl Acad Sci USA.* 1977;74:3171–3175.

Berk AJ. Recent lessons in gene expression, cell cycle control, and cell biology from adenovirus. *Oncogene.* 2005;24:7673–7685.

Carmen IH. A death in the laboratory: the politics of the Gelsinger aftermath. *Mol Ther.* 2001;3:425–428.

DeCaprio JA, How the Rb tumor suppressor structure and function was revealed by the study of adenovirus and SV40. *Virology.* 2009;384:274–284.

de Jong RN, van der Vliet PC, Brenkman AB. Adenovirus DNA replication: protein priming, jumping back and the role of the DNA binding protein DBP. *Curr Top Microbiol Immunol.* 2003;272:187–211.

Mahr JA, Gooding LR. Immune evasion by adenoviruses. *Immunol Rev.* 1999;168:121–130.

Prives C. Signaling to p53: breaking the MDM2-p53 circuit. *Cell.* 1998;95:5–8.

Toth K, Dhar D, Wold WS. Oncolytic (replication-competent) adenoviruses as anticancer agents. *Expert Opin Biol Ther.* 2010;10:353–368. Review.

Viiala NO, Larsen SR, Rasko JE. Gene therapy for hemophilia: clinical trials and technical tribulations. *Semin Thromb Hemost.* 2009;35:81–92.

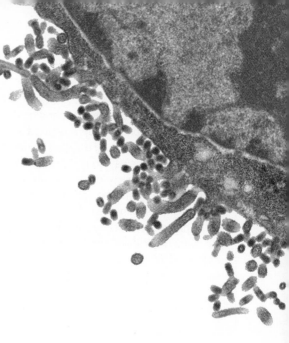

Chapter **40**

Human Papillomaviruses and Warts

Elliot J. Androphy

KEY CONCEPTS

Pathogen: Human papillomaviruses (HPVs) are a group of small, nonenveloped, nonlytic DNA viruses that replicate within squamous epithelial cells.

Encounter: Genital warts are the most common sexually transmitted infection (STI) for which people seek medical attention and the second most common STI, after chlamydia.

Entry: HPVs are spread by direct skin-to-skin contact, sexual transmission, or through contact with contaminated inanimate objects.

Replication and Spread: HPVs initially infect the basal epithelial cells. The virus replicates as an autonomous episome, and the HPV genomes are segregated into daughter cells after cell division. As the cells migrate to the keratinized layer, HPV is amplified, capsids are produced, and virions assemble in the nucleus of keratinocytes. The virus is shed with keratin scales from the skin.

Damage: HPVs cause local infections that may appear as warts (papillomas) at various sites, including the hands, feet, and genital region.

HPVs can cause chronic infections that can lead to malignancy—most frequently, cancer of the cervix.

Diagnosis: HPV infections are usually diagnosed by history and physical findings.

Treatment and Prevention: Treatment includes chemical, surgical, and physical modalities that destroy infected tissue.

HUMAN PAPILLOMAVIRUSES (HPVs) are a large species of genetically related nonenveloped viruses with a small circular DNA genome. Clinical manifestations of warts range from inapparent (subclinical) to large bulky growths. Warts usually appear as **slow-growing bumps** of the skin and mucous membranes. The majority of patients with warts seek medical attention because of physical discomfort or concern about the appearance of a new skin lesion. While most papillomavirus-induced warts are biologically benign, some warts may become cancers. Indeed, **cervical cancer** is one of the most common neoplasms of women and develops from lesions caused by specific types of HPVs.

THE PATHOGEN: HUMAN PAPILLOMAVIRUSES

HPVs belong to the Papillomaviridae family. Particles of these viruses are formed by two tightly packed viral proteins called L1 and L2 and contain a single copy of the circular viral genome (Fig. 40-1). Virus particles are released as the infected epithelial cells are desquamated. Because the viruses do not bud from infected cells, they do not have a lipid **envelope**. The absence of an envelope causes HPVs to be resistant to desiccation, heat, and detergents and surfactants such as Nonoxynol 9. Therefore, these viruses remain infectious in the environment for long periods of time. Because papillomavirus genomes consist of approximately 8,000 nucleotide base pairs, or about one-twentieth the size of herpesviruses, they encode only a few proteins. They do not encode a DNA polymerase to replicate their genome

CASE • As a healthy 26-year-old, Mr. M. was almost in a panic. Four months ago, he noticed a small bump on the shaft of his penis, but he decided to ignore it with the hope that it would go away on its own. When he found two new growths, he and his wife became worried that he had genital warts. The dermatologist he saw immediately confirmed that diagnosis without performing any tests and applied liquid nitrogen to destroy the warts. He told Mr. M. that genital warts are transmissible and that his wife needed to be examined. Mr. M. was anxious about spreading a virus that could cause his wife to develop cervical cancer. The doctor discussed HPV infection and reassured him that with routine gynecological care, his wife should be fine.

This case raises several questions:

1. How and when did Mr. M. acquire the HPV infection?
2. Is Mrs. M. also infected, and what are the clinical implications?
3. What, if any, laboratory tests should be performed on Mr. and Mrs. M.?
4. If Mrs. M. has cervical warts, will they eventually result in cancer?
5. How can Mr. M. and his wife be treated for the HPV infection?

See Appendix for answers.

and thus must rely on host cell DNA replication proteins to reproduce. Nucleoside analogs directed against viral polymerases and used in the treatment of herpesvirus infections (or even HIV) are not effective against warts.

Papillomaviruses are pathogens of humans, monkeys, dogs, cattle, birds, fish, and most other vertebrates. The viruses are species specific, and only HPVs can cause warts in humans. HPVs are subclassified into types on the basis of their **DNA sequences**. If the nucleotide sequence of a short, highly conserved region found in all papillomaviruses varies by more than 10% from all other known HPV sequences, the isolate is defined as a new type, or more accurately, a new genotype. According to that scheme, presently, more than 150 HPV genotypes have

been recognized (Table 40-1). Minor variants that differ by only a few nucleotides have been described within several species, thus expanding the genetic and possibly the biologic diversity of HPVs.

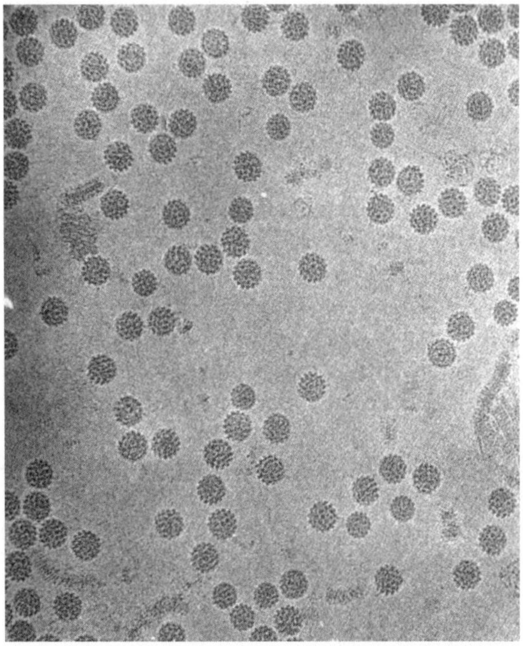

HPV types 1 through 4 were the first to be discovered because they are found in the majority of common **cutaneous warts**. In general, each HPV type is associated with infection of a specific anatomic region or epithelial environment. For instance, HPV-1 is most frequently found in plantar warts. HPV-2 causes common cutaneous warts but has been isolated from genital warts, especially in children. The genital-associated HPV types were identified later because the amount of viral DNA present in genital lesions is very low. **Genital warts**, also called **condyloma**, are usually caused by HPV types 6 and 11. Those HPV types cause warts of the penis, vulva, and anus and can infect the mucosal epithelium of the vagina, cervix, and oropharynx. Genital-type HPVs have been isolated infrequently from cutaneous warts.

ENCOUNTER

HPV particles are present on the surface of warts and the associated keratotic scale. The particles are spread by direct skin-to-skin contact with other people or with oneself—for example, a wart on the side of one finger touching the adjacent finger. However, normal skin is highly resistant to entry. HPVs are not highly contagious, and epidemics are rare, even within a family. Breaks in the epithelial barrier are necessary for entry, so scratching a wart can spread the virus to uninvolved areas. Infection also occurs more readily when the virus comes in contact with mucous membranes or with macerated skin. Despite the low content of virus particles in genital warts, transmission of HPV during sexual contact occurs with high efficiency because the intimate contact disturbs the epithelial barrier. Being nonenveloped, papillomaviruses are quite stable and remain infectious after exfoliation.

FIGURE 40-1. Electron micrograph of purified wart viruses.

TABLE 40-1 Lesions Associated with Human Papillomavirus (HPV) Types

Lesions	HPV Types
Plantar and palmar warts	HPV-1, 4
Common cutaneous warts	HPV-2, 4
Flat warts	HPV-3, 10
Anogenital warts, respiratory papillomatosis, cervical papillomas; "low risk" for becoming malignant	HPV-6, 11, 40, 42, 43, 44, 54, 61, 70, 72, 81
Epidermodysplasia verruciformis; immunosuppression	HPV-5, 8, 9, 12, 14, 15, 17, 19–29
Penile, vulvar, vaginal, and anal warts, Bowenoid papulosis; "high risk" for cervical and anal dysplasia and carcinoma	HPV-16, 18, 31, 33, 35, 39, 45, 51, 52, 53, 56, 58, 59, 66, 68, 73

Therefore, papillomaviruses present on inanimate objects can be a source of infection. Warts of the soles of the feet probably result from implantation of virus present on microabrasions of the feet caused by contact with rough surfaces, like the concrete surfaces of swimming pools.

It is estimated that 20 to 30 million persons are infected with HPV in the United States, with about 3 million new individuals infected each year. Genital warts are the single most common sexually transmitted infection that leads people to seek medical attention and second only to chlamydial infections as the most common sexually transmitted infection. An estimated 600,000 new cases of cervical cancer arise each year on a worldwide basis, leading to more than 250,000 deaths annually, 4,500 of which occur in the United States.

Many people become infected with wart viruses during their lifetime without exhibiting symptoms. Alterations in the epithelium may be so slight that the infection is not recognized. HPVs can lie dormant in the epithelial layers of the skin or mucosa. Compelling evidence of frequent asymptomatic infection derives from polymerase chain reaction (PCR) studies of cervical and vaginal cells obtained from healthy women presenting for routine gynecological care. Prospective studies of college women found that 20 to 60% become HPV DNA positive, although the majority of their cervical cells showed normal histology. Many of those HPV DNA–positive women subsequently become negative on repeat examination several months later. These findings provide evidence that most cervical HPV infections are transient. Although it is assumed that infections resolve due to host cellular immune responses, predictive indicators of susceptibility to HPV persistence are unknown. Since the majority of cervical infections become HPV negative by ultrasensitive nucleic acid detection technologies, this observation implies complete resolution and cure. HPV-negative cervical cancers are rare.

ENTRY

The location of a lesion is determined by the site of virus entry and may be influenced by the HPV genotype involved. The most frequent sites of warts are commonly traumatized skin surfaces such as the fingers, hands, soles, knees, and elbows. Microabrasions that occur with vaginal, anal, or oral sex and the moist, mucosal epithelia promote efficient virus spread to the penis, anus, vulva, vagina, cervix, and, less frequently, the oropharynx and larynx. Rarely, transmission from mother to child occurs during birth with aspiration of HPV. Infection by that route can cause the devastating disease **respiratory papillomatosis** in the infant. There is no consistent evidence of hematogenous spread of papillomavirus.

Host immunity plays an important role in susceptibility and maintenance of HPV infection. Individuals with defective cell-mediated immunity (e.g., transplant recipients receiving immunosuppressive drugs) may have numerous warts that are highly resistant to treatment. Men and women with AIDS are at increased risk for development of HPV-associated carcinomas. In the rare disease **epidermodysplasia verruciformis**, the individual is susceptible to specific HPV genotypes, presumably owing to an inability to mount an immune response to the virus. Widespread and longstanding warts may occur, and if infected with an oncogenic cutaneous HPV type such as type 5 or 8 (see Table 40-1), the individual may develop multiple invasive skin cancers.

Studies using PCR demonstrate that trace levels of HPV DNA are found on skin and in hair follicles from the majority of immunocompetent individuals. The low level of virus may represent the environmental reservoir for the more rare types of HPVs that are usually found in immunocompromised patients. Thus, HPVs can be maintained as subclinical infections in the normal population and arise in an individual when host immune surveillance is decreased.

SPREAD AND REPLICATION

HPVs have a genetic content that is minuscule compared to the human genome. Thus, like all viruses, papillomaviruses must use the host cell machinery to synthesize their macromolecules. To orchestrate these papillomavirus activities, proteins directly or indirectly coordinate the viral life cycle in concert with the cells that they infect. A papillomavirus protein called **E1** maintains the viral DNA as a covalently closed circular molecule or **episome** that does not integrate into the host cell genome. In that form, the viral genome replicates to high numbers at the proper time, independent of cellular DNA. A second viral protein called **E2** binds to a specific DNA sequence within the viral genome. E2 also binds to the E1 protein, and that complex binds with high affinity and specificity to the viral DNA. The E1 protein is a **helicase** that unwinds double-stranded DNA to initiate replication, and it also binds cellular DNA replication proteins and localizes those proteins to the viral episome. The E2 protein is also a **transcription factor** that regulates expression of the viral genes by directing the assembly of cellular transcription factors and RNA polymerase.

Papillomaviruses establish infection in the **basal cell layer** of the epithelium. That layer represents the replicative compartment of the skin, where cells continuously divide to replenish the desquamating surface and heal wounds. Viral entry is a relatively slow process, with the viral L2 capsid protein undergoing cleavage, which triggers conformational changes in the L1 major capsid protein. Heparan sulfated proteins mediate attachment; additional cellular receptors also may be used. After entry, one or at most a few copies of viral DNA are maintained as **extrachromosomal nuclear episomes**. Papillomaviruses are not **lytic**; that is, they do not kill the basal cell upon entry. Therefore, HPVs do not cause any immediate damage to the infected cell. The viral genome is initially replicated as an autonomous episome in synchrony with cellular chromosomes; the replicated viral genomes segregate into daughter cells. As those cells mature and migrate toward the skin surface, the viral genome is transported to upper levels of the epithelium. There, additional viral genes are expressed and viral genome amplification begins.

Virus reproduction occurs in concert with the differentiation program of **keratinocytes**. These cells are destined to form a nonreplicating physical barrier that preserves the integrity of the subcutaneous organs and protects the body from exogenous insults. Experimental evidence indicates that only basal cells in normal tissues are susceptible to HPV infection. As an epithelium differentiates, upper-level epithelial cells are programmed to lose their nucleus and fill with stable, insoluble, structural proteins. The flattened cells are shed as scales into the environment, with fresh cells continually replacing them from below. Papillomaviruses exploit this process for their replication and transmission. After passage near the outer epithelial layer, the virus responds to signals from the differentiated keratinocyte and directs transcription of the late mRNAs that encode its **capsid** proteins **L1** and **L2**. The differentiation-specific cues that trigger viral DNA amplification are unknown. These late proteins are transported into the nucleus of the keratinocyte where they assemble to form hundreds to perhaps thousands of capsids. The newly replicated DNA episomes are packaged into the capsids to form progeny **virions**, which are shed from the surface of the epithelium.

PARADIGM BOX

VIRAL ONCOGENESIS

The recognized human oncogenic viruses include **papillomaviruses, Epstein-Barr virus** (associated with **Burkitt lymphoma** and **nasopharyngeal carcinoma**), **hepatitis B and C viruses** (associated with **hepatocellular carcinoma**), **human herpesvirus 8** (associated with **Kaposi sarcoma**), and **human polyomavirus** isolated from cutaneous **Merkel cell skin cancers** (MCPyV). How and why do viruses transform cells? The paradox of papillomavirus replication is that it occurs in the upper epithelium, which is normally composed of nondividing, differentiated cells. Because papillomaviruses do not encode DNA replication enzymes, they must both prevent exit from the **cell cycle** and activate cellular pathways that replicate DNA.

Many different mechanisms of transformation are used by different viruses, but two recurring themes are inhibition of normal growth regulatory processes and stimulation of cell division. Normal human cells placed in culture do not continuously proliferate and thus are not "**immortal**." Most human cell lines that are serially grown in culture are derived from naturally occurring cancers, although not all cells from human malignancies can be easily propagated. Some oncogenic viruses can induce cell immortalization; that is, the infected cells do not undergo **senescence**, which is characteristic of normal diploid cells in culture. Establishment of the immortal phenotype is an early step in the progression to cancer. Some oncogenic viruses can **transform** established cell lines. **Transformed cells** can be recognized by their altered morphology, loss of contact-inhibited growth, and decreased nutritional requirements. In some cases, transformed cells are malignant; that is, they form tumors when injected into immunodeficient animals.

A common series of molecular events appears to be necessary for neoplastic progression. First, immortalization requires repeated entry into the cell cycle, which is restricted by the cellular **retinoblastoma (Rb)** protein; inactivation of that **tumor suppressor** pathway is found in many types of cancer. Second, the cellular tumor suppressor protein **p53** is often disrupted; p53 induces **programmed cell death (apoptosis)** that would occur following Rb inactivation or damage to the host cell genome. Third, the ends of **chromosomes** must be protected from progressive erosion that normally occurs with each replicative cycle. This process is reversed by the expression of **telomerase**, which protects cells from senescence. Most malignant cells exhibit repeated entry into the cell cycle characterized by loss of Rb function, ability to avoid normal checkpoints that signal DNA damage and activation of the p53 tumor suppressor pathway, mutations in normal growth-regulating genes, or infection with an oncogenic virus.

Tumor induction by high-risk HPVs exemplifies abrogation of these normal control processes. Among the eight proteins encoded by high-risk HPVs, only two, **E6 and E7**, are always expressed in cervical cancer cells. Using in vitro cell-culture assays, the E6 and E7 genes immortalize human keratinocytes and increase their growth rate. E6 and E7 also transform established mouse cell lines. These findings demonstrate that the viral proteins target fundamental growth regulatory pathways.

The molecular details of how high-risk E6 and E7 proteins cause cellular changes are incomplete but are becoming clearer. E7 has amino acid similarities to other viral oncogenes—namely, adenovirus E1A and simian virus 40 (**SV40**) **large T** (tumor) antigen. Those viral proteins form complexes with the **Rb** family member proteins including **p105**, the name reflecting its size (105 kDa). The development of retinoblastoma is associated with the absence of p105-Rb. This protein is a natural suppressor of cell proliferation. By complexing with p105-Rb, viral oncoproteins prevent Rb from exerting its normal check on cell proliferation. Binding to p105-Rb releases a **transcription factor** called **E2F**, which induces expression of a series of genes necessary for DNA synthesis and entry into the cell cycle. E7, E1A, and SV40 large T also bind other Rb family proteins, which activate other E2F members necessary for different stages of cell division. Unlike E1A and SV40 large T, high-risk HPV E7 also induces p105-Rb protein degradation.

The high-risk E6 proteins inactivate the p53 tumor suppressor pathway by using normal cellular mechanisms that **degrade** unwanted and misfolded proteins. High-risk E6 binds to a cellular factor called E6-AP, which is a component of the **ubiquitylation proteolysis pathway. Ubiquitin** is a short polypeptide that can be covalently attached to other proteins to mark them for proteolytic degradation. The E6/E6-AP complexes with p53 and induces its polyubiquitylation and subsequent proteolysis. As a result, levels of p53 are very low, and its effects as a tumor suppressor are inhibited. Interestingly, E6 proteins from low-risk HPV types do not bind p53.

Although high-risk HPV E6 and E7 proteins block the functions of the p53 and Rb tumor suppressors respectively, these viral proteins interact with many other cellular factors. E6 stimulates expression of telomerase and can therefore efficiently induce cell immortalization. Furthermore, inactivation of p53 by E6 allows accumulation of genetic mutations that would normally be eliminated by apoptosis. Such mutations in critical regulatory genes would promote tumorigenesis. The requirement for cellular mutations along with expression of E6 and E7 explains why cervical cancers develop after several years of persistent high-risk HPV infection.

DAMAGE

Papillomavirus-induced alterations in the host epithelium develop slowly and are often clinically inapparent. Changes may not be visible for many months after infection has begun.

Warts look different at different sites. Common warts of the hands and other cutaneous surfaces are elevated, firm, fleshy lesions with a sharp border (Fig. 40-2). On the face, knees, or arms, warts tend to be flat and are more likely to be clustered (Fig. 40-3). On the soles of the feet, they tend to be more deeply embedded and scalier than those on the hands. Anogenital warts (**condyloma**) may be either flat, slightly elevated, or pedunculated. Cauliflower-like lesions may surround the anus, labia, or shaft of the penis (Fig. 40-4). Warts of the uterine cervix are usually flat and may be missed during visual speculum examinations.

Warts of the oropharynx occur in infants and adults. In some cases, these warts lead to progressive impairment of laryngeal function and may compromise the airway. Hoarseness is the usual presenting symptom. Respiratory distress and secondary bacterial pneumonias occur in children and indicate the presence of obstructing lesions in the bronchial tree. The virus types associated with **respiratory papillomatosis** are the same as those that cause anogenital warts and suggest transmission at birth. Oral–genital transmission is usually responsible for newly acquired lesions in adults.

How does the host respond to papillomavirus infection? It is thought that cell-mediated immunity is necessary to restrict HPV. Persons who are deficient in cellular immunity (transplant recipients or those with AIDS) are more likely to have multiple chronic warts that are resistant to treatment. Some individuals fail to mount an

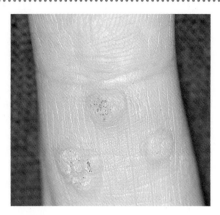

FIGURE 40-2. Common warts.

immune response to only one or a few HPV types and can have extensive warts, often covering the hands and feet. Notably, these individuals do not show susceptibility to other viral or bacterial infections. Epidermodysplasia verruciformis differs in that it is often, but not always, inherited and usually manifests in childhood.

HPV-Related Cancer

The major risk factors for progression of HPV infection to malignancy are the HPV type, persistence of the viral DNA, and host immune status (see the Paradigm). Virtually all high-grade dysplasias (CIN3) and cervical carcinomas contain a subset of so-called **high-risk** HPV genotypes including, but not limited to, types 16, 18, 31, 33, 35, 45, 51, 52, 53, 56, 58, 59, 66, 68, and 73 (see Table 40-1). HPV 16 is the prototype of the group and identified in about 50% of all cervical cancers. Other HPVs found in genital and cervical lesions such as types 6 and 11 are rarely found in cancers and on this basis are called **low-risk**

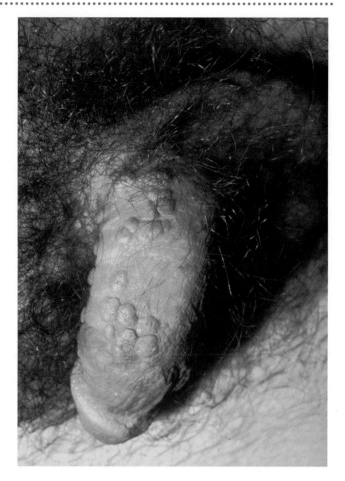

FIGURE 40-4. Penile warts.

types. The high-risk HPVs also have been detected in about 90% of anal cancers, 25 to 30% of penile and vulvar cancers, and 0 to 60% of epithelial malignancies of the head and neck, depending on location.

Although cancers of nonepithelial origin and a variety of cutaneous diseases have detectable HPV DNA using highly sensitive PCR-based techniques, these findings often represent detection of much less than one copy of viral DNA per tumor cell. In malignancies caused by HPVs such as those of the cervix, all tumor cells contain HPV DNA and express the viral E6 and E7 genes. Squamous cell carcinomas of sun-exposed skin in epidermodysplasia verruciformis usually contain high numbers of viral genomes, as do malignancies of skin in immunodeficient individuals. The role of HPV in the pathogenesis of common skin cancers and their predecessors including actinic keratoses is controversial because viral genomes are not identified in all tumor cells and viral proteins may not be expressed. Ultrasensitive PCR methods detect low levels of many different HPV strains, including those in epidermodysplasia verruciformis, in normal skin and even in hair follicles. Therefore, causative etiology is difficult to prove. These results have been reproduced in many laboratories and have led to the understanding that most people are persistently infected with specific strains to

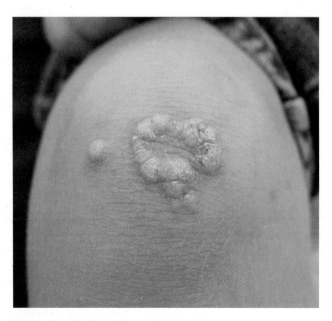

FIGURE 40-3. Multiple flat warts on knee.

which they are susceptible but which their immune function restricts from progressing to a clinically visible lesion.

Cancers of the head and neck are known to contain HPV, primarily type 16. Approximately 25 to 60% of cancers of the tonsils and base of tongue are thought to be induced by HPV infection. HPV-associated oropharyngeal squamous cell carcinomas have a higher rate of 5-year survival than non-HPV tumors.

DIAGNOSIS

The diagnosis of warts is made by clinical history and morphologic appearance. Warts often show plates of thin scale or rough keratotic debris that may form thin fingerlike projections and hence "verrucous." As warts enlarge, dermal capillaries proliferate. When the capillaries become thrombosed, usually because of trauma, they create black dots or "seeds," which can be useful in diagnosing warts. Another diagnostic clue to the identification of HPV infection is the absence of normal skin lines.

Papillomaviruses are not easily cultivated in vitro. Therefore, a skin specimen cannot be tested by inoculating cultured cells. No routine clinical test exists for determining whether HPV is present in a cutaneous lesion, but detection can be performed in a research setting with HPV type-specific nucleic acid probes to specifically amplify viral DNA using PCR. Although exquisitely sensitive, the test is also fraught with problems of sample contamination.

Because of the implications for risk of progression to cervical dysplasia and invasive cancers, sensitive and specific tests have been developed for the detection of high-risk HPV genotypes. These tests are based on detection of either viral RNA or DNA. Repeated identification of a high-risk type in cervical samples implies persistent infection and often requires medical or surgical intervention. Other biomarkers such as overexpression of the tumor suppressor protein p16 are being validated as indicators of risk for development of cervical carcinoma.

Papanicolaou (Pap) smears of exfoliated cervical cells have been used for decades to detect cytological abnormalities typical of HPV infection. This test is not sensitive, with a false-negative rate of about 65%, and it is not specific for HPV. However, when repeated annually or biennially, the Pap smear becomes an effective tool to identify women with precancerous lesions.

TREATMENT

Although it is estimated that perhaps 50% of cutaneous warts in children regress spontaneously within 2 years, new warts also can appear during that time. Because it is not possible to predict which warts will regress and whether new warts will develop, treatment is not always necessary for cutaneous warts. Anogenital warts may be obstructive and raise the concern of sexual transmission and cervical infection. In the uncommon disease respiratory papillomatosis, significant and life-threatening impairment of laryngeal function can occur. Unfortunately, no specific antiviral treatment exists for warts. Nearly all modes of treatment are ablative, such as **liquid nitrogen cryotherapy** and application of **caustic, keratolytic, or cytotoxic chemicals**. These are frequently used and highly effective. **Imiquimod** is thought to act by stimulating immune responses to anogenital HPV infection. **Surgical excision** or **laser ablation** physically destroys infected as well as uninfected tissues. None of these treatments are virus specific, and they may have to be repeated multiple times. Pain at the excision site is common. There is a paucity of placebo-controlled studies with these treatment approaches to evaluate their relative effectiveness and long-term success.

It is not known whether successful treatment of warts actually results in complete viral cure as can occur in the cervix. The risk of spread is reduced since most patients who sustain complete remission do not develop new warts. Because the virus can persist subclinically in apparently normal tissue, only molecular methods can prove whether trace amounts of viral DNA persist. Destruction of a single lesion rarely results in involution of untreated warts, suggesting that the viral infection diminishes local susceptibility to host immune responses.

PREVENTION

The intact skin is an effective barrier to wart virus transmission. Complete avoidance is not practical because papillomaviruses can be transmitted by inanimate objects. There is no definitive evidence that condoms mitigate the risk of transmission of HPV. Women with a history of genital warts should have regular examinations of the external genitalia, vagina, and cervix, including Pap tests. Coating the cervix or other suspected mucosal lesions with 3 to 5% acetic acid whitens HPV lesions, making the papillomas easier to visualize with magnification (colposcopy). Biopsies of suspicious lesions can then be done to detect precancerous changes in time to permit effective treatment. HPV infections can remain clinically inapparent for long periods, which makes it difficult to determine when infection occurred.

Laryngeal warts in the neonate may be prevented if an infected woman is aggressively treated before pregnancy. Some have suggested Cesarean sections for pregnant women with genital warts. However, the risks of surgery are probably greater than the likelihood that the baby will develop respiratory papillomatosis.

Prophylactic vaccines to prevent HPV infection are now available. Synthesis of the L1 protein at high levels in yeast or *Escherichia coli* results in spontaneous assembly of these proteins into viruslike particles (VLPs) that exhibit strain-specific epitopes identical to native infectious virus. VLPs do not contain viral genomes and hence cannot cause disease. Intramuscular injection of VLPs induces high-titer, strain-specific neutralizing antibodies that block viral entry. Gardasil™ (Merck) is composed of

VLPs from HPV 6, 11, 16, and 18 produced in yeast and is 95% effective in reducing the occurrence of new genital warts and cervical dysplasia. Cervarix™ (Glaxo) is made from HPV 16 and 18 VLPs synthesized in insect cells and is similarly extremely effective for preventing new cases of cervical dysplasia caused by HPV 16 and 18. Gardasil is FDA-approved for vaccination of females and males ages 9 to 26 years old and Cervarix in women ages 10 to 25. While these vaccines also have some efficacy against highly related high-risk HPV genotypes such as types 31 and 45, cervical dysplasias and cancer can occur with other high-risk HPV genotypes not included in the current vaccines. There is no evidence that existing HPV disease will remit following vaccination.

CONCLUSION

Papillomaviruses are a large group of related DNA viruses that cause a variety of epithelial lesions ranging from common cutaneous warts to more serious premalignant dysplasias that can progress to frank malignancies. Fortunately, the benign manifestations of HPV infections are by far the most common.

Suggested Readings

Asgari MM, Kiviat NB, Critchlow CW, et al. Detection of human papillomavirus DNA in cutaneous squamous cell carcinoma among immunocompetent individuals. *J Invest Dermatol.* 2008;128(6):1409–1417.

Hazard K, Karlsson A, Andersson K, et al. Cutaneous human papillomaviruses persist on healthy skin. *J Invest Dermatol.* 2007;127(1):116–119.

Kadaja M, Silla T, Ustav E, et al. Papillomavirus DNA replication—from initiation to genomic instability. *Virology.* 2009;384(2):360–368.

Lajer CB, von Buchwald C. The role of human papillomavirus in head and neck cancer. *APMIS.* 2010;118(6–7):510–519.

Lipke MM. An armamentarium of wart treatments. *Clin Med Res.* Dec 2006;4(4):273–293.

Moody CA, Laimins LA. Human papillomavirus oncoproteins: pathways to transformation. *Nat Rev Cancer.* 2010;10(8):550–560.

Palefsky J. Human papillomavirus-related disease in people with HIV. *Curr Opin HIV AIDS.* 2009;4(1):52–56.

Schiller JT, Day PM, Kines RC. Current understanding of the mechanism of HPV infection. *Gynecol Oncol.* 2010;118(1 suppl):S12–17.

Schiller JT, Lowy DR. Vaccines to prevent infections by oncoviruses *Annu Rev Microbiol.* 2010;64:23–41.

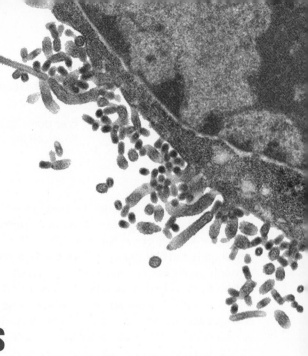

Chapter 41

Alphaherpesviruses: Herpes Simplex Viruses and Varicella-Zoster Virus

Patricia G. Spear

KEY CONCEPTS

Pathogen: Alphaherpesviruses are double-stranded DNA viruses that include herpes simplex virus (HSV) types 1 and 2 and varicella-zoster virus (VZV).

Encounter: There is a high incidence of infections in humans. Almost all individuals become infected with HSV type 1. However, most infections with this virus are asymptomatic.

Entry: HSV is acquired by direct contact. VZV is usually acquired from infectious aerosols.

Replication and Spread: These viruses invariably establish latent infections following primary infection. Latency allows the virus to persist for the life of the infected host and can lead to reactivation of virus replication and recurrent outbreaks of symptoms.

Damage: HSVs cause oral and genital herpes and occasionally encephalitis. VZV causes chickenpox and shingles.

Diagnosis: Diagnosis in humans is accomplished by clinical presentation, virus detection in lesion samples, virus isolation in cell culture, or PCR.

Treatment: Alphaherpesviruses can be treated with antiviral agents such as acyclovir. However, antiviral therapy does not prevent future recurrences.

Prevention: VZV vaccines are available to prevent chickenpox and shingles.

THE TERM HERPESVIRUS refers to many human and animal viruses. The essential physical characteristics of herpesviruses include a large **double-stranded DNA genome**, an **icosahedral nucleo capsid** that encloses the genome, a layer of proteins or tegument that surrounds the nucleocapsid, and an outer envelope derived from a cell membrane but containing predominantly viral glycoproteins (Fig. 41-1). An important biological characteristic of all herpesviruses is the capacity to establish lifelong latent infections, whether or not acute primary disease is evident. Thus, the incidence of infection is cumulative and invariably increases with age. Moreover, reactivation of virus replication can cause recurrent episodes of disease, often with significant morbidity in immunodeficient individuals.

Human and animal herpesviruses are divided into three subfamilies (alpha-, beta-, and gammaherpesviruses) based on their evolutionary relationships and biological properties. The known human herpesviruses and their associated diseases, in order of decreasing frequency, are listed in Table 41-1. The subjects of this chapter are the human alphaherpesviruses, herpes simplex viruses 1 and 2 (HSV-1 and HSV-2) and varicella-zoster virus (VZV). The betaherpesviruses (cytomegalovirus and human herpesviruses 6 and 7) and gammaherpesviruses (Epstein-Barr virus and human herpesvirus 8) are discussed in Chapter 42.

Despite relatively recent public awareness, herpesviruses are not new causes of human disease. Ancient Greek medical texts described oral infections similar to those now recognized as associated with

HSV. The infections are probably what Shakespeare had in mind when he wrote these lines in *Romeo and Juliet* (act 1, scene 4):

> O'er ladies' lips, who straight on kisses dream
> Which oft the angry Mab with blisters plagues

ENCOUNTER

Infection with one or more herpesviruses is inevitable for virtually everyone. Most of us have probably spread HSV-1 by kissing or exchanging saliva. The virus is usually acquired in childhood or during sexual activity, either through oral–oral or oral–genital contact. Nearly two-thirds of adults have antibodies to HSV-1, indicating prior infection. HSV-2 also can be acquired by oral–oral and oral–genital contact, but it is primarily spread by genital–genital contact. Although uncommon before adolescence, HSV-2 infection rapidly becomes more prevalent with increased sexual activity. About one-fifth of all adults are infected with HSV-2, depending on the nature and number of sexual encounters. Neonates are at risk for severe disease caused by HSV-1 or HSV-2 if exposed to virus perinatally, particularly during birth to a mother who experiences primary infection toward the end of pregnancy.

VZV is usually acquired through the respiratory route, but infection by direct contact with vesicular fluid or secretions also can occur. Primary disease caused by VZV is much more contagious than that caused by HSV-1 or HSV-2, in part because direct contact is not required for VZV infection. Prior to the introduction of VZV vaccination, most children became infected with VZV and developed chickenpox. Susceptible adults, who remain unvaccinated and unprotected by childhood disease, can develop more severe symptoms of disease than those usually observed in children. A mild version of chickenpox, called breakthrough disease, can occur in vaccinated individuals, as the vaccine is not 100% effective. Persons with breakthrough disease can transmit the virus to others.

Most infections with HSV-1 or HSV-2 are **asymptomatic**. Perhaps only one-third of the individuals who harbor the virus recognize symptoms from it. However, asymptomatic infected persons can transmit the virus, because **shedding** from epithelial surfaces can occur even if lesions are not large enough to be noticeable. Clinically evident infection with HSV-2 is increasing. Rough estimates suggest about a 10-fold increase occurred between 1965 and 1985. Primary infections with VZV are almost always symptomatic, resulting in chickenpox.

ENTRY

Herpesviruses are fragile and susceptible to drying and inactivation by heat, mild detergent, and solvents. Their susceptibility is imposed by their **membrane envelope**. Because these viruses do not survive well on environmental surfaces, infection with the herpesviruses usually requires direct contact with saliva or other secretions from an infected person, causing inoculation of virus into areas where they can replicate. Mucous membranes of the mouth, eye, genitals, respiratory tract, and anus are the sites most readily infected by HSV-1 or HSV-2. The first line of defense against HSV is the skin, which under normal conditions is not readily penetrated or infected by the virus. It is likely that the thick keratin layer of the superficial epidermis prevents access of HSV to its receptors. Because the mucous membranes do not present such a formidable barrier, those surfaces are more readily infected. Inhalation of VZV contained in **aerosols** is the main way individuals contract chickenpox. However, direct inoculation is possible. Thus, the mucous membranes provide the primary portal of entry for these herpesviruses.

SPREAD AND REPLICATION

The life cycle of herpesviruses resembles that of other large DNA viruses. Infection begins with the attachment of virus particles to susceptible cells (Fig. 41-2). Virions interact with specific cell-surface receptors through glycoproteins that project from the viral envelope. The alphaherpesviruses can bind to cells through the interaction of viral

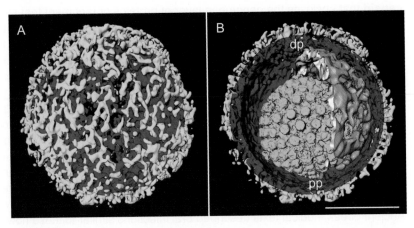

FIGURE 41-1. Cryo-electron tomography of a herpesvirus. A. Outer surface showing the distribution of glycoprotein spikes (*yellow*) projecting from the envelope (*blue*). **B.** Cutaway view of the virion interior showing the nucleocapsid (*light blue*) and the tegument (*orange*) inside the envelope (*blue* and *yellow*): dp, distal pole; pp, proximal pole.

TABLE 41-1 Human Herpesviruses and Associated Diseases

Subfamily	Virus	Diseases
Alphaherpesviruses	Herpes simplex virus 1 (HSV-1)	Gingivostomatitis, pharyngitis, cold sores, fever blisters, keratitis, genital lesions. Rarely, encephalitis, neonatal encephalitis and systemic disease
	HSV-2	Genital lesions, gingivostomatitis, pharyngitis, cold sores, fever blisters. Rarely, meningitis, neonatal encephalitis and systemic disease
	Varicella-zoster virus (VZV)	Chickenpox, zoster (shingles). Rarely, encephalitis, cerebellar ataxia
Betaherpesviruses	Cytomegalovirus (CMV)	Usually asymptomatic. Fetal wastage or developmental abnormalities following intrauterine infections; organ failure in immunosuppressed organ recipients; retinitis and pneumonia in AIDS patients
	Human herpesvirus 6 (HHV-6)	Roseola. Rarely, encephalitis, organ failure in immunosuppressed organ recipients, systemic disease in AIDS patients
	Human herpesvirus 7 (HHV-7)	Roseola
Gammaherpesviruses	Epstein-Barr virus (EBV)	Infectious mononucleosis, Burkitt lymphoma, nasopharyngeal carcinoma, oral hairy leukoplakia, posttransplant lymphoproliferative disorder, Hodgkin disease
	Kaposi sarcoma herpesvirus (human herpesvirus 8 [HHV-8])	Kaposi sarcoma, primary effusion lymphoma, some cases of Castleman disease

glycoproteins with **heparan sulfate** chains on cell-surface proteoglycans. Although this binding is not sufficient for virus entry into the cell, it serves to bring the virus into close proximity to other cell-surface molecules that function as entry receptors. In the case of HSV-1 and HSV-2, several kinds of entry receptors have been identified, any one of which can mediate virus entry. These viruses preferentially use different receptors to infect different cell types at various portals of entry (e.g., cornea, vagina) and in the brain. Entry receptors used by VZV also have been identified, but less is known about how they are used.

As depicted in Figure 41-2, binding of one of the viral glycoproteins to an entry receptor triggers **fusion** of the virion envelope with a cell membrane, either the plasma membrane or the membrane of an endosome. That fusion causes release of the viral nucleocapsid into the cytoplasm. Following transport of the nucleocapsid to nuclear pores, the viral genome is released into the nucleus. If the cell is capable of supporting virus replication, as is true for mucosal epithelial cells, then the viral genes will be transcribed in a temporal fashion, leading to synthesis of viral proteins, replication of the viral genome, and assembly of

CASE • Mr. H., a 26-year-old graduate student, returned home from his first real vacation in years. While on vacation, Mr. H. had engaged in both vaginal and oral sex with Ms. C., who was staying at the same resort. Several days after his last sexual contact with Ms. C., he noted painful, itchy sores on the shaft of his penis and a sore throat. During a difficult telephone call, Ms. C. acknowledged past episodes of genital herpes. "Could I have herpes?" Mr. H. wonders? He had heard about herpes infections and knew that there are several types and that some recur.

This case raises several questions:

1. What tests would be required to confirm Mr. H.'s suspicion that he has genital and oral herpes?
2. Is it likely that Ms. C. would have engaged in sex when she had active herpetic lesions? If she had no lesions, how could she have transmitted herpes to Mr. H.?
3. What are some of the more severe symptoms that can be associated with primary genital herpes?

See Appendix for answers.

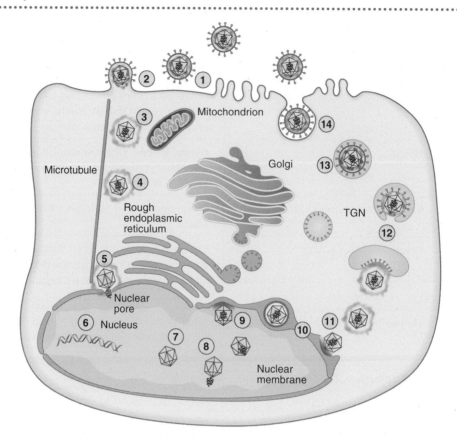

FIGURE 41-2. Alphaherpesvirus replication cycle. After attachment of the virion to a cell surface (*1*) and penetration by fusion (*2*), nucleocapsids are transported to the nucleus (*3*) via interaction with microtubules (*4*), docking at a nuclear pore (*5*) where the viral genome is released into the nucleus. Here, transcription of viral genes and genome replication occur (*6*). Replicated viral genomes are packaged into preformed capsids (*7*), yielding nucleocapsids (*8*), which then leave the nucleus by budding through the inner nuclear membrane (*9*) followed by fusion of these primary virions (*10*) with the outer nuclear membrane (*11*). Final envelopment then occurs in the cytoplasm by budding of the intracytosolic capsids into vesicles of the trans-Golgi network (TGN) (*12*), resulting in an enveloped virion within a cellular vesicle. The virion is transported to the cell surface (*13*) and released from the cell by exocytosis (*14*).

progeny viruses. If the cell is latently infected, then the viral genome circularizes in the nucleus and persists as an episome (analogous to a plasmid) with only minimal transcription of viral genes. In the case of HSV and perhaps VZV, virus gains access to nerve cell endings that extend toward the epidermis and is transported to the nerve cell bodies in peripheral sensory and autonomic ganglia, where latent infections are established (Fig. 41-3).

During productive infection (i.e., an infection in which virus replication occurs), **immediate-early genes** are transcribed with the assistance of transcription factors carried in the virion tegument, the space between the nucleocapsid surface and the envelope. Proteins encoded by the immediate-early genes activate expression of about a dozen **early genes** whose protein products are required to replicate the viral DNA. Following DNA synthesis, the viral **late genes** are expressed. Those genes encode proteins that assemble and comprise the progeny virions. Included among the late proteins are

glycoproteins inserted into cell membranes. As the new viral nucleocapsids are assembled in the nucleus, they bud through the inner nuclear membrane to acquire a temporary envelope, which they then lose by fusing with the outer nuclear membrane. The final viral envelope with the full set of viral glycoproteins is acquired by budding into cytoplasmic vacuoles derived from the Golgi apparatus. These vacuoles transport the mature virions to the cell surface for release by exocytosis (Fig. 41-2).

Unlike many other viruses, newly formed herpesvirus particles are not efficiently released into the extracellular space. Rather, as they are released from the host cell, they immediately attach to and penetrate adjacent cells, a process reminiscent of that used by some bacteria, such as *Rickettsia* and *Shigella*. The process of cell-to-cell spread has several important implications for the pathogenesis of disease associated with each herpesvirus and the host responses to infection by this virus group. For example, diseases induced by HSV are characterized by local spread

A. Primary disease

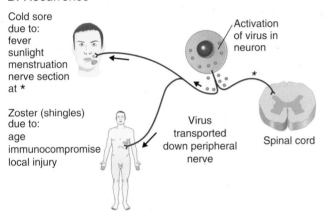

B. Recurrence

FIGURE 41-3. Pathogenesis of primary and recurrent diseases caused by herpes simplex virus (HSV) and varicella-zoster virus (VZV). A. Primary disease with HSV (pharyngitis, gingivostomatitis) is usually localized to the site of inoculation, whereas primary disease with VZV (chickenpox) is systemic. In both cases, sensory nerves become infected, and latent infections are established in sensory ganglia. **B.** Following recovery from primary disease, virus can be reactivated in sensory ganglia and travel to the body surface to cause cold sores or fever blisters (HSV) or shingles (VZV). Some of the precipitating factors are listed. If virus spreads to the central nervous system, encephalitis can result.

and progression of lesions. HSV infection at multiple distant sites is rare and probably requires the circulation of infected cells rather than free virus. HSV rarely spreads systemically, except in newborn infants or severely immunocompromised persons. VZV, on the other hand, causes systemic multiorgan disease—a feature that may be partly the result of its capacity to infect and be transported by circulating leukocytes. Infected leukocytes can deliver virus to multiple organs and to skin by cell-to-cell contact.

HOST DEFENSES

Innate and adaptive immune responses to herpesvirus infections are multifaceted. Host defenses are usually adequate to limit the duration and severity of infection and, in some persons, are capable of preventing symptomatic primary disease or recurrences, at least in the case of HSV-1 and HSV-2. However, host defenses do not prevent latent infections and cannot eliminate latent virus, largely because the latently infected cells apparently do not trigger sterilizing immune responses.

As is true for many viruses, infection with HSV-1, HSV-2, or VZV induces immediate innate responses, such as activation of neutrophils and natural-killer cells and production of interferons and other cytokines. Within several days of infection, antibodies to some of the viral proteins appear in the circulation, and T lymphocytes responsive to viral antigens are amplified in number and activated.

Antiherpesvirus antibodies play a minor role in recovery from primary HSV or VZV disease, perhaps because antibodies develop too late to modify the course of infection. Antibodies also probably have little impact on recurrent disease. In fact, persons who are unable to make antibodies have no particular problems with herpesviruses. The likely reason is that the viruses spread from cell to cell, and their mode of spread provides little opportunity for antibodies to neutralize the viruses. However, antibodies can contribute to prevention of primary disease. The administration of anti-VZV antibodies can prevent or ameliorate infection in immunocompromised children at risk for severe disease. Concordantly, the efficacy of VZV vaccine for prevention of chickenpox partly stems from its capacity to induce antiviral antibodies.

Cell-mediated immune mechanisms are most important for recovery from disease caused by HSV or VZV and prevention or control of recurrent disease. No better proof of the primacy of lymphocyte-mediated immune responses in the control of herpesvirus infections can be found than in the response of severely immunocompromised persons to infections by these viruses. A significant fraction of stem cell transplant recipients experience reactivation of HSV infections within the first month after transplantation. Some of those infections may be severe and destructive. Similarly, children with leukemia and persons with AIDS experience frequent and prolonged HSV infections.

The ability to mount an adequate **cellular immune response** to herpesviruses changes with age. The relevant immune effector cells gradually mature during the first month of an infant's life. Until maturation is complete, herpesvirus infections can be devastating. In fact, neonatal HSV infection is often fatal, in part because of immunological immaturity and perhaps because the cells of developing organs may have greater innate susceptibility to HSV infection. However, by 1 month of age, the infant tolerates the virus well. Some herpesviruses become problematic at the other end of the age spectrum. Reactivation of VZV leading to zoster occurs with increasing frequency as a function of age, perhaps because of senescence of antiviral immune responses. The likelihood

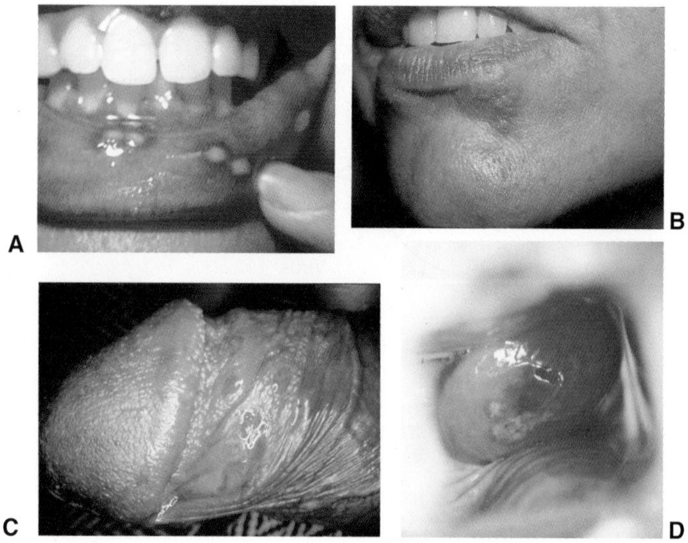

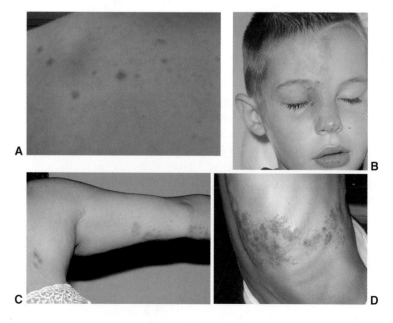

FIGURE 41-4. Mucocutaneous lesions caused by HSV.
A. Primary gingivostomatitis with multiple eroded lesions.
B. Recurrent infection with lesions on the vermilion border of
the lip and beyond. **C.** Multiple grouped erosions on an erythematous base on the penis. **D.** Lesions on the uterine cervix.

of having zoster is about 10 times greater at age 80 years
than at age 8 years.

DAMAGE

Both HSV and VZV destroy the epithelial cells in which
they replicate in skin and mucous membranes, causing
vesicular lesions that rupture, leaving shallow gray-
white ulcers on an **erythematous base** (Figs. 41-4 and
41-5). As virus replication and spread are contained by
immune responses, primarily innate and cell-mediated
responses, the epithelium fully regenerates.

In other ways, HSV and VZV diseases differ in pathology (Fig. 41-3). Both primary and recurrent HSV lesions
are usually localized (Fig. 41-4), with spread of virus
restricted to regional nerves. During primary disease,
there can be sequential crops of lesions, resulting from
reseeding of adjacent epithelial sites by neurons infected

during earlier waves of epithelial replication. Some damage or inflammation of the nerves can occur during the
acute phase of disease, causing symptoms of itching, tingling, burning, or pain. Similar sensations (prodrome)
can indicate that recurrent lesions are about to develop.
Certain factors trigger the reactivation of latent HSV,
including sunburn, systemic infections, immune impairment, emotional stress, and menstruation. It is not known
how seemingly unrelated factors induce viral reactivation. Reactivated HSV travels down the axonal processes
to infect contiguous mucocutaneous epithelial cells. The
usual course of events in HSV infections is summarized
in Table 41-2.

The site of HSV inoculation governs manifestations
of primary and recurrent disease (Table 41-2). Corneal
infections can cause immune responses that damage the
cornea irreparably and cause blindness, necessitating
corneal transplant for recovery of vision. Primary genital

FIGURE 41-5. Skin lesions caused by VZV. A. Chickenpox
lesions on the back of a child (primary disease). **B.** Zoster in a child who presented with 6 days of eye pain and
a rash in the distribution of the ophthalmic branch of the
trigeminal nerve. **C.** A linear eruption of zoster that could
be mistaken for poison ivy. **D.** Zoster around the trunk in an
immunocompromised patient.

TABLE 41-2 Usual Course of Herpes Simplex Virus Infection and Disease

Stage	Events
Acute disease (facial or genital lesions, stomatitis, or keratitis); localized	• Exposure of skin, mucosa, or cornea to secretions containing virus • Replication of virus in epithelial cells, causing vesicular mucocutaneous lesions, stomatitis, or keratitis • Spread to peripheral sensory or autonomic nerve endings and ganglia.
Recovery	• Healing of lesions and establishment of latent infections in neurons
Latency	• Maintenance of latent infections in neurons
Recurrent disease (cold sores, fever blisters, keratitis, or genital lesions)	• Reactivation of latent virus and distal spread (usually localized) • Recurrent lesions caused by virus replication in epithelial cells

herpes, particularly that caused by HSV-2, can progress to meningitis or affect autonomic functions governing urination and defecation. HSV-1 can pass from peripheral nerves to the central nervous system (CNS) to cause life-threatening **encephalitis**, characterized by an unusually progressive and destructive inflammation of a unilateral and focal nature. Persons with no known predisposing risk factors can have CNS involvement. Although rare, encephalitis caused by HSV-1 accounts for about 95% of all cases of sporadic disease in children and adults in developed countries. Newborn infants are especially susceptible to disseminated or neurological disease caused by HSV-1 or HSV-2 and, if they survive, are often developmentally impaired. Persons with inadequate cell-mediated immunity are at risk for developing severe disseminated HSV infections that can spread widely across the skin and to viscera, especially the lungs, esophagus, liver, and brain.

Chickenpox, caused by VZV, is a systemic febrile disease with mucocutaneous lesions (Figs. 41-3 and 41-5). Cells of the lymphatic system are infected at the usual portal of entry in the respiratory tract. The spread of virus-infected leukocytes throughout the lymphatic system induces the types of cytokine responses that result in fever, malaise, and headache. During the course of secondary viremia, circulating leukocytes transmit the virus to epithelial cells of the skin and mucosa, and the characteristic lesions of chickenpox occur. Latent infections are established in peripheral ganglia. Recovery is usually uneventful with no further symptoms from the latent virus unless and until zoster develops years later. Complications of chickenpox include cerebellar ataxia in otherwise healthy children and encephalitis in immunocompromised persons.

Zoster lesions (shingles) are similar to the scattered vesicular lesions of chickenpox except that they appear clustered on the body surface along the dermatome

enervated by the nerve from which VZV was reactivated (Fig. 41-5). The neurological symptoms (primarily pain) associated with zoster are much more severe than for HSV recurrences, probably because there is more viral damage to the affected nerves and supporting cells. The usual course of events in VZV primary disease (chickenpox) and reactivation disease (zoster) are summarized in Table 41-3. As with HSV, VZV can cause severe disseminated disease in immunocompromised individuals.

DIAGNOSIS

The astute clinician will have little difficulty diagnosing oral or genital herpes, chickenpox, and zoster. The patient's clinical presentation, coupled with his or her history, is usually sufficient. To establish the diagnosis, the presence of virus or its components in active lesions can be demonstrated. Scrapings from lesions can be processed for **polymerase chain reaction** with probes for viral DNA or stained directly with specific fluorescein-labeled antibodies that bind to viral antigens. The definitive diagnostic tool, although a more lengthy process, is virus isolation in cell culture. HSV grows well in a wide variety of fibroblast and epithelial cell lines from animals or humans. Replicating viruses induce characteristic changes in cell shape and appearance. The combination of the appearance of cytopathic changes and immunofluorescence establishes a definitive diagnosis of HSV. VZV is more difficult to propagate in cell culture and more fastidious about cell type, but similar methods can be used for definitive diagnosis.

TREATMENT

Some of the first antiviral drugs developed were those for the treatment of HSV infections. The prototype drugs are

TABLE 41-3 Usual Course of Varicella-Zoster Virus Infection and Disease

Stage	Events
Acute disease (chicken pox); asymptomatic incubation period followed by systemic disease with skin lesions	• Exposure of respiratory tract to aerosols containing virus • Replication of virus in regional lymph nodes • Primary viremia (cell-associated virus); replication in liver and spleen • Secondary viremia; transport of virus in mononuclear cells to skin and mucous membranes • Lesions of chicken pox, release of virus from lesions and from respiratory secretions • Spread of virus to sensory and autonomic ganglia
Recovery	• Healing of lesions, recovery from systemic symptoms, and establishment of latent infections in neurons (also possibly in satellite cells)
Latency	• Maintenance of latent infections in neurons
Reactivation disease (zoster or shingles); usually localized, but can spread over large areas of body surface	• Reactivation of latent virus and distal spread • Vesicular lesions along a dermatome enervated by nerve harboring reactivated virus (usually associated with pain)

nucleoside analogs preferentially used by viral synthetic pathways (see Chapter 44). One of the most useful antiviral drugs for several herpesviruses is **acyclovir**. An analog of guanosine, acyclovir is phosphorylated by herpesvirus enzymes, but not cell enzymes, and then incorporated into viral DNA as a chain-terminating nucleotide. Thus, acyclovir is active principally in herpesvirus-infected cells and has little or no toxicity for uninfected cells. **Penciclovir** is a related guanosine analog that can be used topically but has poor oral bioavailability. **Valacyclovir**, a prodrug of acyclovir, and **famciclovir**, a prodrug of penciclovir, have improved oral bioavailability and are often used for the treatment of either HSV or VZV disease in preference to acyclovir.

Use of antiherpesvirus drugs may not be indicated for mild cases of childhood chickenpox or unremarkable primary or recurrent herpetic lesions on the face or genitals. However, antiviral therapy is indicated in severe cases of chickenpox or herpetic lesions, ocular herpes, neonatal herpes, chickenpox in immunosuppressed children or adults, shingles, and any HSV or VZV infections associated with meningitis, encephalitis, or any other neurological manifestation. Acyclovir or related drugs may be administered intravenously or by mouth, depending on the condition being treated. These drugs can prevent the most extreme ravages of disease resulting from viral replication but cannot effect a "cure" because they do not prevent entry of virus into neurons and cannot eliminate latent viral genomes. Therefore, treated patients remain susceptible to later recurrences. Long-term treatment with acyclovir or a related drug will suppress recurrent infections, and such a regimen can be prescribed for

persons with frequent troubling recurrences. Now that successful antiviral treatment has become routine, so has the emergence of drug-resistant viruses. However, resistance is currently a concern only in selected patients with severe immune deficiencies.

PREVENTION

Herpesviruses are ubiquitous, and it is not practical to avoid contact with all infected individuals. In the case of HSV, it is certainly appropriate to avoid sexual contact during active genital herpes infections. This avoidance provides no guarantee of protection because asymptomatic persons can shed HSV and transmit the virus, but it should reduce the probability of transmission. Unfortunately, safe and effective vaccines are not available for HSV, although research directed toward this goal is in progress. Even if an effective vaccine were available, it would probably not help people with existing infections. An effective therapeutic, as opposed to preventive, vaccine would have to induce a better immune response than natural infection, which often does not suffice to prevent recurrence.

Preventive measures for VZV infection are available. Children or adults with chickenpox should be isolated and vaccination offered to family members or other contacts. Exposed immunodeficient children are usually not candidates for vaccination but could be protected by the administration of specific human immune globulin promptly after exposure. A **live**, **attenuated VZV vaccine** prevents chickenpox in normal and some immunologically impaired (leukemic) children (see Chapter 45). The vaccine virus establishes latent infection, just as does the wild-type virus, and reactivations may lead to mild cases of shingles. A new formulation of the VZV vaccine boosts anti-VZV cellular immunity in older individuals and protects them from shingles.

In hospital settings, it is important that patients experiencing primary VZV disease be isolated, because the virus can be transmitted via aerosols. Also, persons with active herpetic lesions should not be allowed contact with newborn infants.

CONCLUSION

Alphaherpesviruses display a wide range of biological properties and clinical manifestations. Key features of their biology and pathogenesis are the capacity to establish latent infections in neurons and activate from the latent state to cause new episodes of clinical disease. Latent infections account for the capacity of these viruses to persist for the lifetime of the host. Infection of neurons and spread to the CNS account for some of the most life-threatening and rare forms of alphaherpesvirus disease. High prevalence of HSV is partly a result of asymptomatic reactivation and shedding of virus, such that healthy people can inadvertently transmit infection. High prevalence of VZV in human populations is principally a result of contagion during primary disease (vari-

cella or chickenpox). Use of the live VZV vaccine has led to replacement of the wild-type virus with the attenuated vaccine virus in originally naïve inoculated populations. Different formulations of the vaccine are effective in preventing chickenpox and shingles. Acyclovir and related drugs are effective at reducing morbidity and mortality resulting from active HSV or VZV replication, but they do not effect cures because latent virus cannot be eliminated by these drugs.

ACKNOWLEDGMENT

Steven E. Straus (deceased) is acknowledged for his contributions to this chapter in previous editions.

Suggested Readings

Cohen JI, Straus SE, Arvin AM. Varicella-zoster virus replication, pathogenesis, and management. In: Knipe DM, Howley PM, eds. *Field's Virology.* 5th ed. Philadelphia, PA: Lippincott Williams & Wilkins; 2007:2773–2818.

Corey L, Wald A. Maternal and neonatal herpes simplex virus infections. *N Engl J Med.* 2009;361(14):1376–1385.

James SH, Kimberlin DW, Whitley RJ. Antiviral therapy for herpesvirus central nervous system infections: neonatal herpes simplex virus infection, herpes simplex encephalitis, and congenital cytomegalovirus infection. *Antiviral Res.* 2009;83(3):207–213.

Chapter 42

Beta- and Gammaherpesviruses: Cytomegalovirus and Epstein-Barr Virus

William J. Britt

KEY CONCEPTS

Pathogens: Beta- and gammaherpesviruses are large, enveloped, double-stranded DNA viruses distinguished by their genomic organization and pathogenesis in humans.

Betaherpesviruses include human cytomegalovirus (CMV), HHV-6, and HHV-7.

Gammaherpesviruses include the lymphocryptovirus Epstein-Barr virus (EBV) and the rhadinovirus HHV-8 (or Kaposi sarcoma herpesvirus).

Encounter: These infections are ubiquitous in human populations with most individuals acquiring infection by young adulthood.

Entry: Viruses attach to cells by low-affinity interactions with cell-surface glycosaminoglycans, followed by high-infinity interactions between a viral envelope glycoprotein and a receptor on the cell surface to induce uptake.

Replication: Viral gene expression is mediated by virus-encoded enzymes in an orderly and sequential manner. Viruses assemble in the nucleus and acquire tegument and envelope layers by sequential passage through the nuclear and plasma membranes. Release occurs by exocytosis or cell lysis.

After primary infection, the virus establishes life-long latency (CMV in myeloid cells; EBV in B cells) with intermittent virus shedding from mucosal surfaces.

Spread: Spread occurs from the primary site of inoculation to multiple organs via the bloodstream.

Damage: CMV is rarely associated with clinical symptoms in normal individuals but can be an opportunistic pathogen in immunocompromised hosts, including the developing fetus, organ-transplant recipients treated with immunosuppressive drugs, and persons with AIDS.

Primary infection with EBV is usually asymptomatic in young children but can be associated with the mononucleosis syndrome during adolescence. In immunocompromised persons, EBV can cause lymphoproliferative syndromes (e.g., posttransplant lymphoproliferative disease [PTLD]), which may progress to malignant lymphoma. EBV is associated with cancers, such as lymphoma, nasopharyngeal carcinoma, and other epithelial-derived neoplasms.

Diagnosis: CMV is detected in biopsy tissue or blood samples by isolating replicating virus or by detecting either viral nucleic acids with PCR or viral antigens with immunoassays.

EBV mononucleosis is diagnosed using heterophile antibody tests (e.g., monospot) or specific EBV serologies. In immunocompromised hosts, the diagnosis of an EBV-related condition is usually made by detecting viral nucleic acids.

Treatment: Antiviral treatment of mononucleosis does not alter the course of illness. Opportunistic infections with CMV can be treated with antiviral agents (e.g., ganciclovir), reduction of immunosuppression, or both modalities.

Prevention: Because of the ubiquity of infection, affected patients are not isolated. There are no vaccines for these viral infections.

THE FAMILY OF HUMAN herpesviruses is divided into subfamilies based on genetic characteristics and biological properties. The beta- and gammaherpesviruses display remarkable differences in the organization of their viral genomes, and, more importantly, the phenotype of human infections associated with each member of these subfamilies is distinct. The prototypic member of the betaherpesvirus subfamily is **human cytomegalovirus (CMV)**; the prototype member of the gammaherpesvirus subfamily is **Epstein-Barr virus**

(**EBV**). Both CMV and EBV are ubiquitous in the human population, and infection with these agents by adulthood is nearly universal in the developing world. In developed countries, particularly in North America and Northern Europe, the epidemiology of infections with CMV and EBV is related to socioeconomic status and exposure to young children. As a result, in some areas of the United States, infections with CMV and EBV occur later in life. Overall, about 50 to 60% of adults in the United States are infected with CMV, and an estimated 90% are infected with EBV. Fortunately, infection with CMV or EBV in normal individuals is self-limited and infrequently leads to disease. In contrast, infection of immunocompromised persons with either of these viruses can result in significant morbidity and, in some cases, fatal disease.

Persistent infection is a hallmark of all herpesvirus infections and, as with other herpesviruses, CMV and EBV persist for the lifetime of the infected host. In the case of EBV, the virus establishes persistent infection of B lymphocytes, and a well-characterized sequence of viral gene expression leads from a state of latency to lytic, productive infection. CMV can establish latent infection of hematopoietic cells of the myeloid lineage. However, the relative contribution of latent CMV infection to CMV persistence is unclear because chronic productive infection in a variety of tissues also is a major source of persistent virus. CMV persistence has not been associated with evidence of organ dysfunction or clinical disease, although persistent CMV infection is associated with a variety of chronic vascular diseases. Intermittent excretion of either virus on mucosal surfaces in the absence of clinical symptoms is common and likely responsible for the spread of these viruses within human populations.

ENCOUNTER

Acquisition of CMV and EBV infection in nonhospitalized patients (community acquired) occurs following exposure of mucosal surfaces including the oropharynx and genital tract to infectious virus. Both viruses can be isolated from secretions collected from the oropharynx and the genital tract.

Early in life, CMV is readily transmitted in breast milk, and infection following ingestion of CMV-infected breast milk is likely the most common mode of infection of infants in many populations in the world. In developed countries, virus acquisition during adolescence is more common and likely results from intimate exposure to oropharyngeal secretions or sexual contact. CMV is a sexually transmitted infection, and near-universal rates of infection are observed in sexually active populations. A third population at risk for CMV infection is the fetus and newborn infant. CMV readily crosses the placenta and infects the developing fetus, giving rise to **congenital (present at birth) CMV infection**. Congenital CMV is the most common viral infection of the fetus in humans resulting in rates of infection of nearly 1% in newborn infants from nearly all regions of the world. Congenital CMV infection can lead to severe disease and permanent neurological damage, including hearing loss.

EBV infection follows a pattern similar to CMV. However, although EBV DNA is detected in breast milk, breastfeeding is not an important route of virus transmission. As with CMV, almost all adults in the developing world have been infected with EBV. In contrast, EBV infection in the United States and Northern Europe is population specific, with infection being more common in the urban poor and less frequent in individuals from middle and upper socioeconomic groups. In populations with limited exposure to EBV during childhood, such as in

CASE

Sore Throat and Swollen Glands in a High School Cheerleader

S., a 16-year-old high school student from a suburban upper-middle-class neighborhood, is a member of her school's cheerleading squad. She recently began dating a 19-year-old student from a nearby college. About 2 months after they began dating, Sally developed a sore throat with a white exudate on her tonsils, swollen but minimally tender lymph nodes in her neck, and a slight yellow tinge to her eyes. She scheduled an appointment with her physician the next day because of worsening symptoms, decreased appetite, and an overall loss of energy. Her new boyfriend had no symptoms. Her physician noted that she had an exudative pharyngitis and icteric sclera. Her spleen was slightly enlarged. Her white blood cell count was 9,500/mm³ with a differential of 30% neutrophils, 55% lymphocytes, 5% monocytes, and 10% atypical lymphocytes. A chemistry panel indicated that her hepatic transaminases were elevated.

This case raises several questions:

1. How was her infection acquired?

2. What is noteworthy about Sally's symptoms and laboratory findings? Does her age together with her clinical presentation suggest a possible diagnosis?

3. How will the physician utilize the laboratory to confirm the diagnosis?

4. Will an antiviral drug alter her symptoms?

See Appendix for answers.

TABLE 42-1 CMV and EBV Infection: Acquisition and Clinical Syndromes Associated with Infection

	Mode of Exposure	Clinical Manifestations
Community Acquired		
Infections in fetus and newborn infant	Intrauterine transmission to fetus (CMV); breast milk transmission (CMV); intrapartum (CMV)	Congenital CMV infection (cytomegalic inclusion disease) with CNS disease, hepatitis, thrombocytopenia; asymptomatic infection with CNS sequelae (hearing loss); asymptomatic infection with prolonged virus shedding
Infections in childhood	Virus-containing saliva (CMV, EBV); urine (CMV)	Asymptomatic infection (CMV, EBV); infrequent mononucleosis-like syndrome (CMV, EBV)
Infections in adolescents and young adults	Virus-containing saliva (CMV, EBV); sexual transmission from virus in genital tract (CMV)	Mononucleosis syndrome (pharyngitis, fever, lymphadenopathy, hepatitis, and lymphocytosis with reactive lymphocytes) (EBV, CMV); asymptomatic infections
Hospital Acquired		
Infections following blood transfusions	CMV, EBV present in white blood cells (acute and latently infected)	Mononucleosis syndrome with more severe symptoms; fever; fatigue
Infections in transplant recipients	CMV and EBV present in allograft; blood transfusion	Mononucleosis syndrome, fever (CMV, EBV); leukopenia; thrombocytopenia (CMV); hepatitis (CMV, EBV); lymphoproliferation (EBV); chronic graft rejection (CMV)

the case of Sally H., infection in adolescence and young adulthood can result in a symptom complex and laboratory features that define **acute infectious mononucleosis**. Primary infection with either CMV or EBV rarely results in symptomatic disease in infants and children, but symptomatic disease following primary infection with EBV in adolescents has been reported to be as high as 30%. A small proportion of mononucleosis is associated with primary CMV infection.

In addition to exposure in the community, specific groups of hospitalized patients are at risk for both CMV and EBV infection. Infection with either virus can follow blood transfusion or transplantation of an allograft from an infected donor. Infection with either CMV or EBV following blood transfusion can result in symptomatic disease and, in the case of immunocompromised persons, can lead to severe and potentially fatal illness. Similarly, transplantation of an allograft from an infected donor results in infection of the recipient.

A summary of modes of acquisition and the types of diseases associated with CMV and EBV is provided in Table 42-1.

ENTRY

CMV and EBV attach to target cells via low-affinity interactions with cell-surface glycosaminoglycans, followed by high-affinity interactions with specific receptors. Both viruses appear to utilize two modes of entry:

(1) interaction with a receptor/coreceptor and fusion at the plasma membrane and (2) interaction with a receptor/coreceptor at the plasma membrane followed by internalization, acid-dependent fusion, and release of the nucleocapsid and tegument proteins from endocytic vesicles. Different viral envelope glycoproteins are apparently required for each form of entry, and acid-dependent or acid-independent mechanisms predominate, depending on the target cell.

The virion envelope glycoproteins (gp) of CMV responsible for attachment remain incompletely defined, as are candidate host cell proteins that serve as receptors. CMV fusion requires gB, gH, and gL, and, in epithelial cells, an additional component consisting of glycoproteins encoded by the UL128 to 131 open reading frames is used. Loss of these glycoproteins limits epithelial cell entry by CMV but not entry into other cell types such as fibroblasts.

EBV infection of B cells is initiated by the attachment of envelope glycoprotein gp350/220 to CD21 (complement receptor 2, CR2). After endocytosis, viral glycoproteins gB, gH, and gL, and the lymphocryptovirus-specific glycoprotein gp42 participate in fusion of the viral envelope and endocytic membrane. In contrast, entry of EBV into epithelial cells occurs at neutral pH and does not require endocytosis. Fusion requires only gB, gH, and gL and, in fact, virions lacking gp42 infect epithelial cells more efficiently than those containing gp42.

REPLICATION

Human CMV and EBV replicate their nucleic acids in the nucleus of infected cells. Both viruses follow a highly regulated and orderly expression of viral genes during lytic virus infection characterized by **sequential expression of immediate-early**, **early**, **and late viral genes**, which are required for the production of progeny virus.

Following fusion and penetration of CMV or EBV, nucleocapsids containing infectious DNA are translocated to the nucleus by a pathway that likely involves microtubular transport. Once the virion DNA has entered the nucleus, the transcriptional program is initiated by interactions between proteins contained within the virion tegument and cellular factors that together activate expression of viral immediate-early genes. Virion tegument proteins also disarm certain host cell–intrinsic antiviral responses.

Expression of the viral immediate-early genes leads to the sequential expression of viral genes required for viral nucleic acid synthesis, including the viral DNA-dependent DNA polymerase, and viral genes that encode virion structural proteins. CMV and EBV also encode viral proteins that limit apoptosis and innate immune responses to virus infection. These viral functions insure host cell survival for an interval sufficient to allow production of progeny virus.

The assembly of CMV or EBV virions includes the processes of nucleocapsid formation, viral DNA packaging, and envelopment that appear to be conserved in all herpesviruses. The pathway of virus assembly involves both nuclear and cytoplasmic steps. Within the nucleus, the viral nucleocapsid shell is constructed around a scaffold generated by a virion capsid protein. This pathway results in the formation of a 130 nm icosahedral nucleocapsid that provides a site for viral DNA packaging.

Viral DNA is synthesized as long chains of genome-length DNA copies (**concatemers**) and cleaved into unit-length genomes during packaging and capsid maturation. Newly replicated viral DNA from both viruses is encapsidated in the nucleus. Nucleocapsids exit the nucleus by sequential budding through the inner and outer leaflets of the nuclear membrane, acquire the **tegument layer** of protein in the cytoplasm, and eventually become enveloped in the secretory pathway. Progeny virions egress from infected cells with a lipid-containing envelope of viral glycoproteins (Fig. 42-1). CMV and EBV virions are large for viruses, measuring between 200 and 300 nm in diameter. Release of infectious virus occurs either through a process of regulated exocytosis or following death of the infected cell. The envelope glycoproteins also elicit protective antiviral antibodies that likely function by neutralization of infectious virions. The complexity of the assembly process of these viruses is illustrated by the finding that CMV virions contain over 100 virus-encoded proteins.

Persistent and Latent Infections

Latent viral infections are characterized by restricted viral gene expression and the lack of progeny virus production. The establishment and maintenance of persistence by CMV is poorly understood. Cell-culture models suggest that the virus can persist as a latent infection in CD34+ myeloid progenitor cells and, following migration to organs such as the liver, these undifferentiated but lineage-committed cells undergo terminal differentiation leading to reactivation of latent infection. The contribution of this mode of

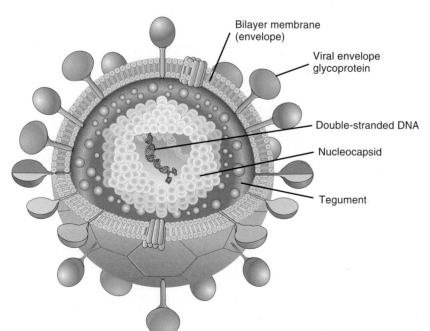

Bilayer membrane (envelope)

Viral envelope glycoprotein

Double-stranded DNA

Nucleocapsid

Tegument

FIGURE 42-1. Schematic of a herpesvirus virion. The virion is shown with double-stranded DNA in the center of the particle surrounded by an icosahedral nucleocapsid. Proteins in the tegument layer are located between the nucleocapsid and lipid envelope with viral envelope glycoproteins inserted through the lipid membrane.

persistence to the overall viral burden in the normal host is unclear, but available evidence suggests that persistence can be explained by chronic productive infection. Latency-associated transcripts are expressed during CMV latency. However, in contrast to members of the alphaherpesvirus family, the role of CMV latency-associated transcripts in the maintenance of latent infection is undefined.

Latent infection by EBV is associated with persistence of the viral genome in the absence of lytic infection and expression of specific viral genes. In the initial phases, viral genes such as **Epstein-Barr nuclear antigen-1** are expressed to insure maintenance and partitioning of the viral genome as a replicating episome during expansion of infected cells. Expression of the latent membrane proteins, **LMP1** and **LMP2a**, provides growth signals to infected cells that drive cellular proliferation. Finally, a minimal number of viral genes and small RNAs are expressed in long-lived nondividing B cells, which serve as a reservoir for EBV in the normal host. By restricting expression of its genome, EBV can maintain its genetic material, while also limiting its recognition by antigen-specific lymphocytes.

Reactivation of EBV from latency in vivo occurs sporadically. B lymphocytes undergoing reactivation can release infectious virus that can subsequently infect epithelial cells, leading to periodic shedding of EBV during the lifetime of the host. Reactivation of latent EBV infection in cultured cells can be accomplished using a variety of nonspecific activators of gene expression. Although reactivation of EBV in infected persons is well documented, specific stimuli that result in productive infection are less well defined. In general, reactivation of EBV is most readily observed in persons with defects in virus-specific T-lymphocyte responses and those undergoing cytotoxic or immunosuppressive therapy.

Small noncoding RNAs (**microRNAs, miRNAs**) that function in posttranscriptional gene regulation serve as a major regulatory mechanism in development, homeostasis, and stress responses, including viral infections. Both CMV and EBV encode a large number of miRNAs that have critical roles in virus replication, including interference with cellular antiviral responses and establishment and maintenance of latent infection. CMV and EBV encode 12 to 16 miRNAs that range in function from inhibition of the expression of immediate-early genes in CMV-infected cells to inhibition of the EBV DNA polymerase during lytic infection. Furthermore, these viruses also induce host cell miRNAs, some of which downregulate cellular antiviral responses. Other cellular miRNAs are upregulated in B-cell malignancies induced by EBV, providing a potential mechanism of EBV-associated B-cell neoplasms.

SPREAD

Although both CMV and EBV can be transmitted between hosts in the form of cell-free virus present in mucosal secretions, it is likely that both viruses disseminate *within* the infected host as cell-associated virus. CMV infects a wide variety of cells in vivo, including epithelial and endothelial cells, blood mononuclear cells, neural progenitor cells, and supporting cells of the central nervous system (CNS). EBV is more restrictive in its cellular tropism and infects B lymphocytes and epithelial cells.

DAMAGE

Host Responses

Cellular effector functions including natural killer (NK) cells and virus-specific cytotoxic CD8+ T lymphocytes serve an essential function in limiting the replication of CMV and EBV. These responses control virus replication during primary infection and provide surveillance during viral latency to limit reactivation. Loss of these responses leads to reactivation, virus dissemination, end-organ infection, and disease. Thus, persons with primary immunodeficiencies that affect NK cell or T lymphocyte function, acquired immunodeficiencies such as human immunodeficiency virus (HIV) infection, or immunodeficiencies associated with therapy to prevent allograft rejection are at risk for development of severe disease following CMV or EBV infection. Biologics used to block inflammatory responses, such as anti-TNF antibodies for the treatment of rheumatologic diseases, are also associated with severe CMV and EBV infections. Clinical trials using passive transfer of ex vivo–expanded CMV- or EBV-specific cytotoxic T lymphocytes into allograft recipients have demonstrated the protective activity of these immune effector cells.

Perhaps one of the most intriguing aspects of the relationship of CMV and EBV with the host cell is the multitude of virus-encoded genes that function to evade innate and adaptive immunity. In the case of CMV, proteins encoded by these genes downregulate and degrade class I and II major histocompatibility complex (MHC) proteins and modulate NK cell receptors and function. In addition, several virus-encoded activities prevent intrinsic cellular responses to infection such as DNA degradation, interferon induction, and apoptosis. CMV encodes a number of functional cytokines, such as interleukin (IL)-8 and IL-10, and chemokine receptors that modulate the inflammatory response to favor virus persistence in the host. These evasion functions contribute to viral persistence by insuring survival of virus-infected cells by limiting the activity of host clearance mechanisms. EBV apparently utilizes similar strategies to evade host immunity, including expression of antiapoptotic functions, induction of immunomodulatory pathways, and inhibition of antigen presentation by MHC molecules. Together, these activities demonstrate that during evolution with their human host, both CMV and EBV have developed multiple mechanisms to facilitate persistence and evasion of host-derived antiviral functions. Many of these strategies are common to other DNA viruses, such as adenoviruses and poxviruses, but, perhaps more than any other family of viruses, they are highly conserved in the herpesviruses. Examples of herpesvirus immune evasion strategies are provided in Table 42-2.

TABLE 42-2 Herpesvirus Proteins that Block Host Antiviral Functions

Host Antiviral Responses	Virus and Viral Protein	Function
Intrinsic	HSV (α-herpesvirus) ICP 34.5	Inhibits host cell antiviral responses leading to translation blockade and cell death
	CMV (β-herpesvirus) UL37	Inhibits caspase activity and prevents apoptosis
	EBV (γ-herpesvirus) BHRF1	Similar activity as cellular *Bcl-2* and prevents apoptosis
Innate	HSV IE genes	Decreased activity of NK cells
	CMV UL83 (pp65); UL16	Inhibition of NK receptor activation
Adaptive	HSV ICP47	Blockade of transporter associated with antigen presentation function resulting in decrease in antigen presentation
	CMV US2, US11	Degradation of class I and class II MHC molecules with resultant decreased antigen presentation
	EBV gp42	Blockade of class II MHC molecule–T-cell receptor interactions

Clinical Syndromes

The vast majority of acute CMV and EBV infections are clinically inapparent, especially in young children. Primary infection in young adults can be associated with an **acute mononucleosis syndrome** that consists of low-grade fever, fatigue, pharyngitis, cervical lymphadenopathy, splenomegaly, and peripheral blood monocytosis with atypical or reactive lymphocytes. Although this presentation is stereotypic for EBV infection, CMV causes up to 20% of illnesses associated with these symptoms but lacking serological evidence of EBV infection (i.e., **heterophile-negative**). The clinical symptoms associated with acute CMV and EBV infections in nonimmunocompromised persons are self-limited, and there is little if any evidence suggesting that antiviral therapy is of value in the treatment of these infections. Indeed, when the mononucleosis syndrome develops, the host immune response is already in full swing. The "atypical" lymphocytes seen in the blood of persons with infectious mononucleosis consist mostly of activated CD8+ T lymphocytes directed against viral antigens on infected cells. These lymphocytes are critical to the control of viral infection, and this host response may be responsible for many of the clinical manifestation of mononucleosis.

Newborn infants infected in utero with CMV can develop significant disease. This infection is acquired following maternal infection with CMV, which is almost always unrecognized by the pregnant woman. The virus is transmitted from the pregnant mother to the developing fetus, presumably following a maternal viremia and infection of the placenta. Infants with congenital CMV infection can exhibit significant multiorgan disease secondary to unrestricted virus replication and a direct viral cytotoxic effect on target organs, perhaps as a result of the developmental immaturity of the fetal immune response. Infants with congenital CMV infection can have CNS involvement, hepatitis, and hematologic abnormalities. CNS disease can include encephalomalacia, hydrocephalus, retinitis, and damage to the auditory system leading to hearing loss (Fig. 42-2). The disease manifestations associated with liver and bone marrow involvement are self-limited, but structural damage to the CNS can result in long-term sequelae. It is estimated that congenital CMV infection results in over 3,000 neurologically impaired infants in the United States each year. Sensorineural hearing loss is the most common sequelae of this infection, occurring in about 12% of infected infants. Remarkably, hearing loss associated with congenital CMV infection is the most common cause of nonfamilial hearing loss in the United States and Northern Europe. In contrast to the other end-organ diseases associated with congenital CMV infection in which the pathogenesis of disease is directly related to virus replication, development of hearing loss can be delayed until 3 to 4 years of age, well after control of virus replication. This observation suggests that mechanisms of tissue injury in addition to lytic virus replication contribute to the illness in some infants.

In adults, persistent CMV infection may have other chronic consequences. For example, studies of patients with atherosclerotic vascular disease suggest a strong association of CMV infection and development of coronary artery disease.

CASE

Betaherpesvirus Infection in an Immunocompromised Renal Transplant Recipient

Mr. K., a 20-year-old man, underwent renal transplantation secondary to end-stage renal disease that developed over a relatively short period. The donor was an unrelated accident victim who was 50 years old. The surgical procedure was uneventful, and Mr. K. tolerated the posttransplant immunosuppressive therapy, which included drugs that significantly decreased CD8+ T lymphocyte function. About 6 weeks after transplantation, Mr. K. developed fever, decreased appetite, cervical lymphadenopathy, and decreased white blood cell count.

After an extensive medical evaluation, a diagnosis was made with the aid of the clinical pathology laboratory.

1. What factors could predispose Mr. K. to infection with either CMV or EBV?

2. Does the limited amount of information included in the case history provide clues to the possible cause of his illness?

3. What laboratory tests were used to make the diagnosis in this patient?

4. Is treatment with antiviral therapy indicated in this patient?

See Appendix for answers.

CMV and EBV Infections in Immunocompromised Hosts

Persistent CMV and EBV infections are associated with chronic inflammatory diseases and human cancers. In contrast to infections associated with CMV and EBV in immunocompetent persons, infection with either virus in immunocompromised individuals can result in organ dysfunction and death. Acute CMV infections in transplant recipients often present as a mononucleosis-like syndrome that includes fever, hematologic abnormalities, lymphadenopathy, and hepatitis. In many cases, these infections are self-limited, but CMV infections in more severely immunocompromised allograft recipients can progress to organ- and life-threatening disease including hepatitis, colitis, and less commonly, pneumonia. The level of morbidity and mortality depends on the level of immunosuppression, particularly on the integrity of CD8+ T lymphocyte responses. In transplant recipients, CMV will establish a chronic productive infection that is associated with an increased risk of chronic graft dysfunction secondary to exaggerated wound healing responses. CMV infection in renal allograft recipients leads to tubular dysfunction secondary to fibrosis and scarring. In hematopoietic allograft recipients, CMV can result in disease early or late (>100 days) after transplantation. Late CMV disease is associated with more severe **graft-versus-host disease** and increased morbidity and mortality.

Prior to the introduction of effective antiretroviral therapy, CMV also was a frequent cause of opportunistic infections in AIDS patients and a major cause of end-organ disease, including colitis, encephalitis, and retinitis. As therapy for HIV has improved, the incidence of CMV

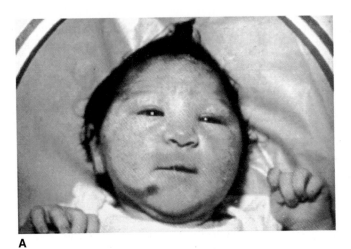

A

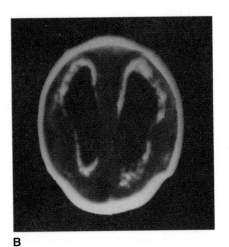

B

FIGURE 42-2. Clinical appearance and radiologic findings of congenital cytomegalovirus (CMV) infection. A. Infant with severe congenital CMV with stigmata of disease including petechial rash, microcephaly, jaundice, and abnormal posture of the upper extremities secondary to central nervous system (CNS) damage. **B.** Computerized tomographic image of an infant with CNS damage secondary to congenital CMV with severe periventricular calcifications (white signal lining ventricles) and ventriculomegaly.

disease has fallen precipitously, providing further support for the importance of cell-mediated immunity in containment of CMV infection.

EBV infection is also an important cause of disease in immunocompromised persons. Among transplant recipients, infection with EBV can occur as a consequence of primary acquisition from a donor organ or blood products in a previously uninfected individual or as a result of reactivation of an existing latent infection in the recipient. Following reactivation, lytic EBV infection in the immunosuppressed transplant recipient can induce lymphoproliferation, leading to a syndrome that is designated **posttransplant lymphoproliferative disease** (**PTLD**). In its most benign form, the virus produces an acute mononucleosis-like syndrome with lymphoid proliferation. Untreated, this initially benign lymphoproliferation can evolve into an oligoclonal neoplasm that in some cases subsequently develops into a lymphoma.

Viral Oncogenesis

There is little doubt that EBV is an oncogenic virus; it is associated with **Hodgkin lymphoma**, **Burkitt lymphoma**, **nasopharyngeal carcinoma**, and more recently **gastric carcinoma**. EBV is present in about 40% of Hodgkin lymphomas, allowing the subclassification of these tumors based on EBV infection status. In addition, the risk of being diagnosed with EBV-positive Hodgkin disease is about fourfold higher in individuals with a history of acute infectious mononucleosis than in those without a history of EBV infection. Furthermore, cytotoxic T cells directed at EBV LMPs induce clinical remission in some patients with EBV-positive Hodgkin disease,

providing additional evidence for a role for EBV in this illness. Burkitt lymphoma at one time was the most common childhood malignancy in certain regions of Africa, primarily those with a high incidence of malaria. It is postulated that chronic malaria leads to immunosuppression in EBV-infected children, which in turns leads to chronic B-cell stimulation with increased opportunity for chromosomal translocations that result in the aberrant joining of genes encoding the immunoglobulin heavy chain and the c-Myc oncogene. This translocation results in the constitutive expression of c-Myc and resultant unregulated cellular proliferation and inhibition of apoptosis. Importantly, the EBV LMPs also drive cellular proliferation while limiting apoptosis, both phenotypes that are commonly observed during carcinogenesis.

CMV has been detected in several different human cancers, including colon carcinoma, prostate carcinoma, cervical carcinoma, and glioblastoma. However, in no case has CMV been etiologically linked to human malignancy.

DIAGNOSIS

CMV and EBV infections can be diagnosed by isolation of the virus in tissue culture, detection of viral antigens or viral nucleic acids in clinical specimens, and assessment of serological responses. Isolation of CMV from urine, saliva, blood, and tissue specimens is readily accomplished. PCR-based assays, both qualitative and quantitative, represent standard approaches for the identification of CMV in clinical specimens. Histopathologic detection of large inclusions ("owl eye" inclusions) in tissue specimens is considered definitive pathological evidence of CMV infection (Fig 42-3). A useful assay for the diagnosis

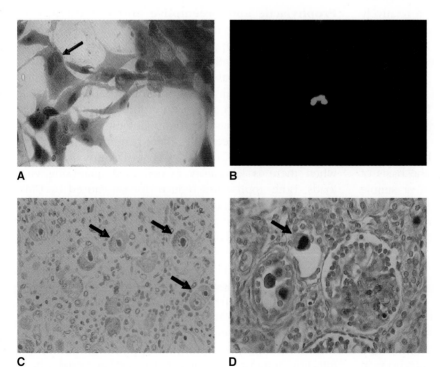

A

B

C

D

FIGURE 42-3. Laboratory findings of CMV infection. A. Extensive cytopathic effect of human fibroblasts infected with CMV. Note rounding of cells and large nuclei (*arrow*). **B.** Fluorescent antibody detection of CMV antigen in circulating polymorphonuclear leukocytes (antigenemia assay) from an allograft recipient. **C.** Nuclear inclusions and cytoplasmic inclusions (*arrows*) in infected alveolar epithelium of an infant with congenital CMV infection. **D.** Immunohistochemical staining of infected cells (*arrow*) in a renal biopsy from a transplanted kidney in a patient with CMV infection.

of CMV infection in immunocompromised patients is the **antigenemia assay**. This technique uses immunofluorescence to detect an abundant CMV antigen in circulating mononuclear and polymorphonuclear leukocytes (Fig. 42-3). Detection of CMV antigens in peripheral blood leukocytes indicates actively replicating CMV and, in transplant recipients, predicts virus dissemination and end-organ disease. Results from the antigenemia assay are used to initiate and monitor antiviral therapy in such persons.

Although EBV can be isolated from clinical specimens, its recovery in tissue-culture systems is arduous and rarely undertaken because freshly obtained human B lymphocytes are required for its cultivation. As with CMV, PCR is a highly sensitive and specific technique for detecting EBV in clinical samples. In the case of EBV, detection of the noncoding nuclear RNAs expressed during EBV infection, called **EBER**s, by in situ hybridization has reasonable sensitivity, perhaps because of the high copy number of these RNAs in EBV-infected cells.

Acquisition of serologic reactivity (or **seroconversion**) is considered a standard approach for the detection of primary infection with both CMV and EBV. The detection of IgM antibodies specific for either CMV or EBV suggests a recently acquired infection in immunocompetent hosts. Detection of IgG antibodies specific for either CMV or EBV in a single serum specimen provides no information about the duration of the infection. In the case of EBV, a peculiar pattern of antibody reactivity for structural and nonstructural virus-encoded proteins has allowed the determination of acute versus longstanding infection by simple serology using a set of EBV-derived antigens. However, serology is of little value in the diagnosis of CMV or EBV infections in immunocompromised persons for two main reasons. First, there is a relatively high incidence of preexisting infection in these individuals. Second, and perhaps more importantly, the underlying immune dysfunction can lead to inconsistent serologic responses.

In acute mononucleosis, EBV infection induces the production of non–EBV-specific antibodies. These anomalous antibodies include some that recognize antigens found on the erythrocytes of heterologous species, such as cows or sheep. They are referred to as **heterophile antibodies**. This serologic reactivity forms the basis of the heterophile antibody or "monospot" test, a simple and rapid agglutination test that is employed in outpatient clinics for the diagnosis of acute EBV mononucleosis. CMV mononucleosis does not induce these anomalous antibodies, so this rapid test will be negative.

TREATMENT

CMV and EBV infections in normal immunocompetent individuals are almost always self-limited and thus, rarely, if ever, require treatment. In contrast, antiviral therapy is indicated in disseminated CMV and EBV infections in immunocompromised patients. Because the viral polymerase enzymes are structurally and biochemically distinct from host cell polymerases, they have been targeted for antiviral drug development much as the polymerases of other viruses such as human immunodeficiency virus and hepatitis B virus. Two agents, **ganciclovir** and **foscarnet**, inhibit CMV replication, and both agents are routinely used in the prevention and treatment of invasive CMV infections. Ganciclovir is a nucleoside analog that is phosphorylated by the virus-encoded phosphotransferase, UL97. The phosphorylated form of ganciclovir blocks virus replication by inhibiting **viral DNA-dependent DNA polymerase** and arresting elongation of newly synthesized viral DNA. Foscarnet also inhibits the viral DNA polymerase, but it works by a different mechanism. Both agents exhibit dose-related toxicity, and resistance to both can develop rapidly.

In contrast to CMV, treatment of EBV infections in the immunocompromised host is difficult. Ganciclovir and the related nucleoside analog, acyclovir, have activity against EBV, and treatment with these agents can limit virus replication. However, treatment of PTLD in EBV-infected transplant recipients with these agents has minimal, if any, efficacy, possibly because the viral genes that are responsible for the lymphoproliferation are expressed in the absence of viral DNA replication. Alternative approaches include passive infusion of EBV-specific antibodies or ex vivo–expanded EBV-specific T lymphocytes. Epithelial malignancies associated with EBV do not respond to treatment with currently available antiviral agents because viral replication is not a prerequisite for oncogenesis.

PREVENTION

Prophylactic and preemptive antiviral therapy of CMV and EBV infections is used to limit disease manifestations. Neither approach is intended to prevent infection. Prophylaxis with antiviral therapy is used in many transplant centers based on the observation that CMV and EBV infections occur during the initial period of intense immunosuppression and that a reduction in viral replication and therefore viral burden will limit viral dissemination and disease. Preemptive therapy relies on monitoring the virologic status of the patient. Therapy is initiated when there is laboratory evidence of increasing viral loads. Both approaches reduce disease caused by CMV in immunocompromised transplant recipients. However, prophylaxis appears to be more commonly associated with late (>100 days posttransplant) disease in hematopoietic allograft recipients, perhaps because viral replication is inhibited during a period when the allograft is generating adaptive immune responses to CMV, which lowers the magnitude of the antiviral immune response. When prophylaxis is discontinued, virus begins to replicate in the absence of T lymphocyte responses, and disease can ensue. The effectiveness of these approaches for EBV infection in transplant recipients has not been established.

Immunoprophylaxis of CMV and EBV infections in transplant patients is now routinely employed. Passive transfer of antiviral antibodies in the form of intravenous immunoglobulin modifies disease in CMV-infected kidney and liver transplant recipients, and, although extraordinarily costly, it is used routinely in some centers. The efficacy of this approach in hematopoietic transplant recipients has not been established. Transfer of ex vivo–expanded virus-specific T lymphocytes protects hematopoietic allograft recipients from severe CMV infections. Similarly, transfer of EBV-specific T lymphocytes diminishes disease associated with EBV infection in hematopoietic and solid organ allograft recipients. Although a number of candidate vaccines to prevent CMV and EBV infection or disease are in development, none have progressed sufficiently to suggest that they will be available in the near future.

CONCLUSION

Beta- and gammaherpesviruses have limited intrinsic pathogenicity and restricted tropism. Members of both subgroups of herpesviruses exhibit more delayed replicative cycles in comparison to the alphaherpesviruses. CMV and EBV establish lifelong persistence in the host. Both viruses enter the host through epithelial surfaces and eventually target reservoirs of persistence. CMV and EBV replication appears to be similar to that of other herpesviruses. Components of host defense that contain CMV and EBV infection include cytotoxic T lymphocytes, NK cells, antiviral antibodies, and soluble effectors such as interferons. These antiviral functions control virus replication, but there is little evidence that they prevent infection. CMV and EBV deploy a complex array of viral functions that limit the effectiveness of host immunity. These include viral gene products that block apoptosis and others that inhibit recognition of infected cells by immune effector cells. Although clinically apparent disease following infection with either virus is rare in normal, immunocompetent individuals, a variety of clinical syndromes can develop in immunocompromised hosts. In some cases, these infections are associated with significant morbidity with organ-threatening and life-threatening disease. Effective antiviral therapy is available for CMV infections, but the value of antiviral agents in immunocompromised persons with EBV infections has not been established. Vaccines to prevent infection with either virus are not currently available.

Suggested Readings

Arvin A, Campadelli-Fiume G, Mocarski E, et al. *Human Herpesviruses: Biology, Therapy, and Immunoprophylaxis*. Cambridge, UK: Cambridge University Press; 2007.

Britt WJ. Cytomegalovirus. In: Remington J, Klein J, eds. *Infectious Diseases of the Fetus and Newborn Infant*. 7th ed. Philadelphia, PA: W.B. Saunders; 2010:706–756.

Reddehase MJ, ed. *Cytomegaloviruses: Molecular Biology and Immunology Horizon Scientific Press*. Norwich, UK: Hethersett; 2005.

Chapter 43

Viral Hepatitis

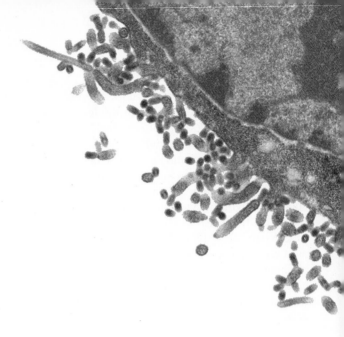

Donald E. Ganem

KEY CONCEPTS

Pathogens: Hepatitis is caused by several viruses (known as hepatitis viruses A through E) that are antigenically and genetically unrelated to each other.

Encounter: Some viruses are acquired by ingestion via the fecal–oral route (hepatitis A and E). Others are primarily bloodborne or sexually transmitted (hepatitis B, C, and delta virus).

Entry: Whatever the portal of entry, all of the hepatitis viruses demonstrate marked tropism for liver cells.

Spread and Replication: Hepatitis A and E viruses produce only a transient infection followed by resolution. In contrast, hepatitis B, C, and delta viruses can produce lifelong persistent infections, with ongoing virus replication in the liver and persistent viremia.

Damage: Viral hepatitis is a clinical syndrome characterized by fever and signs and symptoms of liver injury. The clinical signs are variable and initially indistinguishable among the different hepatitis viruses.

Diagnosis: The specific etiology is identified by testing for the presence of specific viral proteins, specific antibodies against those proteins, or viral nucleic acid associated with the causative agent.

Treatment: Acute hepatitis is not treated, but chronic hepatitis B or C can be treated with specific antiviral drugs to prevent or forestall permanent liver damage.

Prevention: Blood products are routinely screened for hepatitis viruses, so transfusion-related hepatitis is now rare. Effective vaccines can prevent hepatitis A and B infections.

MANY VIRUSES can infect the liver and cause disease. These viruses include adenovirus, cytomegalovirus, Epstein-Barr virus, herpes simplex virus, varicella-zoster virus, and yellow fever virus. However, all of those viruses also infect tissues in addition to the liver and can produce extrahepatic diseases. In contrast, the viruses discussed in this chapter can be thought of as "professional" hepatitis viruses: they have a strong tropism for the liver and preferentially replicate in **hepatocytes**, the predominant cell type of that organ. As a result, the viruses discussed here are associated primarily with liver disease and only rarely produce disease outside that organ.

The professional hepatitis viruses are a diverse group that includes members from five taxonomic families (Table 43-1).

VIRAL HEPATITIS: THE BIG PICTURE
The Liver as a Site for Virus Replication

As the largest organ in the body, the liver represents a major site for virus replication. Approximately 85% of liver cells are hepatocytes, the principal epithelial cell in the liver and the target cell type for most hepatitis viruses. These cells have important roles in human physiology, including (1) the production of plasma proteins like albumin and blood clotting factors; (2) glucose and lipid metabolism; (3) metabolism and detoxification of xenobiotics, toxins, and drugs; and (4) conjugation and excretion of bilirubin, a breakdown product of heme. The liver also is home to many cells of the immune system, including

TABLE 43-1 Properties of Human Hepatitis Viruses

Agent	Size (nm)	Nucleic Acid Composition	Virus Family
Hepatitis A	27	Linear (+) single-stranded RNA	Picornaviridae
Hepatitis B	45	Nicked, circular, mostly double-stranded DNA	Hepadnaviridae
Hepatitis C	~55	Linear (+) single-stranded RNA	Flaviviridae
Hepatitis delta		Circular (−) single-stranded RNA	Deltaviridae
Hepatitis E	27	Linear (+) single-stranded RNA	Caliciviridae

(−), negative-sense polarity; (+), positive-sense polarity.

its innate components (e.g., interferons) and its adaptive responses (e.g., antibodies and cytotoxic T cells [CTLs]). Liver-specific macrophages, known as **Kupffer cells**, are important mediators of inflammatory responses (especially cytokine release), which can aid in the clearance of virus from the liver, either directly or by evoking the influx of additional inflammatory cells from the circulation. The liver also harbors many distinctive populations of T cells, some of which, such as **natural killer T (NKT) cells**, are strikingly overrepresented there. NKT cells belong to the innate immune system and are capable of dramatic cytokine production when activated. The immunology of the liver is a complex and understudied area, and much remains to be learned about how viruses are eradicated from liver tissue and how (in the case of hepatitis B and C viruses) they can sometimes escape immune attack.

When the liver is damaged by viral infection, its normal functions are impaired, resulting in a constellation of symptoms that characterize viral hepatitis. Fever, abdominal pain, nausea, and vomiting are common in mild cases. If liver damage becomes more extensive, **bilirubin** accumulates in the skin, leading to the yellowish discoloration known as jaundice. In still more severe cases, mental function is impaired due to the failure to detoxify toxins absorbed from the gastrointestinal tract, and bleeding can result from diminished production of clotting factors. Laboratory tests show elevations of serum bilirubin and **transaminases**, which are released from damaged hepatocytes. Both tests are frequently ordered by clinicians to gauge the severity of liver injury in viral hepatitis.

Infectious Strategies Used by Hepatitis Viruses

Despite their differing genetic constitutions, the hepatitis viruses display two broad patterns of infection in human hosts (Table 43-2). The simplest is exemplified by **hepatitis A virus (HAV)** and **hepatitis E virus (HEV)**, which are acquired from the environment by oral ingestion. Following uptake in the intestine, HAV and HEV home in on the liver, where replication takes place. Virus is shed into the bile ducts and returned to the intestine, where it can pass out with the feces to contaminate food or drink (this pattern of viral epidemiology is known as fecal–oral spread). Importantly, infected hosts mount an effective immune response that clears the virus from the liver and blood and generates lasting immunity to reinfection. Thus, infection by HAV or HEV produces only a transient, self-limited infection. Although the infection can be severe, fatalities are infrequent and resolution is generally the rule.

In contrast, **hepatitis B virus (HBV) and hepatitis C virus (HCV)** are capable of either transient or persistent infection. They first initiate an acute infection that may or may not result in disease symptoms but always leads to extensive replication of the virus in the liver. However, the immune response that follows is not always effective in clearing the infection. The net result is that, although some infected persons do clear acute infection, many do not and instead develop a persistent infection that frequently is lifelong. **Persistent infection** is characterized by continued virus replication in the liver and release of infectious particles into the bloodstream (Table 43-3). The rate of persistent infection varies widely from virus to virus. In adults infected with HBV, only approximately 5% of infections progress to persistence, while in those infected with HCV, this number is closer to 80%. However, many other factors contribute to the likelihood of persistent infection, for example, the age, sex, and immune status of the infected host.

TABLE 43-2 Transmission of Hepatitis Viruses

Transmission	Hepatitis Virus Type				
	A	B	C	D	E
Fecal–oral	Yes	No	No	No	Yes
Sexual	Yes[a]	Yes	Yes	Yes	Yes[a]
Vertical	No	Yes	Yes	Yes	No
Parenteral	Yes[b]	Yes	Yes	Yes	Yes[b]

[a]From the combined practices of anal and oral sex.
[b]A brief window of viremia exists in which parenteral transmission can occur.

TABLE 43-3 Clinical Comparison of Disease Associated with Hepatitis Viruses

Characteristic	Hepatitis Virus Type				
	A	*B*	*C*	*D*	*E*
Incubation period (d)	15–40	60–180	60–120	60–180	21–42
Asymptomatic infection	Often	Often	Often	Can occur	Often
Chronic infection	No	Yes (5%)	Yes (80%)	Yes	No
Long-term sequelae	No	Yes[a]	Yes[a]	Exacerbation of HBV infection	No

[a]Includes cirrhosis and hepatocellular carcinoma.
HBV, hepatitis B virus.

For HBV and HCV, virus replication in hepatocytes is not directly injurious to the cell. How then does the liver damage of hepatitis result? Current evidence suggests that liver damage is not caused by viral replication but by the **host immune response**. That response generates CTLs directed against viral antigens displayed by major histocompatibility complex class I molecules on the hepatocyte surface. When antiviral CTLs recognize such antigens, the hepatocytes are killed. In addition, cytokines released from T cells promote further inflammation and tissue injury. Therefore, the immune response to hepatitis viruses is a double-edged sword: on the plus side, it kills infected cells and clears the infection; on the minus side, it causes liver injury and results in disease symptoms. If the response is sufficiently robust, the primary infection is resolved, as in HAV or HEV infection. The host immune response clears about 95% of adult HBV infections but only approximately 20% of primary HCV infections. In the remaining cases, the immune response is inadequate to clear the virus and persistent infection results. However, in some cases, this inadequate response continues to injure infected hepatocytes, generating a syndrome of sustained liver damage called **chronic hepatitis**, with signs and symptoms that resemble those of acute hepatitis but that persist. For reasons that are unclear, not all persistently infected persons have liver damage; those who do not are referred to as **asymptomatic carriers** of the virus. Although they are clinically well, they are important reservoirs of infection, from which spread to new hosts occurs.

The liver responds to sustained damage from persistent infection in a stereotypical way, with **regeneration** and, in some cases, with scarring (**fibrosis**). If these two processes are extensive, the resulting disease is **cirrhosis**, in which nodules of regenerating hepatocytes are accompanied by large bands of connective tissue. Cirrhosis usually indicates extensive loss of functioning liver cells (which are not replaced by the regenerative response), and many patients with this disease develop liver failure, a condition that is fatal without liver transplantation. (In fact, chronic HCV infection is the leading indication for liver transplantation in the United States today.) In addition, decades of hepatocyte death and regeneration may lead to liver cancer, most likely due to host mutations that accompany the DNA synthesis process (although additional contributions from viral gene expression also may play a role). Primary cancer of the liver is an important complication of chronic HBV and HCV infections. For example, lifelong HBV infection results in a 100-fold increase in liver cancer risk.

THE INDIVIDUAL HEPATITIS VIRUSES
Hepatitis A Virus

HAV is responsible for most cases of **infectious hepatitis**. HAV is a nonenveloped, single-stranded, positive-sense virus in the Picornaviridae family (see Chapter 32). It is fairly closely related to other picornaviruses, such as poliovirus, and is thought to use a similar overall replication strategy. HAV replication in the liver of humans is quite robust, and virus titers in stool can be enormous: over 10^{11} particles/mL. Although clinical isolates do not grow readily in cell culture, some human HAV isolates have been adapted to cell-culture growth—a development that has greatly facilitated HAV research and made possible the development of a safe and effective vaccine.

HAV is spread primarily through the ingestion of fecally contaminated food or water (Fig. 43-1). Once HAV reaches the intestine, it is thought to be absorbed into the bloodstream and to reach the liver through the portal system. The virus then initiates acute infection of hepatocytes. Newly synthesized virus particles are exported into the bile ducts and from there are eventually excreted into the feces. To a lesser extent, virus is also released into the bloodstream, causing a transient viremia and a brief period in which HAV can be transmitted parentally or by blood transfusion. Virus is present for much longer periods and at much higher titers in stool than in blood, which explains why most HAV transmission is via the fecal–oral route rather than by parenteral spread.

HAV replication in the liver triggers a substantial immune response, both humoral and cell mediated (Fig. 43-1). Neutralizing antiviral antibodies play an important role in clearance of the virus; less is known

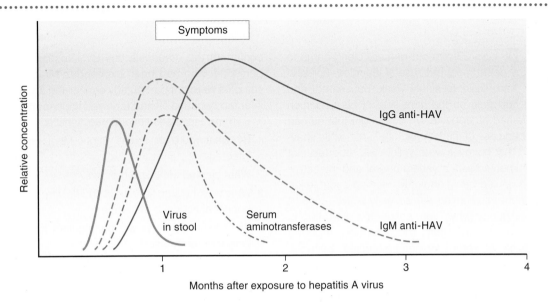

FIGURE 43-1. Typical course of acute hepatitis A virus infection.

about the function of cell-mediated immunity in HAV infection. Symptoms usually appear coincident with the initiation of an immune response, as gauged by the appearance of IgM antibodies specific for the structural proteins of the virus. The extent of illness varies among individuals, but generally, symptoms are more severe in adults than in children. In highly endemic regions where sanitation is generally poor, nearly all children become infected in the first few years of life, although most remain asymptomatic. In contrast, adults from non-endemic regions who become infected are more likely to display symptoms, although death associated with fulminant HAV infection is rare. Following the development of an immune response, the virus is rapidly cleared, and patients are left with lasting immunity to reinfection. As such, *HAV does not cause chronic or persistent infections.*

Prevention and Treatment

At present, there are no effective antiviral drugs for acute HAV infection. An HAV vaccine has been generated by inactivation of cell-cultured-derived HAV particles, much the same way the Salk poliovirus vaccine is prepared. This HAV vaccine has proven to be safe, highly immunogenic, and very effective. Vaccination is now recommended for all children in the United States; for those adults who were not vaccinated as children, vaccination is recommended for members of high-risk groups (e.g., military personnel, frequent travelers to endemic regions, and the staff of child-care facilities and institutions for the severely intellectually disabled).

Persons exposed to HAV (e.g., those who have been served food by an HAV-infected food handler) can be offered administration of serum immune globulin (pooled antibody from normal blood donors), which generally has high titers of anti-HAV antibodies. If given soon after HAV exposure, the anti-HAV antibodies in serum immune globulin can prevent HAV infection or reduce its extent and severity. This form of preventive intervention is known as **postexposure prophylaxis**.

Hepatitis B Virus

HBV belongs to the **hepadnavirus** family, a group of viruses with unusual properties, including a partially double-stranded circular DNA genome and replication via **reverse transcription**. HBV exhibits a marked tropism for human hepatocytes and cannot be grown in cells in culture.

A map of the HBV genome is shown in Figure 43-2. With less than 3,200 nucleotides, HBV has the smallest genome of any human virus (the hepatitis delta virus [HDV] genome is smaller but, as discussed later, it is not a traditional virus). The structure of the HBV DNA is unique: it is a partly double-stranded circular molecule. The minus (i.e., noncoding) strand is nicked, and a polymerase molecule is attached to its 5′ end. The plus strand contains a short RNA oligonucleotide at its 5′ end and is shortened at its 3′ end. Thus, the circular DNA genome has a single-stranded gap (see Fig. 43-2).

The infectious HBV virions are surrounded by an **envelope** and contain only five proteins. The names of the proteins include the letters *HB* and *Ag* as well as various other letters. The **envelope** layer contains three surface antigens, **HBsAg-S, HBsAg-M,** and **HBsAg-L** (the *S, M,* and *L,* are for "small," "middle," and "large"), embedded in a lipid bilayer. Each protein is translated from a different initiator methionine codon on its messenger RNA (mRNA), but the proteins share much of their carboxy-terminal sequences. HBsAg-S is the main constituent of the envelope and required for virion assembly. HBsAg-L, which contains all of HBsAg-S plus additional amino acid sequences at its amino-terminus, is involved in receptor binding and essential for infection. The function of HbsAg-M is unknown.

The HBV capsid is icosahedral and composed entirely of **core proteins (HBcAg)** that surround the viral DNA

CASE • Mr. L., a 23-year-old grocery clerk, came to the emergency department because of jaundice. For several days he had felt increasingly weak, nauseated, and feverish and had pain on the right side of his abdomen and joints. He had no appetite. Mr. L. thought that he had picked up a bad case of the "stomach flu" until, while shaving, he noted that his eyes were yellow. He reported that he had experimented with a variety of oral and injectable drugs, but he denied being addicted. He had a stable job and a girlfriend with whom he was sexually active.

The emergency physician suspected that Mr. L. had contracted HBV infection. The laboratory reported increased levels of serum aminotransferases, bilirubin, and alkaline phosphatase, all indicative of liver injury. Antibodies to hepatitis A and C viruses were absent. A surface antigen associated with HBV, called HBsAg, was detected in his serum, although antibodies directed against that antigen were not found. These findings confirmed the diagnosis of HBV infection. The medical personnel who had been exposed to Mr. L. or his blood samples were not particularly concerned about becoming infected because all had received the hepatitis B vaccine.

This case raises several questions:

1. By what route or routes might Mr. L. have become infected?
2. What caused Mr. L.'s symptoms?
3. What was the significance of finding viral surface antigen but not antisurface antibodies?
4. What follow-up tests will be required to determine his long-term prognosis?
5. What treatment could be instituted?
6. What advice can Mr. L. be given to avoid further transmission?

See Appendix for answers.

and the reverse transcriptase, which is also known as the **Pol** protein. The HBV reverse transcriptase has some properties in common with those of the retroviruses. Both kinds of enzymes can copy RNA into DNA. Furthermore, both enzymes have RNase H domains that digest the RNA template soon after it is copied; once the RNA is removed, the enzyme can copy the remaining DNA strand into duplex DNA. In HBV, this process does not go to completion in the infected cell—this is why the DNA found in the virion is only partially double stranded.

In addition to infectious virions, the blood of HBV-infected individuals contains a 1,000-fold excess of particles with empty envelopes (i.e., lacking the core and genome). The titer of these HBsAg **particles** in the blood can reach 10^{12}/mL. Most of the empty particles are spherical and composed mainly of HBsAg-S. (Filaments enriched for HBsAg-L are found in smaller amounts [Fig. 43-3].)

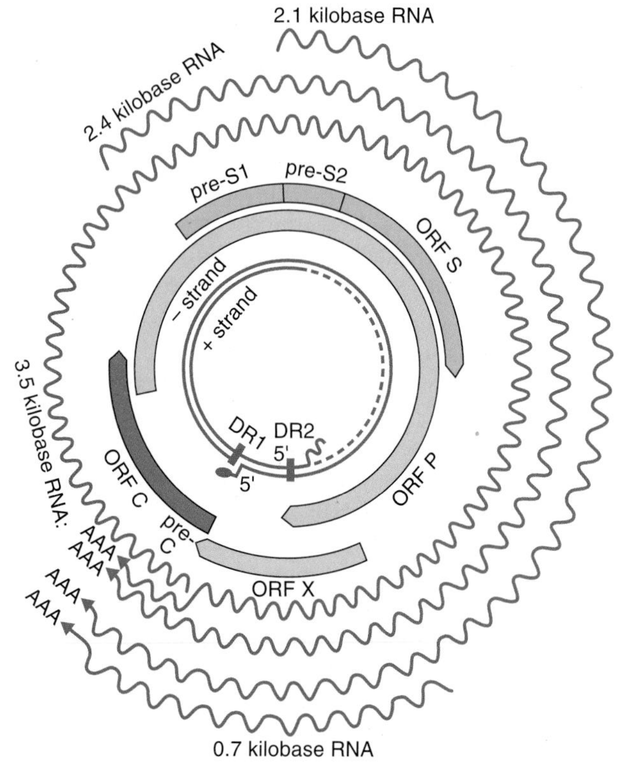

FIGURE 43-2. Hepatitis B virus genome structure and mRNA transcripts. The squiggly line at the 5' end of the plus (+) strand indicates a short RNA oligonucleotide. ORF, open-reading frame; DR, direct repeat.

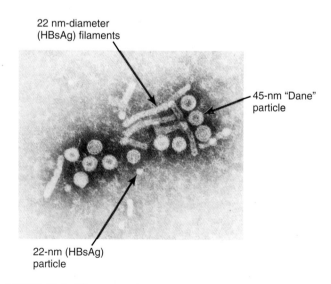

22 nm-diameter (HBsAg) filaments

45-nm "Dane" particle

22-nm (HBsAg) particle

FIGURE 43-3. Electron micrograph of hepatitis B virus. The image includes 22-nm-small, spherical aggregates of hepatitis B surface antigen (HBsAg) particles, 22-nm-wide filamentous aggregates of the antigen, and 42- to 45-nm hepatitis B virus ("Dane") particles.

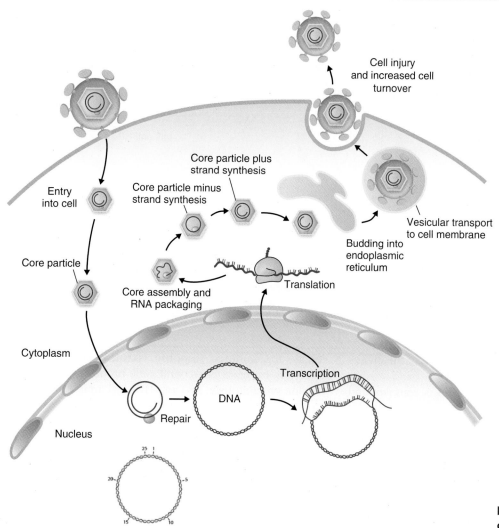

FIGURE 43-4. The replication cycle of HBV.

The role of the empty particles in virus replication and disease is uncertain, but because they are produced in such huge quantities, HBsAg can be readily measured in the blood and is a useful diagnostic marker of HBV infection.

As shown in Figure 43-4, the HBV replication cycle involves several steps:

1. Following its introduction into the bloodstream, HBV travels to the liver and attaches to the surface of hepatocytes. After uptake and uncoating, the viral genome is delivered to the nucleus, where the partially double-stranded nicked viral DNA is converted into a fully double-stranded, covalently closed, circular species (**cccDNA**).
2. The cccDNA serves as template for transcription of viral RNA, which is synthesized by host RNA polymerase II.
3. The single viral RNA that is used for **reverse transcription** is packaged into an immature viral capsid, along with the viral **Pol protein**.
4. Viral RNA is used as template for reverse transcription, resulting in the formation of viral DNA. Viral polymerase itself serves as the primer for first-strand synthesis,

which is why the product DNA is covalently linked to the enzyme.
5. The DNA-laden viral cores then bud through intracellular membranes to pick up their envelope of HBsAg, and progeny virions are released from infected cells.

The Human Biology of HBV

Nearly one-third of the world's population has been exposed to HBV, and more than 300 million people are chronically infected. Patterns of HBV infection are not uniform throughout the world. In the United States, Canada, and northern Europe, HBV infections are common only within certain high-risk groups such as injection drug users and those with multiple sexual partners. In most of Asia and sub-Saharan Africa, HBV infection is far more prevalent in the general population, with approximately 15% of persons in those regions displaying chronic infection. HBV transmission occurs through the exchange of body fluids such as blood, semen, and vaginal secretions. Before effective screening for HBV in donated blood supplies, transfusions were a common route of transmission. Another form of HBV transmission is vertically from

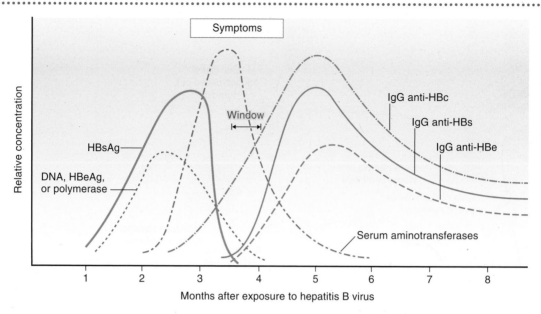

FIGURE 43-5. Typical course of acute hepatitis B virus infection.

mother to infant, probably as a consequence of the child's exposure to maternal blood during birth.

The clinical pattern of HBV infection is complex and can follow several paths. The events can be monitored by determining the presence of viral products and specific antibodies in the patient's blood. The serologic events accompanying primary infection are depicted in Figure 43-5. Primary infection can be asymptomatic or result in liver injury of varying severity. As noted previously, the extent of disease is thought to reflect differences in the magnitude and breadth of antiviral CTL responses, which can damage or kill hepatocytes. Following primary infection, two outcomes are possible. In about 95% of otherwise healthy

adults, the immune response is sufficient to clear the infection. In those cases, viral gene products in the blood decline precipitously, and anti-HBs IgG antibodies appear (see Fig. 43-5); these antibodies provide protective immunity against reinfection. In contrast, about 5% of infected adults progress to chronic infection. Those individuals usually have little or no freely circulating anti-HBs IgG, and viral products such as HBsAg and HBV virions may be found in the blood for decades (Fig. 43-6). The persistence of HBsAg in the blood for 6 months or more confirms the diagnosis of chronic HBV infection. Results of serologic assays for HBV at various stages of infection are summarized in Table 43-4.

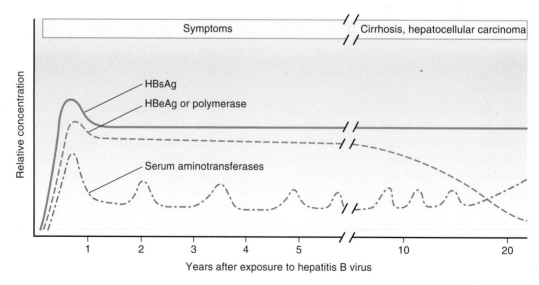

FIGURE 43-6. Typical course of chronic hepatitis B virus infection. After years of undulating symptoms and aminotransferase levels, circulating HBsAg, as well as viral DNA, HBeAg, and polymerase, may decline or even disappear. However, cirrhosis and hepatocellular carcinoma may still develop.

TABLE 43-4 Interpretation of Serologic Assays for Hepatitis B Virus

HbsAg	Anti-HBs	Anti-HBc	Anti-HBe	HBeAg	Interpretation
Neg	Neg	Neg	Neg	Neg	No prior exposure
Neg	Pos	Neg	Neg	Neg	Prior vaccination
Neg	Pos	Pos	Pos	Neg	Prior acute infection, resolved
Pos	Neg	Pos	Neg	Pos	Acute or chronic vinfection
Pos	Neg	Pos	Pos	Neg	Later stage in chronic infection

Neg, negative; Pos, positive.

We know little about why immune responses of some persons can clear the infection, while those of others cannot. Before infection, most chronic carriers display "normal" immune function and have no prior evidence of immune deficiency. However, such persons must have a subtle defect in the way they respond to HBV-specific antigens, although the nature of that defect remains a mystery. As might be expected, rates of chronic infection are much higher for individuals with immature or defective immune responses, like newborn infants or persons with advanced HIV infection. For example, over 90% of exposed babies develop chronic infection.

Once a chronic infection is established, some (but not all) patients suffer from intermittent or persistent episodes of liver injury (termed chronic hepatitis), which is readily demonstrated by elevated serum aminotransferase levels (see Fig. 43-6). After many years of chronic infection, some patients progress to cirrhosis, a potentially fatal condition in which fibrotic scarring of the liver is prominent. In addition, long-term chronic HBV infection predisposes to the development of **hepatocellular carcinoma** (HCC).

Prevention and Treatment

An effective vaccine against HBV is now available. It consists of HBsAg particles prepared from yeast engineered to express HBsAg. HBV vaccine was the first recombinant vaccine approved for use in humans. HBV vaccination is now recommended for all infants in the United States and many other countries. In addition, infants of HBsAg-positive mothers should receive both the vaccine and anti-HBs IgG. Although vaccination programs have reduced the rate of HBV transmission, the virus is far from eradicated. The vaccine requires multiple boosters and is expensive to produce, which has limited its use in some resource-poor countries. However, many countries in Africa and Asia are aggressively vaccinating their populations, and where that has happened, rates of HBV infection and liver cancer are rapidly declining. Nonetheless, since the vaccine is of no benefit to the world's 300 million chronic carriers, much remains to be done before HBV-related diseases disappear.

Treatment options for chronic carriers of HBV are expanding rapidly. For many years, **interferon-α**, a natural antiviral cytokine, was the mainstay of therapy. However, this treatment is expensive, toxic, and of limited efficacy. Most patients who respond to interferon-α have substantial reductions in circulating viral load, although HBsAg remains positive. If these responses are sustained, lasting improvement in liver function results, even though infection has not been eradicated. But for approximately 70% of HBV-infected persons, the benefit of interferon-α treatment is transient, and viral levels rebound following cessation of therapy.

The discovery that HBV replication involves reverse transcription has led to the development of a number of nucleoside analogs that selectively inhibit the viral polymerase. Some of these, like **adefovir, lamivudine**, and **tenofovir**, were initially developed for use against HIV. These drugs also were noted to have activity against the HBV Pol protein. (Interestingly, adefovir is much more active against HBV than HIV and is not approved by the Food and Drug Administration for the treatment of HIV.) Others, including entecavir and telbivudine, were developed specifically for HBV and are relatively selective for that virus. These nucleoside analogs have greatly changed the face of therapy, since they too can reduce viral load and improve liver function, and responses are much more frequent than with interferon-α. In addition, because they are orally bioavailable, they are more convenient and less expensive to use than interferon-based regimens. When used as single agents, resistance does develop to these drugs, albeit rather slowly. To date, combinations of these antivirals have not been firmly established to be more effective than single agents, but this is an active area of investigation.

Hepatitis Delta Virus

HDV is not a true virus but rather a subviral agent incapable of disseminating without help from HBV. The small

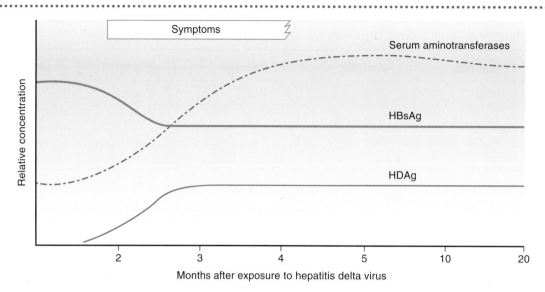

FIGURE 43-7. Course of chronic hepatitis B infection exacerbated by infection with hepatitis delta virus. The levels of aminotransferases may increase, and the liver histology may shift from that of chronic persistent to chronic active hepatitis.

single-stranded circular RNA genome of HDV encodes a single protein, termed hepatitis delta antigen (HDAg), which binds to the viral RNA and is important in viral replication and assembly. HDV does not encode any envelope proteins. Instead, it requires the presence of HBV to provide the envelope proteins (HBsAg-L, HBsAg-M, and HBsAg-S) required for HDV envelopment. As a result of this requirement, HDV only infects persons who are simultaneously infected with HBV (coinfection) or who are already HBV chronic carriers (superinfection). The requirement for a helper virus is a rare property among human viruses. Only one other helper-dependent infectious agent of humans is known (the adeno-associated virus, a parvovirus that requires adenovirus as a helper).

HDV is associated with an increased risk of fulminant hepatitis during the acute phase of hepatitis and likewise tends to increase hepatitis severity during the chronic phase (Fig. 43-7). Not surprisingly, HDV is acquired by the same routes as HBV, but for unknown reasons, HDV is not found at equal rates in all parts of the world where HBV is endemic. HDV-infected persons make antibodies directed against HDAg, and these antibodies are diagnostic of HDV infection.

Prevention and Treatment

As yet, there are no effective antiviral drugs specific for the HDV component of concurrent HBV and HDV infections. However, since the HDV envelope contains HBsAg, successful HBV vaccination protects against the primary acquisition of both HBV and HDV.

Hepatitis C Virus

HCV is responsible for most cases of non-A and non-B hepatitis. The number of persons chronically infected with HCV worldwide is estimated to be about 200 million.

In the United States, roughly 1 to 1.5% of persons have chronic HCV infection. HCV, like HBV, is spread by the exchange of body fluids. Before the elimination of HCV from donated blood supplies, transfusions were a common route of infection. HCV is frequently associated with injection drug use and efficiently transmitted by that route. Sexual spread of HCV occurs, although HCV is much less efficiently transmitted by sexual contact than is HBV. HCV-infected mothers also can transmit the virus to their newborn infants, but the rate of transmission is also much lower than for HBV. HCV infections are diagnosed by the appearance of antibodies directed against viral proteins and by the detection of viral RNA in the blood using a variation of the polymerase chain reaction.

HCV is an enveloped, single-stranded, positive-sense RNA virus in the **Flaviviridae family** (see Chapter 33). Sequencing of HCV genomes from many parts of the world indicates the existence of as many as 11 genotypes, of which genotype 1 is the most prevalent in the United States. Like HBV, clinical isolates of HCV cannot be routinely grown in cultured cells. The only susceptible laboratory animal is the chimpanzee. Much of what is known about HCV replication has been inferred from its sequence and homology to other viruses, from the expression and analysis of recombinant viral proteins, and from the study of viral RNA synthesis in cells transfected with cloned viral RNA. A few isolates of HCV have been found to replicate in cell culture and spread from cell to cell. Thus, the full life cycle of HCV can now be examined in cultured cells.

The main steps in the HCV replication cycle are shown in Figure 43-8. Like other single-stranded, positive-sense RNA viruses, the HCV RNA genome is translated into protein following entry into the cell. HCV RNA is not capped, and HCV has circumvented the cap requirement

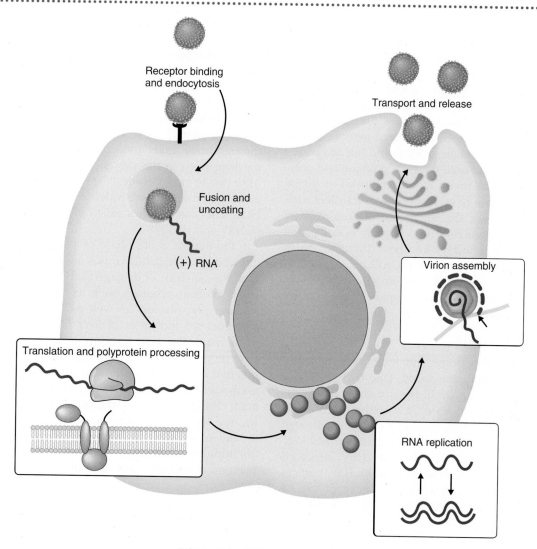

FIGURE 43-8. HCV replication cycle.

by using an **internal ribosome entry site (IRES)** at its 5′ end as a ribosomal binding sequence that directs internal initiation of RNA translation. The product of translation is a single large polyprotein. Within that polyprotein are two protease domains capable of cleaving the polyprotein into a number of functional subunits. The X-ray crystallographic structure of one of the HCV proteases has been determined, which has allowed the design of specific antiviral protease inhibitors (see below). Once the HCV polyprotein is processed, viral nonstructural proteins participate in genome replication. One of those, the viral RNA-dependent RNA polymerase, first copies the positive-sense RNA into a negative-sense RNA intermediate and then copies the negative-sense RNA into more positive-sense RNA. This replicative process is highly error-prone, resulting in a high mutation rate. As a result, an infected individual carries not one unique virus but a whole population of related viruses, termed a **quasi-species** (just as in HIV infection).

The liver diseases caused by HCV are similar to those caused by HBV, although they are often somewhat milder, especially in the early stages of infection. However, the long-term consequences of chronic infection with HCV can be as devastating as those caused by HBV. That fact is particularly ominous because the rate at which acute infections progress to chronic infections in otherwise healthy adults is much higher for HCV than for HBV (80% compared with 5%). Following several decades of chronic HCV infection, the incidence of cirrhosis is approximately 20%, and the risk of HCC is substantial. HCV infection is also associated with extrahepatic diseases, the most notable of which is **mixed cryoglobulinemia**, an immune complex disorder of the kidneys and other sites. In that disease, antiviral antibodies complexed to virions are deposited in affected tissues, triggering inflammatory responses that result in tissue damage.

Prevention and Treatment

Limited treatment options exist for HCV infection, but active research in this area is generating new potential therapies at a rapid rate. Current therapy with **interferon-α** (together with **ribavirin**, an antiviral agent of uncertain mechanism) results in sustained virologic responses in over 30 to 50% of individuals infected with genotype 1 strains but can be up to 70 to 75% with genotypes 2 and 3. Although these responses result in sustained clinical benefit, the regimen is expensive and difficult to tolerate; up to 20% of patients discontinue therapy because of side effects. (Interferon produces fevers, joint and muscle aches, low blood cell counts, and central nervous system depression; ribavirin produces anemia and is teratogenic.) At present, inhibitors of both the HCV protease and polymerase are in clinical trials. When employed as single agents, each new class of inhibitors shows transient antiviral efficacy. However, the emergence of drug-resistant viruses following initiation of monotherapy is as rapid in HCV infection as it is in HIV infection. Therefore, as in HIV, multiple drugs in combination will be required to overcome this problem; until such drugs are available, interferon and ribavirin will likely remain a core component of anti-HCV treatment.

Hepatitis E Virus

HEV is a cause of foodborne and waterborne hepatitis, especially in the developing world. Like HAV, HEV is a nonenveloped, single-stranded, positive-sense RNA virus that causes only acute disease. It resembles HAV in its routes of transmission and associated diseases, although HEV and HAV infections can be distinguished serologically. Symptoms associated with acute HEV infections may be more severe than those induced by HAV, particularly in pregnant women, in whom HEV infection can be life-threatening. Efforts to develop an HEV vaccine are currently under way; preliminary results with a recombinant HEV vaccine have been promising, but commercialization of the vaccine has been slow.

CONCLUSION

The hepatitis viruses are a diverse group of viruses that replicate by a variety of mechanisms. The one attribute shared by hepatitis viruses is a common tissue tropism: each targets the hepatocyte as its focal point for infection. From the standpoint of disease, the hepatitis viruses can be grouped into two categories. Hepatitis A and E viruses are "hit and run" viruses transmitted by the fecal–oral route that replicate prior to the development of an immune response. Ultimately, HAV and HEV are cleared from the liver and thus only cause acute infections. In contrast, hepatitis B, C, and delta viruses are transmitted through body fluids and can cause chronic infections in the liver even in the presence of an immune response. After two or more decades, the resulting chronic infections can have profound consequences, including cirrhosis and HCC. Effective vaccines exist only to prevent the spread of HAV and HBV.

During the acute phase of infection, the symptoms induced by all hepatitis viruses are fairly similar and arise as a consequence of damage to the liver. Elevated serum levels of liver enzymes such as aminotransferases and alkaline phosphatase as well as bilirubin (resulting in jaundice) are indicators of liver damage. Determination of the particular virus responsible for the associated disease requires the use of serological and molecular methods that assay for the presence of specific viral proteins, antibodies directed against those proteins, or viral nucleic acid. Obtaining such a diagnosis is critical for determining the long-term prognosis of the infected individual. Treatment options for chronic HBV and HCV infections are improving, but much work remains to be done in the prevention and treatment of both disorders.

Suggested Readings

Ganem D, Prince A. Hepatitis B virus infection: natural history and clinical consequences. *N Engl J Med.* 2004;350:1118–1129.

Levinthal G, Ray M. Hepatitis A: from epidemic jaundice to a vaccine-preventable disease. *Gastroenterologist.* 1996;4:107–117.

Lindenbach D, Rice C. Unraveling hepatitis C virus replication: from genome to function. *Nature.* 2005;436:933–938.

Pawlotsky JM. Pathophysiology of hepatitis C virus infection and related liver disease. *Trends Microbiol.* 2004;12:96–102.

Taylor JM. Replication of human hepatitis delta virus: recent developments. *Trends Microbiol.* 2003;11:185–190.

Chapter **44**

Antiviral Treatment Strategies

Karen C. Bloch and Julie E. Reznicek

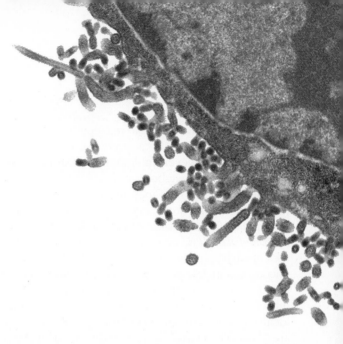

KEY CONCEPTS

- Antiviral drugs block specific steps in virus replication.
- Virus replication relies on, and is intertwined with, essential host cell processes in diverse ways.
- Toxicity of antiviral drugs is often related to drug effects on host cell processes.
- Antiviral drug discovery exploits structural, functional, and genomic information to maximize specific inhibition of virus replication and minimize host cell toxicity.

- Replication of hepatitis B and C viruses, herpesviruses, human immunodeficiency virus (HIV), and influenza viruses is targeted by current antiviral drugs.
- Resistance to antiviral therapy mandates diagnostic testing and ongoing development of new drugs.
- Other advances in antiviral therapy may come from learning how to better detect and minimize virus resistance and how to better exploit cellular mechanisms with specificity for aiding virus replication or evading drug effectiveness.

THE KEY to successful antiviral chemotherapy is specificity against virus replication. An effective antiviral agent must impair the capacity of a virus to replicate while sparing host cells from potentially toxic effects. This chapter describes some of the chemotherapeutic strategies that have proven successful for combating viral infections in humans. Although interferons, which work in part by augmenting innate immune responses, are mentioned here, this chapter focuses on antiviral drugs used to treat viral infections. Approaches used to induce immunity through vaccination, a highly effective and important means of preventing viral infections, are described in Chapter 45.

Antiviral drugs have been sought since the early days of animal virology. Millions of compounds have been screened against viruses in many taxonomic groups. Many substances inhibit virus replication but are also toxic to host cells. A strategy for virus inhibition that uses adverse effects on the host cell to interrupt virus replication, as did some of the earliest empiric efforts, may fail because of drug toxicity. Effective antiviral agents often lead to the emergence of drug-resistant strains through mutations that confer a survival advantage to the virus. This observation is an indication that the agent alters a virus-specific process rather than simply causing host cell toxicity.

Studies of virus–host interactions are increasingly revealing potential points at which viral infections can be interrupted. Researchers have elucidated biochemical targets at which replication of certain viruses may be impaired, including viral polymerases and proteases. Many drugs are safe and effective against some viruses—in particular, hepatitis B and C viruses, herpesviruses, human immunodeficiency virus (HIV), and influenza viruses. No truly "broadspectrum" antiviral drugs yet exist, as they do for bacteria. The diversity of strategies used by viruses to replicate suggests that the development of such agents may not be possible, even as the number of antiviral agents continues to increase. This chapter summarizes the major strategies to inhibit virus replication that have been successfully deployed in the treatment of human viral diseases.

APPROACHES TO ANTIVIRAL DRUG DISCOVERY

Each step and biochemical reaction involved in virus replication is potentially a target for chemotherapeutic intervention. However, inhibition of viral processes that depend on host metabolic pools, host energy sources, and host cell enzymes may result in unacceptable toxicity. Fortunately, *some steps in virus replication differ sufficiently from cellular processes in that they can be inhibited with little or no impact on the host cell.* Examples of such specific processes include virus penetration, uncoating, nucleic acid synthesis, protein processing by virally encoded enzymes, assembly of virus particles, and release of the virus from the infected cell. The steps in an idealized virus growth cycle inhibited by various agents are shown in Figure 44-1. A summary of these agents is provided in Table 44-1. Current drugs and agents in development that affect the virus-specific steps in replication are described here. Drugs also have been identified and developed based on a more empiric approach to screening for inhibitors of virus replication without targeting a particular mechanism or virus process.

Although empiricism remains important in antiviral drug discovery and accounts for some of our current therapeutic armamentarium, the acceleration of advances in antiviral discovery in recent years has come from leveraging knowledge about the structure and function of specific viral target proteins and viral genomics. Following early exploitation of herpesvirus polymerase inhibition based on biochemistry (e.g., acyclovir), many advances occurred in the search for HIV inhibitors. Those advances included additional applications of polymerase

biochemistry for inhibitor development (e.g., HIV reverse transcriptase inhibitors). The first design of specific inhibitors based on viral protein structure also quickly followed the first determination of crystal structures of the HIV reverse transcriptase (e.g., nevirapine) and the HIV protease (e.g., indinavir, nelfinavir, ritonavir, saquinavir, and other HIV protease inhibitors). The design of inhibitors active against specific drug-resistant mutants (e.g., lopinavir) and other viral targets (enfuvirtide, directed against the HIV gp41 membrane fusion apparatus) have emphasized the power of structure-based drug design.

AGENTS DEVELOPED BY AN EMPIRIC APPROACH

Interferon and ribavirin represent two empirically derived agents that are used as primary treatment for hepatitis C virus (HCV) infection. Research is ongoing into the development of more rationally designed pharmacologic agents that specifically target HCV enzymes.

Interferons

Interferons were the first extensively studied antiviral substances. They are not synthetic drugs but rather natural proteins made by the body. The discovery of interferons by Alick Isaacs and Jean Lindenmann in 1957 involved a brilliant and fortuitous observation, somewhat analogous to Alexander Fleming's recognition of the antibacterial effect of certain molds on bacterial cultures leading to the isolation of penicillin. Isaacs was interested in the process of **viral interference**, a phenomenon in which infection by one virus renders a cell resistant to subsequent

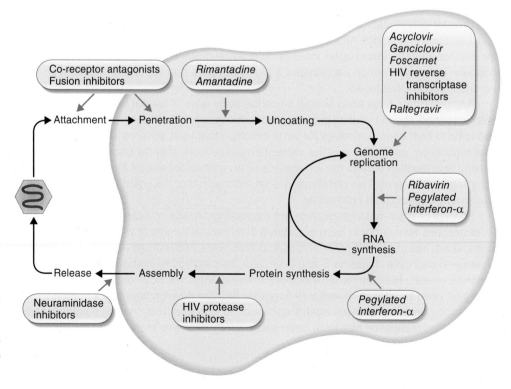

FIGURE 44-1. Viral life cycle. Schematic drawing showing the steps at which replication can be inhibited by antiviral drugs (*in italics*) or classes of drugs (*in regular typeface*). The *light blue area* is the intracellular space.

TABLE 44-1 Summary of Selected Anti-viral Agents

Site of Action	Classes or Drug(s)	Clinically relevant viral targets	Mechanism	Comments
Host cell entry	HIV fusion inhibitor (enfuvirtide)	HIV	Binds to HIV gp41, preventing fusion with the cell membrane	Can only be administered subcutaneously
	CCR5 antagonist (maraviroc)	HIV	Binds to the CD4+ T-cell CCR5 coreceptor, inhibiting HIV gp120 from binding	Coreceptor tropism assay must be performed prior to initiation
Viral disassembly (on cell entry)	Influenza A M2 antagonist (amantidine, rimantidine)	Influenza A	Blockage of influenza A surface protein M2 with inhibition of hydrogen ion influx	No activity among influenza B and some strains of influenza A H1N1 viruses
Viral replication	Herpes thymidine kinase-activated polymerase inhibitor (acyclovir)	HSV, VZV	Nucleoside analog that when phosphorylated inhibits viral DNA polymerase	Only active against replicating (not latent) viruses. Prodrugs include valacyclovir, famciclovir
	HCMV UL97-activated polymerase inhibitor (ganciclovir)	CMV	Nucleoside analog that when phosphorylated inhibits viral DNA polymerase	Major toxicity is host bone marrow suppression. Valganciclovir is a prodrug, available as an oral formulation
	Phosphonate polymerase inhibitor (foscarnet)	CMV	Phosphonate that directly inhibits viral DNA polymerase, without requiring cellular modification	Typically a 2nd line treatment for CMV, used to treat ganciclovir resistant isolates or if bone marrow suppression is a concern
	Nucleoside/nucleotide reverse transcriptase inhibitors (NRTI/NtRTI) (NRTIs: zidovudine, lamivudine; NtRTI: tenofovir)	HIV, HBV	Terminates DNA chain growth, after activation to triphosphate form by cellular enzymes	"Backbone" of HAART, several co-formulations of 2 N(t)RTIs available
	Non-nucleoside reverse transcriptase inhibitors (NNRTI) (efavirenz, etravirine, nevirapine, etc)	HIV	Inhibit the catalytic step in reverse transcription without cellular modification	Low genetic barrier to resistance
	HIV integrase strand-transfer inhibitor (INSTI) (raltegravir)	HIV	Blocks the 'strand-transfer' step of insertion of HIV DNA into cellular genome (integration)	Used in heavily treatment-experienced patients
Viral nucleic acid synthesis	Ribavirin	HCV, RSV	Purine nucleoside analog inhibits RNA and DNA polymerases and mRNA capping	Aerosolized, oral, and intravenous formulations. Typically used in combination with interferon for treatment of HCV
	Interferon	HCV	Nonspecific viral interference & modulation of host immune response	Typically used in combination with ribavirin for treatment of HCV
Virion assembly	Protease inhibitors (darunavir, atazanavir, lopinavir, ritonavir)	HIV, HCV (in development)	Prevent cleavage of precursor peptides to yield mature HIV proteins	Low dose ritonavir given with other protease inhibitors to "boost" the blood level of the latter
Viral release	Neuraminididase inhibitors (oseltamivir, zanamivir)	Influenza A and B viruses	Inhibition of cleavage of sialic acid, preventing release of virus from the infected host cell	Used for prophylaxis or for treatment of influenza infection when started within 48 hours of symptom onset

infection with a different virus. Interference of virus-infected cells allowed, for example, the first laboratory detection of rubella virus; although that virus does not produce visible damage to cells in culture, it does render them refractory to secondary infection with other viruses that can produce cytopathic damage.

In studying viral interference, Isaacs and Lindenmann noted that resistance to viral infection could be transferred to uninfected cultures by the addition of media from infected cell cultures. The cell-free factors that mediated the transferable resistance to virus infection were found to be proteins, which they termed interferons. Two properties of interferons were quickly appreciated. First, interferons released from cells in response to infection by one virus provide resistance to infection by many other viruses; thus, interferons are not virus specific. Second, interferons are present in extremely small amounts, indicating that they are very potent molecules. It was reasoned that if interferons could be purified in sufficient quantities, they might be efficacious therapeutic agents with a broad spectrum of activity. As natural substances, they were likely to be relatively nontoxic, although one might wonder why large amounts are not mobilized spontaneously during infections.

Today, we know that many of the early assumptions about interferons were naive and only partially correct. Large amounts of interferons can be generated by recombinant DNA technology, and their mechanisms of action, biological properties, and therapeutic potencies are relatively well defined. In both animals and humans, the effect of treatment with interferons is more complex than in cell cultures because the compounds not only inhibit virus replication but also modulate host immune responses to infection. Numerous clinical trials have shown that interferons in therapeutic doses, despite being proteins normally produced by humans, cause fatigue, fever, myalgias, bone marrow suppression, and neuropsychiatric problems. In fact, many of the constitutional complaints that accompany common viral infections likely result from interferon-mediated host responses.

Although interferon treatment ameliorates some severe herpesvirus infections, that action is not sufficiently efficacious to make it clinically useful. Nucleoside analogs are much more effective (as discussed in the next section). Similarly, nucleoside analogs such as adefovir and lamivudine are now preferred over interferon for hepatitis B virus (HBV) infection. However, HCV infection responds to recombinant interferon (see Chapter 43). Interferon therapy in persons with HCV infection results in significant improvements in hepatic function. Longer-acting forms of interferon (e.g., **pegylated interferon**), used in combination with ribavirin, have yielded sustained virus clearance in some HCV-infected patients.

Why do interferons not show more dramatic clinical activity for all viruses? Inadequate dosage cannot explain their limitations because circulating levels of the newer recombinant interferon preparations can exceed those produced endogenously in untreated infections. There are two possible explanations for the failure of interferons to provide broad-spectrum antiviral activity. First, the spectrum of production of different interferons may be different in response to different viruses. At least three distinct classes of interferons (α, β, and γ) exist, and some of these have multiple subtypes. It is possible that the exogenously administered formulation does not provide the optimal spectrum of forms. Second, interferons exhibit the most potent activity against RNA viruses, with very limited activity against DNA viruses and retroviruses. Thus, despite their early promise, interferons have limited clinical utility.

Ribavirin

Ribavirin is a purine nucleoside analog with a relatively broad antiviral spectrum in cell culture. It inhibits some DNA viruses and many RNA viruses, including influenza A and B viruses, measles virus, parainfluenza virus, respiratory syncytial virus, and several arenaviruses. Ribavirin appears to inhibit virus replication by several different mechanisms, perhaps explaining its range of activity. The triphosphate form of ribavirin inhibits virus-encoded DNA-dependent DNA polymerases and possibly RNA-dependent RNA polymerases as well. Ribavirin monophosphate inhibits **inosine monophosphate dehydrogenase**, leading to an overall reduction in cellular pools of GTP. That in turn restricts viral (as well as cellular) nucleic acid synthesis. In addition, ribavirin impairs capping of virus-specific mRNA (the addition of methylated guanine nucleotides to the 5′ end of RNA molecules).

The clinical use of ribavirin is limited due to toxicity to host cells at therapeutic doses. Lack of specificity translates into poor clinical activity for most viral infections. Oral and intravenous ribavirin appears useful in the treatment of hemorrhagic fevers caused by Lassa virus. It also has been administered through aerosols for severe respiratory syncytial virus infections in immunosuppressed children and adults. Ribavirin remains useful as an adjunct to pegylated interferon for the treatment of HCV infections.

STEPS IN VIRUS REPLICATION TARGETED BY CURRENT DRUGS AND AGENTS IN DEVELOPMENT

Virus entry into cells, virus genome replication, virus protein processing, and virus release from infected cells are targets of currently available antiviral drugs and new virus-specific inhibitors now in development.

Virus Entry

Virus entry into host cells can be subdivided into attachment of virions to host cell receptors, cell membrane penetration, and virion uncoating or disassembly. These processes differ for different viruses. HIV, for example, binds to target cells such as CD4+ T lymphocytes through adsorption of viral envelope glycoprotein, **gp120**, to CD4 molecules on the cell surface (Fig. 44-2). That binding event leads to conformational changes in gp120 that facilitate additional interactions with one or more coreceptors. Several chemokine

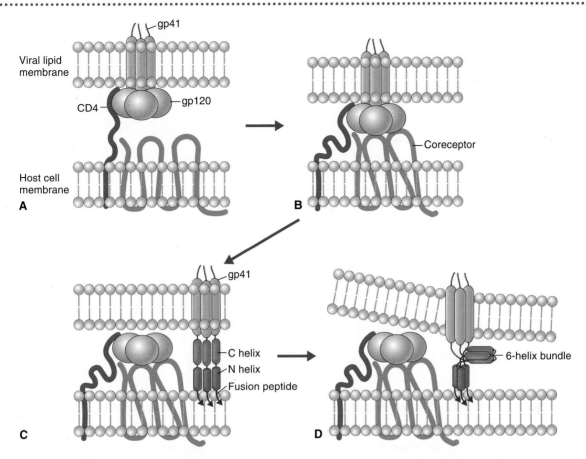

FIGURE 44-2. The process of human immunodeficiency virus (HIV) entry into target cells.
A. Initial attachment of the HIV gp120 envelope protein to the CD4 molecule. **B.** Secondary interaction of HIV gp120 with a chemokine receptor such as CCR5 or CXCR4, which is facilitated by initial CD4 binding. **C.** Stepwise interaction of the HIV gp41 transmembrane protein with the cell membrane, which requires interactions between domains of gp41 that bring membranes of both virus and cell into close proximity for fusion. **D.** Fusion inhibitors, such as enfuvirtide, interact with gp41 intermediates and prevent membrane fusion mediated by gp41 refolding.

receptors serve as **coreceptors** for HIV, the most common of which are **CCR5** and **CXCR4**. The CCR5 receptor antagonist, maraviroc, is approved for use in treatment-experienced HIV-infected persons as part of a combination regimen. Other agents that block the binding of gp120 to CD4 or one of the coreceptors are in development.

After gp120 engages its coreceptor, further conformational changes trigger the HIV transmembrane protein **gp41** to refold, exposing the "**fusion peptide**" to allow fusion of viral and cell membranes. Membrane fusion leads to entry of virion contents into the cytoplasm, where the internalized particle undergoes further uncoating before the initiation of genome replication. One currently available drug, enfuvirtide, specifically interferes with HIV penetration into cells by blocking the conformational changes in the gp41 fusion peptide required to approximate viral and cellular membranes to allow them to fuse.

Maraviroc

Two main chemokine receptors expressed on CD4+ T cells, **CCR5** and **CXCR4**, serve as HIV coreceptors. Although HIV may bind to either of these coreceptors,

host immune status influences which one is used. Persons recently infected with HIV and those with relatively normal CD4+ T-cell counts harbor viruses that almost always bind to CCR5. These are called **R5-tropic viruses**. Alternatively, **X4-tropic viruses** bind only the CXCR4 coreceptor and are found almost exclusively in persons with more advanced disease. **Dual- and mixed-tropic viruses** contain a single envelope glycoprotein that can bind to either coreceptor (dual-tropic) or express a mixture of virus envelope glycoproteins, with some binding to CCR5 and others binding to CXCR4 (mixed tropic). Current diagnostic assays cannot differentiate between dual-tropic and mixed-tropic HIV strains.

Maraviroc inhibits HIV entry by binding to CCR5 to inhibit its engagement by gp120 following its binding to CD4. Maraviroc does not interfere with CD4 binding. It also does not block binding of the CXCR4 coreceptor after CD4 engagement by either dual-tropic or mixed-tropic viruses. Current guidelines recommend that prior to beginning maraviroc, a coreceptor tropism assay should be performed to evaluate whether a CCR5 antagonist would be efficacious.

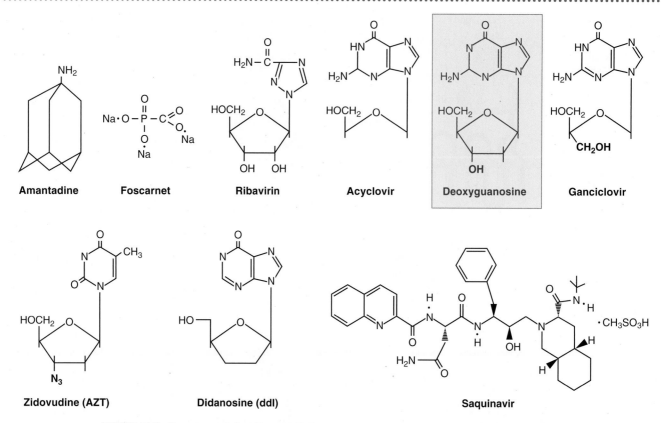

FIGURE 44-3. Structures of selected clinically useful antiviral chemotherapeutic agents. The structure of the physiologic nucleotide deoxyguanosine (*highlighted blue*) is shown for comparison to its analogs.

Enfuvirtide

Enfuvirtide is a peptide that acts extracellularly to bind a specific domain in the HIV gp41 fusion peptide. Following conformational changes in gp120 triggered by receptor and coreceptor interactions (see Fig. 44-2), the gp41 fusion protein brings together the membranes of both virus and cell to facilitate membrane fusion. By occupying a very specific site on gp41, the peptide inhibitor prevents the conformational changes required for membrane fusion, thus inhibiting the penetration step in HIV entry. Given the highly conserved nature of the target motif in gp41, the peptide is effective against a broad range of HIV isolates. It has no known activity against other viruses or cellular proteins. Specific substitutions in the gp41 motif to which enfuvirtide binds mediate antiviral resistance. Although its unique mechanism of action makes it an option for use in patients with multidrug-resistant HIV, its utility is limited by its mode of administration (subcutaneous injection). Therefore, alternative classes of antiretrovirals that are available in oral formulation (including **coreceptor antagonists** and **integrase inhibitors**) have largely supplanted its use.

Amantadine and Rimantadine

The anti-influenza drugs amantadine and rimantadine inhibit the late stages of the entry process of influenza virus A into host cells. Amantadine (Fig. 44-3) and rimantadine (not pictured) are tricyclic amines. Neither has efficacy against influenza B.

The influenza A virion contains a transmembrane protein, **M2**, that is well conserved among human and avian strains (Fig. 44-4). The M2 protein functions as a hydrogen ion channel. Influenza virus enters cells through endosomes, and the M2 protein allows hydrogen ions to move from endosomes into the virion interior during the

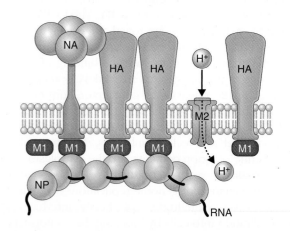

FIGURE 44-4. Structural components of influenza virus. Amantadine and rimantadine block the M2 ion channel and are active only against influenza A. Oseltamivir and zanamivir bind to neuraminidase and inhibit the enzymatic cleavage of sialic acid, thus blocking release of progeny virus from infected cells. These drugs are active against both influenza A and B. NA, neuraminidase; HA, hemagglutinin; H+, hydrogen ion; M1, matrix protein; M2, transmembrane ion channel protein; NP, nucleoprotein.

entry process. The flux of hydrogen ions decreases pH in the virion, promoting conformational changes in the influenza virus nucleocapsid protein that allow movement of the viral ribonucleoproteins (containing the viral genome segments) into the host cell nucleus to establish infection.

Amantadine and rimantadine inhibit the ion channel function of influenza A M2 by physically blocking the flow of hydrogen ions. Failure to establish an acidic environment impedes influenza **virion disassembly** after internalization into endosomes. Resistance to amantadine and rimantadine occurs through single amino acid substitutions in the transmembrane region of M2 that prevent drug binding within the channel. Up to 30% of treated patients may shed drug-resistant virus, although symptoms usually persist only in those who are immunocompromised. Resistant influenza virus strains remain susceptible to neuraminidase (NA) inhibitors (as discussed later in the chapter).

The anti-influenza activity of amantadine was first reported in 1961, but it was not widely used as a treatment for influenza (**therapeutic use**). However, controlled studies of laboratory-induced or naturally occurring influenza A virus infections demonstrated that the drug was beneficial for preventing infection during peak periods of influenza A activity, such as epidemics (**prophylactic use**). When treatment is initiated before exposure to the virus, amantadine and rimantadine prevent clinical disease in more than 75% of cases. In contrast, for patients who begin treatment shortly after the first signs of influenza appear (within 2 days of symptom onset), the reduction in severity of symptoms is only decreased by approximately 50%. When used for prophylaxis, an entire exposed household or risk group (e.g., nursing home residents) should be treated simultaneously to minimize the spread of resistant virus. It is uncertain whether treatment with these agents following confirmed influenza A virus infection reduces complications in high-risk patients.

Both amantadine and rimantadine are fairly well tolerated at therapeutic doses. About 3 to 5% of amantadine recipients (but fewer rimantadine recipients) report mild central nervous system effects, including anxiety, insomnia, and difficulty concentrating. The main use of these drugs has been for prophylaxis in individuals who are at increased risk of severe infection during influenza A virus epidemics. Persons at high risk include the elderly and patients with chronic cardiopulmonary disease. It is also recommended that treatment be initiated in those groups at the onset of endemic influenza in the community. A major limitation of amantadine and rimantadine is that the drugs are not active against influenza B strains or some strains of influenza A H1N1. Moreover, many circulating influenza virus strains are resistant to these drugs. For the most part, amantadine and rimantadine have been supplanted by the newer NA inhibitors.

Virus Genome Replication

Following entry and uncoating, viruses replicate their genomes using virus-specific polymerases. The processes vary among virus families depending on the nature of the genome (DNA or RNA) and the type of enzyme that catalyzes genome replication. However, several drugs specifically inhibit viral polymerases. Acyclovir was the first selective inhibitor of a viral polymerase to be developed, and it remains a model for antiviral drug specificity. Many other compounds are now available that target the HIV reverse transcriptase and the HBV polymerase.

Acyclovir

Acyclovir is the prototype antiviral agent and standard against which all other antiviral drugs are compared. It was the first antiviral drug approved for clinical use that resulted from a rational and directed search for antiviral compounds (see Fig. 44-3). It also illustrates how antiviral drugs can be modified to yield increased activity and improved pharmacologic properties, such as longer half-life or better gastrointestinal absorption.

Acyclovir inhibits the DNA polymerases of several herpesviruses. When its activity against cellular and viral polymerases is compared, acyclovir exhibits a therapeutic ratio (i.e., the ratio of specific therapeutic effects relative to nonspecific toxic effects) that substantially exceeds— by about a thousandfold—that of earlier empirically discovered herpesvirus DNA polymerase inhibitors (e.g., vidarabine). The reason is interesting: For acyclovir to inhibit any DNA polymerase, it must be phosphorylated (Fig. 44-5). Herpes simplex virus (HSV) encodes a **thymidine kinase** that has the unique property of phosphorylating acyclovir far more efficiently than does the thymidine kinase of the host cell. The resulting monophosphate is then further phosphorylated by cellular enzymes to generate acyclovir triphosphate. This moiety inhibits **herpesvirus DNA polymerase** because its incorporation into nascent strands of DNA *blocks further elongation*. Viral DNA polymerase is incapable of attaching bases beyond the point of addition of acyclovir because the drug lacks

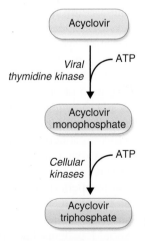

FIGURE 44-5. Activation of acyclovir. Acyclovir must be monophosphorylated by a virus-encoded thymidine kinase. Acyclovir monophosphate is then di- and triphosphorylated by host enzymes to produce the active form of the drug, acyclovir triphosphate. Acyclovir triphosphate is incorporated during viral DNA synthesis, causing premature strand termination and preventing herpesvirus replication.

TABLE 44-2 Typical Concentrations of Acyclovir Required for 50% Inhibition of Herpesvirus Replication In Cell Culture

Virus	µg/mL
Herpes simplex virus 1	0.1
Herpes simplex virus 2	0.3
Varicella-zoster virus	3
Epstein-Barr virus	3
Cytomegalovirus	>40

the 3′ carbon of the sugar ring at which phosphodiester bonds link nucleosides together.

How do the biochemical mechanisms of acyclovir translate into the in vitro potency of the drug for each herpesvirus? HSV types 1 and 2 are effectively inhibited with submicrogram concentrations of acyclovir (Table 44-2). Epstein-Barr virus (EBV) and varicella-zoster virus (VZV) are less sensitive to the drug because their kinases phosphorylate it less effectively; cytomegalovirus (CMV) is even less well inhibited.

The clinical response to acyclovir therapy in humans is similar to the in vitro activity of the drug. The most significant benefits are observed in patients with HSV infections. Clinical responses to acyclovir therapy also are seen in patients with infections caused by VZV, but higher doses are required to treat those infections. Acyclovir has a limited role in the treatment of EBV infections and is not clinically useful in the treatment of CMV infections. The greatest benefit from acyclovir comes in the treatment of prolonged or severe mucocutaneous HSV infections, including primary genital herpes infections of immunocompetent persons or any infection of immunocompromised hosts. Acyclovir speeds the clearing of virus, hastens the resolution of symptoms, and shortens the healing time (Fig. 44-6). A modest reduction in the severity of milder forms of HSV infections can be achieved with prompt administration of oral acyclovir.

Acyclovir does not prevent or terminate herpesvirus latency. Therefore, herpesvirus infections may recur whether or not acyclovir treatment is instituted. Long-term treatment with oral acyclovir is effective in suppressing herpetic recurrences (Fig. 44-7). The suppressive effect of the drug is limited to the period of treatment. Even after years of continuous treatment, recurrences can develop after its termination. This scenario leads to a dilemma for practitioners. Should patients take prolonged treatment for a nonprogressive illness like recurrent genital herpes? An additional source of concern is that the virus may develop resistance to the drug, although this is rare in immunocompetent persons (as discussed later in the chapter). Most practitioners reserve long-term acyclovir

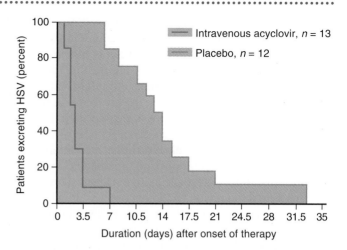

FIGURE 44-6. Comparison of intravenous acyclovir and placebo for inhibition of herpes simplex virus (HSV) 2 shedding in immunocompetent individuals with first episode of genital herpes. Early treatment with acyclovir reduces the median duration of viral shedding to less than 3.5 days, while untreated patients continue to shed infectious virus for a median of 14 days.

suppressive therapy for patients with frequent, painful recurrences of genital herpes.

Ganciclovir

Acyclovir has minimal activity against CMV, a major cause of morbidity and mortality in transplant recipients and persons with HIV infection. In studying modifications of the acyclovir molecule, one compound, ganciclovir, was found to have greatly improved activity against CMV (see Fig. 44-3). Its mechanism of action is similar to that of acyclovir, with preferential phosphorylation by viral

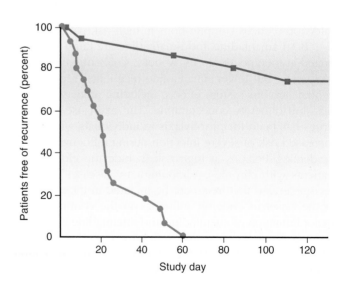

FIGURE 44-7. Comparison of oral acyclovir (*blue*) and placebo (*red*) for suppression of recurrent genital herpes. In this study, greater than 70% of patients with a history of recurrent genital herpes treated with suppressive acyclovir remained symptom-free at 120 days compared to patients treated with placebo, all of whom developed recurrent genital lesions within 60 days.

enzymes and inhibition of the viral DNA polymerase. The CMV-encoded kinase that phosphorylates ganciclovir is much more efficient than the enzymes of other herpesviruses that phosphorylate acyclovir. However, ganciclovir is more toxic than acyclovir possibly because some host cellular polymerases can utilize ganciclovir triphosphate more efficiently than acyclovir triphosphate.

Ganciclovir was the first agent with proven efficacy for the treatment of CMV. CMV-induced retinitis, esophagitis, and colitis in AIDS patients are stabilized by the drug, but reactivation and progressive infections are seen in many patients once treatment is stopped. Therefore, therapy must be continued for the duration of immunosuppression and possibly for life. In some AIDS patients with CMV disease, treatment has to be modified because of the bone marrow toxicity of ganciclovir or the emergence of drug-resistant strains.

Organ and stem-cell transplant recipients are also at risk for serious CMV infections, especially pneumonia. Ganciclovir treatment is less effective in those cases because the disease often causes significant lung injury before it can be diagnosed. A good strategy is to observe transplant recipients closely and screen for infection or reactivation of CMV (e.g., polymerase chain reaction or specific CMV protein detection). When ganciclovir is initiated as soon as an evolving CMV infection is evident from laboratory tests and before any clinical symptoms appear, the likelihood that pneumonia will develop is greatly diminished. That strategy is referred to as **preemptive therapy**.

Other Antiviral Drugs Similar to Acyclovir

Acyclovir and ganciclovir have become standard therapy for a spectrum of herpesvirus infections ranging from relatively common to rare and life threatening. However, the two drugs have important limitations, which have led to focused efforts to improve drug potency and availability. Acyclovir is not very soluble and thus is poorly absorbed from the gastrointestinal tract. Therefore, the maximum serum levels that can be achieved with oral acyclovir are relatively low. **Valacyclovir** is an acyclovir analog that is very well absorbed. It has a valine side chain that is enzymatically removed as the drug traverses the liver, yielding higher and clinically more effective blood levels. Valacyclovir is considered a "**prodrug**" that is converted to an active antiviral compound. A similar modification of ganciclovir to **valganciclovir** has improved the **oral bioavailability** of that drug too. Using the modified drug, immunocompromised patients with persistent CMV infection can be treated with oral rather than intravenous therapy.

Another limitation of acyclovir is its relatively short half-life. After oral administration, acyclovir disappears so quickly from the blood that it must be given five times per day to be most effective. Of the many new antiherpesvirus synthetic compounds, **penciclovir**, which is similar in activity to acyclovir but with a much longer half-life,

was chosen for clinical development. Unfortunately, penciclovir is also poorly absorbed. Therefore, a penciclovir prodrug was designed by adding two acetyl groups that are removed after it is metabolized. The prodrug, called **famciclovir**, is effective when given orally two to three times daily.

Foscarnet

The antiherpesvirus drugs discussed previously are nucleoside analogs that must be phosphorylated before they can inhibit herpesvirus DNA polymerase. Another antiherpesvirus drug, foscarnet, is a phosphonate rather than a nucleoside (see Fig. 44-3). It directly inhibits the enzymatic activity of herpesvirus DNA polymerases. Foscarnet requires intravenous administration and is associated with **nephrotoxicity**.

Drug-resistant herpesvirus strains are relatively uncommon, particularly in the immunocompetent host. There are two major reasons why drug resistance among this class of viruses is limited:

- Most herpesvirus infections (and infections by many other viruses) resolve spontaneously as a result of cellular immune defenses. The goal of antiviral therapy in most instances is to speed resolution. Emergence of drug resistance may lead to delay in virus clearing, but in general, the resistant viruses present a problem mainly for individuals with impaired immune defenses.
- Development of drug resistance may actually reduce the inherent virulence of some viruses. Most acyclovir-resistant strains of HSV have mutations in the gene encoding **thymidine kinase**. However, alterations in thymidine kinase render these strains less virulent in animal models and less likely to establish latent infection in sensory neurons. In fact, patients with strains resistant to acyclovir often do not suffer severe infections. Moreover, recurrences may be associated with reactivation of the original drug-sensitive strains that remain unaltered in sensory ganglia.

Antiviral resistance is a problem for severely immunocompromised persons. The best-studied examples are acyclovir- and ganciclovir-resistant herpesvirus infections in persons with AIDS. Foscarnet, with its completely distinct mechanism of action, may be an option for the treatment of those resistant infections.

Nucleoside/Nucleotide Inhibitors of the HIV Reverse Transcriptase and the HBV Polymerase

The strategy of polymerase inhibition that led to the development of effective antiherpesvirus agents has now been widely exploited, particularly in the search for drugs that inhibit HIV reverse transcriptase. Screening compounds expected to inhibit the enzymatic activity of HIV reverse transcriptase, such as nucleoside reverse transcriptase inhibitors (**NRTIs**) and nucleotide reverse transcriptase inhibitors (**NtRTIs**), identified many candidates for clinical testing. The NRTIs/NtRTIs act as DNA chain terminators after they are converted from their native monophosphate (NRTI) or diphosphate (NtRTI) to the triphosphate form intracellularly. Each lacks a 3′ hydroxyl required for chain elongation and, therefore, these drugs stop chain growth after incorporation by reverse transcriptase. Some NRTIs/NtRTIs are too toxic because they also block cellular polymerases, but several analogs have become mainstays of HIV therapy. However, long-term toxicity of these and other classes of anti-HIV drugs lead most experts to recommend initiation of lifelong therapy only when a certain degree of immunologic impairment is reached. As toxicity of newer agents has decreased, guidelines have recently moved toward earlier initiation of antiretroviral therapy.

Zidovudine (ZDV or AZT) was the first anti-HIV drug to be used clinically (see Fig. 44-3). It inhibits HIV replication at concentrations of 0.1 to 0.5 µg/mL, which are readily achieved following oral or parenteral administration and fall below the cytotoxic level. A series of related nucleosides were developed after AZT that comprise an "alphabet soup" of drug options for HIV-infected persons: abacavir (ABC), didanosine (ddI), emtricitabine (FTC), lamivudine (3TC), and stavudine (d4T). Later, the theoretic advantage of facilitating activation by cellular enzymes to the triphosphate (for faster onset of effect and increased intracellular activity) led to development of the NtRTIs, adefovir and tenofovir (TDF), which require for activation the addition of only one phosphate by cellular enzymes. Each of these drugs has its own toxicity profile, dose schedule, and evolving role in HIV therapy. They are well absorbed after oral administration, and some can be taken once a day. Current practice is to combine two or three NRTIs/NtRTIs with at least one agent from a different class, either a nonnucleoside reverse transcriptase inhibitor (NNRTI) or an HIV protease inhibitor. Certain combinations within the nucleoside class are inappropriate because of additive toxicity (e.g., ddI and d4T) or antagonism based on intracellular metabolism (e.g., d4T and ZDV).

It is noteworthy that HIV variants resistant to NRTIs/NtRTIs can be selected by various mechanisms. Some substitutions in the reverse transcriptase impair binding of the active triphosphate. Other substitutions increase the capacity of the reverse transcriptase to excise the chain terminator and gain a "second chance" to incorporate the natural analog. New analogs are being developed that are more active against viruses resistant to current NRTIs/NtRTIs.

Some analogs also are effective against the HBV polymerase, which in many ways acts like a reverse transcriptase. Adefovir and lamivudine are active at lower doses in vivo against HBV than they are against HIV. Adefovir produces renal toxicity when used at the higher doses required to treat HIV but not at the lower doses required to treat HBV. Adefovir is related to the other current NtRTI, tenofovir, which also has in vitro activity against HBV. Although interferons were formerly used to treat HBV infections, the use of NRTI/NtRTI analogs has supplanted those agents. Other analogs with activity only against the HBV polymerase are in advanced stages of development.

Nonnucleoside Inhibitors of the HIV Reverse Transcriptase

Like the NRTIs/NtRTIs, the **NNRTI**s, including efavirenz, etravirine, and nevirapine, inhibit HIV reverse transcriptase, but they do so by a different mechanism. NNRTIs do not block chain elongation. Instead, they inhibit the catalytic step in reverse transcription by binding to a site on the reverse transcriptase that differs from that bound by nucleoside analogs. Structural studies have elucidated mechanisms of drug resistance for the nonnucleoside inhibitors. These mechanisms have guided development of new second-generation NNRTIs (e.g., etravirine), which are active against variants resistant to the first-generation compounds. Of note, first-generation NNRTIs are active only against HIV-1 and do not inhibit the closely related lentiviruses HIV-2 and simian immunodeficiency virus (SIV). It turns out that the reverse transcriptases of HIV-2 and SIV naturally contain the residues that are selected when HIV-1 develops resistance to the first-generation drugs.

Inhibitors of the HIV Integrase

Because of the essential role of integrase in HIV-1 replication, substantial efforts have been devoted to developing drugs with anti-integrase activity. However, some compounds capable of blocking recombinant HIV-1 integrase activity in vitro failed to inhibit HIV-1 replication in cells. Others were toxic. The breakthrough came from the recognition that integration involves several biochemical steps (see Fig. 44-8): (1) assembly of a complex of integrase bound to specific DNA sequences at the end of the HIV-1 long terminal repeats, (2) removal of the terminal dinucleotide from each 3′ end of the viral DNA, and (3) transfer of the viral DNA 3′ ends to allow covalent linkage to the cellular (target) DNA (**strand transfer**). Development of clinically useful inhibitors of HIV integrase began once it was recognized that molecules capable of binding two metals within the integrase active site could inhibit both recombinant integrase activity in vitro and transfer of a viral DNA strand into cellular DNA in infected cells. **Raltegravir** is the prototype integrase inhibitor and specifically interferes with the strand-transfer step of integration. It is therefore called an **integrase strand-transfer inhibitor** (**INSTI**). Other INSTIs in development might have improved pharmacokinetics or inhibit raltegravir-resistant viruses.

Virus Protein Processing

Following genome replication, production of viral proteins is an essential part of the replication cycle of all viruses. For many viruses, new virus proteins require cleavage by virus-specific proteases to become fully

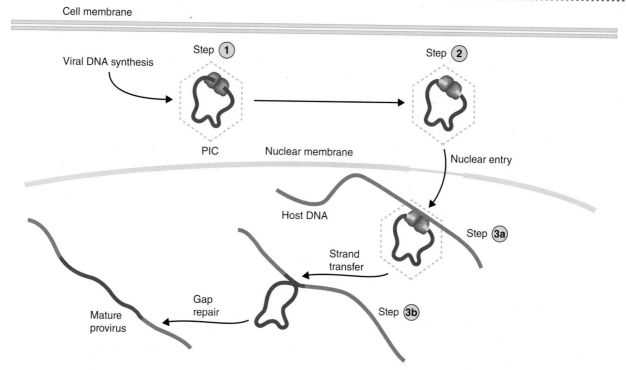

FIGURE 44-8. Integration of the HIV provirus requires multiple steps. Step 1: The viral integrase (*shown in pink*) binds to the ends of the HIV double-stranded DNA reverse transcription product (the provirus, *shown in blue*) within the preintegration complex (PIC). Step 2: The integrase cleaves each end of the viral DNA to leave a single-stranded overhang (*shown in yellow*). Step 3a: The PIC is shuttled from the cytoplasm into the nucleus where other components of the complex help tether the HIV DNA ends to chromosomal DNA (*shown in red*). Step 3b: Strands of HIV DNA are inserted into chromosomal DNA, and the single-stranded ends of host DNA are joined with the overhanging ends of single-stranded HIV DNA. Inhibitors of strand transfer (Step 3b) have been successfully developed as antiviral therapeutics against HIV.

functional. The HIV protease cleaves Gag and Gag-Pol precursor polypeptides to yield the smaller, mature HIV proteins. The cleavage events are triggered when the newly formed virion begins to bud from an infected cell. An understanding of the structure of the HIV protease and modeling of its natural peptide substrates led to the development of **peptidomimetic protease inhibitors**. These pseudosubstrates bind to the protease but are not cleaved themselves, thus preventing cleavage of the natural substrates. HIV protease inhibitors introduced into infected cells before virion budding can block polyprotein cleavage and act to maintain virions in a noninfectious state. Many such compounds are now in clinical use, including atazanavir, darunavir, ritonavir, and saquinavir (see Fig. 44-3).

Some HIV protease inhibitors have unexpected pharmacologic activities that have improved their utility. For example, ritonavir is a very potent inhibitor of **cytochrome P450 3A4**, the enzyme responsible for metabolism of most protease inhibitors. Combining low doses of ritonavir with other protease inhibitors leads to pharmacologic "boosting" of the blood level of the latter, increasing drug effect and half-life. The need for higher blood levels of protease inhibitors, as well as the structure-based design of new agents based on resistance to first-generation protease inhibitors, led to the development of newer coformulations of lopinavir and ritonavir. Specific inhibitors of other essential virus proteases are also being developed, including those required for replication of CMV and HCV.

Since the late 1990s, the standard for anti-HIV chemotherapy has been to use at least three drugs in combination to increase potency and minimize the emergence of drug resistance. This advance is called **highly active antiretroviral therapy** (**HAART**). Unfortunately, the earlier use of single agents and combinations of two drugs has left a legacy of persons who harbor multiple drug-resistant viruses. Treatment decisions are now guided in part by drug resistance testing to determine which resistant mutants are present in an individual patient. Consensus guidelines about HIV therapy are updated frequently. Failure to achieve undetectable viral levels is often the direct result of patient nonadherence, leading to an increased likelihood of development of drug resistance. Fortunately, some contemporary anti-HIV regimens have a higher pharmacologic barrier to resistance, requiring the acquisition of multiple mutations before resistance develops.

Virus Release

Oseltamivir and zanamivir, drugs active against influenza A and B viruses, work by inhibiting NA and preventing extracellular release of viral particles. The influenza virus NA is a virion surface protein that cleaves terminal sialic acid residues (see Fig. 44-4). Another influenza virus protein, hemagglutinin (HA), is used to attach the virion to sialic acid, which serves as the cellular receptor. Removal of sialic acid is essential for release of virus from infected cells and effective spread of virus through the respiratory tract. In the absence of NA-mediated cleavage of terminal sialic acid, newly produced influenza virus aggregates as it buds and cannot spread efficiently from cell to cell. Animal studies indicate that NA activity at the time of virion release is essential for virulence of both influenza A and B virus strains.

Oseltamivir and zanamivir each potently inhibit influenza virus NA; they do not inhibit NAs from cells or other pathogens except at much higher concentrations. Clinical studies have shown prophylactic activity, including activity against influenza viruses resistant to either amantadine or rimantadine. If used within 2 days of symptom onset, symptoms of infections resolve more rapidly, and virus shedding is diminished. Both oseltamivir and zanamivir are effective against most influenza A H1N1 pandemic strains.

CONCLUSION

Antiviral drugs that target a variety of pathogen-specific processes have been successful in the treatment of viral infections. Successful antiviral therapy targets virus entry mechanisms, including attachment, fusion, and uncoating; viral enzymes required for replication, such as polymerases and proteases; and viral enzymes essential for virion release. New advances in antiviral therapy are anticipated as improved methods are developed to detect and minimize virus resistance and interfere with cellular mechanisms required for virus replication.

ACKNOWLEDGMENT

The authors thank Dr. Richard T. D'Aquila for his valuable contributions to this chapter in previous editions of the text.

Suggested Readings

Antiviral drugs for prophylaxis and treatment of influenza. *Med Lett Drugs Ther.* 2006;48:87–88.

Coen DM, Richman DD. Antiviral agents. In: Knipe DM, Howley PM, eds. *Field's Virology.* 5th ed. Philadelphia, PA: Lippincott Williams & Wilkins; 2007:447–485.

Corey L, Wald A, Patel R, et al.; Valacyclovir HSV Transmission Study Group. Once-daily valacyclovir to reduce the risk of transmission of genital herpes. *N Engl J Med.* 2004;350:11–12.

De Clercq E. Antiretroviral drugs. *Curr Opin Pharmacol.* 2010;5:507–515.

Hazuda DJ, Felock P, Witmer M, et al. Inhibitors of strand transfer that prevent integration and inhibit HIV-1 replication in cells. *Science.* 2000;287:646–650.

Hirsch MS, Gunthard HF, Schapiro JM, et al. Antiretroviral drug resistance testing in adult HIV-1 infection: 2008 recommendations of an International AIDS Society-USA panel. *Clin Infect Dis.* 2008;47(2):266–285.

Huang M, Deshpande M. Hepatitis C drug discovery: in vitro and in vivo systems and drugs in the pipeline. *Expert Rev Anti Infect Ther.* 2004;2:375–388.

Panel on Antiretroviral Guidelines for Adults and Adolescents. Guidelines for the use of antiretroviral agents in HIV-1-infected adults and adolescents. Department of Health and Human Services. January 10, 2011; 1–166.

Thompson MA, Aberg, JA, Cahn P, et al.; International AIDS society-USA. Antiretrovial treatment of adult HIV infection: 2010 recommendations of the International AIDS Society-USA panel. *JAMA.* 2010;304:321–333.

Chapter 45

Vaccines and Antisera for the Prevention and Treatment of Infectious Diseases

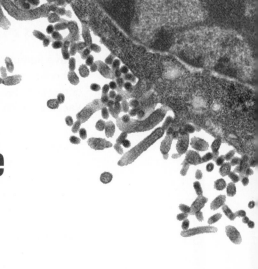

Natasha B. Halasa and H. Keipp Talbot

KEY CONCEPTS

- Either active immunization (the administration of all or part of an infectious agent to induce antibodies or other immune responses) or passive immunization (the administration of exogenously produced antibodies) can be effective in the prevention or treatment of infectious diseases.

- Vaccines can be live, attenuated microorganisms, killed microorganisms, components of microorganisms, or toxoids made from microbial products. In general, live vaccines provide longer immunity than that provided by killed organisms, components of organisms, or toxoids.

- In response to some vaccines, B-cell type-specific protective antibody responses are generated; for other vaccines, T-cell type-specific protective responses are induced.

- Some vaccines elicit secretory immunity at critical sites of microorganism replication or penetration; examples include live, attenuated vaccines against polio, rubella, and cholera.

- Vaccines should be administered to infants, the elderly, and persons at risk for contracting infectious diseases that can be particularly severe in these individuals.

- Vaccines are often administered to healthy persons to prevent disease in immunocompromised individuals.

THE DRAMATIC decrease in the incidence of infectious diseases since the middle of the 19th century is largely due to two factors: improved sanitation and the widespread use of vaccines. The availability of potable water supplies and sewage disposal, along with improvements in housing, has reduced the incidence of disease transmitted by food and water and associated with close living quarters, such as typhoid, cholera, tuberculosis, typhus, and plague. Administration of vaccines directed against a variety of human pathogens also has remarkably reduced the morbidity and mortality associated with infectious diseases. Examples include the use of vaccinia virus to eradicate smallpox, live, attenuated vaccines to prevent polio, measles, rubella (German measles), mumps, and varicella, and toxoid vaccines that have caused an extraordinary decline in cases of diphtheria, tetanus, and pertussis in the United States and abroad. Nevertheless, infectious diseases remain important causes of illness and death in developing countries because of inadequate sanitation or the lack of vaccines. Roadblocks to controlling infectious diseases often represent failures of economics and politics rather than deficiencies in scientific knowledge or public health awareness.

Even in industrialized countries, despite advances in sanitation and the use of vaccines, infectious diseases remain important threats to human health. Vaccines have not been developed for many pathogens, and public health control measures have been difficult to employ for others. Unconquered infections include many viral diseases, particularly those affecting the respiratory and gastrointestinal tracts, sexually transmitted diseases (syphilis, gonorrhea, and chlamydia), and HIV. While rejoicing in the triumphs over many infectious diseases, the health care community should not be complacent about the tremendous tasks ahead in dealing with microbes that continue to attack the human population.

TERMINOLOGY

Active immunization: Administration of all or part of a microorganism or a modified product of that microorganism to evoke an immune response mimicking that of natural infection but presenting little or no risk to the recipient

Vaccine: An immunizing agent derived from microorganisms (or parasites) consisting of the following:

- Live, attenuated microorganisms (e.g., Sabin polio vaccine and measles, mumps, rubella [MMR] vaccine)
- Killed microorganisms or components of microorganisms
- Killed whole agents (e.g., Salk polio vaccine)
- Extracts of microorganisms, such as soluble capsular polysaccharide (e.g., pneumococcal vaccine) or immunologically active subunits (e.g., hepatitis B vaccine)

Toxoid: An inactivated bacterial toxin that has lost its damaging ("toxic") properties but is capable of inducing protective antibody responses; diphtheria and tetanus toxins are inactivated and adsorbed with aluminum salts to produce their respective toxoids

Passive immunization: Administration of exogenously produced or preformed antibodies for the prevention or treatment of infectious diseases

Immune globulin (IG): A mixture of antibodies produced by fractionating large pools of blood plasma

Specific IG: Antibodies produced by fractionating donor blood pools selected for high antibody titer to a specific microorganism

Attenuate: Reduction in the virulence or vitality of a microorganism

Antigen: Molecule recognized by the immune system

Herd immunity: Immunity provided to a population when large numbers of the population are vaccinated

APPROACHES TO IMMUNIZATION

Vaccines to prevent infectious diseases have been enormously successful. The benefits of vaccination include partial or complete protection against infections for both the vaccinated person and society as a whole. Benefits for the individual include protection from symptomatic disease, improved quality of life, and prevention of untimely death. Benefits to society include establishment and preservation of **herd immunity** against communicable diseases, prevention of disease outbreaks, and decrease in health care–related costs. However, no vaccine is completely safe or effective. The risks or side effects of vaccination range from common, minor, and local adverse events to rare, severe, and even life-threatening conditions. Therefore, recommendations for immunization practices must weigh the scientific evidence of the benefits for each person and society at large against the potential costs and risks of the vaccination program.

Several immunization strategies are available to prevent or treat infectious diseases; the choice depends on the infecting microorganism, the age of the host, and the interval of contact between host and pathogen. **Active immunization** with vaccines or toxoids leads to prolonged immunity and is generally preferred to **passive immunization** (administering IGs) for the prevention of infection (see the box entitled "Terminology" for more complete definitions of these and other terms used in this chapter). Vaccines currently licensed for use in the United States are listed in Table 45-1.

The timing of vaccination is an important factor in the effectiveness of a vaccine. As a rule, antibody responses to killed vaccines or toxoids can take several weeks to develop and often require two or three doses at 3- to 4-week intervals to elicit an adequate and persisting immune response. In contrast, *most individuals will develop protective immunity within 2 weeks after administration of a live vaccine.* However, this is not always the case. For example, a small population (<5%) will not respond to one dose of MMR vaccine and require a second dose. Likewise, for varicella vaccine, approximately 20% of persons 13 years of age or older will not respond to the first dose of vaccine, although almost 99% of persons will seroconvert after two doses. To maintain protective antibody concentrations over a lifetime, many vaccines must be readministered as booster doses. For example, booster doses of tetanus and diphtheria toxoids should be given every 5 to 10 years.

Because most infectious diseases have short incubation periods, usually less than 2 weeks, active immunization is often ineffective for use as postexposure control. If available, passive immunization with specific globulins or antitoxins can be used after contact (Table 45-2). Passive immunization can be delivered **transplacentally**, through colostrum, or by injection. Passive immunization

TABLE 45-1 Vaccines Licensed for Use in Humans in the United States

Pathogen		Type of Vaccine	
	Live	*Killed*	*Subunits*
Virus	Measles	Hepatitis A	Hepatitis B (recombinant viral surface glycoprotein)
	Mumps	Influenza (whole virus)	Influenza ("split" vaccine)
	Polio (Sabin)	Polio (Salk)	Human papillomavirus
	Rubella	Rabies	
	Varicella (chicken pox and shingles)	Japanese encephalitis	
	Yellow fever		
	Rotavirus		
	Vaccinia (smallpox)		
	Influenza (cold adapted)		
Bacteria	BCG (tuberculosis)	Cholera	Diphtheria (toxoid)
	Typhoid (oral)	Pertussis (whole cell)	*Haemophilus influenzae* B (HIB) polysaccharide conjugated
		Plague	Meningococcal (polysaccharide and conjugated to protein)
		Typhoid	Pertussis (acellular)
			Pneumococcal (polysaccharide-23 valent and polysaccharide conjugated to protein)
			Tetanus (toxoid)
			Typhoid (VI capsular polysaccharide)

approaches depend on the type of antibody desired, route of administration, and interval after exposure, among other factors. Products for use in passive immunization strategies include IG and specific (hyperimmune) IG administered intramuscularly, IG and specific (hyperimmune) IG administered intravenously, human plasma, and antibodies from animal origin. Pooled intravenous IG (IVIG) is used to treat a variety of immunodeficiencies, inflammatory conditions, and cancers. These illnesses include common variable immunodeficiency, Kawasaki syndrome, chronic B-cell lymphocytic leukemia, bone marrow transplantation in adults, immune-mediated thrombocytopenia, and chronic inflammatory demyelinating polyneuropathy. Importantly, antibody-containing products can inhibit the immune response elicited by live vaccines. Therefore, the administration of live vaccines (e.g., MMR and varicella) should be delayed until passive antibody has decayed, which averages about 11 months.

For diseases that have long incubation periods (e.g., the incubation period for hepatitis B is 6 to 24 weeks)

or variable incubation periods (e.g., rabies and tetanus), both active and passive immunization are used for post-exposure control.

LIVE, KILLED, AND RECOMBINANT VACCINES

Live, attenuated microorganisms, killed microorganisms, or microbial extracts or purified components have been used successfully as vaccines. Influenza, polio, and typhoid vaccines are available in both live, attenuated and killed versions. In general, *immunity generated by a killed vaccine is not as effective or long lasting as immunity stimulated by a live, attenuated vaccine*, which more closely mimics the natural disease. Additionally, live vaccines often elicit both cell-mediated immunity and neutralizing antibodies, which provide prolonged, and often lifelong, immunity. However, killed vaccines are generally easier to manufacture and pose no risk of vaccine-associated

TABLE 45-2 Specific Immune Globulins and Antitoxins

Human Immune Globulins

Botulism (types A, B, E)

Cytomegalovirus

Hepatitis B

Rabies

Respiratory syncytial virus (as both an intravenous and an intramuscular monoclonal antibody preparation)

Tetanus (antitoxin)

Vaccinia (smallpox)

Varicella-zoster

infection. As an example, the advantages and disadvantages of live, attenuated and killed polio vaccines are discussed in Chapter 32 and listed in Table 32-2.

The live, attenuated, intranasal, cold-adapted influenza vaccine (also called the live, attenuated influenza vaccine) offers another live vaccine alternative. It contains a weakened form of live influenza virus instead of killed virus and is administered by nasal spray instead of injection. The term *cold-adapted* indicates that the virus can grow in the nose and throat but not in the lower respiratory tract where the temperature is higher. In comparison to the inactivated influenza vaccine, this vaccine is more efficacious in the prevention of influenza in children.

Attenuation of a virulent pathogen to yield an avirulent vaccine strain can be technically challenging. Even when successful, a small but finite risk exists that the attenuated vaccine strain will revert to a more virulent form in a susceptible host. For example, **vaccine-acquired paralytic poliomyelitis (VAPP)** occurs at a frequency of approximately 1 in every 1 to 3 million doses of live polio vaccine administered. Because wild-type poliovirus transmission was eliminated in the United States in 1979, the only cases of paralytic disease since that time have been due to VAPP. Thus, as a result of this associated adverse event, exclusive use of inactivated polio vaccine was recommended in 1999. However, in other countries where wild-type poliovirus still exists, live, attenuated polio vaccine is the primary vaccine used because of its capacity to elicit mucosal immunity in vacinees and **herd immunity** in the population. Unfortunately, localized outbreaks of paralytic polio have been reported in several countries where the attenuated vaccine strain has reverted to virulence and spread among previously unimmunized persons. Therefore, immunization rates must be kept high to prevent outbreaks.

Another example of adverse events associated with live attenuated vaccines is the previously licensed rotavirus vaccine. After its licensure, this vaccine was found to be associated with an increased rate of **intussusception of the intestine**. As a result, its use was discontinued in 1998. Since 2006, two new live, attenuated rotavirus vaccines have been licensed, and each has a much lower risk of intussusception. Thus, live viral vaccines remain excellent immunogens, but their potential for adverse events must be carefully monitored.

TYPE OF IMMUNE RESPONSE AND CORRELATION OF PROTECTION

The type of immune response, specifically humoral or cellular or both, elicited by a vaccine is dependent on the nature of the vaccine administered. For example, immunization with a live, attenuated organism (e.g., poliovirus) induces B cells, CD8+ T cells, and CD4+ T cells, whereas immunization with inactivated organisms (e.g., rabies and inactivated influenza), protein antigens (e.g., diphtheria, tetanus, and pertussis), and capsular polysaccharide plus a protein carrier (e.g., *Haemophilus influenzae* type B [HIB] polysaccharide linked to a bacterial toxoid) induces B cells and CD4+ T cells. Immunization with capsular polysaccharides (e.g., pneumococcal capsular polysaccharide) induces only B cells.

Immunizing agents can elicit immunity through B-cell proliferation leading to antibody production, with or without helper T cells. For example, pneumococcal capsular polysaccharides (see Chapter 13) and HIB polysaccharide induce B-cell production of antibody without a requirement for T-cell help. These so-called **T-cell–independent antigens** are characterized by low antibody titers, particularly in children less than 18 months of age, with little memory response. By covalently coupling (conjugating) the *H. influenzae* polysaccharide to a protein antigen such as diphtheria toxoid or the outer membrane protein of *Neisseria*, the conjugated HIB vaccine produces a T-cell–dependent antibody response. The conjugate HIB vaccine induces high antibody levels in young infants and primes for strong booster responses following revaccination. The widespread use of the conjugated HIB vaccines has led to a dramatic decrease in the incidence of invasive HIB disease (more than 99%) in comparison to the prevaccine era.

The conjugation of pneumococcal capsular polysaccharides to protein antigens also generates both B-cell– and T-cell–dependent responses in a 7-valent conjugated pneumococcal vaccine, licensed in 2000, and a 13-valent vaccine, licensed in 2010. Since licensure of the 7-valent pneumococcal **conjugate vaccine**, invasive pneumococcal disease caused by the seven vaccine serotypes has decreased substantially in both vaccinated children ages 2 to 59 months and in unimmunized individuals of all age groups, suggesting that herd immunity has been achieved.

Secretory IgA antibodies produced at the mucosal surface offer protection against some mucosal pathogens such as influenza virus, poliovirus, respiratory syncytial virus, rotavirus, rubella virus, *Neisseria gonorrhoeae*, and *Vibrio cholerae*. Live, attenuated vaccines delivered to mucosal sites can induce secretory immunity at the site of initial pathogen contact. Several such vaccines have been produced, including live, attenuated adenovirus, influenza virus, and poliovirus vaccines. Oral typhoid vaccines also induce mucosal immune responses.

The favored approach in vaccine development is to define the "**correlates of protection**," or the host immune responses associated with disease prevention. Vaccines that protect solely or principally by induction of serum antibodies include hepatitis A, polio, rabies, yellow fever, diphtheria, pertussis, tetanus, and extracellular encapsulated bacteria. Both antibody levels and function are important correlates of protection for mumps, rubella, HIB, meningococcal, and pneumococcal vaccines. Secretory antibodies play a role in protection against infections caused by pathogens that must first replicate on mucosal surfaces such as influenza virus, poliovirus, and rotavirus. Lastly, vaccines for which T-cell responses are essential include measles and varicella. Induction of both T-cell immunity and humoral immunity are important goals of current efforts to develop an HIV vaccine.

AGE OF IMMUNIZATION

The age of immunization affects the immunologic response to vaccines and hence the prevention of disease. Because newborns receive serum IgG antibody from their mothers, they have transient protection against some diseases to which their mothers are immune. Breast milk also contains secretory IgA antibodies that provide protection against intestinal and respiratory tract infections to which the mother has developed immunity. This is a type of "passive immunization" that protects newborns from potential pathogens. However, maternal antibody also may prevent responses to live vaccines such as MMR and varicella. Although the humoral immune system is not fully functional at birth and generates poor responses to certain polysaccharide antigens, it generally responds well to protein antigens like those contained in the diphtheria, pertussis, and tetanus vaccines when given at 2 months of age. When given at birth, hepatitis B vaccine is also immunogenic, but repeated doses are required to achieve protective antibody levels.

As with infants, the elderly have reduced antibody and cellular responses to vaccines due to immune senescence. As a consequence, this age group has an increased susceptibility to certain infections such as those caused by influenza virus, pneumococcus, and varicella. Thus, these microbial pathogens are targets for vaccination in elderly persons.

SELECTION OF ANTIGENS

Although infecting pathogens contain an enormous quantity of various types of antigens, immune responses are often directed to surface components that the pathogen uses when it invades. In some instances, a vaccine confers protection against all strains of an infecting organism. In contrast, other infectious agents, such as the pneumococcus, have several distinct capsular polysaccharide types, and immunity to one polysaccharide type does not confer immunity to the others. Thus, pneumococcal vaccines are a mixture of antigens comprising the most common serotypes causing invasive disease.

Another complex problem with antigen selection is seen with influenza virus. The vaccine is formulated annually to protect against the strains anticipated to circulate during the following year. Minor antigenic changes in influenza virus, called **antigenic drift**, occur annually, whereas major antigenic changes, known as antigenic shift, occur approximately every 10 years. Therefore, vaccines must be modified annually to accommodate antigenic drift and shift (see Chapter 36).

Some antigens are not immunogenic due to defects in host immunity. For example, certain HLA haplotypes may not recognize the antigen; neonatal immune systems recognize polysaccharides poorly; immunosuppressive medical regimens (chemotherapy, steroids, etc.) may blunt an immune response; and an aging immune system may be less responsive to certain antigen types.

IMMUNIZATION OF SPECIAL POPULATIONS

Some individuals are at greater risk than others for vaccine-preventable diseases and should be given high priority for immunization. Examples of persons who are at greater risk for morbidity and mortality from influenza (Table 45-3) include persons with underlying heart or lung disease or those greater than 65 years or less than 6 months of age. Some individuals also are at greater risk for disease because specific immune defects reduce their ability to generate adequate immune responses. Because of functional asplenia, persons with sickle cell disease are at risk for infections with encapsulated organisms, particularly pneumococci. After the introduction of the pneumococcal conjugate vaccine, invasive pneumococcal disease in this population decreased substantially. Similarly, persons who are either born without a spleen or who have undergone splenectomy also are at high risk for overwhelming infections with encapsulated organisms, such as those caused by pneumococci, meningococci, and *H. influenzae*. Therefore, such persons should receive the appropriate vaccines. Other special groups that should be targeted for vaccination are the elderly for influenza and pneumococcal vaccines, health care workers for hepatitis B and rubella, and travelers, depending on local health conditions at their destinations.

TABLE 45-3 Immunization of Special Populations

Population	Immunization	Comment
Persons with sickle cell disease; splenectomy	Pneumococcal, meningococcal, and *H. influenzae* vaccines	Infections are often fatal
Elderly	Influenza vaccine, 23-valent pneumococcal polysaccharide vaccine, diphtheria, pertussis, tetanus vaccine, varicella-zoster vaccine	High risk (immunity has waned)
Children with immunodeficiency (including HIV)	Varicella-zoster IG (postexposure)	Chickenpox causes severe, often fatal, disease in this population
Health care workers	Hepatitis B vaccine, measles, mumps, rubella (MMR) vaccine, influenza vaccine, varicella-zoster vaccine	To protect health care workers and patients
Travelers	Hepatitis A and B, yellow fever, rabies, Japanese encephalitis, measles, meningococcal, polio vaccines	Depends on local conditions
Pregnant women	Hepatitis B vaccine, tetanus toxoid, influenza vaccine	Prenatal screening for HbsAg; newborns of carriers receive hepatitis BIG and vaccine;[a] particularly in developing countries to prevent neonatal tetanus;[b] higher risk for morbidity due to influenza, especially in third trimester[c]

[a]Hepatitis B vaccine.
[b]Tetanus toxoid.
[c]Influenza vaccine.

Live, attenuated vaccines generally should be avoided in immunocompromised persons because the attenuated organism may be sufficiently pathogenic to cause disease in those individuals. Clinicians should consult vaccine experts for questions about the safety of live, attenuated vaccines in immunocompromised persons.

DTAP (DIPHTHERIA, TETANUS, ACELLULAR PERTUSSIS) VACCINE: A PROTOTYPE SUBUNIT VACCINE

DTaP vaccine is the oldest and most successful combination vaccine used in children. It consists of a combination of two toxoids (**diphtheria** and **tetanus**) and purified components of *Bordetella pertussis*. The pertussis vaccines consist of inactivated bacterial components. All pertussis vaccines include **pertussis toxin**, and many contain differing amounts of filamentous hemagglutinin, pertactin, and fimbriae. Clinical trials have shown high protection rates and fewer side effects with acellular pertussis vaccines than the previously used whole-cell preparations. The preferred schedule for DTaP vaccination is 2, 4, and 6 months of age, followed by booster doses of vaccine at 15 to 18 months and 4 to 6 years. Thereafter, a booster of tetanus toxoid (full dose) and diphtheria toxoid (reduced dose) is given every 5 to 10 years. In 2005,

two new vaccines comprised of tetanus toxoid, reduced-dose diphtheria toxoid, and pertussis components (Tdap) were licensed in response to the increased incidence of pertussis in adolescents and adults. The American Academy of Pediatrics currently recommends universal vaccination with Tdap for adolescents at 11 to 12 years of age and a catch-up vaccination for older adolescents to boost protection against pertussis. It is also recommended that adults who have been previously immunized with diphtheria–tetanus vaccine should receive Tdap as their next scheduled tetanus booster, and even sooner for adults who have regular exposure to infants.

CONCLUSION

The use of vaccines has had a major impact on the health of many millions of persons throughout the world. The success stories of vaccines are exemplified by the eradication of smallpox and the dramatic decrease in the prevalence of many once common infectious diseases. With success comes controversy: concerns about the safety and side effects associated with vaccines have become a major focus of attention. Those concerns pose challenges for the introduction of new vaccines for the prevention of infectious diseases that remain important causes of morbidity and mortality in humans.

Suggested Readings

Kroger AT, Atkinson WL, Marcuse EK, et al. Centers for Disease Control and Prevention. General recommendations on immunization. Recommendations of the Advisory Committee on Immunization Practices (ACIP). *MMWR Morb Mortal Wkly Rep.* 2006;55(RR15):1–48.

Pickering LK, Baker CJ, Kimberlin DW, et al., eds. *Red Book: 2009 Report of the Committee on Infectious Diseases.* 28th ed. Elk Grove Village, IL: American Academy of Pediatrics; 2009.

Plotkin SA, Orenstein WA, eds. *Vaccines.* 5th ed. Philadelphia, PA: WB Saunders, 2008.

Vaccine and Immunizations. Available at: http://www.cdc.gov/vaccines/.

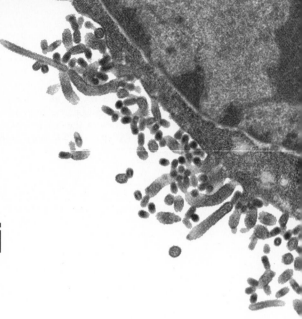

Chapter 46

Introduction to the Fungi and Mycoses

Carol A. Kauffman

KEY CONCEPTS

Fungi:

- Are eukaryotes and constitute a separate kingdom called Fungi
- Can be multicellular filamentous structures (molds) or unicellular forms (yeasts). Some species are dimorphic, that is, they exist in either form depending on environmental conditions.
- Cause superficial, cutaneous, subcutaneous, and systemic infections
- Are typically free living in nature and acquired from environmental sources; some are part of normal human flora.
- Cause disease by eliciting an inflammatory response or through direct invasion or destruction of tissues

FUNGAL infections, or mycoses, are usually classified by the area of the body primarily affected and the type of infection induced, rather than by taxonomic criteria that are not very meaningful clinically.

- **Endemic mycoses** are infections caused by pathogens that are restricted geographically and are true pathogens because they have the ability to cause serious systemic infection in healthy individuals.
- **Opportunistic mycoses** are caused by fungi that cause life-threatening systemic disease almost entirely in immunosuppressed patients.
- **Subcutaneous mycoses** are a group of fungal diseases that involve the skin, subcutaneous tissue, and lymphatics.
- **Superficial and cutaneous mycoses** are common fungal infections limited to the skin and skin structures.

TYPES OF PATHOGENIC FUNGI

Fungi belong to a discrete kingdom, the Fungi, and are classified on the basis of their mode of sexual and asexual reproduction, morphology, life cycles, and, to some extent, physiology. The kingdom Fungi comprises at least 100,000 species found all over the globe. Most exist only in the environment, and far less than 1% cause disease in humans. A crucial role for fungi is to degrade organic waste in the environment; because of this, they cause widespread damage to food and fabrics. Fungi are used commercially in many fermentation processes producing steroid hormone derivatives and antibiotics.

Fungi are **eukaryotes**, with a defined nucleus enclosed by a nuclear membrane, a cell membrane that contains lipids, glycoproteins, and sterols; mitochondria;

Golgi apparatus; ribosomes bound to endoplasmic reticulum; and a cytoskeleton with microtubules and microfilaments. The sterols comprising the cell membrane largely consist of **ergosterol**, whereas mammalian cell membranes are primarily composed of cholesterol. Fungi have **cell walls** predominantly made of chitin, mannan, and glucan; mammalian cells do not have cell walls, and the cell walls of bacteria and plants differ markedly from those of fungi.

In nature, most fungi derive their nutrients from decaying matter. They require an exogenous source of organic carbon for growth. Unlike plants, fungi do not have chlorophyll and do not undergo photosynthesis. Almost all fungi are strict aerobes. Although environmental fungi can tolerate extremes of temperatures, fungi that cause disease in humans favor 35°C to 37°C.

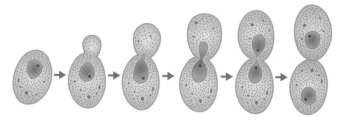

FIGURE 46-1. Yeast cell reproducing by budding. The buds are called blastoconidia.

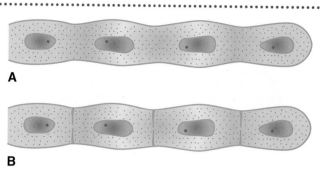

FIGURE 46-3. Hyphae. A. Hyphae that are nonseptate have protoplasm that is continuous and multinucleated. **B.** Hyphae that are septated have protoplasm that is interrupted by cross walls.

The fungi that cause disease in humans have two major forms: **unicellular** forms called **yeasts** and multicellular **filamentous** forms called **molds**. Yeasts are single cells that are ovoid or spherical. Most yeasts divide by budding (asexually), and the bud is called a blastoconidia (Fig. 46-1). On agar, yeasts form moist colonies that appear similar to, but larger than, those of bacteria (Fig. 46-2).

Molds grow as microscopic, branching, threadlike filaments. The filaments, usually 2 to 10 µm in diameter, are called **hyphae**, **and masses of hyphae** are referred to as a **mycelium**. Hyphae are either septate (divided by partitions or cross walls perpendicular to the length of the hyphae) or nonseptate (multinucleate without cross walls; Fig. 46-3). On agar, part of the mycelium grows into the agar to provide nutrients to the aerial hyphae that form a "fuzzy" outgrowth or mold above the surface of the agar (Fig. 46-4). Aerial hyphae provide support for the reproductive structures of molds.

Many pathogenic fungi display both growth forms and can exist as either molds or yeasts. This phenomenon is called **dimorphism**, and the shift frequently occurs when a free-living organism infects a living host. With most fungi that cause systemic infections, the mold form is found in the environment, and the yeast is found in tissues.

Fungi reproduce by either an asexual or sexual process. **Asexual** reproductive structures are termed **conidia**. The appearance of conidia varies enormously and is used for identification of fungi (Fig. 46-5). The conidia can be formed at the tips of the growing hyphae on a specialized structure called a conidiophore, directly off the hyphae, or within the hyphae themselves. **Sexual** reproduction usually occurs through the development of **spores** that often are formed into complex structures. The sexual stages of many of the fungi that cause disease in humans have yet to be described.

ENCOUNTER

The human host encounters infection-causing fungi through two main mechanisms. Most fungi live freely in the environment, and people encounter them incidentally in the course of everyday living. Several important human pathogens are geographically restricted so that only people who enter that habitat are at risk for infection. Others are ubiquitous in the environment, and healthy hosts are continually exposed with no dire consequences. However, markedly immunosuppressed hosts can develop progressive fatal infection after exposure to seemingly innocuous fungi dispersed throughout the environment.

The other source for pathogenic fungi is the normal human flora. Mere colonizers in healthy hosts, these organisms, mostly yeasts, can become pathogenic and cause serious disseminated infection in the immunocompromised host.

ENTRY

The level of innate immunity to pathogenic fungi is high in most humans, as witnessed by the fact that most fungal

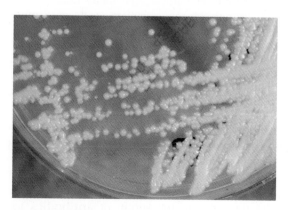

FIGURE 46-2. Colonies of *Candida albicans*, a typical yeast, growing on blood agar.

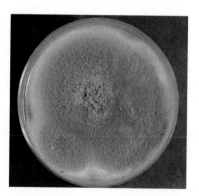

FIGURE 46-4. Growth of a mold on an agar plate. Notice the "fuzzy" growth (aerial hyphae) above the surface of the plate.

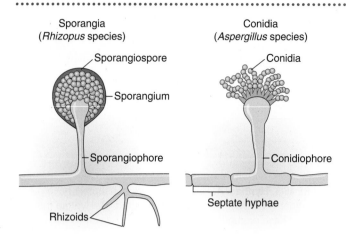

FIGURE 46-5. Mold morphology. Molds can assume various forms, starting with the basic hyphal structure that can then differentiate into various reproductive structures (conidia and spores). Two common molds, *Aspergillus* and *Rhizopus* species, that cause human infection are illustrated.

infections are mild and self-limiting. The intact skin and mucosal surfaces are the primary barriers to infection. Desiccation, epithelial cell turnover, fatty acids, and the low pH of the skin are believed to be important factors in host resistance. In addition, the bacterial flora of the skin and mucous membranes compete with fungi and hinder their unrestricted growth. Alterations in the balance of the normal flora by the use of antibiotics or changes in nutrition allow fungi, such as *Candida albicans*, to proliferate, thus increasing the likelihood of entry and subsequent infection. Violation of the natural barriers by trauma or foreign bodies allows entry of fungi into sterile areas of the body.

SPREAD AND MULTIPLICATION

Tissue reaction to the presence of fungi varies with the species, the site of proliferation, and the duration of infection. Some mycoses are characterized by a low-grade inflammatory response that does not eliminate the fungi; for the most part, however, the organisms are not very virulent and serious disease does not result. In general, nonspecific inflammatory reactions are critically important in eliminating fungi. **Neutrophil phagocytosis and killing** are the primary mechanisms that prevent the establishment of many fungal infections. The extent of disease caused by opportunists, such as *Candida* and *Aspergillus*, is greater in patients with low numbers of neutrophils or with disorders of neutrophil function, such as chronic granulomatous disease.

Fungi that are too large to be ingested are killed by a different mechanism. Instead of "ingesting" and "digesting" filamentous fungi, phagocytic cells line up along the surface of the hyphal structure and secrete lysosomal enzymes that damage the organisms. Antibodies play a role in the elimination of fungi from the body by participating in the extracellular killing of some filamentous fungi and

yeasts by phagocytic cells, but overall, the role of antibodies in host defense is minor.

The most important host defense against most fungi is **cell-mediated immunity**. Several important human pathogens persist within macrophages without being killed until specific T-lymphocyte cell-mediated immunity develops. The clinical observation that AIDS patients with low CD4 lymphocyte numbers are especially prone to invasive and serious systemic fungal disease corroborates the importance of cell-mediated immunity.

DAMAGE

As in all infections, the *outcome is determined by the virulence of the infecting organism, the size of the inoculum, and the adequacy of the host defenses*. Tissue damage varies with each organism and the organ involved but typically results from the direct invasion of the organism with destruction of vital structures, or from toxic effects of the inflammatory response. Fungi that cause invasive disease are not known to secrete toxins that harm the host.

DIAGNOSIS

Fungal infections are diagnosed in the laboratory by **direct microscopy**, **histopathology**, **culture**, **serology**, **and antigen detection**. Some fungi can be identified by **direct examination** of body fluids or purulent material. For direct examination, 10% potassium hydroxide is used to dissolve tissue debris so that the fungi, whose cell walls remain intact, can be observed, or a fluorescent dye, such as calcofluor white, that binds to chitin is used to highlight the fungal cell walls. On **histopathological examination**, special stains are usually needed to detect fungi; morphological characteristics are distinctive enough in some fungi to aid in their identification. That is particularly useful in the diagnosis of serious systemic infections, providing an immediate and reasonably reliable identification of the causative agent.

Pathogenic fungi may be recovered from infected tissues using **culture** procedures. In general, growth of a fungus from a normally sterile body site always implies infection. Culturing clinical specimens does not always result in growth of the organism, and some medically important fungi take weeks to grow. Thus, in a severely ill patient, cultures are used to confirm a diagnosis but cannot be relied on to establish the diagnosis, and therapy cannot be withheld while awaiting culture results. On the other hand, some pathogenic fungi are ubiquitous in the environment or are part of the normal flora of humans; for those fungi, growth in the laboratory does not always establish a diagnosis of infection but may reflect merely contamination or colonization. Once a fungal organism has been grown in culture, the laboratory often uses various morphological characteristics to identify different species.

The detection in the serum of **antibodies** to fungal antigens is helpful in the diagnosis of several of the endemic mycoses but rarely helpful in the diagnosis of opportunistic fungal infections. The detection of fungal **antigens** in body fluids, urine, and serum has proved both sensitive and specific for the diagnosis of some opportunist fungi as well as several endemic mycoses. Polymerase chain reaction techniques will likely prove useful in the future but currently are not readily available.

TREATMENT

Not all fungal infections require treatment. For those that do require systemic antifungal agents, toxicity is a problem because fungi share with mammalian cells many pathways and structures that are targeted by antifungal agents. Compared with antibacterial agents, the number of effective antifungal agents is quite small. Antifungal agents are discussed in Chapter 50.

CONCLUSION

Fungi constitute a separate kingdom composed of at least 100,000 species. They are eukaryotes, which means that they share some metabolic pathways and structural components with mammalian cells. Although most human encounters with fungi do not lead to infection, if the fungal inoculum is large or the human host is immunocompromised, serious and even life-threatening infection can ensue. A variety of diagnostic tests are available to determine if a fungal infection is present.

Suggested Reading

Brandt ME, Lockhardt SR, Warnock DW. Laboratory aspects of medical mycology. In: Kauffman CA, Pappas PG, Sobel JD, et al., eds. *Essentials of Clinical Mycology*. New York, NY: Springer; 2011.

Chapter **47**

Endemic Mycoses

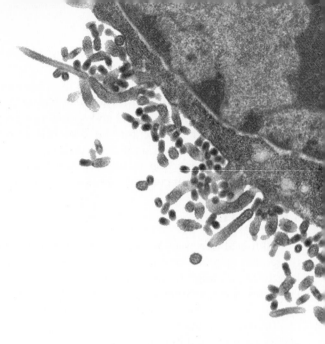

Carol A. Kauffman

KEY CONCEPTS

Histoplasmosis:

- Is caused by *Histoplasma capsulatum*, a mold that grows in soil enriched with bird and bat excreta and transforms into a yeast after being inhaled into the alveoli
- Occurs throughout the Mississippi and Ohio River valleys
- Immunity depends on T cells and activated macrophages
- Causes both acute and chronic forms of pulmonary and disseminated disease
- Is treated with amphotericin B for severe disease and with itraconazole for mild-to-moderate disease

Blastomycosis:

- Is caused by *Blastomyces dermatitidis*, a soil mold that transforms into a yeast after inhalation into the alveoli
- Occurs in the Mississippi River Valley and southeastern and north-central states

- Triggers immunity that depends on both polymorphonuclear leukocytes (PMNs) and T cells and macrophages
- Causes characteristic skin lesions, pulmonary disease, and disseminated infection
- Is treated with amphotericin B for severe disease and with itraconazole for mild-to-moderate disease

Coccidioidomycosis:

- Is caused by two species of *Coccidioides*, *Coccidioides immitis* and *Coccidioides posadasii*, molds that grow in desert soil of the southwestern United States and convert to a large endospore-containing spherule in the body
- Triggers immunity that depends on both PMNs and lymphocytes and macrophages
- Causes a wide spectrum of pulmonary disease, skin and osteoarticular lesions, abscesses, and meningitis
- Is treated with amphotericin B for severe disease and with itraconazole or fluconazole for mild-to-moderate disease; meningitis is treated for life with fluconazole

THE ENDEMIC MYCOSES are due to fungi that are geographically restricted to certain environmental areas and are true pathogens in that they have the ability to infect healthy people, not only those who are immunosuppressed. The diseases that occur in the United States include histoplasmosis, blastomycosis, and coccidioidomycosis. Paracoccidioidomycosis occurs in South America and penicilliosis occurs in Southeast Asia; both of these diseases will be discussed briefly. All the fungi that cause endemic mycoses are dimorphic, existing in the environment as molds and in hosts as either yeasts or spherules.

CASE • An infectious diseases specialist who practiced in the endemic area for histoplasmosis reflected on the varied manifestations of pulmonary histoplasmosis she had seen in the previous week. One patient was a 14-year-old boy from New York City who was spending the summer on his uncle's farm. Approximately 2 weeks after helping his uncle clean out some chicken coops, he developed fever, cough, chest tightness, and malaise. An oral macrolide for a week had provided no benefit, and his cough was worsening. The physical examination was normal; the chest radiograph showed hilar lymphadenopathy and a patchy lower lobe infiltrate (Fig. 47-1). Although the differential diagnosis was broad, she thought that acute pulmonary histoplasmosis was the most likely possibility and ordered acute and convalescent antibody titers to help establish the diagnosis. She did not think that antifungal therapy was warranted and counseled the boy and his uncle that the illness was a self-limited one and would resolve in another few weeks.

The following day, she was consulted on a 58-year-old woman who was in the intensive care unit and had received a kidney transplant 18 months before. She was on prednisone, mycophenolate, and cyclosporine to prevent rejection. She had developed the acute onset of fever, chills, dyspnea, and cough. The Po_2 was 65 mm Hg, white blood cell count was 4,600/mm^3, and creatinine was 1.8 mg/dL. The chest radiograph showed diffuse bilateral infiltrates (Fig. 47-2). A bronchoscopic lung biopsy showed tiny oval, budding, intracellular yeasts in alveolar macrophages, and a test for *Histoplasma* antigen was positive. A diagnosis of severe pulmonary histoplasmosis was made, and therapy

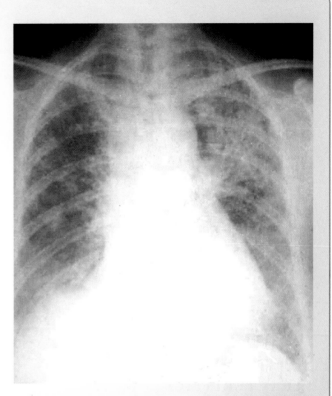

FIGURE 47-2. Kidney transplant recipient with diffuse pulmonary infiltrates that were caused by *Histoplasma capsulatum*.

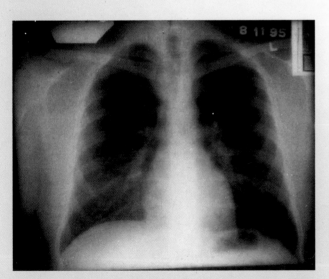

FIGURE 47-1. Patchy pneumonitis and hilar lymphadenopathy typical of acute pulmonary histoplasmosis in an immunocompetent host.

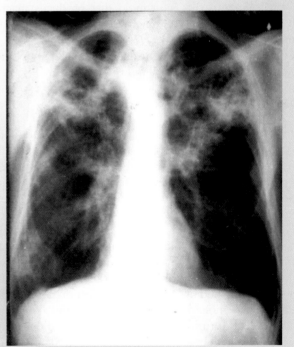

FIGURE 47-3. Chronic cavitary pulmonary histoplasmosis with bilateral cavitary upper-lobe infiltrates and lower-lobe scarring.

continued on page 474

with a lipid formulation of amphotericin B was begun immediately.

Later that week, a 66-year-old man who had a long history of chronic obstructive pulmonary disease (COPD) returned to her office for a follow-up visit. She had initially seen the man 6 months earlier when he came into the hospital with increasing fatigue, dyspnea, fevers, night sweats, anorexia, 20-pound weight loss, and cough productive of yellow sputum mixed with blood. A chest radiograph taken in the hospital had shown extensive upper-lobe cavitary infiltrates (Fig. 47-3). Sputum cultures had grown *Histoplasma capsulatum* after 5 weeks incubation, antibody titers were positive for that organism, and a diagnosis of chronic cavitary pulmonary histoplasmosis had been made. Treatment with itraconazole was begun, and after 1 month, he had noticed improvement in cough and sputum production.

Fevers and night sweats had disappeared, and he began to gain weight by the second month of therapy. The plan was to treat him for 12 to 18 months with itraconazole. At 6 months, he appeared to be responding well to treatment.

These cases raise several questions:

1. What is the main reason that the manifestations of pulmonary histoplasmosis were so different in the three patients?

2. What was the source of *H. capsulatum* that infected each patient? Can a discrete point source be found for most patients?

3. Why was therapy unique for each patient? Do most patients with histoplasmosis require treatment with an antifungal agent?

See Appendix for answers.

HISTOPLASMOSIS
CHARACTERISTICS OF THE ORGANISM

Histoplasma capsulatum is a **dimorphic** fungus that in the environment exists as a mold that produces macro (tuberculate) conidia and microconidia, the infectious form. In the body at 37°C, *H. capsulatum* assumes a yeastlike form, which initially was erroneously thought to have a capsule (hence the name) (Fig. 47-4).

ENCOUNTER

Histoplasmosis occurs primarily in the Mississippi and Ohio River valleys, in Central America, and in some areas of South America (Fig. 47-5). In addition, microfoci occur in caves and other focal areas in several eastern states and elsewhere throughout the world. In the endemic area in the United States, as much as 90% of the population has been infected.

H. capsulatum is a soil fungus whose growth is enhanced by the high nitrogenous content of earth that has been fertilized by bird or bat guano, as might occur under blackbird roosts, around chicken coops, and in caves and old buildings. Clusters of infection occur with spelunking, demolition of old buildings, and construction work that disrupts soil. The largest reported outbreak involved more than 100,000 people infected after the demolition of an old amusement park in Indianapolis.

ENTRY

When *H. capsulatum* enters the lungs, the organism transforms into the yeast phase. That process is complex and not fully understood but clearly is essential for pathogenicity.

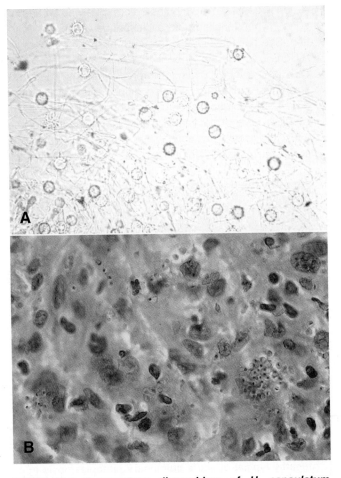

FIGURE 47-4. Temperature dimorphism of *H. capsulatum*.
A. The environmental form is a mold that produces both small microconidia that are inhaled and cause infection and distinctive macroconidia with tuberculate projections on the surface. **B.** The tissue form is a yeast, shown here within macrophages.

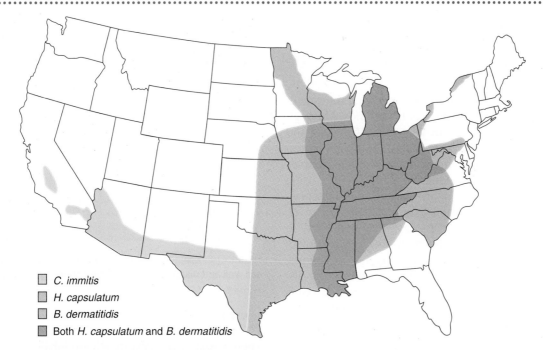

FIGURE 47-5. Geographic distribution of the major endemic mycoses, *H. capsulatum, Blastomyces dermatitidis,* and *Coccidioides* species in the United States.

Legend:
- C. immitis
- H. capsulatum
- B. dermatitidis
- Both H. capsulatum and B. dermatitidis

The yeasts are phagocytosed by macrophages and neutrophils, but killing is problematic.

SPREAD AND MULTIPLICATION

Histoplasmosis should be viewed as *an infection of the reticuloendothelial system.* The organisms remain viable within macrophages by modulating the phagolysosomal pH and capturing essential growth factors from the cell. More than for other fungal organisms, immunity to *H. capsulatum* is mediated through the *cell-mediated immune system of CD4 T lymphocytes and activated macrophages;* antibody appears to play no role in resolution of infection. Only after T-cell sensitization, leading to the release of interleukin-2 and interferon-γ, are macrophages able to kill the intracellular yeasts. That generally takes several weeks, and until then, the organism spreads locally through the lymphatics to the hilar and mediastinal lymph nodes and then hematogenously within macrophages throughout the reticuloendothelial system.

When cell-mediated immunity to *H. capsulatum* is established, the infection is curtailed and resolves. Immunity is lifelong, but reinfection has been noted with exposure to a huge inoculum of *H. capsulatum.* The cell-mediated immune response is reflected in the development of **granulomas** with or without caseation necrosis and a positive skin test to *Histoplasma* antigens. Ultimately, most granulomas calcify. However, yeast cells can remain viable within granulomas for years and are a source for **reactivation infection** should cell-mediated immunity wane.

DAMAGE

The extent of infection and clinical disease manifestations are dependent on both the numbers of conidia inhaled and the cell-mediated immune response. The majority of infected persons have no clinical disease or mild pulmonary and systemic symptoms often ascribed to a viral-like illness. A small proportion of patients will have fever, chills, anorexia, fatigue, and dry cough; **patchy pneumonitis** and **hilar or mediastinal lymphadenopathy** are noted on chest radiograph. With extensive exposure, even in healthy hosts, severe pneumonia can occur, causing bilateral diffuse nodular infiltrates and hypoxemia. Patients who have underlying COPD are at risk for developing **chronic cavitary pulmonary histoplasmosis**, a progressive and eventually fatal infection that mimics reactivation pulmonary tuberculosis.

Dissemination occurs in virtually everyone infected with *H. capsulatum,* but symptomatic disease is uncommon and clearly more likely to occur in people with cell-mediated immune deficiencies, such as AIDS, and those treated with immunosuppressive agents, including corticosteroids and tumor necrosis factor inhibitors. **Acute disseminated histoplasmosis** is characterized by fever, chills, fatigue, mucous membrane ulcers, hepatosplenomegaly, and pancytopenia; in some cases, adrenal insufficiency, sepsis syndrome, and disseminated intravascular coagulation occurs. **Chronic progressive disseminated histoplasmosis** is seen in older adults who have no obvious immune deficiency but for some reason are unable to contain *H. capsulatum.* If not treated, patients with the chronic disease die from progressive infection of the liver, spleen, bone marrow, adrenals, and other organs.

DIAGNOSIS

Histoplasmosis can be diagnosed by growing the organism from sputum, blood, tissues, or body fluids. Although definitive, growth in vitro can take up to 6 weeks and is not successful in many laboratories. Histopathological demonstration of the small intracellular yeasts in samples from bone marrow, liver, lung, or lymph nodes using special stains is rapid and highly suggestive of histoplasmosis. Polysaccharide antigen from the cell wall of *H. capsulatum* can be detected by enzyme immunoassay in urine or serum in most patients with disseminated infection and some with primary pulmonary histoplasmosis, but very few with localized and chronic forms of the disease. The demonstration of antibody to *H. capsulatum* is helpful in the diagnosis of acute and chronic pulmonary and disseminated forms of the disease but not in immunocompromised hosts who cannot mount an antibody response.

TREATMENT AND PREVENTION

Mild-to-moderate pulmonary or disseminated histoplasmosis is treated with **itraconazole**, usually for 3 to 12 months depending on the extent of disease. Patients who have severe infection, generally those with dissemination, should receive **amphotericin B** initially and then can be switched to itraconazole after their condition has stabilized.

Guidelines for prevention of histoplasmosis in the workplace have been issued by the Centers for Disease Control and Prevention. Use of respirators when tearing down old barns and chicken coops or other areas that have housed birds and bats is highly recommended. Immunosuppressed persons should not take part in those activities.

BLASTOMYCOSIS
CHARACTERISTICS OF THE ORGANISM

Blastomyces dermatitidis is a **dimorphic** fungus that in the environment exists as a mold and in the body at 37°C assumes the yeast form. The yeast is large and thick walled and produces a single broad-based bud (Fig. 47-6).

ENCOUNTER

Blastomycosis occurs primarily in the Mississippi River Valley and the southeastern states and extends northward into central Canada and the St. Lawrence River Valley (see Fig. 47-5). The ecology of *B. dermatitidis* is less well known than that of *H. capsulatum*, but soil and decaying wood are presumed sources. Small outbreaks have been described, but most cases appear sporadically.

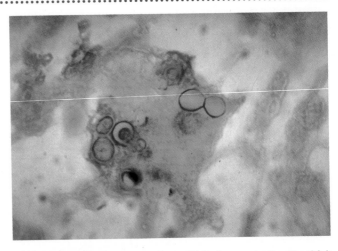

FIGURE 47-6. Yeast form of *B. dermatitidis* demonstrating the thick cell wall and distinctive broad-based budding of the daughter cell.

ENTRY

The conidia of *B. dermatitidis* are inhaled into the lungs, where the organism transforms to the yeast phase. The yeast is phagocytosed by macrophages and neutrophils.

SPREAD AND MULTIPLICATION

B. dermatitidis multiplies initially in the lungs and causes pneumonia. However, skin lesions, which arise as the result of hematogenous dissemination, are extremely common and are often the presenting manifestation of blastomycosis. Cell-mediated immunity is clearly important in eradication of infection, but it appears that neutrophils also play a role in containing the organism. The histopathological picture reflects the **mixed granulomatous and pyogenic response**. As with histoplasmosis, it appears that yeast cells can remain viable within granulomas for years and can be a source for later reactivation.

DAMAGE

Most infected persons have only mild pulmonary infection, and many present only with skin or osteoarticular lesions following a silent pulmonary infection. Those who have more extensive pulmonary disease have fever, chills, anorexia, fatigue, dry cough, and patchy pneumonitis on chest radiograph. With extensive exposure, even in healthy hosts, bilateral diffuse nodular infiltrates, hypoxemia, and acute respiratory distress syndrome can occur. The cutaneous lesions may be single or multiple, have **heaped-up borders** with small central **microabscesses**, or manifest as ulcerated lesions (Fig. 47-7). Other organs can be involved with disseminated infection.

DIAGNOSIS

Blastomycosis is diagnosed by growing the organism from sputum, skin, or other tissues. Unfortunately,

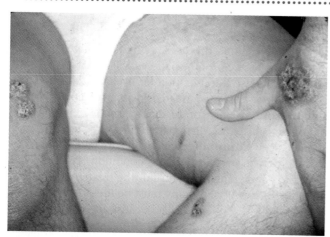

FIGURE 47-7. Skin lesions that had been present for several months in a patient with blastomycosis.

growth in vitro may take weeks. Histopathological demonstration in tissues of large, thick-walled yeasts with single **broad-based buds** is highly suggestive of blastomycosis. Antibody tests for *B. dermatitidis* are not helpful, but a test for *Blastomyces* antigen is useful in more extensive infection.

TREATMENT AND PREVENTION

Mild-to-moderate pulmonary or cutaneous blastomycosis is treated with **itraconazole**, usually for 6 to 12 months depending on the extent of disease. Patients who have severe pulmonary or disseminated infection should receive **amphotericin B** initially and can be switched to itraconazole after their condition has stabilized. Preventative measures have not been established.

COCCIDIOIDOMYCOSIS

CHARACTERISTICS OF THE ORGANISM

There are two *Coccidioides* species, *Coccidioides immitis* and *Coccidioides posadasii*. Both are dimorphic, but the dimorphism is not temperature dependent. In the environment, *Coccidioides* are molds that form **arthroconidia**, the infectious form. In tissues, a large structure called a **spherule**, which is 50 to 100 μm in size, is formed. Inside each spherule are hundreds of **endospores** that, when released, propagate the infection (Fig. 47-8).

ENCOUNTER

Coccidioides species exist primarily in a distinctive ecosystem termed the **lower Sonoran life zone**, which includes Arizona, southern California, the arid interior valleys in California, parts of New Mexico and Texas, and areas in Central and South America (see Fig. 47-5). A semiarid environment fosters the growth of the organism,

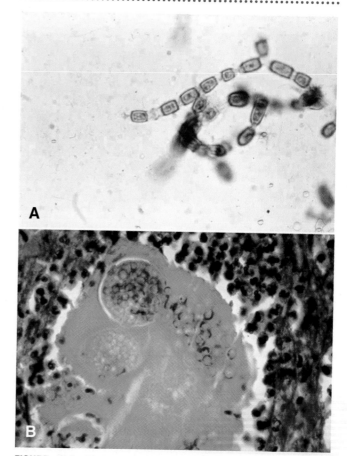

FIGURE 47-8. Tissue dimorphism of *Coccidioides species*. A. Segmented barrel-shaped arthroconidia are found in the environment. **B.** The tissue form, called a spherule, contains hundreds of endospores.

most likely in the burrows of desert animals. When conditions of rainfall, heat, and wind are correct, extensive "blooms" of the organism occur, and outbreaks among humans often follow. In highly endemic areas, as much as 80% of the population has evidence of prior infection with *Coccidioides*.

ENTRY

The arthroconidia of *Coccidioides* are highly infectious and easily inhaled into the alveoli. In the lung, the arthroconidia transform into distinctive large spherules that fill with endospores. Although arthroconidia can be phagocytosed and killed by neutrophils, the spherules resist phagocytosis.

SPREAD AND MULTIPLICATION

The primary target organ for infection with *Coccidioides* is the lung, but in some hosts, the organism spreads hematogenously and infects many different organs. The host response is *a mixture of neutrophils and T lymphocytes and activated macrophages*. Ultimate control of the infection requires development of cell-mediated immunity that leads

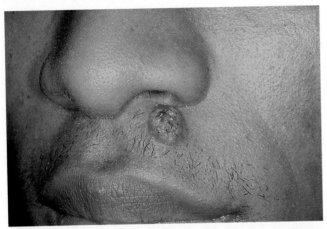

FIGURE 47-9. Patient with coccidioidomycosis and a cutaneous lesion on the face.

to eradication of the spherules. In hosts with deficient CD4 function, such as AIDS patients, severe disseminated infection is frequent. As with the other endemic mycoses, reactivation of an old focus of infection is possible years later.

DAMAGE

Most people with coccidioidomycosis have no symptoms or a mild viral-like illness. Symptomatic **acute pulmonary infection** occurs a few weeks after exposure and is usually manifested by fever, anorexia, fatigue, dry cough, and chest pain. Arthralgias and skin nodules (erythema nodosum) can develop during the illness and reflect the host response to the organism. The syndrome is often called **desert rheumatism** or **valley fever**. For most patients, it is a self-limited illness. However, in a small number of people, disease progresses to **chronic pulmonary infection** that often cavitates and requires antifungal therapy.

Disseminated coccidioidomycosis occurs more often in dark-skinned individuals, pregnant women, and people with cell-mediated immune deficiencies. Cutaneous, subcutaneous, and osteoarticular infections are common (Fig. 47-9), but any organ can be involved. **Chronic meningitis** is the most feared complication because it is fatal if not treated, and those who do respond to antifungal therapy will relapse if therapy is ever stopped.

DIAGNOSIS

The diagnosis of coccidioidomycosis is made by growing the organism, which grows on most media within several days, from involved tissues or body fluids. The laboratory must always be warned that coccidioidomycosis is a possibility because the mold form is highly infectious and has led to outbreaks among laboratory workers. Histopathological demonstration of spherules in tissues is also diagnostic. Various assays for antibodies against *Coccidioides* are quite helpful diagnostically when performed by a laboratory experienced with the assays.

TREATMENT AND PREVENTION

Of all the endemic mycoses, coccidioidomycosis is the most difficult to treat. Some patients will have recurrent and relapsing disease throughout their lives. Mild-to-moderate coccidioidomycosis is treated with **itraconazole** or **fluconazole**, usually for 12 to 24 months depending on the extent of disease. Patients who have severe infection should receive **amphotericin B** initially and then can be switched to an azole after their condition has stabilized. Coccidioidal meningitis can usually be treated successfully with fluconazole, but therapy must be lifelong. Prevention is difficult in the endemic area because the organism is so readily dispersed. Avoiding dust storms may be helpful.

OTHER ENDEMIC MYCOSES

Paracoccidioidomycosis is caused by *Paracoccidioides brasiliensis* and occurs primarily in Brazil and surrounding countries in South America. The most common manifestation is a chronic progressive infection of the lungs and mucous membranes that occurs primarily in older men who are exposed to the organism as rural laborers. An acute form of disseminated infection in young adults and immunosuppressed patients is less common. Treatment is usually with either trimethoprim/sulfamethoxazole or itraconazole, and amphotericin B is reserved for severe infection.

Penicilliosis is caused by *Penicillium marneffei* and is endemic only in Southeast Asia. Infection is usually disseminated, involving the lungs, skin, bone marrow, and other organs and occurs almost entirely in immunosuppressed patients, especially those with AIDS. Depending on the severity of the infection, treatment is with either amphotericin B or itraconazole.

CONCLUSION

The endemic mycoses are common infections that exist within restricted geographical areas. Most persons who are infected are asymptomatic or have only mild self-limited symptoms. Cell-mediated immunity is essential for successful resolution of these infections. Clinical manifestations are unique to each organism, but the lung is prominently involved with all three. Symptomatic disseminated histoplasmosis and coccidioidomycosis are most common in people with deficient cellular immunity. Azoles have revolutionized the treatment of the endemic mycoses; amphotericin B now is required primarily for patients with severe infection.

Suggested Readings

Anstead GM, Graybill JR. Coccidioidomycosis. *Infect Dis Clin North Am.* 2006;20:621–634.

Kauffman CA. Histoplasmosis: clinical and laboratory update. *Clin Microbiol Rev.* 2007;20:115–132.

Pappas PG. Blastomycosis. *Sem Resp Crit Care Med.* 2004;25:113–122.

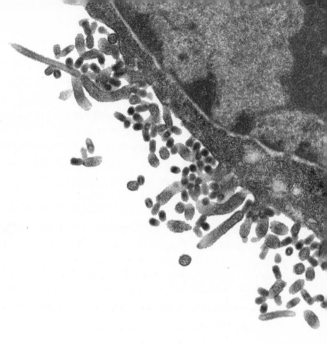

Chapter 48

Opportunistic Fungal Infections

Carol A. Kauffman

KEY CONCEPTS

Candidiasis:

- Is caused by *Candida albicans* and other species of *Candida* that are part of the normal human flora

- Occurs when other members of the normal flora are suppressed and when the host immune response, especially neutrophil function, is diminished

- Presents as either localized mucous membrane infection or invasive infection manifested by candidemia and visceral involvement

- Is treated with topical agents or azoles when involving mucous membranes and azoles, echinocandins, or amphotericin B when candidemia or invasive infection is present

Cryptococcosis:

- Is caused by Cryptococcus neoformans, an encapsulated, environmental yeast that is acquired by inhalation

- Presents most commonly as chronic meningitis because of neurotropism of the yeast

- Is treated with amphotericin B plus flucytosine followed by fluconazole

Aspergillosis:

- Is caused by *Aspergillus fumigatus* and other *Aspergillus* species, which are common environmental molds that have septate hyphae and that are inhaled into the respiratory tract

- Is characterized by angioinvasion, causing hemorrhage and tissue infarction, especially in the lungs

- Is treated with voriconazole, echinocandins, or amphotericin B

Mucormycosis:

- Is caused by Rhizopus, Mucor, and other Mucorales that are ubiquitous environmental molds that have nonseptate hyphae and that are inhaled into the respiratory tract

- Is characterized by angioinvasion, and infection occurs primarily in immunosuppressed patients and diabetics

- Is treated with amphotericin B and aggressive surgical debridement of all involved tissue

Pneumocystosis:

- Is caused by *Pneumocystis jiroveci*, a fungus that cannot be grown in vitro and that occurs in AIDS patients with low CD4 lymphocytes and in other immunosuppressed patients

- Causes pneumonia with hypoxemia as alveoli fill with proteinaceous fluid

- Is treated with trimethoprim/sulfamethoxazole

OPPORTUNISTIC fungi are **not considered true pathogens** because they cause disease only when host defenses are decreased. The group of opportunistic fungi encompasses a variety of disparate organisms. The three most commonly encountered genera are *Candida*, yeasts that are part of the normal flora of humans; *Cryptococcus*, yeasts found in the environment; and *Aspergillus*, molds that are ubiquitous in the environment. This chapter focuses on organisms in those three genera and briefly discusses the molds in the order Mucorales and *Pneumocystis jiroveci*, both of which cause serious infections in immunocompromised patients.

Patients at high risk for opportunistic fungal infections include individuals who are immunosuppressed because of hematological malignancies, solid organ or hematopoietic stem cell transplantation, neutropenia, HIV infection, or corticosteroids or other immunosuppressive drugs. Other risk factors include major burn

CASE • Mrs. D., a 60-year-old woman who had a perforated colon, had been in the intensive care unit for 3 weeks after surgery. She had renal failure and required intermittent hemodialysis. Mrs. D. also had an **ileus** (a nonfunctioning intestinal tract) and was obtaining parenteral nutrition through a central venous catheter. She was on a ventilator and had congestive heart failure. A prior pneumonia had been documented on day 12, and she was treated with piperacillin/tazobactam for that complication. On day 20 in intensive care, Mrs. D. became febrile to 39.3°C, her blood pressure fell to 90/50 mm Hg, and she became less responsive. Cultures of blood, urine, and sputum were obtained, and she was started on meropenem and vancomycin. The catheter was removed, and the tip was cultured. One day later, the laboratory called to report that the blood culture was growing a yeast; the next day, the culture of the catheter tip also showed yeast, and the organism from the blood was noted to be **germ-tube** positive and identified as *Candida albicans*.

This case raises several questions:

1. What factors put Mrs. D. at risk for developing candidemia?

2. Where did the *C. albicans* come from?

3. What does the term "germ-tube positive" mean to the clinician?

See Appendix for answers.

---

wounds, trauma, central venous catheters, broad-spectrum antibiotics, parenteral nutrition, diabetes, renal insufficiency requiring dialysis, and prematurity.

CANDIDIASIS

CHARACTERISTICS OF THE ORGANISM

Candida species are round or oval **yeasts** that reproduce by forming buds or blastoconidia (Fig. 48-1). They have the potential to form **hyphae** in vivo, and that form is seen in invasive infection with some, but not all, species of *Candida*. The most important member of the genus is *Candida albicans*, which is the predominant species colonizing humans and is responsible for most infections. Other species of increasing importance are *Candida glabrata*, which is resistant to some antifungal agents, and *Candida parapsilosis*, which is a common cause of central venous catheter–associated infections.

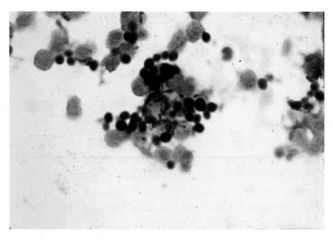

FIGURE 48-1. Budding yeasts typical of *Candida* species.

ENCOUNTER

Candida species normally colonize the gastrointestinal tract from the mouth to the rectum, the vagina, and the skin. Most infections are **endogenous**—that is, derived from the host's normal flora. In addition to immunosuppressed patients, especially those with neutropenia, a major group at risk for developing candidiasis comprises patients in intensive care units. Risk factors include broad-spectrum antibiotics, renal failure requiring dialysis, central venous catheters, and parenteral nutrition.

ENTRY

Candida species do not cause infection unless the ecology of the normal flora is disrupted. The simplest reasons for disruption of normal flora are use of broad-spectrum antimicrobial agents, which allow *Candida* to proliferate on the mucosa, and maceration of the skin, which opens that site to proliferation of the organism. Decreased **T-cell immunity** allows *Candida* proliferation on mucosal surfaces. Circumstances that allow the escape of *Candida* from the gut into the bloodstream include **neutropenia** and use of chemotherapeutic agents that destroy the mucosal barrier of the gut. *Candida* species also gain access into the bloodstream through **central venous catheters**.

SPREAD AND MULTIPLICATION

The main host defense that holds *Candida* in check on mucosal surfaces is **T cell–mediated immunity**. Patients with advanced HIV infection and low CD4 lymphocyte numbers frequently have oropharyngeal and vaginal candidiasis. Despite extensive proliferation of *Candida*, no invasion through the mucosa occurs.

Neutrophils are the main host defense against invasion through the mucosa and subsequent dissemination. Mono-

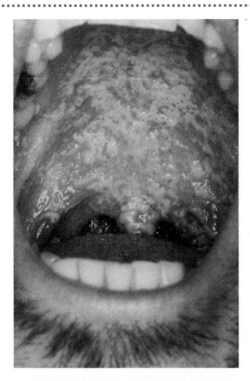

FIGURE 48-2. Extensive thrush on the palate of a patient with AIDS.

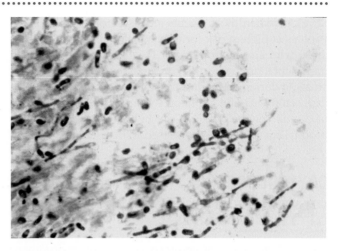

FIGURE 48-3. Biopsy of the esophagus in a leukemic patient who had pain with swallowing, showing tissue invasion with yeast and hyphal forms of *Candida albicans.*

cytes and macrophages play a less important role in phagocytosis and killing of *Candida*. Antibodies do not appear to play a role in host defense. In neutropenic patients, *Candida* spread hematogenously to many organs but especially to the eyes, kidneys, heart, brain, liver, and spleen.

DAMAGE

Mucosal candidiasis is characterized by adherent white plaques on the oropharyngeal and vaginal mucosa (Fig. 48-2). The lesions, often termed **thrush**, are not painful. Proliferation of *Candida* in warm moist areas of the skin, especially in the groin and under pendulous breasts, is termed **intertriginous candidiasis** and, in babies, **diaper rash**. In all circumstances, underlying tissues are not damaged, and patients suffer no long-term consequences.

Disseminated infection can present as unexplained fever, sepsis, or organ dysfunction. **Candidemia** is sometimes the only manifestation of dissemination; when visceral involvement is documented, the usual histopathologic picture is one of multiple **microabscesses** in many organs. The clinical manifestations vary according to the end organ involved. **Meningitis, chorioretinitis** with subsequent **vitritis, hepatosplenic abscesses**, and **vertebral osteomyelitis** are common complications of disseminated candidiasis. **Endocarditis** occurs more often on prosthetic valves.

DIAGNOSIS

The diagnosis of **mucosal candidiasis** is simple. Scrapings of the lesions show budding yeasts and

often pseudohyphae (elongated buds attached one to another), and cultures readily yield *Candida*. **Invasive candidiasis** is more difficult to document. Growth of *Candida* from normally colonized sites is not helpful in the documentation of invasive disease. Culture of blood is the simplest technique to document disseminated infection, but it is not very sensitive. Biopsy of involved tissues will show invasion with a mixture of budding yeast and hyphae that is quite characteristic of candidiasis (Fig. 48-3), and culture of involved tissues should yield the organism.

Candida species readily grow in a few days on blood agar or Sabouraud agar. *C. albicans* can be differentiated from other species in a few hours by the development of **germ tubes** (elongated buds from the yeast) when the yeast is exposed to calf serum. Identification of other species of *Candida* by utilization of sugars can take several more days, but rapid identification methods are increasingly used and allow for more rapid and appropriate choice of antifungal agents.

TREATMENT AND PREVENTION

Mucosal candidiasis and intertriginous candidiasis are treated with local antifungal creams and powders; however, extensive mucosal involvement may require treatment with a systemic antifungal agent. Invasive infection should always be treated with a systemic antifungal agent. The most commonly used agents are **fluconazole** or an echinocandin depending on the species causing infection. **Amphotericin B** also is used for several forms of invasive candidiasis. Candidemia with no obvious end-organ involvement is usually treated for a minimum of 2 weeks; depending on the organ involved, invasive candidiasis may need to be treated for months.

Mucosal infection in AIDS patients can be prevented by prophylaxis with antifungal agents, but resistance develops when those agents are used for many months. Patients at highest risk for disseminated infection, such as those who are neutropenic or have undergone stem cell transplantation, are usually treated prophylactically with an azole during the period of highest risk. In the intensive care setting, careful attention to hand cleansing and care of central venous catheters can help prevent candidemia; prophylaxis is generally not used in that setting.

CRYPTOCOCCOSIS
CHARACTERISTICS OF THE ORGANISM

The etiologic agent of cryptococcosis is an environmental yeast, *Cryptococcus neoformans*, which reproduces by budding. In tissues, but not in the environment, the organism is surrounded by a huge polysaccharide capsule, which helps prevent phagocytosis. *Cryptococcus gattii* is increasingly reported as a cause of human infection, but other species of *Cryptococcus* are generally not pathogenic.

ENCOUNTER

C. neoformans is **found worldwide in soil** contaminated with bird excreta and in a variety of other environmental niches. Patients most at risk for cryptococcosis are those who have **AIDS** or a **hematologic malignancy**, have received an organ or bone marrow **transplant**, or have been treated with **corticosteroids** or other immunosuppressive drugs. In contrast to the situation with most other opportunistic fungi, **about 20% of patients who have cryptococcosis appear to be immunocompetent**.

ENTRY

The yeast is inhaled into the alveoli, initially producing lung infection, which is often asymptomatic. In the alveoli, the organism begins to produce the polysaccharide capsule, a major virulence factor.

SPREAD AND MULTIPLICATION

The host defense against *C. neoformans* is complex. Neutrophils and macrophages are important in initial phagocytosis and killing of the yeast, but as **capsule** production increases, phagocytosis is inhibited. If phagocytosis does occur, the capsule appears to forestall intracellular killing. The capsule also appears to downregulate the development of Th1 mediators. T-cell immunity is crucial to control of infection with *C. neoformans*. A measure of the importance of T-cell immunity is the observation that prior to effective therapy for HIV infection, 5 to 10% of AIDS patients in the United States developed cryptococcosis.

The production of **melanin** by *C. neoformans* also appears to enhance virulence, possibly by providing a kind of "armor" in the fungal cell wall that resists enzyme degradation.

A striking aspect of infection with *C. neoformans* is its **neurotropism**. No explanation currently exists for why the organism preferentially infects the central nervous system. Another unique aspect of infection with *C. neoformans* in some, but not all, patients is the lack of an inflammatory response. Although pulmonary lesions may be granulomatous, the inflammatory response in the central nervous system is minimal.

DAMAGE

Patients most often present with **meningitis**, reflecting the fact that hematogenous spread has occurred from an asymptomatic pulmonary focus of infection. The meningitis is usually subacute to chronic. Symptoms include headache that worsens over days to weeks, fever, cranial nerve palsies, and mental status changes. Signs of **increased intracranial pressure** are often present. Dissemination is common in AIDS patients, who can present with meningitis associated with diffuse pulmonary infiltrates, skin lesions, and widespread visceral infection.

DIAGNOSIS

The diagnosis of cryptococcal meningitis is made by performing a lumbar puncture and examining cerebrospinal fluid for **encapsulated budding yeast** cells that can be highlighted by adding a drop of India ink to the slide (Fig. 48-4). The fluid classically shows a predominance of lymphocytes, a high protein, and a decreased glucose concentration. A **latex agglutination** test for the **capsular polysaccharide antigen** is both sensitive and

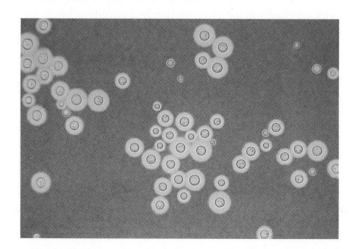

FIGURE 48-4. India ink preparation of cerebrospinal fluid that shows many encapsulated yeast cells, some of which are budding, a finding that is diagnostic of *Cryptococcus neoformans* meningitis.

specific and should be performed on both cerebrospinal fluid and serum. *C. neoformans* grows on many types of agar media in a few days and is easily identified by clinical laboratories.

TREATMENT AND PREVENTION

The initial treatment of cryptococcal meningitis is the combination of **amphotericin B** and **flucytosine** for several weeks followed by consolidation therapy with **fluconazole** for at least several months. Some patients with T-cell defects require lifelong fluconazole suppression to prevent relapse of infection. Other forms of cryptococcosis, such as pulmonary infection, can often be treated with fluconazole as primary therapy.

With the advent of effective therapy for HIV, cryptococcal meningitis has become uncommon as an AIDS-associated infection in the United States, but it remains an important cause of death in AIDS patients in Africa. No prophylactic regimens are currently recommended for AIDS patients or other at-risk populations.

ASPERGILLUS
CHARACTERISTICS OF THE ORGANISM

Aspergillus species are filamentous fungi that form a mycelium of **septate hyphae** and reproduce by forming **conidia** on aerial **conidiophores**. The major pathogenic species are *Aspergillus fumigatus* and *Aspergillus flavus* (Fig. 48-5), but hundreds of species exist in the environment. Species are differentiated by the arrangement of

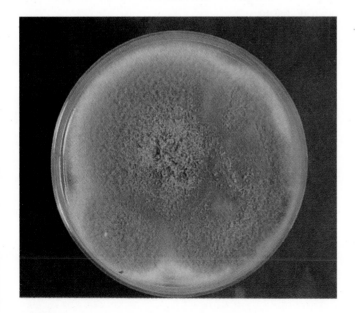

FIGURE 48-5. Colony of *Aspergillus fumigatus*.

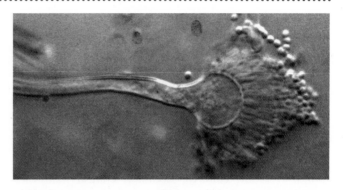

FIGURE 48-6. Distinctive conidia on a conidiophore of *Aspergillus terreus*, an uncommon pathogenic species.

conidia on the conidiophore (Fig. 48-6). *Aspergillus* species are not part of the normal flora of humans.

ENCOUNTER

Aspergillus species are **ubiquitous** in soil, manure, and decomposing vegetation throughout the world and can be cultured from air and water. Outbreaks in hospitals have occurred during construction, which allows wide dispersal of the conidia. The usual hosts are those who are **neutropenic**, are on **corticosteroids** or other immunosuppressive drugs, or are **transplant recipients**.

ENTRY

The **conidia** are inhaled into the upper and lower respiratory tracts. Invasive infection does not occur in the absence of profound immunosuppression. The initial event after entry is **germination** of the conidia into **hyphae**, which then invade into tissues.

SPREAD AND MULTIPLICATION

Neutrophils and macrophages are the main host defense against infection with *Aspergillus*. Pulmonary macrophages phagocytose and kill conidia that reach the alveoli but are unable to kill the hyphal forms. Neutrophils cannot phagocytose hyphae but instead line up along their surfaces and secrete reactive oxygen intermediates that kill the organism. Antibodies and T lymphocytes do not appear to play a major role in host defense against these filamentous fungi. *Aspergillus* is an **angioinvasive fungus**; the hyphae invade through blood vessel walls, causing **tissue infarction, hemorrhage**, and **necrosis**.

DAMAGE

Aspergillosis almost always presents initially as pulmonary or sinus infection. The usual histopathologic picture is one of hemorrhagic infarction and necrosis; with special stains, acutely branching septate hyphae are seen invading through tissues. The clinical manifestations of **invasive pulmonary aspergillosis** include fever, pleuritic chest pain, cough, hemoptysis, and dyspnea. Chest radiograph and computed tomography (CT) scan show multiple pulmonary nodules, hemorrhage around the nodules, and cavitation (necrosis). Acute facial pain is a herald of **sinus invasion**. Dissemination is common because of the propensity of the organism to invade the blood vessels. However, *Aspergillus* species are rarely found in blood cultures. Common clinical manifestations of disseminated aspergillosis include **necrotic skin lesions** and **brain abscess** presenting as stroke, seizures, or mental status changes. At autopsy, multiple areas of hemorrhagic infarction and abscesses can be found in many organs.

DIAGNOSIS

Aspergillus species readily grow on Sabouraud agar in a few days. The major issue is to differentiate contamination from infection as these ubiquitous fungi are frequent laboratory contaminants. Tissue biopsy is important to document tissue invasion (Fig. 48-7) but is not specific for *Aspergillus* because other angioinvasive fungi also demonstrate septate hyphae in tissue biopsies.

TREATMENT AND PREVENTION

The treatment of choice for invasive aspergillosis is **voriconazole**, but in some instances, **amphotericin B**, or an echinocandin is used. Because the mortality rate is very high unless therapy is started before extensive tissue invasion has occurred, empiric treatment is often initiated based on clinical manifestations and CT scan results in a high-risk patient.

Prevention of aspergillosis in high-risk patients is aimed at decreasing exposure by providing filtered air in high-risk units, such as transplant units; decreasing exposure to construction dust; and discouraging patients from activities likely to lead to exposure to these environmental molds. Prophylaxis with antifungal agents, such as voriconazole or posaconazole, is generally used in the highest-risk patients, such as stem cell transplant recipients.

OTHER OPPORTUNISTIC MOLDS

Severely immunocompromised hosts are at risk for infections caused by a large number of opportunistic fungi. Several fungal genera look very much like and behave in a fashion similar to *Aspergillus* species. The Mucorales are molds that differ from *Aspergillus*-like organisms in that their hyphae are broader and have few or **no septae** (Fig. 48-8), but they are similar to *Aspergillus* in their **angioinvasive** properties. The major pathogens in this group are the genera *Rhizopus* and *Mucor*. The patients at risk are those who have **hematologic malignancies, are neutropenic, are on corticosteroids, or have diabetes mellitus**. The reason diabetics are at risk, in part, relates to the adverse effects of acidosis on neutrophil chemotaxis and phagocytosis.

The presentation in diabetics is usually **rhino–orbital–cerebral mucormycosis**, in which the fungi spread from the nares and sinuses into the palate, orbit, and soft tissues of the face and then can invade the cavernous sinus and brain (Fig. 48-9). Pulmonary and disseminated zygomycosis occur more often in leukemics who are neutropenic and mimic invasive aspergillosis. The treatment of mucormycosis is **amphotericin B** and aggressive **surgical debridement** of all infected and necrotic tissue.

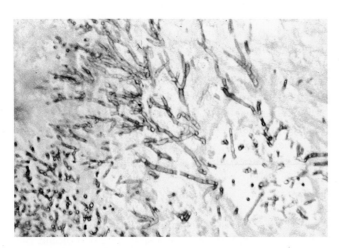

FIGURE 48-7. Invasion of tissue by *Aspergillus* species showing acutely branching septate hyphae.

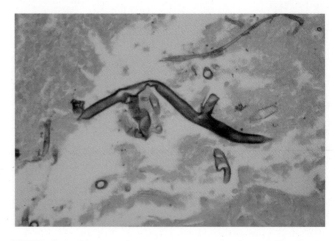

FIGURE 48-8. Biopsy of lung showing invasion of tissues by large, nonseptate hyphae characteristic of the Mucorales.

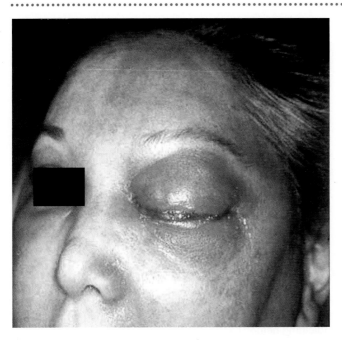

FIGURE 48-9. Rhinocerebral mucormycosis in a diabetic with ketoacidosis.

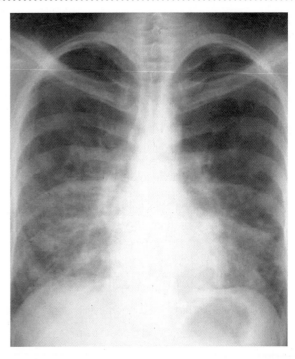

FIGURE 48-11. Diffuse bilateral pulmonary infiltrates in an AIDS patient with pneumocystis pneumonia.

PNEUMOCYSTOSIS

The organism that causes pneumocystosis has **never been grown in vitro**, and this fact has contributed to confusion about its nature. Based on sequence analysis of genes coding for ribosomal RNA and proteins made by the organism, it is clear that this organism is a fungus. *P. jiroveci* is presumably inhaled from the environment, but its ecological niche has not been found. Most people likely have been infected early in life, but disease only occurs when immunosuppression intervenes. The most common risk factor is **T-cell deficiency**, as demonstrated by the fact that pneumocystis pneumonia (PCP) was the most common opportunistic infection in AIDS

patients prior to the advent of effective antiviral therapy for HIV.

The organism only very rarely is found outside the lungs. Histopathologically, the alveoli are filled with **foamy proteinaceous material**, desquamated alveolar cells, and organisms (Fig. 48-10). Patients present with dyspnea, dry cough, fatigue, and mild or absent fever. A chest radiograph shows bilateral **diffuse infiltrates** (Fig. 48-11); hypoxemia, which can be severe, is almost always present. The diagnosis of PCP is made by demonstration of the organism by silver stain (Fig. 48-12), direct fluorescent antibody techniques, or polymerase chain

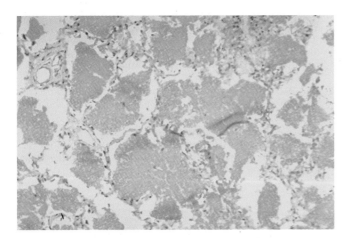

FIGURE 48-10. Lung biopsy stained with hematoxylin and eosin from an immunosuppressed patient with pneumonia caused by *Pneumocystis jiroveci*. Notice the proteinaceous material filling the alveoli.

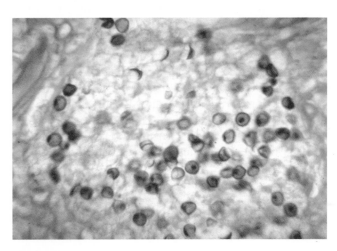

FIGURE 48-12. Silver stain of lung biopsy showing organisms typical of *Pneumocystis jiroveci* in the alveolus.

CASE • Mr. S., a 35-year-old man with acute myelocytic leukemia, had received initial induction treatment with a combination of chemotherapeutic agents that caused severe and prolonged neutropenia and thrombocytopenia. On day 10 of neutropenia, when his absolute neutrophil count was 50 per mm³, Mr. S. had bacteremia with *Klebsiella pneumoniae*, for which he received broad-spectrum antibiotics. On day 21 of neutropenia, while still on antibiotics, Mr. S. developed fever to 39.7°C, complained of pleuritic right-sided chest pain, and developed a cough and shortness of breath. A CT scan showed a nodular lesion in the right lower lobe (Fig. 48-13). A sample obtained by bronchoalveolar lavage revealed acutely branching septate hyphae, and cultures showed a mold that was identified as *Aspergillus fumigatus*.

This case raises several questions:

1. Why was Mr. S. at risk for an opportunistic fungal infection?

2. Why did Mr. S. have pleuritic chest pain?

3. How useful is a bronchoalveolar lavage showing septate hyphae?

See Appendix for answers.

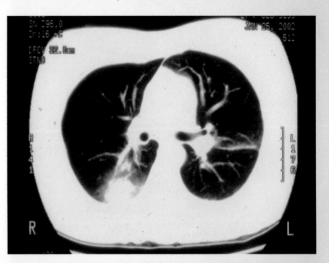

FIGURE 48-13. Chest computerized tomography scan showing a right lower-lobe nodule surrounded by a halo, indicating hemorrhage.

reaction on material obtained by bronchoalveolar lavage or biopsy. The treatment of choice is **trimethoprim/sulfamethoxazole**, which is also a highly effective prophylactic regimen in high-risk populations.

CONCLUSION

Advances in the fields of transplantation of organs and stem cells, treatment of hematologic malignancies and autoimmune disorders, and critical care medicine have resulted in an ever-increasing number of patients at risk for opportunistic fungal infections. Invasive infections caused by *Candida* species occur in patients who are neutropenic and also in those in intensive care. Cryptococcosis and pneumocystosis occur primarily in patients who have defects in T-cell immunity; before effective antiviral therapy for HIV became available, they were prominent opportunistic infections seen in AIDS patients.

Aspergillus species cause invasive infection almost entirely in severely immunosuppressed hosts, while the Mucorales target diabetics as well as the profoundly immunosuppressed population. A large number of molds that occur in the environment and that have not been discussed here have been reported to cause life-threatening infection in patients who are immunosuppressed. Infections with opportunistic fungi constitute increasing diagnostic challenges, are difficult to treat, and have a high mortality rate.

Suggested Readings

Chayakulkeeree M, Perfect JR. Cryptococcosis. *Infect Dis Clin N Am.* 2006;20:507–544.

Pappas PG, Kauffman CA, Andes D. Clinical Practice Guidelines for the Management of Candidiasis: 2009 Update by the Infectious Diseases Society of America. *Clin Infect Dis.* 2009;48:503–535.

Prabhu RM, Patel R. Mucormycosis and entomophthoromycosis. A review of the clinical manifestations, diagnosis, and treatment. *Clin Microbiol Infect.* 2004;10(suppl):31–47.

Segal BH. Aspergillosis. *N Engl J Med.* 2009;360:1870–1874.

Thomas CF, Limper AH. Current insights into the biology and pathogenesis of Pneumocystis pneumonia. *Nat Rev Microboiol.* 2007;5:298–308.

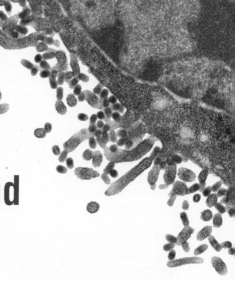

Chapter 49

Subcutaneous, Cutaneous, and Superficial Mycoses

Carol A. Kauffman

KEY CONCEPTS

Sporotrichosis:

- Is caused by *Sporothrix schenckii*, a dimorphic fungus
- Begins with inoculation of the organism from soil, moss, or decaying vegetation
- Presents as an isolated cutaneous ulceration or a series of ulcerated nodules along the lymphatic distribution of the initial lesion
- Is best diagnosed by culture of material from a lesion
- Is usually treated with itraconazole

Mycetoma and Chromoblastomycosis:

- Are seen mostly in the tropics
- Are caused by inoculation of environmental fungi into subcutaneous tissues
- Usually require surgical extirpation

Dermatophyte Infections:

- Are caused by the genera *Trichophyton*, *Microsporum*, and *Epidermophyton*.
- Infect the stratum corneum, hair shafts, and nails
- Cause tinea (meaning wormlike) infections of various skin structures (tinea corporis, tinea pedis, etc.)
- Are treated with local antifungal creams and lotions, except for onychomycosis, which must be treated with systemic antifungal agents

Superficial Mycoses:

- Are caused by *Malassezia* species, normal colonizers of human stratum corneum
- Cause tinea versicolor and seborrheic dermatitis, both of which are treated with antifungal creams or shampoos

FUNGAL INFECTIONS of the skin, skin appendages, and subcutaneous tissues are very common in humans. These infections are classically divided into those, such as sporotrichosis, that invade subcutaneous tissues and uncommonly deeper structures; dermatophyte infections that are restricted to cutaneous structures; and superficial fungal infections that remain localized to the stratum corneum. Sporotrichosis, the subcutaneous mycosis most commonly seen in the United States, spreads regionally through the lymphatics draining the inoculation site. In tropical climates, inoculation of a variety of different fungi that live in the soil or on plants can lead to two different chronic, often disfiguring, subcutaneous infections, mycetoma and chromoblastomycosis. Dermatophyte infections are the most common fungal infections of humans. The dermatophytes are molds that are adapted to live in keratinized tissues and cause annoying, often recurring infections of skin, hair, and nails. Superficial mycoses are caused by yeasts that colonize the stratum corneum of humans.

CASE • Mr. J., a 53-year-old dairy farmer who also raised Christmas trees for a living and whose hobby was raising tropical fish, noticed the appearance of a small nodule on his left hand. The growth enlarged over the next week to about the size of a quarter and then spontaneously opened and began to drain cloudy yellow material. The lesion was not painful or itchy. Mr. J. treated the open sore with an over-the-counter antibiotic ointment. Three weeks later, he noticed two new nodules going up his arm in a line. Those lesions subsequently ulcerated, and several new ones developed proximal to them (Fig. 49-1). At that point, Mr. J. decided to visit his physician.

The physician noted a total of seven nodules along the lymphatic distribution of the original lesion. She saw that the original lesion and several others were ulcerated; the rest were small subcutaneous nodules that were not tender. After taking biopsies of several of the ulcerated lesions for culture and histopathologic examination, Mr. J.'s doctor elected to wait for the results before starting therapy because the lesions could have been manifestations of infection with several different pathogens. The biopsy was read as granulomatous inflammation with no organisms seen, but the culture was reported after 8 days as showing growth of a mold, which was later identified as *Sporothrix schenckii*. Therapy with itraconazole was begun and continued for 4 months until all the lesions had resolved.

This case raises several questions:

1. Where did Mr. J. acquire the organism? Was it related to his dairy farming, raising Christmas trees, or keeping tropical fish?
2. What other infections, besides sporotrichosis, were in the physician's differential diagnosis?
3. Why was Mr. J. treated with itraconazole, which costs approximately 10 times more than the treatment long used for this infection, potassium iodide?

See Appendix for answers.

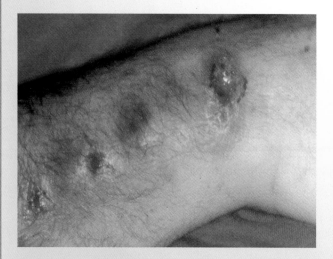

FIGURE 49-1. Multiple ulcerated nodules on the forearm in the distribution of the lymphatic drainage from an initial lesion that occurred on the back of the hand.

SPOROTRICHOSIS (SUBCUTANEOUS MYCOSIS)

CHARACTERISTICS OF THE ORGANISM

Sporothrix schenckii is a **dimorphic fungus**, similar to the fungi that cause endemic mycoses. In the environment, *S. schenckii* exists as a mold whose hyphae produce small conidia that are the infectious form. At body temperature, *S. schenckii* assumes a yeast form.

ENCOUNTER

S. schenckii is found in soil, sphagnum moss, and decaying wood and vegetation throughout the world. Most cases occur in those who have **outdoor vocations or avocations**, such as farming, landscaping, and gardening, that expose them to the fungus and are associated with a risk of penetrating trauma. Most cases are sporadic, but outbreaks have been described among forestry workers, gold miners, and topiary gardeners. An epidemic associated with infected cats is ongoing in Rio de Janeiro, Brazil.

ENTRY

The organism is inoculated into the dermis or subcutaneous tissues by thorns, splinters, or other sharp vegetation. Entry can also occur through animal scratches or just caring for cats that have ulcerated lesions. Most infections are seen on the upper extremities or face. On rare occasions, the organism is aerosolized and inhaled, resulting in pulmonary sporotrichosis.

SPREAD AND MULTIPLICATION

The initial site of inoculation evolves over several weeks into a nonpainful or mildly painful nodular lesion that subsequently ulcerates. In some patients, one cutaneous lesion is the only manifestation of infection (**cutaneous sporotrichosis**), and further spread does not occur. In others, like Mr. J., multiple nodules appear in the distribution of the lymphatics draining the area (**lymphocutaneous sporotrichosis**).

DAMAGE

Sporotrichosis is generally a localized infection with few systemic symptoms. Local tissue necrosis is uncommon, and lesions generally resolve with little scarring following antifungal treatment. However, in immunosuppressed hosts, especially those with AIDS, widespread cutaneous and/or life-threatening visceral infection can occur. Osteoarticular and pulmonary sporotrichosis, often seen in alcoholics, result in significant residual tissue damage.

DIAGNOSIS

Several bacterial infections, especially those caused by *Nocardia* and atypical mycobacteria, mimic lymphocutaneous sporotrichosis. Biopsy of a skin lesion or subcutaneous nodule should be performed for culture and histopathological examination. The characteristic picture is one of **granulomatous inflammation**. The small, cigar-shaped yeasts are rarely seen on histopathological examination, and **culture is the most reliable diagnostic test. Serology currently has no role in diagnosis**.

TREATMENT

Sporotrichosis rarely resolves without antifungal therapy. The treatment of choice is **itraconazole**. It has been known for a century that potassium iodide is effective for cutaneous and lymphocutaneous sporotrichosis, but this agent is poorly tolerated; most clinicians and patients prefer itraconazole. Treatment should be continued until the lesions have resolved completely, usually 3 to 6 months. For the uncommon case of osteoarticular, pulmonary, or disseminated infection, initial therapy with amphotericin B may be required, and itraconazole is subsequently given for 1 to 2 years. Patients who are immunosuppressed may have to remain on itraconazole for life.

OTHER SUBCUTANEOUS MYCOSES

Mycetomas are chronic infections that are characterized by nodules, sinus tracts, and discharge of visible grains that are composed of colonies of microorganisms (Fig. 49-2). Some mycetomas are caused by bacteria, but many are due to soil molds, such as *Madurella mycetomatis,* that are inoculated through the skin. **Chromoblastomycosis** is characterized by chronic nodular, verrucous lesions caused by a variety of different brown-black pigmented soil molds that are inoculated through the skin (Fig. 49-3). In tissues, the organisms are seen as thick-walled, pigmented, septate structures called sclerotic bodies. Mycetomas and chromoblastomycosis occur mostly on the lower extremities in persons living in tropical rural areas. Itraconazole is sometimes helpful

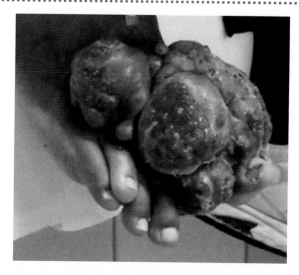

FIGURE 49-2. Extensive fungating mass typical of mycetoma.

but is rarely curative. **Surgical débridement of small lesions is effective, but more extensive infection may require amputation**.

DERMATOPHYTES (CUTANEOUS MYCOSES)

Infection of the skin by dermatophytes is often called **ringworm**, which is a confusing term for patients because there is no connection with worms. A better term is **tinea**, the Latin word for worm. Both words denote the serpentine nature of the lesions that characterize some dermatophyte infections of the skin. The term *tinea* is used in conjunction with the Latin word for the part of the body affected—for example, **tinea capitis** (head), **tinea pedis** (feet), **tinea corporis** (body), **tinea cruris** (crotch), and

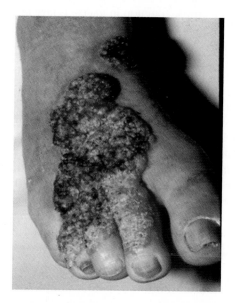

FIGURE 49-3. Chromoblastomycosis involving the foot in a patient from South America.

tinea unguium (nails); however, nail infections are more often called onychomycosis. Other familiar terms often used to describe these diseases include **athlete's foot**, **jock itch**, and **jungle rot**.

CHARACTERISTICS OF THE ORGANISM

Three genera of dermatophytes, *Microsporum, Trichophyton*, and *Epidermophyton*, cause infection in humans. These molds take days to weeks to grow at 25°C in the laboratory, and most are unable to grow at 37°C.

ENCOUNTER

Different species of dermatophytes have different ecological niches. Dermatophytes are not members of the normal skin flora. Some organisms grow in soil, while others are found in association with animals, especially dogs and cats, and still others are found almost exclusively in association with humans. Close contact is usually required for transmission to occur among humans and between animals and humans. The ability of dermatophytes to survive on wet surfaces, such as locker room shower floors, likely contributes to transmission.

ENTRY

For disease to occur, the person must not only be exposed to the fungus but also have breaks in the skin so that the relatively avirulent organisms can gain access. Maceration of tissue, especially common in the feet and groin, contributes to the development of infection. **Genetic and hormonal factors** also are important in the ability of the organism to gain entry and cause infection. For example, the incidence of dermatophyte infections is higher in males than in females, with ratios of 3:1 for tinea capitis and 6:1 for tinea pedis. Tinea cruris, common in males, is rare in females.

SPREAD AND MULTIPLICATION

The dermatophytes spread through the stratum corneum but rarely invade the dermis. The ring shape that is characteristic of dermatophyte lesions is the result of the organism growing outward in a centrifugal pattern. The area of the lesion that yields viable fungal elements is located at the margin. The central area generally has few or no viable fungi. Fungal invasion of nails occurs through the lateral or superficial nail plates and then spreads throughout the nail. When hair shafts are invaded, the organisms can be seen either within the shaft or surrounding it. Keratinases and mannans present in dermatophytes may play a role in invasion of keratinized tissues.

DAMAGE

Tinea infections occur at various anatomic sites, depending on the age of the host. Tinea capitis is most common

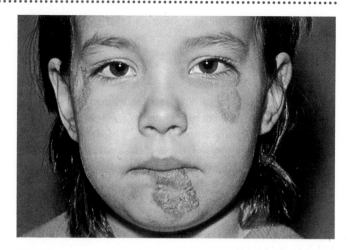

FIGURE 49-4. Typical lesions of tinea corporis (ringworm) in a child. Notice the discrete borders with scaling and central clearing.

in children, with the highest incidence in 3- to 7-year-olds; after puberty, the disease is much less common. Tinea cruris, tinea pedis, and onychomycosis rarely occur in childhood but are common in adults and are especially common in men.

Many of the clinical features of tinea infections are related to the **inflammatory response** in the epidermis and dermis to fungal antigens that diffuse from the site of fungal invasion. Children with **tinea capitis** present with well-demarcated scaly patches in which hair shafts have broken off right above the skin. **Tinea corporis** is manifested by well-demarcated, pruritic (itchy), scaly lesions that undergo central clearing as the lesion expands (Fig. 49-4). Often one or several small lesions are present, but in rare cases, extensive involvement over much of the trunk occurs (Fig. 49-5). **Tinea cruris** presents as a pruritic, erythematous rash with a scaly border in the groin area. **Tinea pedis** causes fissures between the toes and

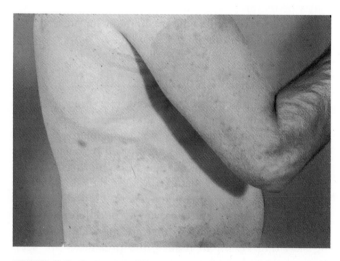

FIGURE 49-5. Extensive tinea corporis in a man who had no underlying medical illness. Notice the well-demarcated border typical of dermatophyte infections. This patient required systemic azole therapy to cure the infection.

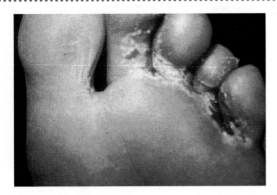

FIGURE 49-6. Maceration in the toe webs due to tinea pedis (athlete's foot).

a scaly pruritic rash along the lateral and plantar surfaces of the feet (Fig. 49-6). Nails infected with dermatophytes become thickened, discolored, and lifted off the nail bed (onycholysis) (Fig. 49-7).

DIAGNOSIS

Scrapings should be taken of the involved area (at the border of skin lesions) and observed under the microscope after treatment with potassium hydroxide. The presence of hyaline, septate, branching hyphae confirms the diagnosis of a dermatophyte infection, but culture is required to identify the specific organism.

TREATMENT

Tinea infections usually respond to treatment with topical antifungal creams and lotions, including tolnaftate, allylamines, and azoles. The exception is **onychomycosis**, which always requires systemic antifungal agents to achieve an effective response. Either terbinafine, which is an allylamine, or itraconazole can be used. For onychomycosis, therapy must be given for a minimum of 3 to 4 months. Relapses are the rule with tinea pedis and tinea cruris. Early institution of topical antifungal agents at the first signs of relapse generally keeps the infection in check.

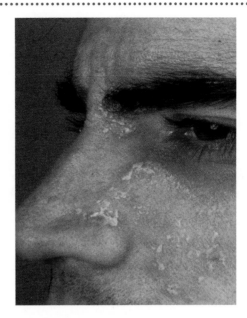

FIGURE 49-8. Seborrheic dermatitis.

SEBORRHEA AND TINEA VERSICOLOR (SUPERFICIAL MYCOSES)

Virtually all adults have colonization of the stratum corneum with the yeast *Malassezia*. Usually no symptoms are associated with colonization. However, this organism can cause **seborrheic dermatitis**, which is characterized by pruritic, erythematous patches with greasy scales in the eyebrows, mustache, and scalp (Fig. 49-8). It is also the cause of **tinea versicolor**, which usually appears on the chest or neck as hypopigmented or hyperpigmented patches with slight scaling. (Although the term "tinea" is used, this condition is not due to dermatophytes.) Superficial mycoses are treated with topical antifungal creams or shampoos.

CONCLUSION

The superficial, cutaneous, and subcutaneous mycoses are the most common fungal infections of humans. They rarely lead to serious disease and in many cases are infections with which patients will live for years. Superficial and dermatophyte infections of the skin are treated with antifungal creams, lotions, or shampoos; infection of the nails must be treated with systemic antifungal agents. Subcutaneous infections require therapy with systemic antifungal agents, and some can be treated only with surgical debridement or amputation.

Suggested Readings

de Berker D. Clinical practice. Fungal nail disease. *N Engl J Med.* 2009;360:2108–2113.

Lichon V, Khachemoune A. Mycetoma: a review. *Am J Clin Dermatol.* 2006;7:315–321.

Ramos-e-Silva M, Vasconcelos C, Carneira S, et al. Sporotrichosis. *Clin Dermatol.* 2007; 25:181–187.

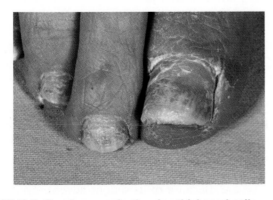

FIGURE 49-7. Onychomycosis showing thickened nails.

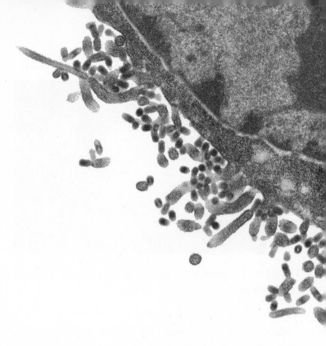

Chapter 50

Antifungal Agents

Carol A. Kauffman

KEY CONCEPTS

- Polyenes interfere with ergosterol synthesis in the fungal cell membrane and have broad antifungal activity, but their use is limited by the high rate of adverse events.

- Allylamines interfere with ergosterol synthesis in the fungal cell membrane but are useful only for superficial fungal infections.

- Azoles target ergosterol in the fungal cell membrane and are relatively safe drugs. Each agent has a unique spectrum of activity and drug interaction profile.

- Echinocandins target the fungal cell wall and have very few side effects; however, they have a limited spectrum of activity.

- Pyrimidine inhibition is the target of flucytosine, an agent with limited use and a high rate of toxicity.

COMPARED with the number of agents available to treat bacterial infections, the drugs available for treating fungal infections seem woefully inadequate (Table 50-1). A major deterrent to the development of antifungal agents has been the shared metabolic and physiologic pathways of eukaryotic fungal and mammalian cells and subsequent risk for toxicity. Several major classes of antifungal agents target the ergosterol pathway in the fungal cell membrane (Fig. 50-1). Although they also target ergosterol synthesis, the azole class of antifungal agents is far safer than the polyenes. With the development of the echinocandins that have a unique mechanism of action on the cell wall, selective inhibition of fungal growth with minimal effects on mammalian cells has been accomplished (Fig. 50-1).

POLYENES

The polyenes act by **binding to ergosterol**, a major component of the cell membrane in fungi. Binding leads to altered membrane permeability, leakage of cell constituents, and cell death. The polyenes also bind, although less avidly, to cholesterol in mammalian cell membranes, thus accounting for their toxicity. Two polyene agents are currently available. **Nystatin** is quite toxic and used only as a topical agent. **Amphotericin B**, introduced in the 1950s, has been the standard of therapy for serious fungal infections until recently.

Amphotericin B is available only as an intravenous formulation and is prepared as a colloidal dispersion with sodium deoxycholate because of its insolubility in water. The drug is highly protein bound to serum lipoproteins and penetrates poorly into cerebrospinal and other body fluids. The half-life is very long (terminal half-life >15 days), and activity can be recovered from urine for several months after discontinuation. Amphotericin B has a very wide **spectrum of activity**. It has excellent in vitro activity against yeasts, including *Candida* species and *Cryptococcus* species; molds, including *Aspergillus* species and the Mucorales; all the endemic mycoses; and most organisms causing subcutaneous and skin infections.

The major drawback to the use of amphotericin B is its **inherent toxicity**. Some degree of nephrotoxicity occurs in almost every patient receiving the agent, anemia is expected with prolonged therapy, and infusion reactions (chills, fever, nausea, myalgias) are common and can be severe. Because of its serious adverse event profile, new formulations have been introduced that mask

TABLE 50-1 Major Classes of Antifungal Agents

Class	Mechanism of Action	Agents	Formulation	Pathogens Treated
Polyenes	Bind to ergosterol causing disruption of cell membrane	Amphotericin B	Intravenous	*Candida, Cryptococcus, Aspergillus,* Mucorales, endemic mycoses, other molds
		Nystatin	Topical	*Candida* (mucous membrane and skin)
Allylamines	Block ergosterol synthesis in cell membrane	Terbinafine	Topical, oral	Dermatophytes
Azoles	Block ergosterol synthesis in cell membrane	Ketoconazole	Oral	Endemic mycoses, dermatophytes
		Itraconazole	Oral	*Candida*, endemic mycoses, *Aspergillus*, dermatophytes
		Fluconazole	Intravenous, oral	*Candida, Cryptococcus*
		Voriconazole	Intravenous, oral	*Aspergillus*, other molds, *Candida*
		Posaconazole	Oral	*Candida, Aspergillus*, Mucorales, other molds
Echinocandins	Inhibit cell wall synthesis	Caspofungin Micafungin Anidulafungin	Intravenous	*Candida, Aspergillus*
Pyrimidine inhibitor	Inhibits DNA and protein synthesis	Flucytosine	Oral	*Cryptococcus, Candida*

much of the toxicity by wrapping the active drug in lipid layers or within liposomes. The introduction of three **lipid-associated formulations of amphotericin B** has ameliorated, but not eliminated, the toxicity of the agent. Many physicians now use the lipid formulations in place of the deoxycholate preparation.

Amphotericin B remains the drug of choice for infection with the Mucorales and is the most appropriate initial therapy for cryptococcal meningitis, severe infections with the endemic mycoses, and some forms of candidiasis. The introduction of new classes of antifungal agents has markedly diminished the need for amphotericin B.

ALLYLAMINES

Terbinafine, the major allylamine agent, inhibits **squalene epoxidase** activity, blocking ergosterol synthesis in the fungal cell membrane. This agent has activity against dermatophytes that cause skin and nail infections, and it has some activity against *Candida albicans*. It is available in both tablet and topical formulations.

The drug is extensively metabolized by cytochrome P450 enzymes in the liver and concentrates in the stratum corneum, hair follicles, and nails. Terbinafine is indicated for the treatment of **dermatophyte** infections of the skin that have not responded to application of creams and for fungal nail infections. It is not indicated for systemic fungal infections.

Terbinafine is usually well tolerated. Changes in taste perception can occur and can interfere with appetite. Hepatic dysfunction and rarely liver failure have been reported with terbinafine.

AZOLES

There are five systemic azole antifungal agents, **ketoconazole, itraconazole, fluconazole, voriconazole, and posaconazole**, currently available. In addition, many topical azole agents are used for localized yeast infections. Voriconazole and posaconazole have a broader spectrum of activity compared with the other agents. All azoles inhibit fungal growth through the same mechanism, inhibition of cytochrome P450–dependent 14α-lanosterol demethylation, a vital step in **cell membrane ergosterol synthesis**. Differences in selectivity for fungal cell membranes compared with mammalian cell membranes predict toxicity of the azoles.

Ketoconazole, the first oral azole, had a significant number of side effects and drug interactions and has largely been supplanted by **itraconazole**, with greater intrinsic activity against many fungi and an improved safety profile. Itraconazole is active against *Candida*

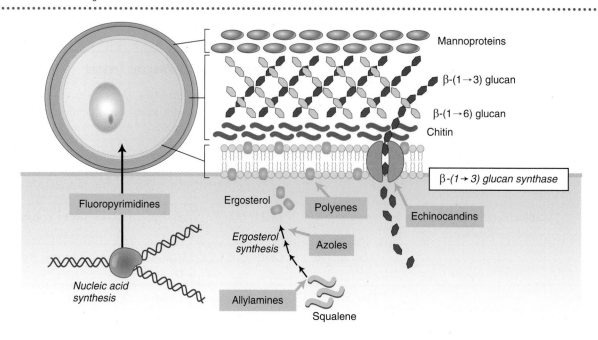

FIGURE 50-1. Graphical representation of the site of action of antifungal drugs in the fungal cell.

species, *Cryptococcus, Aspergillus*, the endemic fungi, and dermatophytes. It is available as capsules and an oral solution. Absorption of itraconazole is problematic in that both food and gastric acid are required for maximum absorption of the capsules. Itraconazole has become the drug of choice for the endemic mycoses, sporotrichosis, and dermatophyte infections.

The antifungal spectrum of **fluconazole** is narrower than that of other azoles. It has excellent activity against most *Candida* species other than *Candida glabrata* and *Candida krusei*, but it is not active against most molds. Fluconazole is water soluble and available in both intravenous and oral formulations. It undergoes less cytochrome P450–mediated metabolism than other azoles, and renal excretion of active drug occurs. Fluconazole is widely used for treatment of *Candida* and *Cryptococcus* infections and for prophylaxis against fungal infections in immunosuppressed patients. It has minimal toxicity.

Voriconazole is a broad-spectrum azole with activity against *Candida, Aspergillus*, and many other molds, and the endemic mycoses. It is not active against the Mucorales. Voriconazole is available as both intravenous and oral formulations and is extensively metabolized by several cytochrome P450 enzymes, leading to many drug interactions. It is the drug of choice for treating aspergillosis.

Posaconazole has the broadest spectrum of activity of all the azoles, having activity against those yeasts and molds that voriconazole is active against plus the Mucorales. It is available only as an oral solution that has to be taken with fatty food for absorption. It has the least cytochrome P450 interactions of all the azoles, and thus, drug interactions are less common. It is approved only for treating thrush and for prophylaxis in high-risk patients. Overall, the azoles are safe antifungal agents. The two most problematic issues are hepatitis, which is an uncommon side effect seen with all azoles, and drug interactions, which differ for each agent and must be monitored carefully to avoid serious and possibly life-threatening reactions.

ECHINOCANDINS

The **echinocandins** have a unique target, the synthesis of β-(1,3)-D-glucan, an essential component of the **fungal cell wall**. Because mammalian cells do not have cell walls, the echinocandins are more selective than the agents discussed earlier that target the synthesis of cell membrane components. β-(1,3)-D-glucan is an important component of the cell walls of all *Candida* and *Aspergillus* species, but it is not present or occurs only in small amounts in other fungi. Thus, the spectrum of activity of the echinocandins is relatively narrow (*Candida* and *Aspergillus*) compared with amphotericin B and the azoles.

There are three echinocandins: **caspofungin**, **micafungin**, and **anidulafungin**. All are available only as intravenous formulations. Hydrolyzed and then acetylated to inactive metabolites, the echinocandins are neither metabolized by nor inhibitors of the cytochrome P450 system.

Given their selective fungal cell wall target, the echinocandins have minimal toxicity. Infusion-related reactions, including rash and headache, have been reported but are uncommon.

The echinocandins have become the drug of choice for certain *Candida* infections, and they have proved useful for treating aspergillosis, either combined with voriconazole or following initial treatment with voriconazole. The three agents are similar enough that they can be used interchangeably.

PYRIMIDINE INHIBITION

The only agent in this class, **flucytosine** (5-fluorocytosine), is an oral fluorinated pyrimidine that is converted to 5-fluorouracil by fungal cells. It interferes with fungal protein and DNA synthesis. Flucytosine is active against *Candida neoformans* and *Candida* species. Because resistance develops quickly, flucytosine is never used alone but must be paired with another antifungal agent. Another major drawback to using this agent is dose-related bone marrow suppression and hepatotoxicity. Flucytosine is used almost entirely only for the initial treatment of cryptococcal meningitis.

OTHER AGENTS

Griseofulvin is an oral agent used only for treatment of superficial dermatophyte infections. The mechanism of action is unique in that it interferes with microtubule function. The use of griseofulvin has largely been supplanted by terbinafine and itraconazole. **Tolnaftate** is another agent used only for dermatophyte infections. The mechanism of action is not known. It is available only in topical formulations.

Potassium iodide has been used for more than a century against cutaneous sporotrichosis, but the mechanism of action remains unknown. It is available as an oral solution. Side effects (metallic taste, thyroid dysfunction, rash, salivary gland swelling) are common.

CONCLUSION

The three major classes of antifungal drugs—polyenes, azoles, and echinocandins—are able to cure many previously fatal fungal infections. All have side effects, but the newer agents are markedly safer than the first systemic antifungal drug, amphotericin B. The host immune response remains the most important determinant of the outcome of infection, even with the new antifungal drugs recently made available.

Suggested Readings

Antoniadou A, Dupont B. Lipid formulations of amphotericin B: where are we today? *J Mycol Med*. 2005;15:230–238.

Dodds-Ashley ES, Lewis R, Lewis JS, et al. Pharmacology of systemic antifungal agents. *Clin Infect Dis*. 2006;43:S28–S39.

Spanakis EK, Aperis G, Mylonakis E. New agents for the treatment of fungal infections: clinical efficacy and gaps in coverage. *Clin Infect Dis*. 2006;43:1060–1068.

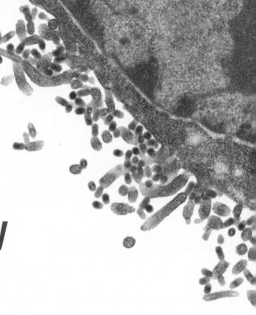

Chapter 51

Introduction to Parasitology

Cary Engleberg

KEY CONCEPTS

Pathogens: Parasites include primarily protozoa and helminths.

Encounter: Local ecology (e.g., climate, arthropods) and socioeconomic factors (e.g., sanitation, housing) govern the geographic distribution of disease by determining whether a particular parasite can complete its life cycle.

Entry: Knowledge of parasitic life cycles is essential to understanding the routes of transmission and the rationales for preventive intervention.

Spread: For many parasitic infections, the capacity to occupy certain tissues (tropism) is an essential feature of the life cycle.

Multiplication: Parasitic protozoa multiply in the human host and cause disease as their numbers increase. Helminth infections generally do not replicate within humans, so their numbers increase only through continued acquisition.

Damage: Many parasites have evolved within human hosts and may cause asymptomatic infections. In helminth infections, symptoms typically result from a high acquired parasite burden or prolonged duration of infection.

Many parasites survive in the human host by evading or subverting the immune response. Damage induced by those pathogens is usually a direct consequence of host hypersensitivity.

Diagnosis: Diagnosis often depends on direct identification of parasitic forms in human samples. Therefore, knowledge of tissue tropisms and modes of transmission determines which samples should be collected and examined.

PARASITIC infections are among the most prevalent infectious diseases worldwide (Table 51-1). Some diseases—malaria, schistosomiasis, and hookworm, for example—cause morbidity and mortality on a massive scale in many tropical countries. In most developed countries, where "tropical diseases" have no potential for transmission, parasites are regarded as strange and exotic. That perception may be misleading, however, because many parasitic infections are cosmopolitan in distribution, occurring in both developed and developing countries. One can theoretically acquire these infections without traveling. Other parasites are geographically restricted to regions where specific conditions for transmission are present (Table 51-2). In either geographical context, infection with many common parasitic infections causes no clinical symptoms. Yet the AIDS epidemic and more advanced immunosuppression for organ transplantation or following cancer treatment have given certain previously benign parasitic diseases new clinical significance.

INFECTION VERSUS DISEASE

As with other agents, parasitic infection must be distinguished from parasitic disease. For example, a large number of adults in the United States are infected with the protozoan *Toxoplasma gondii*, as demonstrated by the prevalence of antitoxoplasma antibodies in the population. However, few people become ill from the infection. Another example is hookworm infection. Hookworms consume small amounts of blood to survive, mate, and release eggs in the human intestine. Because the amount of blood consumed by each worm is small (0.03 to 0.15 mL/d), infections with only a few worms

TABLE 51-1 Worldwide Occurence of Selected Parasitic Infections

A. Prevalence

Infection	Number of Individuals Infected
Ascariasis	1.38 billion
Toxoplasmosis	1–2 billion
Hookworm disease	1.25 billion
Schistosomiasis	200 million
Giardiasis	200 million
Filariasis (skin and lymphatic)	137 million
Pinworm infection	60–100 million
Strongyloidiasis	50–80 million
Trichuriasis	45 million
Trypanosomiasis	15–20 million
Leishmaniasis	12 million

B. Incidence and Mortality

Infection	New Cases per Year	Deaths per Year
Malaria	200–300 million	1–3 million
Amebiasis	48 million	70,000
Leishmaniasis	2 million	80,000
Trypanosomiasis	450,000	145,000

Based on estimates from the 1998 WHO World Health Report.

are clinically insignificant. However, infections with large numbers of hookworms can produce a life-threatening anemia.

Like other infectious agents described in this textbook, parasites have evolved to exploit their hosts in order to grow and procreate. Because they depend on the host for their survival and to complete their life cycle, killing or disabling the host is not to the parasites' advantage. Consequently, disease associated with many parasites is often the consequence of *prolonged, repeated, or unusually burdensome infection*. Parasitic diseases are usually **subacute** or **chronic** and, even if untreated, are rarely fatal over short periods. There are, however, important exceptions, such as malaria caused by *Plasmodium falciparum*, which may be rapidly fatal (within 3 to 5 days in nonimmune hosts). Moreover, parasites that normally produce quiescent, asymptomatic infections in immunocompetent hosts can cause disseminated and potentially lethal diseases in immunocompromised persons (e.g., toxoplasmosis).

PARASITIC INFECTIONS AS ZOONOSES

Several parasitic infections of humans are **zoonoses**; that is, they are caused by agents that infect animals such as birds, reptiles, and other mammals (see Chapter 73 and the Chapter 33 paradigm). Many human parasites require both human and nonhuman hosts to complete their life cycles. For example, people can carry an adult beef tapeworm in the intestinal lumen, but an infected person cannot transmit the parasite to another person. To complete its life cycle, the parasite must undergo larval development in the muscles of cattle (cysticercosis). Humans can become infected with the tapeworm by eating undercooked beef. Both stages (adult and larval) and both hosts (cattle and humans) are required to complete the life cycle of the tapeworm. Other animal parasites do not require a developmental stage in humans but can nevertheless infect humans and cause disease. In those cases, humans are **dead-end hosts**. For example, the blood fluke (schistosome) of birds alternates between birds and snails. Although humans can sometimes "substitute" for birds as vertebrate hosts, the life cycle of the parasite is not completed in humans. The infecting larvae cannot penetrate beyond the skin but die there, causing an irritating dermatitis called "**swimmer's itch**" that resolves spontaneously.

TYPES OF PARASITES AND MODES OF TRANSMISSION
Protozoa

Protozoa are one-celled **eukaryotes**. Protozoal parasites of medical importance include *Plasmodium* species (the agents of malaria) as well as species of *Toxoplasma*, *Giardia*, *Cryptosporidium*, *Leishmania*, and trypanosomes. Infections with any of those pathogens can be initiated by relatively small inocula. Disease is generally a consequence of the replication of the parasites in large numbers within the host. Replication may be intracellular (e.g., plasmodia, which grow within red blood cells, and *Leishmania* species, which grow within macrophages), or it may occur extracellularly, such as in the lumen of the gastrointestinal tract (e.g., amebas and *Giardia* species).

As unicellular organisms bounded by only a cell membrane, many protozoa are unable to withstand desiccation (drying) in the external environment. Consequently, their life cycles usually do not include free environmental stages, and their transmission from one host to another depends on **arthropod vectors**. For example, plasmodia are transmitted by mosquitoes. An alternative strategy used by some protozoa is to alternate between two distinct forms: an active **trophozoite** form that grows and replicates by binary fission with the host, and a dormant, nonreplicating **cyst** form that is

TABLE 51-2 Parasitic Infections by Cosmopolitan Versus Geographically Restricted Range of Transmission

Cosmopolitan	Geographically Restricted
Intestinal and Vaginal Protozoa	
Entamoeba histolytica (amebiasis)	*Isospora belli* (isosporiasis)
Giardia lamblia (giardiasis)	*Balantidium coli* (balantidiasis)
Cryptosporidium parvum (cryptosporidiosis)	
Cyclospora cayetanensis (cyclosporiasis)	
Trichomonas vaginalis (trichomoniasis)	
Blood and Tissue Protozoa	
Toxoplasma gondii (toxoplasmosis)	*Plasmodium vivax, P. falciparum, P. ovale, P. malariae* (malaria)
Free-living amebas (meningoencephalitis, skin and eye infections)	*Leishmania donovani, L. tropica, L. mexicana, L. braziliensis*, etc. (leishmaniasis)
	Trypanosoma brucei (African sleeping sickness)
	Trypanosoma cruzi (Chagas disease)
	Babesia spp. (babesiosis)
Intestinal Helminths	
Ascaris lumbricoides (roundworm)	*Ancylostoma braziliensis* (hookworm)
Enterobius vermicularis (pinworm)	*Necator americanus* (hookworm)
Trichuris trichiura (whipworm)	*Strongyloides stercoralis* (threadworm)
Hymenolepis nana (dwarf tapeworm)	*Taenia solium* (pork tapeworm)
Diphyllobothrium latum (fish tapeworm)	
Blood and Tissue Helminths	
Toxocara canis, T. cati, Baylisascaris spp. (agents of visceral larva migrans)	*Schistosoma mansoni, S. haematobium, S. japonicum*, and others (schistosomiasis)
Trichinella spiralis (trichinosis)	*Echinococcus granulosus, E. multilocularis* (cystic hydatid disease)
Dirofilaria immitis (canine filariasis)	*Wuchereria bancrofti, Brugia malayi* (lymphatic filariasis)
	Onchocerca volvulus, Loa loa (cutaneous and ocular filariasis)
	Dracunculus medinensis (Guinea worm)
	Paragonimus westermani (lung fluke)
	Clonorchis sinensis and others (liver flukes)

adapted for survival in various environmental extremes as it transits between hosts. Protozoal cysts are relatively impermeable because of their double membranes and thus can resist desiccation in the external environment. Protozoa that infect the gastrointestinal tract employ this strategy, and they are transmitted between hosts by the fecal–oral route.

One approach to classifying protozoal pathogens is to group them based on their **life cycles** and **locomotion** (Fig. 51-1):

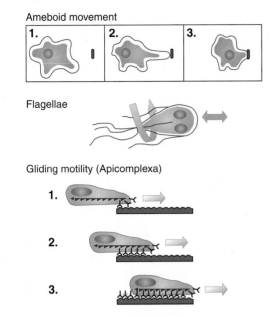

Ameboid movement

Flagellae

Gliding motility (Apicomplexa)

FIGURE 51-1. Mechanisms of protozoal locomotion.

- **Amebas** (or Sarcodina): formless cells that move purposefully by extending **pseudopods** toward an attractive stimulus and then **streaming** their cytoplasm in the desired direction. Amebas are intestinal parasites that alternate between trophozoite and cyst forms.
- **Flagellates**: intestinal and blood protozoa that use one or more flagella for locomotion. Like the amebas, flagellates that infect the gastrointestinal tract form environmentally resistant cysts. Flagellates that infect the tissues or blood are usually transmitted by arthropods.
- **Ciliates**: protozoa covered with tiny cilia that provide locomotion. Pathogenic ciliates are extremely unusual and are not covered in this textbook.
- **Apicomplexans** (or **Sporozoa**): very important pathogens that include the agents of malaria, toxoplasmosis, and several common intestinal parasites. Apicomplexans share the feature of intracellular replication. Based on observations of *T. gondii*, it is thought to move using a "tractor-tread" mechanism of **gliding motility**, and the same mechanism permits its forced entry into host cells (see Fig. 51-1).

Helminths

Helminths (worms) are **multicellular animals** (metazoa) and are considerably larger than protozoa. Because they **reproduce sexually**, productive infections require both male and female worms. However, some tapeworms are **hermaphroditic**, having both male and female reproductive organs. Helminths of medical importance include the following:

- **Roundworms**: circular in cross section. Adult worms of various roundworm species range in size from a few millimeters to 20 cm. One human intestinal roundworm

(*Ascaris lumbricoides*) bears a remarkable resemblance to an earthworm; however, unlike annelids (e.g., earthworms), roundworms have **no visible body segmentation**.
- **Flatworms**: asymmetric in cross section. They comprise two main types:
- **Flukes** (e.g., *Schistosoma, Fasciola*): relatively short flatworms with nonsegmented bodies
- **Tapeworms**: segmented worms that vary in size from millimeters to several meters in length. A tapeworm can be thought of more as a colony than as an integrated multicellular organism. The segments are generated from a germinal worm head that contributes to a growing chain of flat segments, each with its own nutritional and reproductive organs.

Because of their large size, helminths are typically extracellular. However, the larvae of some helminths, such as the roundworm that causes trichinosis (*Trichinella spiralis*) and most tapeworms, develop into dormant cysts. Protected by an impermeable **cuticle**, helminths often have complex life cycles involving environmental or animal reservoirs. With rare exceptions, no helminthic parasite completes its life cycle within a single human host. Therefore, disease is not normally a consequence of helminths growing in number within the host, as it is with protozoa. Instead, the parasitic burden (and the likelihood of pathologic consequences) is directly related to the number of helminthic parasites that the host acquires from the environment.

Vectors

Vectors are living transmitters of disease. Most vectors are **arthropods**. Perhaps the best-known example of a vector is the female *Anopheles* mosquito, which transmits malaria. Other important vectors include tsetse flies, which transmit sleeping sickness; black flies, which transmit the tissue roundworm infection called river blindness; reduviid ("kissing") bugs, which transmit Chagas disease; and ticks, which transmit babesiosis. Arthropods can transmit not only parasites but also bacteria (e.g., the agents of Lyme disease and Rocky Mountain spotted fever) and viruses (e.g., yellow fever, dengue, and encephalitis viruses).

Arthropods are not simply passive agents that transfer parasites from one mammalian host to another. They also are involved in essential steps of the parasitic life cycle. To a large extent, the prevalence of a parasitic disease in a given geographical location may depend on whether the local conditions are favorable to arthropod breeding—for example, stagnant water for mosquito breeding or foliage, moisture, and suitable animal hosts for the propagation of ticks. Because of the obligatory role that arthropods play in the development of some protozoal and helminthic pathogens, their elimination from the environment can theoretically eradicate the respective diseases they cause in humans.

Reservoirs

Reservoirs are sources of parasites in the environment that do not participate directly in transmission to humans. Reservoirs of human parasites include other humans (e.g., for malaria parasites and amebas), other animals (e.g., pigs for trichinosis and pork tapeworm, cattle for beef tapeworm and cryptosporidiosis), and the environment (e.g., soil contaminated with parasitized human feces).

PARASITIC INFECTIONS AND DISEASE

ENTRY

One intriguing aspect of human parasites is the number of strategies they have evolved to enter the host (Table 51-3). Infections can be transmitted by the fecal–oral route (e.g., amebiasis, ascariasis), by the direct penetration of unbroken skin infection (e.g., hookworm, schistosomiasis), or by the bites of arthropod vectors (e.g., malaria, filariasis). With the first two routes of transmission, acquisition usually results from ingestion of *contaminated food or water* or from *inadequate control of human wastes* in soil or water. Although many of the parasites using those routes of transmission live in the gastrointestinal tract, several invade and infect the internal organs or skin, and a few cause disease in both the intestine and deeper tissues.

Most arthropodborne infections are transmitted to humans through bite wounds. Transmission through arthropods can be extraordinarily efficient. In fact, malaria can be acquired from the bite of a single infected mosquito during a stop at an airport in an endemic area. In addition, some arthropodborne infections can be transmitted by the transfusion of blood from asymptomatic infected humans.

TABLE 51-3 Modes of Spread of Some Parasitic Diseases

Mode of Exit	Mode of Entry	Human-to-Human	Animal-to-Human
Feces	Mouth	Cryptosporidiosis	Cryptosporidiosis
		Amebiasis	Toxoplasmosis
		Giardiasis	Visceral larva migrans
		Strongyloidiasis[a]	Echinococcosis
		Ascariasis[b]	
		Trichuris infection[b]	
		Pork tapeworm	
Feces	Skin	Strongyloidiasis	Creeping eruption (dog or cat hookworm)
		Hookworm	Schistosomiasis[c]
Arthropod bite	Arthropod bite	Lymphatic filariasis	Trypanosomiasis (sleeping sickness, Chagas disease)
		Leishmaniasis	Leishmaniasis
		Malaria	
		Onchocerciasis	
None (parasite encysts in muscle)	Ingestion (inadequately cooked meat)		Trichinosis
			Toxoplasmosis
			Beef tapeworm
			Pork tapeworm
			Fish tapeworm

[a]Usually transmitted by fecal–cutaneous route but may also be transmitted by the fecal–oral route.
[b]May require a period outside the human host to be infectious.
[c]Mode of exit may also be urine; development in an intermediate host is obligatory.

SPREAD AND MULTIPLICATION

Inoculum Size

The effective inoculum size has been determined for a few parasites by experimental infections in human volunteers and animals, usually in conjunction with quantitative epidemiologic studies. For example, large inocula are required to cause amebiasis in humans, whereas symptomatic cryptosporidiosis can be produced by the ingestion of relatively few cysts. In most helminthic infections, the severity of the infection is proportional to the inoculum size (or the cumulative inoculum if exposure continues over time).

Parasite Survival Mechanisms in Immunologically Normal Hosts

Like other microorganisms, parasites elicit both antibody- and cell-mediated responses (see the box titled "Parasitic Mechanisms for Evading the Host Immune Response"). However, they are adept at circumventing those host defenses. For example, adult schistosomes (blood flukes) coat themselves with host plasma proteins and are thus not recognized as foreign by the host's immune system. As a result, they are able to persist within the bloodstream for decades without immune-mediated destruction. Trypanosomes elude their hosts' immune systems by varying their surface antigens. In contrast, intracellular parasites are protected by special adaptations. For example, *Leishmania* species, which live in the phagolysosomes of macrophages, secrete a superoxide dismutase that protects them from the toxic superoxide produced in the phagolysosome. Like other protozoal parasites, *Leishmania* species also directly influence the host immune response to their advantage, directing lymphocyte proliferation into the Th2 rather than Th1 pathway.

Species and Tissue Tropisms

The life cycles of parasites are determined by species and tissue **tropisms**, which define the hosts that parasites can infect and the organs and tissues in which they can survive. As yet, very little is known about the biologic basis of tissue tropisms. Thus, it is not clear why the larvae of *Strongyloides* species invade the intestinal wall, whereas those of hookworms remain in the intestinal lumen. Nor is it clear why the pork tapeworm can cause cysticercosis (infection of the deep tissues) in humans but the beef tapeworm cannot. Recent studies have shown that some tropisms depend on specific receptors. For example, the presence of the Duffy factor antigen on the surface of the red blood cell is necessary for the entry of *Plasmodium vivax* malaria parasites (merozoites) into human red blood cells. Thus, subjects whose red blood cells lack the Duffy factor (most Africans) are resistant to *P. vivax* infection.

Temperature also plays an important role in the ability of parasites to infect humans and cause disease. For example, *Leishmania donovani* replicates well at 37°C and causes visceral leishmaniasis (kala azar), a disease of the bone marrow, liver, and spleen. (Note that the temperature of those tissues is, of course, 37°C.) In contrast, *L. mexicana* grows well at 25°C to 30°C but poorly at 37°C and causes infections of the skin (where temperatures are 25°C to 30°C). Temperature changes also induce stage-specific transitions in many parasites. For example, *Leishmania* species change from the promastigote form to the amastigote form when they move from a cooler insect vector to a warmer human host (from 25°C to 37°C). They also synthesize heat shock protein.

DAMAGE

As with other infectious agents, the clinical manifestations of parasitic disease may reflect tissue damage by the parasite, the effects of the host immune response, or both. The pathogenic amebas are examples of pathogens that cause most of their tissue damage by a direct cytolytic effect. For example, amebic liver abscesses are produced by direct destruction of host cells, with the host contributing an ineffective acute inflammatory response. In contrast, many other parasitic infections that involve deep tissues elicit an inflammatory response that may be exclusively responsible for the histopathology. **Chronic inflammation** is the hallmark of diseases such as schistosomiasis

PARASITIC MECHANISMS FOR EVADING THE HOST IMMUNE RESPONSE

- **Antigenic variation**: trypanosomes, *Plasmodium* species, *Giardia* species
- **Intracellular infection**: plasmodia, *Toxoplasma* species
- **Encystation**: amebas, cestodes
- **Camouflage**: schistosomes
- **Cleavage of antibodies or complement components**: amebas, *Leishmania* species
- **Suppression or redirection of the cellular immune response**: plasmodia, *Leishmania* species, schistosomes

and cutaneous filariasis. In these helminthic infections, the adult parasites are innocuous, but their progeny (i.e., microfilaria and eggs of *Schistosoma* species) induce intense inflammatory responses when they degenerate in host tissues. In some parasitic diseases (e.g., trichinosis), the host inflammatory response may cause persistent disease even after the parasites have died. In cysticercosis, the infected individual may remain asymptomatic for a long period until the parasite dies. Then, the leakage of parasite antigens into the tissues may trigger a **hypersensitivity reaction** and produce symptoms in the host.

Eosinophilia

Eosinophils are leukocytes that participate in neutralizing infections with parasitic worms. In helminthic infections, eosinophils may appear in the blood in large numbers. This eosinophilia occurs in response to the parasites' surface glycoproteins and polysaccharides, particularly when the parasites invade or migrate through tissues. Eosinophilia is typically accompanied by increased levels of **IgE** and is driven by elevated levels of **interleukin-5**. Together, eosinophils and IgE play a critical role in killing multicellular parasites. Because eosinophilia and increased levels of IgE occur with helminthic infections and are most striking with helminths that invade the deep tissues, their presence is useful in suggesting a helminth diagnosis. In contrast, eosinophilia is not a feature of most protozoal infections nor of helminth infections that do not involve migration through tissue.

Timing of Clinical Complications

The most important complications of many parasitic diseases occur years after the initial infection. For instance, persons with schistosomiasis typically have bleeding from either the gastrointestinal tract (*Schistosoma mansoni*) or the urinary tract (*S. haematobium*), which continues for years. Decades later, people with heavy, chronic infections may develop complications such as portal hypertension with esophageal varices (*S. mansoni*) or obstructions or cancer of the urinary tract (*S. haematobium*).

Important complications also can occur at distant sites. For example, intestinal pork tapeworm (*Taenia solium*) infections are asymptomatic. However, late complications result if tapeworm eggs are ingested and larval forms of the parasite hatch in the intestine, cross the mucosa, enter the bloodstream, and encyst in the deep tissues as **cysticerci**. The cysts are small (0.5 to 1.5 cm) and produce no signs or symptoms if they lodge in skeletal muscle or the central nervous system. However, when they infect the central nervous system, the cysts may eventually leak their contents into tissue, causing **seizures** or **hydrocephalus** (by blocking the flow of cerebrospinal fluid).

A chronic protozoal infection called Chagas disease (American trypanosomiasis) typically produces a relatively trivial skin lesion at the time of the initial infection. Although in rare cases among young children the initial infection progresses rapidly to death, it is usually asymptomatic or minimally symptomatic. Years later, older persons with chronic infection can develop heart block from damage to the cardiac conducting system or impaired swallowing or defecation from damage to the nerves responsible for the motility of the esophagus or colon. Although late complications are rare, there are no predictors to identify the people at greatest risk of developing them.

Environmental Constraints on Transmission

Examination of the parasitic life cycle often explains why a given parasitic disease is found in one area of the world and not another (see Table 51-2). For example, the transmission of schistosomiasis depends on an intermediate snail host that is not present in North America or Europe. Thus, viable eggs in the stool or urine of infected persons cannot produce the forms infective for humans (**cercariae**) because there are no intermediate snail hosts in which the parasite can mature. For that reason, human schistosomiasis is not endemic in the United States and will not be, unless an intermediate snail host becomes established. It does not matter how many persons infected with schistosomiasis enter the United States and contaminate the environment with infective eggs. In contrast, *Anopheles* mosquitoes capable of transmitting malaria are found in the United States. Therefore, recent immigrants or travelers who acquired malaria in endemic areas may infect the indigenous mosquito pool. Local transmission of malaria by that mechanism occurs a few times each year in the United States (recent cases have occurred in California, New Jersey, and Michigan). Those rare events are diagnostic puzzles because infected individuals typically have no histories of foreign travel. Ongoing malaria surveillance is therefore particularly important when large numbers of people from malaria-endemic areas enter nonmalarious areas where substantial numbers of *Anopheles* mosquitoes are present.

DIAGNOSIS

Most parasitic infections are diagnosed by identifying the parasites or their characteristic progeny (cysts, eggs, or larvae) in clinical specimens. To pursue the most effective diagnostic strategies, it is important to understand the parasite's life cycle (Fig. 51-2). For instance, in the life cycle of hookworms, the adult female lives in the lumen of the human intestine, suggesting that she will release her eggs into the stool. Consequently, examination of the stool for hookworm eggs is an effective and sensitive method for the diagnosis of hookworm infection. In contrast, in the life cycle of *Strongyloides* species, the adult female invades the intestinal wall to release her eggs. Intact eggs are rarely seen in the stool. However, the larvae that emerge from eggs in the intestinal wall can be found in the stool of a person with *Strongyloides* infection, and their presence is diagnostic for that infection.

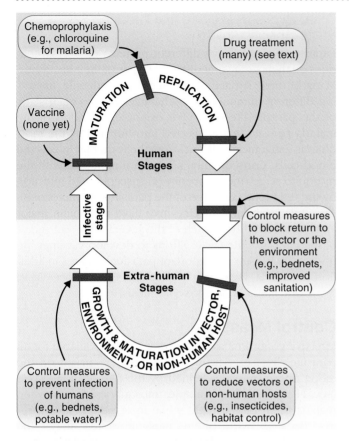

FIGURE 51-2. Idealized (model) parasite life cycle and points of intervention. The human stages of the life cycle are located in the top half of the diagram. The extrahuman stages (in animate or inanimate reservoirs) are in the lower half. When the parasite reaches the infective stage, it invades the human host, matures, replicates, and ultimately completes the life cycle by producing infective forms. The infective forms are taken up by a vector or released into the environment. Control measures interfere with the replication or survival of the extrahuman stages of the parasite. They reduce the incidence of infection by reducing the number of infective stages to which humans are exposed. Immunization (vaccination) prevents symptomatic infection by inhibiting or killing the parasite as it enters (or replicates within) the human host. Chemoprophylaxis is used to inhibit parasite replication and thus prevent symptomatic infection. Neither immunization nor chemoprophylaxis prevents the initial entry of the parasite. Drug treatment is used to prevent death or severe morbidity in persons with established infections.

One species of filarial helminths, *Wuchereria bancrofti*, is transmitted to humans by mosquitoes that bite primarily at night. To maximize their transmission to mosquitoes, the parasites release their microfilaria into the human bloodstream during the late-evening hours. Thus, to examine blood for *W. bancrofti*, samples are typically drawn at midnight.

Traditionally, parasitic infections are diagnosed by visualizing the parasite or its progeny (eggs, cysts, or microfilaria) in clinical specimens. In recent years, immunologic and DNA-based detection of the organisms has assumed new importance because the techniques are both highly sensitive and better adapted for rapid testing of large numbers of samples.

TREATMENT AND PREVENTION

Antiparasite strategies fall into three general categories: (1) drugs for prevention (chemoprophylaxis) and treatment, (2) immunization, and (3) control measures in the field. Eradication programs have generally been effective only when at least two strategies were used simultaneously.

An understanding of the parasitic life cycle is helpful in selecting antiparasitic drugs. For example, different drugs are necessary for the different stages (intestinal and tissue) of the pork tapeworm (*T. solium*): niclosamide is effective against intestinal infection (taeniasis), and praziquantel is used to treat the tissue stage of the infection (cysticercosis).

The parasite life cycle also provides important clues for treatment and control strategies (see Fig. 51-2 and Table 51-3). For example, hookworm larvae from eggs in human stool mature to the filariform stage in the environment; they then cause infection by penetrating unprotected human skin. Therefore, sanitation (appropriate disposal of human waste) and wearing shoes can reduce the transmission of hookworms and thus decrease the number of people infected. Hookworm infection and disease were very common in the southern United States until those preventive measures were instituted on a large scale by the Rockefeller Commission in the 1930s. Sanitation is particularly effective in reducing rates of parasitic infections transmitted through contaminated stool or urine, such as ascariasis, strongyloidiasis, and hookworm infection. Paradoxically, according to the so-called hygiene hypothesis, extremely hygienic environments that help prevent infections with minor intestinal helminth infections among children may also contribute to the development of allergies.

Drugs
Chemoprophylaxis

Drugs used for chemoprophylaxis must meet more stringent requirements than do drugs used only for treatment. Minor drug side effects acceptable for short periods in sick persons (e.g., headache, nausea, or gastrointestinal disturbances) are unacceptable for prolonged periods in persons who are healthy.

One example of successful chemoprophylaxis in the past was the use of chloroquine to prevent malaria. Chloroquine was once effective against all four species of *Plasmodium* that cause malaria in humans. Oral administration once a week produced effective plasma levels of the drug because chloroquine is well absorbed and has a plasma half-life greater than 4 days. Today, most of the strains of *P. falciparum* in most malarious areas of the world have become resistant to chloroquine. The development of resistance is always a concern when relatively lower doses of drugs are used for chemoprophylaxis or incomplete therapy.

Treatment

When does treatment influence the transmission of parasites? Mass treatment may be an effective control strategy for diseases that depend on humans as a reservoir. In contrast, treatment of people with zoonotic and dead-end infections will not influence the occurrence of those diseases. In general, treatment of symptomatic infections is usually an inefficient strategy for controlling transmission because a long delay often occurs between the initial infection and the onset of symptoms (e.g., 10 to 20 years or more for schistosomiasis). During the long asymptomatic interval, infected humans are able to transmit the infection. If treatment is to be effective in reducing transmission, it must be given to all infectious persons, both symptomatic and asymptomatic.

The goal of many treatment regimens for parasitic infection has been to prevent the long-term complications of infection (such as portal hypertension in schistosomiasis or seizures in cysticercosis). In the last 10 years, several new drugs have appeared that represent significant advances in the treatment of parasitic diseases, such as albendazole for cysticercosis, praziquantel for schistosomiasis, ivermectin for onchocerciasis, and difluoromethylornithine for African sleeping sickness. The drugs previously available to treat those diseases were toxic and often ineffective. Prior to praziquantel, no medical treatment existed for cysticercosis (the tissue-invasive form of pork tapeworm infection). Now researchers expect widespread use of the available drugs to significantly decrease seizures and hydrocephalus from cysticercosis, cirrhosis from schistosomiasis, and blindness from onchocerciasis.

Immunity and Immunization

Major Problem in Designing Vaccines: Evasion of the Host Immune Response

Many important parasites survive to produce disease because they can avoid the effects of the host immune response. Schistosomes masquerade as the "self" (host) by covering themselves with host antigens. Because of that protection, circulating antibodies against schistosomal antigens (produced spontaneously or by immunization) are unlikely to bind to the relevant schistosomal antigens and are thus unlikely to be effective against the parasites. Trypanosomes use another strategy to evade the host immune response: they alter their surface antigens (see Chapter 52 and the Chapter 14 paradigm). When the host develops an effective immune response to one antigen, clones of the trypanosomes emerge that express different antigens on their surfaces, leading to successive bouts of high-grade parasitemia. An effective vaccine against all antigenic types seems extremely unlikely.

Other Problems in Designing Vaccines: Stage-Specific Antigens

Parasites typically have different proteins or polysaccharides on their surfaces at different stages of their life cycles. Many of those surface components are antigenic, imparting different immunological characteristics to each stage of the parasite life cycle. For example, the form of the malaria parasite that is injected into humans by the mosquito is antigenically distinct from the form that infects red blood cells. Consequently, a person immunized with the mosquito stage (the sporozoite) is susceptible to infection by the red blood cell stage of the parasite (the merozoite). An effective malaria vaccine may have to contain major antigens derived from each of the several different stages of the parasite's life cycle. Efforts to develop vaccines are under way for several important parasitic diseases in addition to malaria, including schistosomiasis, onchocerciasis, lymphatic filariasis, and toxoplasmosis.

Control Measures

Effective control measures are potentially available for all parasitic diseases. The best measures are based on the mode of transmission defined by the parasite's life cycle (see Fig. 51-2). For example, mosquitoes that transmit malaria often bite at night while most people are sleeping. Because many of the mosquitoes rest under the eaves of houses after biting humans, insecticides such as dichlorodiphenyltrichloroethane (DDT) reduced malaria transmission substantially when sprayed at those sites. Unfortunately, that strategy is limited because many mosquitoes have developed resistance to DDT and the strategy selects for mosquitoes that bite outside the house during daylight hours. Moreover, DDT has been shown to accumulate in human tissues and may have long-term toxic consequences. More effective and safer insecticides are desperately needed.

In developed areas like North America and Europe, transmission of parasitic disease is typically low because sanitation interrupts the parasite's life cycle. However, in developing countries, where the major parasitic diseases are endemic, even simple sanitary methods of interrupting transmission are difficult to implement. Potable water, for example, is unavailable or too expensive in many parts of the world. During the dry season, the transmission of infection by waterborne and fecal–oral routes increases in those regions because the small amounts of water available are used for both washing and drinking.

CONCLUSION

The most striking differences between parasites and other infectious agents are the variety of hosts, vectors, and stages in parasitic life cycles. The life cycles of parasites provide important clues to understanding parasitic diseases and help in diagnosis and in the development of public health strategies. In most cases, the biological basis for the ability of different stages of parasites to invade different hosts and different types of tissues is still unknown.

Although parasitic diseases are more prevalent in areas with inadequate sanitation, they are also found in regions with apparently high sanitary standards, such as Europe and North America. The presence of parasitic diseases in developed countries is frequently related to the susceptibility of immunocompromised patients to the infections. For example, toxoplasmosis is quite prevalent in developed countries but does not produce severe disease in immunologically normal individuals. In immunocompromised patients, some parasites can escape their usual constraints and multiply to high and dangerous numbers.

Suggested Readings

Guerrant RL, Walker DH, Weller PF. *Tropical Infectious Diseases: Principles, Pathogens, and Practice*. London, UK: Churchill Livingston; 1999.

Harries JR, Harries AD, Cook GC. *One Hundred Clinical Problems in Tropical Medicine*. London, UK: Bailliere Tindall; 1987.

Sacks D, Sher A. Evasion of innate immunity by parasitic protozoa. *Nat Immunol*. 2002;3:1041–1047.

Sun T. *Parasitic Disorders: Pathology, Diagnosis, and Management*. 2nd ed. Philadelphia, PA: Lippincott Williams & Wilkins; 1999.

Yazdanbakhsh M, Kremsner PG, van Ree R. Allergy, parasites, and the hygiene hypothesis. *Science*. 2002;296:490–494.

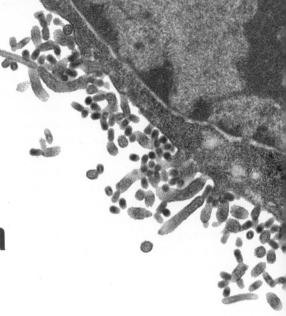

Chapter 52

Blood and Tissue Protozoa

Cary Engleberg

KEY CONCEPTS

Most tissue-invasive protozoa have intracellular stages in their life cycles.

Fever is a cardinal symptom of disseminated protozoal infections. Some species become dormant in tissues and cause prolonged, asymptomatic infection.

Malaria is transmitted among humans by *Anopheles* mosquitoes. Its propagation depends on the presence of a reservoir of partially immune, asymptomatic human carriers. Nonimmune persons (e.g., young children in endemic areas and adult travelers from nonendemic areas) may experience severe, or even fatal, illness. Because it is more virulent and more likely to be resistant to antimalarial drugs, *Plasmodium falciparum* must be distinguished from other plasmodia and treated promptly.

Like malaria, babesiosis is a protozoal infection of erythrocytes, but it is more geographically localized and less prevalent, partly because it is transmitted by ticks rather than mosquitoes.

Cats are the definitive (intestinal) host for *Toxoplasma gondii;* all other animals develop dormant toxoplasmic cysts in their muscles and viscera. Humans acquire infection by ingesting oocysts from cat feces or muscle cysts in undercooked meat. Manifestations in humans include a mononucleosis-like primary infection, chorioretinitis, congenital infection, or mass lesions in the brain (in person with AIDS).

Virulence attributes of various *Leishmania* species determine whether infection results in a chronic skin ulcer at the site of the sand fly bite or a disseminated chronic febrile illness involving the liver, spleen, and lymph nodes.

Long-standing infection with the agent of Chagas disease, *Trypanosoma cruzi,* may result in immunopathologic damage to the heart and the gastrointestinal tract.

The agent of African sleeping sickness, *Trypanosoma brucei,* evades the host immune response by a genetically determined mechanism of antigenic variation.

PROTOZOAL bloodstream infections, such as malaria and babesiosis, typically involve infection and destruction of red blood cells. Protozoa that infect tissues can cause significant damage to the eyes, brain, or heart (toxoplasmosis); to the brain (African sleeping sickness); or to the heart and gastrointestinal tract (Chagas disease). The major blood and tissue protozoa are presented in Table 52-1.

PARASITES OF RED BLOOD CELLS
Plasmodium Species

Malaria is the most important of all protozoal diseases and is said to have caused "the greatest harm to the greatest number" of all infectious diseases. It occurs in many tropical and semitropical regions of the world, with approximately 200 to 300 million cases annually (see Table 51-1). An estimated 2 to 3 million people die of malaria each year, especially malnourished African children. Malaria in humans is caused by four species of the *Plasmodium* protozoa: *P. falciparum, P. vivax, P. ovale,* and *P. malariae.* Infected humans are the only reservoir for these plasmodial species that infect humans; transmission occurs through the bite of infected female anopheline mosquitoes. However, a less common form of human malaria has recently been attributed to a monkey parasite, *P. knowlesi.* These zoonotic

CASE • Ms. M. is a 54-year-old businesswoman from Liverpool who traveled to East Africa (Kenya and Tanzania) on a business trip and then went on a photographic safari. After 1 week in Nairobi, she embarked on a 10-day trip through the wildlife preserves of Serengeti and Ngorongoro, with a final visit to Mombasa on the Indian Ocean. During her flight home, 9 days after leaving the game parks, Ms. M. developed a "flulike" syndrome, with headache, muscle aches, and a temperature of 38°C. After she returned to Liverpool, she saw a physician, who diagnosed influenza. She had returned to England in February during an outbreak of influenza A.

Ms. M. was given acetaminophen, which initially reduced her fever and muscle aches. However, she felt worse the next day. She suddenly developed an intense chill that lasted for about 30 minutes, followed by a fever to 40.2°C that lasted for 6 hours. As the fever abated, Ms. M. became drenched in sweat and felt exhausted and drained. Her symptoms continued to worsen, and she was brought to the hospital unconscious 2 days later. On examination, she had edema of the lungs. She showed no signs of endocarditis, and a lumbar puncture was negative for bacterial meningitis.

The attending physician, drawing on his experience while serving in the armed services abroad, recognized that Ms. M.'s clinical manifestations were typical of a **malarial paroxysm**. The recent history of travel to endemic areas gave credence to his suspicion of the disease, and the diagnosis was confirmed when a Giemsa-stained smear of Ms. M.'s blood revealed large numbers of parasites within red blood cells. The parasites were identified as *Plasmodium falciparum* by their characteristic ring shape. Ms. M.'s hematocrit (packed red cell volume) was 18% (normal is 40 to 45%). Urinalysis revealed dark urine, suggesting extensive hemolysis. Her serum creatinine (a measure of renal function) was 5.4 mg per 100 mL (normal is 1 mg or less per 100 mL).

Because Ms. M. had traveled in Kenya, a country in which drug-resistant malaria is endemic, treatment was begun with intravenous quinidine, which is effective against *P. falciparum* strains resistant to other antimalarial drugs. Ms. M. was also given intravenous glucose as a precaution against hypoglycemia (which can produce coma in patients with severe *P. falciparum* malaria). Hypoglycemia can result both from consumption of glucose by large numbers of parasites and from the direct release of insulin from the pancreas caused by quinidine or quinine. For her pulmonary edema, Ms. M. required artificial ventilation with a respirator. She was given multiple transfusions for her anemia and was put on a dialysis machine because of her kidney failure. She recovered and was discharged after spending 10 days in the intensive care unit.

This case raises several questions:

1. Why did Ms. M.'s fevers occur in paroxysms (episodes) of shaking chills followed by fever and then drenching sweats?
2. Why did she have dark urine?
3. Why did she develop edema of the lungs and an elevation of the serum creatinine?

See Appendix for answers.

---

cases occur in forested areas of Southeast Asia where the other species of human malaria may be absent.

ENCOUNTER AND ENTRY

Malaria is transmitted to humans by the mosquito vector 9 to 17 days after a female *Anopheles* mosquito ingests blood from a person infected with a species of *Plasmodium* that infects humans. Infected persons typically develop malaria symptoms 8 to 30 days later. Most cases of malaria that occur in Europe and North America are acquired in endemic areas and then imported into the nonendemic areas during the incubation period (**imported malaria**). However, mosquitoes that can serve as vectors (*Anopheles*) exist in the United States. Although malaria can no longer take hold in temperate, industrialized countries like the United States, in rare cases, persons who have never traveled abroad have contracted the disease. It is assumed that such cases occur when potential vector mosquitoes feed on blood from a malaria carrier (i.e., an immigrant or traveler from an endemic country) and then survive long enough to become infectious and bite again. Introductions of malaria have occurred when a large number of infected soldiers have returned from war and when a region has received a large number of immigrants at one time. Malaria also can be transmitted by blood transfusion or by the sharing of needles among intravenous drug users (**induced malaria**).

SPREAD AND MULTIPLICATION

The life cycle of the malaria parasite is complex and rich in morphological detail (Fig. 52-1). In the infected mosquito, plasmodia inhabit the salivary glands as **sporozoites**, a stage of the parasite that is infectious for humans. Sporozoites are injected into the human bloodstream when infected mosquitoes bite and feed. These organisms travel through the bloodstream and enter liver cells within 30 minutes of injection. Over the next 8 to 14 days, the parasites multiply and mature inside liver cells to very large numbers. At the end of that period (**the hepatocellular cycle**), they are released once again into the bloodstream in a form that can invade red blood cells (**merozoites**).

TABLE 52-1 Comparison of Major Blood and Tissue Protozoa

Organism	Reservoir	Mode of Transmission	Clinical Manifestations
Blood Protozoa			
Plasmodium species (malaria)	Infected humans	Vectorborne by the female *Anopheles* mosquito	Fever and chills with red blood cell lysis
Babesia species (babesiosis)	Rodents (voles), deer, mice	Vectorborne by the hard-bodied *Ixodes* tick	Fever and chills with red blood cell lysis
Tissue Protozoa			
Toxoplasma gondii (toxoplasmosis)	Sheep, pigs, cattle, cats	Foodborne by the ingestion of inadequately cooked beef or lamb Fecal–oral by the ingestion of infectious oocysts in cat feces	Intrauterine (congenital) infection can cause severe retardation in the neonate Mononucleosis-like illness most common Infection of the brain (encephalitis) or heart (myocarditis) in severely immunocompromised patients
Leishmania species (leishmaniasis)	Infected humans, dogs, jackals, foxes, rats, ground squirrels, gerbils	Vectorborne by infected *Phlebotomus* sand flies	Trivial or mild (self-healing) skin lesions Disfiguring mucocutaneous lesions Systemic illness with involvement of liver, spleen, and bone marrow
Trypanosoma cruzi (Chagas disease, American trypanosomiasis)	Wildlife, domestic animals (zoonosis)	Vectorborne by reduviid bugs followed by rubbing infected feces in the bite wound	Gastrointestinal tract dysfunction from autonomic nerve damage (megacolon, megaesophagus) Cardiac dysfunction from damage to the conducting system (right bundle branch block)
Trypanosoma brucei gambiense or *T. brucei rhodesiense* (West and East African trypanosomiasis, respectively, or sleeping sickness)	Infected humans, wildlife, cattle	Vectorborne by the tsetse fly	Systemic illness with fever, headache, muscle, and joint pains Progresses to central nervous system involvement with altered speech, gait, and reflexes (encephalitis)

Once inside red blood cells, the organisms divide and mature. After 2 or 3 days, the cells burst, liberating a new generation of infective merozoites that infect previously unparasitized red blood cells (the **erythrocytic cycle**).

In the liver and red blood cells, the parasites multiply asexually (i.e., by fission). A minority of the merozoites in the blood develop into forms capable of sexual reproduction, called **gametocytes**. Male and female gametocytes are taken up by biting mosquitoes. In the mosquito gut, the haploid male and female gametes fuse to form a diploid zygote. That event represents the sexual part of the malaria life cycle. After the zygote is formed, the parasite undergoes further changes in the mosquito gut and then divides by meiosis to generate sporozoites. Sporozoites migrate to the salivary glands and once again become infective for humans. All the subsequent asexual stages in the human, up to and including the gametes, are haploid. In each of those stages, the plasmodial cells are morphologically distinguishable (see Fig. 52-1).

The four species of plasmodia that cause human malaria vary in their virulence. One reason for the variation is that different plasmodial species prefer red blood cells

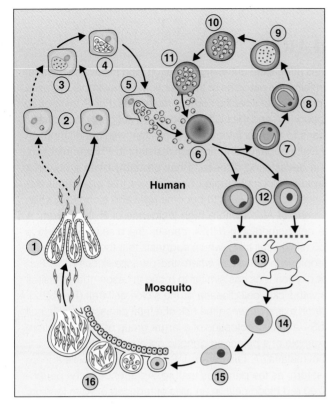

FIGURE 52-1. Life cycle of *Plasmodium* species. Sporozoites released from the salivary gland of the female *Anopheles* mosquito are injected under a person's skin when the mosquito bites (1). They then travel through the bloodstream and enter the liver (2). Within liver cells, the parasites mature to tissue schizonts (3–4). They are then released into the bloodstream as merozoites (5) and produce symptomatic infection as they invade and destroy red blood cells (RBCs). However, some parasites remain dormant in the liver as hypnozoites (see the *dashed lines* from stages 1 to 3). Those parasites (in *P. vivax* and *P. ovale*) cause relapsing malaria. Once within the bloodstream, merozoites (5) invade RBCs (6) and mature to the ring (7–8), trophozoite (9), and schizont (10) asexual stages. Schizonts lyse their host RBCs as they complete their maturation and release the next generation of merozoites (11), which invades previously uninfected RBCs. Within RBCs, some parasites differentiate to sexual forms, male and female gametocytes (12). When gametocytes are taken up by a female *Anopheles* mosquito, the male gametocyte loses its flagellum, producing male gametes. The male gametes fertilize the female gamete (13) to produce a zygote (14). The zygote invades the gut of the mosquito (15) and develops into an oocyst (16). Mature oocysts produce sporozoites, which migrate to the salivary gland of the mosquito (1) and repeat the cycle. The dashed line between stages 12 and 13 indicates that absence of the mosquito vector precludes natural transmission through this cycle. Note that infection by the injection of infected blood bypasses that constraint and permits transmission of malaria among intravenous drug addicts and to persons who receive blood transfusions from infected donors.

of different ages: *P. falciparum* invades erythrocytes of all ages, producing the highest parasitemias and the greatest risk of mortality; *P. vivax* prefers reticulocytes and young red blood cells, while *P. malariae* favors older red blood

cells. Both *P. vivax* and *P. malariae* infect only 1 to 2% or less of red blood cells, thus producing less severe disease. The fourth species, *P. ovale*, is virtually identical to *P. vivax* clinically and morphologically. *P. vivax* and *P. ovale* are also notable for the fact that some infected hepatocytes may harbor latent preerythrocytic parasites for a long period before they are released into the bloodstream. Thus, infection with either species can cause a series of relapses to occur months or even years after the initial episode. Recurrent malaria is prevented by treatment with an antimalarial agent that targets the latent parasites (**hypnozoites**) within liver cells.

The intracellular location of the malaria parasite within the red blood cell has two important consequences:

- The presence of plasmodia within red blood cells makes the cells less deformable. The spleen recognizes and removes older and less deformable red blood cells from the circulation, thus removing parasitized red blood cells from the circulation. Not surprisingly, malaria may cause enlargement of the spleen (**splenomegaly**), and splenectomized people have higher degrees of parasitemia and more-severe infections.
- A red blood cell infected with *P. falciparum* develops special "knoblike" structures on its surface that contain the parasite-derived protein **pfEMP-1**. The protein binds the infected red blood cell to receptors on the endothelial cells of venules and capillaries, such as **intercellular adhesion molecule 1 (ICAM-1)** and CD36. When multiple parasitized red blood cells adhere and accumulate on the endothelium, blood flow through the deep vascular beds is impeded. Thus, *P. falciparum*–infected cells are prevented from circulating to the spleen and being removed from the circulation. However, the obstruction of blood flow in the microcirculation may have dire pathological consequences for the host.

DAMAGE

The main manifestations of malaria are fever, chills, and anemia. The typical malarial paroxysm (as in Ms. M.'s case) coincides with the lysis of many red blood cells and the release of large numbers of merozoites. In the process, parasite molecules, such as membrane molecules, are also released, and some of those molecules, such as membrane **glycophosphatidylinositol (GPI)**, stimulate the production of tumor necrosis factor and interleukin-1 in macrophages. The surge in those cytokines is the stimulus for the sudden chill and fever characteristic of a malaria paroxysm.

Parasite replication can become synchronized so that all infected red blood cells lyse at the same time. As a result, a regular, periodic fever pattern may develop, depending on the length of the intracellular replication cycle: every 2 days with *P. vivax* or *P. ovale* and every 3 days with *P. malariae*. In contrast, the fever pattern is often irregular with *P. falciparum*. Other frequent clinical presentations include a syndrome similar to influenza (fever, muscle aches, and malaise) and gastroenteritis

HUMAN GENETICS AND MALARIA

Genetic polymorphism of several human genes affects the entry, multiplication, and survival of malarial parasites. Genes are also important in determining the outcome of the infection. For example, parasite invasion of red blood cells depends on the presence of specific surface molecules. For *P. falciparum* and *P. vivax,* the surface molecules are glycophorin A and the Duffy blood group antigen, respectively. The variable susceptibility of African Americans to *P. vivax* infection is consistent with the distribution of Duffy antigen. Black Africans are typically Duffy-negative and are thus resistant to *P. vivax* infection.

Because *P. falciparum* malaria is such a devastating disease, it has probably been a powerful selective force in human evolution. Many epidemiological studies have shown that sickle cell disease—a recessive genetic disorder that causes red blood cells to become rigid and elongated when oxygen tension is reduced—is common in areas of Africa with a high incidence of *P. falciparum*. A defective form of hemoglobin, called sickle cell hemoglobin (HbS), causes the disease. Malaria is seldom found in heterozygous carriers of HbS (sickle cell trait), which suggests that the genetic determinant imparts a selective advantage to people living in areas where the parasite is common. Furthermore, in vitro studies have shown that at oxygen tensions similar to those in tissue, the parasites grow poorly in red blood cells from persons with sickle cell disease or the sickle cell trait (Fig. 52-2). Thus, in the Black African population, a trade-off exists between the risk of a fatal disease—sickle cell disease in those who are homozygous for HbS—and the protection of a larger group of the population, the heterozygous HbS carriers. That is an example of a balanced genetic polymorphism.

How does the sickle cell trait protect from malaria? *P. falciparum*–infected red blood cells adhere to the walls of blood vessels using knobs that form as the parasites mature. Adherence to the peripheral microcirculation sequesters the parasitized red blood cells in an area of reduced oxygen tension, which facilitates sickling, potassium loss, and the killing of the parasites.

Other genetic abnormalities that restrict the growth of malarial parasites within red blood cells are glucose-6-phosphate dehydrogenase deficiency (G6PD) and thalassemia. In the case of G6PD, the reduced ability of the red blood cells to produce NADPH via the pentose phosphate shunt is thought to cause an oxidative stress that inhibits parasite growth.

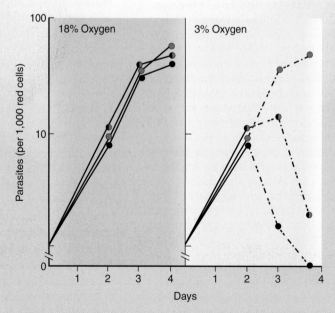

FIGURE 52-2. Effect of hypoxia on parasite growth in sickle hemoglobin red blood cells. In 18% oxygen (**left panel**), *Plasmodium falciparum* grows as well in sickle hemoglobin (SS) red blood cells (*black circles*) as in either heterozygous (SA) red blood cells (*red-black circles*) or normal (AA) RBCs (*red circles*). In contrast, at 3% oxygen, *P. falciparum* parasites grow less well in SS and SA cells than in AA cells (**right panel**).

(nausea, diarrhea, and vomiting). Patients with those signs and symptoms are often misdiagnosed, especially if the physician is not acquainted with malaria or fails to obtain a history of recent travel to an endemic area.

The anemia that occurs in malaria is usually more severe than can be accounted for by the degree of parasitemia alone. Thus, uninfected red blood cells may also be destroyed prematurely, presumably by an immunologically mediated mechanism.

DIAGNOSIS

Malaria is diagnosed in the laboratory by microscopic examination of a Giemsa-stained smear of peripheral blood using the oil immersion objective (Fig. 52-3). Wright stain, which is used more often in the clinical hematology laboratory, stains the parasites less well. If the degree of parasitemia is low, a "thick smear" can be used to increase sensitivity. Because red blood cells are lysed in the preparation of thick smears, this procedure provides no information about the size of the infected red blood cells or about the intracellular location of the parasite within the red blood cells (central or peripheral). Morphological characteristics

that can be seen on a "thin smear" of blood can be used to differentiate among the *Plasmodium* species.

In acutely ill patients, the malarial species is usually either *P. falciparum* or *P. vivax*. In contrast, *P. malariae* most often causes subacute or chronic infections (but can produce acute infections in nonimmune people). *P. ovale* malaria is clinically so similar to *P. vivax* malaria that the distinction of the two species is usually of no practical importance. *P. vivax* can be differentiated from *P. falciparum* on the basis of morphological characteristics. For example, *P. vivax* causes infected red blood cells to progressively enlarge as the parasite matures and produces eosinophilic "stippling" in the red blood cells (**Schüffner dots**). Neither red cell enlargement nor Schüffner dots occur with *P. falciparum*. That distinction is important because *P. falciparum* infection poses a greater risk of death and may be resistant to treatment with chloroquine, whereas *P. vivax* may cause posttreatment relapses caused by slow-growing or dormant parasites in the liver.

Simple rapid antigen detection tests also have been developed and commercialized; however, they are sufficiently sensitive only at relatively high parasite burden (>100 plasmodia/μL). Consequently, they may give falsely

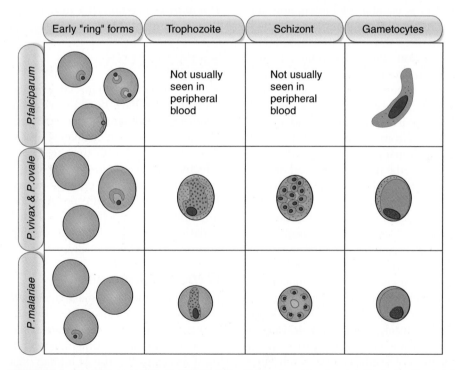

FIGURE 52-3. Malarial parasites in blood cells. This schematic drawing illustrates the most prominent morphological features that distinguish human malarial species in blood smears. The nuclear chromatid bodies of all of the malarial parasites are shaded in dark blue–gray in this diagram but actually appear red in Giemsa-stained preparations. *P. falciparum* usually appears as small, fine, ring forms, sometimes more than one per red blood cell. More-mature forms of the species are not usually seen in the peripheral blood. The gametocyte is characteristically banana shaped. *P. vivax* and *P. ovale* are distinguished by details not illustrated here. Infected cells and ring forms are larger than those of *P. falciparum*. At the trophozoite stage, red Schüffner dots are seen. The schizont contains more than a dozen merozoites before it ruptures. *P. malariae* infects smaller, senescent cells. Schüffner dots are not present. At the schizont stage, 8 to 12 merozoites are arranged peripherally around the central malarial pigment.

negative results in young children or other nonimmune individuals with lower parasitemia. In addition, in many countries with endemic malaria, these tests are not considered cost-effective. Serologic testing is of little value for the diagnosis of malaria in the acutely ill patient, since patients do not develop species-specific antibodies to the parasites for 3 to 5 weeks. Diagnosis using polymerase chain reaction (PCR) is more accurate than microscopy, but it is expensive, takes time, and requires special equipment and expertise (see Chapter 58).

TREATMENT

Natural immunity to malaria is imperfect. Persons who have lived in malarious areas all their lives and who have evidence of humoral and cellular responses to parasite antigens are nevertheless infected on a regular basis. However, their infections tend to be less severe than those of nonimmune persons, suggesting that the immune response plays a significant role in controlling infection. Some researchers have shown that antibodies directed against sporozoites, the form introduced by the insect (see Fig. 52-1), are not sufficient to protect against infection. Unfortunately, the major surface protein of the merozoite stage (**MSP-1**) is capable of undergoing antigenic variation (see Chapter 14 paradigm), an immune evasion mechanism that often thwarts both natural immunity and vaccine production. Protective immunity may involve cell-mediated cytotoxicity of infected liver cells or antibodies against certain surface proteins of the merozoite stage. Consequently, effective future vaccines will probably stimulate cell-mediated immunity and include conserved antigens derived from merozoites and possibly from the other stages of the parasite in humans as well.

Chloroquine was once the most widely used drug for antimalarial chemoprophylaxis and treatment. Chloroquine, and other quinine-based drugs, enter the parasite's food vacuole, where RBC hemoglobin is degraded for the nutrition of the parasite. Normally, toxic heme released by this degradation is detoxified and converted to harmless malarial pigment. Chloroquine blocks heme detoxification and kills the parasite. Chloroquine resistance occurs by mutation of a vacuolar membrane protein that causes chloroquine to be pumped out of the food vacuole and permits heme detoxification to resume. Unfortunately, chloroquine-resistant *P. falciparum* that have a mutation affecting this protein pump are now widespread in most of Southeast Asia, South America, and Africa. This complicates the prophylaxis and treatment of malaria acquired in those geographic areas. Thus, Ms. M. might well have acquired *P. falciparum* infection in East Africa, even if she had been on chloroquine chemoprophylaxis. In contrast, she would have been protected in Haiti, where there is no chloroquine resistance.

Patients infected with chloroquine-resistant *P. falciparum* can be treated with other agents, such as Malarone (a fixed combination of atovaquone and proguanil), Coartem (a fixed combination of artesunate and lumefantrine),

quinine plus doxycycline, or quinidine. At present, *P. falciparum* cases acquired in areas where drug resistance is prevalent are usually treated in the United States with one of the drugs or combinations mentioned above. Mefloquine, a quinine derivative, is also active against chloroquine-resistant strains but is often toxic at treatment doses. However, it is a mainstay for chemoprophylaxis in travelers to most areas with chloroquine-resistant malaria. Unfortunately, resistance to mefloquine has also been detected in parts of Southeast Asia, and travelers to that area are now being advised to take daily doxycycline or Malarone to prevent infection.

Although all of the antimalarials mentioned are effective in controlling acute infection caused by *P. vivax* or *P. ovale*, none is effective against the liver (hypnozoite) stages of those species. **Primaquine**, a derivative of **quinine**, is effective against the hypnozoite stages. It is used with chloroquine to prevent late relapses associated with maturation of the hypnozoite to the tissue schizont stage and the subsequent release of infectious merozoites. However, primaquine is more toxic than chloroquine and causes nausea, vomiting, and diarrhea. In patients with G6PD deficiency, primaquine induces hemolysis. Primaquine is not indicated for either *P. falciparum* or *P. malariae* infections because those parasites do not produce a dormant (hypnozoite) stage in the liver.

PREVENTION

Mosquito control with insecticides and drainage of aquatic breeding sites have been used to control malaria in many countries, resulting in a dramatic decline in the incidence of the disease. Unfortunately, those control measures have some drawbacks: they are expensive and not always effective because mosquitoes can become resistant to some insecticides. In endemic areas, individuals should protect themselves with mosquito netting, house screening, and insect repellents. The best hope for controlling malaria is the development of improved antimalarials and/or an effective vaccine.

Babesia Species

Like the plasmodia of malaria, *Babesia* species are protozoal parasites that cause illness by infecting red blood cells and generating fever on release. Unlike malaria, babesiosis is endemic in the United States. *Babesia microti* is the most recognized cause of human babesiosis in the United States. Interestingly, it is concentrated geographically in the same area as endemic Lyme disease because *B. microti* and *Borrelia burgdorferi* (the bacterial cause of Lyme disease) infect the same animal reservoir—the white-footed mouse—and are transmitted to humans by the same deer tick, *Ixodes scapularis* (see Chapter 25). Cases of babesiosis outside that geographic area (e.g., from the Midwest to the Pacific Coast) appear to be caused by other *Babesia* species more closely related to the principal European species, *B. divergens*, than to *B. microti*.

CLINICAL AND PARASITOLOGICAL FEATURES

Babesiosis is difficult to recognize clinically because the illness it causes is nonspecific. Infected persons experience a flulike illness, with fever, chills, sweats, muscle aches, and fatigue. Because the illness usually occurs in the summer months, when ticks are feeding, babesiosis has been likened to a "summer flu." Illness is usually mild, but as in malaria, more severe disease occurs in splenectomized patients. In a person with an intact spleen, the proportion of infected red blood cells is usually 0.2% or less, but it can rise to more than 10% in a splenectomized patient. In fact, the disease was first detected in postmortem studies of splenectomized patients. As in malaria, the spleen is thought to remove the less deformable *Babesia*-infected red blood cells from the circulation.

The life cycle of *Babesia* species is shown in Figure 52-4. The epidemiology of the disease is restricted by the presence of a suitable tick vector and wildlife reservoir, as well as by human contact with them. Humans are infected accidentally in endemic areas and are not thought to contribute to the maintenance of the parasite's life cycle.

DIAGNOSIS AND TREATMENT

The laboratory diagnosis of babesiosis depends on finding the parasites in Giemsa-stained blood films using the oil immersion objective. The parasites are seen as small rings, often in tetrads. That is the only form of the parasite found in peripheral blood and may be easily missed when parasitemia is low. The ring shape makes the parasites easy to confuse with a similar form of *P. falciparum*. The distinction between the two parasites is important because *Babesia* infections are treated with different chemotherapeutic agents than malaria: clindamycin plus quinine for babesiosis versus a variety of drugs for malaria (as discussed earlier).

Antibodies to *Babesia* species can be detected in most infected persons. However, they often appear too late (3 to 4 weeks after the onset of infection) to be helpful in the diagnosis and treatment of acute babesiosis. PCR-based diagnosis is available in specialized laboratories and is highly accurate.

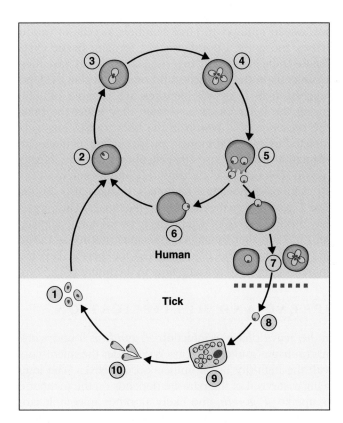

FIGURE 52-4. Life cycle of *Babesia* species. Infectious merozoites are injected under the skin by the hard-bodied tick (*Ixodes*) vector (1) and they invade red blood cells directly (2). Unlike malaria, babesiosis has no intermediate liver stage. Once within the red blood cells, parasites replicate asexually by binary fission (3). *Babesia* species characteristically form tetrads (4), lyse their host red blood cells as they mature (5), and complete the cycle when parasitized red blood cells are ingested by the tick vector (6). The dashed line between stages (7) and (8) indicates that natural transmission does not occur in areas lacking the hard-bodied tick.

TISSUE PROTOZOA
Toxoplasma gondii

Infection with the agent of toxoplasmosis, *Toxoplasma gondii*, is common in humans. However, less than 1% of those infected are ever diagnosed with toxoplasmosis. In the few persons with signs and symptoms of active infection, the clinical presentation of the disease varies. Toxoplasmosis is particularly damaging for immunocompromised patients, such as those with AIDS, and for the developing fetus. *T. gondii* can cause three distinct syndromes:

- A mononucleosis-like syndrome in which tests for the common viral agents of mononucleosis—Epstein-Barr virus and cytomegalovirus—are negative
- A congenital infection that may have severe consequences if acquired in the first trimester of pregnancy (for more detail on the effects of *T. gondii* on the developing fetus, see Chapter 72)
- Infections in immunocompromised hosts (especially people with AIDS), often involving the brain or the heart

ENCOUNTER

People may acquire toxoplasmosis in one of two ways: (1) by eating inadequately cooked meat (e.g., lamb, mutton, or possibly beef) that contains *T. gondii* **tissue cysts** or (2) by ingesting the infectious **oocysts** found in the feces of cats (Fig. 52-5). The first way appears to be the most common, but this is difficult to determine with certainty.

Cats are critical for the propagation of *T. gondii*. Where there are no cats (such as on certain Pacific islands), there is no toxoplasmosis. Cats harbor the sexual cycle of the organisms (analogous to the mosquito in malaria) and

CASE • Mr. H., who is 22 years old, had mild fever, malaise, muscle aches, and headache for 2 weeks. On several occasions he took his temperature orally and found that it ranged from 37°C to 38°C. On physical examination, his physician detected no stiff neck or pharyngitis; however, Mr. H. had several enlarged cervical lymph nodes bilaterally. The liver and spleen were not enlarged on palpation, and the remainder of the examination was normal, including funduscopic examination of the retinas. Routine laboratory tests were similarly unremarkable and included a normal white cell count and normal liver function tests.

Additional history revealed that Mr. H. had no significant contact with animals and no pets at home. He was of Middle Eastern descent and lived with his first-generation immigrant parents. The family occasionally dined on kibbeh, a Middle Eastern dish made with lamb (sometimes raw), bulgur wheat, and spices.

Antibody tests for mononucleosis and cytomegalovirus were negative. However, IgM and IgG serologies for *Toxoplasma gondii* were positive. Mr. H. was advised to rest and to treat fever and muscle aches with acetaminophen. He was given no specific antimicrobial therapy. After 3 weeks, his symptoms were gone, and the lymphadenopathy had receded. A repeat IgG serology for *T. gondii* showed an eightfold increase in titer from the first test.

This case raises several questions:

1. How did Mr. H. acquire the infection?
2. What was the purpose of the second serology?
3. Why was the patient given no treatment?

See Appendix for answers.

---

produce the environmentally resistant infective oocysts in their feces, making them essential to the maintenance of the life cycle.

To complete the cycle, it is also essential that cats ingest small mammals (e.g., rodents) that have become infected by ingesting feline oocysts. In these animals, and in all other nonfeline mammals that acquire toxoplasmosis, parasites that reach the small intestine penetrate the gut wall, invade the bloodstream, and disseminate throughout the body, to the brain, heart, muscles, and other organs. In the first 4 to 6 weeks after the parasites enter the body,

a normal host mount an immune response that controls the infection. However, the parasites are not eliminated but instead multiply to large numbers in cells of various tissues and enter a dormant state, forming **tissue cysts**. Cats become infected by ingesting animals that have these tissue cysts in their muscles and organs. Recent evidence suggests that *T. gondii* parasites are capable of influencing the behavior of rats when they infect the brain. The presence of *T. gondii* in the brain causes rats to be attracted by cat pheromones, an astounding evolutionary adaptation that increases the likelihood that the infected rat will seek out a cat, be captured, and be eaten!

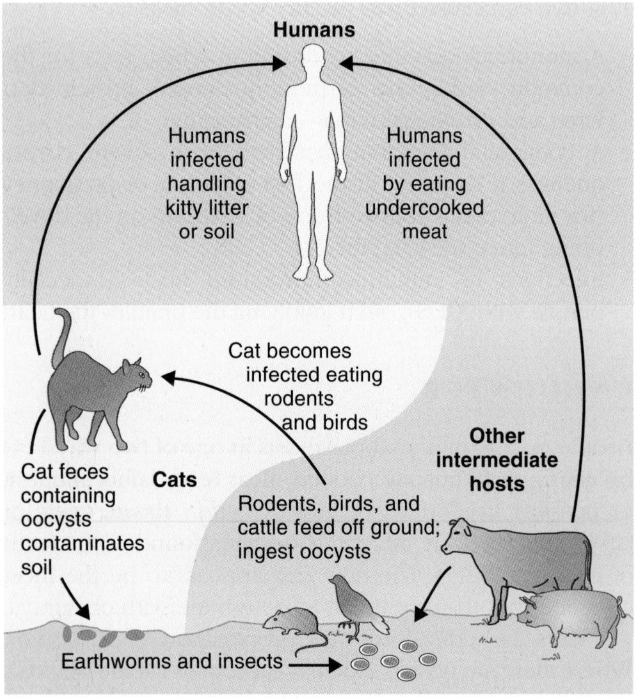

Like other nonfeline mammals, humans also disseminate *T. gondii* from the intestine to the tissues. This process may produce transient symptoms in an immunocompetent person. Thereafter, the infection remains inactive as a dead-end infection in the tissues unless the person becomes immunosuppressed at some time in the future (Fig. 52-6).

SPREAD AND MULTIPLICATION

In the active phase of infection, *T. gondii* is found within macrophages and can be observed under the microscope with the high-dry or oil immersion objectives. The intracellular survival of the parasite depends on the manner of its uptake. *T. gondii*, and likely all other apicomplexans, enters the host cell not by phagocytosis but by active invasion. The secretory and motility functions of the parasite are used to contact the host cell membrane and force the parasite into a membrane-bound vesicle that is devoid of the cellular membrane proteins normally associated with the endocytic pathway. Altering the membrane in that manner has dramatic consequences. Namely, the **parasitophorous vesicle** becomes "invisible" to the host cell and cannot be appropriately targeted to a lysosome by the normal intracellular pathways. In contrast to a resting

FIGURE 52-5. Transmission and spread of *Toxoplasma gondii*.

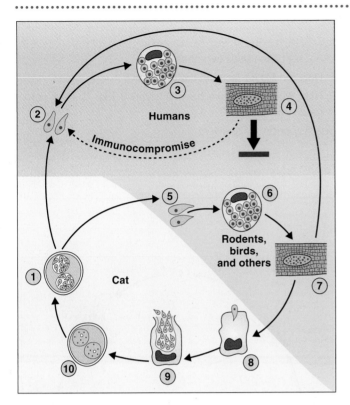

FIGURE 52-6. Life cycle of *Toxoplasma gondii*. Humans and other mammals become infected with *T. gondii* by ingesting inadequately cooked meat containing tissue cysts or by ingesting infectious oocysts excreted in the feces of infected cats (1). Once in the human host, the oocysts mature to tachyzoites (2). Tachyzoites enter the bloodstream and disseminate throughout the body (3). After the initial acute infection, most people mount a successful immune response that eliminates the active infectious (tachyzoite) form of the parasite and leaves only tissue cysts with dormant organisms (4). A similar progression is observed within the cat (I–4), where the parasite also invades intestinal epithelial cells (6). In addition, the organism establishes a sexual cycle (8–9) in the cat, in which infectious oocysts are formed (10) and released (11). The solid line below stage 4 in the upper half of the diagram indicates that human tissue infection is a dead end. Unless an animal or human consumes infected human flesh, human tissue cysts disintegrate after the death of the host.

macrophage or monocyte, activated macrophages can actively phagocytose *T. gondii*. When the macrophage initiates and controls the uptake, the parasite can be appropriately dealt with and killed.

DIAGNOSIS AND TREATMENT

In the immunologically competent host, the diagnosis of acute toxoplasmosis is made by an elevated antibody titer, especially of IgM antibodies. Most previously healthy persons do not need treatment for self-limited, acute toxoplasmosis. Serologic diagnosis is often insensitive in the immunocompromised patient, such as a person with AIDS, who may be unable to produce a diagnostic rise in

antibody titer. Other methods must be used to diagnose toxoplasmosis in immunocompromised patients. The appearance of new neurologic symptoms and the presence of multiple ring-enhancing lesions on a computerized tomography scan or magnetic resonance imaging of the brain should raise suspicion of nervous system toxoplasmosis. On biopsy, the trophozoites associated with acute infection may be difficult to detect morphologically. Staining brain biopsy material with fluorescent or peroxidase-labeled antitoxoplasma antibodies increases the sensitivity of detection. In the absence of an adequate immune response, *T. gondii* causes local inflammation that can result in severe necrosis, tissue damage, and death. Because biopsy of the brain is a complicated and potentially hazardous procedure, most AIDS patients with a suggestive history, positive brain scan, and serological evidence of prior toxoplasmic exposure (e.g., specific IgG antibody) are treated presumptively for cerebral toxoplasmosis. Lifesaving treatment is usually initiated with pyrimethamine plus either sulfadiazine or clindamycin.

T. gondii may be transmitted to a developing fetus if the mother acquires infection during pregnancy. Because most of the potential damage occurs in utero, treatment for congenital infections after the baby is born is usually too late. Therefore, most physicians screen women for antitoxoplasma antibody when they get married or when pregnancy is first detected. Women with preexisting antibodies at the time of pregnancy (indicating prior infection) have virtually no risk of producing a congenitally infected child. Women who are seronegative can be given preventative advice, and those who seroconvert during pregnancy can be counseled, offered therapeutic abortion (if early in pregnancy), or given treatment with experimental drugs, such as spiramycin. The risk of severe complications in the fetus is greatest for women who seroconvert in the first trimester of pregnancy. The frequency of congenital infection is greatest in the third trimester, but most of the children infected late in gestation have no detectable disease at the time of birth. **Chorioretinitis**, which many infants develop early or many years after birth, is sometimes the only manifestation of congenital infection. Unfortunately, various developmental problems may also be seen among initially "asymptomatic" children later in childhood.

Leishmania Species

Leishmania species produce a spectrum of clinical syndromes, from superficial ulcers to severe lesions of the liver, spleen, and bone marrow accompanied by systemic signs such as fever, weight loss, and anemia. Several species are pathogenic for humans. The reason for the wide diversity in clinical disease is not well understood, but it is probably owing in part to the temperature preferences of the various species. Superficial lesions are produced by *Leishmania* species that grow better at lower temperatures (25°C to 30°C), whereas those that invade the viscera grow better at 37°C.

CASE • Ms. Q., a 26-year-old graduate student in anthropology, returned from a 6-month expedition to Peru with a nonhealing 2 × 5-cm lesion on her right shin. A smear taken from the edge of the lesion stained with Giemsa revealed Leishmania-containing macrophages. Ms. Q. was given the antimony-containing, antiprotozoal drug Pentostam for 4 weeks. The lesion began to heal slowly, and she eventually recovered completely.

This case raises two questions:

1. How did Ms. Q. acquire the infection?
2. How would this case have evolved if Ms. Q. had not received treatment?

See Appendix for answers.

ENCOUNTER

Leishmania species are small protozoa that belong to the flagellates because they possess a prominent flagellum during part of their life cycle. The flagellum is connected to an organelle called the **kinetoplast**, which, like the mitochondria, has its own DNA. The protozoa are transmitted by the bite of sand flies—small, short-lived insects that feed on many mammals. The **phlebotomine sand flies** that transmit leishmaniasis are generally found in tropical or subtropical parts of the world, which explains why the disease is rare in North America and Europe. However, phlebotomine sand flies are occasionally found in more temperate regions, and indigenous cases have been reported in the United States. Like malaria, leishmaniasis in the United States is seen mainly among travelers returning from tropical countries and has been observed in military personnel who participated in the 1991 Gulf War. Reservoirs of *Leishmania* parasites include rodents, dogs, other animals, and infected humans.

PATHOGENESIS, DIAGNOSIS, AND TREATMENT

The genus *Leishmania* comprises several species, each with unique tissue tropisms and clinical manifestations. The diseases they cause include localized skin ulcers, mucocutaneous lesions (espundia), disseminated cutaneous leishmaniasis, and disseminated visceral leishmaniasis (kala azar). Ms. Q. had a form of cutaneous leishmaniasis that usually heals poorly and requires treatment.

The life cycle of *Leishmania* species is shown in Figure 52-7. A protein on the parasites' surface binds to one of the complement receptors on macrophages. Phagocytosis then takes place with a minimal degree of oxidative burst. *Leishmania* species also produce superoxide dismutase, which protects them from superoxide produced by the macrophages. After they are taken up into phagosomes, the parasites differentiate into a nonflagellate form, called the **amastigote**. Although the parasite-containing phagosomes fuse with lysosomes, the amastigotes are resistant to killing by lysosomal enzymes. In addition, the amastigotes

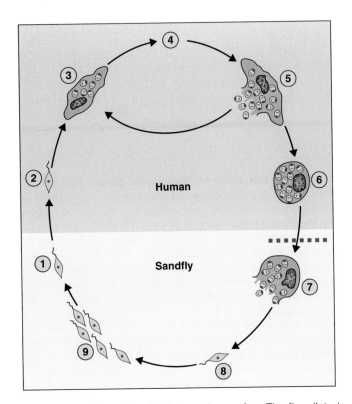

FIGURE 52-7. Life cycle of *Leishmania* species. The flagellated (promastigote) insect form of the parasite (1) is injected under the skin by the sand fly (*Phlebotomus*) vector (2). Once within the human host, the parasite transforms into a nonflagellated (amastigote) form that is more capable of evading the host immune response than the promastigote form (it stimulates less release of H_2O_2 from mononuclear cells than the promastigote and produces its own superoxide dismutase). The parasite then invades lymphoreticular cells (3), replicates (4), lyses the cells (5), and repeats the same sequence in other reticuloendothelial cells (6). In endemic areas, the cycle is completed when previously uninfected sand flies acquire infectious leishmanial amastigotes by biting infected humans (7). The amastigotes then transform into flagellated promastigotes (8) and replicate in the gastrointestinal tract of the sand fly (9). Infective promastigotes are injected under the skin of another human when the parasitized sand fly takes a blood meal (1–2). The dashed line between stages 6 and 7 indicates that transmission is blocked at this point in nonendemic areas such as the United States because the sand fly vector is not present.

depend on the low pH of the phagolysosomes for the uptake of nutrients such as glucose and proline.

Immunity against leishmaniasis involves cell-mediated mechanisms and the induction of interferon-γ (a Th1 response; see Chapter 7). It is thought that the parasite may facilitate its own survival by possessing immunodominant antigens that preferentially induce a Th2 response, which is not protective. Patients with AIDS, who lack coordinated cell-mediated immunity altogether, may develop severe *Leishmania* infections. In fact, leishmaniasis is one of the most common causes of unexplained fevers in persons with AIDS who live in the Mediterranean region.

Leishmaniasis is best diagnosed by histologic examination of biopsy material using the high-dry objective. However, the various species look alike and cannot be distinguished morphologically. *Leishmania* species can be distinguished by culturing them in special media and then analyzing patterns of isoenzymes. That is done in only a few specialized reference laboratories. Alternatively, PCR has become a more practical and rapid technique for both diagnosis and speciation.

A variety of drugs are used to treat leishmaniasis, especially the invasive forms of the disease. Antimony-containing compounds are modestly successful. However, disease of deep organs, such as the bone marrow, may produce fatal anemia and granulocytopenia, despite treatment. Some forms of cutaneous leishmaniasis can be treated with allopurinol or ketoconazole.

Trypanosoma cruzi

Chagas disease, caused by *Trypanosoma cruzi*, occurs throughout Latin America. Overt disease is much less common than infection, but the reasons for the difference are poorly understood.

PATHOGENESIS

The life cycle of *T. cruzi* is shown in Figure 52-8. In the endemic areas of South and Central America, most persons are infected by *T. cruzi* in childhood by the bite of an infected **reduviid bug** (or "kissing bug"). A chancre or tissue and lymph node swelling may develop at the bite

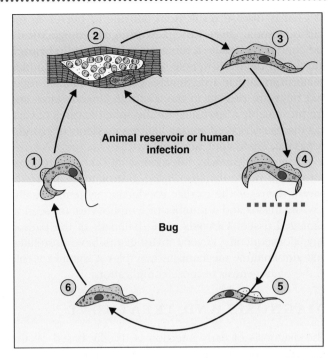

FIGURE 52-8. Chagas disease (American trypanosomiasis). The reduviid bug vector deposits feces containing infectious trypomastigotes on the skin (1). The human host rubs the itching bite wound, allowing the parasites to enter the bloodstream. In the human host, the trypomastigote transforms into an amastigote (analogous to the leishmanial amastigote) as it invades tissue such as muscle (2). Cells containing large numbers of amastigotes often rupture, liberating large numbers of trypomastigotes (3). Trypomastigotes invade other host cells (*arrow* from 3 back to 2) or may be taken up by the vector to complete the cycle (4). In the vector, the parasite replicates as an epimastigote (5) and produces additional infectious trypomastigotes (6). The *dashed line* below stage 4 indicates that natural transmission does not occur in areas lacking the reduviid bug vector. Although reduviid bugs are present in the southern United States, indigenous cases are rare.

site. Although some persons develop serious (even fatal) illness, most develop a relatively mild disease with fever, recover spontaneously, and remain asymptomatic. A small proportion of individuals infected with *T. cruzi* develop complications 10 to 20 years later. The complications

CASE • Mr. S., a 58-year-old Brazilian businessman, was admitted to a hospital in Sao Paulo for the evaluation of chronic constipation. Radiologic examination of his gastrointestinal tract revealed a large, dilated colon (megacolon) and a somewhat less-dilated esophagus (megaesophagus). A blood sample revealed antibodies to *Trypanosoma cruzi*. Because no drugs are effective after the onset of complications, Mr. S. was not given antiparasitic treatment. His chronic constipation was treated symptomatically with a high-fiber diet. A few years

later, Mr. S. was hospitalized for treatment of cardiomyopathy with congestive heart failure. Although that complication was adequately compensated with medical therapy, Mr. S. expired suddenly at home 1 year later.

This case raises two questions:

1. What does the case reveal about Mr. S.'s past?

2. Why were antiparasitic drugs not given?

See Appendix for answers.

of Chagas disease result from damage to nerves in the gastrointestinal tract (**megaesophagus**, **megacolon**), the conducting tissue in the heart (**right bundle branch block**), or the heart muscle (**cardiomyopathy**). Sudden death from cardiac arrhythmia is common. Infected reduviid bugs are present in the southern United States and are presumably responsible for the sporadic cases of Chagas disease observed among lifelong residents of Florida, Louisiana, Mississippi, and California.

It is not clear why infection with *T. cruzi* produces autonomic nerve damage in the gastrointestinal tract or why it damages the cardiac conduction system. Usually, few organisms and a number of lymphocytes are seen in damaged tissue. **Fibrosis** is the hallmark of the pathology. Consequently, several investigators have postulated that autoimmune mechanisms may play a significant role in the pathogenesis of those complications.

DIAGNOSIS AND TREATMENT

The diagnosis of early infection is usually based on the appearance of the patient. Organisms often are found in the blood if it is cultured in an appropriate medium. Early infection can also be diagnosed by detecting infection in reduviid bugs that have purposely been allowed to feed on the patient. Antibodies appear in acutely ill patients within several weeks. Antibody titers usually remain positive for years. The diagnosis of chronic infection with complications is based on a positive antibody titer or history of exposure plus a known complication.

Patients with early acute Chagas disease may respond to treatment with either **nifurtimox** or **benznidazole**. However, no effective treatment is available for patients with late complications, perhaps because the critical damage has already occurred and is no longer reversible.

Trypanosoma brucei

African sleeping sickness is caused by *T. brucei* (Fig. 52-9). The disease is endemic in Africa and transmitted by the bite of infected tsetse flies. *T. brucei* was one of the first microorganisms found to undergo **antigenic variation** of its immunodominant surface antigen, a process now known to occur in several parasitic pathogens.

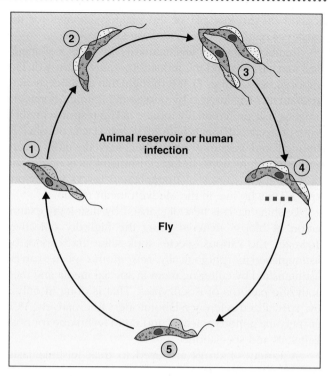

FIGURE 52-9. Sleeping sickness (African trypanosomiasis). The tsetse fly vector inoculates infectious trypomastigotes under the skin (1) when it bites humans or other mammals. Once inside the new host (2), the parasite replicates in the bloodstream by binary fission as a trypomastigote (3). Unlike *Leishmania* species and the trypanosome that causes Chagas disease, the trypanosomes that cause African sleeping sickness do not have promastigote or amastigote forms. The rate of movement of trypomastigotes from the bloodstream and lymph nodes to the central nervous system defines the point at which the illness changes from a systemic (hemolymphatic) infection to an encephalitis. Circulating trypomastigotes (4) taken up anew by tsetse flies complete the cycle. Within the tsetse fly, the parasites replicate in the gastrointestinal tract and transform into epimastigotes (5). The *dashed line* below stage 4 indicates that natural transmission does not occur in countries such as the United States where the tsetse fly vector is not present.

T. brucei and its vectors differ in several biological characteristics from *T. cruzi* (the agent of Chagas disease) and its vectors. For example, *T. brucei* resides in the salivary glands of tsetse flies and is transmitted directly by

CASE • Mr. B., a 32-year-old student from Senegal living in Canada, had fevers of 38°C and swollen lymph nodes at the back of his neck for 8 months. Two weeks ago, he developed a severe headache, stiff neck, and an aversion to light (photophobia). Trypanosomes were seen on Giemsa-stained specimens of blood and cerebrospinal fluid under the oil immersion objective. Mr. B. was treated with eflornithine for both the hemolymphatic and central nervous system infection. He recovered after 6 weeks of treatment.

This case raises two questions:

1. How did a parasite survive in Mr. B.'s blood for 8 months? Is he immunocompromised?
2. How would Mr. B.'s illness have been different if he had immigrated from South Africa rather than West Africa?

See Appendix for answers.

bites. *T. cruzi*, on the other hand, grows in the intestine of reduviid bugs and is transmitted when feces deposited by the biting insect are introduced into the bite by scratching.

PATHOGENESIS AND DIAGNOSIS

The spread of African trypanosomiasis is restricted by the distribution of its tsetse fly vector (*Glossina*) and of its animal reservoirs. In East Africa the main reservoirs are wild game animals (such as impalas); West African reservoirs are infected humans and domestic animals, such as cattle. Several weeks to months after the initial infection, a patient develops a systemic illness with fever and swollen lymph nodes, and trypanosomes are present in the bloodstream. After several months (in the East African form) or years (in the West African form), the parasites invade the central nervous system and infect the brain and spinal fluid.

During months or years of chronic bloodstream infection, patients undergo bouts of parasitemia (Fig. 52-10). During each bout, the parasite changes its dominant surface antigen (**variable surface glycoprotein**), thus avoiding immune destruction by the host. As with bacterial pathogens that undergo similar antigenic variation, the basis for variability is **genetic rearrangement**. Each parasite expresses only one glycoprotein gene from an "expression locus," but it also carries a repertoire of numerous alternative versions of the gene that are not expressed. When one of those "silent copies" recombines into the expression locus, the parasite expresses an immunologically distinct surface glycoprotein. For a full discussion of antigenic variation, see the Chapter 14 paradigm.

TREATMENT

In addition to eflornithine, several drugs (e.g., pentamidine and suramin) are useful in the systemic stage of the infection. However, treatment is much more difficult after the central nervous system becomes involved.

Free-Living Amebas

In this section, we discuss only the amebas that do not have human or animal reservoirs. Amebas with human or animal reservoirs, such as *Entamoeba histolytica,* are discussed in Chapter 53. A number of protozoa, principally

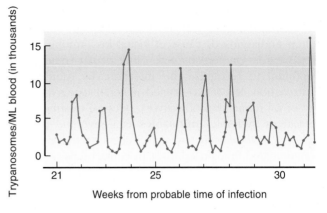

FIGURE 52-10. Periodic fluctuation in the number of *Trypanosoma brucei* in the blood of a patient with African trypanosomiasis.

Naegleria, Acanthamoeba, and *Hartmannella,* have no known animal reservoirs but may cause rare but serious systemic diseases.

There are two types of amebic meningoencephalitis. The first is a usually fatal disease caused by *Naegleria fowleri* that, as in E.'s case, typically occurs in young, previously healthy people. That form of amebic meningoencephalitis is associated with exposure to warm, freshwater lakes that harbor the amebas. The second form is a disease caused by *Acanthamoeba* or *Hartmannella* and is typically seen in older patients who are immunocompromised (such as those with lymphoma or diabetes). Both types of disease, once clinically apparent, tend to progress despite treatment. Although recovery using multiple drugs (amphotericin B, miconazole, and rifampin) has been reported, the regimens have not proven to be reproducibly effective.

In the meningoencephalitis caused by *N. fowleri*, the parasite is thought to enter the central nervous system through the cribriform plate along the olfactory nerve tracts. That site is the area in which the nervous system is in nearest proximity to the exterior; it can thus serve as a unique portal of entry into the central nervous system. *Acanthamoeba* or *Hartmannella*, on the other hand, are thought to spread to the central nervous system through the bloodstream, as suggested by the postmortem finding of foci of infection at distant sites, such as the lung.

CASE • E., a healthy 6-year-old girl living in rural Virginia, swam in a lake in the month of August. Two days later she developed a severe headache, neck stiffness, and eye pain on exposure to light (photophobia). Spinal fluid obtained a day later had 300 mononucleated cells/mm3 and a few neutrophils. Many of those cells were actively motile in a wet mount, suggesting that they were not leukocytes but amebas. Despite treatment with antimicrobial drugs, E. died 3 days later.

This case raises a question:

1. How did amebas get into E.'s central nervous system?

See Appendix for answers.

Infection of the cornea (keratitis) is produced by *Acanthamoeba* and is an increasingly important (often undiagnosed) cause of visual loss among contact lens wearers or persons with other ocular trauma. It is important to recognize this infection (by morphologic examination of Giemsa-stained material using the high-dry or oil immersion objectives), because treatment with topical or systemic **imidazoles** can save the patient's sight. *Acanthamoeba* can gain access to the eye from contaminated fluids used to clean contact lenses.

CONCLUSION

The global morbidity and mortality associated with tissue-invasive protozoal infections is staggering. Malaria is a leading cause of death in young children in endemic regions. Toxoplasmosis is estimated to affect more than 1 billion people and is cosmopolitan in its distribution. Although public health measures to control vectors, mass treatment programs, and chemoprophylaxis (for malaria and toxoplasmosis) have dramatically reduced the impact of some diseases in countries that can economically support such measures, the best hope for worldwide eradication rests on the development of effective vaccines.

Suggested Readings

Baird JK. Effectiveness of antimalarial drugs. *N Engl J Med.* 2005;352:1565–1577.

Greenwood BM, Bojang K, Whitty CJ, et al. Malaria. *Lancet.* 2005;365:1487–1498.

Magill AJ, Grogl M, Johnson SC, et al. Visceral infection due to *Leishmania tropica* in a veteran of Operation Desert Storm who presented 2 years after leaving Saudi Arabia. *Clin Infect Dis.* 1994;19:805–806.

Miller LH, Baruch DI, March K, et al. The pathogenic basis for malaria. *Nature.* 2002;415:673–679.

Moorthy VS, Good MF, Hill AV. Malaria vaccine developments. *Lancet.* 2004;363:150–156.

Sacks D, Sher A. Evasion of innate immunity by parasitic protozoa. *Nat Immunol.* 2002;3:1041–1047.

Sibley LD. No more free lunch. *Nature.* 2002;415:843–844.

Vernick KD, Waters AP. Genomics and malaria control. *N Engl J Med.* 2004;351:1901–1904.

Zambrano-Villa S, Disney RB, Carrero JC, et al. How protozoan parasites evade the immune response. *Trends Parasitol.* 2002;18:272–278.

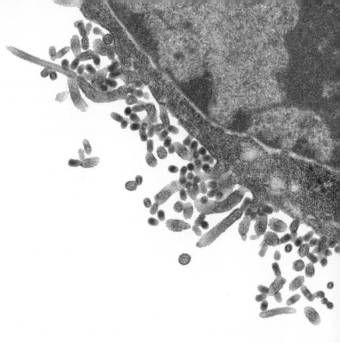

Chapter 53

Intestinal and Vaginal Protozoa

Cary Engleberg

KEY CONCEPTS

Pathogens: Include the ameba, *Entamoeba histolytica*; the flagellate, *Giardia lamblia* (aka *G. intestinalis*); and the apicomplexans, *Cryptosporidium parvum*, *Cyclospora cayetanensis*, and *Isospora belli*.

Encounter: *E. histolytica* relies on a population of infected humans who pass infective cysts in the feces.

G. lamblia and Cryptosporidium are zoonoses but may also be traced back to human sources on occasion. The role of animals in transmission of the other apicomplexa species is less clear.

Entry: Intestinal protozoa are acquired by ingestion of cysts by the fecal–oral route of transmission, usually involving contaminated food or water. Gastric acid is typically the trigger for the transmissive (i.e., cyst) form of the protozoa to release the vegetative forms (i.e., replicating trophozoites).

Spread: Only *E. histolytica* has the capacity to invade tissues beyond the intestinal tract, with portal parasitemia that may carry it to the liver.

Multiplication: *E. histolytica* and *G. lamblia* multiply extracellularly. The apicomplexans replicate intracellularly in the apical regions of intestinal mucosal cells.

Damage: *E. histolytica* lyses cells in the colon and feeds on their contents, resulting in colonic ulcerations and dysentery (diarrhea with blood and mucus).

Giardiasis induces acute watery diarrhea but may also produce a chronic inflammatory response resulting in the loss of intestinal villi, malabsorption syndrome, and weight loss.

The apicomplexans protozoa infect the small intestine and cause noninflammatory, watery diarrhea that can last for days or weeks; however, persons with AIDS and other immunodeficiencies may experience intractable cholera-like diarrhea.

Diagnosis: Diagnosis traditionally involves finding recognizable forms of the parasite in the feces (or other intestinal fluids). Recently, fecal immunoassays have proven to be more sensitive and specific.

Treatment: Both amebiasis and giardiasis respond to metronidazole. Cyclosporiasis and isosporiasis can be treated with trimethoprim/sulfamethoxazole, but cryptosporidiosis is highly resistant to most antiparasitic drugs.

Prevention: Measures that isolate raw foods and potable water from fecal contamination will interrupt the cycle of transmission.

Trichomoniasis is a common form of sexually transmitted vaginitis and urethritis that requires treatment of all contacts to ensure that reinfection will not occur.

THE PROTOZOA are classified according to their motility and their replicative cycles. The intestinal and vaginal organisms discussed in this chapter are a varied group: an **ameba** (*Entamoeba histolytica*), two **flagellates** (*Giardia lamblia* and *Trichomonas vaginalis*), three **apicomplexans** (genera *Cryptosporidium*, *Cyclospora*, and *Isospora*), and Microsporidia (a group of organisms that are difficult to classify because they possess features of both protozoa and bacteria; Table 53-1). The sporozoans (also known as apicomplexans) are intracellular parasites that reproduce by alternating sexual and asexual cycles (as do *Toxoplasma gondii* and malaria parasites; see Chapter 52).

Between 5 and 10% of all people in developing countries harbor ameba in their stool. In the United States, amebiasis is extremely rare. *Giardia* and *Cryptosporidium* species are zoonoses that are more frequent in the United States. Both have caused large waterborne outbreaks, but their prevalence varies considerably among US regions. The *Cyclospora* genus was recognized as a human pathogen during the last two decades, when it was implicated in a series of foodborne outbreaks. The genera *Isospora* and the Microsporidia are most serious when they affect persons with AIDS. Other protozoa that live in nonintestinal tissues include *Trichomonas vaginalis*, a common agent of vaginitis that is usually transmitted sexually.

CASE • Two years ago, 26-year-old Mr. A. was discharged from the U.S. Army after 6 years of service. He was stationed abroad for 3 years, on tours of duty in Korea, Panama, and Germany. During the last 2 years, he developed intermittent diarrhea, with blood and mucus visible in the stool (i.e., dysentery). Sigmoidoscopy (endoscopic examination of the colon) and a radiographic study of the intestine following a barium enema revealed pseudopolyps consistent with inflammatory bowel disease. He was diagnosed with ulcerative colitis, an inflammatory bowel disease of unknown cause, and was treated with steroids.

At the time of admission to the hospital, 4 months after beginning steroid therapy, Mr. A. reported a weight loss of about 24 pounds (down to 147 pounds) and a recent increase in bloody stools and abdominal pain. He had no fever (probably because he was medicated with large doses of steroids). Examination of his stool under the microscope showed many white and red blood cells but no amebas. However, a serological test for *Entamoeba histolytica* antibodies in serum (indirect hemagglutination) revealed a high titer (1:2,000). A computerized tomography scan showed an 8-cm abscess in the right lobe of the liver.

He had a stormy hospital stay with several episodes of bacteremia (secondary to disruption of the intestinal mucosa by the parasite). He finally recovered after the steroids were tapered and he was treated with the antiamebic agent metronidazole.

This case raises two questions:

1. Why were no amebas seen in Mr. A.'s stool?
2. What was the role of steroids in this case?

See Appendix for answers.

ENTAMOEBA HISTOLYTICA

Entamoeba histolytica causes a disease called **amebiasis**. As its species name indicates, *E. histolytica* may cause destruction of host tissue, especially in the colon. The lesions start as small ulcerations of the intestinal epithelium. Amebas within the lesions spread laterally as they encounter the deeper layers of the colon, sometimes producing **flask-shaped ulcers** that undermine the mucosal epithelium. Organisms may also spread through the portal circulation to produce abscesses in the liver and less commonly in the lung, brain, or other organs. Despite their pathogenic potential, organisms in the intestinal tract often cause few or no symptoms. In addition, many humans carry nonpathogenic amebas that are morpho-

---

TABLE 53-1 Comparison of Major Intestinal and Vaginal Protozoa

Organism	Reservoir	Modes of Transmission	Clinical Manifestations
Entamoeba histolytica (amebiasis)	Infected humans	Fecal–oral transmission by the ingestion of feces containing infectious cysts	Bloody diarrhea (dysentery), distant abscesses (especially liver), asymptomatic intestinal infection
Giardia lamblia (giardiasis)	Infected humans and other mammals	Fecal–oral transmission by ingestion of feces containing infectious cysts	Watery diarrhea; may also cause steatorrhea and malabsorption
Cryptosporidium parvum (cryptosporidiosis)	Infected humans and a wide variety of other animal hosts (zoonosis)	Fecal–oral transmission by the ingestion of feces containing infectious cysts	Watery diarrhea; intractable diarrhea in people with AIDS
Cyclospora cayetanensis	Unknown	Foodborne and waterborne; person-to-person spread unlikely	Watery diarrhea
Isospora belli	Infected humans	Foodborne and waterborne	Watery diarrhea; intractable diarrhea in people with AIDS
Microsporidia	Unknown	Unknown	Watery diarrhea, biliary tract infection, etc.

logically indistinguishable from *E. histolytica*. The species name *Entamoeba dispar* is used to designate the avirulent strains, which can be identified only by biochemical or nucleic acid–based techniques.

ENCOUNTER AND ENTRY

E. histolytica is transmitted from person to person through the fecal–oral route. The protozoan has a simple life cycle with two forms: the actively growing, vegetative **trophozoite** and the dormant but highly resistant **cyst** (Fig. 53-1). The critical factors responsible for the transformation from trophozoites to cysts and vice versa are not understood. The transmission of *Entamoeba* and *Giardia* has a paradoxical aspect. Patients with diarrhea pose only a minor threat of transmission because they excrete the actively growing yet labile trophozoites; this form of the parasite is easily destroyed by drying in the environment and, if ingested, by acid in the stomach. Conversely, asymptomatic carriers excrete the durable cyst form of the parasite, which survives well in the environment and remains intact through the stomach. Asymptomatic carriers thus represent the greatest danger of transmission. That paradox illustrates the biological principle that successful parasites generally do not harm the host. When amebas are in balance with their host, they do not cause symptoms but are excreted as cysts, thus ensuring their transmissibility.

Because the parasite is infectious in the cyst stage and does not require a period of maturation in the environment, transmission of amebiasis is not restricted to warm climates. In fact, *E. histolytica* can even be transmitted in polar regions. The only requirement for transmission is that contaminated feces of the carrier be ingested with food or water. Sexual transmission (anal–oral or oral–genital) is also important, particularly among homosexual men.

SPREAD, MULTIPLICATION, AND DAMAGE

E. histolytica are frequently found in the human colon in persons without symptoms of disease. The amebas must adhere using a critical surface protein (or **lectin**) to specific receptors on host cells containing digalactose residues (i.e., Gal–galNAc). In experimental models, attachment to cells is inhibited by adding galactose. Attachment is also inhibited by intestinal mucus, which suggests that disruption of the mucus layer may be a critical event in the pathogenesis of amebiasis.

Damage to host cells requires intimate cell-to-cell contact and takes place in three steps: (1) receptor-mediated attachment to the mammalian target cell via the Gal–galNAc binding lectin; (2) contact-dependent killing, probably by insertion of pore-forming proteins (**amebapores**) into the host cell membrane; and (3) ingestion of the killed host cell by the ameba.

Phagocytic cells do not control amebic infection in nonimmune hosts: pathogenic strains of amebas actually kill neutrophils and nonactivated macrophages (notice the reversal of the usual "phagocyte ingests invader" theme). The situation is different in immune hosts, in whom the most important line of defense appears to be cell-mediated immunity. This was suggested by the finding that amebas can be killed in vitro by activated macrophages. Furthermore, persons given steroids (which suppress cell-mediated immunity) tend to have disseminated infection despite high titers of antibodies, as was the case with Mr. A. Thus, circulating antibodies may not play a critical role in protection against amebic infection. Amebas are known to produce a **cysteine proteinase** that digests secretory IgA, IgG, and other proteins involved in the humoral immune response.

DIAGNOSIS

The traditional method of diagnosis involves the microscopic identification of trophozoites in freshly passed dysenteric stool or in scrapings from colonic ulcers obtained

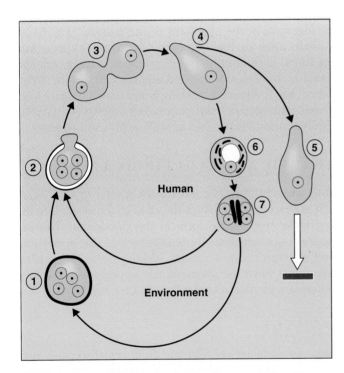

FIGURE 53-1. Life cycle of *Entamoeba histolytica*. Humans acquire amebic infection by oral ingestion of the cyst form of the parasite (*1*). Viable cysts may be ingested from the external environment (where they remain stable and infectious for prolonged periods after excretion), from the stool of other infected persons, or from the stools of the patients themselves (the *arrow* from *7* to *2*). In the upper gastrointestinal tract, the parasite excysts after passing through the stomach (*2*), replicates asexually by binary fission (*3*), and transforms to the potentially pathogenic trophozoite form (*4*), which is typically found in the large intestine. Trophozoites die rapidly when they are shed into the external environment (*5*; *solid line* represents dead end). When conditions in the gastrointestinal tract are unfavorable, trophozoites transform into cysts (*6*, *7*), which can remain dormant for long periods of time in the host and the environment.

through a sigmoidoscope. On a warm microscopic slide, organisms demonstrate ameboid movement. *E. histolytica* may contain ingested red blood cells. However, *E. histolytica* trophozoites without internalized red blood cells and cysts are indistinguishable from the nonpathogenic ameba *E. dispar*. Consequently, microscopic examination of stool from a patient without characteristic clinical features and colonic ulcers may be misleading. In that case, alternative diagnostic methods may be helpful. In particular, a **stool immunoassay** for *E. histolytica* antigen may be more sensitive than microscopic examination and, in some formats, capable of distinguishing *E. histolytica* from *E. dispar*. Isoenzyme analysis of cultured organisms or PCR is required to make the definitive distinction. Alternatively, serological diagnosis may be useful. Ameba serology is positive in 10 to 15% of asymptomatic carriers, in more than 80% of people with invasion of the intestinal mucosa, and in 96 to 100% of persons with metastatic infection (e.g., liver abscess). However, since antiameba antibodies persist for several years after infection, serology does not distinguish current from past infection and is therefore not useful in countries where amebiasis is endemic. However, in the United States, where less than 1% of the general population has antibodies to *E. histolytica*, a strongly positive serology can be taken as evidence of active infection. *E. dispar* infections produce very weak or no antibody response.

TREATMENT

The drug of choice for active amebic infection is **metronidazole**, the same antimicrobial used to treat infections caused by anaerobic bacteria. Pathogenic amebas carry out anaerobic metabolism and convert metronidazole to its active form in the same way as do species of *Bacteroides* (see Chapters 3 and 15). The drug is particularly effective for invasive infections because it penetrates well into most tissues, including the brain. Because metronidazole is less efficient at killing amebas within the intestinal lumen, a second drug is given to eradicate the luminal forms. Drugs such as diloxanide, paromomycin, and diiodohydroxyquin are used for that purpose and can also be used to treat asymptomatic carriers of pathogenic strains.

GIARDIA LAMBLIA

Giardia lamblia (also known as *Giardia intestinalis*) is the intestinal protozoan that causes **giardiasis**. *G. lamblia* is distributed all over the world. Giardiasis is a zoonosis, and it may be acquired by ingestion of water contaminated by feces from animal or human carriers. Because *Giardia* cysts are resistant to chlorine, waterborne outbreaks associated with municipal water systems have occurred in the United States and around the world. In the United States, giardiasis is sometimes transmitted in settings with problematic sanitation such as in day care centers, where there is frequent opportunity for direct fecal–oral transmission. Giardiasis is also an important infection among homosexual males. *Giardia* infection typically produces a mild but persistent diarrheal illness, with organisms often localized to the duodenum and jejunum. Occasionally, chronic infection causes intestinal malabsorption.

ENCOUTER AND ENTRY

As with *E. histolytica* infection, giardiasis is acquired by ingestion of the cyst form of the parasite (Fig. 53-2). *Giardia* cysts are highly resistant in the environment and are found in ostensibly "pure" mountain streams contaminated by the feces of infected animals or humans. When asked, Ms. P. admitted drinking water drawn directly from a mountain stream. Like pathogenic amebas, *G. lamblia* can be transmitted in cold as well as in warm climates.

SPREAD AND MULTIPLICATION

Stomach acid does not kill *Giardia* cysts. In fact, stomach acid actually stimulates the cysts to transform into the vegetative trophozoite form in the duodenum. *Giardia* trophozoites attach to the epithelium of the duodenum and jejunum using a ventral sucking disk. The vegetative forms have the characteristic appearance of a face adorned with mustachelike flagella (see Fig. 53-2).

DAMAGE

Signs of malnutrition resulting from malabsorption may occur as a result of extensive, prolonged infection. In those

---

CASE • Thirty-six-year-old Ms. P. visited Colorado for 10 days of backpacking 2 months before seeing her physician. One week after returning, she developed abdominal bloating, belching, and diarrhea with three to five watery stools per day. The stool contained no pus or blood, and she had no fever or chills. A stool examination was positive for *Giardia lamblia*. Ms. P. was treated with metronidazole and improved markedly over a 7-day period. Subsequently,

symptoms recurred and the organisms were again found in her stool.

This case raises two questions:

1. How did Ms. P. acquire *Giardia* infection?
2. What prompted the physician to check for a parasite rather than to culture for agents of bacterial gastroenteritis?

See Appendix for answers.

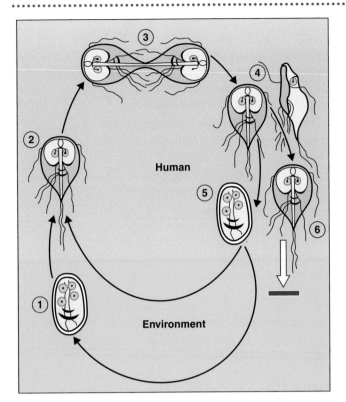

FIGURE 53-2. Life cycle of *Giardia lamblia*. Humans acquire giardiasis by ingesting the cyst form of the parasite (*1*). After contact with the gastric contents, the parasite excysts and transforms to a trophozoite in the upper gastrointestinal tract (*2*), where it replicates asexually by binary fission (*3*). Trophozoites cause disease by attaching to the epithelium of the small intestine via a ventral sucking disk (*4*). As indicated by the *solid line* and *open arrow* below stage *6*, trophozoites are not infectious for others because they are readily killed by drying in the external environment. As in amebiasis, humans acquire infection by ingesting cysts from the external environment (*1*), from the stools of other patients, or from their own stool (*arrow* from stages *5* to *2*).

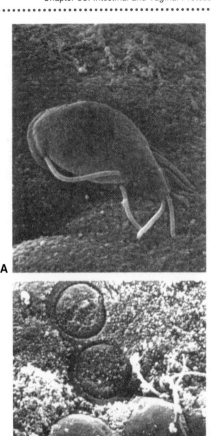

FIGURE 53-3. Scanning electron micrograph of *Giardia lamblia*. **A.** *G. lamblia* adhering to the gastrointestinal epithelium using its ventral sucking disk. Patients with giardiasis may have a significant reduction in the amount of absorptive surface available because of the large number of adhering parasites. **B.** On detaching from the intestinal epithelium, the organisms often leave a clear impression on the microvillous surface (*upper circles*).

cases, the organisms literally cover the mucosal surface of the small intestine (Fig. 53-3). Unlike *E. histolytica*, *G. lamblia* is not invasive and does not produce bloody diarrhea or metastatic infection. However, the host responds to *Giardia* infection with a submucosal infiltrate of chronic inflammatory cells (mostly lymphocytes) and an effacement of the normal intestinal villi. With the loss of villi, the total absorptive area of the intestine is significantly diminished. In particular, malabsorption of fats can lead to greasy, foul-smelling stools; diarrhea associated with unabsorbed fatty acids in the lumen; deficiencies of fat-soluble vitamins (i.e., A, K, D, and E); and weight loss.

DIAGNOSIS

The classic approach to diagnosis of giardiasis is direct identification of parasites in stool or in duodenal aspirates. Trophozoites are actively motile in fresh specimens by virtue of their multiple flagella. Cysts are small, ovoid, nonmotile bodies with four nuclei. Trophozoites are rarely seen

in direct stool examinations, and it may take three or more stool examinations to find cysts in an infected patient or carrier. Fortunately, an antigen detection assay for giardiasis is now available. This test is more sensitive than a single microscopic stool examination for diagnosing giardiasis.

TREATMENT AND PREVENTION

In the United States, giardiasis can be treated with metronidazole, but relapses can occur. Alternative antimicrobial agents with a similar mechanism of action include **tinidazole** and **nitazoxanide**. Hikers and campers can prevent unpleasant episodes of diarrhea by boiling or filtering their drinking water or by treating it with adequate amounts of iodine or chlorine.

CASE • Mr. W., a 40-year-old homosexual with HIV infection, lives on a farm in rural Michigan. Despite a low CD4 count and periodic episodes of oral candidiasis, he had been well and had refused treatment. Six weeks ago, he began to have watery stools three to eight times a day. He denied fever or chills, and no blood or pus appeared in the stools. A microscopic examination of his stool after an acid-fast stain revealed the presence of acid-fast spherical organisms that were slightly smaller than erythrocytes. Although Mr. W. was treated with oral rehydration and a synthetic hormone that reduces intestinal secretion, he continued to have persistent watery diarrhea. He eventually agreed to treatment with a four-drug combination of antiretroviral agents and noted improvement in the frequency of diarrhea over the subsequent months.

This case raises several questions:

1. How did Mr. W. acquire cryptosporidiosis?
2. What other significant pathogens might be seen on an acid-fast stain of the stool?
3. Why was antiretroviral therapy given to control the diarrhea instead of an antiparasitic agent?

See Appendix for answers.

CRYPTOSPORIDIUM

Cryptosporidia cause a zoonosis first discovered among veterinary students and animal handlers who acquired it from calves they were treating for diarrhea. It is now clear that cryptosporidiosis is an important diarrheal disease in both developed and developing countries.

ENCOUNTER

Cryptosporidiosis is often acquired in rural areas because of greater contact with animals, particularly with cattle. However, it can also spread from person to person in crowded urban environments such as day care centers. It is now recognized as a frequent cause of diarrhea in Great Britain and the United States, and it has been identified as a potential cause of diarrhea in travelers to developing countries. Cryptosporidiosis is particularly troublesome in patients with advanced AIDS who lack the immune mechanisms necessary to resolve the infection.

ENCOUNTER AND ENTRY

Recent attention has focused on outbreaks associated with public water systems. *Cryptosporidium* oocysts can be found in most surface waters in this country, and most public utilities draw on these sources to provide public water service. Several outbreaks of cryptosporidiosis have involved drinking water or swimming pools. The largest single waterborne outbreak of *Cryptosporidium* infection in the history of the United States occurred in Milwaukee, Wisconsin, in 1993. More than 400,000 persons were affected, and more than 4,000 people were hospitalized after contamination of the municipal water supply. More recently, outbreaks at swim clubs have followed fecal accidents in swimming pools by infected children. Cryptosporidia oocysts are highly resistant to chlorine, and the infectious particles are expelled in huge numbers in watery stool. Thus, even standard chlorination methods and massive dilution of the fecal organisms in the entire pool volume do not prevent transmission to swimmers who inadvertently swallow pool water. Currently, the only recourse in that situation is to close and drain the contaminated pool.

SPREAD AND MULTIPLICATION

Cryptosporidium parasites resemble *Toxoplasma* species in that infectious oocyst forms are produced in the intestine and spread to other animals. However, unlike *Toxoplasma* species, cryptosporidia do not invade past the intestinal mucosa, nor do they disseminate to produce systemic infection. They carry out their entire life cycle among the microvilli of the small intestine where they multiply at the apical end of the epithelial cells and are released back to the luminal surface (Fig. 53-4). In immunocompetent individuals, the life cycle takes place only once or twice, resulting in a single episode of diarrhea that usually lasts 2 weeks or less. In immunocompromised patients (e.g., persons with AIDS), the life cycle of the organism is repeated many times and is associated with persistent and often intractable watery diarrhea.

DIAGNOSIS AND TREATMENT

The diagnosis of cryptosporidiosis can be made by identifying characteristic acid-fast cysts in the stool. A commonly used alternative is a stool antigen detection assay for cryptosporidia, which is less labor intensive than making stained smears of stool.

Nitazoxanide appears to have activity against cryptosporidia in immunocompetent hosts, but treatment with that agent has not resolved the problem of persistent diarrhea in AIDS. Supportive therapy with rehydration and antimotility agents is the mainstay in that setting. In addition, successful treatment with antiretroviral therapy and restoration of cell-mediated immunity can result in significant improvement of symptoms.

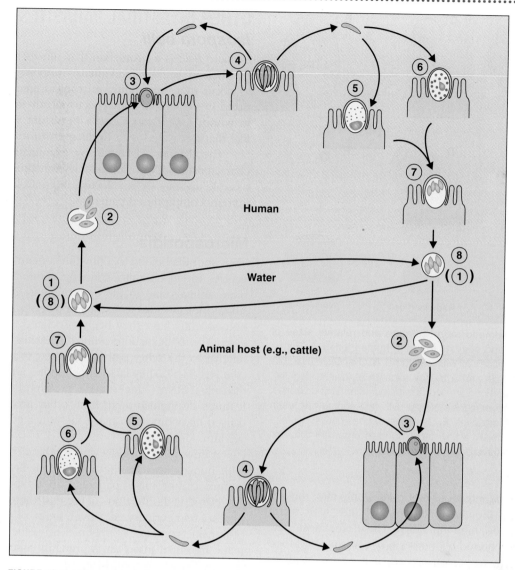

FIGURE 53-4. Life cycle of *Cryptosporidium* species. Humans acquire infection by ingesting infectious oocysts (*1*) after direct contact with infected animals or humans or by ingesting water or food contaminated with human or animal feces. Autoinfection can also occur. Once inside the human host (*2*), sporozoites are released from the oocyst, enter the epithelial cells of the gastrointestinal tract and develop into trophozoites (*3*). Trophozoites develop into structures containing individual merozoites (*4*). The trophozoites can either recapitulate the asexual cycle (*3*) or evolve into one of two sexual gametes (*5, 6*). The gametes join and form oocysts (*7*). When mature and released, oocysts are the infectious form of the parasite that is excreted in the feces (*8*). Identical events take place in the reservoir.

CYCLOSPORA CAYETANENSIS

Cyclospora cayetanensis is a protozoal parasite that resembles *Cryptosporidium* species in producing acid-fast cysts in stools, although the *Cyclospora* cysts are roughly twice the size of those caused by cryptosporidia (Fig. 53-5).

ENCOUNTER

In the late 1980s and early 1990s, *C. cayetanensis* was increasingly recognized as a cause of epidemic diarrhea in the United States and chronic diarrhea in developing countries around the world. In 1996, more than 40 outbreaks

of cyclosporiasis occurred in several states. Most of those outbreaks were linked to ingestion of raspberries imported from Central America. In Lima, Peru, species of *Cyclospora* were found in the stools of 6 to 18% of young children, often associated with diarrhea. The species *C. cayetanensis* is named for the Peruvian University (Cayetano Heredia) where those observations were made.

ENTRY

Unlike *Entamoeba* and *Giardia* cysts, *Cyclospora* oocysts are not infectious when excreted in human feces. The

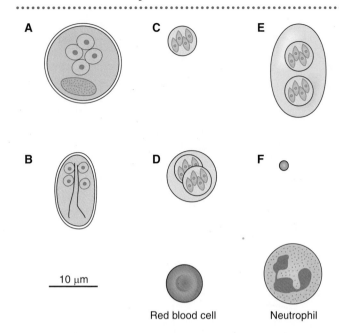

FIGURE 53-5. Schematic representation and relative sizes of protozoal cysts and oocysts found in human feces. A. Round *Entamoeba histolytica* cyst with four nuclei. **B.** Oval *Giardia lamblia* cyst with four nuclei and a central axostyle (encysted flagella). **C.** *Cryptosporidium parvum* oocyst with four internal sporozoites. **D.** *Cyclospora cayetanensis* oocyst with two sporocysts, each containing four sporozoites. **E.** Oval *Isospora belli* oocyst containing two sporocysts. **F.** A tiny microsporidian organism with few distinguishing features by light microscopy.

parasites become infectious (sporulate) only after days to weeks of incubation in environmental sites with warm temperatures and high humidity. Therefore, most new infections are acquired by ingestion of contaminated food or water. Person-to-person spread, if it occurs at all, is probably very rare.

SPREAD, MULTIPLICATION, AND DAMAGE

C. cayetanensis follows a life cycle in the intestine that is similar to the closely related *Cryptosporidium* spp. with intracellular infection of the apical intestinal epithelial cells. Organisms do not invade beyond the intestinal mucosa. Infection with *C. cayetanensis* causes watery diarrhea that may be associated with loss of appetite, bloating, cramps, nausea and vomiting, fatigue, muscle aches, and low-grade fever. The illness may last for only a few days, or it may persist for a month or longer. Relapses are common.

DIAGNOSIS AND TREATMENT

Diagnosis depends on the identification of the large acid-fast oocyst in the stool. Treatment with trimethoprim/sulfamethoxazole relieves symptoms and shortens the course of infection.

OTHER INTESTINAL PARASITES
Isospora belli

Isospora belli is a protozoan that causes transient watery diarrhea in healthy individuals. *Isospora* infection tends to occur more frequently in tropical areas. Cases recognized in the United States occur mostly in AIDS patients, in whom *I. belli* can cause a persistent watery diarrhea, like that associated with *Cryptosporidium* species.

The diagnosis is made by examination of stool for characteristic oocysts. Fortunately, trimethoprim/sulfamethoxazole appears to be effective in controlling infection in immunocompromised patients.

Microsporidia

Microsporidia belong to a phylum containing almost 1,000 species found ubiquitous among vertebrate and invertebrate animals and in the environment. They have been studied for decades as causes of insect and fish diseases; only recently have they been associated with human disease. The obligate intracellular parasites are very small relative to the other pathogens discussed in this chapter (see Fig. 53-5). They lack mitochondria and possess small ribosomal RNA, suggesting a prokaryotic origin. Those features distinguish them from other protozoa and have caused taxonomists to place the parasites into their own phylum, Microsporidia.

A few Microsporidia species have been associated with human diseases, particularly but not exclusively in immunocompromised patients. Various species have been associated with infections of the gastrointestinal tract, respiratory tract, urinary tract, liver, brain, or eye. The modes of transmission have not been clearly elucidated. Symptomatic intestinal infection is primarily associated with the species *Enterocytozoon bieneusi*.

E. bieneusi is believed to cause transient diarrhea in healthy hosts but a protracted watery diarrhea in AIDS patients. The organism infects the mucosal epithelial cells and, in AIDS patients, can also disseminate to distant sites. Thus, *E. bieneusi* may ascend into the biliary tree and cause symptoms of cholangitis. The diagnosis can be made by microscopic examination of stool or intestinal biopsy material after special staining procedures. Optimal treatment has not yet been found; common antibacterial and antiprotozoal drugs are not very effective. Oddly, the antihelminthic drug **albendazole** and a compound isolated from the fungus *Aspergillus fumigatus*, **fumagillin**, have been used with some success.

TRICHOMONAS VAGINALIS

Trichomonas vaginalis is a common inhabitant of the vagina and is found in 15% or more of women, in whom it occasionally causes vaginitis. Less common and less pathogenic species of *Trichomonas* are found in the gastrointestinal tract (*T. hominis*) or the mouth (*T. tenax*).

ENTRY, MULTIPLICATION, AND DAMAGE

T. vaginalis infection is transmitted by sexual intercourse. Vaginitis is typically associated with a frothy creamy discharge. Most male partners of symptomatic women become infected; however, the majority of infections in men are asymptomatic. Symptoms sometimes seen among men include mild urethritis, epididymitis, or prostatitis.

DIAGNOSIS AND TREATMENT

It is usually possible to see these flagellates moving vigorously in wet preparations of vaginal secretions from infected women. Infection of male partners can be assumed. Single-dose metronidazole or tinidazole treatment is recommended by most investigators. In pregnant women, trichomoniasis is associated with adverse pregnancy outcomes. Such patients require careful counseling, and single-dose metronidazole therapy is thought to be safe and effective. Male sexual partners must also be treated to prevent "ping-pong" relapses, a common feature of many sexually transmitted diseases.

CONCLUSION

Most intestinal protozoa produce self-limited illness with watery diarrhea, abdominal cramps, and characteristic protozoal forms in the stool. Amebiasis is unique among these diseases because it involves direct destruction of tissues and occasionally disseminates to vital organs. Accordingly, the clinical features of amebiasis may include bloody stools (dysentery), fever, or abscess formation in the liver and elsewhere. Amebiasis is also distinct from the other protozoa in that the transmission depends on a reservoir of asymptomatic human carriers, rather than nonhuman sources. Thus, infection always results from a failure to dispose of human feces safely, in contrast to giardiasis and other intestinal protozoal infections, which may result from contamination of food and water at its source. Understanding the pathophysiologic differences among these parasites aids in the diagnosis of diarrheal illness, and an appreciation for their epidemiology may direct attention to the circumstances and source of infection.

Suggested Readings

Ali SA, Hill DR. *Giardia intestinalis. Curr Opin Infect Dis.* 2003;16:453–460.

Centers for Disease Control and Prevention. Protracted outbreaks of cryptosporidiosis associated with swimming pool use—Ohio and Nebraska, 2000. *MMWR Morb Mortal Wkly Rep.* 2001;50:406–410.

Chalmers RM, Davies AP. Minireview: clinical cryptosporidiosis. *Exp Parasitol.* 2009;124:138–146.

Herwaldt BL, Ackers ML. An outbreak in 1996 of cyclosporiasis associated with imported raspberries. The Cyclospora Working Group. *N Engl J Med.* 1997;336:1548–1556.

Katz DE, Taylor DN. Parasitic infections of the gastrointestinal tract. *Gastroenterol Clin North Am.* 2001;30:797–815.

Loftus, et al. Amoebiasis: a well-tuned genome. *Nature.* 2005;433:865–868.

Madico G, McDonald J, Gilman RH, et al. Epidemiology and treatment of *Cyclospora cayetanensis* infection in Peruvian children. *Clin Infect Dis.* 1997;24:977–981.

Marshall MM, Naumovitz D, Ortega Y, et al. Waterborne protozoan pathogens. *Clin Microbiol Rev.* 1997;10:67–85.

Petri WA Jr. Therapy of intestinal protozoa. *Trends Parasitol.* 2003;19:523–526.

Petri WA Jr, Haque R, Mann BJ. The bittersweet interface of parasite and host: lectin-carbohydrate interactions during human invasion by the parasite *Entamoeba histolytica. Ann Rev Microbiol.* 2002;56:39–64.

Stanley SL Jr. Amoebiasis. *Lancet.* 2003;361:1025–1034.

Tanyuksei M, Petri WA, Jr. Laboratory diagnosis of amoebiasis. *Clin Microbiol Rev.* 2003;16(4):713–729.

Ximenez et al. Reassessment of the epidemiology of amebiasis: State of the art. *Infect Genet Evol.* 2009;9:1023–1032.

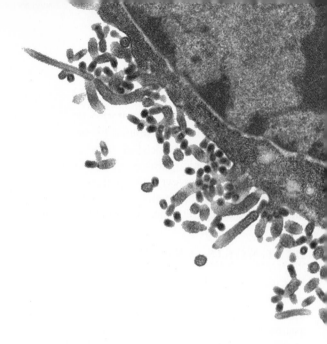

Chapter **54**

Intestinal Helminths

Cary Engleberg

KEY CONCEPTS

Pathogens: The common intestinal helminthic infections are caused by nematodes (roundworms) and cestodes (tapeworms).

Encounter: The life cycles of helminths require indiscriminate handling of human wastes leading to fecal helminth eggs contaminating soil, foodstuffs, animal feeds, and other materials.

Entry: Nematode infections are acquired by ingestion of eggs (e.g., *Ascaris, Trichuris, Enterobius*) or by direct penetration of soil larvae through the skin (e.g., *Strongyloides*, hookworm).

Three species of tapeworm can cause infections when people ingest encysted worm larvae in undercooked tissues of beef, pork, or fish.

Spread and Multiplication: Adult intestinal helminths remain in the intestinal tract and do not replicate within an infected host; that is, the worm burden is increased only by reexposure to infectious eggs or larvae. However, sustained autoinfection is a unique feature of strongyloidiasis, and

immunosuppressed individuals may develop a syndrome of *Strongyloides* hyperinfection with diarrhea, pneumonitis, rash, and eosinophilia.

Damage: Infections are usually asymptomatic unless the worm burden is very large. Pathologic features include intestinal obstruction (*Ascaris*), rectal prolapse (*Trichuris*), anal itching (*Enterobius*), and iron deficiency anemia (hookworm).

Fish tapeworms may successfully compete for vitamin B_{12} and cause anemia in the host. Beef or pork tapeworms rarely produce systemic signs or symptoms.

Diagnosis: Diagnosis of intestinal helminths relies on identifying the characteristic eggs, larvae, or adult worms (or segments) in feces.

Treatment: Albendazole, ivermectin, and praziquantel are anthelmintic agents that can kill intestinal parasites.

Prevention: Sanitary disposal of human waste (nematodes) and avoidance of undercooked meat and fish (tapeworms)

THE HELMINTHS, or worms, are multicellular animals. They include many free-living, harmless species as well as some pathogenic species that infect a high proportion of all people on earth (see Table 51-1). Helminth infections are sometimes mistakenly considered a problem only for people living in the tropics. In fact, some infections are common in temperate zones; others are relatively rare but have major consequences when they go unrecognized, especially in immunocompromised persons.

Helminths are the largest parasites that affect humans, ranging in size from 10-yard-long tapeworms to barely visible pinworms. The three groups of helminths are **roundworms** (nematodes), **tapeworms** (cestodes), and **flukes** (trematodes). Each group is generally distinguished by its shape. Examples of each type of worm are discussed in this and the next chapter. However, the number and range of all helminths is beyond the scope of this text, and specialized parasitology textbooks should be consulted for details. From the point of view of human disease, helminths can be divided into the **intestinal helminths** and the **tissue and blood helminths** (see Chapter 55). The generalities about helminths mentioned here apply to both intestinal and tissue-invasive helminths.

In small numbers, helminths often cause chronic infections that are well tolerated by their human host. They reproduce sexually. Therefore, humans must harbor both a male and female worm for an infection to produce fertilized eggs or larvae that can propagate infection to other hosts. A few species (tapeworms) are hermaphroditic, enabling a single parasite to produce eggs. In massive numbers, intestinal parasites can cause disease by contributing to the malnutrition of their host, occluding the intestinal lumen, or triggering a symptomatic immune response (Tables 54-1 and 54-2). Tissue-invasive helminths in large numbers cause disease by immunopathologic mechanisms or by creating an obstructing mass in vessels or organs (see Table 54-1).

Critical developmental stages of some helminths (e.g., hookworms) take place outside the human body, sometimes involving insect vectors and/or animal reservoirs. In these complex life cycles, the hosts that harbor the adult, sexual form of the parasites are called **definitive hosts**, and the animal hosts that harbor the developmental stages are called **intermediate hosts**. Because multiple steps are required for infectivity, direct transmission from human to human does not occur with these species. However, for some helminths (e.g., *Enterobius* infections), an infected patient may pass feces containing eggs or larvae that are immediately infectious for other humans. Person-to-person transmission, or **autoinfection**, is then possible. In all these species, however, the total number of parasites does not increase during the course of infection because the life cycle cannot be completed entirely within the human body. As a result, the intensity of infection, called the **worm burden**, is determined by the size of single or repeated inocula (i.e., the number of eggs or larvae acquired from the external environment).

A few helminthic species (e.g., *Strongyloides*) can carry out their entire life cycle within the human body. A continuous reinfection cycle prolongs the duration of the infection long beyond the life span of a single worm. In infections of these species, the host immune system may provide a check on the continuous propagation of worms, but an immunocompromised individual may experience uncontrolled growth of the worm burden.

In general, established adult worm infections are not eliminated by the host immune response. Most helminth infections resolve spontaneously when the adult parasites reach senescence (after a few months or years, they die of old age). Longevity differs by species. In some infections, immunity to progressive stages of the parasite may develop to keep continuous acquisition in check. Unfortunately, in most helminthic infections, the major contribution of the host immune response is to cause the pathophysiologic features of the disease. Most of the pathologic features of these infections do not result from the direct action of the parasite on tissues but rather on the host's response to the products of parasites (eggs, larvae, and soluble antigens).

Eosinophilia is often regarded as a characteristic host response to parasitic infection. Indeed, specific antibodies together with eosinophils can adversely affect some parasites. However, a significant systemic eosinophilia occurs only when parasites are invading or migrating through host tissues. Although some intestinal parasites have stages of migration through the tissues and lungs that may provoke eosinophilia, worm infections confined to the intestinal lumen do not cause that systemic response.

CASE • T., a 4-year-old-boy living in rural Georgia, had been well until 3 weeks before a visit to the doctor, although he had always been small for his age (height and weight at the 10th percentile). His parents reported that he passed "earthworms" with his stool. For the previous 2 to 3 weeks, he had vague abdominal pain with nausea. His appetite had been poor, his abdomen was distended, and he had not had a bowel movement for 5 days. Radiographs of his abdomen were consistent with intestinal obstruction. Stool examination revealed large numbers of *Ascaris* eggs.

He was given mebendazole and placed on intravenous fluids. One day after beginning treatment, he passed large numbers of *Ascaris*. Three days later, his abdomen was no longer distended, he was able to eat and drink, and he had a normal bowel movement.

This case raises two questions:

1. How did T. acquire the worms?
2. Is T.'s case typical of *Ascaris* infections?

See Appendix for answers.

INTESTINAL NEMATODES (ROUNDWORMS)

The comparative life cycles of intestinal roundworms (nematodes) are summarized in Figure 54-1. Some of these parasites enter the body through the mouth when eggs are ingested. Others develop into larvae that penetrate through intact skin. The species discussed here infect large numbers of people and cause infections that range from asymptomatic to severe.

Nematode Infections Acquired by Ingestion: *Ascaris*

Ascaris is one of the largest of the human parasites, up to 30 cm in length, and one of the most frequently encountered

TABLE 54-1 Pathophysiologic Mechanisms in Helminth Diseases

Mechanism	Example
Mechanical Obstruction or Mass Effect	
Intestinal obstruction	_Ascaris_ ("worm ball")
Lymphatic obstruction	Lymphatic filariasis (elephantiasis)
Displacement of normal tissue	Echinococcosis (cystic hydatid disease), cysticercosis
Facilitating Bacterial Invasion into Normally Sterile Spaces	Strongyloidiasis
Anemia	
From consumption of blood	Hookworm
From vitamin B_{12} depletion	Fish tapeworm
Chronic Inflammation	Schistosomiasis, onchocerciasis

worldwide. It affects perhaps one-quarter of the human population, including a substantial number of people in the southern United States. A few _Ascaris_ are generally well tolerated, but a large worm load can cause serious illness.

ENCOUNTER AND PATHOBIOLOGY

After excretion in the stool, _Ascaris_ eggs require several weeks in a warm environment to mature to the infective stage (Fig. 54-2). For that reason, ascariasis, like hookworm disease, is restricted to warm climates and to areas where the soil is contaminated by untreated human feces. The eggs must be ingested to complete the cycle. Ingestion occurs by placing soiled hands in the mouth or by eating food contaminated with soil-containing eggs. Fruits and vegetables growing near to the ground become contaminated by direct contact with fecally contaminated soil, either inadvertently or deliberately (as when human feces are used as fertilizer).

Once ingested, the eggs hatch in the small intestine and release larvae, which penetrate the mucosa and

TABLE 54-2 Main Intestinal Helminths

Example	Reservoir	Clinical Manifestations
Acquired by Passage Through the Skin		
Roundworms		
Strongyloides stercoralis	Infected humans	Gastrointestinal manifestations that can mimic peptic ulcer or gallbladder disease; disseminated infection (hyperinfection syndrome)
Hookworms (_Necator americanus, Ancylostoma duodenale_)	Infected humans	Iron deficiency anemia from chronic gastrointestinal blood loss
Acquired by Ingestion		
Roundworms		
Ascaris lumbricoides	Infected humans	Often asymptomatic except for passage of 25- to 30-cm worms; may produce biliary obstruction or peritonitis from intestinal perforation
Enterobius vermicularis (pinworm)	Infected humans, especially children	Itching of the perianal or genital region
Trichuris trichiura (whipworm)	Infected humans	Often asymptomatic; damage to intestinal mucosa; malnutrition and anemia if severe
Tapeworms		
Taenia solium	Pigs	Intestinal infection (taeniasis) is typically asymptomatic; for cysticercosis, see Table 55-1
Taenia saginata	Cattle	Intestinal infection (taeniasis) is typically asymptomatic
Diphyllobothrium latum	Fish	Intestinal infection is typically asymptomatic but may lead to vitamin B_{12} deficiency

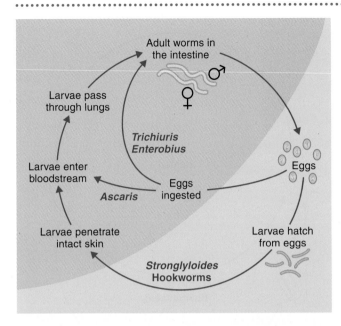

FIGURE 54-1. Comparative life cycles of intestinal nematodes.

submucosa and enter venules or lymphatics. The parasites travel to the lung and migrate up the trachea to the pharynx, where they are swallowed to access the gastrointestinal tract. The worms mature in the intestinal lumen, and the females release their eggs into the stool.

Large numbers of larvae (from many ingested eggs) can produce a transient pneumonia as they cross from the bloodstream into the lungs. That reaction may be particularly severe if the patient has been sensitized by a previous *Ascaris* infection. Later, if adult worms are present in large numbers in the intestine, they may form a large mass (worm ball) and produce intestinal obstruction, as in T.'s case. Occasionally, individual worms produce biliary obstruction (by migrating up the bile duct and occluding it) or peritonitis (by perforating the intestinal wall). Small or moderate intestinal worm burdens, on the other hand, can be totally asymptomatic.

Humans can also be infected by ingesting ascarid worms native to dogs, cats, or raccoons. Transmission is also by the fecal–oral route. The resulting infection is known as **visceral larva migrans**. Animals are the definitive hosts for these worms, which are unable to complete their cycle in humans. After leaving the intestine, dog or cat ascarid worms wander randomly through the tissues rather than crossing the lung to the trachea. Enlargement of the liver and spleen (**hepatosplenomegaly**) may result from the inflammatory response to the worms. **Eosinophilia** is usually marked because the worms invade the deep tissues. Because the worms cannot complete their life cycle in humans, humans are considered **dead-end hosts** for these animal infections. The aborted nature of human infection by parasites of other primary hosts (dog or cat *Ascaris* in visceral larva migrans; dog or cat hookworms in creeping eruption) is a vivid reminder of the specificity of host–parasite interactions.

DIAGNOSIS AND TREATMENT

Usually, ascariasis is readily diagnosed by stool examination using low-power (×100) magnification, because each adult female worm releases approximately 200,000 eggs per day into the intestinal lumen. The number of eggs in the stool can be used to estimate the number of worms present.

Mebendazole, albendazole, ivermectin, nitazoxanide, and several other drugs are effective in treating *Ascaris* infection of the gastrointestinal tract. Medical treatment with the anthelmintics typically relieves intestinal obstruction without surgical intervention.

Nematode Infections Acquired by Ingestion: *Enterobius* (Pinworm)

Pinworm infection is common in both temperate and tropical regions, affecting at least 200 million people worldwide. It is most prevalent among small children, who typically infect their siblings and parents, and among institutionalized persons. Pinworms seldom produce serious disease but may cause considerable discomfort.

ENCOUNTER AND PATHOBIOLOGY

Pinworm eggs do not require a period of maturation outside the body; therefore, the infection can be transmitted readily by anal–oral contamination (Fig. 54-3). The eggs also resist drying and may be transmitted from an infected person to other members of a household from

CASE • D., a healthy 3-year-old girl, was brought to the pediatrician because she had developed what the mother considers "unacceptable behavior"—she frequently scratched herself in the anal and vulval areas.

This case raises two questions:

1. What caused D.'s anal itching?
2. Should her mother be concerned that D. may become reinfected after being treated?

See Appendix for answers.

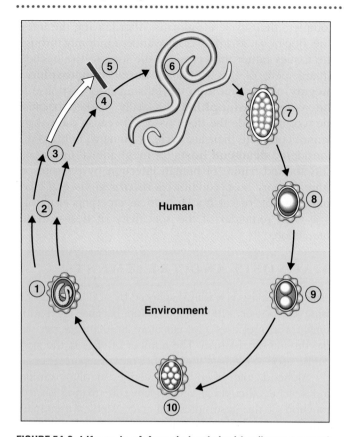

FIGURE 54-2. Life cycle of *Ascaris lumbricoides* (human roundworm) and dog or cat roundworm (visceral larva migrans). Humans acquire these infections by ingesting embryonated roundworm eggs from the environment (*1*). After ingestion, the parasites hatch in the upper intestine (*2*), cross the bowel wall (*3*), and enter the bloodstream. The human *Ascaris* (innermost set of *arrows* in the top half of the diagram) enters the lung by crossing into the alveolus (*4*). It then travels up the trachea, is swallowed, and reenters the gastrointestinal tract to develop to a mature adult (*6*). The *open arrow* and *solid line* on the diagram indicate that neither dog nor cat *Ascaris* worms are able to enter the lung from the bloodstream. As a result, the parasites wander aimlessly through deep tissues and cannot return to the gastrointestinal tract (*5*). Stool examinations are therefore negative in patients with visceral larva migrans and positive in patients with human *Ascaris* infection (*7*). In the environment, fertilized *Ascaris* eggs (*8*) germinate and divide (*9*) and produce embryonated eggs (*10*) that are infectious on oral ingestion. That process takes several weeks and requires a warm, moist climate. In visceral larva migrans the infectious eggs are shed by infected dogs or cats rather than humans.

bed clothes or dust. After oral ingestion, the eggs hatch in the duodenum and jejunum. The larvae mature in the ileum and large intestine. Gravid females migrate out of the rectum to the perianal skin to deposit eggs. The most typical symptom of pinworm infection is perianal itching, which may be caused by dermal sensitivity to parasite egg antigens. Scratching facilitates the spread of the infection because infective eggs can be spread to the same person (**autoinfection**) or to others by putting contaminated fingers into the mouth. Other moist areas, such as the

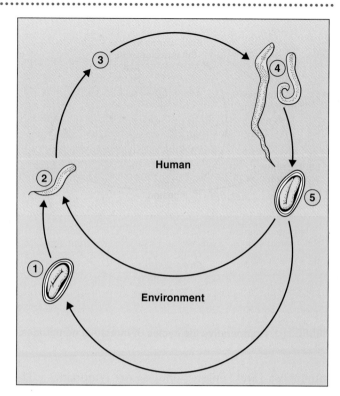

FIGURE 54-3. Life cycle of the pinworm (*Enterobius vermicularis*). Humans acquire pinworm infection by the ingestion of embryonated eggs (*1*). After ingestion, the eggs hatch in the small intestine (*2*), mature to adults in the large intestine (*3*, *4*), and produce eggs (*5*). Because the gravid female lays her eggs in the perianal area, the eggs may be shed into the environment (lower half of diagram) or inadvertently ingested by patients or their close contacts when fingers used to scratch the perianal area are licked or used to prepare food.

vagina, may also be affected. Occasionally, the parasite is found in the lumen of the appendix, although it rarely produces **appendicitis**.

DIAGNOSIS AND TREATMENT

Pinworm infection is easy to diagnose using the microscope. The buttocks are gently separated, and a microscope slide covered with Scotch tape (adhesive side out) or its commercially prepared paddle version is placed between them before the patient arises in the morning. Pinworm eggs are captured on the adhesive surface and are large enough to be identified by direct microscopic examination using low-power (×100) magnification.

Several anthelmintics, including albendazole, mebendazole, and pyrantel pamoate, are effective in the treatment of pinworm infection. Because one untreated person can easily infect others, the entire family must be treated (including relatives who live with or visit the infected child, baby sitters, and other children at the day care center).

CASE

Hookworm Infection

V., a 4-year-old boy, underwent a routine medical examination and immunizations after immigrating to the United States from a rural town in a central African country. The physical examination revealed pallor of the conjunctivae, and the examining physician ordered a blood count, which showed a hematocrit of 28%. On a peripheral smear, V.'s erythrocytes were hypochromic and microcytic, suggesting **iron deficiency**. The astute physician also ordered a stool examination for ova and parasites, which was positive for eggs of *Ancylostoma duodenale*, a hookworm. Treatment of the hookworm infection with mebendazole and the iron supplementation resulted in a return of the hematocrit to 45% at a 3-month follow-up visit.

Intestinal Nematodes That Penetrate the Skin: Hookworms and *Strongyloides*

Hookworms

Hookworm disease is caused by two species of roundworms: *Necator americanus* and *Ancylostoma duodenale*. Human hookworms penetrate human skin as larvae of a particular stage, that is, **filariform larvae**. Thus, transmission of the parasites does not require the ingestion of contaminated feces; typically, transmission is through the fecal–cutaneous route, not the fecal–oral route.

ENCOUNTER AND ENTRY

People become infected with hookworms by contact with soil contaminated by human feces and subsequently filled with mature filariform larvae. As larvae penetrate the skin at the time of initial infection, they may cause local manifestations of itching and irritation ("**ground itch**"). In human hookworm infections, dermal manifestations are brief and resolve when the larvae enter the bloodstream and lymphatics. However, people can also become infected with cat and dog hookworm larvae, a condition known as "**creeping eruption**" (or **cutaneous larva migrans**). Unlike those of the human hookworm, the filariform larvae of dog or cat hookworms cannot find their way from the skin into the circulation. Instead, they migrate randomly in the skin until they die. This process can produce an intensely itchy, red, serpentine track around the site of penetration that can persist for weeks.

Human hookworm larvae enter the circulation through the bloodstream or lymphatics, traverse the right side of the heart, and become trapped in the lungs. In the lungs, the larvae mature and then break through the alveolar wall into the alveolar lumen. They are coughed up and then swallowed into the gastrointestinal tract where they continue their life cycle as adults (Fig. 54-4), primarily in the duodenum and jejunum. Female worms shed fertilized eggs into the stool. If the eggs hatch in a warm environment (usually soil in warmer climates), they yield larvae that mature by molting into the infective filariform stage. That process requires a significant period of incubation outside the human host. Consequently, transmission of hookworms requires contamination of the soil with untreated human feces and subsequent exposure of unprotected human skin to the larvae that develop from

CASE

Strongyloides Infection

Ms. C., a 57-year-old-woman, was hospitalized for her fourth episode of unexplained Gram-negative bacteremia. The only other pertinent medical history was that the patient had recently begun treatment with corticosteroids for asthmatic bronchitis. Paradoxically, her cough worsened with that therapy, and she began to experience abdominal pain and diarrhea. Likewise, the other episodes of bacteremia followed the initiation of steroid therapy.

A resident of Michigan, Ms. C. had lived in rural eastern Kentucky as a child and teenager. She was treated with antibiotics for the organism causing her bacteremia. Because a computerized tomography scan of Ms. C.'s abdomen showed a thickened intestinal wall, she underwent a small intestinal biopsy that revealed the presence of helminth parasites attached to the mucosa. Subsequently, examination of the patient's stool revealed numerous immature, **rhabditiform larvae** of *Strongyloides stercoralis*. More-developed larvae were identified in the patient's sputum.

These two cases raise several questions:

1. How did these patients acquire adult helminths in their intestinal tracts?

2. Why did V. have anemia, while Ms. C. presented with recurrent Gram-negative sepsis?

3. Can these patients transmit their infections to other people?

See Appendix for answers.

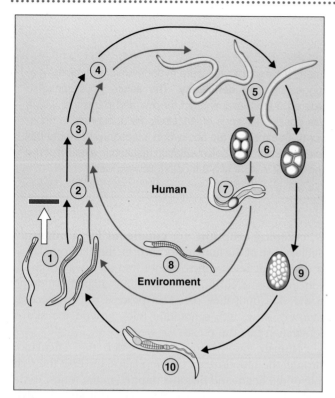

FIGURE 54-4. Life cycle of *Strongyloides* species and human hookworm. The invasive filariform larvae of these parasites penetrate unbroken human skin (*1*). Once inside the host, *Strongyloides* and human hookworm larvae migrate through the subcutaneous tissues to the bloodstream (*2*), enter the lung by crossing into the alveoli (*3*), travel up the trachea, and are coughed up and swallowed into the gastrointestinal tract (*4*). In contrast to *Strongyloides* and hookworm, the filariform larvae that cause creeping eruption (the larvae of dog or cat hookworms) are unable to enter the bloodstream and migrate to the lung. Instead, they wander through the subcutaneous tissues causing cutaneous larva migrans. The *solid line* and *open arrow* (above and to the left of stage *1*) indicate that the larvae of the parasite are unable to complete their normal life cycle in a human host. The larvae of *Strongyloides* and the hookworm mature (*5*) within the upper gastrointestinal tract. As shown on the right side of the diagram, female hookworm larvae remain within the lumen of the gastrointestinal tract, releasing their eggs into the stool (*6*), which then pass into the environment (*9*). Because the female *Strongyloides* larvae enter the bowel wall, their eggs do not appear in the stool (left side of stage *6*), and only the larvae (*7*) are normally found in the stool. Occasionally, the larvae mature to the filariform stage in the gastrointestinal tract (*8*) to produce endogenous reinfection (autoinfection). Because hookworm larvae require maturation in the environment to become infectious (*9, 10, 1*), autoinfection cannot occur in this disease.

the infected feces. Hookworm infection can be prevented by improved sanitation (using indoor or outdoor toilets or treating feces used for fertilizer) or by protecting the skin from contaminated soil, for example, by wearing shoes. Hookworm infection was common in some areas of the southern United States, where poor sanitary conditions were common until the early part of the last century.

DAMAGE

Hookworms produce chronic anemia by hanging onto the intestinal mucosa with their teeth, secreting an **anticoagulant**, and sucking the host's blood. That mode of attachment results in a slow, steady blood loss (0.03 mL per worm per day for *Necator americanus* and 0.15 mL for *Ancylostoma duodenale*). Hookworms affect some 800 to 900 million people throughout the globe; it has been estimated that the total loss of human blood to hookworms is at least 1 million L daily. The severity of the anemia is proportional to the worm burden. Severe infections in children can produce chronic anemia, which may lead to developmental delays.

DIAGNOSIS AND TREATMENT

The adult female hookworm releases 10,000 to 20,000 eggs per day into the bowel lumen, which makes it easy to diagnose significant hookworm infections by stool examination using low-power (×100) magnification. In fact, it is possible to estimate the number of worms present and the average daily blood loss by quantitating the number of eggs in the stool.

Albendazole, mebendazole, and pyrantel pamoate can be effectively used to treat hookworm infection. Emergency treatment is not required because hookworms produce chronic but not acute or invasive disease. Patients with hookworm disease may require dietary supplementation with iron and folic acid to produce sufficient numbers of red blood cells to correct their anemia.

Strongyloides stercoralis

Strongyloidiasis is prevalent in tropical areas of the globe but may also be found elsewhere. In large numbers, *Strongyloides stercoralis* worms may cause intestinal malfunction. They can perforate the intestinal wall, resulting in serious bacterial septicemias. In addition, they can reinfect the same host, especially one who is immunocompromised, to produce a lethal systemic disease.

ENCOUNTER AND ENTRY

The life cycle of *Strongyloides* species does not require an external soil phase (see Fig. 54-4). Consequently, in areas of poor sanitation, the worm may be transmitted directly through human feces and regardless of climate and soil temperature. Thus, outbreaks of strongyloidiasis have been reported from institutions for the mentally retarded in temperate zones, from Eskimo settlements north of the Arctic Circle, and from the tropics. In past decades, strongyloidiasis was a common infection in the Appalachian region of the United States. Like hookworms, *Strongyloides* infects humans by direct penetration through intact skin. Their route of migration to the intestines is identical to that of hookworms (see Fig. 54-4).

DAMAGE

After accessing the general circulation, *S. stercoralis* passes through the lungs, where it can elicit a transient response characterized by coughing, wheezing, and fever. Many people infected with *S. stercoralis* carry only a small number of the worms in the intestine, and few of those people have any clinical manifestations. However, if the worm burden is large, the infection may cause pain, vomiting, and diarrhea when the number of worms becomes large. Those symptoms occur because, unlike the other intestinal roundworms, the female *S. stercoralis* can invade the bowel wall to lay its eggs. That invasion may cause severe disease, because the early **rhabditiform larvae** that hatch from the eggs can cross the intestinal wall into the peritoneum and cause intestinal perforations, permitting intestinal bacteria to follow and producing peritonitis. As a result, strongyloidiasis can produce acute clinical syndromes (such as peritonitis) or mimic chronic abdominal problems such as peptic ulcer or gallbladder disease.

Because the female *S. stercoralis* lays her eggs in the bowel wall instead of the intestinal lumen, the larvae hatch and mature while still in the body. Reinfection may then occur from larval invasion of the perianal skin, even if the patient has not been exposed to new external sources of infection. *Strongyloides* **autoinfection** produces a characteristic snakelike (serpiginous) urticarial rash (**larva currens**), typically located near the anus.

Strongyloides infections may become chronic and produce symptoms for several decades. Persistent infections lasting more than 40 years have been described among former prisoners of war (from World War II). Those individuals often have chronic syndromes that are misdiagnosed as peptic ulcer or gallbladder disease and fail to respond to medical or surgical treatments for those conditions. Patients in whom autoinfection has been controlled can develop urticarial skin lesions from the migration of larvae at the surface of the skin.

In immunocompromised patients, the process of endogenous reinfection may produce a **hyperinfection syndrome** that is sometimes fatal. Ms. C. may have acquired the infection as a youth in rural Kentucky. She apparently maintained an asymptomatic *Strongyloides* infection by the mechanism of autoinfection. With the administration of corticosteroids later in life, the infection was no longer controlled, and she experienced respiratory and abdominal symptoms.

IMMUNOSUPPRESSION AND STRONGYLOIDIASIS

Patients immunosuppressed by malnutrition or drugs have a much greater risk of dissemination and progression to **hyperinfection syndrome**. In fact, strongyloidiasis is a major cause of death in kidney transplant recipients in the tropics. Presumably, those patients could control the infection before transplantation. However, they become unable to control the infection when their cell-mediated immunity is compromised by the immunosuppressive drugs used to prevent rejection of the transplanted kidney.

Because the hyperinfection syndrome is often seen in patients with impaired cell-mediated immunity, it seems likely that this kind of immunity is the critical factor in the control of strongyloidiasis. The relative role of mononuclear cells and eosinophils is not yet known.

DIAGNOSIS

Strongyloidiasis is often difficult to diagnose. Because the worms lay their eggs in the bowel wall, the eggs (which closely resemble hookworm eggs) are rarely found in the stool. It is more typical to diagnose *Strongyloides* by identifying rhabditiform larvae in the stool.

Patients with strongyloidiasis typically have a marked eosinophilia (10 to 20% of white blood cells, >10,000 to 20,000 eosinophils/μL of blood). However, lack of eosinophilia does not exclude the disease. The magnitude of the eosinophilia in persons with the hyperinfection syndrome may be limited by the basic T-cell defects predisposing to the syndrome, the outpouring of neutrophils resulting from secondary bacterial infection, and corticosteroid therapy. Patients thought to have strongyloidiasis should be studied first by stool examination. Even if three or more stool examinations reveal no larvae, examination of the duodenal contents or duodenal biopsy could be positive.

TREATMENT

Albendazole and ivermectin are the drugs of choice for strongyloidiasis. **Albendazole** is thought to act by binding to β-tubulin of the parasite. **Ivermectin** paralyzes the worms by blocking γ-aminobutyric acid (GABA)–mediated neuromuscular transmission. The latter drug is nontoxic for humans because GABA-mediated synaptic transmission in mammals is found only in the central nervous system, and ivermectin does not cross the blood–brain barrier.

INTESTINAL TAPEWORMS

As the name suggests, tapeworms are long and ribbonlike and are composed of chains of rectangular segments. An individual tapeworm is actually an animal colony, because each segment (known as a **proglottid**) is a self-contained unit capable of reproduction, metabolism, and food uptake (a tapeworm has no common gut). A tapeworm attaches to the intestinal wall by a head (**scolex**) that has sucking disks or grooves (Fig. 54-5). In their intermediate animal host, tapeworms penetrate deep tissues and develop into infective, cystic larval forms.

CASE • Mrs. N., the wife of a high-ranking government official, accompanied her husband on a trip to the Near East. During a diplomatic reception, they were served steak tartare (highly seasoned raw beef), a traditional dish in that region. Three months later, she noticed thin, white, rectangular segments in her stool (~1 × 2 × 0.2 cm). She experienced nausea, apparently brought about by seeing the worms in her stool. Laboratory studies revealed that the segments were proglottids of *Taenia saginata*. The stool also contained eggs of the worm.

Mrs. N.'s physician assured her that the infection was unlikely to have clinical consequences in a healthy person. On the other hand, he could understand her revulsion at seeing the worm segments in her stool and visualizing the rest of the worm inside her. The physician prescribed niclosamide, which eliminated the rest of the tapeworm.

This case raises two questions:

1. How could this infection have been prevented?
2. What would have happened to Mrs. N. had she been given no treatment?

See Appendix for answers.

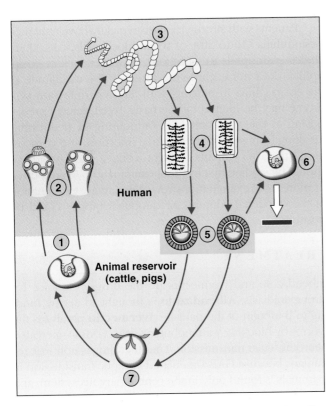

FIGURE 54-5. Life cycle of intestinal tapeworms *Taenia solium* (pork tapeworm) and *Taenia saginata* (beef tapeworm). Humans acquire intestinal tapeworm infections by ingesting the tissue stage of the parasite (cysticercus) in inadequately cooked meat (*1*). The parasite then hatches in the intestine (*2*) and matures to an intestinal tapeworm (*3*). The pork tapeworm (outside diagram) has a crown of spines on its head and fewer pairs of lateral uterine branches in its proglottids (segments) than the beef tapeworm (*4*). The eggs of both tapeworm parasites are identical morphologically (*5*). As shown in the diagram, only the pork tapeworm (*T. solium*) produces human cysticercosis (*6*). When human feces containing viable eggs are ingested by either pigs or cattle, the eggs hatch (*7*) and produce the tissue (cysticercal) stage of the infection in those animals (*1*) to complete the cycle.

The most common human tapeworms are acquired by eating uncooked or inadequately cooked beef (*Taenia saginata*), pork (*Taenia solium*), or fish (*Diphyllobothrium latum*). Tapeworms cause two types of disease:

- Intestinal infection (**taeniasis**) is caused by ingestion of larval cysts in undercooked pork, beef, or fish. The clinical picture of intestinal infection is generally mild and is essentially the same for all tapeworms.
- Deep tissue infection is caused by ingestion of eggs from the pork tapeworm (cysticercosis) or the canine tapeworm (echinococcosis or cystic hydatid disease). Tissue-invasive infections are discussed in detail in Chapter 55.

The two types of disease are very different and must be distinguished. Unfortunately, confusion is possible because one tapeworm (pork tapeworm) can produce both taeniasis and deep tissue infection in the same patient.

ENCOUNTER AND ENTRY

The life cycle of beef tapeworm requires both humans (definitive host) and cattle (intermediate host) (see Fig. 54-5). Cattle become infected by ingesting human feces containing the parasite's eggs; humans become infected by eating beef that contains larvae (**cysticerci**). The eggs hatch in the intestine of cattle and enter the bloodstream to lodge in peripheral tissues, where they develop into cysticerci (see Chapter 55). Beef tapeworm infection only exists in areas where infected humans defecate in grazing areas for cattle. Those areas, however, are found in most countries of the world.

All human intestinal tapeworm infections correlate with gastronomic preferences: They are found mainly among people who consume their meat undercooked or raw (as in the case of Mrs. N.). Transmission also clearly depends on lack of sanitation. These diseases are common in many parts of the world but are infrequent in Western

Europe and the United States. Cooking effectively destroys the larvae, but cooks have been known to become infected by tasting raw food during preparation. For example, fish tapeworm infection is said to be an occupational hazard of Jewish or Scandinavian women in the north-central United States who make gefilte fish or lutefisk.

DAMAGE

The infectious tissue larvae from the intermediate host (beef, pork, fish) hatch in the human small intestine and mature into adult tapeworms. The worms can live in the human intestine for several decades and attain lengths of up to 10 m, which has given rise to the popular but mistaken notion that they increase a person's appetite by consuming a significant amount of their food intake.

Most patients are asymptomatic, but some have nausea, diarrhea, and weight loss. The infection is usually noted only because of the presence of tapeworm segments (**proglottids**) in the stool. Almost half the people infected with fish tapeworm have low levels of vitamin B_{12}, leading to serious **megaloblastic anemia**. The B_{12} deficiency appears to be the result of competition between the host and the parasite for that vitamin in the diet. The intestinal disease caused by tapeworm is very different from the tissue disease (see Chapter 55).

DIAGNOSIS

Most tapeworm infections are readily diagnosed by stool examination. The proglottids are macroscopic and can be seen by the naked eye. The eggs are large enough (31 to 43 μm in diameter) to be seen using low-power (×100) magnification. Although the eggs of pork and beef tapeworms are identical, their proglottids can be distinguished by the experienced observer (those of *T. solium* have uteri with fewer pairs of lateral branches).

TREATMENT

Most patients (>90%) with intestinal tapeworms are cured with a single dose of **niclosamide**. Those who are not cured often have nausea or vomiting with their first treatment and typically respond to a second treatment with the drug. Patients with cysticercosis require a different approach to therapy (see Chapter 55).

CONCLUSION

Intestinal helminthic infections are usually benign but can cause significant illness if the worm burden is very large. With the exception of *Strongyloides*, helminthic parasites have no capacity to increase their numbers in the infected host. Therefore, the worm burden in infections other than those caused by *Strongyloides* is directly related to the size of the ingested inoculum (or the accumulation of repeated inocula). Because *Strongyloides* infection can be asymptomatic and sustained, the hyperinfection syndrome can occur during immunosuppression decades after the initial exposure.

Suggested Readings

Adedayo O, Grell G, Bellot P. Hyperinfective strongyloidiasis in the medical ward: review of 27 cases in 5 years. *Southern Med J.* 2002;95:711–716.

Brooker S, Bethony J, Hotez PJ. Human hookworm infection in the 21st century. *Adv Parasitol.* 2004;58:197–288.

Crompton DW. Ascaris and ascariasis. *Adv Parasitol.* 2001;48: 285–375.

Hotez PJ, Brooker S, Bethony JM, et al. Hookworm infection. *N Engl J Med.* 2004;351:799–807.

Keiser PB, Nutman TB. *Strongyloides stercoralis* in the immunocompromised population. *Clin Microbiol Rev.* 2004;17:208–217.

Phillis JA, Harrold AJ, Whiteman GV, et al. Pulmonary infiltrates, asthma and eosinophilia due to *Ascaris suum* infestation in man. *N Engl J Med.* 1972;286:965–970.

Weber M. Pinworms. *N Engl J Med.* 1993;328:927.

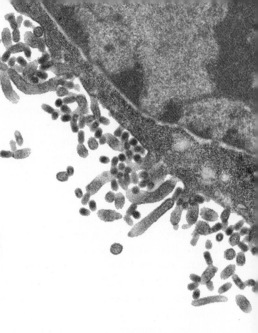

Chapter 55

Tissue and Blood Helminths

Cary Engleberg

KEY CONCEPTS

Pathogens: Helminths that invade tissue include roundworms (e.g., *Trichinella spiralis*, filaria), flatworms (e.g., *Schistosoma* spp.), and tapeworms (e.g., *Taenia solium, Echinococcus* spp.).

Encounter: Trichinosis is maintained by a "cycle of carnivorism" in which predators and scavengers feed on each other and acquire larvae encysted in muscles. Humans usually acquire infection from undercooked meat from pigs or carnivorous game animals.

Invasive cestode infections occur when humans ingest tapeworm eggs (*Taenia solium*, or pork tapeworm, eggs from human feces or *Echinococcus granulosum* eggs from canine feces).

Schistosomiasis is prevalent in geographic areas where (1) fresh surface waters are used for bathing or washing, (2) waters are contaminated with human feces or urine, and (3) certain types of snails are present to host the intermediate stages of the parasite.

Entry: Tissue-invasive helminths enter humans by ingestion (*Trichinella spiralis*, or invasive cestodes), penetration through the skin (schistosomes), or arthropod bites (various filariae).

Spread, Multiplication, and Damage: *Trichinella* larvae disseminate from the intestine and encyst in skeletal muscles; fever, severe muscle pain, and intense eosinophilia occur when larvae disseminate to human skeletal muscles.

Cestode larvae that emerge from ingested eggs migrate to and encyst within the brain (*T. solium*) or in the liver or lungs (*E. granulosum*). Symptoms develop after prolonged infection because of pressure effects of the enlarging cysts or hypersensitivity to released parasite antigens.

Adult **schistosomes** localize to the mesenteric or pelvic veins. Disease manifestations are caused by granulomatous reaction to helminth eggs that are trapped in tissues (e.g., intestine, bladder, liver).

Lymphatic filariasis results from chronic obstruction of lymph channels by adult worms and progressive swelling of extremities or genitals (e.g., elephantiasis). Adult worms are often inapparent in **cutaneous filariasis,** but their microfilaria (larvae) disseminates subcutaneously and produces chronic hypersensitivity reactions, which can lead to chronic dermatitis or blindness (e.g., onchocerciasis or "river blindness").

Diagnosis: Parasitological diagnosis can be made by visualizing characteristic forms of each helminth in body fluids or tissues. Serologic assays are available but do not distinguish recent from past infection and are therefore most useful for diagnosis of visitors to an endemic region.

Treatment: Anthelmintic drugs are effective against schistosomiasis (e.g., praziquantel) and invasive cestodes (e.g., albendazole). Treatment of trichinosis may shorten the course of illness by killing adult worms in the intestine to prevent ongoing larval dissemination. Antifilarial drugs (e.g., ivermectin) eliminate microfilariae but not adult worms. Corticosteroids are sometimes used to prevent hypersensitivity reactions to dying worms in tissues.

Prevention: Prevention of acquisition, treatment of carriers, and blocking return of parasites to the environment are strategies for interrupting the cycles of helminth transmission.

HELMINTHS cause a variety of diseases by establishing residence in deep tissues. As with the intestinal helminths, some are acquired by ingestion and others by penetration of the skin, either by direct entry of the parasites or by insect bites. The diseases they produce almost invariably involve chronic inflammation and thus are caused in part by the host immune response to the parasite. As with the intestinal helminths, when the worm burden is low, infections are rarely symptomatic. Because many worms are long lived in humans, they may gradually accumulate in large numbers as the consequence of repeated encounters. When present in sensitive target organs, helminths can produce severe disease and even death. Helminths that cause deep tissue infections include members of all three helminth groups: roundworms, tapeworms, and flukes (Table 55-1).

TABLE 55-1 Main Tissue and Blood Helminths

Examples	Reservoir	Mode of Transmission	Clinical Manifestations
Acquired by Ingestion			
Tapeworms			
Cystic hydatid disease (*Echinococcus granulosus*)	Sheep, cattle, horses	Fecal–oral (eggs)	Tissue-displacing and invasive lesions, most common in liver but seen in lung, CNS, and elsewhere
Cysticercosis	Pigs	Foodborne	Tissue-displacing lesions, most critical in CNS (*Taenia solium*)
Roundworms			
Visceral larva migrans (*Toxocara canis* and *T. catis*)	Dogs and cats (respectively)	Fecal–oral (eggs)	Systemic illness with malaise, eosinophilia, often enlarged liver and spleen
Trichinosis (*Trichinella spiralis*)	Pigs (and other carnivores)	Ingesting contaminated food	Mild infection produces malaise, mild diarrhea, and periorbital edema; severe infection may be life threatening, with CNS and heart involvement.
Guinea worm (*Dracunculus medinensis*)	Infected humans (larvae)	Ingesting contaminated water	Malaise, fever, other systemic symptoms when the adult worm emerges 1 y after initial infection
Flukes			
Lung fluke (*Paragonimus westermani*)	Animals, possibly humans	Ingesting contaminated food (metacercariae in crabs)	Cysts rupture in lung, leading to secondary bacterial infection, chronic bronchitis, and tuberculosis-like picture.
Liver fluke (*Clonorchis sinensis*)	Fish, animals, humans	Ingesting contaminated food (metacercariae in freshwater fish)	Often asymptomatic; if worm load is high, can lead to biliary stones, chronic inflammation, and liver cancer
Acquired by Passage through the Skin			
Blood Flukes			
Schistosomes (*Schistosoma mansoni, S. haematobium, S. japonicum, S. mekongi*)	Infected humans	Skin contact with contaminated water (cercariae)	Symptoms vary with the intensity of infection, from asymptomatic to hematuria and bladder cancer (*S. haematobium*), to blood in stool and portal hypertension (*S. mansoni* and *S. japonicum*).
Roundworms			
Cutaneous larva migrans (hookworms of dogs, cats, and other animals)	Dogs, cats	Skin contact with contaminated feces (filariform larvae)	Superficial skin lesions progressing at a rate of 2 cm/d
Filaria			
Lymphatic filariasis (*Wuchereria bancrofti, Brugia malayi*)	Infected humans (larvae)	Mosquito bite	Vary from asymptomatic to massive enlargement of the legs, scrotum, and breasts with recurrent filarial fevers
Onchocerciasis ("river blindness") (*Onchocerca volvulus*)	Infected humans (larvae)	Black fly bite	Subcutaneous nodules (adults) and itching (microfilariae); blindness from reaction to microfilariae in the anterior chamber of the eye

CNS, central nervous system.

CASE • Mr. Y., a 45-year-old immigrant from Laos living in Iowa, had been well until a few days after a family celebration that featured a highly seasoned but undercooked pork dish made from an animal raised on his family farm. Two days after the celebration, he developed diarrhea and abdominal pain. About a week after the onset of diarrhea, he developed severe muscle pain, swelling around the eyes, and headache. Physical examination revealed "splinter" hemorrhages in his fingernails. Laboratory studies demonstrated a marked eosinophilia ($12,000/mm^3$). Biopsies of Mr. Y.'s tender muscles and of the splinter hemorrhages revealed *Trichinella spiralis* larvae.

This case raises several questions:

1. How did Mr. Y. acquire this illness?
2. What caused Mr. Y.'s diarrhea and abdominal pain?
3. Why was his eosinophil count elevated?
4. How could the illness have been prevented?

See Appendix for answers.

TISSUE HELMINTHS ACQUIRED BY INGESTION

The main helminths that invade tissue and are acquired by ingestion are the roundworm *Trichinella spiralis* and the deep tissue–invading tapeworms.

Trichinella spiralis

The presence of *T. spiralis* larvae in the heart, skeletal muscle, brain, or gastrointestinal tract causes trichinosis. Most infected people are asymptomatic and are not seriously ill. Only a few hundred clinically significant cases occur in the United States each year.

ENCOUNTER AND PATHOBIOLOGY

The life cycle of *T. spiralis* is illustrated in Figure 55-1. After the ingestion of meat containing viable encysted *T. spiralis* (usually undercooked pork), the infective larvae hatch and mature in the small intestine of pigs or humans. After a few days, the adult worms release larvae that cross the mucosa to enter the intestinal lymphatics and the bloodstream (producing diarrhea and pain in the process). The larvae are then carried to all parts of the body through the bloodstream. The larvae encyst in striated and cardiac muscle fibers and produce a marked initial inflammatory response. The cysts usually calcify, although the worms can remain viable for up to 30 years. The life cycle of the parasite is completed in nonhuman vertebrates when their muscle (meat) containing viable larvae is eaten by another carnivore. Thus, the propagation of *T. spiralis* infection depends on a "cycle of carnivorism" (Fig. 55-2).

The US incidence of trichinosis, judged by the prevalence of *T. spiralis* cysts at autopsy, declined dramatically during the middle 20th century. This decline occurred partly because of legislation prohibiting the use of uncooked garbage for feeding pigs and partly because of increased public awareness about the danger of eating undercooked pork. Clinically significant trichinosis is now very rare in the United States and typically occurs in settings associated with noncommercial pig husbandry and pork preparation (as in the case of Mr. Y). Alternatively, in Arctic regions, *T. spiralis* cycles among carnivorous animals such as wild pigs and bears, including polar bears, have caused several outbreaks among hunters and in Eskimo communities.

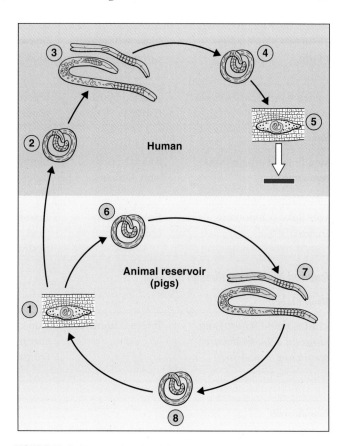

FIGURE 55-1. Life cycle of *Trichinella spiralis*. Humans acquire trichinosis by eating undercooked pork containing viable encysted *T. spiralis* larvae (*1*). After ingestion, the larvae hatch in the intestine (*2*), mature to adults (*3*), and release larvae that invade the intestinal wall and enter the bloodstream (*4*). The larvae then encyst in striated or cardiac muscle (*5*). As indicated by the *open arrow* and *solid line* below stage *5* on the diagram, human infection is normally a dead end in the natural transmission of trichinosis. Similar phenomena are observed in the pig reservoir and in other carnivores that harbor *T. spiralis* larvae (*6–8*).

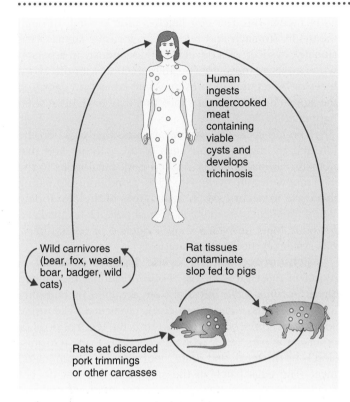

FIGURE 55-2. Epidemiology of trichinosis. In temperate climates, the infection is maintained in the food chain of wild carnivores by a "cycle of carnivorism." Carnivorous rodents contaminate garbage that is fed to domestic pigs, and humans become infected by eating undercooked pork or game meats. In arctic climates, indigenous peoples commonly become infected by eating undercooked bear, walrus, or seal meat. In the tropics, bush pigs and warthogs are potential sources.

The manifestations of trichinosis correlate with the load of worms in tissues and range from asymptomatic to fatal. Several studies suggest that larger inocula (ingestion of many viable larvae) result in more severe disease with a shorter incubation period (2 to 3 days vs. 10 days or more). Patients with 1,000 to 5,000 larvae/g of tissue may die from involvement of the heart or central nervous system. Studies in experimental animals suggest that cell-mediated immunity is important in the control of *T. spiralis* infection.

DIAGNOSIS AND TREATMENT

A rise in antibody titer is diagnostic. However, the increase typically occurs 3 to 4 weeks or more after the initial infection and is thus useless for the management of severely ill patients (in whom the incubation period may be as short as 2 or 3 days). In severely ill patients like Mr. Y., muscle biopsy often reveals *T. spiralis* larvae under low-power (×100) magnification and permits a definitive diagnosis long before serologic testing.

Treatment of trichinosis is problematic. In the early stages of infection, anthelmintic drugs (albendazole, mebendazole) are useful because they kill adult parasites in the intestine and may prevent ongoing production of invasive larvae. In contrast, anthelmintic agents are of little therapeutic value against the encysted larval forms and may actually provoke symptoms. Bed rest and anti-inflammatory agents (such as aspirin) are most useful for controlling symptoms. Corticosteroids have been used for their anti-inflammatory effects in severely ill patients with myocarditis and/or encephalitis.

CASE

Cysticercosis

Ms. F., a 33-year-old nurse, had been a Peace Corps volunteer in Thailand 10 years earlier. While in Thailand, she had occasionally passed tapeworm segments (proglottids) in her stool, but she was never treated. Eight years after her return to the United States, Ms. F. developed multiple subcutaneous nodules across her chest and arms and began having headaches. After two generalized seizures, she was brought to the emergency room. A computerized tomography (CT) scan of her brain revealed numerous lesions consistent with cysticerci (tapeworm larvae). After treatment with praziquantel, Ms. F.'s headaches worsened. She then received corticosteroids to reduce brain swelling and antiepileptic drugs to control her seizures, and she was able to complete the praziquantel treatment. One year later, Ms. F. was withdrawn from the antiepileptics and had no additional seizures.

Echinococcosis

A 39-year-old Navajo sheep farmer living in Arizona, Ms. K. was examined for abdominal pain. Two years previously,

she had first noticed a sensation of fullness in the right upper quadrant of her abdomen. Since then the sensation has increased, and she now has an obvious swelling (8 × 10 cm) in the area of the liver. Stool examination revealed no tapeworm eggs. A CT scan of the liver revealed a large (12-cm diameter) encapsulated lesion consistent with a hydatid cyst. Serologic testing revealed antibodies against *Echinococcus granulosus*. Because of the size of the liver lesion, the mass was removed surgically, using liquid nitrogen to freeze it and prevent its contents from spilling into the peritoneum.

These two cases raise several questions:

1. How did the two patients acquire their infections?
2. Why did Ms. F. have an intestinal tapeworm at some point but Ms. K. did not?
3. Can these patients be treated and cured?

See Appendix for answers.

Infections by Tissue Forms of Tapeworms

The larvae of a few species of tapeworms infect deep tissues of humans and cause diseases that may have severe manifestations. Illness caused by the tissue form of the pork tapeworm is known as **cysticercosis**; that illness caused by tapeworms of canines is known as **echinococcosis**. The life cycle of *Echinococcus* species is illustrated in Figure 55-3.

ENCOUNTER

Human **cysticercosis** is acquired by ingesting *Taenia solium* eggs from the feces of humans who harbor an

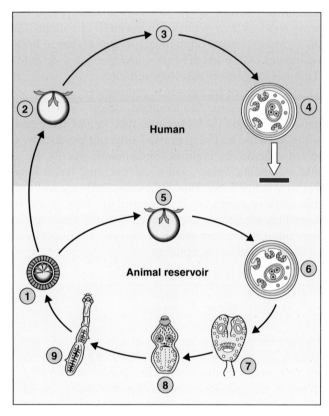

FIGURE 55-3. Life cycle of *Echinococcus* species. Humans acquire infection by ingesting eggs in the feces of infected carnivores, such as dogs or wolves (*1*). After ingestion, the eggs hatch in the intestine (*2*). The larvae cross from the gastrointestinal tract to the tissues (*3*), where they develop into cysts containing daughter cysts and scolices (heads) from which tapeworms can develop under the appropriate circumstance (*4*). As indicated by the *open arrow* and *solid line* below step 4, this infection is a dead end in humans. However, domestic animals (e.g., sheep and goats) may acquire infection by grazing in fecally contaminated pastures (see Fig. 55-4). The tissue cysts that develop in the animals are identical to those in humans (*5*, *6*), but when the animals eventually die in the pasture (often from unrelated causes), dogs or wolves may eat their remains and ingest the tissue cysts. In the canine intestine, the ingested heads (scolices) may develop into adult tapeworms (*7–9*), which eventually produce eggs (*1*) to complete the cycle.

adult tapeworm. The egg hatches after passing through the acidic stomach and releases an invasive larva. Occasionally, cysticercosis develops endogenously in a person who carries a tapeworm (by autoinfection with their own feces or by regurgitation of intestinal tapeworm eggs into the stomach). Endogenous infection may have been what happened to Ms. F.

The life cycle of *T. solium* requires that pigs become infected by ingesting the eggs of the parasite and that humans eat inadequately cooked pork (analogous to the beef tapeworm life cycle; Fig. 55-4). Conditions permitting this cycle to occur exist in many areas of the developing world. In Mexico, as many as 15% of persons hospitalized for neurologic problems show evidence of central nervous system cysticercosis at autopsy.

Echinococcosis, or **cystic hydatid disease**, is found in most areas of the world, including the United States. *Echinococcus* infections are acquired by ingesting infectious eggs, rather than tissue cysticerci. The usual source of *Echinococcus granulosus* is the feces of dogs or other carnivores (e.g., wolves, coyotes). Thus, transmission is by the fecal–oral route, not by eating contaminated meat. The eggs hatch in the small intestine but do not reside there. Rather, they penetrate the intestinal wall and form so-called **hydatid cysts** in many organs.

The life cycle of *Echinococcus* species is maintained between sheep and sheep-herding dogs in the southwestern United States (see Fig. 55-4). Native Americans who keep sheep in that region are sometimes victims of the *E. granulosus* infection. A "sylvatic" cycle is also present in the northern United States and Alaska, with wolves as the carnivores and elk and other large game as the herbivores. *Echinococcus multilocularis* is an analogous parasite in colder climates, for which foxes and cats are the carnivore hosts and mice and voles are the herbivores.

PATHOBIOLOGY

The sequence of events in echinococcosis and cysticercosis is generally similar. The parasites lodge under the skin or within internal organs, such as the brain or liver, and develop a cyst wall surrounded by a fibrous capsule of host origin. In echinococcosis, the hydatid cysts are lined internally by a germinal membrane that generates numerous embryonic tapeworm heads (each of which has the potential to develop into a tapeworm in the canine intestine). Most hydatid cysts occur in the liver or the lung. They usually produce few symptoms until they reach 8 to 10 cm or more in diameter, which may take years or even decades. The growing mass may produce symptoms by compression of vital structures, or the cysts may leak or rupture and pose a significant risk of death from anaphylactic reactions.

Tapeworm larvae (cysticerci) each contain only one potential tapeworm head. The cysts are generally more numerous than hydatid cysts but rarely grow larger than

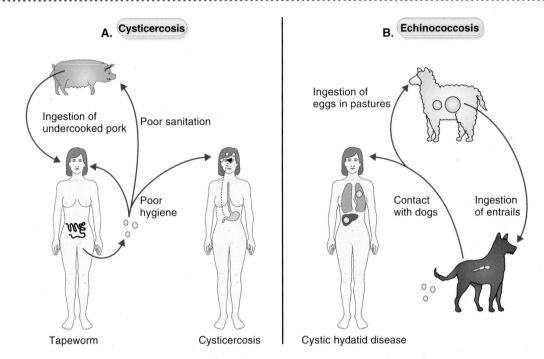

FIGURE 55-4. Comparative epidemiology of two tissue-invasive tapeworm infections: cysticercosis (caused by the pork tapeworm *Taenia solium*) and echinococcosis, or cystic hydatid disease (caused by *Echinococcus granulosus*). A. In pork tapeworm, the definitive host is the human, not the pig, because only humans harbor the adult tapeworms. Pigs are an intermediate host, since they develop only the tissue invasive form of infection (cysticercosis) after ingestion of eggs from feces of infected humans. Humans also develop the tissue-invasive stage of infection after ingesting eggs from human feces. Although tapeworm carriers can infect themselves with eggs from their own feces, many humans acquire cysticercosis directly by ingestion of fecally contaminated food and never actually harbor tapeworms themselves. **B.** The definitive host for the tapeworm that causes echinococcosis is the canine (dog, wolf, or fox). Intermediate hosts that harbor the tissue-invasive forms become infected by ingesting eggs from canine feces. In humans, tissue-invasive disease with either tapeworm is considered a dead-end infection, since humans are rarely cannibalized (to complete the *Taenia* life cycle), and human remains are buried or incinerated in most cultures (making completion of the echinococcal life cycle improbable).

1 or 2 cm. When a cyst dies, its contents leak into the surrounding tissues and induce a host inflammatory response. Cysts outside the central nervous system rarely produce symptoms. However, even small cysticerci in the brain can cause cerebral dysfunction, including seizures, increased intracranial pressure, and blindness. Cysticerci thus provide a good example of the correlation between the location and the severity of a disease. Cysticerci may cause symptoms when the parasites die and displacement of normal tissue is magnified by the host inflammatory response. That typically occurs 5 to 10 years after infection, but symptoms may not become apparent until as much as 50 years after the initial infection.

DIAGNOSIS AND TREATMENT

Because cysticerci can be present in patients without evidence of intestinal infection, *T. solium* cysticercosis is usually diagnosed by its deep tissue manifestations (including lesions visible by CT scan or by a "soft"

radiographic technique in the long axes of skeletal muscles). A positive serologic test for antibodies to *T. solium* is helpful, especially among persons who live in Europe, the United States, or other areas of low incidence. The test is typically negative in persons with intestinal *T. solium* infection only.

Praziquantel and albendazole are both effective in the treatment of cysticercosis. Drug treatment kills the organism and decreases the size of the lesions. The fluid-filled cysts collapse, and the parasite is ultimately resorbed by the host or calcified. During treatment, central nervous system symptoms may transiently worsen because of the inflammatory response to dying cysticerci. As with Ms. F., the concomitant use of steroids typically alleviates the headaches and seizures that the treatment can cause.

The anthelmintic drug albendazole administered over a period of weeks can kill growing echinococcal cysts as well. Alternatively, surgical removal of a large cyst can cure the infection, although great care must be taken to avoid spillage and dissemination of the infection. For the same

---

CASE

Schistosoma mansoni Infection

Ms. U., a 48-year-old woman from Egypt, had noticed for many years that she had dark stools. During the past year she had two episodes of vomiting blood. Examination of her esophagus and stomach with a fiberoptic gastroscope revealed dilated veins in the esophagus that were oozing large amounts of blood. Because viable eggs of *Schistosoma mansoni* were found in her stool, she was treated with praziquantel.

---

reason, it is unwise to attempt blind needle aspiration of a cystic structure that may be a hydatid cyst. Nevertheless, and despite the potential hazard of needle puncture, procedures for aspiration of cysts have been developed that are safe and effective. Quite often, patients with echinococcosis are discovered after their cysts have died. In those cases, the cysts appear calcified in radiographs or CT scans, and no treatment is needed (Fig. 55-5).

TISSUE HELMINTHS THAT PENETRATE THROUGH THE SKIN

Two types of helminths enter the host through the skin: worms that can cross the skin directly (the schistosomes or blood flukes) and those that penetrate via insect bites (the filariae, which are members of the roundworms).

Schistosomes

Schistosomiasis is an important and common disease in tropical regions. It is estimated that about 200 to 300 million people are infected worldwide. Schistosomiasis produces a variety of clinical syndromes, depending on the anatomic location of the adult worms and the eggs they release. The three main pathogenic species of the genus *Schistosoma*—*S. haematobium*, *S. mansoni*, and *S. japonicum*—are mostly found in warm climates. However, each species has a unique geographic distribution that depends on the presence of the snail intermediate host (Fig. 55-6). The schistosomal life cycle is illustrated in Figure 55-7.

ENCOUNTER AND PATHOBIOLOGY

The life cycle of schistosomes requires development in certain species of freshwater snails, which are their intermediate hosts. The infective stage of the parasite emerges from the snails and swims in water until it finds a suitable host. Because these snails are not present in the United States, schistosomiasis cannot be transmitted in the United States, despite the migration of infected persons from Africa and the Middle East. Suitable snails are present in parts of the Caribbean.

The infective forms released from the snails are called cercariae. They are capable of burrowing through the skin of people standing, swimming, or walking in infected water, like the rice paddies in which Mr. G. worked. In the human body, the cercariae lose their tails and change into forms called schistosomula, which can enter the bloodstream. The parasites then pass through the pulmonary circulation to the portal venous system, where they mature. After several weeks, pairs of male and female adults move to the venous plexuses of the large intestine (*S. mansoni*), small intestine (*S. japonicum*), or bladder (*S. haematobium*). The mating worms remain locked together, copulating in the venous system for 10 years or more. The eggs they release may be excreted via the stool (*S. mansoni, S. japonicum*) or the

---

CASE

Schistosoma haematobium Infection

Born and raised in Europe, Mr. G., 38 years old, had worked in West Africa for 10 years on a rice-growing irrigation scheme. During the past year, he noticed blood in his urine. Under the microscope, his urine showed the presence of *Schistosoma haematobium* eggs. At cystoscopy, his bladder had a cobblestone pattern, consistent with the granulomatous changes seen in schistosomiasis. Typical eggs were seen in the bladder biopsies taken during cystoscopy. He was treated with a single dose of praziquantel.

These cases raise two questions:

1. What caused the granulomatous changes associated with these infections?
2. Why was infection with *S. mansoni* associated with bleeding from the stomach, whereas *S. haematobium* was associated with blood in the urine?

See Appendix for answers.

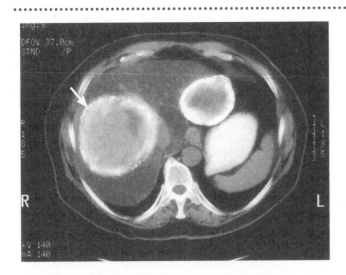

FIGURE 55-5. Abdominal computerized tomography (CT) scan of an asymptomatic 55-year-old Lebanese woman. The patient was scheduled to have surgery for an unrelated problem. A routine, preoperative chest radiograph showed a large calcified mass. The CT scan shows two large calcified structures in the liver that represent dead hydatid cysts (*arrow*).

urine (*S. haematobium*). The life cycle is completed when the eggs are released into fresh water, where they hatch and penetrate the appropriate snail intermediate host.

S. mansoni and *S. japonicum* adult worms reside in the venous plexuses of the intestine. There they release eggs that migrate to the intestine and the liver. Eggs

trapped in host tissues induce the formation of granulomas (Fig. 55-8A). The granulomas eventually undergo fibrosis. Over many years of infection, that process results in the pathological changes of schistosomiasis, such as periportal fibrosis in the liver (Fig. 55-8B), which can lead to portal hypertension and thus to dilated collateral veins in the esophagus (esophageal varices, as in the case of Ms. U.). *S. haematobium* adults live in the venous plexus of the urinary bladder and produce blood in the urine (hematuria), granulomatous inflammatory changes in the bladder, and sometimes bladder carcinoma. Fibrotic changes in the bladder and ureters can cause ureterovesical obstruction and recurrent secondary bacterial infections of the bladder, leading occasionally to Gram-negative septicemia.

As in other helminthic infections that invade the tissues, eosinophilia and elevated IgE levels are common in persons with schistosomiasis. Two important anomalous host–parasite interactions are central to the pathogenesis of schistosomiasis:

- Profound fibrotic reactions to schistosome eggs, probably mediated by cytokines, account for the important pathology of the disease and its long-term complications.
- Lack of an effective immune response to the male and female adult worms, which can reside in the vascular system for decades without being eliminated by the host. Studies have shown that adult worms adsorb host proteins (including serum albumin and HLA antigens) on their surfaces. Essentially, the parasite camouflages itself with those host proteins to evade the host immune response.

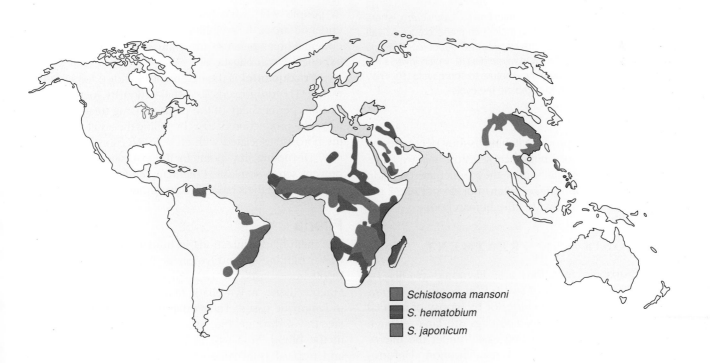

FIGURE 55-6. Geographical distribution of human schistosomiasis.

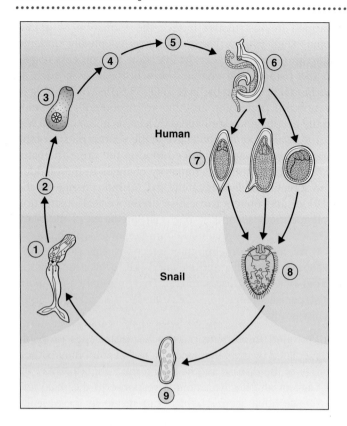

FIGURE 55-7. Life cycle of *Schistosoma* species. Humans acquire schistosomiasis by exposure of unprotected skin to water containing infectious cercariae (*1*). The cercariae penetrate unbroken skin (*2*), lose their tails, and become schistosomula (*3*). They then travel throughout the bloodstream, cross the lungs (*4*), and mature (*5*) in the venous system of the liver to adult worms (*6*). After a period of 6 to 8 weeks, pairs of adult worms travel to the venous plexuses of the bladder (*S. haematobium*), the large intestine (*S. mansoni*), or the small intestine (*S. japonicum*), where they remain for decades releasing their characteristic eggs (*7*, left to right: *S. haematobium*, *S. mansoni*, and *S. japonicum*). Eggs released into fresh water hatch to miracidia (*8*), which invade the snail intermediate host where they mature to sporocysts (*9*). They then release cercariae (*1*) to complete the cycle.

Cercariae often produce itching as they penetrate the skin. The cercariae of nonhuman schistosomes (of birds and fish) also cause itching as they penetrate the skin (swimmers' itch, clam diggers' itch) but do not enter the bloodstream or mature within the human body.

DIAGNOSIS AND TREATMENT

Most schistosome infections are diagnosed readily by microscopic examination of stool (*S. mansoni, S. japonicum*) or urine (*S. haematobium*) or by biopsy of a rectal valve (*S. mansoni*). Schistosome eggs are large enough (90 to 210 μm) to be identified easily under the microscope with low-power (×100) magnification. Unfortunately, it can be difficult to find schistosome eggs in the stool or urine of patients who are chronically infected

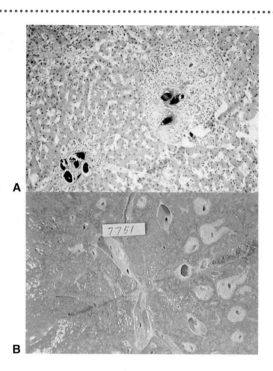

FIGURE 55-8. Liver sections from patients infected with *Schistosoma* species. A. *S. japonicum* infection shows egg granulomas in two portal areas. **B.** "Pipe stem" fibrosis of the portal tracts characteristic of schistosomiasis.

and at risk of developing long-term complications. In such patients, serologic testing for antischistosomal antibodies may be valuable. However, a positive serologic test does not distinguish between recent and old or mild and severe infections. Serologic testing is most useful in people who have had single, defined exposures in endemic areas. It is of little use for lifelong residents of endemic areas because most are seropositive but not all experience complications.

Praziquantel is the treatment of choice for schistosomiasis. The drug exerts its lethal action by increasing the calcium permeability of the parasite. Drug treatment eliminates the production of eggs by killing the adult worms, but the fibrosis associated with chronic infection is not reversible. Disrupting any point in the parasitic life cycle can prevent schistosomiasis. Potentially effective public health measures and their rationales are shown in Table 55-2.

Filaria

The main filarial infections in humans are onchocerciasis ("river blindness") and lymphatic filariasis (elephantiasis). In onchocerciasis, the adult filarial worms live in subcutaneous tissue; in lymphatic filariasis, the adult larvae live in lymphatic tissue. Their offspring, known as microfilariae, travel through the subcutaneous tissue or circulate in the blood. Some 17 million persons in Africa, Asia, and tropical Latin America have onchocerciasis. Unless they are treated, about 10% of those infected will become blind from the disease, and approximately 30% will have

TABLE 55-2 Control of Human Schistosomiasis

Rationale	Method of Control
Reduce carriers	Mass treatment program
Eliminate snail hosts	Molluscicides
	Destroy snail habitats
	Snail-eating fish
Prevent contamination of water	Provide latrines and sewage systems.
	Public health education
Prevent human exposure	Provide clean water systems for washing, bathing, drinking, and recreation.

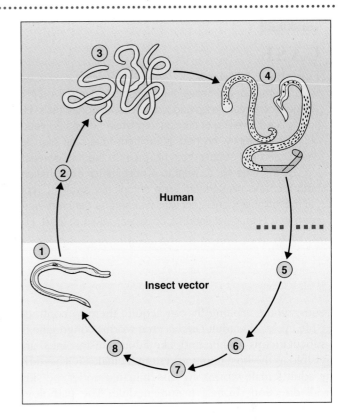

FIGURE 55-9. Life cycle of filariae (*Onchocerciasis*, lymphatic filariasis). Humans acquire infection with the filariae that cause onchocerciasis or elephantiasis from the bite of black flies or mosquitoes, respectively. After third-stage larvae (*1*) are injected under the skin by the vector, the larvae mature (*2*) to adult worms (*3*) that release microfilariae in the subcutaneous tissue (onchocerciasis) or in lymphatics (lymphatic filariasis; *4*). Microfilariae ingested by the insect vector during feeding mature through a series of stages (*5–8*) to infectious third-stage larvae (*1*) within approximately 2 weeks.

visual impairments. In some West African villages, most people become blind from onchocerciasis by the time they reach adulthood. Lymphatic filariasis affects more than 100 million people in tropical regions, especially in Asia. The disease leads to tissue swelling, sometimes to elephantine proportions (hence the name elephantiasis). Neither disease is endemic in the United States. The life cycle of filariae is illustrated in Figure 55-9.

ENCOUNTER AND PATHOBIOLOGY

The regional distribution of the vectors and infected human reservoirs limits the geographic distribution of filarial diseases. Onchocerciasis is transmitted by *Simulium* black flies, and lymphatic filariasis is transmitted by mosquitoes. Neither infection is transmitted within the United States; no reservoir of infected humans serves as a source of infection for susceptible insect vectors, and in the case of onchocerciasis, there are no competent *Simulium* vectors. With both diseases, filarial larvae enter the host during a bite by an infected insect.

The typical manifestations of lymphatic filariasis are low-grade fever and inflammation of lymphatics and lymph nodes induced by the adult worms (usually in the inguinal or pelvic nodes). With repeated episodes, the lymphatics become occluded and fluids leak into tissues, producing severe swelling. After many years, the lower limbs and the scrotum may swell to gigantic size. The diurnal cycle observed in lymphatic filariasis facilitates transmission because the microfilariae are more prevalent in the bloodstream at night, when mosquitoes bite more frequently.

In contrast, the microfilariae of onchocerciasis and other skin-dwelling filariae invade the subcutaneous

CASE

Onchocerciasis

Mr. L. is 32 years old and lives in a small Nigerian village near a rapidly running stream where men fish and hunt. Like many of his neighbors, Mr. L. began to lose his vision in his late twenties. He was prompted to go to a hospital in a nearby town for an evaluation because he had three nodules (2 × 3 × 2 cm) on his trunk. Skin snips revealed microfilariae of *Onchocerca volvulus*. He was treated with a single oral dose of ivermectin.

CASE

Lymphatic Filariasis

Mr. J., a 48-year-old native of a Philippine island, lived in a village where many men and women had elephantiasis. He first noticed swelling of his right leg when he was 20 years old. Subsequently, he had intermittent fevers as high as 39.0°C and red streaks from his groin to the foot on each leg. By the time Mr. J. went to a hospital for examination, both feet and his scrotum were chronically swollen. Typical microfilariae consistent with *Wuchereria bancrofti* were seen in a Giemsa-stained blood smear taken at 2 AM. His recurrent episodes of lymphangitis were treated with an antimicrobial effective against streptococci. The antifilarial drug diethylcarbamazine was given but discontinued when it produced shock and hypotension.

These cases raise two questions:

1. Why did Mr. L. became blind, while Mr. J. developed swelling?

2. How did these patients acquire the infections?

See Appendix for answers.

---

tissues, where a biting fly can acquire them to continue the life cycle. The adult *Onchocerca* worms congregate in a subcutaneous nodule and, like adult schistosomes, are invisible to the host immune system. Females released by the adult female worms are disseminated under the skin in all directions from a mature nodule. The pathology of the disease is caused by a type III hypersensitivity reaction to antigens released from dying microfilariae (see Chapter 7). Thus, the clinical manifestations include chronic dermatitis and loss of eyesight (caused by nodules on the head with migration of microfilariae into the anterior chamber of the eye).

DIAGNOSIS AND TREATMENT

Infections that release microfilariae into the bloodstream (lymphatic filariasis) are diagnosed by examining smears of peripheral blood. The microfilariae may be scarce and difficult to find. The sensitivity of the method can be increased by lysing red blood cells and concentrating the remainder of the specimen and by sampling blood at night for microfilariae with nocturnal periodicity (e.g., with *Wuchereria bancrofti*). Onchocerciasis is diagnosed by examining for microfilariae in a superficial "skin snip." In all these specimens, microfilariae are identified with Giemsa stain under the high-dry or oil immersion objectives. Recent studies suggest that antigen detection using antifilarial antibodies may be a more sensitive and convenient method.

The treatment for lymphatic filariasis is less than ideal. The drugs diethylcarbamazine and ivermectin reduce the number of circulating microfilariae but do not eliminate the adult worms. In any form of filariasis, diethylcarbamazine can produce systemic reactions, presumably resulting from the sudden release of filaria antigens from damaged microfilariae (as in Mr. J.'s case). In heavy infections with *Onchocerca*, diethylcarbamazine can cause severe reactions, including sudden blindness,

vascular collapse, or even death. Ivermectin is less likely to produce those effects and is the preferred treatment for severe disease. This drug has been used in preemptive mass treatment campaigns in parts of the world where there is significant morbidity and blindness. Surgical resection of subcutaneous nodules in onchocerciasis removes the source of microfilariae and may thus decrease the risk of blindness. However, it is impossible to be sure that all nodules have been removed because they are often in deep tissue and not palpable.

A recent observation that *W. bancrofti* adult worms require colonization by a natural symbiont, *Wolbachia*, to maintain normal health and fertility has raised the possibility of treating the parasite infection by eradicating the symbiont. The *Wolbachia* bacteria are similar to rickettsiae and are susceptible to tetracycline. Initial trials treating *W. bancrofti* infection with tetracycline have shown promising results. It is still too early to say whether this approach will be useful for other treatment-resistant parasites.

Prevention of filarial diseases relies mainly on vector control. Unfortunately, the flies that transmit onchocerciasis breed in clean, fast-running streams and rivers. Although they can be controlled readily with insecticides, effective spraying may be difficult in those areas.

CONCLUSION

Tissue-invasive helminths are a diverse group of pathogens with distinct and complex life cycles. To diagnose and treat infections of these parasites, it is essential to know where they reside within the human host and which tissues, body fluids, or excreta harbor the characteristic eggs or larvae. Anthelmintic drugs are active against the parasites; however, infections of long duration with high worm burdens can produce chronic, fibrotic changes that are irreversible with treatment. To control infections in endemic regions, it is necessary to understand the parasitic life cycles and to know what environmental conditions, vectors, or intermediate hosts enable the tissue-invasive parasites to deliver their progeny from one human to the next.

Suggested Readings

Clausen MR, Meyer CN, Krantz T, et al. *Trichinella* infection and clinical disease. *Q J Med.* 1996;89:631–636.

Garcia HH, Del Brutto OH, Nash TE, et al. New concepts in the diagnosis and management of neurocysticercosis (*Taenia solium*). *Am J Trop Med Hyg.* 2005;72:3–9.

Golemanov B, Grigorov N, Mitova R, et al. Efficacy and safety of PAIR for cystic echinococcosis: experience on a large series of patients from Bulgaria. *Am J Trop Med Hyg.* 2011;84(1):48–51.

Gryseels B, Polman K, Clerinx J, et al. Human schistosomiasis. *Lancet.* 2006;368(9541):1106–1118.

Hise AG, Gillette-Ferguson I, Pearlman E. The role of endosymbiotic *Wolbachia* bacteria in filarial disease. *Cell Microbiol.* 2004;6:97–104.

Rajan TV. Natural course of lymphatic filariasis: insights from epidemiology, experimental human infections, and clinical observations. *Am J Trop Med Hyg.* 2005;73(6):995–998.

Taylor MJ, Hoerauf A, Bockarie M. Lymphatic filariasis and onchocerciasis. *Lancet.* 2010;376(9747):1175–1185.

Theis JH, Ikeda RM, Ruddell CR, et al. Apparent absence of *Sarcocystis* and low prevalence of *Trichinella* in artificially digested diaphragm muscle removed during post-mortem examination at a Sacramento (California) medical center. *Am J Trop Med Hyg.* 1978;27(4):837–839.

Tisch DJ, Michael E, Kazura JW. Mass chemotherapy options to control lymphatic filariasis: a systematic review. *Lancet Infect Dis.* 2005;5:514–523.

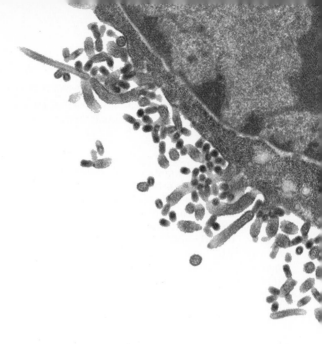

Chapter **56**

Prion Diseases

C. Alan Anderson and Kenneth L. Tyler

KEY CONCEPTS

Pathogen: Prions consist of a pathologic isoform of a normal host protein. They contain no nucleic acid.

Encounter and Entry: Prion diseases may occur as sporadic, iatrogenic, hereditary, or transmissible diseases. They include Creutzfeldt-Jakob disease (CJD), variant CJD ("mad cow disease"), and others.

Spread and Multiplication: Prions do not multiply in the conventional sense. Instead, they increase in number by inducing a conformational change in the related normal host protein so that the latter assumes the prion isoform. These progressive changes occur primarily in the central nervous system (CNS).

Damage: Accumulation of prions in the CNS is usually associated with dementia, abnormal movements, ataxia, and neuropsychiatric features.

Diagnosis: Diagnosis depends on clinical features and neuropathological findings.

Treatment: These diseases are uniformly fatal. There are no effective treatments.

Prevention: Sporadic diseases cannot be prevented, but transmission of prions can be avoided by special decontamination procedures for neurosurgical equipment or neural tissues used therapeutically.

PRION DISEASES are rare, fatal, rapidly progressive neurodegenerative diseases that occur in humans and other animal species. In all species, they share common and recognizable neuropathologic features, namely the presence of small vacuoles within the neuropil, which produces a **spongiform** appearance, neuronal loss, and glial cell proliferation, which occur in the absence of an inflammatory response. These features were first recognized in a fatal neurodegenerative disease of sheep, called **scrapie**. As the prototype for prion diseases, scrapie was shown to be a transmissible disorder in the 1930s when the disease was successfully passed from a sheep to a goat. Because of the very long incubation period, measured in months or years, researchers originally thought that prion diseases were caused by a "slow virus" infection.

Subsequently, a human disorder with similar neuropathology was observed among the Fore people of Papua New Guinea. Known as **kuru**, the disorder was thought to be transmitted by a form of ritual cannibalism that involved eating the brains of deceased relatives. Consistent with the idea that the ingestion of human neural tissue transmitted the disease, kuru has disappeared now that the cannibalistic rituals have been discontinued. However, the spongiform histopathologic changes seen in the brains of kuru victims resemble another established neurodegenerative disease that occurs in humans worldwide, Creutzfeldt-Jakob disease (CJD). Since the 1930s, CJD has occurred both sporadically and in familial clusters. However, cases of iatrogenic transmission among humans through contaminated neurosurgical instruments, surgical grafts of dura mater, injections of human pituitary extracts, or even corneal transplantation also have been documented. Dura mater transplants and injections of human pituitary extracts account for most of the iatrogenic cases, but even these mechanisms are rare, with fewer than 200 cases each. In the late 1960s, both kuru and CJD were transmitted from humans to chimpanzees, confirming that both are associated with a transmissible agent. The most puzzling aspect of these disorders is the absence of any appreciable nucleic acid in the material capable of transmitting the diseases.

Prion diseases are now known to be associated with the accumulation in the central nervous system of an abnormal form of the normal cellular isoform of the **prion protein (PrP^C)**. The "infectious agent" is not a virus but rather an *abnormally folded, degradation-resistant form of the PrP^C protein*. Several prion diseases have been identified in animal species (Table 56-1). In addition, five human prion diseases are currently recognized (see the box entitled "Human Prion Diseases"). Although all are theoretically transmissible under appropriate circumstances, only kuru and variant CJD among the human diseases are thought to be predominantly acquired exogenously—that is, by ingestion of or contact with the prion protein from another human (kuru) or animal (CJD) source.

PRIONS

The term *prion*, (pronounced "pree-on" and derived from "proteinaceous infectious particle") refers to a small infectious agent that consists of protein but lacks nucleic acid. A host protein, PrP^C, appears to be the sole constituent of prions. The gene encoding PrP^C (*PRNP*) is found in the genomes of all humans and animals. It is expressed in most human tissues, with the highest levels in the central nervous system. Studies suggest that PrP^C is a copper-binding protein that may be involved in the cellular response to oxidative stress. It also might play a role in long-term memory, regulation of cellular immunity, synaptogenesis, and peripheral myelin maintenance. The pathological protease-resistant form of PrP^C isolated from the brains of animals with scrapie has been designated **PrP^{Sc}** (PrP^{Sc} also refers to the conformationally altered isoform of PrP^C in other prion diseases besides scrapie). Transgenic mice that cannot make PrP^C cannot develop prion disease, indicating that host PrP^C must be present for the development of illness.

Prion diseases appear to result from the **accumulation of abnormal isoforms** of PrP^C, which depends on the conversion of normal PrP^C into PrP^{Sc}. That conversion is not a chemical modification but a **conformational change** in PrP^C from a predominantly α-helical form to one that contains predominantly β-sheet. In the sporadic forms of prion disease (e.g., most cases of CJD), the first molecule of PrP^{Sc} seems to appear spontaneously, triggering the conversion of other PrP^C molecules to PrP^{Sc}, resulting in the assembly of long strands of polymerized proteins, or **amyloid** fibrils (Fig. 56-1). That process may be analogous to crystallization in solution in which a single seed crystal serves as a nidus for the continued growth of the crystal. A conformational change in PrP^C appears to be the necessary pathogenic first step in all forms of illness.

A common polymorphism (valine or methionine) at codon 129 of the *PRNP* gene product appears to play an important role in determining susceptibility to acquiring prion disease. Most patients with sporadic and iatrogenic CJD, and all patients reported to date with variant CJD, are homozygous for methionine at codon 129. This polymorphism may influence other features of prion disease, including incubation time and clinical features of the illness. A lysine substitution at codon 219 may confer resistance to prion disease. Other polymorphisms or inherited mutations in PrP^C explain how prion diseases may be sporadic (by spontaneous PrP^C to PrP^{Sc} conversion), heritable (by enhanced conversion because of an unfavorable, inherited PrP^C allele), or transmissible (by exogenous acquisition of PrP^{Sc}).

TABLE 56-1 Animal Prion Diseases

Disease	Animals Affected
Bovine spongiform encephalopathy	Cattle
Scrapie	Sheep and goats
Chronic wasting disease	Deer and elk
Transmissible mink encephalopathy	Farmed mink
Feline spongiform encephalopathy	Zoological and domestic cats
Transmissible spongiform encephalopathy	Zoological ruminants and nonhuman primates

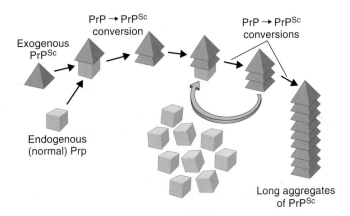

FIGURE 56-1. One possible model for the conversion of normal PrP^C to PrP^{Sc} with subsequent polymerization and accumulation of amyloid.

HUMAN PRION DISEASES

Kuru
Creutzfeldt-Jakob disease (CJD)
Variant Creutzfeldt-Jakob disease (variant CJD)
Gerstmann-Straussler-Scheinker (GSS) syndrome
Fatal familial insomnia (FFI)

CREUTZFELDT-JAKOB DISEASE
Sporadic and Iatrogenic CJD
ENCOUNTER

Prion diseases are rare, but CJD is the most common human prion disease, accounting for 85% of all human prion diseases, with an annual incidence of approximately one case per 1 million population worldwide. Its occurrence is mostly sporadic (90 to 95%), but familial clusters of CJD have been described. Men and women are at equal risk. The age at disease onset is usually between 55 and 65 years, although rare cases of patients under 30 and over 80 years of age have been described. In the 1990s, the appearance in Great Britain of numerous patients in their twenties led physicians to conclude that a variant of CJD was emerging.

ENTRY

In sporadic prion disease, a spontaneous conversion of the normal PrP^C protein to the abnormal PrP^{Sc} isoform is assumed to set in motion a continuous refolding and polymerization of normal PrP^C. Thus, no "entry" actually occurs. However, rare cases of iatrogenic CJD are associated with inoculation of PrP^{Sc} directly into the central nervous system. That may occur with corneal transplants, liver transplants, cadaveric human pituitary hormone, dural graft transplants, and the use of contaminated neurosurgical instruments or stereotactic depth electrodes.

SPREAD AND MULTIPLICATION

The incubation period for sporadic CJD is unknown. In the case of iatrogenic disease, a better estimate is possible based on the timing of the inciting event (e.g., dural graft placement or initiation of hormonal therapy). One study of human growth hormone recipients with CJD found that most developed illness 8 to 12 years following exposure. The time to presentation is much shorter with transmission through contaminated neurosurgical instruments. In that case, the mean incubation time is approximately 18 months.

DAMAGE

The cardinal clinical manifestations of CJD are rapidly progressive dementia and myoclonus. The clinical features correlate with the distribution of PrP^{Sc} in the brain, and it is assumed that the abnormal accumulations of those proteins contribute to the focal neurologic features. Thus, most cases present with visual, cerebellar, thalamic, or striatal signs and symptoms, reflecting the distribution of PrP^{Sc} in those sites.

Attentional problems, memory loss, and judgment difficulties are frequent early signs. Cognitive disturbances involving language, visuospatial function, and other aspects of executive function emerge during the course of illness. Apathy and depression are common; less often, euphoria, emotional lability, and anxiety can occur. As the disease progresses, dementia becomes prominent in most patients and advances rapidly. Death usually occurs within 1 year after the onset of symptoms.

Myoclonus (sudden involuntary jerking movements), especially provoked by loud noise or sudden movement, eventually occurs in more than 90% of patients, although in some cases, presentation is late in the disease course. CJD should be considered in the differential diagnosis of a patient showing myoclonus and rapidly progressive dementia. Extrapyramidal signs, such as **hypokinesia** (reduced or slow movement) and **cerebellar signs** (nystagmus and ataxia), occur in most patients. The motor system also may be involved, with patients displaying weakness and, on examination, **hyperreflexia**, extensor plantar responses (Babinski sign), or spasticity.

Cranial nerve abnormalities, sensory abnormalities, and peripheral nervous system involvement, although occasionally present in CJD, should raise the suspicion of an alternative diagnosis, especially if those findings are a prominent part of the presentation. Sensory abnormalities are common in variant CJD but rare in other human prion diseases (as discussed later in the chapter).

DIAGNOSIS

No definitive diagnostic test for CJD is available, other than brain biopsy, but supportive evidence for the diagnosis is usually obtainable. Routine laboratory tests are generally

CASE • Mr. I., a 22-year-old native of England who had lived in Florida for 10 years, sought medical attention in November 2001 for depression and memory loss that was interfering with his work performance. He was referred to a psychologist for his complaints. However, in December, he developed involuntary muscle movement, difficultly walking and dressing, and incontinence. In January 2002, he went to a local emergency room where a computerized tomography (CT) scan of the brain was found to be normal, and he was treated for an anxiety attack.

Later that month, at his mother's urging, Mr. I. returned to the family home in England. By then his symptoms had worsened: he experienced falls and could not shower or dress himself, recall his home phone number, or do simple arithmetic. An evaluation for variant CJD was conducted: an electroencephalogram (EEG) was normal, and magnetic resonance imaging (MRI) of the brain showed high signal intensity in the pulvinar and dorsomedial thalamus bilaterally. Subsequently, a tonsil biopsy was performed. Tonsillar tissue was examined by immunoblotting and immunohistochemical staining for the protease-resistant form of prion protein (PrP^Sc). Both were positive and consistent with variant CJD. Sequencing of the patient's PrP^C genes showed homozygosity for methionine at position 129 but no mutations. Mr. I. had no history of transfusions, transplants, or major surgery.

In spite of an attempt at experimental therapy with quinacrine, the patient's decline continued. By September 2002, he was bedridden and unable to eat or communicate. (Adapted from Centers for Disease Control and Prevention. Probable variant Creutzfeldt-Jakob disease in a U.S. resident—Florida, 2002. *Morb Mortal Wkly Rep.* 2002;51:927–929.)

This case raises several questions:

1. What features of Mr. I.'s case are characteristic of variant CJD?
2. How and when did he acquire the disease?
3. Should he be isolated to prevent transmission of the disease to others?
4. What are his chances for recovery?

A discussion of the circumstance and expression of Mr. I.'s case of variant CJD requires an understanding of how the sporadic form of CJD arises.

See Appendix for answers.

---

normal, and the cerebrospinal fluid (CSF) contains no cells and has normal concentrations of glucose and protein. Elevations of certain normally occurring central nervous system proteins may serve as a marker of CJD. For example, an elevated CSF level of the **14-3-3 protein** has been suggested as a potential diagnostic test for the disease, although the protein may be a marker of brain cell death in general rather than of CJD in particular. Importantly, a negative test does not exclude the diagnosis of CJD, especially in persons with possible familial or variant CJD, and a positive test can occur in a variety of nonprion diseases, such as herpes simplex virus encephalitis, cerebral metastases, hypoxic encephalopathy, and metabolic encephalopathies. Thus, the CSF level of the 14-3-3 protein should be considered an adjunctive rather than a definitive test for CJD. Genetic testing should be considered for patients with atypical presentations, younger age at onset, or a family history suggestive of prion disease.

The **electroencephalogram (EEG)** finding of periodic synchronous biphasic or triphasic sharp wave complexes is present in more than two-thirds of patients with sporadic CJD at some point during the course of the illness. Although helpful in making the diagnosis, that EEG pattern is also not specific for CJD, and the finding can be masked by some neuroactive drugs and may not be seen in the initial or terminal stages of the disease.

As with the EEG, neuroimaging findings are not specific for CJD but can support the diagnosis. The **computerized tomography (CT) scan** is generally normal and serves mainly to exclude other diagnoses. **Magnetic resonance imaging (MRI)** is more informative. The most common MRI finding is increased T2 signal intensity in the putamen and head of the caudate (Fig. 56-2A). Less often, T2 hyperintensity is seen in the hemispheric white matter, globus pallidus, thalamus, and cerebellar cortex. Ribbonlike hyperintensities are observed in the cerebral cortex (Fig. 56-2B). MRI diffusion-weighted imaging (DWI)

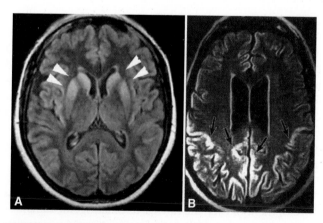

FIGURE 56-2. Magnetic resonance imaging of a patient with Creutzfeldt-Jakob disease. A. Increased signal intensity in the putamen and head of the caudate (*arrowheads*). **B.** Bilateral parietooccipital cortical hyperintensity (*arrows*).

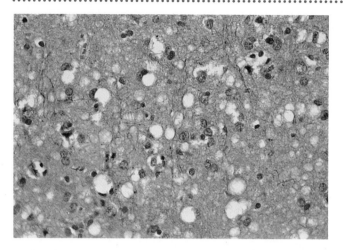

FIGURE 56-3. Pathologic specimen from a patient with CJD demonstrating spongiform changes and neuronal loss.

measures the mobility of water molecules in tissue and provides a physiological assessment of brain function not seen with standard MRI. DWI has lower spatial resolution than conventional MRI but may be more sensitive to the cortical ribbon hyperintensity and facilitate early diagnosis. In contrast to standard MRI, DWI changes can be apparent as early as 3 weeks after the onset of symptoms.

The typical neuropathological changes of CJD are **spongiform vacuolation**, **neuronal degeneration**, and **glial proliferation** (Fig. 56-3). The definitive test for diagnosis is the presence of PrP^{Sc} as determined by immunohistochemical testing of brain tissue.

Testing for the 14-3-3 protein in CSF, gene sequencing to identify mutations or clinically relevant polymorphisms in *PRNP*, and pathological examination of brain tissue from biopsy or autopsy is available through the National Prion Disease Pathology Surveillance Center at Case Western Reserve University.

TREATMENT

Currently, there is no specific treatment that alters the course of CJD. The disease remains inexorably progressive and invariably fatal. As with all prion diseases, care for CJD patients is supportive. Various antiviral, antibacterial, and immunomodulatory agents have been tested but found ineffective. Despite the capacity of chlorpromazine and quinacrine to inhibit PrP^{Sc} formation in tissue culture, human trials of the drugs have not been encouraging thus far.

PREVENTION

Although there is no strategy to prevent the spontaneous development of CJD, the rare cases of iatrogenic transmission can be prevented. Fortunately, no evidence exists that CJD has been transmitted by blood transfusion. The majority of iatrogenic CJD cases followed either dural graft transplants or use of cadaveric pituitary hormones. Those iatrogenic routes of transmission have been dramatically reduced by changes in the process employed to prepare dural grafts and the use of recombinant-derived pituitary hormones.

One of the characteristic features of prions is their resistance to routine sterilization and decontaminating procedures. Therefore, special care and handling techniques are required for neuropathological specimens from patients with suspected prion diseases. Similarly, neurosurgical instruments used on patients with suspected prion diseases may be contaminated and require quarantine until a pathological diagnosis is established. If the patient is determined to have a prion disease, the surgical instruments used for the procedure must be cleaned following special decontamination protocols or discarded. PrP^{Sc} is resistant to processes affecting nucleic acids, such as hydrolysis or shearing. However, agents that digest, denature, or modify proteins do have activity against prions. PrP^{Sc} can be inactivated by prolonged autoclaving (at 121°C and 15 psi for 4.5 hours) or immersion in 1 N NaOH (for 30 minutes, repeat three times) or concentrated solutions of guanidine thiocyanate (more than 3 M). However, certain cautions prevail; it appears that inadequate autoclaving can establish heat resistant subpopulations that fail to diminish with a further cycle of autoclaving. Stainless steel instruments also may retain infectivity even after treatment with 10% formaldehyde.

Variant CJD

Considerable evidence supports the hypothesis that variant CJD represents bovine-to-human transmission of **bovine spongiform encephalopathy** (**BSE**), known popularly as "**mad cow disease**." For example, PrPs derived from different prion diseases and species differ in their glycosylation patterns and electrophoretic mobility. Evidence in favor of an association of variant CJD with BSE includes a pattern of glycosylation and electrophoretic mobility that has not been seen in other prion diseases. In addition, inoculating bovine PrP^{Sc} into transgenic mice expressing the human PrP^{C} gene can produce a disease resembling variant CJD.

Because of the unusual source of transmission of variant CJD, the initial reports in 1996 of cases of the disease focused intense interest on human prion diseases. Unique epidemiologic, clinical, and neuropathologic features of the illness led to the early recognition that the disease was indeed a "new variant" distinct from sporadic CJD.

ENCOUNTER

The variant form of CJD appeared in the late 1990s following an epizootic of BSE in Great Britain in the early 1990s (Fig. 56-4). Changes in the rendering process for bovine by-products and the subsequent use of the products in cattle feed (a form of forced cannibalism) may have amplified the epidemic in animals. Variant CJD was initially reported in a 16-year-old girl from Great

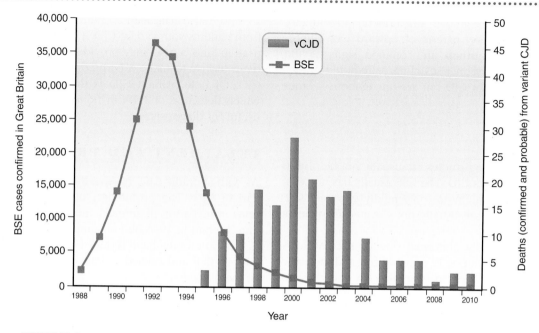

FIGURE 56-4. Annual frequency of bovine spongiform encephalopathy and variant CJD in Great Britain, 1988 to 2010.

Britain in 1995. As of November, 2011, 225 cases of variant CJD have been reported worldwide, with 176 from Great Britain, 25 from France, five from Spain, four from Ireland, three each from the Netherlands and the United States, two each from Italy, Portugal, and Canada, and one each from Japan, Saudi Arabia, and Taiwan.

The average age at onset for variant CJD is about 30 years (ranging from 16 to 48 years) compared with 65 years for sporadic CJD. The variant form has a slower progression than sporadic CJD, with a mean survival of 14 months for variant CJD compared with 5 months for the sporadic form.

ENTRY

Although considerable experimental evidence links BSE and variant CJD, scant epidemiological evidence associates variant CJD with the consumption of beef or any particular beef products. The assumption is that the PrP^Sc is ingested, but the exact circumstances of exposure are not known. Three cases of variant CJD potentially related to a blood transfusion from an affected donor have been reported.

The majority of BSE cases have occurred in Great Britain, with spread to Europe, Asia, and the Middle East. A small number of infected animals have been identified in Canada, and two infected animals (one from a Canadian herd and the other from a native herd) have been identified in the United States. A third cow in the United States was determined to have a heritable form of BSE associated with a polymorphism in the PrP^C gene. Humans have consumed an estimated 50,000 BSE-infected cattle. Fortunately, considering the number of persons exposed to BSE, the incidence of human cases has remained relatively low. Possible reasons include the following:

- Low levels of PrP^Sc in milk and meat, the main bovine products consumed by humans
- Inefficient transfer of PrP^Sc to the nervous system from ingested food
- Biologic barriers to transmission of disease between species
- Low incidence (about 30%) of homozygosity at PrP^C codon 129 in the human population

SPREAD AND MULTIPLICATION

As with sporadic CJD, the progression and specific manifestations of variant CJD depend on the locations of PrP^Sc accumulation in the nervous system. All forms of CJD are uniformly fatal; however, in variant CJD, the interval between the onset of symptoms and death is much longer than in sporadic CJD. In addition, the distribution of high-intensity signals by MRI scanning differs, which correlates with the differences in clinical presentation.

DAMAGE

Unlike patients with sporadic CJD, those with variant CJD commonly have prominent **sensory disturbances** (dysesthesias and paresthesias of the face, limbs, and torso) and psychiatric symptoms. Many cases of variant CJD in Great Britain presented with psychiatric symptoms, with depression being the most common. For example, Mr. I.'s first symptoms were diagnosed and treated as a psychiatric disorder. Apathy, anxiety, intermittent delusions, and psychosis also have been described. Once neurologic signs (typically ataxia) appear, the progression of the illness accelerates. Cognitive impairment, involuntary movements, immobility, paresis of upward gaze, unresponsiveness, and **mutism** are common signs as the disease advances. Abnormalities of gaze are noted in 50% of patients with variant CJD but are uncommon in other forms of CJD.

DIAGNOSIS

Laboratory and imaging studies are usually not helpful in the diagnosis of variant CJD. The CSF usually has no cells, and levels of CSF protein are only mildly elevated. CSF 14-3-3 protein levels are usually not elevated in patients with variant CJD.

An EEG is usually abnormal due to excess slowing. However, the pattern is nonspecific, and periodic discharges like those seen in sporadic CJD rarely occur. While an MRI can be normal in a patient with variant CJD, recent studies indicate that many patients have signal **hyperintensity in the pulvinar** (Fig. 56-5A) or in the pulvinar combined with the dorsomedial thalamus ("hockey stick sign") (Fig. 56-5B). As with sporadic CJD, an abnormal scan supports the diagnosis of variant CJD, but a normal MRI does not exclude the diagnosis. PrP^C mutations are not present in variant CJD, but like Mr. I., nearly all patients tested to date are homozygous for a methionine at codon 129 in PrP^C, suggesting that host factors play a role in determining disease susceptibility.

The neuropathology of variant CJD also differs from that of sporadic CJD. The most striking difference is the presence of **plaques**, which stain intensely for PrP^{Sc}, throughout the cerebrum and cerebellum and, to a lesser degree, the basal ganglia and thalamus. The plaques have an eosinophilic center and a pale periphery and are surrounded by spongiform changes. The cerebellum is commonly involved in variant CJD but only occasionally affected in sporadic CJD.

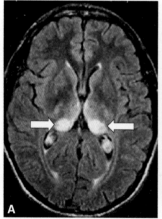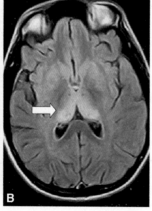

FIGURE 56-5. Magnetic resonance imaging of a patient with variant CJD. A. Increased signal intensity in the pulvinar ("pulvinar sign"). **B.** Increased signal intensity in the pulvinar and dorsomedial thalamus ("hockey stick sign").

PrP^{Sc} also has been identified in tonsil biopsy tissue from patients with variant CJD. That approach, which was used in Mr. I.'s case, may provide a less invasive way than brain biopsy to make a pathological diagnosis of variant CJD. Of note, variant CJD is the only prion disease in which detection of PrP^{Sc} in nonneural tissue is currently useful for diagnosis.

TREATMENT AND PREVENTION

As with sporadic CJD, no specific therapy is available for variant CJD. The prohibition on ruminant-derived proteins in feeds for all animals and poultry in Great Britain and the ban in 1996 on consumption of animals over the age of 30 months have reduced the risk of human exposure to BSE and caused a dramatic decline in new cases of the disease.

OTHER HUMAN PRION DISEASES

Gerstmann-Straussler-Scheinker syndrome (GSS) is a rare human prion disease with an autosomal dominant pattern of inheritance and essentially complete penetrance. The incidence of GSS is 1 to 10 cases per 100 million population each year. GSS presents with progressive cerebellar degeneration accompanied by various degrees of dementia in patients entering midlife (mean age 45 years). The illness gradually progresses with a mean survival of 5 years after symptoms develop. Because the majority of cases are familial, all patients with definite GSS have PrP^C mutations.

Fatal familial insomnia (FFI) is a rapidly fatal midlife disease with a mean survival of 13 months following onset of symptoms. The disease presents with progressive insomnia, often associated with a dream-like confusional state during waking hours. Inattention, memory loss, confusion, and hallucinations occur, but overt dementia is rare. Myoclonus, ataxia, and spasticity can occur late in the disease. FFI is the only prion disease to produce dysautonomia (hyperhidrosis, hyperthermia, tachycardia, and hypertension) and endocrine disturbances (decreased adrenocorticotropic hormone secretion, increased cortisol secretion, and disturbances in growth hormone, melatonin, and prolactin secretion).

CONCLUSION

Prion diseases are a unique group of illnesses resulting from a conformational change in a normal human protein. Occurring as sporadic, iatrogenic, hereditary, and transmissible forms of disease, they are relentlessly progressive and uniformly fatal. Ongoing concern about animal-to-human transmission has focused both popular and scientific attention on prions. Prion research may yield new insights into cellular physiology as well as treatments and methods of prevention for these unusual diseases.

Suggested Readings

Aguzzi A, O'Connor T. Protein aggregation diseases: pathogenicity and therapeutic perspectives. *Nat Rev. Drug Discovery.* 2010;9;237–248.

Aguzzi A, Calella AM. Prions: protein aggregation and infectious diseases. *Physiologic Rev.* 2009;89;1105–1152.

Bosque PJ, Tyler KL. Prions and prion diseases of the central nervous system (transmissible neurodegenerative diseases), chapter 178. In: Mandell GL, Bennett JE, Dolin R, eds. *Principles and Practice of Infectious Diseases.* 7th ed. Philadelphia, PA: Churchill Livingstone; 2010:2423–2438.

Brown P. Transmissible spongiform encephalopathy in the 21st century: neuroscience for the clinical neurologist. *Neurology.* 2008;70;713–722.

Stewart LA, et al. Systematic review of therapeutic interventions in human prion disease. *Neurology.* 2008;70;1272–1281.

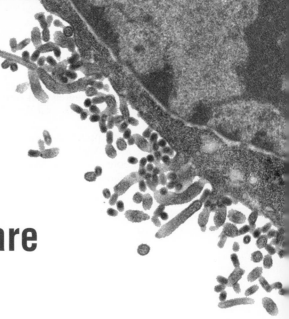

Chapter 57

Biological Agents of Warfare and Terrorism

Sandro K. Cinti and Philip C. Hanna

KEY CONCEPTS

General concepts about bioterrorism:

- Biological agents provide a convenient and inexpensive way for rogue nations or organizations to foment terror.

- The National Institutes of Health and the Centers for Disease Control and Prevention have identified probable agents of bioterrorism and have grouped them into three categories for priority research.

- It is speculated that terrorists would attempt to disperse the most infectious agents in aerosol form.

Features of select agents:

- Anthrax causes a deadly hemorrhagic mediastinitis, septicemia, and meningitis when *Bacillus anthracis* spores are inhaled; however, the most common naturally acquired form of the disease in humans is an ulcerative skin lesion. It is not transmitted from person to person.

- Plague is a zoonosis naturally acquired from infected fleabites and causes suppurative lymphadenitis. However, *Yersinia pestis* can spread to the lungs to cause a pneumonia that can be transmitted among humans by droplets.

- Tularemia is a zoonosis usually acquired from contact with or ingestion of an infected animal. The typical infection involves skin and regional lymph nodes, but *Francisella tularensis* can also cause a serious pneumonia when inhaled.

- Smallpox (variola virus) is acquired by droplets spread from an infected individual. It causes a scarring, vesicular rash with high fever. Vaccination is an effective means of prevention but has not been widely used since the disease was declared eradicated.

- Hemorrhagic fever viruses (e.g., Ebola virus, Lassa fever, Marburg virus, and yellow fever) spread among humans mostly by contact. Features of the diseases vary but generally include fever, disseminated intravascular coagulation, and hemorrhagic manifestations.

- *Clostridium botulinum* toxin interferes with the release of acetylcholine at the neuromuscular junction and results in flaccid muscular paralysis without fever or changes in mental status.

BIOTERRORISM is the malevolent use of bacteria, viruses, or toxins against humans, animals, or plants in an attempt to cause harm and to create fear. Although concern about bioterrorism has always existed (see the box titled "Bioterrorism in History"), the 2001 anthrax attack in the United States that killed five people and prompted preemptive treatment of more than 10,000 others has focused attention on bioterrorism as an imminent threat to national security. An understanding of the concern requires familiarity with the pathogens that are most likely to be used in any future attack and awareness of the available methods for detecting and responding to such an event. Consider how the following case—the first fatal case in the 2001 attack—came to light.

Biological weapons, unlike other weapons of mass destruction, are inexpensive to make. Nuclear and chemical weapons programs are 800 and 600 times more costly to develop, respectively, than a comparable biological weapons program. The pathogens are relatively available, and the materials and equipment for producing biological weapons are the same as those used for peaceful purposes. For example, the organism that causes anthrax is present in the soil in many countries and can be grown in standard laboratory culture medium. The *Salmonella* species used in the Oregon attack described in the box titled "Bioterrorism in History" was easily obtained by a member of the Rajneeshee cult. The necessary culture media, incubators, and milling equipment are available for

BIOTERRORISM IN HISTORY

The use of biological agents for warfare has a centuries-long history, predating even the concept of germ theory. The first documented case was in 1346 when the Tartars, frustrated after years of laying siege to the Black Sea city of Kaffa, catapulted plague victims over the unassailable city walls. The Black Death epidemic that followed and eventually spread from Kaffa wiped out almost half of Europe. In 1763, Sir Jeffrey Amherst, the commander of British troops in America, sanctioned the use of smallpox-infected blankets as germ warfare implements against the American Indians who were highly susceptible to the deadly virus.

During World War I, the Germans infected cattle destined for consumption by Allied forces with anthrax and glanders. That act resulted in the 1925 Geneva Protocol, which prohibited the use of biological weapons. In spite of that agreement and the 1972 Biological and Chemical Weapons Convention, several nations continued to produce biological weapons. Biopreparat, the Russian biological weapons program, was the largest in the world, with 10,000 scientists working in 50 production facilities. In 1979, an accidental release of weaponized anthrax from a production plant in Sverdlovsk resulted in 66 deaths downwind of the facility. The program was dismantled in 1992 after Boris Yeltsin finally admitted that it existed.

Aum Shinrikyo, a Japanese cult, attempted several unsuccessful biological attacks with anthrax and botulinum toxin before releasing sarin gas in the Tokyo subway in 1995. The most successful biological attack in the United States was perpetrated by a religious cult, the Rajneeshees. In 1984, in an attempt to affect elections in a small Oregon town, the cult poisoned 10 restaurant salad bars with *Salmonella typhimurium* and sickened more than 700 people.

During the 2001 anthrax attacks in the United States, 22 people were infected with anthrax that was placed in mailed envelopes, and 5 died of inhalational anthrax. Most of the infected victims were mail workers in Washington, DC, but cases also occurred in Florida, New York, and Connecticut. On February 19, 2010, the U.S. Department of Justice (DOJ) named Dr. Bruce Ivins, an anthrax researcher at the United States Army Medical Research Institute of Infectious Diseases (USAMRIID), as the sole perpetrator of the 2001 anthrax attacks. In the 92-page report, the DOJ laid out the following summary of evidence implicating Dr. Ivins:

- Dr. Ivins' lab at USAMRIID maintained an anthrax strain, RMR-1029, that was the parent strain to the anthrax used in the attacks.
- The anthrax vaccine program that Dr. Ivins oversaw was in jeopardy of being cut before the anthrax attacks, and it was rejuvenated after the attacks.
- Dr. Ivins had a history of mental health problems and "a history dating to his graduate days of homicidal threats, actions, [and] plans," and that a prior psychiatrist "called him homicidal [and] sociopathic with clear intentions."
- Envelopes used in the attacks were part of a batch distributed, among other places, to a post office in Frederick, MD, several blocks from Dr. Ivins' home where the researcher had a post-office box.
- The language used in the anthrax letters is similar to language used by Dr. Ivins in e-mails he sent to colleagues in September 2001 before the first anthrax case occurred.
- Dr. Ivins demonstrated a guilty conscience. He submitted questionable samples of the RMR-1029 anthrax strain to the FBI.
- Dr. Ivins had a history of disguising his identity and going on long rides to mail letters. He was known to use pseudonyms when communicating with others.
- Dr. Ivins had a history of obsessive behavior toward a particular sorority and would drive hours and stand in front of the sorority house for minutes. One of the anthrax letters was sent from a mailbox in front of the sorority.
- Dr. Ivins could not explain his late hours prior to the anthrax attacks, and he could not explain why he had given questionable anthrax samples to the FBI.

Dr. Ivins committed suicide before the above investigation was complete.

CASE • On October 2, 2001, Mr. O., a 63-year-old photo editor at a Florida newspaper, awoke early with nausea, vomiting, and confusion. He was taken to a local emergency room for evaluation. Mr. O. had experienced malaise, fatigue, fever, chills, anorexia, and sweats beginning on September 27 during a trip to North Carolina. He denied headache, cough, chest pain, myalgias, dyspnea, abdominal pain, diarrhea, or skin rash. Medical history included hypertension, cardiovascular disease, and gout. He did not smoke.

On physical examination, Mr. O. was alert and interactive but spoke nonsensically. His temperature was 39.2°C, his heart rate was 109 beats per minute, and his blood pressure and respiratory rate were normal. Initial pulmonary, heart, and abdominal examinations were normal, and his neck was not stiff. Mr. O. was not oriented to person, place, or time.

Laboratory testing included a normal total white blood cell (WBC) count, but the platelet count was low. A chest radiograph showed prominence of the superior mediastinum and a possible small left pleural effusion (Fig. 57-1). A spinal tap was performed, and the cerebrospinal fluid (CSF) showed a WBC count of 4,750/mm³ with 81% neutrophils, red blood cell count of 1,375/mm³, glucose of 57 mg/dL (simultaneous serum glucose

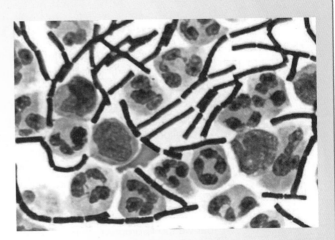

FIGURE 57-2. Gram stain of cerebrospinal fluid obtained from patient infected with _Bacillus anthracis_.

was 174 mg/dL), and protein of 666 mg/dL. Microscopy examination of the CSF showed many Gram-positive bacilli (Fig. 57-2). Anthrax was suspected. After only 7 hours of incubation of the CSF culture, _Bacillus anthracis_ was isolated, and blood cultures were positive within 24 hours of incubation.

Mr. O. received a single dose of cefotaxime and was admitted to the hospital with a diagnosis of meningitis. Shortly after admission, he had generalized seizures; an endotracheal tube was placed for airway protection. Initially he received multiple different intravenous antibiotics, but by day 2, Mr. O.'s ongoing therapy consisted of penicillin G, levofloxacin, and clindamycin. In spite of that combination therapy, he remained febrile and became unresponsive to deep stimuli. His condition progressively deteriorated, with hypotension and worsening renal function. Mr. O. died on October 5. A postmortem examination revealed hemorrhagic inflammation of the mediastinal lymph nodes, and immunohistochemical staining showed disseminated _B. anthracis_ in multiple organs. (Adapted from Jernigan JA et al. Bioterrorism-related inhalation anthrax: the first 10 cases reported in the United States. _Emerg Infect Dis._ 2001;7(6):933–944.)

This case raises several questions:

1. Why was anthrax considered early as a probable diagnosis in this case?

2. Why was bioterrorism suspected?

3. Why did antibiotic therapy fail to save Mr. O.'s life?

See Appendix for answers.

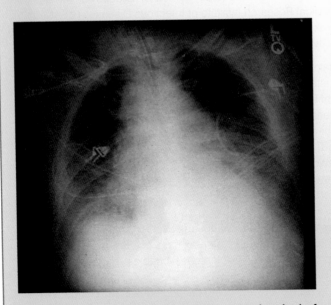

FIGURE 57-1. Chest radiograph (anterior–posterior view) of patient infected with _Bacillus anthracis_.

purchase, and information on cultivating the organisms and on generating antibiotic-resistant strains is available in the scientific literature and from the Internet.

Biological weapons produce fear and panic, as was apparent in the 2001 anthrax attack. The weapon can be released covertly, and its effects only become apparent days later when the terrorist is gone. Unlike that of chemical and nuclear events, the point of release of a biological agent may not be apparent. If it is a contagious agent, the uncertainty about who has been exposed could lead to widespread panic. Finally, the lethality of a biological attack could exceed that of other weapons of mass destruction. By one governmental estimate, 50 kg of powdered anthrax similar to that used in the 2001 attack released over a city of 500,000 people would cause death in 95,000 and incapacity in 125,000.

EPIDEMIOLOGY OF A BIOTERRORIST ATTACK

A bioterrorist attack will have features that are similar to any naturally occurring epidemic of the involved disease. However, *certain epidemiologic features should increase suspicion that a biological agent has been released deliberately* and prompt further investigation (Table 57-1). For example, *B. anthracis* is found in soils around the world; however, naturally occurring anthrax in humans is uncommon. It is now so rare in the United States that any case, regardless of its clinical manifestations, should be investigated as a bioterrorist act. Thus, in the case of Mr. O., a deliberate biological attack was an early consideration.

ENCOUNTER WITH BIOLOGICAL WEAPONS

Biological weapons can be released by aerosolization, contamination of food, contamination of water, person-to-person transmission of a contagious agent, or release of infected insect vectors. **Aerosolization**, the dispersion of organisms into the environment, is the most feared and potentially lethal method of releasing biological agents. As mentioned earlier, a very small amount of weaponized anthrax (50 kg) could result in very high casualties (95,000). The Russian bioweapons program spent considerable resources developing effective methods of aerosolizing biological agents, especially anthrax, tularemia, and smallpox. Both the 1979 Sverdlovsk outbreak of anthrax and the 2001 anthrax attack in the United States involved the release of finely powdered anthrax into the environment. Means of aerosolizing an agent include spraying devices (crop dusters), air-handling systems in buildings, incendiary devices (bombs), and the postal system (infected mail). However, aerosolization of a biological agent is not easy. Infectious particles **must be precisely the right size (0.5 to 5 μm) to enter and infect the lungs**. Furthermore, radiation from sunlight, shear forces from sprayers, or

TABLE 57-1 Clues That Raise Suspicion for a Deliberate Release of a Bioterrorism Agent

Clue	Potential Source or Circumstance
A large number of ill persons presenting at the same time with a similar disease, especially the following syndromes:	
Flaccid paralysis	Botulinum toxin
Hemorrhagic fevers (HFs)	Ebola virus, Lassa fever
Vesicular/pustular rash with considerable mortality	Smallpox
Flulike illness associated with a widened mediastinum on chest radiograph	Anthrax and/or meningitis
Pneumonia with painful lymphadenopathy	Plague
Illness in animals and humans concurrently	Anthrax, encephalitis
A large number of unexplained deaths, especially in young healthy adults	Various agents
A single case of an uncommon organism	Smallpox, pulmonary anthrax, Ebola virus
Multiple disease entities presenting in one patient	Multiple agents released
An unusual disease presentation	Pneumonic instead of bubonic plague
An unusual geographic distribution	Ebola virus in the United States
An unusual seasonal pattern	Influenza in the summer
An illness that fails to respond to usual antimicrobials or vaccines	Engineered antibiotic- or vaccine-resistant anthrax
Clusters of a similar illness in noncontiguous areas, domestic or foreign	Various agents

explosions from incendiary devices would likely destroy most of the released organism.

Contamination of the food or water supply with biological agents is another method of dissemination. The *Salmonella typhimurium* contamination of salad bars in Oregon restaurants is an example of a successful attack (see the box titled "Bioterrorism in History"). The most likely agents to be disseminated in this fashion include botulinum toxin, anthrax, and diarrheal agents including *S. typhimurium*. However, contamination of food and water would be difficult given inspection criteria, water purification, and filtering systems and increased security at water reservoirs and food distribution centers.

Dissemination through **person-to-person transmission** is a likely means of dispersing a contagious agent such as smallpox. As few as 100 smallpox-infected people could start an epidemic in a nonimmune population. The fear, panic, and quarantine measures that would result from such an epidemic could rapidly overwhelm health care resources and destabilize affected countries.

Zoonotic delivery, or the use of **insect vectors** to disperse a biological agent, is an unlikely method of bioterrorism because it is inefficient and unpredictable. The most likely agent to be delivered by zoonosis would be *Yersinia pestis* (plague) or viral hemorrhagic fevers (HFs) (Ebola virus, Lassa fever).

The characteristics of an ideal agent for bioterrorism include *accessibility, durability, infectiousness, and communicability*. Although hundreds of agents and toxins may qualify, the Centers for Disease Control and Prevention (CDC) has developed **categories A, B, and C** *based on the perceived threat*. The characteristics of the pathogens in the CDC categories are listed in the box titled "Characteristics of Priority Biological Agents in Categories A, B, and C." Category A agents pose the greatest threat, and these agents are discussed individually in this chapter. A complete list of the pathogens listed in categories A, B, and C is included in the electronic supplement to this chapter.

CATEGORY A AGENTS
Anthrax

Anthrax, a disease most associated with grazing herbivores, has been reported throughout human history. It is believed to have been one of the Egyptian plagues at the time of Moses and was described in detail by the ancient Roman poet Virgil. Anthrax bacilli were used by Robert Koch to prove his theory that "germs" cause disease, and Louis Pasteur's celebrated public demonstration of the first attenuated vaccine showed protection of farm animals against anthrax.

Bacillus anthracis is a Gram-positive bacterium that forms stable endospores when nutrients are limited. These spores are extremely robust and capable of remaining dormant in the soil for decades or longer. *The spore is the infectious particle*. The natural stability of anthrax spores, their longevity and resistance to destruction, and their ability to cause lethal infections are likely reasons they were chosen as weapons. The "**weaponization**" of anthrax spores by drying and milling generates a unit spore size capable of reaching the recesses of the lung. In addition, spores prepared in this manner are easier to disperse in aerosols and remain airborne longer. Anthrax is **not known to spread from person to person**.

The virulence of *B. anthracis* depends on the presence of its **two large plasmids**. Plasmid pXO2 encodes the synthesis genes for an **antiphagocytic poly-D-glutamic acid capsule**. Plasmid pXO1 encodes for **two binary exotoxins** that act as potent enzymes in the cytoplasm of host cells. **Edema toxin** contains **edema factor**, a **calmodulin-dependent adenylate cyclase** that increases cellular cyclic adenosine monophosphate and upsets cellular water balance. Edema toxin probably contributes to the massive edema seen in anthrax infection. **Lethal toxin** contains **lethal factor**, a **zinc metalloprotease** that cleaves a variety of cytoplasmic substrates and inactivates the signal-transducing enzyme MAPKK. Inoculation of purified lethal toxin kills test animals.

In addition to edema factor and lethal factor, each toxin has a second, shared subunit called **protective antigen**. Protective antigen is the binding subunit that mediates entry into host cells. Neither toxin is active without it, and the protective antigen subunit is the main ingredient of the anthrax subunit vaccine, underscoring the importance of exotoxins in the production of disease manifestations.

The **three main clinical forms** of anthrax are classified by the route of entry of the spores into the body: cutaneous, gastrointestinal, and inhalation (Table 57-2). **Cutaneous anthrax is by far the most common** and mildest form. Naturally acquired cases of cutaneous anthrax occur after contact with infected animals or their by-products. However, during the postal attacks of 2001, half the people infected had the cutaneous form of disease. In cutaneous infections, spores enter the skin through minor cuts or abrasions, germinate to form growing bacilli, and cause local ulceration of the skin. The primary skin lesion is usually a painless itchy papule that appears 3 to 5 days after contact. In 24 to 36 hours, the lesion forms a vesicle that undergoes central necrosis and drying, leaving a typical smooth-edged, painless black crust, or **eschar**, surrounded by edema and a number of **purplish vesicles**. Cutaneous anthrax can be self-limiting, but antibiotic treatment is recommended to prevent any dissemination into the bloodstream. When treated, cutaneous anthrax heals completely and usually without scarring.

Gastrointestinal anthrax is extremely rare in developed countries. Symptoms appear 2 to 5 days after ingestion of spore-contaminated meat from diseased animals. They include fever and diffuse abdominal pain and tenderness, and patients often report either

TABLE 57-2 Disease Manifestations of Category A Agents

Primary Clinical Feature	Pathogen	Mode of Entry	Communicable Among Humans?
Pneumonia	*Yersinia pestis*	Inhalation	Yes
	Francisella tularensis	Inhalation	No
Single skin ulcer	*Bacillus anthracis*	Abrasion of skin	No
	F. tularensis	Arthropod bite or abrasion of skin	No
Lymphadenitis			
Mediastinal	*B. anthracis*	Inhalation	No
Regional	*Y. pestis* (bubo)	Arthropod bite	No
	F. tularensis	Arthropod bite or abrasion of skin	No
Eye infection with lymphadenitis	*F. tularensis*	Direct inoculation of conjunctiva	No
Meningitis	*B. anthracis*	Inhalation, dissemination	No
Necrotizing intestinal infection	*B. anthracis*	Ingestion of spores	No
	F. tularensis	Ingestion of bacteria	No
Multiple skin vesicles	Smallpox	Respiratory droplet	Yes
Fever with hemorrhaging	*Y. pestis*	Dissemination from skin or lung	Yes
	HF viruses	Arthropods, penetration through abraded skin, unknown inhalation	Yes (some agents)
Paralysis	*Clostridium botulinum toxin*	Ingestion, inhalation	No

Gray highlighting indicates potential bioterrorist scenario.

constipation or diarrhea and black or bloody stools or vomitus. Ulceration and inflammation of the gastrointestinal tract is typically accompanied by massive edema, mucosal necrosis, and spread to the mesenteric lymph nodes. Mortality from gastrointestinal anthrax is very high and is associated with blood loss and shock, intestinal perforation, or spread of the organism into the bloodstream.

Inhalation anthrax occurs after aerosolized spores are inhaled and thus represents the greatest concern as a bioweapon. Though extremely rare, naturally occurring disease has been reported in persons working with spore-contaminated furs or wools (thus the name "**woolsorter's disease**"). Although the airways are the initial site of contact, inhalation anthrax is *not a true pneumonia*, and in most cases, no bacteria are found in the lungs. Rather, spores reaching the alveoli are engulfed by phagocytes and *transported to the mediastinal and peribronchial lymph nodes*, germinating en route. Illness may begin 1 to 6 days after exposure or after several weeks because of smaller inocula or delays in spore internalization by alveolar phagocytes.

Early symptoms of inhalation anthrax are "flulike" and include **fever**, **myalgia**, and **malaise**. As the bacilli multiply, **hemorrhagic mediastinitis** and **widening of the mediastinum** become visible on chest radiograph or computerized tomography scan (see Fig. 57-1). Symptoms of shortness of breath, strident cough, and chills develop at that point and are followed quickly by massive pleural effusions, sepsis, shock, and death as bacilli spread throughout the body in high numbers. Anthrax **meningitis** occurs in up to 50% of inhalation cases and is almost always fatal in spite of intensive antibiotic therapy. Meningitis resulting from anthrax causes extensive hemorrhage of the leptomeninges, giving them a dark red appearance on autopsy, sardonically described as "**cardinal's cap**."

Anthrax can be successfully treated with antibiotics if they are administered prophylactically after spore exposure or early in the course of infection. During the anthrax outbreak of 2001, 6 of the 11 victims of inhalation anthrax survived with aggressive hospital care and multiple intravenous antibiotics. *B. anthracis* is naturally susceptible to fluoroquinolones, tetracyclines, and most other antibiotics. There is also an **anthrax vaccine** that is currently

CHARACTERISTICS OF PRIORITY BIOLOGICAL AGENTS IN CATEGORIES A, B, AND C

Category A (e.g., anthrax, smallpox)

The most dangerous agents with the highest research priority for the following reasons:

- Can be easily disseminated or transmitted from person to person
- Result in high mortality rates and have the potential for major public health impact
- Might cause public panic and social disruption
- Require special action for public health preparedness

Category B (e.g., *Salmonella* species, viral encephalitis)

Represent a secondary priority for the following reasons:

- Are moderately easy to disseminate
- Result in moderate morbidity rates and low mortality rates
- Require specific enhancements of the CDC's diagnostic capacity and enhanced disease surveillance

Category C (e.g., multidrug-resistant tuberculosis, influenza)

Represent emerging pathogens that pose less of an immediate threat but may be genetically engineered in the future to produce more lethal disease or disease resistant to current antibiotics and/or vaccines for the following reasons:

- Are readily available
- Can easily be produced and disseminated
- Have a potential for high morbidity and mortality rates and major health impact

administered to military personnel, researchers, and some animal and human health care providers; however, it is not clear how well the current vaccine protects humans against inhalation anthrax.

Physicians will face many challenges during an anthrax outbreak. It is a disease with a rapid progression to death but manifesting vague early symptoms that are flulike and delay patients from seeking medical attention. Once the disease progresses and high numbers of organisms are disseminated to the blood, organs, and tissues, anthrax is difficult to treat and often requires intensive care with mechanical assistance for breathing.

Plague

Plague has been the cause of several pandemics; the most famous of which, the Black Death, began in 1346 and killed 30 million people in Europe. Although pandemics of plague have ceased with the advent of antibiotics and improved rodent control, outbreaks around the world continue to account for 1,700 cases per year, including a few each year in the southwestern United States. The bacterium that causes plague, *Yersinia pestis*, has several advantages as a biological weapon:

- It is relatively stable in the environment and can survive up to 1 hour in aerosolized form.
- The pneumonic form is contagious.

- Mortality from pneumonic plague is 100% without treatment.
- The mention of plague elicits considerable panic.
- Plague is highly infective, requiring only 100 to 500 organisms to cause infection.

The most feared method of disseminating plague is through aerosolization. Although the Japanese attempted to infect the Chinese by dropping plague-infected fleas during World War II, that method of delivering plague is inefficient and unpredictable. The Russian bioweapons program, Biopreparat, produced an aerosolized form of plague, 50 kg of which could have infected up to 100,000 persons and caused 36,000 deaths.

Y. pestis is a **Gram-negative coccobacillus**. The virulence of the organism depends on several factors:

- An **envelope antigen F1** is antiphagocytic.
- A **plasminogen activator** degrades fibrin and facilitates spread of the organism.
- **V and W antigens** are antiphagocytic and allow the organism to survive and reproduce in host cells.
- **Yops proteins** are antiphagocytic and prevent an effective inflammatory response.

In addition, *Y. pestis* produces a **lipopolysaccharide (LPS) endotoxin**, which causes most of the clinical manifestations of plague.

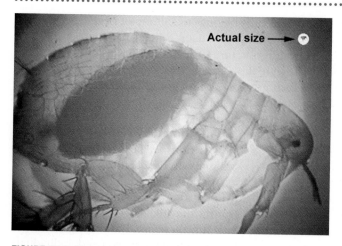

FIGURE 57-3. Flea engorged with blood.

Plague is a **zoonotic infection of rodents**. In urban areas, the animal reservoir is usually the rat, whereas in sylvatic areas, squirrels, mice, or prairie dogs can carry the disease. In any case, infection is transmitted among rodents by the bites of their fleas (Fig. 57-3). Natural transmission to humans occurs when an infected rodent flea attempts to feed on a human (see Table 57-2). After biting the host, the inoculated bacteria migrate to lymph nodes, where they associate with mononuclear cells and multiply. An incubation period of 2 to 8 days results in the bite victim developing fever, chills, and a swollen tender lymph node, or **bubo**, the cardinal feature of **bubonic plague** (Fig. 57-4). Buboes are usually found in the groin, axilla, or cervical region and are often so tender that the affected individual cannot move the affected limb. If left untreated, bubonic plague can spread to the lungs (**pneumonic plague**) or disseminate in the bloodstream (**septicemic plague**). A biological attack with aerosolized *Y. pestis* would most likely present as primary pneumonic plague without buboes.

Pneumonic plague can be primary or secondary. Secondary pneumonic plague results from the hematogenous spread of *Y. pestis* in untreated bubonic or septicemic plague. Primary pneumonic plague results from direct inhalation of plague bacilli from other humans or animals, particularly cats, with pneumonic plague. Clinically, patients have signs of pneumonia including fevers, chills, shortness of breath, and hemoptysis (coughing of blood).

Septicemic plague is characterized by **disseminated intravascular coagulation** (**DIC**), necrosis of small vessels, and hemorrhages in the skin causing large purple or black lesions (**purpura and ecchymoses**). The skin lesions and necrosis of the fingers and toes that occurred in terminally ill persons during the 14th century plague pandemic are the features that inspired the name Black Death. The mortality rate of septicemic plague approaches 100% without treatment.

The diagnosis of plague from a biological attack would be difficult because most cases would present as primary pneumonic plague without the characteristic bubo present in naturally occurring plague. A chest radiograph would show a **bronchopneumonia**, and laboratory data would be nonspecific and consistent with a systemic inflammatory response. Sputum Gram stain (and possibly blood smear) might show Gram-negative bacilli with characteristic **bipolar staining**. Although *Y. pestis* would eventually grow on culture, identification could take 6 days.

Treatment of pneumonic plague must be started *within 24 hours of onset of symptoms*, or mortality approaches 100%. Naturally occurring *Y. pestis* is sensitive to aminoglycosides, such as streptomycin and gentamicin; doxycycline; and fluoroquinolones. Because pneumonic plague can spread from person to person by droplet transmission, patients with this form of disease must be treated in respiratory isolation. In addition, persons in close contact with the affected individuals should receive prophylactic antimicrobial therapy.

Tularemia

Tularemia, the disease caused by the Gram-negative bacterium *Francisella tularensis*, occurs naturally throughout North America and Eurasia. Animal reservoirs of infection include rabbits, hares, voles, and squirrels. As with plague, transmission of the infection among those animals occurs through the bites of ticks, flies, and mosquitoes. Human infection is acquired by arthropod bites, handling infectious animal tissue, ingestion of contaminated food or water, and inhalation of aerosols.

F. tularensis is an intracellular pathogen that infects macrophages, hepatocytes, and epithelioid cells. Virulence factors include an **antiphagocytic capsule** and the enzyme **citrulline ureidase**. Although *F. tularensis* does produce an LPS endotoxin, the activity of the LPS is a thousandfold less than that of *Escherichia coli*. **Cell-mediated immunity** is the major host response to infection and results in a characteristic granulomatous infiltrate

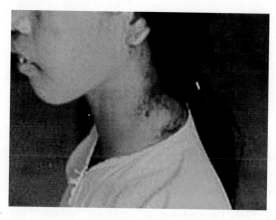

FIGURE 57-4. Bubo of the neck of a young woman with bubonic plague.

of the lymph nodes, liver, lung, spleen, and bone marrow. Tularemia can be misdiagnosed as tuberculosis if granulomas are caseating.

Tularemia also has a history as an agent of bioterrorism. The Japanese studied the disease in their bioweapons program in Manchuria (1932 to 1945), and the Russian Biopreparat program developed aerosolized forms of *F. tularensis* that were engineered to be resistant to antibiotics and vaccines.

In humans, *tularemia can present in various ways depending on the route of transmission and the site of entry into the body* (see Table 57-2). A bioterrorism attack would most likely involve aerosolized *F. tularensis*, with the predominant manifestations being pneumonic, typhoidal, septicemic, and possibly oropharyngeal. It has been estimated that one or two organisms are enough to produce infection. The mortality rate of untreated pneumonic or septic tularemia is as high as 60%. With treatment, the case fatality rate is less than 2%. Isolation is not recommended for tularemia patients, given the lack of human-to-human transmission.

The diagnosis of a bioterrorist attack with tularemia would be difficult given the nonspecific presentation. Lymphadenopathy, the hallmark of naturally occurring tularemia, may not be present, and standard microbiological testing of sputum could miss *F. tularensis* or delay it by days to weeks.

The treatment of choice for pneumonic, septic, or typhoidal tularemia is an aminoglycoside antibiotic. Ciprofloxacin and doxycycline are also effective and would be preferred in a mass casualty setting. A live, attenuated *F. tularensis* vaccine is available for laboratory workers exposed to tularemia; however, in volunteer studies, the vaccine did not protect all subjects from an aerosolized challenge.

Smallpox

The last naturally occurring case of **smallpox** was diagnosed in 1977 in Somalia. In 1980, 13 years after initiating an eradication program, the World Health Organization (WHO) certified the world free of smallpox and recommended discontinuation of the smallpox vaccine. Only two official repositories maintained the deadly **variola** (smallpox) virus, the Institute of Virus Preparations in Moscow and the CDC in Atlanta, Georgia. Thus, a case of smallpox anywhere in the world today could only arise as a result of a clandestine laboratory accident or a bioterrorist attack. Russia's now-dismantled Biopreparat program produced large amounts of smallpox as a biological weapon, and there is concern that some of those stocks may have fallen into the hands of rogue nations. A bioterrorist could initiate a smallpox epidemic by aerosol release or by sending intentionally infected individuals into an unsuspecting population. In a world that is no longer immune to the disease, the infection would spread rapidly from person to person. In its most pathogenic form, variola causes *disfiguring skin eruptions, fever, and a mortality rate of 30% or more* in unvaccinated persons.

Variola virus belongs to a group of large **DNA viruses** called the **orthopoxviruses**. Natural infection occurs when virus from respiratory droplets or skin lesions comes into contact with the oropharyngeal or respiratory mucosa. The infectious dose is thought to be very small, but historical outbreaks suggest that close contact is usually required to spread the disease. After migration to regional lymph nodes, an **asymptomatic viremia** transmits virus throughout the body. A nonspecific **prodrome** of fever, malaise, and prostration with headache and backache follows an incubation period that averages 12 to 14 days (ranging from 7 to 17 days). Abdominal pain and delirium also can occur. During the initial febrile prodrome, the patient is not contagious; therefore, monitoring for fevers is an excellent way of identifying exposed individuals who need to be isolated.

Within 2 to 4 days of fever onset, the patient develops a maculopapular rash on the mucosa of the mouth, pharynx, face, and arms that spreads to the trunk and legs. The patient is highly contagious at that point. Over the next several days, the rash becomes vesicular and then pustular as it covers the whole body (Fig. 57-5). If the patient survives, lesions form crusts after 2 weeks and leave disfiguring scars. The patient is most contagious during the first week of rash, but transmission continues to occur until all scabs have fallen off (about 3 weeks). Mortality is usually associated with **toxemia**, probably the result of circulating immune complexes and soluble variola antigens, or, less often, encephalitis or secondary bacterial pneumonia.

Differentiating smallpox (variola) from the more common chickenpox (varicella) can be challenging, but several discriminating features make accurate diagnoses possible (Table 57-3). Because laboratory testing for smallpox requires high-level containment facilities, suspected samples of vesicular or pustular fluid or scabs must be sent to the CDC for testing and cultivation. The

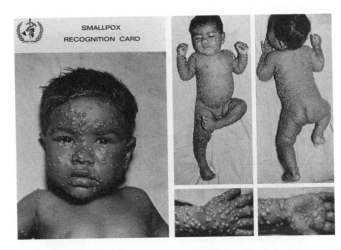

FIGURE 57-5. Progression of smallpox lesions. Note early involvement of the face, hands (including the palms), and feet (including the soles).

TABLE 57-3 Features That Distinguish the Rash of Smallpox (Variola) and Chickenpox (Varicella)

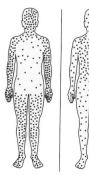

Smallpox   Chickenpox

	Smallpox	**Chickenpox**
Fever	Occurs 2–4 days before rash onset	Occurs at the time of rash, if at all
Rash		
• Distribution	More lesions on the face and extremities; lesions on palms and soles	More lesions on the body; no lesions on palms and soles
• Appearance	Large, deep-seated vesicles or pustules in the same stage of development	Small, shallow vesicles in various stages of development
• Course	Lesions resolve over 14–21 days	Lesions resolved within 7–10 days
Mortality	10–30%	Very uncommon

large, brick-shaped virions of orthopoxviruses can be easily identified by electron microscopic examination (Fig. 57-6). Two other orthopoxviruses, cowpox and vaccinia, can be ruled out from the patient's history or the appearance of the lesions.

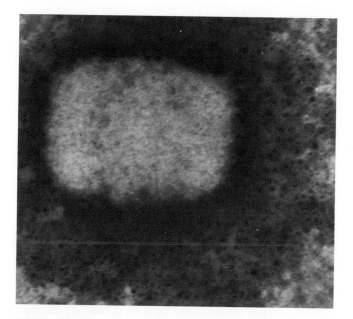

FIGURE 57-6. Electron micrograph of a variola virion.

No antiviral therapy has been established for smallpox. One antiviral drug, **cidofovir**, has some activity against poxviruses, but it is toxic to the bone marrow and kidneys. Vaccination with live vaccinia virus has been the best way to prevent smallpox disease since the late 1700s, and mass vaccination would most likely occur in a widespread outbreak.

During an outbreak, infection control measures would be of paramount importance in preventing the spread of smallpox. All health care workers caring for smallpox patients would be vaccinated as soon as possible, and patients with suspected infection would be placed in high-level isolation. Vaccine administered within 4 days of exposure to smallpox can significantly decrease morbidity and mortality. Public health officials would immediately begin contact tracing to identify other potential cases and candidates for vaccination.

Viral Hemorrhagic Fevers

In nature, humans are infected with HF viruses from the bite of an infected arthropod (mosquito), from aerosols of rodent excreta, or from direct contact with an infected animal. Person-to-person spread of **Ebola virus** has been the cause of several devastating outbreaks in Africa. **Marburg virus** and possibly **Lassa fever** also spread through person-to-person contact, although aerosol spread was implicated in an outbreak of Lassa fever in Nigeria in 1969.

Several distinct groups of RNA viruses can produce a viral HF syndrome. The pathogenesis of the syndrome is poorly understood. After an incubation period of 2 to 21 days, infected persons develop *fever, myalgias, headache, retro-orbital pain, and prostration*. A maculopapular rash and/or conjunctivitis may be present with Lassa fever and yellow fever. **Jaundice** is a hallmark of yellow fever and Rift Valley fever. In its most severe form, viral HF syndrome manifests as **hemorrhagic complications**, including diffuse bleeding in the skin and gastrointestinal tract. DIC and shock may be present. The mortality rate varies from less than 1% for Rift Valley fever to more than 70% from Ebola or Marburg virus.

The HF viruses—Ebola, Marburg, Lassa, Junin, and Machupo—were developed as aerosolized biological weapons in Russia until 1992. The US developed Rift Valley fever and yellow fever viruses as biological weapons before the US program was dismantled in 1969. The most likely route of dissemination in a bioterrorist attack would be aerosolization.

Rapid diagnosis of HF viruses is problematic at present. Tests for a specific HF virus, including antigen detection by antigen-capture enzyme-linked immunosorbent assay (ELISA), IgM antibody detection by antibody-capture ELISA, and reverse transcription polymerase chain reaction are done in specialized laboratories. Viral culture should be attempted only at the CDC or the U.S. Army Medical Research Institute of Infectious Diseases.

Because of the potential for person-to-person transmission of some HF viruses (e.g., Ebola virus), infected individuals must be cared for in isolation rooms. Although the U.S. Food and Drug Administration has not approved any drug for viral HF syndrome, **ribavirin**, a nucleoside analog, has reduced mortality from Lassa fever in some small trials. Ribavirin has no activity against Ebola virus, Marburg virus, or yellow fever. Except for yellow fever, there is no vaccine for any of the HF viruses.

Botulinum Toxin

Botulinum toxin, produced by the spore-forming anaerobe *Clostridium botulinum*, is the most potent toxin known to humans. It has already been used as a biological weapon by the Japanese cult Aum Shinrikyo, which attempted aerosol dispersions on US military installations in Japan on three occasions between 1990 and 1995. Large amounts of weaponized botulinum toxin were also produced in the former Soviet Union and in Iraq. Methods of dispersion include aerosolization and poisoning of the food supply. Contamination of the water supply with botulinum toxin is impractical given that large amounts of toxin would be required, and standard water purification methods (e.g., chlorination) rapidly inactivate the toxin.

C. botulinum is ubiquitous in the soil and can be easily isolated in culture. Botulinum toxin exists in seven distinct antigenic forms (A through G) that make convenient epidemiologic markers in an outbreak. Most natural foodborne outbreaks of botulism occur with toxins A, B, and E. The lethal dose of botulinum toxin for a 70-kg human is 0.09 to 0.15 µg intravenously, 0.70 to 0.90 µg inhaled, and 70 µg orally. Therapeutic BoTox contains only 0.3% of the lethal inhalational dose and 0.005% of the lethal oral dose. Botulinum toxin does not permeate intact skin.

Botulinum toxin acts at the neuromuscular junction to prevent release of acetylcholine, a neurotransmitter that stimulates muscle contraction (Fig. 57-7). The clinical symptoms that result are manifestations of impaired muscle contraction. Symptoms typically appear 12 to 72 hours after ingestion of toxin, but inhalation botulism is likely

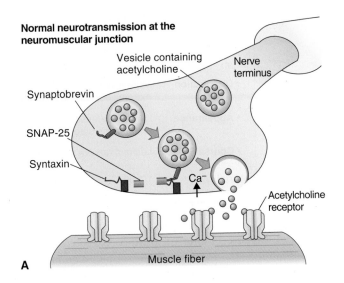

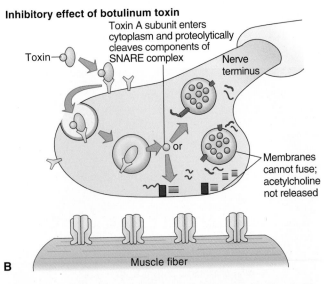

FIGURE 57-7. Mechanism of action of botulinum toxins. A. The assembly of the SNARE mechanism that mediates fusion of acetylcholine-containing vesicles with the cell membrane and release of acetylcholine into the neuromuscular junction after normal excitatory stimuli. **B.** The actions of botulinum toxins: proteolytic cleavage of either synaptobrevin, syntaxin, or SNAP-25 (the main components of the SNARE complex).

to present within hours. The classic triad of botulism is (1) descending flaccid paralysis with prominent bulbar signs, (2) normal body temperature, and (3) normal mental status. The patient remains lucid because the toxin does not penetrate the brain. The bulbar signs include the "4 Ds": **diplopia** (double vision), **dysarthria** (difficulty forming words), **dysphonia** (difficulty intoning words), and **dysphagia** (difficulty swallowing). Paralysis may progress to involve the muscle of respiration, in which case, death results from asphyxiation or secondary infection (aspiration pneumonia).

In addition to foodborne botulism (see Chapter 76), the toxin can also be released from *C. botulinum* growing in wounds (**wound botulism**) or in the intestinal tracts of infants (**infant botulism**), particularly those fed honey.

Treatment of botulism consists of supportive care (e.g., **mechanical ventilation** is required in 20% of foodborne cases) and the administration of **equine antitoxin**. Antitoxin must be administered early because it will not reverse existing paralysis.

CONCLUSION

Several virulent bacterial and viral pathogens are potential agents for a bioterrorist attack. Some have already been used for that purpose. Certain terrorist groups or rogue nations may favor using these agents over nuclear or chemical weapons of mass destruction because they are relatively easy to obtain, cheap to produce in large quantities, and highly effective in creating human morbidity and panic. The category A agents are considered the most dangerous. A major release of these pathogens in a terrorist attack would likely involve large quantities of the agent released in aerosol form. Physicians of the future must be familiar with the clinical diseases caused by these pathogens, even though they are rarely seen today in clinical practice. In addition, physicians must be aware of the clues that signal that a terrorist attack may be under way.

Suggested Readings

Barlett J, Borio L, Radonovich L, et al. Smallpox vaccination in 2003: key information for clinicians. *Clin Infect Dis.* 2003;36:883–902.

Borio L, Inglesby T, Peters CJ, et al.; Working Group on Civilian Biodefense. Hemorrhagic fever viruses as biological weapons: medical and public health management. *JAMA.* 2002;287:2391–2405.

Centers for Disease Control and Prevention. Bioterrorism agents/diseases. Available at: http://www.bt.cdc.gov/agent/agentlist.asp. Accessed August 16, 2011.

Centers for Disease Control and Prevention. Recognition of illness associated with the intentional release of a biologic agent. *MMWR Morb Mortal Wkly Rep.* 2001;50:893–897.

PART III

Pathophysiology of Infectious Diseases

Chapter 58

Diagnostic Principles

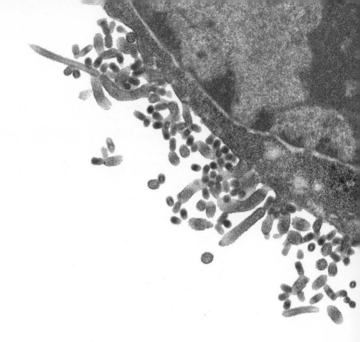

Cary Engleberg

THE ROLE of the clinical microbiology laboratory is to determine whether potential pathogens are present in tissues, body fluids, or secretions of patients and if present, to identify them. This service is indispensable to the modern clinician because information about a pathogen's identity is of critical importance in predicting the course of an infection and in guiding the selection of appropriate therapy. This information can be generated in four ways:

1. Microscopic examination of patient samples.
2. Cultivation and identification of microorganisms from patient samples.
3. Measurement of a pathogen-specific immune response in the patient.
4. Detection of pathogen-specific macromolecules in patient samples.

The extent and reliability of the information that the laboratory can provide vary depending on the nature of the pathogen. Some pathogens (e.g., *Staphylococcus aureus*) are easily detected, cultivated, identified, and characterized; others (e.g., *Toxoplasma gondii*) require extraordinary measures merely to establish their presence. However, thanks to technological advances in molecular biology, the capabilities of the modern clinical microbiology laboratory are continually expanding. New diagnostic procedures are being introduced into clinical practice at an ever-increasing pace. Clinicians need to understand the principles underlying both the new and old methods to make an informed and critical assessment of their value and reliability and to use them wisely.

ASSESSING THE PERFORMANCE OF LABORATORY TESTS

No laboratory test is perfect. Therefore, to interpret the results of tests, clinicians must have a sense of how reliable they are. When a microbiologic test correctly predicts the presence of a pathogen, the result is called **true positive**. Similarly, a negative test obtained in the absence of the pathogen is **true negative**. Inaccuracies occur either because the laboratory test is negative in the presence of the pathogen (**false negative**) or positive in the absence of the pathogen (**false positive**).

The terms *sensitivity* and *specificity*, defined in Figure 58-1, are commonly used to describe the performance and value of all diagnostic tests. The **sensitivity** of the test is the likelihood that it will be positive when the

pathogen is present. The **specificity** of the test measures the likelihood that it will be negative if the pathogen is not present.

In clinical practice, diagnostic tests with 100% sensitivity and 100% specificity do not exist. If available, a combination of tests often yields a higher level of diagnostic certainty. In addition, clinicians can use less-than-perfect tests to their advantage. Thus, a test that is very sensitive but not particularly specific can be useful in screening for the presence of an infection. For example, the so-called rapid plasma reagin (RPR) test or the Venereal Diseases Reference Laboratory (VDRL) Test is commonly used to screen patients for syphilis, even though several other infectious and noninfectious conditions can cause those tests to be false positive. However, nearly all patients who have syphilis have positive RPR tests or VDRLs after the

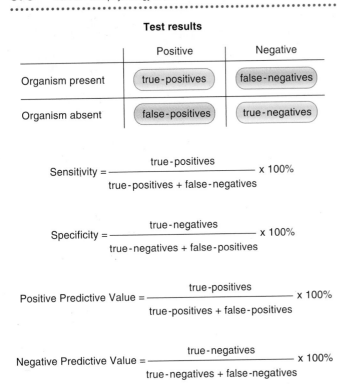

Test results

	Positive	Negative
Organism present	true-positives	false-negatives
Organism absent	false-positives	true-negatives

$$\text{Sensitivity} = \frac{\text{true-positives}}{\text{true-positives} + \text{false-negatives}} \times 100\%$$

$$\text{Specificity} = \frac{\text{true-negatives}}{\text{true-negatives} + \text{false-positives}} \times 100\%$$

$$\text{Positive Predictive Value} = \frac{\text{true-positives}}{\text{true-positives} + \text{false-positives}} \times 100\%$$

$$\text{Negative Predictive Value} = \frac{\text{true-negatives}}{\text{true-negatives} + \text{false-negatives}} \times 100\%$$

FIGURE 58-1. Definitions of terms used in evaluating diagnostic tests.

primary (chancre) stage. Therefore, either test has few false negatives and is useful to "rule out" the diagnosis of syphilis. If the RPR test or VDRL is positive, then a second, confirmatory test must be employed to determine whether syphilis is actually present. In contrast to a screening test, a confirmatory test used to "rule in" a suspected diagnosis must be highly specific. Consider the example of a patient found to have a positive enzyme immunoassay (EIA) screening test for HIV after a blood donation. A more specific (and costly) confirmatory test, the immunoblot (or "Western blot") is used to determine whether the patient actually has HIV infection or whether the screening test result was false positive.

The predictive value of a diagnostic test is influenced by the frequency of the infection in the population being tested. Because the specificity of the EIA for HIV is 99.8%, it will register as false positive in one of every 500 negative individuals tested. If less than one person in 500 in a given population is infected with HIV, then there will be more false-positive tests than true-positive tests, and the positive predictive value will be poor (see Fig. 58-1). For example, HIV infection is extremely rare among elderly women with no apparent risk factors, and a positive result in such a patient is most likely to be false positive. In contrast, in populations with a high prevalence of HIV infection—among intravenous drug users, for instance—the proportion of true-positive tests will be higher. The lesson is this: the interpretation of a laboratory test result depends not only on the technical accuracy of the method used but also on the prevalence of the infection in the

population to which the patient belongs. The positive and negative predictive values are measurements that incorporate this consideration. In contrast, the sensitivity and specificity are measurements of the accuracy of a test independent of the patient population in which it is used.

DIAGNOSING INFECTIONS BY MICROSCOPY

Because they possess characteristic morphologic features, staining properties, or movement, some pathogens can be accurately identified by direct microscopic examination of clinical material. For certain infections, microscopic diagnosis is highly sensitive and specific. It is also a rapid technique that sometimes permits the physician to initiate treatment without waiting for the results of a culture.

Most helminth and protozoal infections are routinely diagnosed by microscopy. Many fungal pathogens also have characteristic morphologic features. Notably, *Cryptococcus neoformans* meningitis is diagnosed rapidly by finding encapsulated yeast in cerebrospinal fluid (CSF). By staining the CSF background with India ink, the transparent capsule of the yeast is visualized (see Fig. 48-4). In contrast, the morphology of most bacteria is too simple to permit microscopic identification; however, a few exceptions exist. Syphilis can easily be diagnosed by observing the characteristic helical form and bending motions of spirochetes from fresh scrapings of primary or secondary lesions. Although viruses cannot be seen in the light microscope, virus-induced changes in host cell morphology may be diagnostic. Examples include the multinucleated giant cells in scrapings from herpes simplex or varicella-zoster virus lesions (the Tzanck smear) and the specific intracellular inclusion bodies in tissues that are actively infected with cytomegalovirus.

Stains

Although a species identification is rarely possible, bacterial pathogens may be visualized and assigned to morphologic and functional groups using special stains. The basic principles of the **Gram stain** and the **acid-fast stains** were described in Chapter 3. The Gram stain is both rapid and simple to perform and can be carried out on virtually any body fluid or tissue sample. It can yield clinically useful information of three kinds:

1. The presence of bacteria in a normally sterile body fluid (e.g., CSF, pleural fluid, urine)
2. Staining properties and morphology of the organisms in a sample or culture that can direct further efforts at species identification or the empirical selection of antibiotics for the patient
3. For certain clinical specimens, a diagnosis. For example, the presence of Gram-negative diplococci inside the leukocytes of urethral pus is highly specific for gonococci. The same morphologic type seen in samples of CSF is nearly always the meningococcus.

The Gram stain is much less useful when a sample is obtained from a nonsterile body site and thus contains normal microbiota. Considerable experience and skill are required to interpret Gram stains of coughed sputum specimens because they are typically contaminated with oropharyngeal bacteria that are indistinguishable from respiratory pathogens. In contrast, acid-fast bacteria (i.e., mycobacteria) are not normally found in the respiratory tract, and seeing them in a coughed sputum suggests pulmonary tuberculosis. In general, acid-fast bacteria in smears of sputum or normally sterile tissues are assumed to be *Mycobacterium tuberculosis* until proven otherwise.

A variety of other stains are used to visualize pathogens. Among the most commonly used stains are the **Giemsa stain** for systemic protozoal infections (e.g., malaria), iodine stains for intestinal helminths, and silver stains for systemic fungal pathogens. Special stains can be used to visualize the characteristic cysts of *Pneumocystis jiroveci* in a sample of bronchial fluid from an immunocompromised patient.

Antibody-Based Identification

The accuracy of microscopic identification of bacterial and viral pathogens is enhanced when **specific antibodies** are used in conjunction with direct microscopy. These procedures generally involve the attachment (or conjugation) of a detectable substance to antibody molecules so that the microscopist can see where the antibodies bind. For example, in a **direct fluorescent antibody (DFA) test** for *Cryptosporidium* protozoa, a monoclonal antibody has been conjugated to a fluorescent compound. To diagnose the infection, stool is fixed to a slide and then treated with the conjugated antibodies. After washing, the slide is examined using a **fluorescence microscope**. *Cryptosporidium* cysts appear as bright yellow–green, glowing spheres when illuminated with light of the appropriate wavelength. Because the organisms are so distinct against the dark background, they are easy to pick out when scanning the slide. The DFA technique can be used to identify any pathogen to which specific antibodies can be produced.

Clearly, the specificity of antibody-based identification of pathogens depends on the specificity of the antibodies used. Most antisera are polyclonal mixtures of antibodies that bind to different domains of different antigenic molecules (Fig. 58-2). Therefore, when polyclonal antiserum is used in a diagnostic test, the likelihood is high that unwanted cross-reactions with other microorganisms will occur. The specificity of the test may be enhanced with the use of monoclonal (monospecific) antibodies, as suggested in Figure 58-2. The principles illustrated in the figure apply to all antibody-based methods of diagnosis, including the serologic antigen detection tests described in the next few sections of this chapter.

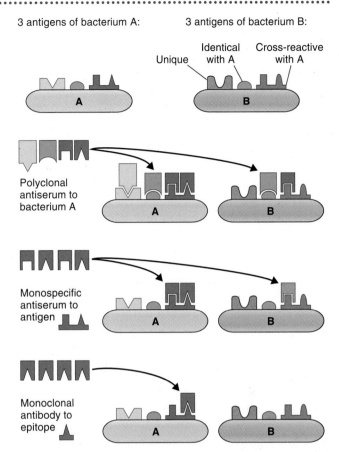

FIGURE 58-2. The cross-reactivity of three types of immunoglobulin preparations. Antibodies raised to react with bacterium A may cross-react with bacterium B. Polyclonal antisera are cross-reactive because bacteria A and B have protein antigens in common. Additionally, monospecific antiserum raised against a single antigen of bacterium A is also cross-reactive, because one of the antibody-binding sites (epitopes) on this antigen is shared by an antigen of bacterium B. However, a monoclonal antibody against an epitope on this antigen was found to be unique to bacterium A and to have no cross-reactivity.

DIAGNOSING INFECTIONS BY CULTURE

Culturing is usually the most specific way to establish the presence of a particular pathogen in a patient sample. However, in many situations, culturing may not be sensitive or clinically practical. Culture is routine for most bacterial and fungal infections but is rarely performed for helminthic and protozoal pathogens. Some microorganisms cannot be cultured at all in clinical microbiology laboratories (e.g., hepatitis viruses, *Treponema pallidum*, *Mycobacterium leprae*, and *P. jiroveci*), either because the necessary conditions for their cultivation in vitro are not yet known or because the available culture systems are inefficient and impractical. Because chlamydiae and viruses are obligate intracellular pathogens, they can be propagated and identified only in appropriate cell cultures. Cultivation of other pathogens, such as rickettsiae and mycoplasmas, is shunned by most clinical laboratories because of the hazards involved in handling the microorganisms.

General Principles

In general, the choices of culture method and medium are tailored to the nature and source of the specimen and the question that the culture is meant to address. For example, when a specimen of pus from a brain abscess is cultured, the implied question is, "What microorganisms are present in the abscess?" The assumption is that any organisms present are causative and that chemotherapy directed against them will be beneficial. To look for the etiologic agents, the sample is cultured on a variety of agar-based media and in a broth medium under both aerobic and anaerobic conditions. The culture strategy is to recover all microorganisms that might inhabit a brain abscess.

In contrast to that open-ended approach, other cultures are performed primarily to determine whether a particular pathogen is present or not. An example is the throat culture for *Streptococcus pyogenes* in cases of exudative pharyngitis, because that is the common culturable bacterial agent for which treatment is indicated. Throat swab specimens are inoculated only onto nutrient sheep's blood agar plates, which not only support the growth of streptococci but also show the characteristic β-hemolysis of *S. pyogenes*.

Cultures from nonsterile body sites present yet another problem: the inhibition or obscuring of the pathogen's growth by an abundant normal microbiota. Thus, **selective media** are needed for those cultures. An example of a selective medium is Thayer-Martin medium, used to culture gonococci. Thayer-Martin is a **chocolate agar** (made with boiled blood, not chocolate) containing antibiotics that inhibit the growth of members of the normal microbiota in the genitourinary tract but not gonococci. Selective and semiselective media are also used to cultivate enteric pathogens from the bacteria-rich stool specimens or respiratory pathogens from sputum. One disadvantage of selective media is that they can inhibit the growth of some strains of the pathogen of interest. Therefore, selective media should be used only for specimens that are likely to contain contaminating normal organisms.

As with all diagnostic methods, culture results require interpretation by the physician. In some situations (e.g., meningitis, urinary tract infection), a negative culture is quite reassuring that the etiology of the patient's problem is not a bacterial or fungal infection. In other situations, the sensitivity of culture diagnosis is relatively poor. For example, a negative culture for pneumococci does not rule out the agent as the cause of a bacterial pneumonia, because the sensitivity of sputum culture for this fastidious pathogen may be 50% or lower in some clinical settings.

Positive cultures always raise the question of whether the isolate is the actual cause of the patient's illness. In cultures from nonsterile body sites, the problem is whether the isolate represents normal microbiota (colonization) or an etiologic agent (infection). In cultures from normally sterile body sites, contamination can occur when patient samples are obtained using faulty sterile technique. Typically, specimens obtained by needle puncture are contaminated with normal skin microbiota (e.g., *Staphylococcus epidermidis*, diphtheroids, streptococci). Because these bacteria can occasionally cause true infections, the physician must consider the clinical circumstances of the individual patient to judge whether the isolate is a contaminant. In many cases it is necessary to reisolate the same organism by repeated cultures to be convinced of its significance. As another example, almost all voided urine collections have some degree of contamination; true infection is associated with a relatively high concentration of bacteria in the specimen. However, a urine sample that sits at room temperature for hours becomes grossly contaminated as the microorganisms in the specimen start growing.

Blood Culture

The simplest blood culture involves the direct inoculation of a blood sample into nutrient broth, followed by incubation at 37°C and periodic checks for an indication of microbial growth. In the past, turbidity was used as an indicator of microbial growth. However, the development of visible turbidity can take days. Modern automated blood culture systems periodically assay culture bottles for a byproduct of microbial growth (e.g., CO_2). Using such sensitive techniques, growth of organisms can be detected long before visible turbidity develops. Once growth is detected, microorganisms from cultures are transferred to agar plates, or **subcultured**, to permit species identification.

Another method that works well for fungi, mycobacteria, and certain fastidious pathogens is the **lysis–centrifugation technique**. In this method, blood is collected directly into a tube containing a solution that lyses blood cells. The remaining dense material, which includes any microorganism, is pelleted by centrifugation to the bottom of the tube, where it is removed and inoculated directly onto an appropriate agar-based medium. In addition to its increased sensitivity for some pathogens, this technique has the advantage of bypassing the usual subculture step, because the isolates grow directly as colonies on agar plates.

Culture Identification

Classically, bacteria cultured from clinical specimens are identified by determining **phenotypic properties**, such as motility; utilization of various nutrient substrates; and production of enzymes, toxins, or byproducts of metabolism. Because regrowth is required for many of the tests on bacteria, definitive identification typically requires an extra day or more.

Microorganisms in culture are sometimes identified more rapidly using **antibody-based techniques**, which are discussed in more detail in the next section. Viruses are frequently identified in culture by their reaction with specific antiviral antibodies or by the ability of a specific antiserum to neutralize them when inoculated into fresh tissue culture.

Antimicrobial Sensitivity Testing

Perhaps the most important advantage of culturing is that the isolate can be tested for susceptibility to antimicrobial agents, often the most important piece of therapeutically related information to be obtained. Antibiotic sensitivity testing of bacteria is discussed in Chapter 30. Fungal and viral pathogens can also be tested for drug susceptibility, but those tests are beyond the capabilities of most clinical microbiology laboratories.

MEASURING THE ANTIBODY RESPONSE TO INFECTION

Serologic tests measure the patient's humoral immune response to an infection. Because human serum contains many antibodies, serologic tests are designed to measure only those directed at specific microbial antigens. Some of the common formats for **serology** of infectious diseases (i.e., agglutination, complement fixation, neutralization, and indirect fluorescent antibody tests) are discussed in the electronic supplement to this chapter. In those tests and others, the amount of specific antibody present in the patient's serum is quantified by testing dilutions of the patient's serum. The highest dilution of the patient's serum that still can exert the measured function, or **endpoint**, is the positive **titer** for that assay.

Later generations of serologic tests do not measure the activity of specific antibody but measure their presence directly. Most of these tests are **solid-phase assays**, which use either the pathogen or antigens from the pathogen fixed to a solid support, such as the wells of a microtiter plate, porous membrane, or inert beads. Patient serum is added to the system, and specific antibodies are bound and immobilized to the fixed antigen. All nonreacting antibodies and serum components are washed away. The presence of the bound specific antibody is typically detected by adding a labeled antibody directed against human immunoglobulin molecules (raised in animals by immunization with human antibodies). A popular format for these tests is the **ELISA**, or **EIA** (Fig. 58-3). In an EIA, the "second antibody" is conjugated to an enzyme, such as peroxidase or alkaline phosphatase, which catalyzes the production of visibly colored compounds from colorless precursors and makes the detection far more sensitive. In addition, the second (conjugated) antibody may be made specific for IgG, IgM, or other immunoglobulins, permitting the assay to measure only antibodies of a certain class.

The specificity of a serologic test is determined largely by the character and purity of the antigen used to capture the patient's antibodies. An **immunoblot** (or **Western blot**) is one of the most specific serologic methods available because the antigens to which the patient's serum reacts are specified. In this test, the antigenic molecules from a pathogen are first separated according to their size using **electrophoresis**. The whole series of antigens is then "blotted" onto a solid support and incubated with the patient's serum (Fig. 58-4). It is then possible to determine whether the patient's antibodies are directed against pathogen-specific or cross-reactive antigens. That additional level of analysis allows the discrimination of specific and nonspecific reactions. Western blotting has become a mainstay for confirming the diagnosis of HIV infection first detected by EIA.

Serological tests for particular infectious diseases can be both sensitive and specific, but their utility in clinical management is often limited. Because the tests depend

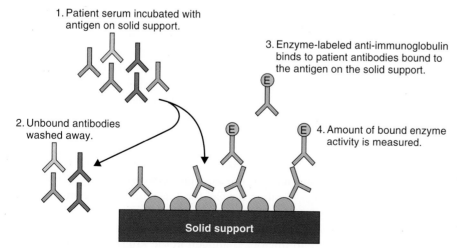

1. Patient serum incubated with antigen on solid support.

2. Unbound antibodies washed away.

3. Enzyme-labeled anti-immunoglobulin binds to patient antibodies bound to the antigen on the solid support.

4. Amount of bound enzyme activity is measured.

Solid support

FIGURE 58-3. Direct ELISA serology for the detection of specific antibodies in patient serum. (See the online supplement to view a narrated animation of this process.)

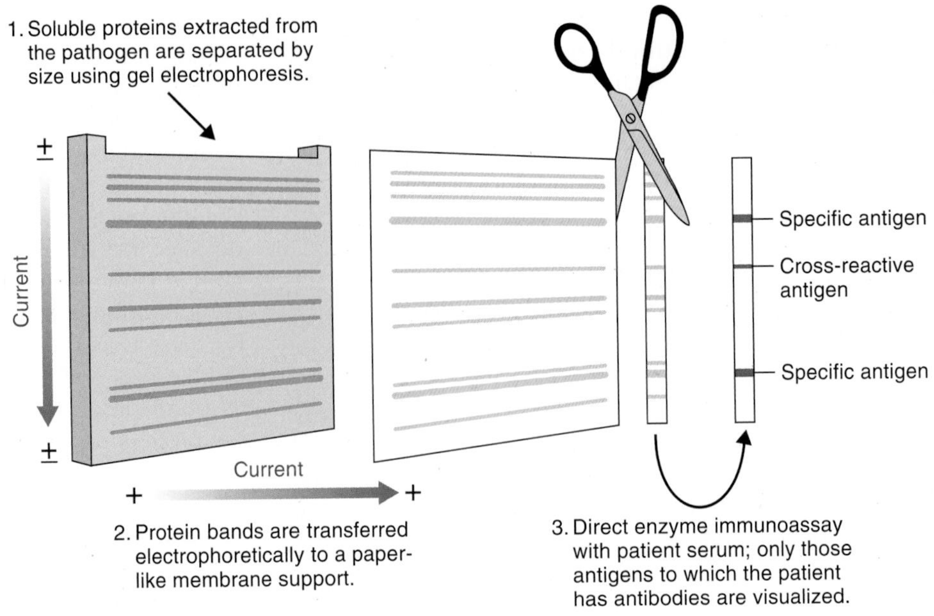

1. Soluble proteins extracted from the pathogen are separated by size using gel electrophoresis.

Current

Current

Specific antigen

Cross-reactive antigen

Specific antigen

2. Protein bands are transferred electrophoretically to a paper-like membrane support.

3. Direct enzyme immunoassay with patient serum; only those antigens to which the patient has antibodies are visualized.

FIGURE 58-4. Western blot. By noting the antigens ("bands") with which the patient serum reacts, it is possible to determine whether the reactivity is owing to specific or cross-reactive antibodies.

on the immune response to infection, they have limited use in the early diagnosis of acute infections, before the patient develops specific antibodies. Serology is typically more useful in determining whether infection with a particular pathogen has occurred in the past. The physician must decide whether the positive serology is the result of the patient's current illness or an infection that took place months or years earlier. There are two ways to make this determination. First, the patient's specific antibody titer can be measured at two points in time, usually several weeks apart (**acute and convalescent titers**). A significant increase in the amount of antibody indicates a recent or ongoing infection with the pathogen. The second way to diagnose a recent infection serologically is to measure specific **IgM antibodies** against the pathogen. In the course of most infections, IgM antibodies appear first and tend to disappear a few months after onset.

DIAGNOSING INFECTION BY DETECTING MICROBIAL MACROMOLECULES

In the investigation of a crime, a detective looks for traces left by the perpetrator. Similarly, the microbial culprit associated with an infection can often be identified by recognizing its products or parts, provided those parts are as specific for the pathogen as fingerprints are for a criminal. Identifications may be made either by detecting an **antigen** or a **nucleic acid sequence** that is specific for a pathogen. As you know from recent, celebrated criminal cases, prosecutors also use laboratory methods when traces of blood or body fluids are the available clues.

Macromolecular detection tests have inherent disadvantages and advantages compared with standard culture diagnoses. Among the disadvantages are the imperfect specificity, the inability to further study the infecting pathogen (e.g., for antimicrobial sensitivity, strain typing), and the need to perform separate tests for each suspected pathogen. Advantages include the capacity to diagnose the infection within hours rather than days and greater sensitivity in certain settings (e.g., the detection of a pathogen after treatment with antimicrobials has rendered the culture negative).

Detecting Microbial Antigens

Antigen detection tests are like serologic tests in reverse; instead of using the microbial antigen to capture antibodies from patient serum, specific antibodies are used to capture microbial antigens from a patient sample. In most of these assays, the "capture" antibody is bound to a solid support. Certain antigens, such as capsular polysaccharides, can be detected by a simple agglutination assay (Fig. 58-5). Several widely performed tests use antibody-coated latex beads (**latex agglutination tests**) to detect capsular material from *C. neoformans*, meningococcus, pneumococcus, *Haemophilus influenzae*, and others.

For many antigens, the presence of the "captured" molecule is detected using a second antibody (e.g., in the **enzyme immunoassay**; Fig. 58-6A); this test is analogous to the EIA test for antibody detection. The sample is incubated with an antibody-coated solid support, and the unbound material in the sample is washed away. An enzyme-labeled second antibody, which is also directed against the microbial antigen, is then added, forming a "**sandwich**" of the antigen between two layers of antibody. Another format for this test is the **competitive assay** (Fig. 58-6B). In these systems, the sample is coincubated with an enzyme-labeled antigen that competes with an unlabeled antigen in the sample for binding to a

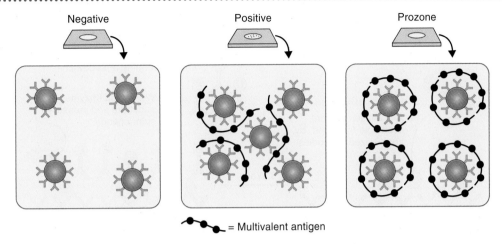

Negative   Positive   Prozone

= Multivalent antigen

FIGURE 58-5. Detection of a polyvalent antigen by particle agglutination. Particles are coated with specific antibodies. If a multivalent antigen is present in the patient sample, bridges form between the particles, causing clumping. When there is much more antigen than antibody in the mixture, a false negative, or prozone phenomenon, may occur because no bridges between beads can form. Paradoxically, a serum sample that is negative because of a prozone reaction becomes positive when it is diluted. (See the online supplement to view a narrated animation of this process.)

fixed amount of specific antibody. A positive test is one that fails to develop an enzymatic color reaction. These basic formats have been adapted to simple kits to test for several pathogens in office practice (e.g., influenza) or at home (e.g., pregnancy tests detecting human chorionic gonadotropin).

Nucleic Acid–Based Diagnosis of Infection

DNA is composed of two separate strands held together by hydrogen bonding between complementary bases. Because they are bound by relatively weak hydrogen bonds, the two strands of DNA can be separated into single strands by heating. When the temperature is again lowered, the complementary strands reconnect (or **hybridize**), reforming double-stranded DNA. Hybridization occurs only when the two strands are a genuine **complementary pair**. A short, single-stranded DNA sequence (or **probe**) can be chosen so that it hybridizes *only* to a perfectly complementary "**target**" **sequence**. The precision of this interaction accounts for the high degree of specificity of nucleic acid–based tests.

The **DNA probe test** was the first nucleic acid–based test to be used. Typically, a single-stranded DNA probe is labeled with a radioisotope, enzyme, or other detectable label, and the patient's sample is treated so that microorganisms are disrupted and DNA and RNA are released and then heat denatured (i.e., converted to single strands). The mixture of labeled probe and sample is incubated, and the amount of probe hybridized to nucleic acids is measured. The bound and unbound probes are distinguished, commonly by using probes attached to a solid support, as in the separation steps in antibody and antigen detection tests. On the microscopic level, **in situ hybridization** may be performed on tissue sections. DNA probe tests have also been used to confirm the identity of an organism grown in culture; however, they tend to be insufficiently sensitive for direct testing of patient samples for pathogens.

Nucleic Acid Amplification

In many instances, the amount of specific nucleic acid in a sample is insufficient for direct detection with a DNA probe. In such cases, it may be possible to use **nucleic acid amplification methods**, such as the **polymerase chain reaction** (**PCR**). To design a PCR test, a specific sequence of microbial nucleic acid must be known. Two short DNA probes, or **primers**, are then chemically synthesized so they will hybridize to the opposite strands of the target DNA sequence at a given distance (Fig. 58-7). In the assay, three components are added to DNA extracted from the patient's specimen: the two primers, deoxyribonucleotides (deoxynucleotide triphosphates, or dNTPs), and a heat-stable DNA polymerase. The reactants are subjected to repeated cycles of temperature shifts that result in denaturation of DNA (heating), hybridization of the primers (cooling), and DNA synthesis. In each cycle of the reaction, the DNA spanned by the two primers is duplicated. With the synthesis of each new strand of DNA, new primer-binding sites are generated. Consequently, each new strand becomes a new template for subsequent rounds of primer-initiated synthesis.

With every cycle of the PCR, the number of copies of the DNA segment between the primers doubles, thus

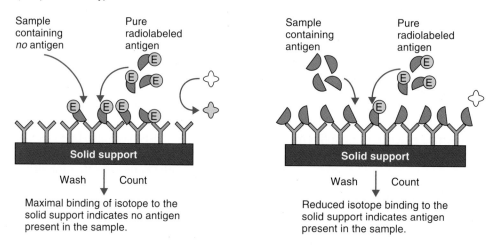

A. ELISA for antigen detection
(direct "sandwich" assay)

1. Add patient sample.

2. Any antigen present in sample "captured" by immobilized antibodies.

3. Wash.

Solid support

4. Enzyme-conjugated specific antibody added; binds to antigen, forming a "sandwich."

5. Wash; add enzyme substrate and measure color change.

Solid support

B. Enzyme immunoassay for antigen detection
(competitive assay)

Sample containing *no* antigen

Pure radiolabeled antigen

Solid support

Wash | Count

Maximal binding of isotope to the solid support indicates no antigen present in the sample.

Sample containing antigen

Pure radiolabeled antigen

Solid support

Wash | Count

Reduced isotope binding to the solid support indicates antigen present in the sample.

FIGURE 58-6. Enzyme immunoassays for microbial antigen detection. A. In the "sandwich" assay format of the test, "capture" antibody bound to a solid support binds antigen from the patient sample. Nonspecific contents of the sample are washed away. The presence of the captured antigen is detected using a second, specific antibody conjugated to an enzyme. Lastly, the activity of the enzyme bound to the solid support is measured using a color-producing substrate; color production signals the presence of the antigen, which is sandwiched between the two antibodies. **B.** In the competitive assay format, the patient sample is coincubated with a measured, small amount of purified, enzyme-labeled antigen over the same captured antibody solid support. If the patient sample contains no antigen, all the labeled antigens will complex with the antibody, and all the added enzyme-labeled antigen will be bound in immune complexes. If the patient sample contains antigen, it will compete with the labeled antigen for binding to the available antibody, and there will be minimal enzyme associated with immune complexes. (See the online supplement to view a narrated animation of this process.)

doubling the templates for further synthesis. This "chain reaction" results in the geometric increase in the amounts of target DNA. In this respect, PCR is analogous to the biological process of DNA replication that occurs in populations of dividing cells; however, in PCR, the exponential synthesis is limited to the DNA segment bounded by the two synthetic primers. In early version of PCR, the amplified sequences (or **amplicons**) were analyzed by gel electrophoresis as fragments of a predicted size or "captured" and detected by conventional DNA probe hybridization. Commercial nucleic acid amplification assays now in common use include tests to detect the presence of *M. tuberculosis* in a sputum sample, *Pneumocystis* in respiratory secretions, herpes simplex virus or enterovirus in CSF, and *Chlamydia trachomatis* or *N. gonorrhoeae* in a urine specimen or cervical swab, among others.

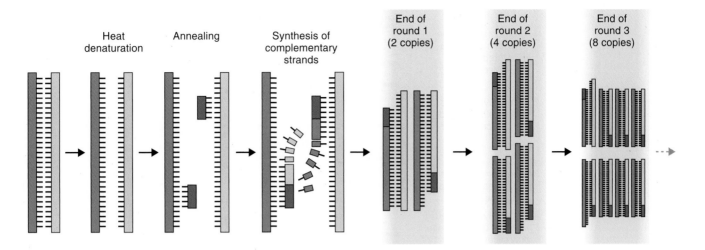

FIGURE 58-7. Nucleic acid amplification: the polymerase chain reaction (PCR). The patient sample is mixed with specific primers, deoxynucleotide triphosphates (dNTPs), and a thermostable DNA polymerase enzyme. The reaction involves three steps repeated in sequence: (1) heat denaturation, which permits complementary strands of the target DNA to separate; (2) annealing, as the primers hybridize to opposite strands of the targeted sequence when the temperature is lowered; and (3) synthesis, as the polymerase incorporates the dNTPs into a new complementary strand of DNA, in a sequential and unidirectional manner, beginning at each hybridized primer. Note that synthesis from either primer generates a new site to which the opposite primer can hybridize in the next cycle. Each time this cycle is repeated, the number of double-stranded target DNA sequences available to bind the two primers doubles. One target DNA molecule subjected to 30 repetitions of the PCR would result in 2^{30} copies of the target sequence. The products of the reaction are detected by gel electrophoresis or by a gene probe specific for the sequences between the two primers. (See the online supplement to view a narrated animation of this process.)

The detection of PCR products has been simplified in a quantitative version of the assay, called "**real-time**" **PCR** or **qPCR** (i.e., quantitative PCR). One popular version of the technique employs a fluorescent-labeled probe that hybridizes to the newly synthesized amplicons (Fig. 58-8A). The typical result of this method and others is that the intensity of the fluorescence in the reaction vessel increases as more amplicons are generated. Thus, qPCR adds two important features to the process: First, it combines the steps of amplification and amplicon analysis into a single process, simplifying the analysis of the amplicons. Second, it offers the possibility of quantifying the target nucleic acid sequence in the original sample by measuring the number of cycles required to reach a threshold of fluorescence detection (Fig. 58-8B). Quantitative PCR is now routinely used to detect and measure viruses in human fluid samples (e.g., HIV, cytomegalovirus, Epstein-Barr virus, hepatitis viruses).

The great power of PCR is its sensitivity. Theoretically, the chain reaction can be initiated by a single copy of the target sequence. However, the procedure's exquisite sensitivity is also its major drawback as a clinical diagnostic tool. A serious potential for cross-contamination (microcontamination) exists in laboratories that process many similar samples every day. The prevention of false-positive PCR results is a matter of great concern to physicians and lawyers because no equally sensitive, alternate method may be available to verify a positive PCR result. The most celebrated example of that pitfall occurred in the murder trial of O. J. Simpson, in which questions about mishandling of specimens and cross-contamination of evidence may have influenced the verdict. To avoid cross-contamination in clinical diagnostic laboratories, specimen preparation and amplification are performed in separate areas. Another strategy is to incorporate modified nucleotides in the PCR so as to render the products (amplicons) susceptible to enzymatic degradation should they contaminate a patient sample.

Microarrays

A disadvantage of nucleic acid–based tests and antigen detection assays is that they can tell the physician only whether a particular pathogen is present in a sample. As a diagnostic tool, bacterial culture has an advantage over those methods because it does not require the physician to guess which pathogens may be present and to test for each individually. One culture can detect an enormous variety of pathogenic organisms by a single method. Advances in microchip technology have created the possibility of using nonculture diagnostics in a similar manner. A microchip can be printed to contain hundreds of oligonucleotide probes bound in an array no bigger than a microscopic slide.

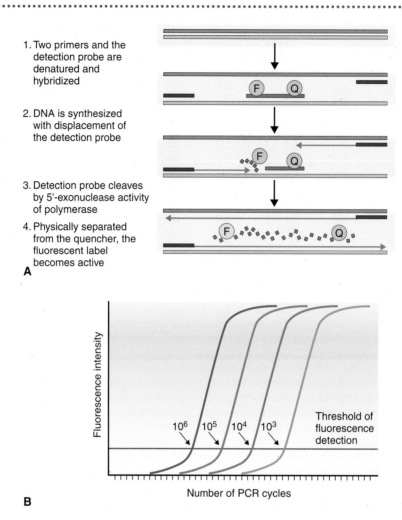

1. Two primers and the detection probe are denatured and hybridized

2. DNA is synthesized with displacement of the detection probe

3. Detection probe cleaves by 5'-exonuclease activity of polymerase

4. Physically separated from the quencher, the fluorescent label becomes active

A

B

FIGURE 58-8. Real-time PCR. A. In the TaqMan (Applied Biosystems) procedure for confirming and quantifying PCR products, the PCR vessel contains target DNA (*pink and lavender*), primers (*dark purple*), and a DNA detection probe that hybridizes specifically to the amplified sequence (*blue*). Conjugated to this detection probe are a fluorescent dye and a fluorescence quencher in close proximity to one another, such that the fluorescence from the dye is quenched and is undetectable. As DNA synthesis proceeds, the 5'-exonuclease activity of the polymerase digests the detection probe, releasing the fluorescent dye and the quencher. As they separate from one another, the fluorescent dye becomes active and emits a signal. With each round of PCR, more detection probes hybridize and are cleaved, increasing the fluorescent signal geometrically until all of the primers and probes are exhausted. **B.** Fluorescent signals obtained with real-time PCRs beginning with decreasing quantities of target DNA. As the number of copies of target DNA decrease, the fluorescence curve shifts to the right. For quantitative PCR, a standard curve can be generated by determining how many cycles of PCR are required to exceed a predetermined threshold for fluorescence detection (purple horizontal line). By reference to these standards, the number of target nucleic acid molecules in a patient sample can be determined. (See the online supplement to view a narrated animation of this process.)

Since bacteria have many conserved sequences (e.g., 16S ribosomal RNA) with intervening, nonconserved regions, it is theoretically possible to design PCR primers that will amplify a product from any bacterial species, albeit with different amplified sequences between the primers. Imagine that DNA extracted from a patient sample is incubated with these primers in a PCR. The products of such a reaction could then be hybridized with a microarray containing the known intervening sequences from hundreds of bacterial species. It would then be possible to determine which one (or ones) is (are) present in the patient sample (Fig. 58-9).

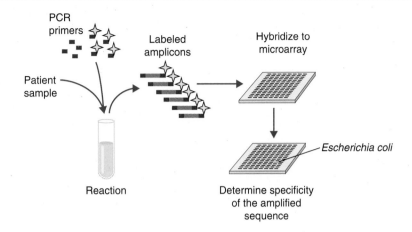

FIGURE 58-9. Oligonucleotide microarray analysis to identify specific products of a nonspecific PCR amplification. In this theoretical assay, PCR is conducted using primers that bind to all bacterial chromosomes but amplify intervening sequences that are different in each species. During the amplification process, the amplicons are labeled with a fluorescent dye–conjugated primer. Finally, the amplicons are hybridized to a microarray that has bound oligonucleotides representing the inventing sequences from hundreds of bacterial species. In this case, the amplicons bind to the sequences characteristic of *Escherichia coli*, identifying *E. coli* as the bacteria in the original sample.

CONCLUSION

Many techniques are available to establish the presence of a pathogenic microorganism in an ill patient. All methods have the potential for inaccuracy, either in failing to detect a pathogen or immune response when present or in signaling their presence when the pathogen or the immune response is absent. Some tests are more sensitive or more specific than others, and those measures of performance determine how and when they are used. However, even when a test accurately analyzes a given sample, the simple presence of a microorganism in the specimen or of antibodies against a pathogen in patient serum does not always indicate active infection, nor does it necessarily establish the cause of illness. Therefore, interpretation is always necessary with any microbiologic test, regardless of its technical performance characteristics. In the final analysis, there is no substitute for the interpretive skills of the clinician in placing microbiologic test results into the context of the patient's illness.

Suggested Readings

Andreotti PE, Ludwig GV, Peruski AH, Tuite et al. Immunoassay of infectious agents. *Biotechniques*. 2003;35:850–859.

Bodrossy L, Sessitsch A. Oligonucleotide microarrays in microbial diagnostics. *Curr Opin Microbiol*. 2004;7:245–254.

Boehme CC, Nabeta P, Hilleman D, et al. Rapid molecular detection of tuberculosis and rifampin resistance. *N Engl J Med*. 2010;363:1005–1015.

Relman DA. Microbial genomics and infectious diseases. *N Engl J Med*. 2011;365:347–57.

Tenover FC. Developing molecular amplification methods for rapid diagnosis of respiratory tract infections caused by bacterial pathogens. *Clinic Infect Dis*. 2011;52(suppl 4):S338–S345.

Winn WC, Allen SD, Janda WM, Koneman EW, et al. eds. *Koneman's Color Atlas and Textbook of Diagnostic Microbiology*. 6th ed. Philadelphia, PA: Lippincott Williams & Wilkins; 2005.

Chapter 59

Principles of Epidemiology

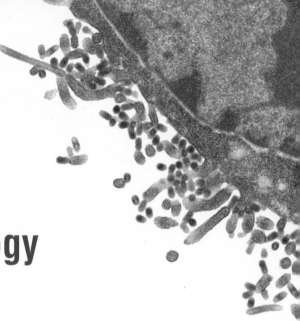

Christian B. Ramers

EPIDEMIOLOGY is the study of the determinants of disease in a population. Epidemiologists deal with both infectious and noninfectious etiologies. When infectious agents are involved, the aim is to understand their mode of transmission and what predisposes a population to a particular agent. The practical purpose of epidemiology is to control the spread of disease in a population, either by limiting microbial transmission or by altering the susceptibility of a population through public health interventions. Common control measures include removing the source of the agent, active surveillance of suspected cases, control of transmission through quarantine or personal protective measures, and protection of the population through immunization or prophylactic treatment with antibiotics.

This chapter considers epidemiological concepts and methods through the examination of an epidemiological "case," the investigation of a new disease. Following the case discussion, the chapter considers general epidemiological issues. However, before considering a case, the reader should review some of the key terms that are commonly used in the field of epidemiology (Table 59-1).

EPIDEMIOLOGICAL METHODOLOGY

This group of Connecticut epidemiologists undertook what is known as an **epidemic investigation**, the study of the extent, characteristics, mode of transmission, and etiology of a cluster of cases of a specific disease. It is one of the most useful methods of infectious disease epidemiology, but it is by no means the only one. Others, including **case–control studies**, **cohort studies**, and **epidemiological interventions**, used in investigating both infectious and noninfectious diseases are discussed later in this chapter.

An epidemic investigation is typically undertaken when the number of cases of a disease increases over what is considered to be the norm or standard. In the Connecticut study, it was necessary to determine first if the arthritis cases did indeed represent an epidemic.

CASE • In October 1975, the Department of Health of Connecticut received separate calls from two mothers living on rural roads in the towns of Lyme and Old Lyme. They reported that several children in their households and their neighborhoods had what appeared to be arthritis. They had voiced their concern to local physicians and were not deterred by being told that arthritis is "not infectious."

This case raises several questions:

1. Were the cases reported in the two towns related?

2. Did any other people in either town have similar symptoms?

3. Did the children have an infectious form of arthritis?

4. What steps should epidemiologists take, and what principles should they apply to studying the reported cases, after discussions with the parents and local physicians?

See Appendix for answers.

TABLE 59-1 Terms Used in Epidemiology

Term	Definition	Example
Attack Rate	The proportion of persons who are exposed to a disease agent who become clinically ill from that agent, such as during an epidemic	Some pathogens transmitted by the respiratory route such as measles and varicella have a very high attack rate among vulnerable hosts.
Bias	Any trend in the collection, analysis, interpretation, publication, or review of data that can lead to conclusions that are systematically different from the truth	Clinical trials that are not blinded and do not use placebo controls may be biased because researchers and patients may expect to get better with a certain treatment.
Case-fatality rate	The proportion of persons with a particular condition (cases) who die from that condition	Rabies has one of the highest case-fatality rates of any infection, since only a few individuals have ever survived.
Case-control	A type of observational analytic study that enrolls "cases" that have a disease and "controls" that do not have the disease. Characteristics such as previous exposures are then compared between cases and controls.	Outbreak investigations are a form of case–control study since usually characteristics of disease cases are compared with healthy controls to figure out which exposure contributed to the outbreak.
Cohort	A type of observational analytic study in which a well-defined group of people with common exposures are followed through time. Disease, death, or other health-related outcomes are then ascertained and compared.	The Framingham cohort is a large study that has followed individuals from Framingham, MA, for many years to determine the incidence of many diseases such as cardiovascular disease.
Epidemic	The occurrence of more cases of disease than expected in a given area or among a specific group of people over a particular period of time	An unusually high number of *Cryptosporidium* cases in Milwaukee, WI, in 1993 alerted public health officials of an epidemic related to contaminated water.
Epidemic curve	A histogram that shows the course of a disease outbreak or epidemic by plotting the number of cases by time of onset.	See Figure 59-1 for the epidemic curve of a disease in Lyme, CT.
Incidence	The frequency of new cases of illness in a population over a period of time	In the United States, the incidence of new HIV infections was ~48,100 in 2009.
Incubation period	A period of subclinical or inapparent pathologic changes following exposure, ending with the onset of symptoms of infectious disease	Toxin-mediated food poisoning has a much shorter incubation period than invasive disease because often the toxin is preformed in the food that is consumed.
Pandemic	An epidemic occurring over a very wide area (several countries or continents) and usually affecting a large proportion of the population	In 2009, the World Health Organization declared an H1N1 influenza pandemic, in which nearly every country identified cases.
Prevalence	The amount of a particular disease present in a population at a single point in time	The prevalence of HIV infection in the United States is roughly 1.1 million individuals.
Risk factor	A personal behavior, lifestyle, exposure, or inherited characteristic that is associated with an increased occurrence of disease or other health-related event or condition	The use of injection drugs is an important risk factor for Hepatitis C infection.
Vector	An animate intermediary in the indirect transmission of an agent that carries the agent from a reservoir to a susceptible host	The *Anopheles* mosquito is the vector for malaria transmission.
Zoonosis	An infectious disease that is transmissible under normal conditions from animals to humans	Brucellosis is a zoonosis that can be transmitted through unpasteurized goat or sheep milk.

The determination of an epidemic depends solely on the background incidence of the disease in the population and not on an absolute cutoff point. For example, before the advent of the polio vaccine in the 1950s, about 50,000 cases of the disease occurred in the United States annually. After the vaccine was put into widespread use, the number of cases dropped dramatically to about 10 per year. Therefore, one or two cases of polio after widespread vaccination might be considered an epidemic.

In addition to epidemics, epidemiologists study **endemic** and **pandemic** diseases. An endemic infectious disease is one that is consistently found in the population, such as dental caries, gonorrhea, or athlete's foot. A pandemic is a worldwide epidemic; examples are the current global AIDS pandemic and the H1N1 influenza "swine flu" pandemic of 2009.

Case Definition

The investigators of the cases of arthritis in Connecticut began by asking whether other individuals had the same disease. They first had to establish a set of clinical criteria known as the **case definition**. After all, many people have arthritis. From the mothers, physicians, and school nurses in the area, they obtained a list of other individuals who may have had the same symptoms. After examining those people and taking careful histories, the epidemiologists included, as fitting the case definition, individuals with the following clinical picture: a sudden onset of swelling and pain in a knee or other large joint lasting a week to several months, several attacks that recurred several times at intervals over a few months, and/or fever and fatigue.

Time, Place, and Personal Characteristics of Patients

Armed with a usable case definition, the investigators found other cases in Old Lyme and two adjacent towns. The best sources of additional cases were the two determined mothers who had made the original phone calls. From current and past episodes, the investigators collected 51 cases that conformed to the case definition. They could now try to identify the risk factors for the clinical syndrome by carefully determining what epidemiologists call the time, place, and personal characteristics of the cases. The **time characteristics** include the **time of onset** of the disease and its **duration**. As shown in the **epidemic curve** in Figure 59-1, many of the Connecticut cases clustered in the summer and early fall. The duration of each bout of the disease varied from a week to a few months, and 69% of the patients had recurrences of the symptoms. Not knowing at the time the etiology of the disease, the investigators could not determine another important time characteristic, the **incubation period**, or the interval from exposure to the first onset of symptoms.

Place characteristics are primarily the site of residence and the area in which the patients lived. For occupation-related illnesses, the workplace is another location to

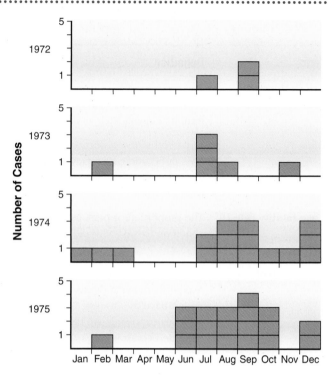

FIGURE 59-1. Clustering of cases of Lyme disease in three towns in Connecticut (Lyme, Old Lyme, and East Haddam) between 1972 and 1975.

consider. The Connecticut cases were concentrated in three adjacent towns on the eastern side of the Connecticut River. Most of the patients lived in wooded areas near streams and lakes. **Personal characteristics** include the age and sex of the patients and any possible genetic predisposition to the disease. Of the 51 Connecticut cases, 39 were children, nearly evenly divided by gender. No familial pattern was discerned, arguing against a genetic etiology.

Using the information they gathered on time, place, and personal characteristics, the epidemiologists listed the cases by times of onset and constructed what is called an **epidemic curve (Fig. 59-1)**. They dubbed the outbreak Lyme arthritis, although that name was later modified to Lyme disease.

The epidemiologists now posed other questions. Was the outbreak a surveillance artifact resulting from the many questions about arthritis that were being asked by outsiders? Did they introduce **bias** by drawing so much attention to this area? The simplest way to assess that possibility was to go elsewhere and ask the same questions. By surveying towns on the other side of the Connecticut River, the investigators determined that increased interest did not result in an increase in the number of cases of arthritis reported. In their early investigation, the epidemiologists wondered how common Lyme disease might be. Assessing the **attack rate** of an epidemic disease requires knowing the total number of cases (the numerator) and the total number of people who are "at risk" (the denominator). In the context of many confined outbreaks, it is possible to make that calculation. For example, if

25 of 125 guests who attended a wedding later developed staphylococcal food poisoning from eating the potato salad, the attack rate is 20% (i.e., 25 divided by 125).

In the first Lyme disease investigation, neither the total number of cases nor the number of at-risk persons was known. However, surveillance for the infection in subsequent years has yielded case reports from each state that can be used to calculate the local risk of Lyme disease in the United States. Those data can be reported as an **incidence** (the number of cases during a defined time period divided by the population of the state during that time) or as a **prevalence** (the total number of cases at any given time). For example, we now know that the annual incidence of Lyme disease in Connecticut (from 1992 to 1998) was 68 per 100,000 population, whereas in neighboring Massachusetts, the annual incidence was only 5 per 100,000 population, an almost 12-fold lower risk.

Is Lyme Disease Communicable?

The investigating team then asked, "Is this an infectious disease?" The most common arthritic conditions of childhood, such as juvenile rheumatoid arthritis, are collagen vascular problems and are not known to be infectious. Nonetheless, the clustering of cases in the summer or early fall, and most patients living in wooded areas along lakes or streams, suggested transmission through a **vector** such as an insect or tick. If so, the investigators wondered, "Is the disease new?" Many infectious diseases, like measles, polio, and tuberculosis, are **communicable**. Others, like a ruptured appendix, urinary tract infections, or osteomyelitis, are not. Was Lyme disease communicable, or did it merely affect susceptible individuals? To answer that question, the investigators attempted to trace contacts; but even in families with several affected members, the onset of illness had usually taken place in different years. When they tried to identify a common exposure, they could not find any. However, an intriguing clue surfaced. About one-quarter of the patients had reported that the symptoms of arthritis were preceded by an unusual skin rash. The rash had started as a red spot that spread to form a 6-inch ring. What was the connection? An astute dermatology consultant remembered that similar rashes had been described in 1910 in Sweden and had been attributed to tick bites. The rash went by the impressive name of erythema chronicum migrans.

The investigators undertook a **case–control study** in 1977, in which the cases are matched with a similar group of control or unaffected persons. Note that case–control studies are always **retrospective**; that is, they begin by defining groups of ill or well subjects and then look to the past for potential exposures or **risk factors** that were more common among the ill than the well subjects. After matching for age, sex, and any other relevant factors, the epidemiologists found that those affected by Lyme disease were more likely to live in households with pets and thus were more likely to come in contact with the ticks that dogs and cats picked up in the woods of that region. In a roundabout way, that clue became more credible when the investigators remembered the suggestive clinical finding of the Swedish researchers.

So far, the connection between the rash and Lyme disease depended on **retrospective evidence**, which is subject to more **bias** because it depends on collecting exposure data from people who already know they are ill. To make the connection stronger, it became appropriate to ask if patients with the signs of erythema chronicum migrans progressed to develop Lyme disease. In 1977, the team set up a **prospective study**, looking for patients with the rash and observing them **prospectively** for some time. That type of study is referred to as a **cohort study** since the individuals included in the cohort have specific characteristics in common but have not yet developed the disease of interest. In contrast to the case–control approach, a cohort study defines subjects by their clinical characteristics and exposures and then follows the subjects to determine who becomes ill and who remains well. In the Connecticut study, 19 of 32 new cases of erythema chronicum migrans progressed to Lyme disease.

Meanwhile, the "tick connection" became even more plausible after a thorough entomological survey. After collecting insects and ticks from Lyme and the surrounding areas, the investigators found that adult ticks were 16 times more abundant on the east side of the Connecticut River than on the west side. That finding corresponded roughly to the incidence of cases of Lyme disease in the two areas. In addition, many more tick bites were reported by the arthritis patients than by their neighbors without the disease. Thus, the tick–rash–arthritis connection seemed more and more plausible. The final proof of the investigators' scheme awaited the discovery of the etiological agent and the direct demonstration of its transmission by ticks.

At the same time, a **surveillance network** had been set up in Connecticut and parts of the adjacent states to gather information about other cases. A careful study revealed that, contrary to the early reports, the disease was more frequent in adults than in children. It was easier to recognize arthritis as an unusual occurrence in children. Many arthritis patients had serious manifestations, such as neurological dysfunction and myocarditis. Thus, the disease turned out to be considerably more complex than described by the original case definition. That illustrates an important epidemiological point: an early case definition is, by necessity, tentative and may be modified when the full spectrum of the disease becomes known. As an example of a complex case definition, consider the one developed for AIDS.

Search for the Etiological Agent

So far, the investigators hypothesized that Lyme disease was an infection, most likely transmitted by ticks. It appeared to be a new clinical entity. However, the search for the etiological agent had proved unproductive. Despite many attempts, no laboratory had succeeded in isolating a virus, which at the time seemed to be a good candidate for being the agent of the disease. On the other hand, the investigators collected anecdotal evidence that tetracycline, erythromycin, and penicillin were clinically effective. With time, more physicians reported the beneficial effects of antibiotics, making a bacterial etiology more likely. At about that time, in 1979 and 1980, entomologists and microbiologists at the Rocky Mountain Public Health Laboratory in Montana, who were experts in tickborne diseases, examined ticks sent from the affected area and found that the gut of many specimens contained unusual spirochetes. Were those the agents of Lyme disease?

Using a culture medium that supports the growth of tickborne or louseborne spirochetes, the microbiologists succeeded in growing a newly recognized spirochete. Soon thereafter they isolated the spirochete from human cases, and the immune responses of patients were linked to that organism. The spirochete was classified in the *Borrelia* genus, a group that includes the agent of another tickborne disease also found in the United States, relapsing fever. The agent of Lyme disease was given the name *B. burgdorferi*, in honor of the entomologist who discovered the organism in the ticks.

Once the organism was identified, a diagnostic test of exposure to the infection was developed. Investigators in many parts of the world could carry out serological surveys, or **serosurveys**, to determine the proportion of persons with antibodies to *B. burgdorferi*. In general, serosurveys enable investigators to recognize a wide range of clinical manifestations, from asymptomatic cases to full-blown disease. That recognition is important because in most infectious diseases, there are many more asymptomatic than clinically overt cases. The use of serosurveys has led to diagnoses of Lyme disease in other parts of the United States, especially on both coasts, as well as in Canada, Europe, Asia, and Australia. It is considered a serious disease, mainly because of its important and chronic neurological manifestations.

Prevention Strategies

After the agent was confirmed, investigators set about attempting to develop a vaccine against disease. That process was complicated and required knowledge of the immunology of infection and the role of the outer membrane proteins of *B. burgdorferi* and the establishment of animal models of infection with demonstrated protection. As with many infectious agents, a vaccine would be one way to prevent future cases of Lyme disease. In fact, a vaccine against the disease was developed and was shown to be effective, but manufacturers have stopped development because of concern about the potential risk of arthritis resulting from vaccine administration. Liability issues led to the vaccine becoming unavailable. Alternative prevention strategies, such as public health awareness of exposure, examination for tick bites or tick attachment, and use of a short course of antibiotics after exposure,

have been shown to be effective in diminishing the risk of infection. Reducing the overabundant deer population through authorized deer hunting has been a controversial means of indirectly controlling *B. burgdorferi* transmission.

The puzzle of "Lyme arthritis" had been solved. A few years after the original phone calls, a new disease was described, its agent and mode of transmission were identified, and preventive and therapeutic measures had been instituted. Note that it took the joint efforts of epidemiologists, clinicians, entomologists, microbiologists, and alert and determined members of the public.

ROUTES OF TRANSMISSION
Humans as Reservoirs

We now turn from a specific example to a more general consideration of epidemiological principles. These principles include the routes of transmission, incubation periods, communicability, and individual susceptibility. The first is the mode of transmission (Table 59-2). **Transmission from human to human** may take place from parent to offspring or between mature individuals. **Vertical transmission** refers to the passage of an agent from an infected mother to her fetus or infant. Examples of such congenitally acquired diseases are syphilis and rubella. A newborn can also pick up chlamydiae, gonococci, cytomegalovirus, or hepatitis B virus during passage through the birth canal. Other organisms are transmitted through breast milk.

Horizontal transmission can be among individuals in close proximity and involves sexual intercourse, hand-to-hand contact, and spread via droplet or aerosol (e.g., coughing, sneezing) The actual path of an organism from one person to another depends on the way the agent exits the body of the donor. Thus, bacteria or viruses that infect the respiratory tract are often expelled as aerosols during coughing and even talking, and may be inhaled by bystanders. If the organism is resistant to drying, as is the case with the tubercle bacillus, the danger of inhalation can persist for a long time. Intestinal pathogens often cause diarrhea, which increases their distribution in the environment through oral–fecal contact and, under conditions of poor sanitation, results in contaminated drinking water and foodstuffs.

Some diseases are acquired by breaching the skin or mucous membranes by trauma, insect bites, blood transfusions, or contaminated hypodermic needles. Agents transmitted in this fashion include the HIV or hepatitis B and C viruses. Many of the agents that are transmitted by insect **vectors** have different life cycles in the vector and in the host. Note that some of these organisms may be transmitted by more than one of these routes. For example, HIV infection can be transmitted vertically from mother to child, by sexual intercourse, or by the use of needles.

TABLE 59-2 Modes of Transmission

Mode	Example	Factor	Route of Entry
Direct Contact			
Respiratory aerosol	Influenza	Crowding?	Lung
	Tuberculosis	Household	Lung
Nasal secretions	Respiratory syncytial virus	Household, nosocomial	Upper respiratory tract
Droplets	Meningococcus	Crowding	Nasopharynx
Skin	*Streptococcus* (impetigo)	Crowding	Skin
Semen	HIV	Sexual contact	Mucous membrane
Transplacental	Hepatitis B	Carrier	Mother
Indirect Contact			
Blood	Hepatitis B	Transfusion, needlestick	Blood
	HIV	Transfusion	Blood
Stool	Hepatitis A	Ingestion	Gastrointestinal tract
Animal	*Salmonella* infection	Ingestion	Gastrointestinal tract
Inanimate	*Legionella* infection	Water contamination	Respiratory tract
Arthropod Vector			
Tick	Lyme disease	Bite	Skin, blood
Mosquito	Malaria	Bite	Blood

Nonhuman Reservoirs

Other diseases are acquired from **nonhuman reservoirs**. These include the **zoonoses** (Chapter 73), in which the reservoir is an animal. Transmission from the animal may be direct, as in the bite from a rabid dog, or through insect vectors, as in the plague or the viral encephalitides. Lyme disease is another zoonosis; its natural reservoir is mice, and the infection is transmitted to humans by a tick that feeds on mice, deer, and a variety of other mammalian hosts. Indirect transmission can result from contact with a contaminated environment, such as with rodent excreta in the hantavirus outbreak in the southwestern United States.

In other diseases, the reservoir is the **inanimate environment** and the organisms live freely in nature. For example, *Clostridium tetani*, the bacteria that causes tetanus, can be found in soil and is encountered whenever dirt enters a deep wound. In addition, humans or animals can contribute to the frequency with which the agents are found in nature. The cholera bacilli grow naturally in warm estuaries, probably on the surface of shellfish, but contamination from human feces can help the organisms become established in a previously unaffected area.

INCUBATION PERIODS AND COMMUNICABILITY

The length of the **incubation period** differs considerably among infectious diseases, from a few hours to months and years (Table 59-3). Many host and exposure factors can influence the incubation period. For example, a large infective dose can shorten it, and a small one can lengthen it. To epidemiologists, the incubation period is particularly important because some diseases can be transmitted from asymptomatic patients during that time. Control of transmission may therefore rely on special surveillance methods that include infected but asymptomatic persons. The periods of incubation and of communicability are not always the same. For example, the incubation period in hepatitis A usually ranges from 2 to 6 weeks. However, individuals can transmit the virus for only 1 or 2 weeks before the onset of the disease.

The period of communicability may extend long after the disease symptoms abate, as in the case of a **chronic carrier**. For example, hepatitis B carriers can usually transmit the virus for the length of time they carry it. Many of the preceding chapters have discussed the carrier state at some length (see Chapters 14, 17, 27, 38, 41, and 42).

TABLE 59-3 Incubation Periods

Disease	Range of Period
Staphylococcal food poisoning	1–6 h
Clostridial food poisoning	12–24 h
Hepatitis A	14–42 d
Hepatitis B	30–180 d
Gonorrhea	2–9 d
Salmonellosis	0.5–3 d
Epstein-Barr virus infection	21–49 d
Mycoplasma pneumoniae infection	8–21 d
Varicella-zoster virus	10–21 d
AIDS	21 d to 5 y or more
Leprosy	7 mo to 5 y

INDIVIDUAL SUSCEPTIBILITY

Humans differ in their susceptibility to infectious diseases. For instance, some individuals seem more prone to respiratory or intestinal infections than are most people. Often, the reason for this variability is unknown or related to the subtle and complex genetic variability that makes us each a unique individual with a unique immune system. However, there are several specific immunodeficiencies of which the clinician should be aware, as they may portend specific patterns of risk for infection. When the immune deficiency becomes more severe and the risks more evident, the specific etiology is often easier to ascertain.

Epidemiologists must be aware of the various susceptibilities of members of the general population. Age, sex, nutritional status, previous exposure, and immune competence all influence susceptibility to a particular infectious disease. For instance, children and older persons frequently are more likely to contract bacterial pneumonia or intestinal infections. The incidence of the carrier state of hepatitis B is greater in males than in females. It is also more frequent among individuals with Down syndrome or those receiving hemodialysis.

Genetic factors are also known to play a role in susceptibility, although the mechanisms by which specific genes contribute are just now being determined. Why do some colonized patients develop overwhelming meningococcal disease, for instance, and others do not? The importance of genetic factors is often difficult to differentiate from a myriad of socioeconomic factors that might contribute to the state of health and nutrition. Nonetheless, the role of genetic factors has been well established in certain diseases. It has been shown, for example, that

among identical twins living apart, when one twin contracted tuberculosis, the other had a greater chance than average of getting the disease. Nonidentical twins did not show that pattern. One of the most intensively studied genetic effects is the decreased susceptibility to malaria of persons with the sickle cell trait (see Chapter 52). It is also well established that nonwhites are more prone to the disseminated form of the fungal disease coccidioidomycosis than are whites.

PRACTICAL ASPECTS OF EPIDEMIOLOGY

In our global society, epidemiology has become extremely important in monitoring disease incidence and responding quickly to new and unexpected outbreaks. The practicing physician and all members of the health care team must be aware of the public health implications of a given patient's infectious disease. To safeguard both the public interest and individual rights to privacy, a considerable body of local and national laws has been developed in most countries of the world. For instance, in the United States, **certain communicable diseases are notifiable**; that is, physicians are obliged to report cases to the U.S. Public Health Service. Typically this is accomplished through case-report forms that are collected and monitored by a local health department. The Centers for Disease Control and Prevention (CDC) is our national public health entity in the United States. CDC reports statistics on notifiable diseases of interest in a publication called the ***Morbidity and Mortality Weekly Report (MMWR)***. In addition, each state has its own surveillance mechanism and reporting requirements for the study of communicable diseases within its borders. Each has a **state board of health** and a **reference laboratory** equipped to carry out special diagnostic tests that are often outside the scope of hospital laboratories. Of course, most outbreak investigations and the discovery of new infectious agents usually start at the bedside of an individual patient and physician. It is therefore crucial for practicing clinicians to be aware of reporting requirements and state laboratory support resources and to remain ever alert for the next new outbreak.

CONCLUSION

Epidemiology sometimes appears to be a remote "nonclinical" discipline practiced mainly by public health officials. However, in reality it pervades all forms of medical practice and furnishes particularly important clues to the diagnosis of infectious diseases. Inquiry into time and place characteristics is not only the foundation of outbreak investigation but should be part of the usual process of taking a clinical history. Epidemiological information reveals how people encounter disease agents and helps reduce the exposure and spread of infectious diseases.

Suggested Readings

Esdaile JM, Feinstein AR. Lyme disease: a medical detective story. In: Bernstein, E. ed. *1985 Medical and Health Annual*. Chicago, IL: Encyclopedia Britannica; 1984:267–271.

Giesecke J. *Modern Infectious Disease Epidemiology*. 2nd ed. Westminster, CA: Arnold Publications; 2001.

Gordis L. *Epidemiology*. 3rd ed. Philadelphia, PA: WB Saunders, 2004.

Morens DM, Folkers GK, Fauci AS. Emerging Infections: a perpetual challenge. *Lancet Infect Dis*. 2008;8(11):710–719.

Rothman KJ. *Epidemiology: An Introduction*. Oxford, UK: Oxford University Press; 2002.

Sackett DL, Haynes RB, Guyatt GH, et al. *Clinical Epidemiology: A Basic Science for Clinical Medicine*. 2nd ed. Boston, MA: Little, Brown, 1991.

Steere AC, Malawista SE, Snydman DR, et al. Lyme arthritis: an epidemic of oligoarticular arthritis in children and adults in three Connecticut communities. *Arthrit Rheum*. 1977;20:7–17.

Chapter 60

Digestive System Infections

David Acheson and James M. Fleckenstein

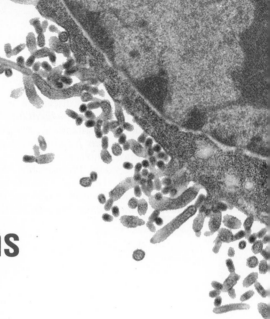

HUMAN BEINGS have coevolved in a complex mutual relationship with the tremendous number of bacteria that we harbor in our intestines, estimated to be 10 times greater than the total number of eukaryotic cells in our bodies! The numbers of organisms in the gastrointestinal (GI) tract are astounding, with bacteria in the colon present at approximately one-tenth the theoretical limit of packing cells into a defined space (about 10^{12} bacteria/g). Interestingly, while more than 50 phyla of bacteria exist, 4 phyla predominate in the human GI tract and constitute our "microbiota" (Fig. 60-1). Collectively, these phyla represent a community of well over 400 distinct species of bacteria, in addition to a few fungi and protozoa, and form the normal resident flora of the GI tract.

In essence, the microbiota residing in our intestinal tracts have evolved to consume materials in our diet that we otherwise would be incapable of digesting and, in return, supply fermentation products that provide energy or raw materials (such as vitamin K). Likewise, both innate and adaptive immune responses in our intestine keep the microbiota in check, permitting this **symbiotic relationship** (see Chapter 2) to occur without allowing these beneficial organisms to overstep their bounds. Effective enteric pathogens must compete with the beneficial flora and subvert or avoid host responses to gain a foothold in this environment.

The frequency of infections of the digestive system varies from the most prevalent human infectious disease, dental caries, to fairly common diarrhea and food poisoning, to unusual opportunistic infections of immunocompromised persons. Diarrheal diseases are a far greater cause of morbidity and mortality worldwide than are the more familiar diseases of the industrialized nations (heart disease, cancer, and strokes). Unfortunately, infants and young children are disproportionately affected, especially in developing countries with poor nutrition and environmental sanitation. Although diarrheal diseases do not usually cause fatalities in the United States, diarrhea remains among the most common complaints of people seen in general medical practice. Of the estimated 48 million cases of foodborne disease in the United States each year, much of the burden of illness can be attributed to gastroenteritis.

Intestinal infections range in severity from mild diarrhea (e.g., most rotavirus infections) to life-threatening loss of fluid and electrolytes (e.g., cholera) and severe mucosal ulceration complicated by intestinal perforation (e.g., bacillary dysentery). This variation in clinical manifestations is not surprising when one considers the striking local differentiation in the alimentary tract and the tremendous variation in virulence genes among different pathogens.

ENTRY

Barriers to Infection

Because the human GI tract presents potential pathogens with an estimated 200 to 300 m² of potentially vulnerable surface area, each portion of the alimentary tract possesses special anatomical, physiological, and biochemical barriers to infection (Fig. 60-2). One very effective barrier to enteric pathogens is **stomach acid**. The low pH of the normal stomach (usually ≤4 in healthy individuals) provides an effective first line of host defense that limits replication of ingested organisms (and thus explains the increased risk to infections when gastric acidity is compromised).

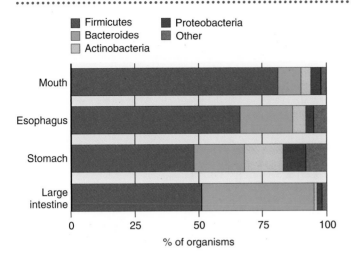

FIGURE 60-1. **Distribution of bacterial phyla within the normal human gastrointestinal (GI) tract.** Although four phyla predominate throughout, each region harbors vastly different numbers of organisms as well as a wide variety of distinct bacterial species. While the stomach generally is home to fewer organisms, these are adapted to the acid environment and, therefore, the normal stomach is not "sterile."

Another general impediment to infective agents is the **mucosal epithelium** lining the alimentary system. Normally, sophisticated intracellular junctional complexes maintain the integrity of this lining. However, disruption of the mucosa by ionizing radiation or cytotoxic cancer chemotherapy can lead to mucositis (superficial ulcerations of the mucosa of the entire GI tract) and penetration of normal flora into deep tissues followed by life-threatening bacteremias and dissemination through the bloodstream to other organs.

A variety of local defense mechanisms, such as **mucus formation** and **gut motility**, hinder adhesion of microorganisms to the epithelial wall (Fig. 60-3). Within GI mucous are mucins, complex glycoproteins that occur in both secreted and membrane-complexed forms. Commensal organisms can reside in the mucous layer using the complex carbohydrates as an energy source, whereas enteric pathogens must surmount this barrier in order to adhere to intestinal epithelial cells and potentially gain access to those cells and beyond. Some enteric pathogens have co-opted binding to these proteins or modulate their production (for instance, *Clostridium difficile* toxin

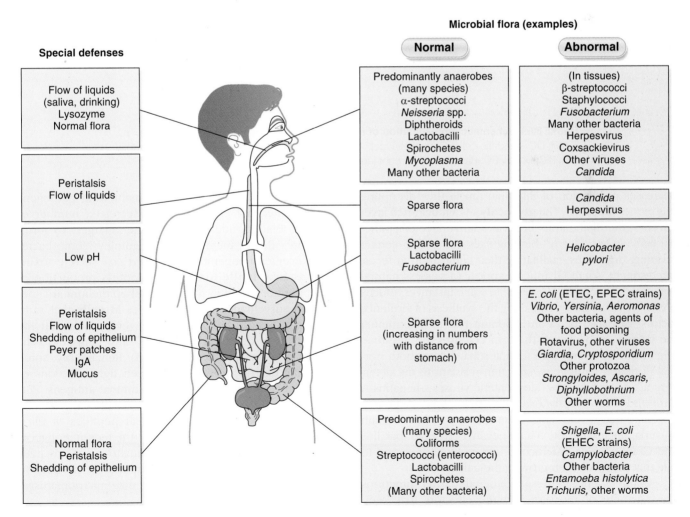

FIGURE 60-2. **Microbiological overview of the digestive system.**

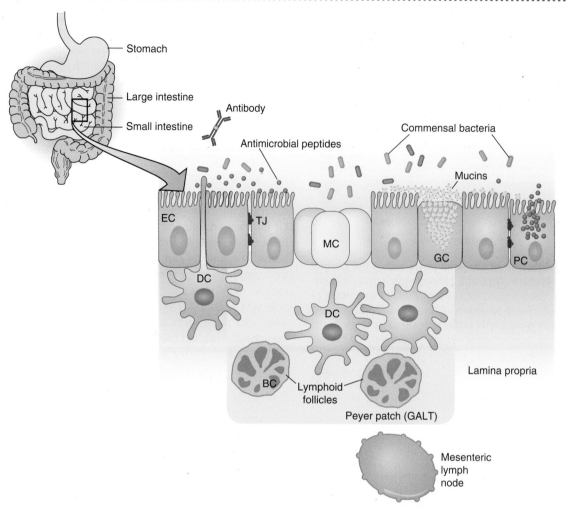

FIGURE 60-3. Schematic representation of host barriers faced by intestinal pathogens. BC, B cell; DC, dendritic cell; EC, epithelial cell; GALT, gut-associated lymphoid tissue; GC, goblet cell; MC, M cell; PC, Paneth cell; TJ, tight junction.

decreases production of intestinal mucin thus disrupting this barrier function). The **glycocalyx** is a mucin-rich layer covering the filamentous brush border surface of epithelial cells. It has "decoy" binding sites that entrap certain invading organisms, facilitating their elimination in feces. Interestingly, some GI mucins appear to possess natural antimicrobial activity. However, in some instances, mucus promotes virulence by triggering the synthesis of virulence factors. **Bile** also plays an important role in determining the bacteria and viruses that can colonize the intestine. Organisms that survive in the intestinal lumen, both normal flora and pathogens, are often resistant to the detergent action of bile salts. Most enteric viruses—hepatitis A virus and poliovirus, for example—lack a lipid-containing envelope that would make them sensitive to bile. Certain bacteria, including the Gram-negative typhoid bacillus and Gram-positive enterococci, are so highly resistant to bile that they can even grow in the gallbladder.

Complementing these epithelial barrier functions are a variety of mucosal immune effectors that keep both commensal organisms and marauding pathogens at bay. Intestinal epithelial cells secrete a number of antimicrobial peptides that kill bacteria largely by forming pores in the membrane. Intriguingly, some bacteria like enterotoxigenic *Escherichia coli* secrete toxins such as **heat-labile toxin** that suppress production of these peptides. Within the intestinal epithelium are specialized surveillance cells known as **M cells** that sample antigens and microbes for delivery to subepithelial collections of dendritic cells (DCs) and lymphoid cells known as Peyer patches (Fig. 60-3). Remarkably, some DCs may extend processes between tight junctions of epithelial cells to directly sample luminal antigens. Pattern recognition receptors on DCs or epithelial cells may activate production of antimicrobial peptides or elicit the expression cytokines that in turn recruit polymorphonuclear cells and other inflammatory cells to neutralize microbes. Lymphocytes respond by production of secretory IgA, which may neutralize microorganisms or their products.

Establishment of Infectious Disease in the Digestive System

Infectious diseases of the alimentary tract represent the end result of pathogen–host interactions in which the pathogen overcomes host barriers to infection or in which normal defenses are altered in favor of the microbe. The latter include:

- *Anatomic alterations*: Obstructions to the flow of secretions remove one of the most powerful defense mechanisms of the hollow organs. Thus, stones in the gallbladder or the common bile duct that impede the flow of bile predispose the biliary tree to infections. Surgery may create **intestinal "blind loops"** that are isolated from the moving stream of intestinal contents. Bacterial overgrowth can occur in the blind loop and result in malabsorption.

- *Changes in stomach acidity*: Alteration of the acid barrier of the stomach by disease, surgery, or drugs (even "over-the-counter" drugs such as antacids) dramatically increases the survival of various pathogens in this organ, allowing some ingested organisms greater access to the lower GI tract. Thus, in persons with impaired gastric acidity, bacterial infection in the lower intestinal tract can occur after ingestion of smaller numbers of pathogens. This scenario occurs with infections by acid-sensitive bacteria like *Vibrio cholerae* or *Salmonella* species but not in infections by *E. coli* O157:H7 or *Shigella* species, which are naturally resistant to acid.

- *Alterations to the normal flora*: In regions of the digestive tract that are most heavily colonized, the mouth and the colon, changes in the density or composition of the flora may permit pathogens to become established. The most frequent cause of such an alteration is the use of **broad-spectrum antibiotics**.

- *Encounter with specific pathogenic agents*: Certain viruses, bacteria, protozoa, and helminths cause disease even in the absence of predisposing host factors. At each site in the GI tract, pathogens must be able to resist the specific local defenses. Because microorganisms face different survival problems in the mouth, stomach, small intestine, and colon, they must possess different attributes to infect a specific site.

DAMAGE

The signs and symptoms of infections related to the digestive system are caused by several general mechanisms:

- *Pharmacologic action*: Some bacteria produce toxins that alter normal intestinal function without causing lasting damage to their target cells. Typical examples are the **enterotoxins** elaborated by *V. cholerae* or some strains of *E. coli* (such as enterotoxigenic *E. coli*), which provoke copious watery diarrhea. Because the

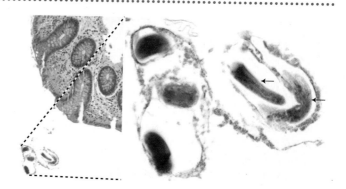

FIGURE 60-4. *Strongyloides stercoralis* **larvae discovered on colonic biopsy.** Filariform larvae of *Strongyloides* may penetrate the intestinal mucosa or the skin of the perianal region (autoinfection), sustaining infections in patients who have not been in endemic regions for several years. (H&E stain, courtesy of Dr. Pamela Sylvestre.)

small bowel is primarily responsible for absorbing most of the 9 to 10 L of fluid that passes through the gut each day, even small reductions in its absorptive capacity cause large amounts of fluid to enter the colon, overwhelming its relatively modest absorptive function. The excess unabsorbed fluid results in diarrhea, which can rapidly lead to dehydration, electrolyte loss, depletion of the intravascular volume, and shock, as seen in cholera.

- *Local inflammation*: In certain areas of the alimentary tract, an inflammatory reaction can occur as a consequence of microbial invasion. Often, the invasion is limited to the epithelial layer, but it can spread to contiguous tissue and beyond. In the mouth, usually the gums, infections with anaerobic bacteria cause inflammation in the gingival pocket (**periodontitis**). In the large intestine, inflammation due to *Shigella* infection of the lamina propria can result in bloody diarrhea or **dysentery**.

- *Deep tissue invasion*: Some organisms are able to invade the GI tract and enter the circulation. Examples are the protozoan *Entamoeba histolytica* and the worm *Strongyloides* (Fig. 60-4), which are capable of burrowing through the intestinal wall, and *Salmonella*, which penetrates the lamina propria and eventually reaches the bloodstream. Interestingly, *Strongyloides* itself is often colonized by gut bacteria; as a result, invasion by the worm can cause a polymicrobial bacteremia.

- *Perforation*: When the mucosal wall is **necrotic** or perforated, the normal flora can spill into the usually sterile peritoneal cavity and invade the bloodstream, often with serious consequences. Thus, rupture of an inflamed appendix can lead to **peritonitis**, and traumatic perforation of the esophagus results in mediastinitis.

The variety of infectious agents and the intestinal diseases that they can cause is daunting. This chapter is organized by the principal sites of infection: the mouth, stomach, biliary tree, and intestine.

INFECTIONS OF THE MOUTH

Virtually all the pathogens of the alimentary tract enter through the mouth. Because most of these pathogens come from the stools of infected persons, their route is known as **fecal–oral transmission**. The organisms reach the mouth by hitching a ride aboard food, fluids, or fingers.

The specific defenses of the mouth include:

- *Nonpathogenic resident flora*: Among the normal flora of the mouth are bacteria, fungi (e.g., *Candida*), and protozoa (e.g., the ameba *Entamoeba gingivalis*). These organisms resist the establishment of newcomers by occupying suitable sites and repelling other organisms, presumably by the production of acids and other metabolic inhibitors.
- *Mechanical actions of saliva and the tongue*: We produce more than a liter of saliva per day. With assistance from the tongue, saliva mechanically dislodges and flushes microorganisms from mucosal surfaces. If salivary flow is reduced, as with dehydration or during fasting, the bacterial content of saliva increases markedly.
- *Antimicrobial constituents of saliva, notably secreted antibodies and lysozyme*: **Secretory IgA** selectively inhibits the adherence of certain bacteria to mucosal cells or to tooth surfaces. **Lysozyme** is effective mainly against Gram-positive bacteria.

Several properties allow bacteria to evade host defenses. Some can stick to teeth or mucosal surfaces. Attachment to teeth is not direct; rather, bacteria adhere to a coating of sticky macromolecules, mainly proteins, called the **dental pellicle**. The bacteria themselves produce polysaccharides that help in adherence. For example, *Streptococcus mutans* transforms sucrose into polysaccharides that are particularly sticky. They are layered on the pellicle to form a matrix that allows adherence of other organisms. The result is **dental plaque**, one of the densest collections of bacteria in the body. Microbial metabolism in plaque transforms dietary sugar into acids, mainly lactic acid, which are responsible for **dental caries** (cavities). Other bacteria, especially strict anaerobes, reside in the **gingival crevices** between the tooth and gum, where they evade the washing effects of saliva and normal tooth brushing.

The bacteria of the indigenous oral flora are not highly virulent, but when a break occurs in the mucosal barrier, such as with advanced **gingivitis** (periodontal disease), these organisms may invade surrounding healthy tissue. The mouth is also the likely portal of entry of α-hemolytic streptococci that cause subacute bacterial endocarditis in persons with rheumatic heart disease. A synergistic cooperation between several types of bacteria, both aerobic and strictly anaerobic, also can lead to a severe and rapidly advancing mixed infection of the soft tissues surrounding the oral cavity. **Ludwig angina**, a polymicrobial infection of the sublingual and submandibular spaces that arises from a tooth (often the second and third mandibular molars), is a cellulitis—an inflammation of submucosal or subcutaneous connective tissue—that can progress rapidly, press against the airway, and compromise respiratory airflow and threaten the affected individual with asphyxiation.

CANDIDIASIS
PATHOBIOLOGY

In the case of A., the white patches adhering to the oral mucosa consisted of "**pseudomembranes**" made up of the yeast *Candida* mixed with desquamated epithelial cells, leukocytes, oral bacteria, necrotic tissue, and food debris. *Candida albicans* and related species are yeasts

CASE • A., a 7-month-old girl, was treated by her pediatrician for a middle ear infection. She was prescribed a 10-day course of amoxicillin, which cleared the infection within 4 days. On the sixth day of antibiotic therapy, her mother noticed that the child was irritable and feeding poorly. During a follow-up visit, her pediatrician noted several creamy white, curdlike patches on the tongue and buccal mucosa. When scraped, they were clearly painful and left a raw, bleeding surface. Microscopic examination of the exudate scraped from the affected areas revealed

yeast. Thrush, or oral **candidiasis**, was diagnosed. Antibiotics were stopped, a topical antifungal solution was administered, and the patches disappeared within 2 days.

This case raises two questions:

1. What aspects of normal physiology prevent the development of thrush?
2. Should A. be evaluated for an immune deficiency?

See Appendix for answers.

found in the environment that establish themselves in the alimentary tract early in life (see Chapter 48). The adult vagina is commonly colonized with these organisms, and they may be acquired by infants during delivery. Small numbers of *Candida* live harmlessly in the alimentary tract until the balance between indigenous bacterial flora and host defenses is upset. A.'s antibiotic therapy killed many of the normal oral bacteria and allowed *Candida* to proliferate.

Candida exploits changes in the normal host flora to multiply locally. If the number or function of neutrophils is decreased, or if defects in cellular immunity are present, they may invade beyond the mucosal surface. Predisposing conditions for oral and other forms of candidiasis include diabetes, malnutrition, malignancy, immunosuppressive drugs, genetic abnormalities of the immune system, and human immunodeficiency virus (HIV) infection. The prolonged use of inhaled steroids for asthma also can predispose to candidal overgrowth in the mouth. In more severe forms of immunodeficiency, the organism can disseminate through the bloodstream and infect virtually any organ system but most commonly the liver, lung, and kidney.

Candida can invade the esophagus, an organ that is rarely prone to infection. Candidal esophagitis is seen in persons with specific T-cell abnormalities, such as **chronic mucocutaneous candidiasis** or AIDS. The differential diagnosis of esophagitis in immunocompromised patients includes infection by cytomegalovirus (CMV) and herpes simplex virus type 1 (HSV-1). Those infections can cause particularly troublesome mucosal ulcerations, with severe pain and difficulty swallowing.

DIAGNOSIS

Thrush is characteristic in appearance, and the diagnosis is usually suspected on oral inspection. It is confirmed by examination of the exudate using a microscope and detection of characteristic yeast forms. Culture is not necessary and often misleading, because *Candida* is a **commensal** and can be cultured from the mouths of some healthy persons.

PREVENTION AND TREATMENT

Because candidal colonization of the GI tract is frequent, prevention and treatment consist primarily of correcting the reversible predisposing factors and avoiding the unnecessary use of antibiotics. Candidiasis of the mouth is usually superficial and responds to oral antifungal agents such as nystatin. If the infection extends more deeply than the mucosa, it may be necessary to use an absorbed oral antifungal agent, such as fluconazole, or intravenous amphotericin B.

STOMACH INFECTIONS

Until recently, the stomach received little attention as a locus of infections of the alimentary tract because it was considered insusceptible to infection. Rather, research focused on the important role the stomach plays in protecting the gut from infection further downstream by its secretion of acid. The majority of oral or foodborne bacteria, washed with saliva into the stomach, are destroyed by acid secreted by the stomach.

In some individuals, the stomach is indeed sterile, and in most others, the concentration of bacteria is very low, generally less than 10^3/mL. The predominant bacteria found in the stomach are acid-resistant Gram-positive organisms, like *Lactobacillus*, *Peptostreptococcus*, *Staphylococcus*, and *Streptococcus*. The normal stomach contains very few enteric Gram-negative rods, *Bacteroides*, or *Clostridium*, organisms that are usually associated with the lower GI tract.

Helicobacter pylori, involved in the pathogenesis of gastritis and peptic ulcers, is particularly well adapted for colonization of the stomach (Fig. 60-5). This pathogenic lifestyle requires the expression of multiple virulence genes including those involved in urease production to neutralize stomach acid and motility via its flagella to allow organisms to penetrate the mucous layer of the stomach lining. Remarkably, it is estimated that this ubiquitous pathogen infects nearly half of the human population worldwide (see Chapter 22).

By contrast, most bacteria, including many pathogens, are not adapted to survive the harsh environment of the stomach, but under the right conditions, they can survive and enter the small intestine alive. Survival of pathogens during transit through the stomach may depend on buffering effects of food or may be favored in persons who do not produce normal amounts of gastric hydrochloric acid because of disease, partial or total gastrectomy, drug therapy (e.g., histamine-2 receptor [H2] or proton pump blockers), or antacid consumption. For example,

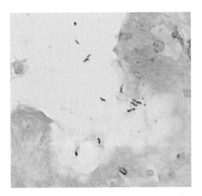

FIGURE 60-5. *Helicobacter pylori* in gastric biopsy specimen. (Steiner stain, courtesy of Dr. Pamela Sylvestre.)

the infective dose of cholera bacilli or salmonellae in human volunteers is 10,000 times lower when the organisms are administered with 2 g of sodium bicarbonate. Low levels of *Salmonella* in foods such as chocolate and peanut butter have been associated with human illness, which raises the possibility that these high-fat foods are somehow protecting *Salmonella* from the harsh environment of the stomach.

Low or absent acid production, known as **hypochlorhydria** or **achlorhydria**, often leads to colonization of the stomach and upper small intestine by enteric Gram-negative rods. That colonization can have two important consequences: (1) development of a disease called bacterial overgrowth syndrome (discussed later in the chapter) and (2) regurgitation of abnormal gastric flora, which becomes a source of nosocomial (hospital-acquired) aspiration pneumonia (see Chapter 62).

INFECTIONS OF THE BILIARY TREE AND LIVER

Infections of the gallbladder (**cholecystitis**) are a frequent complication of obstruction to the flow of bile caused, for example, by gallstones migrating into the cystic duct or common bile duct. The clinical presentation is often sudden and dramatic, with the obstruction leading to increased pressure and distention. Mechanical, chemical, and bacterial inflammation caused by enterococci, *E. coli*, *Klebsiella pneumoniae*, *Staphylococcus aureus*, or *Clostridium perfringens* can result. The hallmark of cholecystitis is **pain in the right upper quad-**

rant of the abdomen, which may build to a crescendo and then subside, only to recur rapidly. That pattern is called **biliary colic**. Nausea and vomiting usually accompany the pain and may be intractable. The majority of patients with common bile duct obstruction have shaking chills, high spiking fever, jaundice, and tenderness over the gallbladder. Biliary colic, jaundice, and chills and spiking fever, known as **Charcot triad**, are characteristic of acute cholecystitis.

Inflammation and infection can cause ischemia of the gallbladder wall, sometimes progressing to gangrene and perforation, which can lead to contamination of the peritoneal cavity with bacteria and abscess formation. The spread of infection from the biliary ducts to the liver, known as **ascending cholangitis**, is common in this situation. With complete obstruction, the combination of pus and increased pressure leads to abscess formation, bacteremia, and symptoms of septic shock.

Primary bacterial infections of the **liver parenchyma** are not common, partly because of the defensive capacity of the phagocytic Kupffer cells. Liver abscesses can develop from portal vein bacteremia from an infected intra-abdominal site, from systemic bacteremia via the hepatic artery, from ascending cholangitis, and from contiguous infections. Intracellular pathogens that survive in macrophages can cause granulomatous infections. Examples are the agents of typhoid fever, Q fever, brucellosis, and tuberculosis.

Infectious diseases of the liver are not discussed in detail here. The most important diseases stem from hepatitis viruses (see Chapter 43). The liver also is the site of several parasitic infections, including leishmaniasis

---

CASE • Ms. F., an obese 48-year-old mother of eight with a vague history of intermittent "stomach problems," awoke with moderate midepigastric pain. Approximately 2 hours before going to bed, she had eaten a large meal of fried chicken and mashed potatoes. The pain soon shifted to her right upper quadrant and was occasionally felt in the area of the right scapula. She vomited several times and felt better but had residual pain for several days with numerous similar but less intense attacks. By the sixth day, she felt sick again and developed jaundice and a shaking chill. In the emergency department, she was in obvious pain and had a temperature of 40°C. Her skin was slightly yellowish. The right upper quadrant of her abdomen was markedly tender to palpation. An 8-cm tubular mass was felt under the margin of the right ribs. Her white blood cell count was elevated (14,000/mm³), suggesting a bacterial

infection. Her serum bilirubin and alkaline phosphatase levels were elevated, suggesting biliary obstruction.

Blood was cultured and antibiotic therapy begun. An ultrasound examination showed that her gallbladder was markedly distended and contained several stones. The diagnosis of acute cholecystitis was made. Within 36 hours of admission, the pain improved and the fever resolved. The blood cultures grew enterococci and *E. coli*. Ms. F. was scheduled for surgery to remove the affected gallbladder and stones.

This case raises two questions:

1. What risk factors contributed to the development of cholecystitis in Ms. F.?

2. What are the possible complications of this disease?

See Appendix for answers.

(see Chapter 52), amebiasis (see Chapter 53), and schistosomiasis (see Chapter 55), among others. An important, although clinically silent, part of the life cycle of malarial parasites also takes place in the liver.

Cholecystitis and Cholangitis
PATHOBIOLOGY

Infections of the gallbladder (**cholecystitis**) and the bile duct (**cholangitis**) are secondary consequences of obstruction. The process begins with obstruction and distention, resulting in inflammation of the gallbladder wall. The disease may not progress, but the process increases the risk of infection caused by the small number of bacteria normally present in bile. Patients with cholecystitis commonly have a history of recurrent attacks of biliary colic resulting from obstruction of the biliary outlet. It is possible that Ms. F.'s vague "stomach problems" of the past were episodes of mild biliary colic caused by transient or partial obstructions of the duct by gallstones. In the most recent episode, infection developed, and the character of her illness changed.

Once bacterial infection becomes established, tissue damage may be accelerated by the resulting inflammatory response. Healing is unlikely to occur without surgical or spontaneous relief of the obstruction and specific antimicrobial therapy.

A particularly rapid and severe form of gallbladder infection can occur in patients with compromised arterial blood supply to the gallbladder wall, such as those with diabetes or the elderly. If the infecting organisms invade the gallbladder wall, they may produce a condition called **emphysematous cholecystitis**. The condition is distinguished by rapid clinical onset, extensive gangrene, presence of gas in the gallbladder wall (when gas-forming species, such as clostridia or *E. coli*, are present), and a high mortality rate. Surgical removal of the gallbladder (**cholecystectomy**) is required because of the frequent occurrence of gangrene, perforation, and extensive peritonitis.

The usual clinical presentation of cholangitis is similar to cholecystitis, as in Ms. F.'s case, but is often accompanied by high spiking fever, chills, jaundice, and constant pain. The most common obstructing causes are gallstones and neoplasms, but, occasionally, a helminthic infection, such as *Ascaris lumbricoides*, is responsible. Considerable pressure within the duct seems to be a prerequisite for infection. Experiments in dogs have shown that the normal common duct pressure of 70 mm H_2O must be raised to 250 mm H_2O before *E. coli* injected into the bloodstream produces infection in the gallbladder. It is not known why the resulting distention facilitates bacterial invasion of the duct wall, but microscopic tears or ischemic damage are obvious possibilities.

Organisms that infect the gallbladder and bile duct are usually derived from the GI tract, *E. coli* being the most frequent agent. Approximately 40% of infections in the gallbladder and bile duct are caused by a mixed facultative and strictly anaerobic flora that ascends from the duodenum.

Typhoid bacilli have an unusual predilection for the gallbladder (see Chapter 17). The organisms may persist for a prolonged period within gallstones, where they are protected from the effects of antibiotics. They produce little or no inflammation, and the infected person may not be aware that he or she is a carrier. All carriers, cognizant or not, shed the typhoid bacteria into the environment and can infect other people.

DIAGNOSIS

When the clinical presentation of cholecystitis is typical, as in Ms. F.'s case, a tentative diagnosis can be made on clinical grounds. Unfortunately, the disease is prone to misdiagnosis because it often presents in an atypical form. Abdominal ultrasound is a useful test to establish the diagnosis of cholecystitis; the imaging technique can reliably visualize obstruction or distention in the biliary system. Direct culture of the infected bile is rarely performed because it is difficult to obtain a specimen; therefore, antibiotics are chosen empirically on the basis of expected flora.

PREVENTION AND TREATMENT

Patients with suspected cholangitis should receive antibiotics appropriate for the expected mixed bacterial species typically present, even before the diagnosis is confirmed. However, correct antibiotics are not sufficient. To effect a definitive cure, the underlying obstruction must be relieved. Relief of the obstruction may occur spontaneously or with surgery. The timing and need for surgery to remove stones and an inflamed gallbladder is controversial, and the surgeon's decision depends on many factors specific to each patient.

INFECTIONS OF THE SMALL AND LARGE INTESTINE

The diseases discussed here illustrate the diversity of infectious problems of the gut, based on host factors and virulence attributes of the causative organisms. Examples of other classic infections of the intestines caused by bacteria are discussed in Chapters 16 and 17; examples

CASE • At the age of 63 years, Mr. O. had an operation to remove a tumor that obstructed his stomach outlet. The surgeon excised part of the stomach and duodenum and connected the remainder of the stomach with the jejunum (gastrojejunostomy), bypassing the unresected duodenum. Two years later, Mr. O. developed chronic diarrhea, and his weight dropped from 139 to 97 pounds. Because his food intake was adequate, anorexia could not account for his weight loss. The diarrhea had recently become bulky, smelly, and greasy. Mr. O. felt fatigued, was short of breath on exertion, and had numbness and tingling in his hands and feet. On examination he was extremely thin and appeared ill with a pale complexion.

Laboratory tests showed a severe anemia with large red blood cells (i.e., megaloblastic anemia) and leukopenia with many neutrophils with extranuclear lobes. Serum levels of vitamin A and its precursor, carotene, were depressed, and vitamin B_{12} was undetectable, although intrinsic factor was present in his gastric juice. Specific tests of intestinal function revealed malabsorption. The diagnosis of bacterial overgrowth syndrome was made. (Although not done in this case, intubation of the small bowel might have revealed approximately 10^9 *Bacteroides fragilis* and 10^6 *E. coli* per mL of small bowel content.) Fat-soluble vitamins and vitamin B_{12} were replaced, and Mr. O. was treated with a course of ciprofloxacin. The diarrhea resolved, and tests of absorptive function improved. He continued to receive antibiotic therapy, and after several months, he returned to his normal weight and felt entirely well.

This case raises two questions:

1. What is the underlying cause of the numbness and tingling experienced by Mr. O.?
2. What is the mechanism of the diarrhea that Mr. O is experiencing?

See Appendix for answers.

of intestinal infections caused by animal parasites are described in Chapters 53 and 54.

The anatomy and physiology of our alimentary tract ensure that our bodies have first crack at the food we eat (Fig. 60-3). Thanks to the sterilizing power of the stomach and the defenses of the small intestine, we absorb most of our nutrients without microbial competition. The upper intestinal contents, rich in unabsorbed sugars, fats, and other nutrients, do not normally come in contact with large numbers of bacteria.

The presence of a large microbial biomass in the absorptive small intestine leads to competition for certain vitamins and malabsorption of fats and produces a disease known as **bacterial overgrowth syndrome**. The study of bacterial overgrowth in the small intestine has helped us understand the normal relationship of the gut flora to gut function.

Bacterial Overgrowth Syndrome
PATHOBIOLOGY

Prior surgery left Mr. O. with a loop of small bowel diverted from the main flow of intestinal contents. The result of this "blind loop" was **stasis of the intestinal contents** caused by the absence of the continuous flushing action of the intestinal secretions. Bacterial proliferation occurred, leading to impaired absorption of fats and fat-soluble vitamins.

Bacterial overgrowth in the small intestine can arise from other causes, such as motor abnormalities that depress **peristalsis** (e.g., diabetic neuropathy, scleroderma, or gastric atony) or **gastric achlorhydria**, which permits large bacterial inocula to reach the proximal small bowel. Under those conditions, bacterial overgrowth begins. As stagnation progresses, the small number of bacteria normally present increases dramatically. Careful anaerobic sampling of the small intestines of patients with depressed peristalsis has revealed bacteria counts as high as 10^{10}/mL, which are comparable to levels in the colon. By far, the most numerous bacteria and those most likely to be responsible for the physiological derangement are strict anaerobes, mainly *Bacteroides* species.

DAMAGE

Bacterial overgrowth in the small intestine may have the following effects:

- *Increased fecal fat, or steatorrhea*: Malabsorption of fat resulting from depletion of the bile acid pool is the primary cause of steatorrhea. Why is the pool depleted? Bile acids such as cholic acid are normally conjugated with glycine or taurine in the liver, secreted in the bile, and reabsorbed in the terminal ileum in the conjugated form. The bacterial overgrowth flora can deconjugate those compounds, making them unavailable for reabsorption and ultimately depleting the bile salts needed to form fat micelles necessary for fat absorption in the proximal gut.

- *Deficiency of vitamin B₁₂*: Normally, vitamin B_{12} (or cobalamin) is bound to intrinsic factor from the stomach, and this complex is absorbed from the terminal ileum. With bacterial overgrowth, dietary B_{12} is used by bacteria, making it unavailable for uptake by the host. With prolonged B_{12} malabsorption (longer than 1 year), endogenous stores are depleted. Cellular systems with a high rate of turnover and DNA synthesis (e.g., bone marrow, central nervous system, and gut epithelium) are severely impaired, possibly leading to megaloblastic anemia or structural gut abnormalities. The epithelial villi are shortened with decreased enterocyte turnover and atrophy, reducing the absorptive area. Thus, bacterial overgrowth sets off a cascade of malabsorptive events. Vitamin B_{12} also is required for myelin synthesis, and its deficiency results in degeneration of myelin sheaths, producing the classic neurological syndrome of pernicious anemia.

- *Diarrhea*: Defined as an increase in fecal water and electrolyte excretion or increased frequency of bowel movements above normal amounts, diarrhea occurs in all patients with bacterial overgrowth. In this situation, it usually results from the degradation by the normal flora of malabsorbed oligosaccharides reaching the colon. When the concentration of osmotically active solutes increases and water moves across the mucosa to maintain iso-osmolarity, the result is **osmotic diarrhea**. Deconjugated bile salts in the colon also can cause osmotic diarrhea.

- *Malabsorption of vitamins A and D*: Poor absorption of fat-soluble vitamins (A, D, E, and K, but particularly A and D) causes severe visual disturbance (night blindness) and softening of the bones (osteomalacia). Interestingly, vitamin K deficiency is rare. The reduced absorption of that fat-soluble vitamin is offset by the markedly increased vitamin production by the plentiful bacteria, ordinarily our main source of vitamin K.

CASE

Amebic Colitis

Ms. T., a 46-year-old woman who had recently worked as a missionary in Guatemala, presented to her internist with complaints of intermittent low-grade fever, cramping abdominal pain, and intermittent diarrhea with occasional blood in her stool. She noted that while in Guatemala, she frequently ate food prepared by street vendors and that she experienced several episodes of bloody diarrhea prior to returning to the United States. However, several routine stool cultures for enteric pathogens were unrevealing, as were repeated samples submitted for examination of ova and parasites (O&P). Ms. T.'s symptoms continued unabated over the course of several months, and she was referred to a gastroenterologist. Concerned that she might have inflammatory bowel disease, the gastroenterologist scheduled her for a colonoscopy, which revealed several flask-shaped ulcerations in the rectal and colonic mucosa. Pathologic examination of the lesions obtained by biopsy revealed few inflammatory cells but multiple amoeboid cells containing ingested red blood cells consistent with *Entamoeba histolytica* infection (Fig. 60-6). Ms. T. immediately received treatment for amebic colitis using oral metronidazole and a nonabsorbable antibiotic, paromomycin, instead of the immunosuppressive therapy that was anticipated for inflammatory bowel disease.

This case raises several questions:

1. What placed Ms. T. at risk for amebiasis?

2. Why is it necessary to treat intestinal amebiasis with two different antibiotics?

3. What might have happened if the biopsy had failed to reveal *E. histolytica*, and the patient had been started on immunosuppressive therapy instead?

See Appendix for answers.

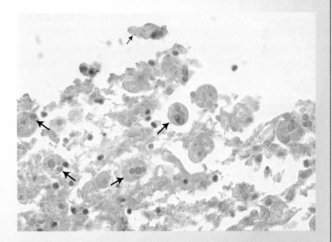

FIGURE 60-6. Amebic colitis. Biopsy of a colonic ulcer demonstrates multiple trophozoites of *Entamoeba histolytica* with characteristic erythrophagocytosis (*large arrows*) and a single nucleus with central nucleolus and thin peripheral chromatin (*small arrow*).

CASE

Giardiasis

Mr. G. is a 24-year-old graduate student who returned from a backpacking trip in Colorado several weeks ago. While camping, he had assumed that cold mountain stream water would be pure and safe to drink. After developing profuse watery diarrhea, he began to wonder if he might have "picked something up" by drinking unfiltered stream water. He continued to have intermittent diarrhea, which was subsequently accompanied by anorexia and weight loss of about 10 pounds. His stools were foul smelling and floated on the surface of the water in the toilet. Frequent trips to the bathroom and uncontrollable flatulence at work finally prompted him to seek medical attention. After learning his history, his physician ordered several stool studies for ova and parasites (O&P), which were negative. However, a subsequent endoscopy with biopsy of the duodenum revealed the cause of his suffering (Fig. 60-7).

This case raises two questions:

1. How might the student have avoided infection?
2. Why was the diagnosis missed by O&P tests?

See Appendix for answers.

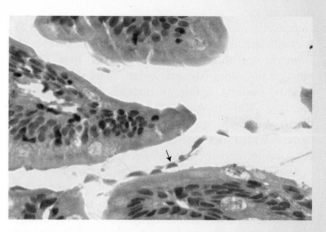

FIGURE 60-7. Giardiasis. Small intestinal biopsy from a patient with giardiasis. Giardia trophozoites typically appear pear- or sickle-shaped (*arrow*).

DIAGNOSIS AND TREATMENT

Bacterial overgrowth syndrome is usually diagnosed when malabsorption and nutritional deficiencies are present together with predisposing anatomic or physiological conditions, such as intestinal blind loops. Noninvasive breath tests are available to document the presence of the overgrowth flora in the proximal small bowel. Treatment requires correction of the surgical or medical predisposing condition in conjunction with careful nutritional repletion and, most importantly, broad-spectrum antibiotic therapy. Relapse can occur, and repeated courses of therapy may be necessary.

Diarrhea and Dysentery

Diarrhea is the final common pathway of intestinal responses to many inciting agents, both infectious and noninfectious (see Chapter 16). **Dysentery**, in contrast,

CASE

Rotavirus Infection

A., a 9-month-old girl, had been enrolled in a child-care facility for the past month. Usually a satisfied and happy child, she suddenly became irritable, began to vomit, and had a low-grade fever. She also developed mild upper respiratory symptoms, with cough, nasal discharge, and pharyngitis. Watery diarrhea, without blood or leukocytes, developed and persisted for 2 days. The infant was brought to the pediatrician, who made the clinical diagnosis of rotavirus gastroenteritis. An enzyme-linked immunosorbent assay (ELISA) to detect **rotavirus** antigen in the stool was positive. The pediatrician prescribed an oral rehydration solution to be given at home, and A. made an uneventful recovery by the sixth day.

This case raises two questions:

1. How did A. become infected with rotavirus?
2. Is there a vaccine to prevent rotavirus disease?

See Appendix for answers.

CASE

Hemolytic–Uremic Syndrome

L., a 3-year-old girl, became ill with cramps, fever, and mild watery diarrhea 24 hours after eating a hamburger at a fast-food restaurant. Her pediatrician advised giving fluids but did not prescribe antibiotics. The diarrhea turned bloody on day 3, and the child was hospitalized. Laboratory tests revealed moderate leukocytosis but no other abnormalities.

On day 5, *E. coli* O157:H7 was isolated from the initial stool culture. Laboratory studies the next day revealed a leukocytosis of 27,000 with 85% neutrophils and 5% bands, anemia (hematocrit of 30%), thrombocytopenia (34,000 platelets/mm³), and an elevated creatinine of 8.8 mg/dL. Erythrocyte fragments characteristic of red cell damage secondary to endothelial cell injury (**microangiopathic hemolytic anemia**) were seen on the blood smear.

Over the next 2 days, L.'s anemia, thrombocytopenia, and uremia progressed, without evidence of consumptive coagulopathy. Those signs established the diagnosis of **hemolytic–uremic syndrome** (**HUS**). L. required a week of hemodialysis for oliguria, hypertension, and uremia. She also received transfusions of red cells and platelets. She was discharged after 3 weeks, and by 3 months, all laboratory tests had returned to normal. L. remained well after 2 additional years of follow-up.

This case raises several questions:

1. What was the source of the *E. coli* that led to L.'s disease?
2. What is the basis for the renal manifestations of HUS?
3. Should antibiotics have been administered to L.?

See Appendix for answers.

---

is a distinctive syndrome involving the colon, in which an inflammatory response results in abdominal pain and **small-volume stools consisting of blood, pus, and mucus** (see Chapter 17). Dysentery has a distinctive pathophysiology and association with specific microorganisms, usually *Shigella* species. Therapy is directed toward elimination of the pathogen using antibiotics, an issue now complicated by multiple antibiotic resistance.

In recent years, foodborne outbreaks of bloody diarrhea due to *E. coli* that produce toxins related to Shiga toxin (STX) (from *Shigella dysenteriae* type 1) have emerged. These organisms, known as enterohemorrhagic *E. coli* (EHEC), constitute a variety of serotypes with O157 being the most common. However, there are many non–O157 EHEC that have been associated with human illness. Approximately 10 to 15% of EHEC infections result in more systemic complications such as hemolytic–uremic syndrome (HUS). HUS results from toxin-mediated damage to endothelial cells, leading to thrombus formation in multiple organs including the kidneys and brain.

CASE

Yersinia Infection

Mr. D. took his family to southern Sweden to visit his parents who were dairy farmers outside Malmö. S., a 5-year-old boy, and I., a 12-year-old girl, enjoyed helping their grandparents care for the many domestic animals on the farm and loved the home-cured meat and fresh raw milk served to them. Between 7 and 10 days after arrival, all members of the D. family became ill. S. developed watery, mucoid diarrhea with occasional flecks of blood, low-grade fever, and diffuse abdominal pain, all of which resolved spontaneously after 4 days. I.'s episode began similarly but worsened after 3 days, when her pain localized to the right lower quadrant and became associated with high fever and leukocytosis. She was brought to the local hospital, and a tentative diagnosis of acute appendicitis was made. During surgery, her appendix was found to be normal. However, the terminal ileum was inflamed, with many **enlarged mesenteric lymph nodes**.

Cultures of stool obtained on admission were incubated at 25°C and after several days grew *Yersinia enterocolitica*. By that time I. had made a nearly complete recovery. Mr. D., like S., developed an acute mucoid diarrhea, abdominal pain, and fever that remitted by the fourth day. Three weeks later Mr. D. developed painful swelling of several joints and a painful raised rash over his shins (**erythema nodosum**). Although he had no gastrointestinal (GI) symptoms, his stool tested positive for *Y. enterocolitica*, and he was treated with trimethoprim/sulfamethoxazole. The rash and arthritis slowly resolved, returned several months later, and then spontaneously remitted, not to return again.

This case raises two questions:

1. Why did the clinical manifestations of *Yersinia* infection differ in S. and I.?
2. Describe the pathogenesis of the arthritis and rash that developed in Mr. D.?

See Appendix for answers.

The cases presented here illustrate distinctive ecological features of the pathogens and their interactions with the host.

ENCOUNTER

The list of intestinal pathogens is expanding as well-known organisms appear in unexpected frequency and in new settings and as new organisms are recognized (Table 60-1). Other chapters discuss some of the more common agents of intestinal infections (see Chapters 16, 17, 37, 51, 53, 54, and 76). This chapter adds a few more to the list. *Campylobacter jejuni*, formerly thought to be a rare cause of diarrhea in the United States, has now emerged as one of the most common. It is usually transmitted by poultry, which are almost always colonized by the organism. Within the last several years, *Aeromonas hydrophila* and *Plesiomonas* species have become established as occasional agents of waterborne or shellfish-associated outbreaks. Other common agents of diarrhea in the United States and abroad include the protozoan *Cryptosporidium* (see Chapter 53), which was responsible for a massive waterborne outbreak in Milwaukee, Wisconsin, in 1993 involving almost one-half million people, and a newly described foodborne coccidian parasite,

Cyclospora cayetanensis (transmitted in a 1996 US outbreak by contaminated imported raspberries; see Chapter 53). Another protozoal group, **microsporidia** (including *Enterocytozoon bieneusi* and *Septata intestinalis*), can cause chronic diarrhea in persons with AIDS. Viral diarrhea is common in all age groups. Agents of viral diarrhea include enteric adenovirus, astrovirus, norovirus, and rotavirus, among others, in normal young children and adults as well as viruses associated with diarrhea and inflammatory enteritis in immunocompromised persons (e.g., CMV and HSV). As the list of enteric pathogens lengthens and an understanding of how they produce disease emerges, the practical challenge of diagnosis and treatment increases.

In areas endemic to cholera, infected persons can transport the bacteria to other areas and initiate epidemics of cholera where water and food cannot be protected and environmental sanitation is poor. Those events occurred in Latin America in early 1993, resulting in more than one million cases of cholera over the subsequent 2 years and approximately 5,000 to 10,000 deaths. Interestingly, *the segment of DNA that encodes cholera toxin is actually contained on a filamentous bacteriophage* (called CTX) that infects the cholera bacteria. The possibility that a functional set of cholera toxin genes can be acquired by phage transduction raises questions about the safety of cholera vaccines based on deletions of the toxin gene. Attesting to the constant evolution of microbes and emerging diseases, a previously unknown epidemic serotype of *V. cholerae*, designated O139 (Bengal), was first detected in India in 1992 and spread in epidemic fashion beginning in 1993 (see Fig. 16-1). The new strain resulted from deletion of O1 lipopolysaccharide (LPS) synthesis genes and insertion of new LPS synthesis genes into the current pandemic serogroup O1 cholera strain. The O139 strain causes severe disease and continues spread in Asia.

In contrast, *Shigella* infection is found only in close association with humans. Relatively few organisms are required to cause shigellosis (also known as bacillary dysentery). As a result, the disease spreads readily among persons in close contact. It is most commonly a disease of children and, in the United States, the most common species, *S. sonnei*, is a frequent cause of self-limited watery diarrhea in infants and children in child-care centers. *S. flexneri* is no longer common in the United States but remains an important cause of infection in developing countries where *S. sonnei* is rare. *Y. enterocolitica* has yet another ecological characteristic; it is often zoonotic (acquired from infected animals; see Chapter 73) and may be transmitted by drinking raw milk or consuming undercooked meat such as pork.

Diarrhea affecting children who are younger than 2 years of age is most likely of viral etiology, with rotavirus by far the most common cause. In temperate regions, rotavirus diarrhea is seasonal and produces **"winter vomiting disease"**; in tropical zones, it occurs

TABLE 60-1 Some Etiologic Agents of Diarrhea

Organism	Source
Escherichia coli	Food contaminated with human feces
Salmonella species	Contaminated food, especially poultry products
Shigella species	Fecal–oral
Campylobacter species	Farm animals, contaminated food (e.g., raw eggs)
Yersinia enterocolitica	Animal products
Vibrio cholerae	Water and shellfish
Vibrio parahaemolyticus	Seafood (e.g., sardines, shellfish)
Bacillus cereus	Contaminated food (e.g., reheated rice)
Clostridium perfringens	Contaminated food (e.g., reheated meat)
Entamoeba histolytica	Fecal–oral and water
Giardia lamblia	Fecal–oral and water
Cryptosporidium and *Cyclospora* species	Fecal–oral and water

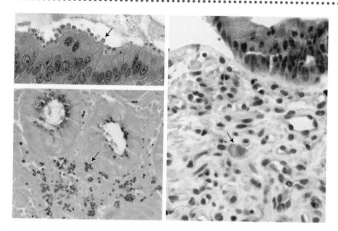

FIGURE 60-8. GI pathology images from AIDS patients who presented with diarrheal illness. (Clockwise from top left) Cryptosporidia trophozoites (*arrow*) attached to the luminal surface of enterocytes in the intestine of a patient with advanced HIV disease. Cytomegalovirus (CMV) infection in the intestine demonstrating classic large "owl's eye" viral inclusion body (*arrow*) from which CMV derives its name (H&E stain). Histoplasma fungal elements (*arrow*) in an intestinal biopsy of an AIDS patient presenting with fever and chronic diarrhea (Gömöri methenamine silver stain).

year-round. Adults may be infected when a child introduces the virus into the household, but adults often do not experience symptoms, presumably because of pre-existing immunity. In areas where malnutrition is prevalent, severe diarrhea is also associated with measles, which is highly contagious and kills large numbers of infants. The use of the measles vaccine in those populations would reduce the incidence of this life-threatening complication.

A distinct group of enteric infections is seen in men who have sex with men (MSM). Anal intercourse permits infection of the distal bowel with pathogens typically associated with sexually transmitted diseases. Proctocolitis due to *Chlamydia trachomatis*, HSV, *Neisseria gonorrhoeae*, or *Treponema pallidum* has been observed in men who practice anal receptive intercourse. Likewise, MSM are also at increased risk for *E. histolytica* infections due to fecal–oral transmission. These infections have declined in frequency with modification of sexual practices initiated following the onset of the AIDS epidemic.

A number of infections of the GI tract are more common and more severe in persons with advanced immunosuppression due to HIV infection. These include a variety of bacteria, parasites, and fungi (Fig. 60-8).

PATHOBIOLOGY AND DAMAGE

The diarrheal disease pathogens have distinctive sets of virulence properties and preferentially infect specific areas of the bowel (Table 60-2). Therefore, this chapter considers the small and large intestine separately.

Infections of the Small Intestine The mechanisms involved in diarrhea arising in the small intestine differ according to the type of pathogenic agent:

- *Viruses that cause death or dysfunction of intestinal epithelial cells*: The main agents are the rotaviruses (the case of A.) and noroviruses. These viruses *cause diarrhea by destroying or altering the function of enterocytes at the villi, but they do not affect those in the crypts*. Villus cells are sodium-absorbing cells, whereas crypt cells secrete chloride ions. One theory of virus-induced diarrhea is that damage of villus cells leads to decreased sodium and water absorption, which results in net accumulation ("secretion") of fluid in the lumen and damage to the disaccharidase-containing microvillus membranes, leading to sugar malabsorption. Instead of being hydrolyzed locally and absorbed, these sugars enter the colon where they are metabolized by the bacterial flora to osmotically more active products. As a result, fluid is drawn into the lumen, which worsens the diarrhea. It is also partly responsible for a postenteritic syndrome seen in children, in whom mild diarrhea persists for a considerable time after the infection is resolved. These mechanisms are more fully discussed in Chapter 37.

- *Bacteria that colonize the small intestine* (e.g., enterotoxigenic *E. coli* and *V. cholerae*): In enterotoxigenic *E. coli* infections and cholera, diarrhea is secondary to the production of toxins by the organisms. The *toxins activate the enzymes responsible for synthesis of cyclic nucleotide mediators* (cyclic adenosine monophosphate and cyclic guanosine monophosphate), which in turn stimulate **net chloride secretion** and inhibit **sodium uptake**, resulting in fluid loss. These mechanisms are described in detail in Chapter 9.

- *Protozoa* (e.g., *Giardia* and *Cryptosporidium*, which infect the small bowel) (see Chapter 53): It is not known if a toxin is involved in these infections or precisely how the organisms colonize or invade the gut epithelium. However, clues are beginning to emerge as the genomes of these organisms are sequenced, yielding novel putative surface-expressed or secreted molecules that may participate in host interactions and pathogenesis. Interestingly, individuals with hypogammaglobulinemia are at increased risk for giardiasis. Conversely, *Giardia* express a variety of surface proteins to avoid neutralization by secretory IgA, explaining its ability to persist in the intestine of normal hosts for extended periods of time.

- *Bacteria that cause true food poisoning*: This form of diarrhea occurs when toxigenic bacteria (e.g., *Bacillus cereus* and *S. aureus*) multiply in food before it is eaten. As a result, toxins accumulate and are ingested along with the food. Because the signs and symptoms of food poisoning are not caused by bacterial multiplication in the body, the effects are often felt within a few hours after the tainted meal is consumed. Examples are discussed in Chapter 76.

TABLE 60-2 Clinical Features of Diarrheal Disease

Pathogen	Location	Clinical Features	Sequelae or Extraintestinal Complications
Helicobacter pylori	Stomach	Peptic ulcer disease, gastritis	Gastric cancer
Rotavirus	Small intestine	Watery diarrhea	
Noroviruses	Small intestine	Watery diarrhea, vomiting	
Giardia lamblia	Small intestine	Diarrhea, bloating	Malabsorption
Cryptosporidium parvum	Small intestine	Watery diarrhea	
Cyclospora	Small intestine	Watery diarrhea	
Vibrio cholerae	Small intestine	Watery diarrhea	
Enterotoxigenic *E. coli* (ETEC)	Small intestine	Watery diarrhea	Growth delays in children
Enterohemorrhagic *E. coli* (EHEC)	Large intestine	Bloody diarrhea	Hemolytic–uremic syndrome (HUS), hemorrhagic colitis
Shigella spp.	Large intestine	Bloody diarrhea, tenesmus	HUS
Campylobacter jejuni	Large intestine	Fever, diarrhea	Guillain-Barré syndrome
Yersinia enterocolitica, Yersinia pseudotuberculosis	Terminal ileum	Fever, diarrhea, RLQ abdominal pain	Erythema nodosum, uveitis, arthritis, mesenteric adenitis
Salmonella spp.	Small intestine	Fever diarrhea, fecal leukocytes	Septicemia, metastatic complications

Clearly not all infections of the small intestine produce a secretory diarrhea. Some organisms such as *C. jejuni* or *Y. enterocolitica* (as illustrated by the D. family) may infect the terminal ileum, producing watery, sometimes bloody, stools. The varied presentations of illness in the D. family also illustrate the age-related differences in disease caused by a single organism. *Y. enterocolitica* is unique in that respect, and little is known about the reasons for the diversity. *Y. enterocolitica* infects primarily the terminal ileum and colon in all patients, but in children who are younger than 5 years of age, infection manifests as watery diarrhea. In older children, like S., bacteria from the intestine invade the mesenteric lymph nodes and cause focal inflammatory responses. Interestingly, diarrhea may be minimal or absent, and the mesenteric adenitis can mimic acute appendicitis. Many adults infected with *Y. enterocolitica* develop reactive arthritis within weeks after the onset of diarrhea. The same symptoms occur after *C. jejuni*, *S. flexneri*, and nontyphoidal *Salmonella* gastroenteritis. **Reactive arthritis** is probably an immunological phenomenon driven by molecular mimicry because organisms are not found in the joint fluid. Interestingly, individuals affected most severely by arthritis often possess the major histocompatibility antigen **HLA-B27**.

Infections of the Large Intestine   Bacterial pathogens that infect the large intestine tend to produce epithelial damage, mucosal inflammation, and bloody diarrhea, known as the dysentery syndrome. The major pathogens that invade the large bowel and cause dysentery are *Shigella* species and the ameba, *E. histolytica*. Because inflammation in shigellosis is prominent and usually located in the distal large bowel, pain often worsens with bowel movements, a symptom known as **tenesmus**. The mucosa is easily damaged and looks ulcerated when examined by proctoscopy. The stools may be watery and initially substantial but later decrease in volume and consist of blood, mucus, and pus. White blood cells are usually scarce in amebic dysentery because they are lysed by a toxin produced by the amebic trophozoites present in the lesions. Certain bacteria (e.g., species of *Campylobacter*, *Salmonella*, and *Yersinia*) produce inflammatory pathology in the terminal ileum. The inflammation is associated with bloody diarrhea containing leukocytes and occasionally extends to the colon, resulting in dysentery.

Enterohemorrhagic *E. coli* (EHEC) colonize the intestine of cattle as well as other ruminants (e.g., sheep, goats, and deer). Interestingly, cattle do not become ill from EHEC infection as they lack a critical receptor for the

STX molecules. Contaminated beef products, most often ground beef, are a common source of infection by *E. coli* O157:H7 and other EHEC serotypes. However, a diverse variety of other sources such as water and fresh produce (e.g., lettuce and spinach) have been linked to outbreaks of EHEC. Following infection of the large bowel, these organisms adhere to colonic epithelial cells, causing a characteristic lesion in which the brush border is effaced by a dramatic change in cytoskeletal structures beneath the attached organism. Bloody diarrhea usually develops in most patients 2 to 3 days after onset of the illness, a syndrome known as **hemorrhagic colitis**. This syndrome may result from the action of STX on the colonic endothelium or as a result of mesenteric ischemia from circulating toxin. A different disease is caused by *Clostridium difficile* and its toxins. *C. difficile* infection usually arises after administration of antibiotics, which deplete or alter the resident flora. This infection is characterized by an adherent **pseudomembrane** with considerable mucosal inflammation and damage but without tissue invasion (see Chapter 20).

Serious complications arise occasionally from infection of the colon by invasive organisms. Shigellosis may be associated with severe malnutrition, leading to a protein deficiency syndrome in children known as **kwashiorkor**. Shigellosis sometimes results in rectal prolapse or in a frequently fatal distention of the colon known as toxic megacolon, with a complete cessation of colonic peristalsis. Systemic complications also can occur, leading to **HUS** (at least with the STX–producing *S. dysenteriae* species), leukemoid reactions with high white blood cell counts, encephalopathy, and other consequences. Amebiasis may cause intestinal perforation or obstruction, or the organisms may spread to produce abscesses in other organs, especially in the liver.

EHEC infections are associated with the production of STXs. While there are multiple variants of the toxins, there are two main types called **STX1 and STX2** (also called Shigalike toxins or verotoxins). These toxins appear to cross the intestinal mucosa and injure the endothelium of the intestinal lamina propria, the glomeruli, and the brain. The toxins cause HUS in children and a more prominent neurological disease in older adults called **thrombotic thrombocytopenic purpura** (TTP). HUS is associated with an immediate mortality rate of 5 to 10% and an unknown frequency of renal failure after many years. In the past, TTP was usually fatal, but the mortality rate has dropped to 20% with improved therapy and the use of exchange transfusion.

OTHER GASTROINTESTINAL INFECTIONS
Infections of Gut-Associated Lymph Tissue

A different type of enteric infection is exemplified by typhoid fever (see Chapter 17). It is characterized by *Salmonella typhi* invasion of the gut-associated lymph tissue of the small bowel. From there, the organisms disseminate to the liver and spleen where they proliferate. When the number of organisms is sufficient, they enter the bloodstream, causing the **persistent bacteremia** and fever characteristic of **enteric fever**. Diarrhea may be absent or transient; some patients may even complain of constipation. Other characteristic findings are a low white blood cell count in relation to fever and enlargement of the liver and spleen. With sustained bacteremia, the organisms invade the lymphatic tissue of **Peyer patches** and may cause severe inflammatory lesions, bleeding, and perforation. The mortality rate is high if the disease is untreated. Early use of effective antibiotics curtails the acute illness but predisposes to relapse, presumably by interfering with the protective immune response.

Surgical Complications of Intestinal Infections

Perforation of the wall of either the small or the large intestine may be caused by certain intestinal infections that induce inflammatory responses and tissue damage. Trauma, such as a penetrating knife injury or motor vehicle collision, can also cause perforation of the wall of the bowel. Perforation results in spillage of intestinal contents into the normally sterile peritoneal cavity. The severity of the resulting peritonitis is generally related to the volume of the spill, its spread in the abdomen, and the capacity of the omentum to wall off (contain) the abscess. A small amount of fecal contents may be handled by the defenses in the peritoneum, but a large inoculum can easily overwhelm them; the presence of blood worsens the response. The ensuing peritonitis is usually severe and, if untreated, is often life threatening. Peritoneal infections are most often caused by a mixture of strict anaerobes, in particular, *Bacteroides fragilis* and facultative Gram-negative bacteria of the *Enterobacteriaceae* family. The pathogenic mechanisms are discussed in Chapter 15.

DIAGNOSIS

Most patients with acute diarrhea have a mild and self-limited course and never seek medical attention. It is not practical or necessary to search for enteric pathogens in all patients with diarrhea. In a large percentage of cases, it is sufficient to replenish fluids and electrolytes, usually by oral rehydration, and avoid the use of intravenous fluids unless the patient is in hypovolemic shock. A careful history of symptoms is the most important part of the investigation and often narrows the diagnostic possibilities. The clues that suggest disease requiring specific therapy (e.g., antimicrobial drugs) include fever, tenesmus, and persistent or severe abdominal pain (the triad of dysentery), weight loss, blood in the stool, recent antibiotic use, raw seafood meals, male homosexual practices, foreign travel, especially to developing countries, and prolonged duration of symptoms.

Culturing of stool samples for enteric pathogens is primarily intended to isolate *E. coli* O157:H7 and species of *Campylobacter*, *Salmonella*, and *Shigella*. Isolation or identification of other enteric pathogens requires special culture techniques, evaluation of serotype, or tests for toxin production that are not part of routine laboratory practices (see Chapter 58). Animal parasites, protozoa, or helminths are detected by various methods including enzyme immunoassays or direct microscopy of fresh or appropriately preserved stools, but the specimens may require special concentration or staining procedures. Therefore, it is important to narrow the list of possible organisms that are sought. For example, if cholera is suspected, the laboratory should be instructed to inoculate **thiosulfate-citrate-bile salt-sucrose agar**, which is not used in routine stool cultures. Similarly, if *E. coli* O157:H7 is suspected, the laboratory should inoculate **sorbitol-containing MacConkey agar** (**SMAC**) because that serotype of *E. coli* usually does not ferment sorbitol and stands out from the other sorbitol-fermenting *E. coli* of the normal flora. However, the SMAC test does not distinguish the non–O157:H7 STX–producing *E. coli*, which are an important group of organisms that cause a disease similar to that caused by *E. coli* O157:H7. An enzyme immunoassay is available to detect the STXs in stool produced by any STX–producing *E. coli*.

If nonbloody diarrhea persists or remains unexplained, tests for protozoa, especially *Cyclospora* species and *Giardia lamblia*, are indicated. If the patient is infected with HIV, samples should be examined for *Cryptosporidium parvum*, *Isospora belli*, and microsporidia species. Immunoassays to detect antigens of *Cryptosporidium* and *Giardia* are also available. *Cryptosporidium*, *Cyclospora*, and *Isospora* infections can be readily diagnosed in stool or in biopsy specimens because the organisms are visible when stained by the acid-fast technique used for mycobacteria, an unusual feature among protozoa.

The clinical value of a particular test depends on whether the results will affect the management of the patient. Sometimes the information is used not for treatment of the individual but to determine if special isolation measures are warranted. Thus, the presence of rotavirus in A.'s stool did not materially change the treatment plan. However, the positive ELISA test for rotavirus suggested that if she were hospitalized or near other susceptible infants, she would have to be isolated.

TREATMENT

Most acute infectious diarrheas are mild, self-limited, and best treated with oral fluid replacement and continued feeding. The decision to employ specific antimicrobial or more aggressive intravenous fluid replacement therapy is determined by the severity or duration of diarrhea or the presence of shock or dysenteric symptoms. In general, infections caused by toxigenic and invasive *E. coli*, *Shigella* species, and *V. cholerae* are improved with antibiotics, but those infections often resolve before the diagnosis is made. In contrast, the use of antibiotics for the treatment of EHEC (e.g., *E. coli* O157:H7) can *increase* the risk for developing HUS. The disadvantage of treating all infections with antibiotics is that the organisms may develop drug resistance. Furthermore, rather than altering the disease course, antibiotic treatment could increase the risk of inducing a carrier state, with the potential of increased spread of the infection, as with *Salmonella*. Other specific antimicrobials are prescribed for *Cyclospora*, *E. histolytica*, *G. lamblia*, and *Isospora*. To date, *Cryptosporidium* species defy truly effective therapy.

Antidiarrheal agents can reduce the stool frequency and improve their consistency, but no evidence suggests that the drugs shorten the course of illness or (with the exception of loperamide) reduce the volume of fluid lost. In fact, by decreasing gut transit time, antimotility agents may impair pathogen clearance, thereby prolonging the infection and enhancing its severity. In addition, anticholinergics or opiates can produce toxic megacolon, especially in children and those with inflammatory diarrhea.

An important medical breakthrough has been the development of **oral rehydration therapy** for mild-to-moderate diarrhea. Following the discovery that sodium and glucose transport are coupled in the small intestine, it was observed that the oral administration of glucose with essential electrolytes dramatically accelerates absorption of sodium, with water following passively (i.e., without the expenditure of energy) to maintain osmolality. Moderate dehydration associated with cholera or other small bowel diarrheas should now be corrected with oral replacement. Even in severe dehydration, which requires rapid intravenous fluids to correct or prevent shock, oral rehydration may later be used alone for maintenance of adequate hydration. The impact of this simple concept on worldwide mortality from dehydration cannot be overstated, especially in the poorest areas of the world where the problem is prevalent and severe. In those areas, the use of intravenous therapy is too expensive, and trained personnel are too scarce to provide it to more than a small proportion of affected persons. Nonmedically trained people can be taught to mix the proper ingredients (sometimes using bottle caps as measuring devices) or dissolve prepackaged mixtures. The recipe for oral rehydration is remarkably simple.

To 1 L of water, add the following:

1/2 teaspoon salt (3 g)
1/4 teaspoon bicarbonate (1.5 g)
1/4 teaspoon KCl (1.5 g)
4 tablespoons sugar (20 g)

CONCLUSION

With approximately 48 million cases of foodborne disease in the United States each year resulting in more than 100,000 hospitalizations, many of which are due to gastroenteritis, upsets to the digestive system are a major burden on the health care system. These numbers do not include persons with peptic ulcer disease, gallbladder disease, and other disorders of the alimentary tract that may be related to infection. One key point to remember in relation to many of the agents discussed in this chapter is that foodborne disease is generally preventable by careful handling and appropriate cooking of food combined with proper personal hygiene. Thus, many GI illnesses can be avoided.

Generally, the intestinal system is well designed to defend against pathogenic microbes, but with the growing number of persons who are either immunocompromised or taking medications that alter gastric acidity, physicians must take care to provide advice about preventative strategies to avoid infections of the GI tract. Because a properly functioning digestive system is important for good nutrition, and good nutrition is critical for the prevention of many other diseases, it is important to understand infectious diseases of the intestine and the measures employed in their diagnosis and treatment.

Suggested Readings

Angulo FJ, Swerdlow DL. Bacterial enteric infections in persons infected with human immunodeficiency virus. *Clin Infect Dis.* 1995;21:S84–S93.

Ankarklev J, Jerlström-Hultqvist J, Ringqvist E, et al. Behind the smile: cell biology and disease mechanisms of Giardia species. *Nat Rev Microbiol.* 2010;8:413–422.

Artis D. Epithelial-cell recognition of commensal bacteria and maintenance of immune homeostasis in the gut. *Nat Rev Immunol.* 2008;8:411–420.

Bäckhed F, Ley RE, Sonnenburg JL, et al. Host-bacterial mutalism in the human intestine. *Science.* 2005;307:1915–1920.

Berg RD. Bacterial translocation from the gastrointestinal tract. *Trends Microbiol.* 1995;3:149–154.

Blaser MJ, Atherton JC. *Helicobacter pylori* persistence: biology and disease. *J Clin Invest.* 2004;113:321–333.

Dethlefsen L, McFall-Ngai M, Relman DA. An ecological and evolutionary perspective on human-microbe mutalism and disease. *Nature.* 2007;449:811–818.

Greenough WB. The human, societal, and scientific legacy of cholera. *J Clin Invest.* 2004;113:334–339.

Haque R, Huston CD, Hughes M, et al. Amebiasis. *N Engl J Med.* 2003;348:1565–1573.

Kawakubo M, Ito Y, Okimura Y, et al. Natural antibiotic function of a human gastric mucin against *Helicobacter pylori* infection. *Science.* 2004;305:1003–1006.

Liévin-Le Moal V, Servin AL. The front line of enteric host defense against unwelcome intrusion of harmful microorganisms: mucins, antimicrobial peptides, and microbiota. *Clin Microbiol Rev.* 2006;19:315–337.

Mahon BE, Mintz ED, Greene KD, et al. Reported cholera in the United States, 1992–1994: a reflection of global changes in cholera epidemiology. *JAMA.* 1996;276:307–312.

Merrell DS, Falkow S. Frontal and stealth attack strategies in microbial pathogenesis. *Nature.* 2004;430:250–256.

Montecucco C, Rappuoli R. Living dangerously: how *Helicobacter pylori* survives in the human stomach. *Nat Rev Mol Cell Biol.* 2001;2:457–466.

Oldfield EC III. Evaluation of chronic diarrhea in patients with human immunodeficiency virus infection. *Rev Gastroenterol Disord.* 2002;2:176–188.

Petri WA, Miller M, Binder HJ, et al. Enteric infections, diarrhea, and their impact on function and development. *J Clin Invest.* 2008;118:1277–1290.

Sutton FM, Graham DY, Goodgame RW. Infectious esophagitis. *Gastrointest Clin North Am.* 1994;4:713–729.

Thielman NM, Guerrant RL. Clinical practice. Acute infectious diarrhea. *N Engl J Med.* 2004;350:38–47.

Viswanthan VK, Hodges K, Hecht G. Enteric Infection meets intestinal function: how bacterial pathogens cause diarrhoea. *Nat Rev Microbiol.* 2009;7:110–119.

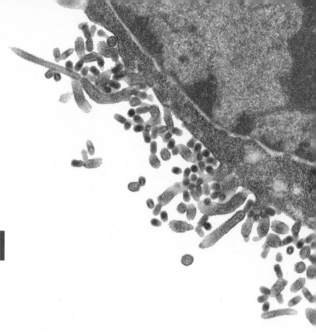

Chapter **61**

Infections of the Central Nervous System

Roberta L. DeBiasi and Kenneth L. Tyler

HUNDREDS of pathogens are capable of infecting the human central nervous system (CNS), including viruses, bacteria, mycobacteria, fungi, protozoa, and parasites. The involvement of specific anatomical structures results in distinct clinical presentations of CNS infection, including meningitis, encephalitis, myelitis, and focal suppurative infections such as brain abscess and empyema. CNS infections are among the most serious diseases affecting humans, causing significant morbidity and mortality even when diagnosed and treated appropriately. Antimicrobial therapies have reduced the overall mortality attributable to many CNS infections to less than 10%, but that rate is still unacceptably high. **Neurologic sequelae** resulting from these diseases may lead to significant impairment in daily functioning and have the potential to greatly alter normal cognitive and motor development when occurring in childhood. Prompt diagnosis of CNS infection is essential to maximize the likelihood of a positive response to therapy.

ANATOMIC DEFINITIONS AND THE BLOOD–BRAIN BARRIER

The brain and spinal cord are suspended in **cerebrospinal fluid** (**CSF**) and are surrounded by three layers of meninges: the **pia mater** and **arachnoid mater**, which together constitute the **leptomeninges**, and the **dura mater** or **pachymeninges** (Fig. 61-1). From a microbiological point of view, the brain and spinal cord have distinct features that simultaneously afford significant protection from infection, but some features place a person at risk for serious consequences should infection occur. A significant degree of mechanical protection and isolation is provided by the skull and vertebral column, but the intracranial and intravertebral spaces are restrictive, and inflammation and swelling of the brain or spinal cord can lead to dramatic changes in intracranial pressure, resulting in irreparable damage or even death. The **blood–brain barrier**—including the endothelial cells that line brain capillaries and are cemented together by intercellular tight junctions—provides an important barrier to the passage of microorganisms and toxic substances into the brain and CSF. However, the blood–brain barrier also impedes the passage into the CSF of protective components of

the humoral and cellular immune system and reduces the penetration of many antimicrobial drugs, resulting in decreased efficacy of available therapeutic agents.

CLINICAL DISEASE DEFINITIONS

Infections of the CNS can be categorized by the anatomic part of the brain affected. Infection of brain parenchyma results in **encephalitis** or **brain abscess**, infection of meninges causes **meningitis**, and infection of spinal cord tissue leads to **myelitis**. That categorization of CNS infections is somewhat artificial, because all areas of the brain are in anatomic communication with each other and can be infected simultaneously. In addition to direct injury from pathogens, CNS disease can result from postinfectious immune-mediated injury. Postinfectious encephalitis (**acute disseminated encephalomyelitis**, **ADEM**) occurs weeks after acute viral infection and is thought to result from immune-mediated cross-reactivity against components of the normal brain, such as myelin, rather than from direct injury of brain tissue by an infecting virus. In addition to acute infections, some organisms produce chronic or persistent infections. "Slow virus disease" (such as subacute sclerosing panencephalitis caused by measles

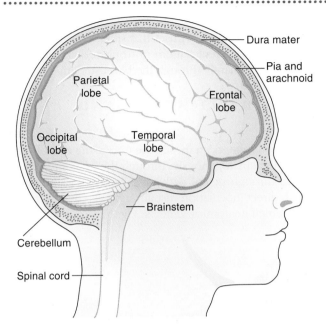

FIGURE 61-1. Gross anatomy of the cranium. The brain is located within a closed space, surrounded by the meninges (pia mater, arachnoid mater, and dura mater) in close approximation to mucosal surfaces containing commensal flora (the nasopharynx)

virus) is thought to result from viral persistence within the CNS in conjunction with altered immune mechanisms that facilitate persistent infection, leading to a slowly destructive process occurring over years following infection (see Chapter 34). Other types of chronic progressive, uniformly fatal CNS infections (such as bovine spongiform encephalopathy and kuru) are caused by **prions**, which are a novel class of infectious agents consisting of abnormally folded proteins (see Chapter 56).

MICROBIOLOGY

CNS infections are caused by viruses, rickettsiae, bacteria, mycobacteria, fungi, amebae, or parasites. The most frequent etiologic agents and the types of disease with which they are most commonly associated fall into distinct categories (Table 61-1). For example, certain bacteria (e.g., *Streptococcus pneumonia*, *Haemophilus influenzae*, and *Neisseria meningitidis*) classically cause meningitis but rarely cause infections of brain parenchyma, whereas others (e.g., *Staphylococcus aureus* and anaerobic streptococci) commonly cause brain abscesses but seldom cause meningitis. Some viruses are more likely to cause encephalitis (e.g., herpes simplex virus, or HSV), whereas others more commonly cause meningitis (e.g., enteroviruses).

Not all pathogens that infect humans can invade the CNS; organisms capable of CNS invasion possess special characteristics enabling them to infect cells of the nervous system, a property called **neurotropism**. Certain viruses show marked **tropism** for certain neural cell types (e.g., poliovirus for motor neurons of the spinal cord and

TABLE 61-1 Categorization of Central Nervous System Infections and Frequent Etiologic Agents

Acute Meningitis

Bacteria
Streptococcus pneumoniae
Neisseria meningitidis
Haemophilus influenzae type b
Group B streptococci
Escherichia coli

Viruses
Arboviruses
Enteroviruses
Herpes Simplex Virus

Chronic Meningitis

Bacteria
Mycobacterium tuberculosis

Fungi
Cryptococcus neoformans
Others

Acute Encephalitis

Viruses
Arboviruses
Enteroviruses
Herpesviruses

Acute Brain Abscess

Bacteria
Staphylococci
Mixed anaerobic and aerobic flora
Group A or D streptococci

Chronic Brain Abscess

Bacteria
Mycobacterium tuberculosis

Fungi
Cryptococcus neoformans

Parasites
Taenia solium (cysticercosis)
Toxoplasma

medulla and mumps viruses for ependymal cells lining the ventricles in the fetal brain). The basis for such tropism is probably the distribution of viral receptors on specific neural cells. An example of a microbiologic attribute conferring the capacity of bacteria to infect the CNS is encapsulation. Over half the strains of *Escherichia coli* that infect the CNS have a capsule composed of **K1 antigen**, suggesting that neuropathogenic strains have been selected from the many antigenically distinct strains of *E. coli*. In contrast to other *E. coli* capsular antigens, K1 is a polysaccharide rich in **sialic acid**, as are capsular polysaccharides of group B streptococci. Polysaccharides containing sialic acid assist in bacterial adherence to the meninges and resultant bacterial growth. K1 antigen also possesses antiphagocytic properties and inhibits activation of the alternative complement pathway, resulting in impeded clearance of the organism. Additional factors that can influence tropism include the

site of entry of a pathogen into the host and its mechanism of spread. For example, viruses that spread through neural routes have a different pattern of tropism than those that spread predominantly through the bloodstream.

ENTRY, REPLICATION, AND SPREAD

An infectious agent can invade the CNS using one of three routes: (1) hematogenously, through the systemic circulation; (2) through neural pathways; or less commonly (3) through direct inoculation (usually associated with trauma or congenital anatomical defects; Fig. 61-2).

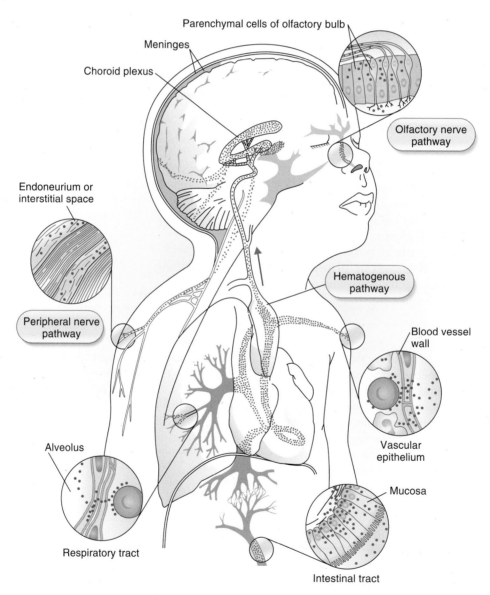

FIGURE 61-2. Pathways of entry of agents causing central nervous system (CNS) infections. In bloodborne infections, agents from the respiratory tract, gut, or vascular endothelium enter via the choroid plexus. Inside the CNS, microorganisms can spread either by contiguous dissemination from cell to cell or through extracellular spaces. Some neurotropic viruses reach the brain through peripheral nerves or olfactory nerve endings.

Hematogenous Route

Most cases of CNS infection are caused by entry of microorganisms from the **circulation** (see Fig. 61-2). Pathogens can gain access to the bloodstream by various routes, such as following colonization and penetration of the respiratory epithelium (e.g., meningococci), the bite of an arthropod (e.g., West Nile virus), the bite of a mammal (e.g., rabies virus), or transplacentally (e.g., rubella virus). Once an organism is in the bloodstream, the precise mechanism by which it penetrates the blood–brain barrier is not well understood. Some organisms enter the CNS at sites where the blood–brain barrier is less restrictive because of the lack of tight junctions between endothelial cells, such as the choroid plexus. Choroid plexus infection in turn provides direct access to the CSF within the ventricular system. Infection spreads sequentially from the blood to the choroid plexus to the ventricular CSF to ependymal cells lining the ventricles to periventricular brain tissues. Other viruses, including many arboviruses, have the capacity to directly infect endothelial cells, including those of the microvascular circulation of the brain. Regardless of the route of entry to the CNS, the likelihood of infection increases in relation to the microbial load in the bloodstream.

Neural Route

Although many neurotropic viruses reach the CNS through the bloodstream, a few use special neural pathways (see Fig. 61-2). For example, following inoculation by the bite of a rabid animal, rabies virus enters the axons of peripheral nerves and travels inside nerve axons via axoplasmic transport to reach nerve cell bodies in sensory ganglia and the spinal cord. HSV spreads through nerves from sites of primary infection in the oropharynx (HSV-1) or genital area (HSV-2) to infect trigeminal (HSV-1) or sacral (HSV-2) ganglia, where the virus becomes latent in sensory neurons (see Chapter 41). Reactivation results in spread of virus along sensory nerves to mucosal surfaces, producing recurrent herpes labialis (cold sores) or herpes genitalis. Following chicken pox, which results from primary infection with varicella-zoster virus (VZV), virus spreads from the skin through sensory nerves to become latent in neurons in sensory ganglia. Reactivation results in spread of virus through sensory nerves to produce zoster or shingles.

Some viruses and other infectious agents can penetrate the body through olfactory nerve endings, which are the only elements of the nervous system in direct contact with the external environment. Experimental studies suggest that herpesviruses can reach the brain by this route, and nasal infections occur with rabies virus and some arboviruses under conditions with high airborne concentrations of virus, as in caves filled with infected bats. The freshwater ameba *Naegleria fowleri*, which causes a rare but lethal meningoencephalitis, is thought to penetrate the CNS through traumatic gaps in the cribriform plate, allowing access to the olfactory bulbs, perhaps induced when a person dives into water containing the organism.

LOCAL IMMUNE RESPONSES

The CNS is a sequestered compartment with more restricted immunological defense mechanisms than most other regions of the body. For example, complement levels are low in the CSF, apparently owing to both poor penetration from the blood and the presence of substances that can inactivate complement. Therefore, complement-dependent lysis or phagocytosis of bacteria does not readily occur in the brain, the meninges, and the CSF. However, the CNS is not as immunologically restricted as was once thought. The CNS possesses an intrinsic immunological surveillance mechanism in the **microglia**. Microglial cells have many cell type–specific markers identical to those of peripheral blood monocytes, suggesting that microglia are derived from blood monocytes that enter the CNS and differentiate. In addition, the CNS has a lymphlike system consisting of the **Virchow-Robin spaces** (the perivascular sheaths surrounding the blood vessels as they enter the brain). These spaces contain macrophages and lymphocytes and are thought to be sites where those cells enter the CSF. In certain CNS infections, the host immune response maintains the infecting microorganisms in a latent state; active disease results only when immune mechanisms are compromised by drugs, HIV infection, or other forms of immunosuppression. Examples of such infections include tuberculosis and toxoplasmosis.

Immunodeficient persons are at risk for more severe or unusual presentations of CNS disease not seen in immunocompetent individuals. For example, persons with acquired immunodeficiency (e.g., Hodgkin disease and other lymphomas, AIDS, patients receiving immunosuppressive drug regimens) can develop **progressive multifocal leukoencephalopathy** (**PML**). PML is caused by reactivation of a polyomavirus called **JC virus**, which is usually acquired in early childhood. Acute infection with JC virus is either asymptomatic or results in self-limited mild illness before becoming latent within the CNS. However, immunosuppression allows reactivation and replication of latent virus, leading to progressive CNS destruction.

EPIDEMIOLOGY

The most important epidemiological determinants of CNS infection are the age and geographic location of the affected individual and the time of year. For example, certain bacteria are more likely to cause meningitis in persons of defined age groups (Table 61-2). That information is important to consider when choosing empiric antimicrobial therapy while awaiting CSF culture results. Thus, in newborn infants, bacterial meningitis is most commonly caused by

TABLE 61-2 Etiology and Empiric Therapy of Bacterial Meningitis by Patient Category

Bacterial Pathogen

Age	Underlying Disease	Most Common	Other	Initial Empiric Therapy
Birth to 3 mo	None	*Streptococcus agalactiae* (group B)	*Escherichia coli*	Ampicillin and cefotaxime (or gentamicin)
			Listeria monocytogenes	
			Other Gram-negative organisms	
3–60 mo	None	*Streptococcus pneumoniae*	*Neisseria meningitidis*[a]	Vancomycin and cefotaxime (or ceftriaxone)
			(*Haemophilus influenzae* type b)[b]	
>60 mo	None	*Streptococcus pneumoniae*	*N. meningitidis*[a]	Vancomycin and cefotaxime (or ceftriaxone)
			L. monocytogenes	
			Other Gram-negative organisms	
Any age	Cranial surgery	*Staphylococcus aureus*	*Staphylococcus epidermidis*	Vancomycin and cefepime (or ceftazidime)
			Gram-negative organisms, including *Pseudomonas aeruginosa*	
Any age	Immunosuppression (malignancy, drug induced, AIDS)		*L. monocytogenes*	Ampicillin (or vancomycin) and cefepime (or ceftazidime)
			Gram-negative organisms, including *P. aeruginosa*	

[a]Occurs in epidemics.
[b]Only in unimmunized populations.

group B streptococci (*Streptococcus agalactiae*) and *E. coli*. Likewise, *Listeria monocytogenes* is a more frequent cause of bacterial meningitis in neonates and the elderly than in other age groups. The season in which clinical illness develops also can suggest which specific pathogens are the most likely causal organisms (Table 61-3). For example, spread of arboviruses by mosquito and tick vectors occurs more commonly in summer months, when mosquito breeding and likelihood of exposure is greatest, and wanes in winter months (see Chapter 33). Enteroviral infections usually peak in the late summer and fall. On the other hand, some pathogens do not have specific seasonal variation and occur with equal frequency throughout the year; among these pathogens is HSV, the most common cause of sporadic viral encephalitis in adults. The geographic distribution of several arboviruses is suggested by their names (e.g., California encephalitis virus, St. Louis encephalitis virus, and West Nile virus), although they often misrepresent the

modern host ranges of the viruses. For example, although St. Louis encephalitis virus was named for the city in which it was first isolated from patients with encephalitis, it occurs throughout the United States. Similarly, although West Nile virus was first isolated from the West Nile Valley in Uganda, it is now widely distributed throughout the United States and many other regions of the world. West Nile virus also provides a dramatic example of how the host range of an infectious agent can change dramatically over a relatively short period: the range of the virus expanded across the entire 48 contiguous United States in just 5 years from 1999 to 2004 (see Chapter 33).

DAMAGE

Tissue dysfunction resulting from CNS infection occurs by several mechanisms. Death of CNS cells can result from the action of bacterial toxins, lytic cycles of viral replication,

TABLE 61-3 Viruses Causing Encephalitis

Virus	Virus Type	Geographic Location	Major Age Group	Predominant Season	Notable Features
Herpes simplex viruses 1 and 2	DNA	All	All	None	Focal symptoms and signs
West Nile virus	RNA	All	Older adults	Summer through fall	Weakness, movement disorders, poliomyelitis syndrome
St. Louis encephalitis virus	RNA	All	Older adults	Summer through fall	Most cases mild
Eastern equine encephalitis virus	RNA	Atlantic and Gulf coasts, Great Lakes	Children	Summer through fall	High mortality (50–80%) and morbidity (80% with neurologic sequelae)
Western equine encephalitis virus	RNA	Western United States and Canada	Infants and older adults	Summer through fall	Higher mortality (10–20%) and morbidity in infants (50%)
California (La Crosse) virus	RNA	Midwest and Northeast United States, southern Canada	Older children	Summer through fall	<1% mortality and rare encephalitis morbidity
Enteroviruses	RNA	All	Infants and children more than adults	Summer	Severity inverse to age
Rabies virus	RNA	All	All	All	Animal bite (bats)
Varicella-zoster virus	DNA	All	Children and immunocompromised adults	Winter	Rare
HIV	RNA	All	Adults more than children	All	Dementia in persons with AIDS

or intracellular growth of bacteria and fungi. However, in most infections, some component of cell death and tissue destruction results from the host immune response. Multiplication and spread of microorganisms within the CNS elicits an inflammatory response similar to but generally less intense than that produced in other areas of the body. Infiltration of microglia and proliferation of **astrocytes** are characteristic of the inflammatory response within the CNS. As in other parts of the body, the CNS inflammatory response has both humoral and cellular components. Inflammation can lead to vasogenic edema caused by increased capillary permeability. Neutrophils and macrophages then infiltrate the area and phagocytize microorganisms and dead cells. Lysis of infiltrating neutrophils releases enzymes, leading to further tissue destruction.

Swelling of the brain resulting from inflammation within the closed cranial vault (cerebral edema) can produce neurologic symptoms as a consequence of decreased capillary perfusion of brain tissue. More severe forms of cerebral edema can cause herniation of the temporal lobe through the falx or the brainstem into the foramen magnum, producing severe brain damage or death. Thus, neurological symptoms that arise during infection of the CNS can be caused by focal tissue destruction that produces specific functional deficits or by cerebral edema that leads to global loss of cortical function.

The localization of specific functions in different areas of the brain, combined with differences in the capacity of microorganisms to infect those areas, provides clues to the diagnosis of specific infections. For example, psychosis, impairment of memory, and seizures suggest HSV encephalitis (because of the preferred involvement of the frontal and temporal lobes); stiffness of the neck without severe impairment of cerebral function is characteristic of enteroviral meningitis; and flaccid paralysis of the lower extremities suggests injury to the motor neurons of

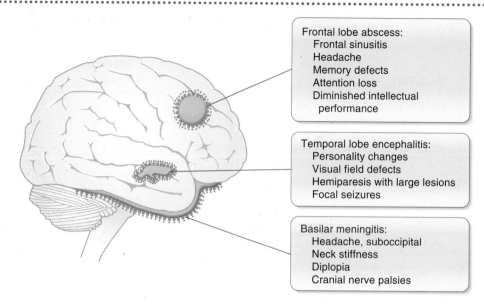

Frontal lobe abscess:
  Frontal sinusitis
  Headache
  Memory defects
  Attention loss
  Diminished intellectual
    performance

Temporal lobe encephalitis:
  Personality changes
  Visual field defects
  Hemiparesis with large lesions
  Focal seizures

Basilar meningitis:
  Headache, suboccipital
  Neck stiffness
  Diplopia
  Cranial nerve palsies

FIGURE 61-3. Anatomic basis of localization of symptoms in central nervous system infections. Focal involvement of the cerebral cortex produces specific signs and symptoms depending on the primary function of that part of the brain. In contrast, pyogenic meningitis produces global cerebral cortical dysfunction as a result of diffuse cerebral edema.

the spinal cord from poliovirus or West Nile virus. Focal symptoms likely to result from specific CNS infections are shown in Figure 61-3.

The following case histories and discussion describe characteristic infections of the CNS and their diagnoses. They include cases of acute bacterial meningitis, acute viral (aseptic) meningitis, chronic tuberculous meningitis, acute viral encephalitis, and brain abscess.

MENINGITIS

Most cases of meningitis can be classified in the following manner:

- By clinical presentation: acute, subacute, or chronic
- By etiology: bacterial, viral, or fungal
- By epidemiology: sporadic or epidemic

Acute meningitis is usually characterized by the rapid onset of symptoms, occurring within hours of contact with the infectious agent and possibly days before presentation for medical evaluation. Acute meningitis is usually bacterial or viral in etiology. In all cases of suspected bacterial meningitis, antimicrobial therapy must be administered immediately. The predominant etiology of acute bacterial meningitis varies with the age of the patient. In infants younger than 3 months of age, acute bacterial meningitis is caused chiefly by group B streptococci, *E. coli*, or *L. monocytogenes*. The most common etiologic organisms in children more than 3 months of age, adolescents, and adults are *S. pneumonia* (pneumococci) and *N. meningitides* (meningococci), *H. influenzae*

type b was once the most common cause of bacterial meningitis in children. However, with the introduction of effective *H. influenzae* conjugated vaccines in the mid-1980s, in which *H. influenzae* type b capsular carbohydrate is covalently linked to a protein carrier (tetanus or diphtheria toxoids), that type of bacterial meningitis has been nearly eradicated in immunized populations. Children who are not immunized or only partially immunized remain susceptible to infection with *H. influenzae* type b. Meningitis also can be caused by nontypeable *Haemophilus* species, but those organisms are seen less often than are other causes of bacterial meningitis. With the advent of routine universal pneumococcal vaccination of children in 2000, marked reductions in the rates of invasive pneumococcal disease, including meningitis, have been observed in this population. However, pneumococcal strains that are not represented in currently available vaccines continue to cause invasive disease. Acute viral meningitis (the most common etiology of the clinical entity referred to as aseptic meningitis) is usually caused by enteroviruses and occurs most frequently in the late summer and fall in annual epidemics.

Subacute or chronic meningitis is most commonly caused by fungi (such as *C. neoformans*) or mycobacteria (such as *Mycobacterium tuberculosis*), organisms that cause chronic, inflammatory, granulomatous tissue reactions. Persons with subacute or chronic meningitis often present with weeks to months of less fulminant clinical symptoms than those associated with acute meningitis, but an acute worsening could prompt the decision to seek medical evaluation.

CASE

Bacterial Meningitis

One week after arriving at the Army recruit camp at Fort Ord, California, Pvt. W. became the first of three cases of meningitis. He had the precipitous onset of fever and headache and felt a pain in his neck when he moved his head. When he arrived at the infirmary, he had a petechial rash on his lower extremities. On lumbar puncture, his opening pressure was slightly elevated at 220 mm H_2O (normal range is <180 mm H_2O). CSF cell count revealed white blood cells (WBCs) at 500/mm³ (80% polymorphonuclear cells), the CSF glucose was 30 mg/dL (decreased), and protein was 100 mg/dL (increased). A smear of the CSF revealed small Gram-negative coccobacilli and numerous leukocytes (Fig. 61-4).

Antimicrobial therapy was instituted immediately with intravenous vancomycin and ceftriaxone, pending culture results. Twenty-four hours later, the CSF culture grew *N. meningitides*. Vancomycin was discontinued, and following 10 days of intravenous ceftriaxone therapy, Pvt. W. recovered completely. Pvt. H. had developed the same symptoms 24 hours after Pvt. W. When Pvt. B. was diagnosed the next morning with the same illness, the other soldiers in

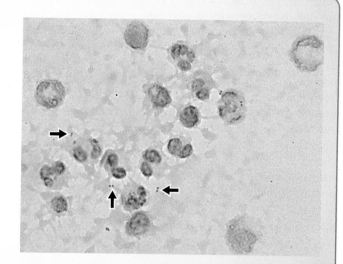

FIGURE 61-4. Gram stain of CSF from a patient with meningococcal meningitis. Gram-negative coccobacilli (*arrows*) and neutrophils are evident.

the camp became alarmed. Their fears calmed when the medical corps personnel explained that further spread of infection could be halted by the prophylactic administration of antibiotics to all close contacts of the infected cases.

Acute Bacterial Meningitis
ENCOUNTER AND ENTRY

The two most common agents of acute bacterial meningitis, pneumococci and meningococci, are acquired by the respiratory route through inhalation of aerosol droplets from asymptomatic human carriers. It is likely that in the meningococcal outbreak at Ford Ord (see Case: Bacterial Meningitis), most of the recruits were exposed to the organism from another individual, because meningococci are found in the oropharynx of about 10% of healthy people. However, the frequency of colonization does not always correlate directly with outbreaks, because individual strains of meningococci vary considerably in

CASE

Viral Meningitis

While Privates W., H., and B. were being treated for their infections, Pvt. E. left the Fort Ord camp for his assignment at Fort Leonard Wood, Missouri. When he arrived, he had a fever, severe headache, and some nausea. The next day, when putting on his boots, he noticed that his neck was stiff. He also became very sensitive to bright sunlight. When he was evaluated at the infirmary, a lumbar puncture was performed. The CSF opening pressure was 90 mm H_2O (in the normal range). The CSF contained 76 WBCs/mm³ (90% lymphocytes), 70 mg/dL of protein (mildly increased), and 66 mg/dL of glucose (normal). He was observed in the hospital for 2 days, without institution of antibiotics, pending results of CSF bacterial and viral cultures and CSF enterovirus polymerase chain reaction (PCR). The CSF cultures were negative, but the enteroviral PCR returned positive 36 hours after admission. His symptoms resolved without antimicrobial therapy, and he was discharged from the hospital with a diagnosis of aseptic meningitis caused by enterovirus.

These cases raise two questions:

1. Why did meningococcal meningitis, the etiology of Pvt. W.'s illness, produce alarm and warrant aggressive treatment and measures to prevent spread of infection, whereas viral aseptic meningitis, the etiology of Pvt. E.'s illness, did not require specific therapy?

2. How do the CSF findings in Pvt. W.'s case (bacterial meningitis) compare with those in Pvt. E.'s case (viral meningitis)?

See Appendix for answers.

virulence. The reason so many people become colonized but only a few get sick is not well understood. The best clue comes from the observation that susceptible individuals lack antibodies against the meningococcal capsular antigen, whereas carriers have protective antibodies, possibly induced by colonization of the upper respiratory tract with nonpathogenic neisserial species. Moreover, a striking association has been made between congenital deficiency in the late components of the complement cascade and neisserial infection, particularly with meningococci. Those findings suggest that the immunological status of an individual plays a role in determining whether disease develops.

SPREAD, MULTIPLICATION, AND DAMAGE

Acute bacterial meningitis can be an isolated clinical event or part of overwhelming bacterial septicemia. In the latter case, the symptoms of meningitis only add to an already grave clinical picture; the presence of large numbers of organisms in the blood causes severe nonneural manifestations, such as shock and disseminated intravascular coagulation. In the case of meningococcal disease, those signs reflect the high blood content of Gram-negative endotoxin.

The clinical manifestations of acute meningitis, caused by meningococci or other bacteria, include fever, stiff neck (nuchal rigidity), headache, and occasionally global or focal CNS dysfunction. These symptoms are caused by the inflammatory response to meningeal invasion. The extent of inflammation caused by pathogens varies and is influenced by the intrinsic virulence of the organism and the immune response of the patient. Pus in the subarachnoid spaces can spread over the brain, the cerebellum, and the spinal cord. Pneumococcal infections

and those caused by members of the *Enterobacteriaceae* family are marked by particularly thick accumulations of pus that block CSF flow and readsorption, leading to elevated intracranial pressure. In meningococcal meningitis, the CSF pressure is usually only mildly elevated. Increased intracranial pressure from cerebral edema invariably leads to nausea and vomiting, severe headache, and progressive depression in the level of consciousness.

In general, the incidence of neurologic sequelae is lower when bacterial meningitis is caused by meningococci than it is when the cause is some other bacteria. *H. influenzae* meningitis often results in deafness, intellectual disability, or both in affected patients. Neurologic sequelae from pneumococcal meningitis also tend to be severe and frequent.

DIAGNOSIS

Acute bacterial infection of the CNS is a medical emergency. Appropriate antibiotic therapy must be initiated immediately after a patient arrives in an emergency department or physician's office. Fortunately, examination of a Gram stain of the CSF obtained by lumbar puncture can rapidly yield a presumptive diagnosis. Examination of the CSF is absolutely necessary when acute meningitis is suspected. The characteristic patterns of inflammation in the CSF in the setting of various CNS infections are summarized in Table 61-4.

The elements of the inflammatory response in the CSF also can help in determining whether the infection is likely to be bacterial or viral and may even point to a specific etiological agent. A large number of neutrophils suggests bacterial infection, whereas a predominance of lymphocytes or mononuclear cells suggests a nonbacterial (most commonly, but not always, viral) etiology. Gram stain examination of the CSF should be a routine

TABLE 61-4 Usual Composition of Cerebrospinal Fluid in Various Central Nervous System Infections

Factor	Normal	Acute Bacterial Meningitis	Chronic Mycobacterial and Fungal Meningitis	Acute Viral Meningitis	Viral Encephalitis	Brain Abscess
Leukocytes (per mm³)	0–6	>1,000	100–500	10–1,000, usually <300	10–500	10–100
% Neutrophils	0	>50	<10	May predominate in first 24 h, then <50	May predominate in first 24 h, then <50	<50
Red blood cells (per mm³)	0–2	0–10	0–2	0–2	10–500 (HSV)	0–2
Glucose (mg/dL)^a	40–80	<30	≤40	40–80	40–80	40–80
Protein (mg/dL)	20–50	>100	50–100 (fungal), >100 (mycobacterial)	50–100	50–100	50–100

^{a}Diagnostic values are best interpreted as the ratio of glucose levels in CSF compared with those in serum. Ratios <0.4 are considered diminished.

procedure because it reveals infecting bacteria in about 60 to 90% of the cases of bacterial meningitis.

Culture of CSF can definitively establish the etiology of bacterial meningitis and guide the choice of antibiotic therapy. Rapid tests based on identification of bacterial antigens are unreliable, with unacceptably low sensitivity and specificity to be useful in diagnosis. PCR testing for enterovirus has excellent sensitivity and specificity (>95% each), with results often available in less than 24 hours. PCR tests for bacteria are not yet widely available beyond research applications.

TREATMENT

To treat bacterial meningitis effectively, antibiotics to which the bacteria are susceptible must penetrate the CSF in an active form. **β-Lactam antibiotics** are frequently used to treat bacterial meningitis. These drugs are highly polar and have relatively low penetration through blood–brain and blood–CSF barriers. The average drug concentration normally achieved in CSF is about 15% of that in serum. Nevertheless, these antibiotics are drugs of choice because they have a very high therapeutic index (i.e., toxic levels are much higher than therapeutic levels). Consequently, they are tolerated at serum levels that are high enough to produce therapeutic CSF levels. In addition, β-lactam drugs also enter the CSF through capillary leaks that are enhanced by inflammation. β-lactam antibiotics, such as **cefotaxime** and **ceftriaxone**, are very potent and produce CSF concentrations that exceed those required to kill bacteria by 20 times or more. Since we cannot rely on the immune response in meningitis to clear bacterial infection, acute meningitis is treated only with antibiotics that are bactericidal, at bactericidal levels.

In recent years, β-lactam resistance has emerged among pneumococcal isolates in the United States. Up to 50% of isolates are partially or completely resistant in many parts of the country. This development makes it imperative to use combination therapy with vancomycin (a glycopeptide antibiotic with a mechanism of action that differs from that of β-lactam drugs) for empiric therapy of bacterial meningitis, until resistance to cephalosporins has been definitively excluded by culture and susceptibility testing.

An important aspect of the treatment of meningitis is the control of increased intracranial pressure. Cerebral edema can further decrease the already diminished cerebral blood flow and depress oxidative glucose metabolism. Death from compression of the brainstem into the foramen magnum (i.e., herniation) is possible. Supportive measures must ensure that the patient is adequately oxygenated and that the blood glucose is in the normal range. Dexamethasone, a glucocorticoid with potent anti-inflammatory activities, decreases the incidence of deafness as a consequence of *H. influenzae* meningitis in children greater than 3 months of age. In adults, the role of steriods in improving outcomes in acute bacterial meningitis remains uncertain.

PREVENTION

Vaccines are currently available for *N. meningitides*, *S. pneumoniae*, and *H. influenzae* type b, the most common causes of bacterial meningitis (see Chapter 45). Routine vaccination against meningococci was previously limited to high-risk groups, such as military recruits. However, since 2005, a quadrivalent (serogroups A, C, Y, and W135) meningococcal vaccine has been included as part of the routine immunization schedule for 11- to 12-year-old children. It is not currently possible to induce antibodies against type B meningococci with vaccine, because the molecular structure of this capsule type (polysialic acid) mimics human glycoproteins. Chemoprophylaxis with rifampin, quinolone antibiotics, or ceftriaxone effectively eradicates nasopharyngeal carriage of meningococci in the majority of recipients and is indicated for all close contacts of index cases. A multivalent polysaccharide pneumococcal vaccine is available for persons older than 2 years of age who are at risk for acquiring invasive pneumococcal disease (asplenic persons and those with certain forms of primary immunodeficiency). Conjugated pneumococcal vaccine is now recommended as part of the routine immunization schedule for all children in the United States beginning at 2 months of age. Widespread pneumococcal immunization has led to a much lower incidence of pneumococcal meningitis in the last decade, as has been observed following widespread use of the *H. influenzae* type b vaccine among children.

Viral Meningitis
PATHOBIOLOGY

Viruses are the most common cause of the syndrome known as aseptic meningitis. In its traditional sense, the term "aseptic" is a misnomer because it refers only to the fact that the CSF of patients with the syndrome is sterile on routine bacteriological culture. However, aseptic meningitis also results from infections caused by various agents that do not grow on standard bacteriological media (e.g., fungi, leptospira, borrelia, and *Treponema pallidum*). In addition, aseptic meningitis can result from noninfectious etiologies, such as cancer or autoimmune disease.

DIAGNOSIS AND TREATMENT

Compared with bacterial meningitis, viral meningitis produces a milder disease with low to moderate inflammatory reaction in the CSF consisting primarily of lymphocytes. Pvt. E. had the clinical disease and CSF findings typical of viral meningitis (chiefly, a mildly increased number of CSF leukocytes and normal glucose level; see Table 61-4). Therefore, he did not receive antibiotics and was observed in the hospital. His improvement without antibacterial treatment further supported a viral etiology. The positive CSF PCR test for enterovirus confirmed the diagnosis of the most common etiology of viral

CASE

Tuberculous Meningitis

Ms. G., a 32-year-old native of South America, immigrated to the United States 2 months ago with her husband and three children. Four weeks following her arrival, her oldest child returned from child care with chicken pox. Two weeks later, Ms. G. and the rest of her family developed the disease. All recovered uneventfully. However, as Ms. G.'s rash faded, she developed a headache and again had fever. Over the next week, she lost her appetite and vomited a few times. Those symptoms persisted for another week, and she became apathetic. When she developed stupor 4 days later, she was taken to a local hospital.

On physical examination, Ms. G. was noted to have impaired eye movements. A chest radiograph showed right upper lobe pneumonia. A cranial computerized tomography (CT) scan showed enlarged ventricles suggestive of acute hydrocephalus. A lumbar puncture revealed an opening pressure of 310 mm H_2O (highly elevated), and the CSF showed 350 WBCs/mm³, of which 87% were lymphocytes. The CSF protein was 168 mg/dL (increased), and the glucose was 20 mg/dL (decreased) with coincident serum glucose of 120 mg/dL. Gram stain and acid-fast stain of the CSF did not show organisms.

Additional studies of the CSF included detection of tuberculostearic acid and a positive mycobacterial PCR, which led the physician to diagnose tuberculous meningitis (see Chapter 23). Subsequently, *M. tuberculosis* grew from her CSF and was found to be susceptible to isoniazid, rifampin, pyrazinamide, and streptomycin. Ms. G. was treated with urgent ventricular drainage, the four antituberculosis drugs tested, and steroids for 2 months. With resolution of her symptoms, ventricular drainage was discontinued and she was discharged to receive 10 additional months of therapy with isoniazid and rifampin.

This case raises several questions:

1. What is the explanation for Ms. G.'s eye movement abnormalities?
2. How do the CSF findings in tuberculous meningitis compare with those in viral and bacterial meningitis?
3. Why are multiple drugs required for the treatment of tuberculous meningitis?

See Appendix for answers.

---

meningitis. However, many other viruses can cause the disease, including arboviruses (such as West Nile virus, WNV) and the herpesviruses (HSV-1, HSV-2, and VZV). Although viral meningitis can be confirmed by isolating a virus by culture from the CSF, that process is time consuming, and many viruses cannot be cultivated. Isolating a virus known to cause aseptic meningitis from the throat or stool of a patient with appropriate symptoms suggests, but does not prove, that the suspect virus is the cause of aseptic meningitis. If the enterovirus PCR had been negative, and Pvt. E. had not improved, other causes for his symptoms and the presence of leukocytes in the CSF would have been pursued.

In infants less than 1 year of age, it is often difficult to distinguish bacterial from aseptic meningitis. The newborn has a limited set of immune responses when the CNS is infected, and the relative immaturity of the reticuloendothelial system at that age may not permit an adult-type inflammatory response. As a result, most infants with symptoms of acute meningitis and leukocytes in the CSF are treated empirically with intravenous antibiotics while bacterial cultures are pending, even if a viral etiology is suspected.

Chronic Meningitis
PATHOBIOLOGY

Ms. G. came from a geographic region in which pulmonary tuberculosis is endemic. During primary pulmonary infection, tubercle bacilli may be deposited in multiple organs (including the brain), where they are contained within granulomas and remain quiescent (termed latent tuberculosis). Ms. G.'s chicken pox suppressed her cell-mediated immunity, enabling the tubercle bacilli to multiply and cause inflammation. In the brain, granulomas located near the ventricles may spill tubercle bacilli into the CSF. The organisms then spread throughout the subarachnoid space and characteristically become most prevalent in the basilar cisterns. As cell-mediated immunity returns, it elicits an intense delayed-type hypersensitivity reaction to the organisms. Granulomas and inflammation around cranial nerves cause them to malfunction. In Ms. G.'s case, the nerves affected were cranial nerves III and VI, as indicated by the impaired eye movements. Inflammation of the base of the brain compromises CSF circulation from the fourth ventricle into the cisterna magna, which causes acute hydrocephalus and increased intracranial pressure, leading to stupor and the possibility of coma.

DIAGNOSIS

Ms. G.'s CSF findings (lymphocytic pleocytosis, decreased glucose, and increased protein) and indolent course are consistent with chronic meningitis. Both fungi and *M. tuberculosis* are potential etiologies that should be considered in such cases. Acid-fast stain of CSF has poor sensitivity for the diagnosis of tuberculous meningitis, being positive in only 5 to 25% of cases. Thus, the test cannot be used to exclude disease. Mycobacterial culture may require up to 6 weeks for growth and identification of the organism. The presence of a **tubercular lipid** (tuberculostearic acid) in the CSF made the diagnosis of tuberculous meningitis likely in the case of Ms. G. The diagnosis was later confirmed by PCR amplification of mycobacterial DNA and isolation of *M. tuberculosis* from the CSF.

Because the diagnosis of tuberculous meningitis is so important, many research groups are working to develop sensitive and specific DNA-based methods to detect mycobacteria in the CSF, employing PCR primers specific for certain genes of *M. tuberculosis*. Although PCR of CSF has not yet achieved adequate sensitivity or specificity to replace more standard methods, it may be useful as an adjunctive diagnostic method. An intradermal skin test using purified protein derivative may or may not be positive in fulminant tuberculosis, but it should be positive when repeated after weeks to months of effective antituberculous therapy.

TREATMENT

The emergence of drug-resistant strains of *M. tuberculosis* in most parts of the world makes combination therapy with at least three and preferably four drugs with different mechanisms of action the standard of care for the treatment of active tuberculosis, particularly with involvement of the CNS. If the organism is isolated from the CSF (which may take up to 6 weeks), susceptibility testing should be performed to verify selection of the proper drug regimen for long-term therapy (usually 12 months).

Steroids are used for treatment of CNS disease because the intense inflammatory response to the organism is a major component of neural dysfunction and damage to the brain and meninges. With successful treatment, CSF cultures should become sterile within 1 month and CSF glucose should become normal by 1 to 2 months. CSF cell counts and protein may take 1 year to normalize.

ACUTE VIRAL ENCEPHALITIS
PATHOBIOLOGY

Approximately 20,000 cases of encephalitis occur in the United States each year, almost all of which are caused by viruses. The hallmark of encephalitis is the acute onset of a febrile illness accompanied by headache and **altered mental status**. The presence of altered mental status (e.g., disorientation, hallucination, or behavioral disturbances) and focal or diffuse neurologic signs (e.g., hemiparesis or seizures) help distinguish encephalitis from meningitis. HSV is the most frequent etiology of sporadic encephalitis in the United States, accounting for approximately 10% of cases annually. Arboviruses, including West Nile virus, are the most important cause of epidemic encephalitis (see Table 61-3 and Chapters 33 and 41).

HSV-1 (and rarely HSV-2) is usually associated with severe focal encephalitis in adolescents and adults. Untreated, the disease carries a 70% mortality rate, and 97% of untreated survivors are left with permanent neurologic deficits. Fibers emerging from the trigeminal ganglia, in which HSV-1 resides in the latent state following primary infection, innervate the dura of the middle and anterior fossae and the meningeal arteries of the area.

CASE

HSV Encephalitis

Mr. R., a 60-year-old man, was brought to the hospital with confusion, right-sided weakness, and fever. His daughter, who was visiting him, reported that when she arrived, he thought "there were devils in the room." On the way to the hospital, he hallucinated intermittently, telling her that he smelled roses. Three days previously, he had complained of mild nausea and vomited once. When he arrived at the emergency department, Mr. R. had a generalized seizure.

A CT scan of the head was normal, but a magnetic resonance imaging (MRI) scan documented T1-hypointense and T2-hyperintense signal in the cortex and gray–white matter junction in the left temporal lobe. CSF obtained by lumbar puncture contained 50 WBCs/mm³ (90% mononuclear cells) and 300 RBCs/mm³, glucose in the normal range (70 mg/dL), and elevated protein (100 mg/dL). CSF was sent for bacterial and viral culture and enterovirus and

HSV PCR. An electroencephalogram (EEG) revealed periodic high-voltage spike wave activity from the left temporal region.

Intravenous acyclovir was started immediately. By the next day, the CSF enterovirus PCR was negative and the HSV PCR was positive. Mr. R. continued to receive intravenous acyclovir for 3 weeks, which halted the progression of his neurological symptoms. However, he had many residual signs of neurological impairment and required extensive rehabilitation therapy.

This case raises two questions:

1. What is the best single diagnostic method to establish a diagnosis of HSV encephalitis?

2. What is the prognosis for patients who survive HSV encephalitis?

See Appendix for answers.

HSV may use this route to spread to the meninges and meningeal arteries and, from there, to the contiguous cortex. That postulated pattern might explain the frequent localization of HSV in the temporal and frontal lobes.

Five to 50% percent of newborns who acquire HSV (usually HSV-2), either transplacentally or at the time of delivery from the maternal genital tract, develop CNS infection. CNS disease occurs predominantly in two forms: (1) nondisseminated neuronal transmission, with disease limited to the CNS or (2) hematogenous dissemination with multiorgan involvement, including the CNS. Many of the manifestations of HSV encephalitis result from the destruction of neurons, especially within the temporal and frontal lobes, accompanied by inflammation with infiltration of mononuclear cells from the perivascular sheaths (Virchow-Robin spaces). Portions of the temporal lobe responsible for the sense of smell may be affected, resulting in olfactory hallucinations (e.g., smelling roses in the case of Mr. R.).

DIAGNOSIS

The diagnosis of herpes encephalitis is suspected if adult patients have fever and focal cerebral cortical lesions, particularly in the frontal and temporal lobes. CSF abnormalities are generally similar to those found in viral meningitis. Modest pleocytosis (predominantly mononuclear) occurs in 95% of cases, along with the presence of red blood cells in 75% of cases. Increased CSF protein occurs in 90% of cases but rarely exceeds 200 mg/dL; CSF glucose is almost always normal. EEG abnormalities also can provide diagnostic clues because 90% of patients have focal or generalized slowing. The presence of periodic sharp wave complexes in the temporal leads superimposed on a slow amplitude background is highly suggestive of HSV encephalitis. MRI scans show abnormal areas involving the temporal lobes and orbitofrontal cortex in more than 90% of cases of herpes encephalitis. MRI scans are much more sensitive than CT scans early in the illness, but eventually, more than 60% of patients will show some abnormality on CT scans. The pattern of brain parenchymal involvement in HSV disease is often distinct from that seen in arboviral encephalitis, in which deep nuclear structures are commonly affected, or ADEM, in which white matter is primarily involved (Fig. 61-5).

In the past, cerebral biopsy with virus isolation was employed as the standard for diagnosis of HSV encephalitis. However, biopsy has been replaced by detection of HSV DNA in the CSF by PCR. If performed with optimal techniques in an experienced laboratory, specificity is 100% and sensitivity is 95%. However, recent reports indicate that PCR performed on HSV-infected CSF within the first 48 hours of illness may have decreased sensitivity. The frequency of positive PCR tests also declines with treatment and duration of illness. The CSF PCR becomes negative

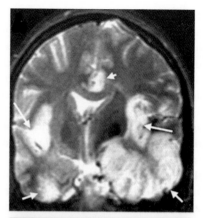

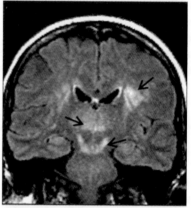

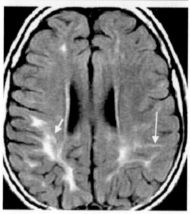

FIGURE 61-5. Magnetic resonance imaging of patients with viral encephalitis and acute disseminated encephalomyelitis (ADEM). Top: Herpes simplex virus encephalitis. Abnormal signal and edema in the left temporal lobe (*short bottom arrow*), insula (*long arrow*), and cingulate gyrus (*arrowhead*), with mass effect compressing the left lateral ventricle and uncal herniation; also note increased signal in the right inferomedial temporal lobe (*short bottom arrow*) and insular cortex (*long arrow*). **Middle:** West Nile encephalitis. Deep-seated structures characteristically involved subcortical white matter (*top arrow*), thalami (*middle arrow*), and substantia nigra (*bottom arrow*). **Bottom:** ADEM or postinfectious encephalomyelitis after virus infection. Subcortical white matter lesions (*short arrow*) involving subcortical U fibers with tangential lesions (*long arrow*).

for HSV in the majority of treated patients within 14 days. Therefore, negative PCR results should be interpreted based on the timing during illness and the clinical setting. HSV is rarely cultured from CSF in patients with encephalitis.

TREATMENT

Early recognition of HSV encephalitis is essential because effective antiviral therapy (acyclovir) is available, and prompt treatment can significantly decrease the morbidity and mortality of the disease. Acyclovir acts by inhibiting the viral DNA polymerase, thus interfering with viral replication (see Chapter 44). In adults with HSV encephalitis, acyclovir has reduced mortality from 70 to 19%. However, even in treated patients, neurologic impairment can occur in 40 to 60% of survivors. Outcome is related to the severity of disease at the time antiviral therapy is begun, hence the urgency to begin treatment as soon as the diagnosis is considered. Intravenous therapy should be continued for 14 to 21 days. As with bacterial meningitis, supportive

care must be instituted, including close attention to seizure control, monitoring for hyponatremia secondary to the syndrome of inappropriate antidiuretic hormone secretion, and treatment of increased intracranial pressure. Neurologic sequelae can include seizures, paralysis, and cognitive impairment (e.g., memory loss and difficulty with speech, concentration, and attention).

BRAIN ABSCESS
PATHOBIOLOGY

A **brain abscess** is a focal infection of the brain parenchyma, which may be caused by bacteria, fungi, or parasites. Microorganisms that cause brain abscesses reach the brain by direct extension from a contiguous focus of infection (such as the paranasal sinuses, middle ear, or mastoids), hematogenous dissemination (as in acute bacterial endocarditis or cyanotic congenital heart disease), or direct penetration (following skull fractures or surgical

CASE

Acute Abscess Caused by a Bacterial Infection

Twenty-nine-year-old Ms. M. complained of earache. She had had many such episodes in the past, especially involving the left ear, but the most recent episode was associated with a headache that made her nauseated. She vomited once. After 4 days of those symptoms, she was driven to the hospital because she had developed a large blind spot in her right field of vision. At the hospital, Ms. M. had a temperature of 38.1°C. A CT scan of her head revealed a 4×3-cm mass in her left occipital lobe, consistent with an abscess (Fig. 61-6).

A neurosurgeon performed a needle aspiration of the abscess under CT guidance. A smear of the aspirate revealed Gram-positive cocci and Gram-negative rods. The abscess fluid was sent for culture under both aerobic and anaerobic conditions. She was empirically treated with broad-spectrum antibiotics, including ceftriaxone, metronidazole, and vancomycin, while awaiting the results of the culture. The aspirate grew only *S. aureus*, which was susceptible to methicillin. She was treated with intravenous nafcillin (to cover *S. aureus*) and metronidazole (to cover anaerobic bacteria) for 6 weeks. During that period, serial CT examinations showed the abscess to be shrinking. She recovered completely, but a small blind spot remained in her right visual field.

This case raises two questions:

1. Why was antimicrobial therapy with both nafcillin and metronidazole continued even though no anaerobic bacteria grew from culture?
2. What was the relationship between Ms. M.'s earache and the location of her brain abscess?

See Appendix for answers.

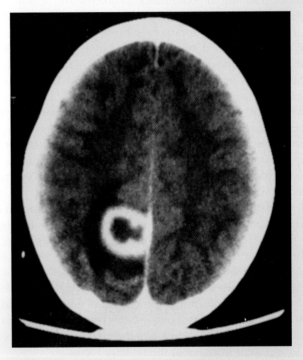

FIGURE 61-6. Contrasted computerized tomography scan of a patient with left occipital brain abscess. The necrotic material in the abscess center appears dark (hypodense). The white rim surrounding the abscess is its wall, which is visualized because of its vascularization and contiguous vasodilation. There is surrounding hypodensity, representing edema.

procedures involving the brain or spinal column). In the case of infections of the middle ear, mastoid, or sinuses, veins that bridge the surrounding bony structures and the cerebral cortex can become infected (septic thrombophlebitis), leading to a decrease in local blood supply and providing a reservoir of bacteria.

Abscesses can appear at many locations within the brain parenchyma and the subdural or epidural meningeal spaces. Infarction of the superficial cerebral cortex during meningitis can produce a subdural abscess that is poorly localized, a condition called **subdural empyema**. If an empyema is not completely drained, it slowly resolves, as do abscesses in other parts of the body. In contrast with intracerebral abscesses, **epidural abscesses**, located external to the dura mater, are invariably related to contiguous infection of bone, sometimes secondary to infection of the paranasal sinuses or mastoids. A spinal epidural abscess can be a complication of epidural anesthesia.

The symptoms caused by brain abscesses are the result of increased intracranial pressure and tissue destruction at specific locations. When the frontal lobe is involved, diminished intellectual performance, memory deficits, drowsiness, and perhaps some memory loss can occur (see Fig. 61-6). Temporal lobe involvement can result in visual field defects and occasionally in difficulty speaking. In some patients, mastoiditis predisposes to cerebellar abscess, resulting in coordination problems and ataxia.

Acute abscesses in the CNS are frequently caused by a mixed bacterial flora consisting of strict and facultative anaerobes. That mixture is similar to the combination of bacteria found in the mouth or a parameningeal focus such as an infected middle ear, mastoid, or sinus. Because anaerobic bacteria are particularly difficult to culture, most patients should receive empiric therapy for anaerobes, regardless of culture results. Staphylococci are more likely to be isolated from brain abscesses in the setting of septic emboli from infected heart valves, trauma, or surgical procedures. Nosocomial Gram-negative organisms also can cause postsurgical brain abscesses.

Chronic abscesses are located in either the meninges or brain tissue. The most common causative agents are mycobacteria, *Cryptococcus* species, and other fungi. Although chronic abscesses are invariably the result of metastatic spread from foci elsewhere, the CNS manifestations sometimes are the first indication of the presence of infection. Usually running a course of remission and relapse, chronic abscesses are often associated with loss of cell-mediated immunity, when the causative agents are no longer kept in check at the primary focus.

DIAGNOSIS

Diagnosis of a brain abscess is aided by imaging techniques. Cranial CT scans classically demonstrate a mass with a central hypointense nonenhancing center, surrounded by a faint ring that becomes hyperintense with contrast, surrounded by nonenhancing hypointense edema. T1-weighted MRI scans often demonstrate similar findings, whereas T2-weighted scans show the inverse. Lumbar puncture is inadvisable in a person suspected of having a brain abscess because the increased intracranial pressure could cause brainstem herniation with lumbar decompression. Furthermore, a lumbar puncture is rarely diagnostic, unless the abscess has ruptured into the ventricular space to produce acute ventriculitis and meningitis.

Aspiration of the abscess cavity yields material for cytological analysis, Gram stain, and culture. Anaerobes are common in brain abscesses, and the aspirate should be cultured using both aerobic and anaerobic conditions. Often a smear will show the presence of many Gram-positive cocci, Gram-positive rods, and perhaps a few Gram-negative rods, yet only S. *aureus* will grow in culture. The bacteria that failed to grow can be assumed to be oxygen-sensitive anaerobes.

TREATMENT

Like abscesses elsewhere in the body, brain abscesses usually must be drained to effect resolution. In addition, aspiration of the contents of an abscess helps lower the intracranial pressure and improves CNS function. Focal symptoms due to tissue destruction will not improve, but the lesion can be contained from further increase in size by the administration of antibiotics. Antibiotic therapy is not always effective in the treatment of brain abscesses. Inflammation of the meninges is usually too slight to enhance penetration of antibiotics into the CSF. In addition, most antibiotics function poorly in an abscess. Ideally, an antibiotic should be chosen based on the susceptibility of organisms isolated from the abscess cavity, but aspiration of material for culture and susceptibility testing is not always practical. Usually, an antimicrobial agent with activity against methicillin-susceptible and methicillin-resistant strains of staphylococci (e.g., vancomycin) and oral flora and Gram-negative enteric organisms (e.g., ceftriaxone or cefotaxime) are administered in combination with an agent active against anaerobes (e.g., metronidazole). Antimicrobial therapy can be tailored based on the organisms recovered, except that anaerobic coverage should be maintained regardless of whether anaerobes are successfully cultured. Mortality from brain abscess remains high at 10 to 20%, with the majority of deaths occurring in patients who present in coma or have a major complicating illness that is the source of the brain abscess organism (e.g., endocarditis).

CONCLUSION

Anatomic and physiological protective mechanisms effectively limit access of microorganisms into the CNS. However, once a microbe gains access to the CNS, various serious consequences may result, including meningitis, encephalitis, and brain abscess. The most frequent infections of the CNS are caused by relatively few agents. Encephalitis is almost exclusively caused by viruses, acute meningitis by viruses and bacteria, and chronic meningitis by tubercle bacilli and fungi. Brain abscesses, in contrast, are frequently caused by a mixture of bacteria derived from the microbiota of the mouth and oropharynx.

Infections of the CNS are often severe and life threatening. Many require immediate action based on rapid and accurate clinical assessment in conjunction with appropriate application of radiographic and microbiologic testing. The single most helpful diagnostic procedure in many cases of CNS infection is evaluation of the CSF for cell counts, chemistries, and the presence of microorganisms. Rapid and sensitive diagnostic tests, such as PCR, have improved the speed and reliability of specific diagnoses, as is the case for enteroviral meningitis and herpes encephalitis. Improved diagnostic methods have allowed more effective application of antimicrobial therapies with proven efficacy in reducing the high mortality and morbidity associated with these diseases.

Suggested Readings

DeBiasi RL, Tyler KL. Molecular methods for diagnosis of viral encephalitis. *Clin Microbiol Rev.* 2004;17:903–925.

Honda H, Warren DK. Central nervous system infections: meningitis and brain abscess. *Infect Dis Clin North Am.* 2009;23:609–623.

Kennedy PG. Viral encephalitis: causes, differential diagnosis, and management. *J Neurol Neurosurg Psychiatry.* 2004;75(suppl 1):i10–i15.

Rotbart HA. Viral meningitis. *Sem Neurol.* 2000;20:277–292.

Saez-Lorenz X, McCracken GH Jr. Bacterial meningitis in children. *Lancet.* 2003;21:2139–2148.

Thigpen C, Whitney CG, Messonnier NE, et al. Emerging Infections Programs Network. Bacterial meningitis in the United States, 1998–2007. *N Engl J Med.* 2011;364:2016–2025.

Thomson RB Jr, Bertram H. Laboratory diagnosis of central nervous system infections. *Infect Dis Clin North Am.* 2001;15:1047–1071.

Tyler KL. Neurological infections: advances in therapy, outcome, and prediction. *Lancet Neurol.* 2009;8:19–21.

Ziai WC, Lewin JJ III. Update in the diagnosis and management of central nervous system infections. *Neurol Clin.* 2008;26:427–468, viii.

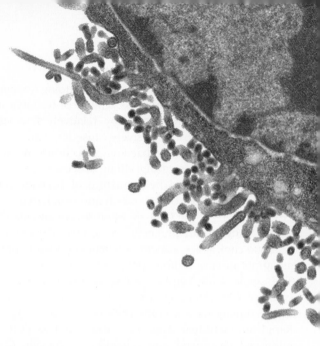

Chapter 62

Respiratory System Infections

Melissa A. Miller and Kevin R. Flaherty

THE RESPIRATORY TRACT is the most common site for infection by pathogenic microorganisms. Because respiratory infections are so common and typically mild, their impact is often underestimated; however, they represent an immense disease burden on our society. Upper respiratory infections (URIs) account for more visits to physicians than any other diagnosis. It has been estimated in the United States that pharyngitis alone accounts for 40 million physician visits annually. Furthermore, some respiratory infections can have severe consequences, especially in immunocompromised individuals. Pneumonia, the most severe form of respiratory infection, is the sixth leading cause of death in the United States and the most common cause of death from infectious diseases.

The frequency with which the respiratory tract becomes infected is not surprising, as it represents the greatest epithelial surface in continuous contact with the external environment of any human organ. Nevertheless, most microorganisms do not cause infection unless other factors interfere with host defenses.

The clinical syndromes and common pathogens associated with infection at various locations within the respiratory tract are shown in Figure 62-1. Infections of the middle ear and the paranasal sinuses are included because these areas are contiguous with the respiratory tract and are lined by respiratory epithelium. Several important diseases of the respiratory system are also discussed in other chapters (see Chapters 13, 19, 23, 27, 29, 32, 34, 36, and 68). The clinical manifestations of respiratory tract infections depend on the causative agent. Viruses can often invade the upper respiratory tract and account for most cases of pharyngitis. Bacteria are commonly implicated in otitis media, sinusitis, pharyngitis, epiglottitis, bronchitis, and pneumonia. Fungi and protozoa rarely cause serious respiratory tract infections in healthy individuals but are important causes of pneumonia in immunocompromised hosts.

ENTRY AND SPREAD

Pathogens can enter the respiratory tract by one of five routes: (1) direct inhalation, (2) aspiration of upper airway contents, (3) spread along the mucous membrane surface, (4) hematogenous spread, and, rarely, (5) direct penetration. Of these, inhalation and aspiration are the most common. Hematogenous spread and direct penetration are rare but important sources of infection of the lung parenchyma.

DEFENSE MECHANISMS

The defense of the respiratory tract begins in the nose, where specialized hairs, known as **vibrissae**, filter large particles suspended in inhaled air (Fig. 62-2). Large particles (>10 μm in diameter) tend to settle at points where abrupt changes in the direction of airflow occur, such as the posterior nasopharynx. Smaller particles (<3 μm in diameter) are likely to elude those barriers and reach the terminal bronchioles and alveoli. Additionally, the structure of the larynx and the cough reflex provide protection against gross aspiration of upper airway and gastric contents, preventing transmission of associated bacteria to the lower respiratory tract.

The respiratory epithelium itself has specialized defenses against infection. Epithelial cells from the nose to the terminal bronchioles are covered with **cilia** that beat coordinately. Overlying these cilia is a covering of mucus

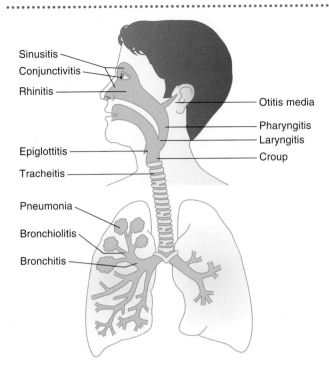

Sinusitis
Conjunctivitis
Rhinitis
Otitis media
Pharyngitis
Laryngitis
Epiglottitis
Croup
Tracheitis
Pneumonia
Bronchiolitis
Bronchitis

FIGURE 62-1. Clinical syndromes associated with infection at different locations within the respiratory tract.

containing antimicrobial compounds such as **lysozyme**, **lactoferrin**, and **secretory IgA** antibodies. The cilia move the overlying mucus layer upward toward the larynx; together,

they are called the mucociliary escalator. Many patients with impaired ciliary function have frequent respiratory infections that ultimately lead to **bronchiectasis** (permanent abnormal dilation of the small airways). Evidence suggests that in patients with cystic fibrosis, abnormal sodium and chloride transport in the respiratory epithelial cells decreases the volume of the mucous layer and impairs ciliary function. Impaired clearance of mucous predisposes these patients to chronic infection and inflammation, making them particularly susceptible to infections with *Staphylococcus aureus* and pseudomonas species.

The final lung defenses are found in the alveoli. The alveoli contain IgA antibodies, complement components, and most importantly, alveolar macrophages. These phagocytic cells function as active scavengers, ingesting and killing invading pathogens. When they cannot contain infection by themselves, they are helped by other phagocytic cells that do not normally reside in the lungs, especially neutrophils. Macrophages and neutrophils are especially important in fighting bacterial infections. In viral infection, histopathological studies of the lungs (or other affected tissues) show infiltration by large numbers of lymphocytes and plasma cells, suggesting that viral infection stimulates the recruitment of lymphoid cells rather than neutrophils. Lymphocytes contribute to host defense by producing antibodies and attacking infected cells through cytotoxic T lymphocytes, naturalkiller cells, and antibody-dependent cell-mediated cytotoxicity.

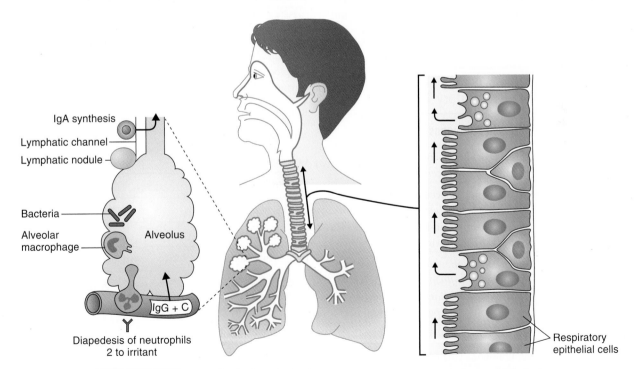

IgA synthesis
Lymphatic channel
Lymphatic nodule
Bacteria
Alveolar macrophage
Alveolus
IgG + C
Diapedesis of neutrophils 2 to irritant
Respiratory epithelial cells

FIGURE 62-2. Defense mechanisms of the respiratory tract. Aerodynamic factors include the presence of vibrissae in the nasal passage and abrupt changes in the direction of flow of the air column. The epiglottis and cough reflex prevent introduction of particulate matter into the lower airway. The ciliated respiratory epithelium propels the overlying mucus layer (*red*) upward toward the mouth. In the alveoli, macrophages, humoral factors (including immunoglobulins and complement), and neutrophils (when inflammation is present) assist in preventing or clearing infection.

CASE

Group A streptococcal pharyngitis

F., a 5-year-old boy who had been in good general health, was brought to the pediatrician because of fever and sore throat that began 2 days earlier. On examination, F. had a temperature of 38.3°C. His oropharynx was erythematous. His tonsils were enlarged and coated with patchy white exudates. His anterior cervical lymph nodes were also enlarged and tender. The remainder of the examination was unremarkable. A throat culture was positive for

group A streptococcus. F. was treated with intramuscular penicillin, and his symptoms resolved over the next week.

This case raises two questions:

1. What common organisms cause pharyngitis?
2. Why is it important to distinguish streptococcal pharyngitis from other forms of the disease?

See Appendix for answers.

INFECTIONS OF THE NOSE AND THROAT

Group A streptococcal pharyngitis is most frequently seen in school-aged children during the winter. Although no clinical features are diagnostic for a specific etiologic cause of pharyngitis, fever, tonsillar exudates, and tender cervical adenopathy increase the likelihood of group A streptococcal infection, whereas conjunctivitis, cough, coryza, and diarrhea decrease the likelihood. It can be difficult to differentiate between viral and bacterial pharyngitis on the basis of clinical findings; therefore, a throat culture or a rapid diagnostic test should be performed to detect group A streptococci, which can be associated with several complications, including peritonsillar and retropharyngeal abscesses, otitis media, sinusitis, pneumonia, acute glomerulonephritis, and rheumatic fever (Table 62-1).

The next most common causes of pharyngitis are the respiratory viruses, including rhinoviruses, adenoviruses, coronaviruses, influenza viruses, and parainfluenza viruses (Table 62-2). The presence of conjunctivitis suggests infection by adenovirus. In adolescents and young adults, Epstein-Barr virus is a common cause of pharyngitis, one of the manifestations of infectious mononucleosis. The enteroviruses, especially the group A coxsackieviruses, sometimes produce small vesicles on the mucous membrane of the throat, a clinical picture known as **herpangina**.

TABLE 62-1 Pathogens Producing Disease at Various Levels of the Respiratory Tract

Location	Common Pathogens
Nasopharynx	Rhinovirus, coronavirus, other respiratory viruses, *Staphylococcus aureus*
Oropharynx	Group A streptococcus (*Streptococcus pyogenes*), *Corynebacterium diphtheriae*, Epstein-Barr virus, adenovirus, enterovirus
Middle ear and paranasal sinuses	*Streptococcus pneumoniae, Haemophilus influenzae, Moraxella (Branhamella) catarrhalis*, group A streptococcus (*Streptococcus pyogenes*)
Epiglottitis	*Haemophilus influenzae*
Larynx–trachea	Parainfluenza viruses, *S. aureus*
Bronchi	*S. pneumoniae, H. influenzae, Mycoplasma pneumoniae*, influenza viruses, measles virus
Bronchioles	Respiratory syncytial virus (RSV)
Lungs	See Table 62-3

TABLE 62-2 Common Causes of Pharyngitis

Agent	Relative Importance
Streptococcus pyogenes (group A β-hemolytic)	+ + + +
Rhinovirus	+ +
Adenovirus	+ +
Coronavirus	+ +
Epstein-Barr virus	+ +
Herpes simplex virus	+
Parainfluenza virus	+
Influenza virus	+
Coxsackie virus	+
Chlamydia pneumonia	+
Mixed anaerobic bacteria	+
Neisseria gonorrhoeae	+
Corynebacterium diphtheriae	+
Corynebacterium hemolyticum	+
Mycoplasma pneumoniae	+
Unknown	+ + + +

CASE

Acute epiglottitis

P., an unvaccinated 3-year-old girl, was put to bed by her parents with a low-grade temperature. In the middle of the night, she awoke crying, and her parents found that her fever was higher and that she was having trouble breathing. The family pediatrician told the parents to take P. immediately to the local hospital. On examination in the emergency department, P. had a temperature of 38.9°C. She appeared anxious, sitting upright, and drooling. Nasal flaring was noted. A presumptive diagnosis of epiglottitis was made, and the child was taken to the operating room, where an endotracheal tube was inserted. A radiograph of the lateral neck that had been taken on the way to the operating room revealed swelling of the epiglottis (Fig. 62-3). When her throat was examined as she was being intubated, her epiglottis was noted to be quite erythematous (red) and edematous (swollen). She was treated with nafcillin, which is effective against *Haemophilus influenzae* type b. The next day, the laboratory reported that blood and epiglottis cultures grew *H. influenzae*. She responded promptly to treatment and recovered completely.

This case raises one question:

1. Why was P. started on therapy for *H. influenzae* type b before culture results had returned?

See Appendix for answer.

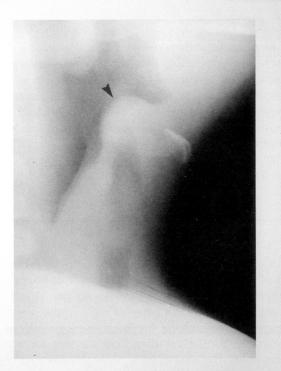

FIGURE 62-3. Radiograph of the neck taken in a lateral projection reveals marked swelling of the epiglottis (*arrow*).

In approximately one-third of patients with pharyngitis, a pathogen cannot be identified despite extensive evaluation. Recent studies suggest that *Chlamydophila pneumoniae* (formerly *Chlamydia pneumoniae*) may be a common cause of pharyngitis. Non-group A β-hemolytic streptococci account for a small proportion of cases, as do gonococci in sexually active individuals. Another organism, *Arcanobacterium haemolyticum*, has been found to cause some cases of pharyngitis in older children and young adults. *Mycoplasma pneumoniae*, although more commonly an agent of bronchitis and pneumonia, can cause pharyngitis as well. All of these agents can be easily overlooked or difficult to detect in a routine throat culture.

Infections of the nasopharynx are generally caused by viruses and give rise to the signs and symptoms known collectively as the common cold. **Approximately 40 to 50% of colds are caused by the rhinovirus group** (see Chapter 32). **Coronaviruses** are the next most common group of agents, accounting for approximately 10% of colds. The agents of the remaining percentage of colds are various respiratory viruses, including parainfluenza viruses, respiratory syncytial virus (RSV), influenza viruses, and adenoviruses. Although the patient with a cold may experience a "scratchy" throat, nasal symptoms are usually more prominent. Bacterial infection of the nose occurs occasionally but is not common.

INFECTIONS OF THE EPIGLOTTIS

Acute epiglottitis, also called supraglottitis, is probably the most serious form of URI. This distinct clinical syndrome can lead to rapid swelling of the epiglottis and surrounding structures and can be rapidly fatal if the airway is compromised due to this swelling. Acute epiglottitis occurs most often in children 2 to 7 years of age, with the most common cause being *Haemophilus influenzae* type b. Fortunately, since immunization of infants against *H. influenzae* type b has become universal, this feared clinical entity has become less common. In adults, *H. influenzae* type b is still occasionally pathogenic, but other etiologic agents, such as *Streptococcus pneumoniae* and group A streptococci, are more commonly implicated than they are in children. Despite the current rarity of this condition, the practitioner must remain vigilant because early recognition of acute epiglottitis can make the difference between life and death. Why *H. influenzae* type b displays a marked tropism for the epiglottis is not well understood.

CASE

Laryngotracheitis

H., a 19-month-old boy, developed a runny nose, hoarseness, cough, and a low-grade temperature. His pediatrician diagnosed a viral URI and prescribed no specific treatment. That night, H. had a **barking cough**. His breathing was forced and noisy, especially with inspiration. Alarmed, the parents called the pediatrician, who told them that the child probably had a viral infection called croup. He advised them to take H. into the bathroom and to fill the room with steam by running the hot water in the shower.

He also advised them to call back 15 minutes later if the respiratory difficulty worsened. In fact, it subsided, and H. fell back to sleep. A similar but milder episode occurred the next night. Over the next few days, all the symptoms gradually resolved.

This case raises one question:

1. Why did the pediatrician suspect a viral pathogen?

See Appendix for answer.

If a child presents with the characteristic manifestations of epiglottitis as described in the case of P., ensuring maintenance of the airway should be the physician's first priority. If a patient presents early in the course of diagnosis, radiographs of the lateral neck may show an enlarged epiglottis protruding from the anterior wall of the hypopharynx (see Fig. 62-3). In adults, nasopharyngolaryngoscopy can aid the diagnosis. If airway compromise is suspected, the first and most important intervention is securing the airway with endotracheal intubation. Epiglottitis usually responds readily to treatment with antibiotics, and the outcome is generally good if appropriate support has been implemented.

INFECTIONS OF THE LARYNX AND TRACHEA

Laryngotracheitis in small children, referred to as **croup**, is characterized by the sudden onset of a barking cough and difficult respiration, which may also resolve suddenly. Mucous membrane edema is more likely to result in narrowing of the tracheal lumen in children due to their smaller airways and the presence of nonexpandable rings of cartilage present in the tracheal wall. This narrowing is more significant during inspiration and results in inspiratory stridor. Almost all cases are caused by viruses, especially the parainfluenza viruses. Infection with parainfluenza virus types 1 through 3 is common in young children, and repeated infections can occur. In rare cases, bacteria, particularly *Staphylococcus aureus*, can cause clinical findings similar to those of viral croup. Typically, mild upper respiratory symptoms such as nasal discharge and dry cough are present days before the signs of airway obstruction become evident. In most cases, the illness is self-limited and resolves after 5 to 7 days. No specific drug treatment for parainfluenza virus infection currently exists. Management of croup consists of providing oxygen and supporting the airway as needed. Although there is no direct antiviral therapy, corticosteroids and inhaled aerosolized epinephrine can be used to reduce airway tissue inflammation and edema.

In adults, the major clinical manifestation of infection of the larynx is **hoarseness**. As in children, most acute laryngeal infections in adults are self-limited conditions caused by respiratory viruses. *Moraxella catarrhalis* and *H. influenzae* have also been reported to cause acute laryngitis in adults. Although antibiotic therapy can sometimes shorten the duration of illness, the hoarseness generally resolves over the course of a week, regardless of therapy.

CASE

Acute tracheobronchitis

Dr. V., a 28-year-old physician, developed symptoms of cough, myalgias (aches and pains in the muscles), headache made worse by coughing, substernal chest pain, and high fever. She suspected influenza because an outbreak was in progress and she had recently cared for several patients with similar symptoms. During the next 3 days, she was bedridden because of weakness and a persistent

temperature of 38.9°C. The symptoms gradually resolved over the next few days without specific treatment. After 10 days, Dr. V. was able to resume her usual activities. A viral throat culture she took on the first day of illness confirmed the diagnosis of influenza.

This case raises one question:

1. Do most cases of tracheobronchitis resolve on their own, or are antibiotics usually required?

See Appendix for answer.

INFECTIONS OF THE LARGE BRONCHI

Acute tracheobronchitis is one of the most common causes of office visits to family practitioners. Infection is the major cause, but inhalation of irritants can also lead to this clinical syndrome. Viruses that have been implicated include rhinoviruses, coronaviruses, RSV, influenza viruses, and adenoviruses. Bacterial infections that can cause bronchitis include *M. pneumoniae*, *Chlamydophila pneumoniae*, and *Bordetella pertussis*. *B. pertussis* causes **whooping cough**, which is a highly contagious disease characterized by paroxysmal, productive coughs occurring primarily in infants and young children (see Chapter 19). In the United States, the disease occurs infrequently because of vaccination, although its incidence is increasing, with a disproportionately high number of cases occurring in adolescents and adults in whom vaccine-induced immunity has waned over time.

In general, acute tracheobronchitis tends to run a short, self-limited course requiring only symptomatic treatment. The role of antibiotics in patients with no underlying lung disease has been controversial because most cases result from viral infections. Studies have shown little to no benefit from antibiotics, yet antibiotic prescriptions for acute bronchitis account for a significant percentage of all prescriptions written in adult practice. Patient education is an important first step in decreasing the use of unnecessary antibiotics.

An important distinction should be made between bronchitis in otherwise healthy patients and those with underlying structural lung disease. Patients with chronic obstructive pulmonary disease (a disease usually related to smoking) may have excessive sputum production, also known as chronic bronchitis. Acute infection in these patients can lead to **acute exacerbation of chronic bronchitis (AECB)**, a clinical diagnosis based on the patient's history of increased cough and sputum production, increased sputum purulence, and increased shortness of breath. The presence of at least two if not all three of these symptoms increases the likelihood of a bacterial infection as the etiology, particularly in the presence of sputum purulence. The role of bacterial infection as the causative agent of AECB has been controversial; however, when viewed collectively, studies show a modest but significant improvement in clinical recovery for patients treated with antibiotics. Thus, treatment for AECB usually includes supportive care and antibiotics effective against *H. influenzae*, *M. catarrhalis*, and *S. pneumoniae*. In selected patients, coverage of Gram-negative enteric pathogens may be important.

INFECTIONS OF THE BRONCHIOLES

Bronchiolitis is a common clinical syndrome in the first 2 years of life and is usually associated with **respiratory syncytial virus**. This topic is covered in depth in Chapter 34.

INFECTIONS OF THE LUNGS

Pneumonia, infection of the lung parenchyma, represents a variety of diseases that share a common anatomic location. Many diverse pathogens can cause pneumonia, and clinical manifestations can vary greatly. Although pneumonias can be categorized in various ways, this chapter uses clinical and epidemiological classification (Table 62-3). Because its perspective is from that of the clinician, this classification can form the basis for managing the patient's illness even before a specific microbiologic cause has been proven.

The first important distinction that the classification makes is between **acute pneumonia** and **subacute or chronic pneumonia**. Acute pneumonia is characterized by fairly sudden onset with progression of symptoms over a very few days, whereas subacute or chronic pneumonia occurs in those cases in which infection is present for weeks or months before presentation. Among the acute pneumonias, a second important distinction is made between community- and hospital-acquired (nosocomial) pneumonias. Hospital-acquired pneumonias (HAPs) are classified separately because the responsible pathogens are usually different from those that produce pneumonia in nonhospitalized individuals.

Most of the common forms of **acute community-acquired pneumonia (CAP)** are caused by pathogens transmitted from person to person. Transmission is typically airborne over short distances or by contaminated secretions or fomites. On encountering some pathogens—*S. pneumoniae*, *H. influenzae*, and *S. aureus*, for example—most individuals become colonized, but only a few develop disease directly or after a variable period of colonization. Another group of pneumonia pathogens, encountered less frequently, have animal or environmental reservoirs. These pathogens are often not easily detected with routine testing. In many cases of pneumonia caused by these agents, diagnosis is difficult unless the physician seeks out the circumstances of exposure (e.g., exposure to a parrot leading to psittacosis). CAPs in infants and young children are usually grouped separately as they have a distinctive etiological spectrum.

Several forms of subacute and chronic pneumonias can be distinguished. These forms include tuberculosis, fungal pneumonia, and anaerobic lung abscesses. Although this classification is based on the common clinical patterns of disease, exceptions do occur. For example, patients with tuberculosis, histoplasmosis, or lung abscesses sometimes experience acute, rapidly progressing disease. Physicians must also be aware that immunocompromised patients are at risk for a more severe and fulminant presentation of both acute and subacute pneumonias. Additionally, they may be susceptible to opportunistic pathogens, those which usually do not cause disease in immunocompetent individuals.

TABLE 62-3 Classification of Pneumonia Syndromes

Acute

Community Acquired

Person-to-Person Transmission

Streptococcus pneumoniae, *Mycoplasma pneumoniae*, *Haemophilus influenzae*, *Chlamydia pneumoniae*, *Staphylococcus aureus*, *Klebsiella pneumonias*, and other enteric Gram-negative rods, *Moraxella. catarrhalis*, *Neisseria meningitides*, *Streptococcus pyogenes*, influenza viruses

Animal or Environmental Exposure

See Table 62-4

Pneumonia in Infants and Young Children

Chlamydia trachomatis, RSV, and other respiratory viruses, *S. aureus*, group B streptococci, cytomegalovirus, *Ureaplasma urealyticum* (?), *Pneumocystis jiroveci* (?), *S. pneumoniae*, *H. influenzae* type b

Hospital Acquired (Nosocomial)

S. aureus, Enterobacteriaceae species, *K. pneumonia*, *Escherichia coli*, *Serratia marcescens*, *H. influenzae*, *S. pneumoniae*, *Pseudomonas aeruginosa*, *Acinetobacter* species, influenza A, *Legionella* species, *Aspergillus*

Subacute or Chronic

Pulmonary Tuberculosis

Mycobacterium tuberculosis and nontuberculous mycobacteria

Fungal Pneumonia

Histoplasma capsulatum, *Blastomyces dermatitidis*, *Coccidioides immitis*, *Cryptococcus neoformans*

Aspiration Pneumonia and Lung Abscesses

Mixed anaerobic and aerobic bacterial organisms

Pneumonia in Immunocompromised Patients

P. jiroveci, cytomegalovirus, atypical mycobacteria, *Nocardia*, *Aspergillus*, *Phycomycetes*, *Candida*

CASE • Thirty-six-year-old Ms. T., who has a history of smoking 20 packs of cigarettes a year, presented to the emergency department of her local hospital after 3 days of fevers to 39.2°C, chills, cough, and pain on her left side, which was worse with breathing. On examination, her respiratory rate was elevated at 22 breaths per minute and her pulse oximetry was normal at 96%. Auscultation of her lungs revealed rales in her left lower lung field. A chest radiograph showed an infiltrate in her left lower lobe consistent with pneumonia. Her blood work revealed an elevated white blood cell count of 16,000 per mm³. Ms. T. was diagnosed with a CAP, prescribed a course of antibiotics, and discharged. Over the next several days, her fevers resolved, and within 2 weeks, her symptoms had disappeared. A chest radiograph performed at her physician's office 3 months later was normal.

This case raises two questions:

1. How did the physician differentiate bronchitis from pneumonia?

2. What organisms should a physician be concerned about when treating CAP?

See Appendix for answers.

Acute Pneumonias

Community-Acquired Pneumonia

Community-acquired pneumonia (CAP) afflicts between 4 and 6 million people in the United States each year, nearly 1 million of whom require hospitalization. In elderly and chronically ill patients, CAP can be associated with prolonged hospitalizations and high mortality. Presenting symptoms frequently include fever and cough. Sometimes the patient complains of chest pain, frequently pleuritic (exacerbated by respiratory motion). Patients with extensive involvement of the lungs may have shortness of breath, rapid respiration, and **cyanosis** (bluish tinge to the skin indicative of hypoxemia). Auscultation may reveal **crackles** (also called **rales**) and peripherally auscultated bronchial breath sounds, which are usually indicative of alveolar disease.

Both bacteria and viruses cause CAPs, as outlined in Tables 62-3 and 62-4, although in approximately one-half of patients, an organism is never identified. Traditionally, organisms have been divided into two groups, typical and atypical, based on the belief that the clinical and radiographic features of presentation suggest certain etiologic agents. A typical presentation is characterized by high fever, shaking chills, chest pain, and lobar consolidation on chest x-ray. An atypical presentation is characterized by less severe illness, dry cough, headache, and other systemic complaints. Although studies have shown that it is very difficult to predict an etiologic agent based on presentation, the classification of organisms as typical and atypical persists. *S. pneumoniae* is the most common cause of CAP, and along with *H. influenzae*, *S. aureus*, and other Gram-negative bacteria, these agents are classified as typical organisms. *M. pneumoniae*, *C. pneumoniae*, and *Legionella pneumophila* are among the atypical organisms.

Although considerable overlap exists in the clinical manifestations of pneumonia, certain pathogens tend to be associated with characteristic presentations or to affect certain patient populations. For instance, *M. pneumoniae* and *C. pneumoniae* are seen with higher frequency in patients with less severe presentations of pneumonia. Pneumococcal pneumonia can occur at any age, but it has a predilection for the very young and the elderly, particularly those with **chronic obstructive pulmonary disease (COPD)**. It usually has a rapid onset and an acute course. Patients with a history of COPD also have an increased risk for infection with *H. influenzae* and *M. catarrhalis*. Compared to the general population, alcoholics are more susceptible to *S. pneumoniae*, *Klebsiella pneumonia*, *S. aureus*, and anaerobic pathogens (by aspiration). Nursing home residents, immunocompromised patients, and people with underlying structural lung disease are at higher risk for pneumonia due to *Pseudomonas aeruginosa*, Gram-negative enteric bacteria (derived from the gut), and *S. aureus*.

Several pneumonias result from agents found in animals or in the environment (Table 62-4). Infection by these agents is usually associated with a unique exposure. For example, *Chlamydia psittaci*, a common cause of disease in birds, can lead to psittacosis (**parrot fever**) in humans and may be acquired by inhalation (see Chapter 27). This illness is difficult to diagnose unless the physician obtains the history of contact with birds. Another example is **Q fever**, caused by the rickettsia *Coxiella burnetii* and usually acquired from sheep, goats, or cattle. The organism is stable in the environment, and infection can occur after exposure to contaminated material from infected animals. As with psittacosis, diagnosis of Q fever is difficult unless the physician elicits the history of exposure to animals or their environment. Another agent of CAPs, *L. pneumophila*, is associated with contaminated environmental water sources that produce aerosols, such as showers, fountains, sprayers, air conditioners, and water-cooling towers.

Viruses such as influenza, RSV, parainfluenza, and adenoviruses can also cause pneumonia. The clinical course is usually milder, with spontaneous recovery, although rarely, some viral pneumonias can lead to severe respiratory disease. Severe acute respiratory syndrome virus and influenza have been associated with acute respiratory distress syndrome. Additionally, bacterial

TABLE 62-4 Community-Acquired Pneumonias (CAPs) Transmitted by Animals or Environmentally

Disease	Causative Organism	Source
Psittacosis	*Chlamydia psittaci*	Infected birds
Q fever	*Coxiella burnetii*	Infected animals
Histoplasmosis	*Histoplasma capsulatum*	Infected soil, bats
Coccidioidomycosis	*Coccidioides immitis*	Soil
Cryptococcosis	*Cryptococcus neoformans*	Soil, pigeons
Plague	*Yersinia pestis*	Infected animals, insect vectors
Melioidosis	*Pseudomonas pseudomallei*	Soil
Tularemia	*Francisella tularensis*	Infected animals, ticks
Legionnaires disease	*Legionella pneumophila*	Contaminated water

superinfection can occur with viral pneumonia (especially influenza), causing a more severe clinical picture. RSV can cause severe lung disease in young children, especially premature infants, sometimes with long-term sequelae such as wheezing and asthma. In children under 2 years of age, the agents of acute pneumonias are more often viruses than bacteria. In other age groups, viruses are infrequent causes of CAP.

Diagnosis of CAP is generally based on appropriate clinical history and chest radiographs. The most important diagnostic finding is a chest radiograph that reveals a shadow, or **infiltrate**. The radiographic pattern may suggest particular pathogens, although this is not definitive. Focal lobar consolidation is more commonly seen with *S. pneumoniae*, *K. pneumoniae* (a Gram-negative rod), and infections caused by aspiration (with a predilection for the lower lobes because of lung anatomy). Diffuse interstitial infiltrates can be seen with infections of *M. pneumoniae*, *C. pneumoniae*, and *P. carinii*. Organisms that tend to cavitate include *S. aureus*, aerobic Gram-negative bacteria, and *Mycobacterium tuberculosis*. Skilled interpretation is important because other processes, tumors, pulmonary edema, or pulmonary hemorrhage can produce radiographic changes very similar to those of pneumonia.

The decision to admit a patient to the hospital for CAP treatment rather than to administer outpatient therapy can be a difficult one, but factors such as severity of illness and medical comorbidities are used as general guidelines. Several prediction rules have been proposed to identify patients at increased risk of a complicated course. These are generally based on identifying host factors associated with more virulent organisms or an impaired response to infection.

In most cases, the choice of antibiotic therapy is empiric based on the patient's risk factors for certain organisms and the severity of illness. A patient with relatively mild illness managed outside the hospital usually does not undergo sputum Gram stain and culture tests, whereas these tests are performed for patients admitted to hospitals. In addition, in about half of cases of pneumonia, a microbiologic cause is not identified. Opinion-based recommendations by multispecialty experts have been published to provide guidance for empiric antimicrobial therapy based on clinical scenarios and host factors (Table 62-5). Increasing antimicrobial resistance among respiratory pathogens, especially *S. pneumoniae*, has altered initial antimicrobial therapy recommendations. Risk factors for drug-resistant *S. pneumoniae* (DRSP) include recent respiratory infection; recent antimicrobial use; advanced age; medical comorbidities, including being immunocompromised; and living in a high-risk area (e.g., a residential institution, a daycare center). Additionally, some geographic areas have a higher prevalence of DRSP. Patients at risk for DRSP should be treated with antibiotics with expanded activity against *S. pneumoniae*.

Hospital-Acquired Pneumonia

Hospital-acquired pneumonia (**HAP**) is defined as a new parenchymal lung infection appearing 48 or more hours after admission to the hospital. It is the leading cause of death from hospital-acquired infections, with an estimated mortality of 20 to 50%. Symptoms suggesting a diagnosis of HAP include fever, cough, purulent sputum production, shortness of breath, and pleuritic chest pain. Physical exam may reveal fever, **tachycardia** (elevated heart rate), and **tachypnea** (elevated respiratory rate). Signs of consolidation on physical exam include crackles and bronchial breath sounds. **Tactile fremitus** and **dullness to percussion** may also be present.

Microaspiration of bacteria from the oropharynx is considered the most common route of infection. Factors influencing the risk of pneumonia are the types of bacteria colonizing the pharynx and prior exposure to antibiotics. The oropharynx of hospitalized patients can become colonized with Gram-negative bacteria within several days of admission. Furthermore, illness and medications can disrupt the gastric pH, leading to colonization of the stomach with bacteria. Aspiration of bacteria-contaminated gastric contents can increase oropharyngeal colonization and heighten the risk of HAP. Patients with advanced age; poor nutrition; history of smoking, alcoholism, or intravenous drug use; or other underlying chronic illnesses are also at increased risk for developing nosocomial pneumonia.

One important type of HAP is **ventilator-associated pneumonia** (**VAP**). In patients requiring mechanical ventilation, the endotracheal tube can provide a conduit from the outside environment to the lower airway by circumventing the defenses of the upper airway and allowing direct passage of oropharyngeal secretions, gastric contents, and associated bacteria down the course of the tube itself into the lower respiratory tract.

The bacteria which most commonly cause HAP are enteric Gram-negative rods and *S. aureus*. Common Gram-negative rods include members of the Enterobacteriaceae family, *K. pneumonia*, *Proteus* species, and *Escherichia coli*. Mechanically ventilated patients frequently are infected with multiple organisms. Other organisms reported include *H. influenzae*, *Serratia marcescens*, and *S. pneumoniae*. In patients who have more severe infections, who have been exposed to broad-spectrum antimicrobial agents, or have had more prolonged hospitalizations, *P. aeruginosa* and *Acinetobacter* species are more common. Rare etiologic agents include influenza A, RSV, *Legionella* species, and *Aspergillus* species.

Diagnosis of HAP in clinical practice can be difficult. Fever, elevated white blood cell count, and purulent sputum are suggestive but not definitive. Chest radiograph showing a new infiltrate is sensitive but not specific because other conditions (e.g., congestive heart failure and pulmonary embolus) can cause similar radiograph abnormalities. Sputum Gram stain and culture are frequently obtained, but unfortunately, the

TABLE 62-5 Initial Empiric Antimicrobial Therapy for CAP in Immunocompetent Adults

Clinical Scenario	Preferred Therapy
Outpatient	
Previously Healthy	
No recent antimicrobial therapy	Macrolide or doxycycline
Recent antimicrobial therapy	Respiratory fluoroquinolone
	Advanced macrolides plus high-dose amoxicillin
Comorbidity	
No recent antimicrobial therapy	Advanced macrolides plus high-dose amoxicillin/clavulanate
Recent antimicrobial therapy	Advanced macrolides or respiratory fluoroquinolone
Suspected aspiration with infection	Respiratory fluoroquinolone
Influenza with bacterial superinfection	Advanced macrolides plus β-lactam
	Amoxicillin/clavulanate or clindamycin
	β-lactam or respiratory fluoroquinolone
Inpatient	
Medical Ward	
No recent antimicrobial therapy	Respiratory fluoroquinolone or advanced macrolides plus β-lactam
Recent antimicrobial therapy	Advanced macrolides plus β-lactam or respiratory fluoroquinolone alone
Intensive Care Unit	
Pseudomonas infection unlikely	β-lactam plus either advanced macrolides or respiratory fluoroquinolone
Pseudomonas infection unlikely and patient has β-lactam allergy	Respiratory fluoroquinolone, with or without clindamycin
Pseudomonas infection possible	Antipseudomonal agent plus ciprofloxacin, or antipseudomonal agent plus aminoglycoside plus respiratory fluoroquinolone or macrolides
Pseudomonas infection possible and patient has β-lactam allergy	Aztreonam plus levofloxacin, or aztreonam plus moxifloxacin or gatifloxacin, with or without an aminoglycoside

Adapted from Mandell LA, Bartlett JG, Dowell SF, et al. Update of practice guidelines for the management of community-acquired pneumonia in immunocompetent adults. *Clin Inf Dis.* 2003;37:1405–1433.

microscopic examination of sputum has limitations. Some patients cannot produce sputum, or they produce sputum contaminated by oropharyngeal contamination. The presence of squamous epithelial cells in large numbers indicates contamination by oropharyngeal contents, and a culture of such a specimen can yield misleading information. Finding a predominant organism in the Gram stain may point toward the etiological agent; however, if an organism is cultured, it can be difficult to differentiate a colonizing organism from one causing active disease.

Bronchoscopic sampling of the lower airways by bronchoalveolar lavage may be more helpful in establishing an etiologic agent but is an invasive procedure generally reserved for immunocompromised patients, individuals with severe disease, and those with illness not resolving with standard therapy.

As with CAP, the choices in initial antibiotic therapy for HAP are generally empiric, based on severity of illness and patient risk factors. Antibiotic therapy is based on the likelihood of infection with **multidrug-resistant (MDR)**

CASE • At 52 years of age, Mr. L., who had a history of chronic alcoholism, was admitted to the hospital for an emergent appendectomy. The procedure went well, but on postoperative day 3, he was noted to have a fever of 38.5°C, an elevated heart rate of 115 beats per minute, pulse oximetry of 89%, a cough productive of green sputum, and increased shortness of breath. Examination revealed an ill-appearing patient in moderate respiratory distress. In his left lung base, he had bronchial breath sounds on auscultation. Chest radiograph revealed a large left-sided infiltrate (Fig. 62-4). The patient was started on oxygen therapy by nasal cannula. Gram stain and sputum culture were performed. Broad-spectrum antibiotic therapy was begun. The sputum culture eventually showed heavy growth of *K. pneumoniae*, one of the Enterobacteriaceae. Mr. L.'s 3-week hospital course was stormy, and he required mechanical ventilation for 4 days. He was discharged to a chronic care hospital and eventually recovered.

This case raises two questions:

1. How do most patients in the hospital contract pneumonia?
2. Which patients are at increased risk for developing HAP?

See Appendix for answers.

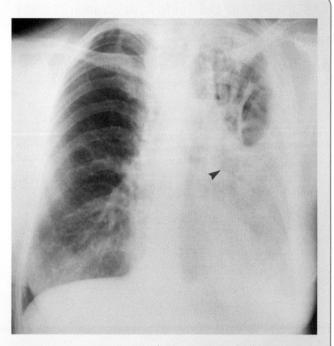

FIGURE 62-4. Pneumonia caused by *Klebsiella pneumoniae*. Chest radiograph shows extensive consolidation of the left lower lobe. Cavity formation is apparent within the involved area *(arrow)*.

pathogens. Risk factors for infection with MDR pathogens include antimicrobial therapy in the preceding 90 days, current hospitalization of 5 days or more, high frequency of MDR organisms in the community or hospital unit, immunosuppressive disease and/or therapy, and the presence of risk factors for health care–associated pneumonia such as chronic dialysis, home infusion therapy, or a family member with an MDR pathogen. If risk factors for infection by MDR pathogens are present, broad-spectrum agents are generally used; if not, more limited-spectrum therapy is generally recommended. With appropriate therapy, many patients display improvement 48 to 72 hours after treatment is initiated. However, many patients with severe infections may develop complications and require mechanical ventilation, sometimes for prolonged periods. Patients with pleural effusion associated with pneumonia (**parapneumonic effusion**) should have the fluid evaluated for evidence of infection of the pleural space. Pus in the pleural space is called an **empyema** and requires surgical drainage.

Subacute Pneumonias

A common cause of subacute pneumonia is the lung abscess, often a consequence of gross aspiration of oropharyngeal or gastric contents. The typical lung abscess represents a polymicrobial infection with multiple species of bacteria. The bacteria most commonly involved are anaerobes and microaerophilic organisms from the normal flora of the mouth. Lung abscesses can also result from infection with other organisms that destroy lung tissue, including *S. aureus*, *K. pneumoniae*, mycobacteria, and others. The resulting infection has a number of distinguishing features. The clinical course tends to be less acute than that of most other forms of bacterial pneumonia. Patients may be ill for several weeks or even months before seeking medical attention. Definitive diagnosis is usually made on the basis of a chest radiograph. Prolonged antibiotic therapy is generally required. If not treated promptly, lung abscess can spread to involve the pleural space, resulting in empyema.

Other causes of infectious subacute pulmonary diseases are fungi and mycobacteria. Fungi that affect the lungs include *Histoplasma capsulatum*, *Blastomyces dermatitidis*, *Coccidioides immitis*, and *Cryptococcus neoformans* (see Chapters 47 and 48). *H. capsulatum* and *B. dermatitidis* are dimorphic fungi found in the soil and are endemic to the midwestern and south-central United States, although *B. dermatitidis* extends farther north. *C. immitis* is found in the deserts of the southwestern United States and *C. neoformans* in areas frequented by pigeons. The latter is frequently but not exclusively found in individuals who are immunocompromised. Other causes of subacute pneumonias include infections with *M. tuberculosis* (see Chapter 23), nontuberculous mycobacteria such as *M. avium intracellulare*, actinomycosis, and nocardiosis.

CASE ● Mr. A., who is 46 years old with a poorly controlled seizure disorder, was brought to a physician after 2 weeks of coughing, fever, and weight loss. Physical examination revealed an ill-appearing man with a temperature of 38.3°C and foul-smelling breath. He had amphoric breath sounds (resembling those produced by blowing across the mouth of a bottle), suggestive of a lung cavity. A chest radiograph showed a large cavity in the left midlung with extensive surrounding inflammation (Fig. 62-5). Mr. A. was admitted to the hospital and treated with high-dose intravenous penicillin. He began to feel better almost immediately, his fever disappeared over the course of a week, and he was then discharged. He was then treated for 3 months with oral penicillin before his infection was deemed fully resolved.

This case raises one question:

1. Which organisms can cause cavitary lung lesions?

See Appendix for answer.

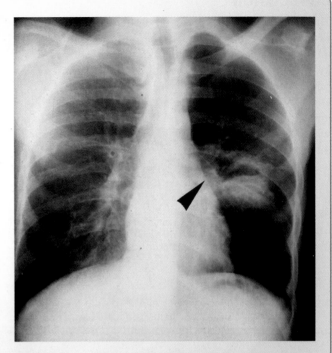

FIGURE 62-5. Lung abscess. Chest radiograph showing a cavitary lesion (*arrow*) with surrounding infiltrate.

CASE ● Mrs. S., who is 53 years old and has HIV infection, presented to her internist with a 1-month history of low-grade fevers, cough, and fatigue. On examination, her temperature was 37.7°C, and she was not in respiratory distress. Her pulse oximetry was 94% on room air but dropped with exertion to 88%. Auscultation and percussion of the chest were normal. Chest radiograph revealed a diffuse, bilateral interstitial infiltrate. Sputum was induced by inhalation of nebulized hypertonic saline. PCR of the sputum confirmed the diagnosis of *P. jiroveci*. Mrs. S. underwent a 3-week course of trimethoprim and sulfamethoxazole. Repeat chest radiograph 2 months later showed no infiltrate, and Mrs. S.'s energy level returned to normal.

This case raises one question:

1. Which patients are at increased risk for developing *P. jiroveci* pneumonia?

See Appendix for answer.

Pneumonia in the Immunocompromised Patient

Pneumonia is a common occurrence in immunocompromised individuals, including individuals who undergo cancer chemotherapy, have HIV infection, are taking immunosuppressive medications, or have congenital immunodeficiencies (see Chapters 69 and 70). In addition to being at higher risk for contracting the same kinds of infections to which individuals with normal immune systems are susceptible, immunocompromised patients can become infected with opportunistic pathogens that rarely cause infections in normal individuals. Examples include *Pneumocystis jiroveci* (previously *Pneumocystis carinii*), which is typically seen in patients with HIV whose CD4 lymphocyte count is less than 200 cells/mm^3, and the fungus *Aspergillus fumigatus* and the cytomegalovirus, which can be seen in patients receiving immunosuppressive therapy for organ transplants. The etiologic agent in patients who develop pneumonia in the setting of an immunosuppressed status depends, in part, on the basis of the defect in the host immune system. Some of these infections can be diagnosed only by carrying out invasive procedures such as bronchoscopy or lung biopsy.

CONCLUSION

The respiratory tract is in continuous exposure with the external environment and is therefore at high risk for infection. However, most microorganisms do not cause infection unless other factors impair host defenses. Respiratory tract infections can become very serious if they affect the patency of a patient's airway or the ability of the lungs to exchange oxygen and carbon dioxide. Familiarity with the spectrum of pathogens that affect each part of the respiratory tree and knowledge of pathogenic predilections for certain patient populations can help physicians make rapid, rational decisions regarding treatment of infections of the respiratory system. Awareness of the natural course of infections and their potential complications will help the physician identify patients needing immediate attention and treatment.

Suggested Readings

American Thoracic Society. Guidelines for the management of adults with hospital-acquired, ventilator-associated, and healthcare-associated pneumonia. *Am J Respir Crit Care Med.* 2005;171:388–416.

Balter MS, La Forge J, Low DE, et al.; Chronic Bronchitis Working Group on behalf of the Canadian Thoracic Society and the Canadian Infectious Disease Society. Canadian guidelines for the management of acute exacerbations of chronic bronchitis. *Can Respir J.* 2003;10(suppl B):3B–32B.

Bisno AL. Acute pharyngitis: etiology and diagnosis. *Pediatrics.* 1996;97:949–954.

Chakinala MM, Trulock EP. Pneumonia in the solid organ transplant patient. *Clin Chest Med.* 2005;26:113–121.

Denny FW, Clyde WA Jr. Acute lower respiratory infections in non-hospitalized children. *J Pediatr.* 1986;108:635.

Dick EC, Jennings LC, Mink KA, et al. Aerosol transmission of rhinovirus colds. *J Infect Dis.* 1987;156:442–448.

Ewig S, de Roux A, Bauer T, et al. Validation of predictive rules and indices of severity for community acquired pneumonia. *Thorax.* 2004;59:421–427.

Green GM. In defense of the lung. *Am Rev Respir Dis.* 1970;102:691–703.

Huxley EJ, Viroslav J, Gray WR, et al. Pharyngeal aspiration in normal adults and patients with depressed consciousness. *Am J Med.* 1978;64:564–568.

Mandell LA, Bartlett JG, Dowell SF, et al. Update of practice guidelines for the management of community-acquired pneumonia in immunocompetent adults. *Clin Inf Dis.* 2003;37:1405–1433.

Marrie TJ, Poulin-Costello M, Beecroft MD, et al. Etiology of community-acquired pneumonia treated in an ambulatory setting. *Resp Med.* 2005;99:60–65.

Marston BJ, Plouffe JF, File TM Jr, et al. Incidence of community acquired pneumonia requiring hospitalization. *Arch Intern Med.* 1997;157:1709–1718.

Mason CM, Nelson S. Pulmonary host defenses and factors predisposing to lung infection. *Clin Chest Med.* 2005;26:11–17.

Niederman MS, Mandell LA, Anzueto A, et al.; American Thoracic Society. Guidelines for the Management of Adults with Community-acquired Pneumonia. *Am J Respir Crit Care Med.* 2001;163:1730–1754.

Pennington JE, ed. *Respiratory Infections: Diagnosis and Management.* New York: Raven Press; 1983.

Sande MA, Hudson LD, Root RK, eds. *Respiratory Infections.* New York: Churchill Livingstone; 1986.

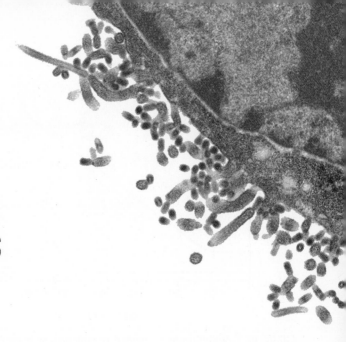

Chapter **63**

Urinary Tract Infections

Lindsay E. Nicolle

URINARY tract infection (UTI) is the most common bacterial infection in humans (Fig. 63-1). This problem occurs in a substantial proportion of otherwise healthy women, is common in both men and women with structural or functional abnormalities of the genitourinary tract, and is a frequent cause of both community- and hospital-acquired infection. At least 20% of all women experience an episode of UTI by the age of 30 years, and over 50% have one or more lifetime UTIs. One in ten women experience frequent recurrent infections for at least some period. An estimated 3 million office visits for this complaint take place each year in the United States. Nosocomial or hospital-acquired UTI accounts for about 40% of all infections acquired in acute care facilities. From 25 to 50% of nursing home patients have bacteriuria at any time.

DEFINITIONS

UTI may be at any site in the urinary tract, including the bladder, kidneys, and, in men, the prostate. Urethritis is infection of the urethra and characteristic of some sexually transmitted diseases such as *Neisseria gonorrhea* and *Chlamydia pneumoniae* (see Chapters 14 and 27). **Acute uncomplicated urinary tract infection** is a UTI presenting as acute cystitis (bladder or lower-tract infection) in otherwise healthy women. **Acute nonobstructive pyelonephritis**, also called acute uncomplicated pyelonephritis, is kidney infection (renal or upper-tract infection) that occurs in this same group of otherwise healthy women. **Complicated urinary tract infection** occurs in individuals with underlying structural or functional abnormalities of the genitourinary tract. It may be infection limited to the bladder, or it may affect both the bladder and kidneys. **Asymptomatic bacteriuria** is bacteria present in the urine without symptoms or signs attributable to UTI. **Bacterial prostatitis** is bacterial infection of the prostate gland. **Acute bacterial prostatitis** is a severe infection of acute onset. **Chronic bacterial prostatitis** is the persistence of bacteria in the prostate causing recurrent or persistent pelvic or urinary symptoms in men. **Renal abscess** is uncommon but may occur as a complication

of pyelonephritis or following bacteremic spread of infection from other body sites.

An individual who experiences one episode of UTI is usually at risk for recurrent episodes. Recurrent infection is considered **reinfection** when a new organism is isolated or if a previously isolated organism is reintroduced into the urinary tract from the colonizing gut or genital flora. **Relapse** is recurrent infection with bacteria that persist within the urinary tract, usually the kidney or prostate, despite antimicrobial therapy. Chronic bacterial prostatitis is a frequent source for relapsing UTI in older men.

PATHOGENESIS

UTI usually occurs when colonizing flora from the periurethral area or, in women, the vagina, ascend up the urethra into the bladder. Factors that promote ascension and subsequent persistence of bacteria in the bladder include host and organism variables (Fig. 63-2).

Source of Infecting Organisms

Bacteria causing UTI usually originate from the normal gut flora. The greater frequency of UTI in women is

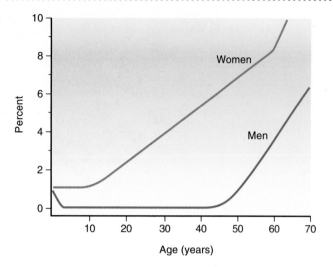

FIGURE 63-1. Variation in estimated prevalence of bacteriuria with age and for different sexes.

thought to be attributable to the shorter female urethra, allowing easier access of bacteria to the bladder. Most bacteria that ascend to the bladder will be removed with the next normal voiding. For infection to occur, bacteria must be able to persist and reproduce in the bladder. Pyelonephritis occurs when organisms further ascend from the bladder to the kidneys. This may be facilitated by adhesins produced by the infecting organism or reflux of urine from the bladder up the ureter in individuals with incompetent ureteral sphincters. Bacterial infection of the prostate gland also occurs primarily through ascension of organisms from the urethra into the prostate ducts. This is facilitated by turbulent urine flow, which is common in men with prostate hypertrophy.

Occasionally, UTI occurs following bacteremic dissemination of organisms through the bloodstream from another infected site. The characteristic pathologic feature of hematogenous dissemination is one or more renal cortical abscesses. Some microorganisms, including *Staphylococcus aureus* and *Candida* species, are more common with infection following hematogenous spread.

Microbiology

The most important uropathogen is *Escherichia coli*. However, a wide spectrum of other organisms may be isolated, depending on the clinical syndrome.

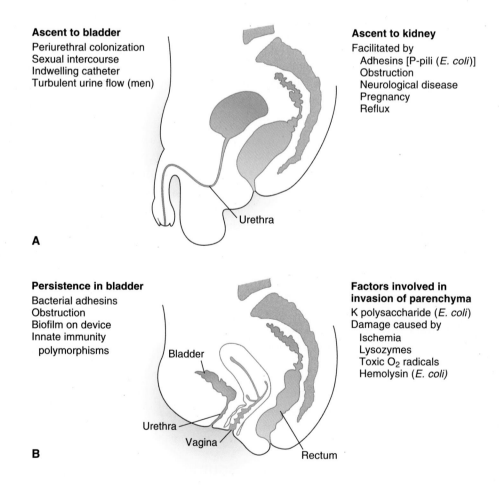

FIGURE 63-2. Pathogenesis of urinary tract infections. A. Male urinary tract. **B.** Female urinary tract.

INFECTIONS OF THE URINARY TRACT
Uncomplicated Urinary Tract Infection

E. coli is isolated from 80 to 85% of episodes of acute uncomplicated cystitis. An essential *E. coli* virulence characteristic for acute cystitis is expression of the **mannose-sensitive fimbria** or ***FimH***. This protein receptor facilitates adherence of *E. coli* to bladder uroepithelial cells through attachment to mannosylated glycoproteins that line the bladder mucosa. This adhesin, however, is widespread and present in more than 80% of all *E. coli* strains, including fecal strains. Additional factors must also contribute to establishing bladder infection. *Staphylococcus saprophyticus*, a Gram-positive organism, is isolated from 5 to 15% of the remaining episodes of acute cystitis. This organism shows a temporal variation, being isolated more frequently in the fall than other times of year. Organisms such as *Klebsiella* spp., *Proteus* spp., and group B streptococcus are isolated from the few remaining episodes.

E. coli is also isolated from 85 to 90% of episodes of acute nonobstructive pyelonephritis. The organism virulence factor most highly associated with this clinical presentation is another adhesin, the **P fimbria**. The receptor for this adhesin is the **glycosphingolipid Gal(α1–4) Galβ disaccharide**. Attachment of *E. coli* to renal cells mediated by this adhesin enhances bacterial persistence and inflammation in the urinary tract. Additional *E. coli* virulence factors associated with pyelonephritis include **aerobactin** (which scavenges for iron that the bacteria need to grow) and **hemolysin** (which may lyse host cells). These virulence factors may occur together on "**pathogenicity islands**" on the *E. coli* chromosome. Other factors are also likely involved as certain *E. coli* serotypes are more frequently associated with pyelonephritis.

Complicated Urinary Tract Infection

E. coli is also the most common pathogen isolated from patients with complicated UTI but is isolated from a lower proportion of these infections compared with uncomplicated UTI. *E. coli* strains isolated from complicated renal infection are characterized by a lower frequency of virulence factors than organisms isolated in uncomplicated infection. This is consistent with the concept that host rather than organism factors are the principal determinants of complicated infection.

A wide variety of organisms other than *E. coli* are also isolated. These include Enterobacteriaceae such as *Klebsiella* spp., *Enterobacter* spp., and *Citrobacter* spp. and nonfermenting Gram-negative organisms, particularly *Pseudomonas aeruginosa*. Urease-producing organisms such as *Proteus mirabilis*, *Morganella morganii*, and *Providencia* spp. are common. These organisms have additional pathogenic potential as the urease metabolizes urea to ammonia and may lead to struvite formation. The ammonia produced damages the kidney directly and facilitates stone formation, which may cause obstruction and further damage. *Enterococcus* species and coagulase-negative staphylococci are the most common Gram-positive organisms. Yeast species are occasionally isolated. *Candida albicans* is the most common, and other species such as *C. tropicalis*, *C. glabrata*, and *C. parapsilosis* may also occur.

Bacteria isolated from patients with complicated UTI are also characterized by an increased prevalence of antimicrobial resistance. This is largely attributable to repeated antimicrobial exposure with prior recurrent infection. Many of these patients also undergo invasive genitourinary interventions to assess or manage underlying abnormalities. These procedures may be associated with nosocomial acquisition of organisms, which are likely to be of increased resistance.

Individuals with complicated UTI often have indwelling urologic devices, such as an **indwelling urethral catheter**, **ureteric stent**, or **nephrostomy** tube. The devices become coated with a **biofilm** when periurethral organisms or bacteria contaminating the drainage bag grow along the exterior or internal catheter surface, ultimately ascending to the bladder. The biofilm consists of microorganisms, extracellular substances produced by the organisms, and urine components such as Tamm-Horsfall protein, calcium, and magnesium. When devices remain in situ for several weeks, three to five different organisms are usually present in the biofilm. Organisms that exist in this environment are relatively protected from both antibiotics and host immune defenses and are difficult to eradicate without removal of the device. They are a frequent source for relapsing infection.

Asymptomatic Urinary Tract Infection

The spectrum of organisms isolated from persons with asymptomatic UTI generally mirrors the spectrum isolated from symptomatic infection in the same patient group. Thus, *E. coli* is most common in otherwise healthy women, and *E. coli* and a wide variety of other organisms may be isolated from individuals with complicated UTI. *E. coli* strains isolated from individuals with asymptomatic bacteriuria are characterized by a low prevalence of potential virulence factors. Gram-positive organisms of low virulence such as enterococcus species and coagulase-negative staphylococci are also frequently isolated from patients with asymptomatic UTI.

Prostatitis

Acute bacterial prostatitis is an uncommon infection, primarily caused by *S. aureus* or *E. coli*. The prevalence of virulence factors of *E. coli* in prostate isolates is intermediate between strains isolated from acute cystitis and from pyelonephritis. Chronic bacterial prostatitis is associated with many different organisms. Prostate stones form in men with aging, providing a nidus for organisms to persist in the prostate and a source of bacteria for relapsing cystitis.

HOST FACTORS

The most important host defense preventing UTI is periodic, complete, normal voiding. This removes bacteria in the bladder as well as desquamated uroepithelial cells to which bacteria may adhere.

Host Factors in Uncomplicated Urinary Tract Infection

Women who experience acute uncomplicated UTI have normal voiding. Access of organisms to the bladder and subsequent persistence are facilitated by both genetic and behavioral factors. Women with recurrent acute uncomplicated UTI are more likely to have first-degree female relatives—mothers, sisters, daughters—who also experience recurrent infection. Some of this genetic predisposition is mediated through being a *nonsecretor of the ABH blood group antigens*. These antigens are secreted at mucosal surfaces and bind to receptors on bacterial cells to prevent attachment to the uroepithelium. Persons who are nonsecretors, about 20% of the population, have bacterial cell surface receptors that remain exposed, allowing attachment of bacteria to host uroepithelial cells. Other genetic variation promoting infection may include polymorphisms affecting the innate immune system such as endogenous antimicrobial peptides in the urine or toll-like receptors.

The most important behavioral risks for acute cystitis in premenopausal women are *sexual intercourse and spermicide use for birth control*. Sexual intercourse mechanically facilitates the ascension of organisms from the periurethral area into the bladder. Bacteria enter the bladder in about 30% of episodes of intercourse. These are usually cleared with the next voiding, but if they persist, symptomatic or asymptomatic infection can occur. An increased frequency of intercourse is associated with an increased frequency of symptomatic episodes. The normal **lactobacillus** flora of the vagina maintains an acidic pH that prevents colonization by potential uropathogens such as E. coli. **Spermicide disrupts this normal flora**, and uropathogens such as E. coli may then colonize the vagina and become a source of infecting organisms.

Other behavioral risk factors of less importance include having a new sexual partner, diaphragm use without spermicide, and recent antimicrobial therapy. A new sexual partner increases exposure to new strains of E. coli, some of which are uropathogens. Diaphragm use may obstruct the urethra and impair complete bladder emptying. Diaphragms are usually used with spermicide, however, and this remains the major determinant of infection in these women. Condom use without spermicide or use of birth control pills does not increase the risk of infection. Recent antimicrobial therapy may also suppress normal colonizing flora, leading to overgrowth of potential uropathogens. Behavioral factors not associated with an increased risk for UTI include voiding practices prior to or following intercourse, wiping practices after toileting, use of douches or tampons, types of underwear, or bathing rather than showering.

The genetic propensity for acute uncomplicated UTI persists throughout a woman's lifetime, from girls to postmenopausal women. Older women may also have additional risk factors such as cystoceles or diverticula, which are abnormalities consistent with complicated UTI. Estrogen deficiency may increase the likelihood of infection for some women, but further study of this association is needed. Uncomplicated UTI occurs rarely in healthy young men. Risk factors for men include having a new sexual partner and anal sex. This syndrome is so uncommon in men, however, that any infection occurring in a man is generally presumed to be complicated UTI.

Host Factors in Complicated Urinary Tract Infection

Patients with complicated UTI have structural or functional abnormalities of the genitourinary tract that compromise voiding or promote entry of bacteria into the urinary tract, irrespective of age or gender. The specific defects include, singly or in combination, obstruction to urinary flow, decreased clearance of organisms in protected environments such as stones or biofilm, or increased access of organisms through reflux or catheters. UTI in pregnant women is also sometimes considered complicated, as urine stasis attributed to hormonal effects on autonomic muscles and ureteric obstruction from pressure of the fetal head at the pelvic brim both likely promote pyelonephritis.

Host Response to Infection

The host immune and inflammatory response in UTI is not fully described but includes both innate and adaptive components. The role of cell-mediated immunity is unclear. Women with acute cystitis have an inflammatory response in the urinary tract characterized by local cytokine production such as **IL6**, **IL8**, and **IL10** and recruitment of leukocytes. This is likely initiated through activation of TL-4 receptors on the bladder epithelium by lipopolysaccharide. A limited local IgA and IgG antibody response specific to the infecting organism also develops. The natural history of untreated acute uncomplicated cystitis is resolution for about 50% of episodes by 2 to 4 weeks, but the contribution of the immune response to resolution is not known. The limited **local immunity** that develops with an episode of acute cystitis *does not protect from subsequent episodes*.

For acute pyelonephritis, the initial local response is again inflammatory, manifested by **pyuria**, or leukocytes in the urine, and cytokine production. A systemic inflammatory response includes fever, leukocytosis, and elevated C-reactive protein. Subsequently, systemic antibodies develop, with IgM antibodies predominating for the first infection and IgG antibodies in subsequent infections. IgG antibodies to lipid A correlate with severity of renal infection. The inflammatory response in the kidney likely contributes to tissue damage and renal scarring. The degree of protection for subsequent renal infection provided by this host response is unclear.

The host immune response is not well studied in individuals with complicated UTI. The inflammatory and immune responses are likely similar to uncomplicated infection, varying with the site of infection in the bladder or kidney. Spontaneous resolution of bacteriuria is less frequent in individuals with complicated UTI, although replacement by another organism is common.

Patients with asymptomatic bacteriuria also usually have pyuria. If pyuria is not present, spontaneous resolution may be more likely to occur. Less virulent organisms, such as enterococcus species and coagulase-negative staphylococci, are less often accompanied by pyuria. Some individuals with asymptomatic bacteriuria also manifest a local immune response, with elevated urinary IgG and IgA antibodies and local cytokine production, but the significance of this response is uncertain.

DIAGNOSIS

The definitive diagnosis of UTI requires isolation of bacteria from the urine. However, the clinical presentation characterizes the site of infection, identifies some underlying host factors, and determines the initial management approach.

Clinical Presentation

Uncomplicated Cystitis or Pyelonephritis

Acute cystitis in women presents with lower-tract irritative symptoms such as dysuria (pain on voiding), frequency (frequent urination), urgency (need to void immediately once the urge is felt), and suprapubic discomfort. Some women also experience gross hematuria. These symptoms vary in intensity from mild to severe in different patients and for different episodes in the same patient. If vaginal symptoms such as discharge or irritation are present, an alternate diagnosis of vaginitis or a sexually transmitted disease must be considered. The physical examination is normal in most women presenting with acute cystitis.

Women with acute uncomplicated pyelonephritis present with costovertebral angle pain and tenderness due to renal inflammation. This is usually unilateral, but bilateral renal involvement can occur. The systemic inflammatory response accompanying pyelonephritis manifests with fever and, in severe cases, nausea, vomiting, and hemodynamic instability consistent with sepsis syndrome. Pyelonephritis may also be accompanied by lower-tract irritative symptoms. Some patients with only lower-tract symptoms also have bacteria present in the kidney. This is referred to as subclinical pyelonephritis and is of uncertain clinical significance.

Complicated Urinary Tract Infection

Individuals with complicated UTI present with symptoms consistent with either acute cystitis or pyelonephritis, depending on the level of urinary tract involvement. If an indwelling catheter is present, UTI may present with fever alone. Some patients with neurologic impairment have altered clinical presentations. Spinal cord injury patients may complain of increased spasticity of the lower limbs or, with high cervical injury affecting the brainstem, autonomic dysreflexia. Multiple sclerosis patients may complain of increased fatigue and a deterioration of neurologic symptoms.

Prostatitis

Acute prostatitis presents with severe local and systemic symptoms, including **high fever**, **pelvic pain**, and **urinary retention**. Physical examination reveals a swollen and tender prostate, but digital rectal exam is discouraged as it may precipitate bacteremia. Chronic bacterial prostatitis is usually characterized by recurrent episodes of acute cystitis from relapses of bacteria persisting in the prostate. Complaints of chronic pelvic discomfort and voiding symptoms, however, are attributed to chronic bacterial prostatitis in only 10% of men with this presentation.

Urine Culture

The microbiologic diagnosis of UTI requires isolation of bacteria from the urine in appropriate quantitative counts (Table 63-1). When voided urine specimens are obtained for culture, external secretions from the periurethral area and, in women, the vagina may contaminate the specimen, leading to false-positive cultures. Urine collection methods must limit such contamination. For men, a clean-voided or clean-catch specimen collected during the middle of voiding is adequate. Contamination is more common for women, but a clean-catch midstream urine specimen is also usually adequate. If a woman is unable

TABLE 63-1 Quantitative Criteria for Identification of "Significant Bacteriuria" in Selected Groups

Population	"Significant Bacteriuria"
Asymptomatic bacteriuria	
• Women	$\geq 10^5$ CFU/mL, usually in two consecutive specimens
• Men	$\geq 10^5$ CFU/mL
Acute pyelonephritis	$\geq 10^5$ CFU/mL[a]
Women with acute dysuria	$\geq 10^2$ CFU/mL, with pyuria
Specimens collected by in and out catheter	$\geq 10^2$ CFU/mL

[a]Five percent of episodes may have counts 10^4–10^5.

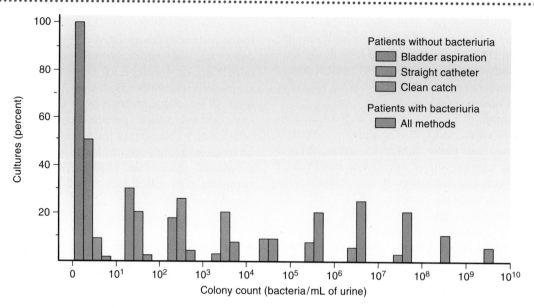

FIGURE 63-3. Quantitative colony counts isolated from urine specimens of patients with bacteriuria and without bacteriuria, using different collection methods.

to cooperate for voiding, a urine specimen may be collected by in and out catheter.

Infecting and contaminating bacteria are distinguished by quantifying the number of organisms growing from the urine specimen. *Colony counts of contaminants in voided specimens are low, while infecting organisms achieve high concentrations* (Fig. 63-3). However, small numbers of bacteria in urine grow well at room temperature, so specimens must be promptly forwarded to the laboratory following collection. A single organism is isolated from most patients with UTI. Some patients with complicated UTI have more than one organism isolated, particularly when chronic urethral catheters or other chronic devices are present.

Urine specimens collected through biofilm-coated devices will sample the microbiology of the biofilm as well as the urine. The biofilm usually has both a greater number and higher quantitative count of organisms. Patients with a chronic indwelling catheter should have the catheter replaced and a urine specimen collected through the new biofilm-free catheter before instituting antimicrobials. This specimen samples bladder urine and is representative of the infecting organisms.

Any quantitative count of a potential uropathogen (e.g., *E. coli, K. pneumoniae, S. saprophyticus*) is consistent with UTI for women with acute uncomplicated UTI (Table 63-1). About 70% of these women will have counts of greater than or equal to 10^5 colony-forming units (CFU)/mL, and 30% have lower counts. For acute pyelonephritis or complicated UTI, greater than or equal to 10^5 CFU/mL is the appropriate quantitative count. Asymptomatic bacteriuria in women is usually identified by two consecutive urine specimens with greater than or equal to 10^5 CFU/mL. If an initial specimen is positive at that quantitative count, a second consecutive voided specimen remains positive in about 80% of women.

Any quantitative count of organisms isolated from a urine specimen obtained by in and out catheterization is consistent with infection. Symptomatic patients with indwelling catheters usually have greater than or equal to 10^5 CFU/mL isolated; the frequency of lower counts in these patients is not well described.

Occasional patients, such as those experiencing diuresis from diuretics, renal failure, or frequent voiding, may have lower quantitative counts isolated because organisms do not have sufficient time to grow to high concentrations in bladder urine. In these patients, quantitative urine culture results must be interpreted in the context of the clinical presentation. Rarely, the urine culture from an infected patient is negative. This occurs with complete ureteric obstruction and infection proximal to the obstruction. Fastidious organisms, such as *Haemophilus influenzae* and *Ureaplasma urealyticum*, infrequently cause infection but are not isolated with routine laboratory methods. The most common reason for a negative urine culture, however, is that the specimen was obtained after initiation of antimicrobial therapy.

Other Laboratory Tests

Pyuria is measured by microscopic examination of the urine or a dipstick leukocyte esterase test. Although pyuria is a consistent finding in patients with symptomatic UTI, the majority of persons with persistent asymptomatic bacteriuria also have pyuria. Pyuria is not specific for UTI. It occurs with noninfectious conditions, such as interstitial nephritis and diabetic nephropathy, and with contamination from vaginal secretions. Thus, pyuria does not diagnose UTI or differentiate symptomatic from asymptomatic infection. The absence of pyuria in a urine specimen, however, is good evidence for the absence of UTI.

TABLE 63-2 Approaches to Treatment of Urinary Tract Infections (UTIs) for Different Clinical Presentations

Type of Infection	Treatment	Rationale
Cystitis	Short course (3 d) preferred	Effective for bacterial cystitis; will not be effective in patients with early pyelonephritis or resistant bacteria—detected by symptomatic relapse posttherapy
Pyelonephritis	7–14 d full doses; initial empiric antimicrobial therapy reassessed when susceptibility tests are available	Requires antimicrobials that achieve high concentrations in renal tissue as well as urine
Asymptomatic bacteriuria	Indicated only for pregnant women or patients about to undergo instrumentation of the urinary tract	• 24–40% of pregnant women with asymptomatic bacteriuria develop pyelonephritis if not treated. • Bacteremia and sepsis likely following instrumentation
Recurrent infection		• Eradicates colonizing flora
Frequent reinfection	Prophylaxis: long term (6–12 mo), low dose, or postintercourse (for uncomplicated UTI only)	• Repeatedly sterilizes urine
Relapse	Long-term treatment (e.g., 4–8 wk or longer)	• Suggests structural abnormality and merits investigation

Patients presenting with severe systemic manifestations or with urinary obstruction may have bacteremia, and blood cultures should be obtained. The peripheral leukocyte count gives information about the severity of illness and may be used to monitor response to therapy. These patients should also have renal function assessed, initially with a blood urea nitrogen and creatinine measurement.

TREATMENT

The treatment of UTI requires antimicrobial therapy directed at the presumed or known infecting organism. Antimicrobials with urinary excretion should be used for therapy; some agents achieve very high urinary levels.

For cystitis, which is considered a superficial mucosal infection, only urinary antibacterial activity is needed. For pyelonephritis, treatment requires adequate antimicrobial levels in both urine and tissue. Other variables considered in selecting therapy include patient tolerance, renal and hepatic function, potential adverse effects, drug interactions, and cost (Table 63-2).

Acute uncomplicated cystitis is usually treated empirically. When the presenting symptoms are consistent, a pretherapy urine culture is not routinely obtained. Women who experience recurrent acute cystitis are 95% accurate in self-diagnosis based on their symptoms. In addition, the microbiology of acute cystitis is highly predictable, and the urine culture results are not available for 48 to 72 hours. As short-course therapy of 3-day

CASE • A 23-year-old woman presents with a 48-hour history of dysuria, frequency, and gross hematuria. She had a similar episode about 8 months ago. Currently, she has a single sexual partner and uses a condom with spermicide for birth control.

1. What is the most likely diagnosis in this woman?

2. What factors have contributed to this episode of infection?

3. Should a urine specimen for culture be obtained?

4. What is the optimal antimicrobial treatment of this episode?

5. What might prevent further episodes of infection?

See Appendix for answers.

duration is preferred for treatment, antimicrobial therapy will often be complete by the time the culture result is available. A pretherapy urine specimen for culture should be obtained, however, in women with atypical symptoms, when empiric therapy is not effective, if there is an early (<1 month) symptomatic recurrence posttherapy, and for any woman who is pregnant.

Considerations in selecting empiric therapy include efficacy for UTI, patient tolerance, and local prevalence of resistance in community *E. coli*. Trimethoprim/sulfamethoxazole (TMP/SMX) or trimethoprim (TMP) are the drugs of first choice for 3-day therapy. Second-line choices include a fluoroquinolone given for 3 days or nitrofurantoin for 5 days. Amoxicillin is not used for empiric therapy because resistance rates of *E. coli* approach 30 to 50%. Cephalosporins are not generally recommended because they share with other β-lactam antibiotics a somewhat lower efficacy, especially with short-course therapy. These agents are useful, however, for treatment of pregnant women, as they are safe for the fetus. Fosfomycin trometamol as a single dose is also available for acute cystitis but is likely somewhat less effective than other agents.

Acute Uncomplicated Pyelonephritis

A urine specimen for culture should be obtained prior to initiating antimicrobial therapy whenever pyelonephritis is a diagnostic consideration. The potential seriousness of this infection means the infecting organism and susceptibilities must be identified to facilitate appropriate antimicrobial therapy. A peripheral leukocyte count, serum creatinine, and blood and urine cultures should be obtained. The severity of illness is assessed clinically by the presence of fever, hemodynamic status, and other systemic symptoms. Other important information also includes whether the patient can tolerate oral therapy, presence of conditions such as diabetes or pregnancy that require closer monitoring, or likelihood of structural abnormalities requiring investigation or intervention. Based on the clinical assessment, a decision is made whether to manage the patient as an outpatient with oral therapy, hospital admission for initial parenteral therapy and monitoring, or short-term observation with an initial dose of parenteral therapy in the emergency department. Empiric therapy is initiated, and antimicrobial management is reassessed once urine culture results are available, usually after 48 to 72 hours. For oral therapy, TMP/SMX, TMP, or a fluoroquinolone may be used depending on anticipated local susceptibilities. For parenteral therapy, an aminoglycoside, extended-spectrum cephalosporin, or fluoroquinolone is appropriate. Generally, 7 to 14 days of therapy is recommended. If there is no convincing clinical improvement by 48 to 72 hours, urinary obstruction, abscess, or other abnormality should be excluded by appropriate diagnostic imaging studies.

Complicated Urinary Tract Infection

The wide variety of potential infecting organisms and greater likelihood of antimicrobial resistance means a urine specimen for culture should be obtained prior to antimicrobial therapy for every episode of complicated infection. When symptoms are mild, antimicrobial therapy should be delayed until the culture results are available so specific therapy can be prescribed. If symptoms are severe, empiric therapy selected on the basis of patient tolerance and anticipated organism susceptibilities is initiated and then reassessed when urine culture results are available. Patients who are significantly ill with high fever, nausea and vomiting, or hemodynamic instability, or with highly resistant organisms, may require hospitalization and initial parenteral therapy. The genitourinary abnormality must be characterized for all patients. This may require additional or repeated diagnostic imaging or urologic investigations.

Asymptomatic Bacteriuria

Asymptomatic bacteriuria is common in many populations, including nursing home residents. In most cases, it should not be screened for or treated, as benefits with treatment of asymptomatic bacteriuria have not been shown. In fact, there are negative outcomes including adverse drug effects and emergence of antimicrobial resistance. The majority of patients will experience reinfection, so the urine cannot be sterilized permanently

---

CASE • A 32-year-old nonpregnant woman presents with fever, rigors, back pain, nausea, vomiting, and mild dysuria. Symptoms have increased in severity over 48 hours. The patient describes two or three previous episodes with a clinical presentation consistent with cystitis. The temperature is 39.2°C, and right costovertebral angle tenderness is present.

1. What is the most likely infecting organism, and what virulence factor is characteristic?
2. What initial investigations should be obtained to confirm the diagnosis and assess the clinical status of this woman?
3. What antimicrobial regimen should be initiated?

See Appendix for answers.

CASE • A 39-year-old male, T6 paraplegic for 8 years, has bladder emptying managed by condom drainage. He presents with complaints of increased bladder and lower-leg spasms, which he attributes to urinary tract infection (UTI). He has had two similar episodes in the past year. A urine specimen for culture grows Klebsiella pneumoniae of greater than or equal to 105 CFU/mL, resistant to fluoroquinolones and aminoglycosides.

1. Why is this man experiencing UTI?

2. Why is the isolate resistant to some antimicrobials?

3. How will you select antimicrobial therapy to treat this infection?

4. What additional management should be considered for this patient with complicated UTI and a recent increase in infection frequency?

See Appendix for answers.

or even for an extended time. An important exception, where treatment is always indicated, is a pregnant woman. A woman with asymptomatic bacteriuria identified in early pregnancy who is not treated has a 20 to 30% risk of pyelonephritis later in pregnancy. Pyelonephritis occurs most frequently at the end of the second trimester or early in the third trimester, when hormonal effects are maximal. Any febrile illness at this gestation may be associated with premature labor and delivery and is a risk for the fetus. Identifying and treating asymptomatic bacteriuria in early pregnancy can prevent this complication. A second patient group for whom identification and treatment of asymptomatic bacteriuria is recommended is those undergoing a urological procedure with potential mucosal trauma and bleeding. Bacteriuric patients are at high risk for bacteremia and sepsis following mucosal injury, and this is prevented by treatment of bacteriuria immediately prior to the procedure.

Recurrent Urinary Tract Infection

The more difficult clinical problem in the management of UTI is not treatment of a single episode but management of patients who have recurrent infection, including some with very frequent recurrences. Prolonged antimicrobial therapy may occasionally be indicated. This is characterized as prophylactic therapy to prevent reinfections or, less frequently, suppressive therapy to prevent symptomatic relapse when a cure is not possible.

Acute Uncomplicated Urinary Tract Infection

For women with frequent symptomatic reinfections, generally defined as two episodes every 6 months or three every year, prophylactic antimicrobial therapy can prevent 90 to 95% of acute symptomatic episodes. This is given as long-term low-dose therapy daily or every other day, or postintercourse. For pregnant women, prophylaxis is indicated following two documented infections, either symptomatic or asymptomatic. Prophylactic antimicrobials appear to be effective through at least two mechanisms. Antimicrobials such as TMP/SMX, TMP, and fluoroquinolones reduce aerobic Gram-negative colonizing flora in the gut, vagina, and periurethral area, preventing reinfection with these organisms. Nitrofurantoin is as effective as these antimicrobials but has no impact on colonizing flora. It is likely effective through intermittent sterilization of the urine with high urinary antimicrobial levels. Probiotics, including yoghurt, have not been found to be effective in preventing recurrent infection. Daily cranberry juice or tablets decrease the frequency of infection by about one-third. The mechanism of action is thought to be binding of *E. coli* adhesins by proanthocyanidins in cranberry, which are excreted in the urine.

Complicated Urinary Tract Infection

Management of recurrent infection for these patients focuses on characterization and correction of the

CASE • An 87-year-old female nursing home resident with chronic incontinence had a urine specimen sent for culture by the nursing staff because the patient appeared somewhat lethargic and was noted to have cloudy urine. The culture result returned 5 days later and was reported as E. coli of greater than 105 CFU/mL. She was no longer lethargic, but the urinalysis also showed pyuria, with white cells too numerous to count.

1. What is the diagnosis in this woman?

2. What antimicrobial treatment should be given for the *E. coli* grown in the urine culture?

See Appendix for answers.

underlying abnormalities that promote infection. Suppressive therapy may be indicated, infrequently, for patients with recurrent symptomatic infection where bacteria cannot be eradicated because of persistent urologic abnormalities. Prolonged antimicrobial therapy may be associated with emergence of more resistant organisms, so suppressive therapy is used only for highly selected patients where alternate approaches are not possible.

CONCLUSION

UTIs are important bacterial infections affecting all ages and both sexes. An appreciation of the epidemiology, pathogenesis, and management is necessary to understand the difference between individuals with normal or abnormal genitourinary tracts. The approach to effective management requires appropriate specimen collection and interpretation of urine cultures, as well as addressing host factors that contribute to the occurrence of infection.

Suggested Readings

Gupta K, Hooton TM, Naber KG, et al. International clinical practice guidelines for the treatment of acute uncomplicated cystitis and pyelonephritis in women: An update. *Clin Infect Dis.* 2011;52(5):e103–e120.

Nicolle LE, Bradley S, Colgan R, et al. IDSA guideline for the diagnosis and treatment of asymptomatic bacteriuria in adults. *Clin Infect Dis.* 2005;40:643–654.

Nicolle LE. Urinary tract infection in the elderly. *Clin Geriatric Med.* 2009;25:423–436.

Schaeffer AJ. Chronic prostatitis and chronic pelvic pain syndrome. *N Engl J Med.* 2006;355:1690–1698.

Stamm WE, ed. Urinary tract infections. *Infect Dis Clin North Am.* 2003;17. Philadelphia, PA: WB Saunders.

Chapter 64

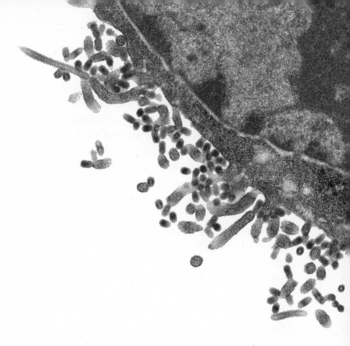

Infections of the Skin and Soft Tissue

Dennis L. Stevens

INFLAMED HANGNAILS, infected cuts, and athlete's foot occur so frequently that we scarcely notice. Those mild and usually inconsequential conditions represent one extreme of the infections of the skin. The other extreme comprises less frequent but more serious diseases like herpes zoster, candidiasis, and certain bacterial infections, such as cellulitis, necrotizing fasciitis, and gas gangrene. Infections of the skin may be caused by viruses, fungi, or bacteria. In addition, many diseases that affect other organs have cutaneous manifestations. Visible skin lesions may indicate systemic infections by viruses (e.g., smallpox, measles, chickenpox), fungi (e.g., cryptococcosis, blastomycosis), or bacteria (e.g., syphilis, tuberculosis, scarlet fever, meningococcemia, endocarditis).

Primary infections of the skin and systemic infections with cutaneous manifestations are discussed throughout this book in the context of specific agents: staphylococci (see Chapter 11), streptococci (see Chapter 12), *Pseudomonas aeruginosa* (see Chapter 18), paramyxoviruses (see Chapter 34), warts (see Chapter 40), and fungal infections (see Chapter 49). This chapter is limited to bacterial skin infections and emphasizes those with important pathobiological implications. This chapter also recognizes that these infections frequently involve the soft tissues underlying the skin, subcutaneous fat, and superficial fascia.

ANATOMY AND PHYSIOLOGY OF THE SKIN

An understanding of the pathogenesis of skin and soft tissue infections requires knowledge of skin anatomy and physiology. The skin is divided into three distinct layers: the epidermis, dermis, and fat layer. The **epidermis** is a thin, self-renewing epidermal sheet that covers the body. It is about the thickness of two sheets of this book (0.1 mm) in most places and devoid of vessels and nerves. The basal cells of the epidermis, the **keratinocytes**, divide, differentiate, mature, and are eventually sloughed from the skin surface. As they rise from the basal layer to the skin surface, they become more stratified and produce a cornified layer of dead cells, the **stratum corneum**. This outermost epidermal layer consists of dead keratinocytes rich in the tough fibrous protein **keratin** and is held together by intercellular neutral lipids. The stratum corneum is the major physical barrier preventing environmental chemicals and microorganisms from entering the body. In addition to the keratinocytes, the epidermis contains the **Langerhans cells** and the pigment-containing **melanocytes**. Langerhans cells are fixed tissue macrophages. They represent a distant outpost of the immune system and process antigens that breach the stratum corneum.

Skin appendages, including hairs, sebaceous (oil) glands, and sweat glands, originate from the basal layer of the epidermis. They invaginate into the dermis and exit at the surface through the epidermis. Bacteria may bypass the stratum corneum by traversing these conduits.

The **dermis** is several millimeters thick and separated from the epidermis by a basement membrane. The fibrous proteins **collagen** and **elastin** are embedded in a glycoprotein matrix and constitute the strong supportive dermal structure. A rich plexus of blood vessels and lymphatics courses through the dermis. Interruption of dermal blood flow predisposes to infection by restricting access of humoral and cellular immune defenses against invaders and by compromising oxygen delivery and nutrition of the epidermal barrier.

Subcutaneous fat, the third layer of the skin, consists predominantly of lipid cells. Those cells serve as heat insulators, shock absorbers, and depots of caloric reserves. The final layer is **superficial fascia** that separates skin from muscles. Any or all of these layers of soft tissue may be involved in a given infectious process.

ENCOUNTER

The skin is sterile in utero and during birth, but it is soon colonized by both anaerobic and aerobic bacteria ranging from 10^2 to 10^4 colony-forming units (CFUs) per square centimeter of surface. Many factors affect the distribution, composition, and density of these microorganisms. These factors include not only the environmental climate, which differs throughout the world, but also the microclimates of the body. The intertriginous areas of the axilla and groin are markedly different from the drier areas of the back, forearms, and calves of the leg.

The two properties that make the skin hostile to bacterial growth are **exfoliation** and **dryness**. The constant sloughing of the stratum corneum dislodges many of the bacteria that adhere to its surface. The importance of dryness can be seen when occlusive dressings are applied: Within 2 or 3 days, bacteria counts may increase from 10^2 to more than 10^7 CFU/cm². Accordingly, bacteria counts are much higher in the moister areas of the skin than in the drier regions. Other factors that help limit bacterial growth are low pH, low temperature, and chemical composition. The skin has a pH of approximately 5.5, the result of hydrolysis of sebum lipids by the skin bacteria themselves. Growth of some microorganisms is further hindered by the skin's low temperature, which averages about 33°C. The saltiness of some parts of the skin, the result of the evaporation of sweat, may encourage the growth of salt-resistant species, such as *Staphylococcus epidermidis*. In addition, some organisms are inhibited by the lipid content of the skin surface.

The bacterial microbiota of skin, like that of mucous membranes, also helps protect the host from invasion by pathogens; skin infections are more likely to occur when the microbiota is wiped out. The precise mechanisms involved in the skin-protecting ability of the normal microbiota are not known but may include saturation of binding sites, competition for nutrients, and production of bacteriocins and other inhibitory chemicals by endogenous microbes.

Members of the resident microbiota of the skin are of low virulence and rarely cause significant infections. Included in the microbiota are **resident bacteria**, which multiply on the skin and are regularly present, and **transient bacteria**, which survive on the skin for only a short period. Members of the transient microbiota are deposited on the skin from either mucous membrane sites or the environment. Specific adhesins are required for bacterial adherence to the skin, and these molecules are a prerequisite for colonization.

The dry and exposed areas of the skin are normally colonized with Gram-positive bacteria (including *S. epidermidis*, micrococci, anaerobic Gram-positive cocci, and both anaerobic and aerobic diphtheroids). *Propionibacterium acnes*, a Gram-positive rod, thrives in the sebaceous areas. Facultative and anaerobic Gram-negative rods more often colonize the axilla and groin regions and other moist areas, such as the webs of the toes. For unknown reasons, the skin of bedridden patients with serious medical illnesses often has increased colonization of Gram-negative bacilli.

The most important organisms of the transient microbiota are the common pathogens of cutaneous infections, *Staphylococcus aureus* and *Streptococcus pyogenes*. These organisms are found more often on exposed skin than on areas normally protected by clothing. *S. aureus* is found commonly in the nose and on the face and upper body rather than on the trunk and legs, probably because the upper respiratory tract is the reservoir for the organism. The box entitled "Members of the Skin Microbiota and the Infections They Cause" lists some of the important pathogens that transiently colonize the skin and cause infections.

MEMBERS OF THE SKIN MICROBIOTA AND THE INFECTIONS THEY CAUSE

Resident Microbiota

- *Propionibacterium acnes*
- *Staphylococcus epidermidis*: infection around foreign bodies (percutaneous catheters, prosthetic devices, etc.)
- Micrococci
- Anaerobic Gram-positive cocci
- Aerobic Gram-negative bacilli (low numbers)
- *Pityrosporum ovale* (a yeast)

(*continued*)

Transient Microbiota

- Bacteria
  - Frequent:
    - *Staphylococcus aureus*: folliculitis, furuncles, carbuncles, toxic shock syndrome, and bacteremia
    - *Streptococcus pyogenes*: cellulitis, lymphangitis, impetigo, erysipelas, necrotizing fasciitis, and toxic shock syndrome
  - Infrequent:
    - *Haemophilus influenzae*: cellulitis
    - *Clostridium* species: gas gangrene
    - *Francisella tularensis*: tularemia
    - *Bacillus anthracis*: anthrax
    - *Pseudomonas aeruginosa*: infections resulting from hot-tub use
    - *Burkholderia cepacia*: foot infection ("foot rot")
    - *Mycobacterium marinum*: "fish tank cellulitis"
- Fungi
  - *Candida albicans*: diaper rash, chronic paronychia
  - Dermatophytes: tinea infections (ringworm)
- Viruses
  - Frequent:
    - Herpes simplex virus 1 and 2: perioral ("cold sore") and genital infection
    - Papillomaviruses: warts
  - Infrequent:
    - *Molluscum contagiosum*: wartlike lesions

ENTRY

Infectious agents enter the skin and its underlying soft tissues by two routes:

- **From the outside**: through cuts, wounds, insect bites, skin disease, or other breaks in the integrity of the stratum corneum
- **From within**: through underlying tissue or carried by blood or lymph

Once microorganisms penetrate the skin, they spread locally and invade the lymphatics or the bloodstream. As a result, infections originally confined to the skin and soft tissues may ultimately cause disease in other parts of the body.

SPREAD AND MULTIPLICATION

The spread of some bacteria is associated with specific virulence factors; an example is **hyaluronidase** (also called **spreading factor**), an extracellular enzyme made by both *S. aureus* and *S. pyogenes*. Other enzymes, such as hemolysins, lipases, collagenase, and elastases, are elaborated by cutaneous pathogens and probably play important roles in pathogenesis (see Chapter 9). In general, *S. aureus infections tend to localize*, forming abscesses, for example, whereas *S. pyogenes infections spread more extensively through tissues*, causing cellulitis.

What is the role of cellular and humoral immunity in the skin? Neutrophils are attracted to the infected area by chemoattractants elaborated by bacteria, tissue macrophages, and activation of complement through the alternative pathway. A local antimicrobial effort is mounted by epidermal macrophages, the Langerhans cells, through the elaboration of cytokines. Persons with acquired and congenital immunodeficiencies have an increased frequency of certain skin infections (e.g., candidiasis), suggesting that cellular immunity is an important component of skin defenses. When microorganisms breach the stratum corneum and multiply, the host's defenses are mobilized to the skin. When the defenses are defective, infections of the skin become frequent events, and more extensive infection may be manifest.

DAMAGE

Cellular damage to the skin and soft tissues can be mediated by toxins, degradative enzymes, and the induction of host defense mechanisms that destroy tissues. The manifestations of infection caused by the invasion of microorganisms in the skin depend on the level of penetration, the virulence factors of the microbe, and the host response. Infections of skin and soft tissue are divided into three groups:

- **Exogenous infections** resulting from direct invasion from the external environment

- **Endogenous infections** caused by invasion from an internal source, such as the blood or an infected organ
- **Toxin-induced infections** produced by toxins formed at a distant site

EXOGENOUS INFECTIONS

Controversy exists about whether virulent pathogens directly penetrate the normal skin when present in high concentrations or whether they enter through imperceptible microscopic lesions. Without a noticeable break in the skin, high numbers of virulent pathogens are required to produce exogenous skin and soft tissue infection. Experimental studies show that colonization of the skin by *S. aureus* at a density of more than 10^6 CFU/cm^2 is required to cause skin infections. Normally, bacteria grow to densities of that magnitude only under special circumstances, such as when the skin is dirty or kept moist for prolonged periods. Once the skin barrier is broken from trauma, surgery, or a foreign body such as suture material, a sliver, or an intravenous catheter, *S. aureus* infection can be caused by as few as 10 to 100 CFU/cm^2. Thus, a number of conditions predispose to skin invasion, including excessive moisture, trauma, introduction of a foreign body, pressure, and compromised blood supply.

Excessive moisture can result from the use of occlusive dressings or from wet diapers on babies. Obese people accumulate moisture in their intertriginous folds. **Immersion infection** is seen in people who spend long periods in wet or swampy areas and cannot allow their footwear to dry out, such as troops during training or combat. Moisture induces skin **maceration** and breakdown of the stratum corneum. It is estimated that among US foot soldiers in Vietnam, disability was more often associated with skin infections than with combat-associated wounds. Staphylococci and streptococci are frequently responsible for immersion infections, but waterborne Gram-negative bacteria also can be involved. Bathing in hot tubs containing high numbers of *Pseudomonas aeruginosa* is another mechanism of immersion infection (see Chapter 18).

Trauma is the most common factor leading to skin and soft tissue infection. Trauma may be mild, as in a torn hangnail or cracks in the skin caused by athlete's foot. Major forms of trauma that place persons at risk for skin invasion include surgery (considered "organized trauma"), gunshot wounds, crush injuries (e.g., automobile accidents), or burns. Infections in surgical wounds are a major cause of morbidity in postoperative patients. Infection also is the primary cause of mortality in burn victims.

Many procedures used in the hospital breach the skin. The most common procedure is the use of **percutaneous** ("through the skin") **catheters**. The list of such devices is enormous and includes central venous lines, peritoneal dialysis catheters, tubes to drain body cavities, temporary pacemaker lines, chemotherapy infusion lines, and parenteral nutrition lines. Indeed, the most common reason for premature removal of percutaneous catheters is bacterial

infection. Another type of skin infection in hospitalized patients is the **decubitus ulcer**, the cutaneous lesion that develops secondary to pressure injury informally referred to as a bed sore. Constant pressure against the skin of a paralyzed or immobile person leads to skin necrosis and frequently to secondary infection.

Any condition that compromises the blood supply predisposes the skin to invasion by causing barrier breakdown and limiting host defenses. Blood supply compromise can occur acutely following trauma or chronically as a result of peripheral vascular disease, as in persons with diabetes or vasculitis, or in elderly people. In the diabetic patient, compromise of the vascular supply is often accompanied by peripheral sensory neuropathy, which limits the patient's awareness of traumatic damage to the skin. Secondary infections also can follow certain noninfectious skin diseases such as **atopic dermatitis** or **pemphigus vulgaris**.

The skin responds to invading microorganisms in a limited number of ways that fall into three general categories:

- **Spreading infections**: called **impetigo** when confined to the epidermis, **erysipelas** when involving the dermal lymphatics, and **cellulitis** when the major focus is the subcutaneous fat layer
- **Abscess formation**: known as folliculitis, boils (furuncles), and carbuncles
- **Necrotizing infections**, including fasciitis and gas gangrene (myonecrosis)

The organisms commonly implicated in exogenous infections are listed in Table 64-1. Cellulitis is illustrated in the following case.

TABLE 64-1 Frequent Exogenous Infections of the Skin and Soft Tissues

Disease	Organisms
Folliculitis	Staphylococci, *Pseudomonas* species
Carbuncles, furuncles	Staphylococci
Impetigo	Streptococci, staphylococci
Erysipelas	Streptococci
Lymphangitis	Streptococci
Cellulitis	Streptococci, staphylococci, *Haemophilus influenzae* (in unimmunized children)
Synergistic cellulitis	Streptococci, enteric bacteria, anaerobes
Gas gangrene	Clostridia
Necrotizing fasciitis	Streptococci, enteric bacteria, anaerobes

CASE • Ms. W., a 27-year-old emergency medical technician, was evaluated by a physician for an infection around the nail of her left index finger (called a **paronychia**). The physician drained the lesion, and a culture of the pus grew a group A β-hemolytic streptococcus (*S. pyogenes*). Ms. W. was not given antimicrobial therapy because the physician thought that drainage was sufficient. Five days later, Ms. W. complained of fever and severe pain in the forearm, which had become swollen and red (erythematous). Her temperature was 40.2°C, and she was hot and sweaty. A patchy rash extended from her left upper arm to her shoulder. Lymph nodes in the axilla were enlarged and tender. Ms. W. was admitted to the hospital with a diagnosis of **streptococcal cellulitis**. She was treated successfully with high doses of penicillin. Blood cultures obtained before starting antimicrobial therapy also yielded *S. pyogenes*.

This case raises several questions:

1. What risk factors predisposed Ms. W. to the development of cellulitis?

2. What virulence determinants are expressed by *S. pyogenes*?

3. What antibiotic should have been administered at the time of the incision and drainage?

See Appendix for answers.

Streptococcal Cellulitis, Impetigo, Erysipelas, and Lymphangitis

Cellulitis is an acute inflammatory process that involves subcutaneous tissue, characterized by areas of redness, induration, heat, and tenderness (Fig. 64-1). The borders of these areas are usually indistinct. Cellulitis can spread rapidly and is often accompanied by lymphangitis and inflammation of the draining lymph nodes. More than 90% of cases are caused by *S. aureus* and group A streptococci, while the rest are attributed to a variety of bacteria. In unimmunized children, infection with *Haemophilus influenzae* type b is an important cause of periorbital cellulitis, and it may be characterized by a blue tint of the overlying erythema. Cellulitis associated with bites or scratches from cats or dogs is often the result of *Pasteurella multocida* infection (see Chapter 73). A normal inhabitant of the oral microbiota of many domestic and wild animals, *P. multocida* spreads rapidly and causes painful cellulitis when inoculated into human skin through a bite or scratch.

The pathological processes in cellulitis develop rapidly and may progress within 24 to 48 hours from a minor injury to severe septicemia. Characteristically, the tissues contain few organisms but undergo a marked inflammatory response, probably caused by toxins elaborated by the invading bacteria and products of inflammation such as cytokines and prostaglandins. The capacity of group A streptococci to spread through the tissues is aided by hyaluronidase and other virulence factors that promote tissue invasion and dissemination.

Impetigo is a characteristic infection of the epidermis, manifested by intraepidermal vesicles that are filled with exudate and eventually become weeping and crusting lesions (Fig. 64-2). Caused by either group A streptococci or staphylococci, impetigo is a common disease of children seen mainly in exposed areas of the body during warm, moist weather. Although not usually associated with systemic signs or symptoms, impetigo caused by nephrogenic group A streptococci can lead to post-streptococcal glomerulonephritis.

Erysipelas is a more serious disease characterized by tender, superficial erythematous and edematous

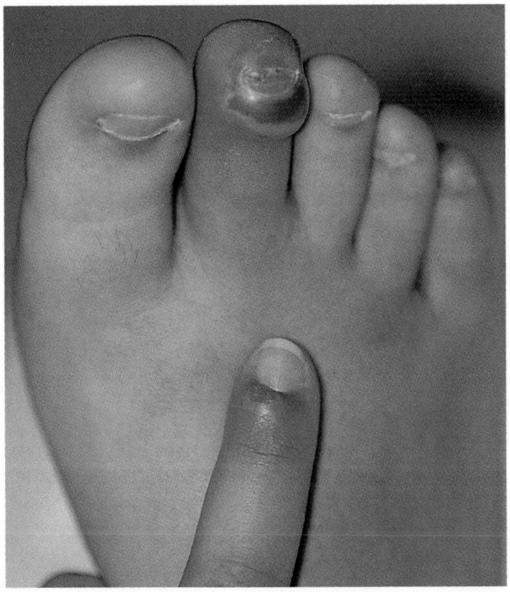

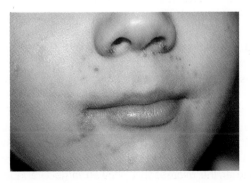

FIGURE 64-1. Cellulitis of the toe. The infection began adjacent to the nail as a paronychia and spread proximally to involve the shaft of the toe as cellulitis.

FIGURE 64-2. Streptococcal impetigo. Weeping and crusting lesions are typical of impetigo.

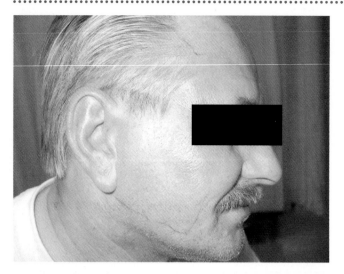

FIGURE 64-3. Erysipelas. The rash on the right side of the face is confluent and salmon red in color.

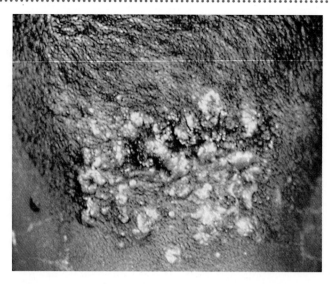

FIGURE 64-4. Staphylococcal carbuncle. The posterior shows multiple follicular abscesses discharging purulent material.

lesions. The infection spreads primarily in the superficial lymphatics of the dermis (Fig. 64-3). The rash is usually confluent, salmon red in color, and sharply demarcated from the surrounding, normal skin. It is seen most frequently in adults with edema of the extremities and often occurs on the face. The most common organisms that cause erysipelas are group A streptococci. Infection of the deep lymphatics, or **lymphangitis**, also is caused by group A streptococci. Erysipelas used to be one of the most serious complications of surgery (see Chapter 12), and it carried a high mortality rate. Its severity and incidence have markedly decreased over the last few decades. The decline can be explained only partially by the widespread use of penicillin to treat streptococcal infections.

Folliculitis, Furuncles, and Carbuncles Caused by *Staphylococcus aureus*

Cutaneous abscesses usually begin as superficial infections in and around hair follicles, which is called **folliculitis**.

Folliculitis is a pustular eruption usually associated with *S. aureus*. In the follicle, bacteria are somewhat sequestered from defense mechanisms and can form microabscesses. If not controlled, the abscesses enlarge to become **furuncles**, better known as **common boils**. If a number of boils cluster together to form a large multifocal infection, the lesion is called a **carbuncle** (Fig. 64-4). Furuncles may be a recurring and frustrating problem in some individuals, especially young people who are chronic nasal carriers of virulent *S. aureus*. Although the lesions are confined to the skin, they can be a source of bacteremia and systemic disease.

The pathological processes leading to abscess formation include a massive influx of neutrophils and sequestration of the infected site. That process is caused by deposition of fibrin (fostered by staphylococcal coagulase) and stimulation of fibroblasts to produce a fibrous capsule. The result is a well-organized infection containing necrotic white blood cells and huge numbers of

CASE • Mr. C., a 37-year-old roofer, came to the emergency department with fever and a painful swelling on the left side of his neck. He had previously been healthy except for occasional boils. Three days before, he had noted a minor irritation around some whiskers. The lesion progressed to the size of a walnut, which prevented him from buttoning his shirt. Physical examination revealed a healthy man in mild distress. His temperature was 38.8°C. A 2- to 3-cm mass with a soft center was noted on his left anterior neck at the beard line, surrounded by erythema. Needle aspiration of the mass yielded about 1 mL of pus that, under the microscope, showed large Gram-positive

cocci in clusters and many neutrophils. A culture grew *S. aureus*. The abscess was incised and drained, and he was successfully treated with antibiotics.

This case raises several questions:

1. What was the source of the *S. aureus* in the case of Mr. C.?

2. Should the physician suspect any underlying immune deficiency?

3. What should be suspected if the infection fails to respond to β-lactam antibiotics?

See Appendix for answers.

CASE • Mrs. S., a 57-year-old woman with type II diabetes mellitus, came to the emergency department slightly feverish after 2 days of pain in her right foot. When the pain started, she noted tenderness and serous (watery) discharge between her third and fourth toes. She had been bothered before by an ulcer on the sole of her foot, apparently caused by constant scraping against her shoe. On physical examination, she appeared ill and had a temperature of 39.8°C. Her right foot was swollen with patchy erythema, cyanosis, and signs of necrosis. Crusting and oozing were evident around her third and fourth toes.

Cultures of the exudate and blood were obtained, and Mrs. S. was treated with antibiotics. After 24 hours, she showed no clinical improvement, and the infection continued to ascend proximally. She was taken to the operating room, and multiple incisions revealed necrotic fascia extending to the upper thigh. As much of the necrotic tissue was removed as possible. Cultures from the wound grew the anaerobic Gram-negative rod, *Bacteroides fragilis*, and an enteric bacterium, *Enterobacter*. Her blood cultures were negative. Mrs. S. slowly recovered and underwent a second operation for closure of her wound.

This case raises several questions:

1. How does diabetes mellitus predispose to the development of skin infections?
2. Would antibiotics alone have been effective in eradicating this infection?

See Appendix for answers.

---

bacteria (i.e., pus). Steps that lead to abscess formation include tissue destruction by the invading organisms and massive release of lysosomal enzymes from lysing neutrophils, as well as the deposition of fibrin (see Chapter 11). The unique physicochemical characteristics of abscesses are discussed in Chapter 30. Therapy of an abscess is usually two pronged: removal of pus by incision and drainage and, when patients have systemic evidence of infection, treatment with antimicrobial agents.

Necrotizing Soft Tissue Infections

The case of Mrs. S. is an example of **necrotizing fasciitis**, probably started by the entry of bacteria through the ulcer on the sole of her foot. Persons with diabetes frequently suffer from poor skin circulation and lack of local sensation, which may have been the reason for the development of the ulcer. The infection spread rapidly along the superficial fascia that separates subcutaneous fat and muscle. The vessels and nerves that supply the skin course through that fascia, and their destruction leads to the patchy necrosis and cutaneous anesthesia that characterize such a rapidly spreading and dangerous infection.

Although tissue necrosis occurs to some extent in most infections, the term **necrotizing (or gangrenous) infection** is reserved for one in which extensive necrosis is the outstanding characteristic. Mrs. S.'s case illustrates a necrotizing fasciitis caused by multiple bacteria (i.e., polymicrobial). In addition to diabetes, loss of integrity of mucous membranes of the gastrointestinal or genitourinary tract can lead to necrotizing fasciitis of the perineum (Fournier gangrene), which also is caused by mixed aerobic and anaerobic bacteria colonizing those sites. Gas from bacterial metabolism is sometimes found in lesions from Fournier gangrene.

Necrotizing fasciitis can be caused by monomicrobial etiologies, such as group A streptococci, *Aeromonas hydrophila*, or *Vibrio vulnificus*. Necrotizing infection of muscle is called myonecrosis, and when caused by gas-producing *Clostridium* bacteria, *C. perfringens*, *C. septicum*, *C. histolyticum*, or *C. sordellii*, the illness is called gas gangrene (see Chapter 20). **Myonecrosis** also is found in about 50% of patients with necrotizing fasciitis caused by group A streptococci. If a necrotizing infection is suspected, the diagnosis should be confirmed by inspection of the fascia and muscle by surgical exploration. Interestingly, Gram stains of wound drainage or debrided tissue show few, if any, white blood cells but large numbers of bacteria in deep infections caused by clostridia (large Gram-positive rods) and group A streptococci (Gram-positive cocci in chains).

The major factors that predispose to clostridial infection are interruption of the blood supply from penetrating trauma, such as a crush injury, gunshot wound, or stabbing, and contamination of the wound with soil or dirty clothing. Injection of black tar heroin into the skin also has been associated with a variety of skin infections, including necrotizing fasciitis and myonecrosis. Thus, traumatic wounds, particularly those grossly contaminated with dirt, should be meticulously cleaned, debrided, irrigated copiously with normal saline, and left open to heal by secondary intention. Infection can be caused by vegetative bacilli or endospores that germinate only under anaerobic conditions. Antibiotic treatment alone is rarely successful, probably because of the compromised blood supply; extensive surgical debridement is mandatory. Antibiotics also are ineffective against spores. Clostridia produce potent toxins such as hemolysins and phospholipases that cause rapid tissue destruction. Experimental studies suggest that suppression of toxin production by antibiotics that inhibit

CASE • Fifty-two-year-old Mr. A. underwent chemotherapy with cytotoxic agents for an aggressive form of lymphoma. As a result of chemotherapy, his white blood cell count fell to fewer than 100/mm³. Suddenly, Mr. A. developed shaking chills and fever and noted pain over his left shoulder. Examination of the area showed an erythematous round area with a central vesicle (Fig. 64-6). Because of the suspicion of Gram-negative bacteremia, Mr. A. was treated with broad-spectrum antibiotics. Within a few hours, the area on the left shoulder developed a necrotic center with surrounding erythema, a lesion known as **ecthyma gangrenosum**. A biopsy of the lesion showed an infarcted blood vessel teeming with bacteria. Cultures of the biopsy material and the blood grew *P. aeruginosa*. Mr. A. responded to the antimicrobial therapy with resolution of fever and clearing of the skin lesions.

This case raises several questions:

1. What alteration in host defense most directly contributed to the development of *P. aeruginosa* bacteremia in Mr. A.?
2. What is the pathogenesis of the skin lesions?
3. Why was antibiotic therapy initiated prior to obtaining culture results?

See Appendix for answers.

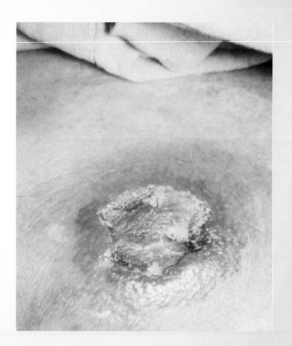

FIGURE 64-6. Ecthyma gangrenosum, a necrotic skin lesion caused by *Pseudomonas aeruginosa*.

protein synthesis (e.g., clindamycin) in combination with β-lactam antibiotics is more efficacious than treatment with β-lactam antibiotics alone (see the section on toxic shock syndromes later in this chapter).

Endogenous Infections

The skin can become infected by microorganisms that spread from another infected site, either by direct extension from an underlying focus or through the bloodstream. Such secondary infections occur in both immunocompetent and immunosuppressed hosts but with different degrees of incidence and severity. Some types of skin infections that occur from within are listed in the box entitled "Sources of Endogenous Skin Infections." Systemic infections are manifested in various ways. **Abscesses** can result from intravascular infections such as endocarditis, particularly when caused by *S. aureus*. **Necrosis** seen in chronic meningococcemia or overwhelming meningococcal septicemia can involve large areas of the skin. Called **purpura fulminans**, the confluent necrosis is the skin manifestation of disseminated intravascular coagulation (Fig. 64-5). Milder forms of necrosis are also seen, for example, in disseminated gonorrhea.

Immunocompromised hosts like Mr. A. are susceptible to a unique skin lesion called **ecthyma gangrenosum**, usually seen with *P. aeruginosa* septicemia. One of the characteristics of endogenous infection with this organism is vasculitis resulting in infarction of the skin from vascular insufficiency. *P. aeruginosa* grows in the infarcted area and causes necrosis by the production of exotoxin A and other toxins (see Chapter 18). In Mr. A.'s case, biopsy of the necrotic area revealed no neutrophil infiltrate because of the patient's granulocytopenia. Instead, infarction of blood vessels by bacterial **emboli** occurred, with destruction of the arterial wall and bacterial invasion of the surrounding tissues.

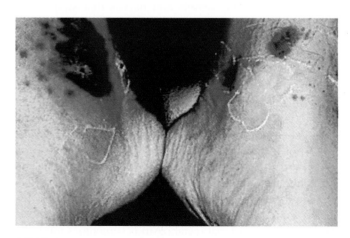

FIGURE 64-5. Purpura caused by disseminated intravascular coagulation.

SOURCES OF ENDOGENOUS SKIN INFECTIONS

Direct Extension

- Osteomyelitis: draining sinus
- Septic arthritis: draining sinus
- Lymphadenitis
  - Tuberculosis
  - Atypical mycobacteriosis
  - Streptococcal or staphylococcal infection
- Oral infection: dental sepsis (Ludwig angina)
  - Actinomycosis (lumpy jaw)
  - Mixed cellulitis
- Intra-abdominal: necrotizing infection
- Herpes simplex virus
- Varicella-zoster virus

Hematogenous Spread

- Bacteremia
  - Meningococci
  - Staphylococci
  - *Pseudomonas aeruginosa*
- Endocarditis
- Fungemia: candidiasis
- Viremia
  - Measles virus
  - Varicella-zoster virus
- Rickettsioses
  - Rocky Mountain spotted fever
  - Epidemic or endemic typhus

Besides *P. aeruginosa*, other Gram-negative rods such as *Klebsiella* and *Serratia* species also may be involved, and occasionally, *S. aureus* can cause these manifestations. Disseminated fungal infections, including those due to *Aspergillus* and *Cryptococcus*, can produce the same characteristic lesions. It is imperative that the physician treats an ecthyma gangrenosum early, before bacteriological confirmation, because the mortality rate in untreated granulocytopenic patients with Gram-negative bacteremia is 50% within 24 hours.

Exanthems, or rashes, are seen in a large variety of infections caused by *Rickettsiae*, other bacteria, and viruses. They are subdivided into hemorrhagic rashes, often accompanied by necrosis (as in meningococcemia; see the box entitled "Sources of Endogenous Skin Infections"), and macular (spotted) rashes (as in typhoid fever or Rocky Mountain spotted fever). Rashes prominent in several viral infections, such as measles and rubella, are known as the **viral exanthems** (see Chapter 34 and Table 64-2).

Many cutaneous lesions are themselves **noninfectious** but rather occur as a consequence of septicemia or other systemic infections. They include hemorrhages, petechiae, and special manifestations of subacute bacterial

TABLE 64-2 Some Viral Diseases with Cutaneous Manifestations

Disease	Etiological Agent	Principal Cutaneous Manifestation
Herpes labialis	Herpes simplex virus (most often HSV-1)	Vesicles on the lip ("cold sores")
Herpes genitalis	Herpes simplex virus (most often HSV-2)	Vesicles in the genital area
Shingles (zoster)	Varicella-zoster virus	Vesicles over specific dermatomes
Chickenpox (varicella)	Varicella-zoster virus	Vesicles, becoming purulent, then dry, crusted lesions
Measles	Measles virus	Maculopapular rash
German measles	Rubella virus	Maculopapular rash
Smallpox (eradicated)	Smallpox virus	Uniform pustular vesicles

CASE • At the age of 24 years, Mr. N. had an operation to repair an inguinal hernia. Five days later, he developed shaking chills and cool extremities. He became progressively more ill over the next 48 hours and developed a rash on his trunk and face. The rash was accompanied by a sore throat, headache, myalgias (muscle pains), vomiting, diarrhea, and postural dizziness (dizzy when upright, suggesting low blood pressure). On physical examination, Mr. N. had a diffuse rash with some blanching on pressure. His eyes were inflamed with conjunctivitis, and he had an erythematous pharynx and a "strawberry" tongue. His inguinal wound was draining a brown, odorless material. Laboratory examination revealed a high white blood cell count and an elevated serum creatinine value (5.7 mg/dL), indicating acute renal failure. A Gram stain of the material from the wound showed Gram-positive cocci in clusters and grew *S. aureus.* The organism tested positive for the toxic shock syndrome toxin-1 (TSST-1). The patient ultimately showed desquamation of his hands and trunk (Fig. 64-7). He was treated with antibiotics and eventually recovered.

This case raises several questions:

1. What conditions place persons at risk for the development of toxic shock syndrome?

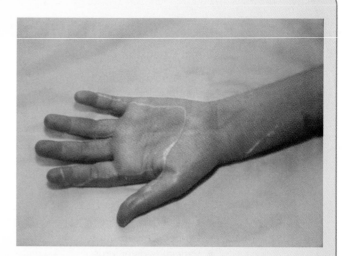

FIGURE 64-7. Desquamation of the skin of the palm in a patient with staphylococcal toxic shock syndrome.

2. What other organisms can cause this disease?
3. How does TSST-1 cause shock and organ failure?

See Appendix for answers.

---

endocarditis called Janeway lesions and Osler nodes. These skin manifestations are caused by vasculitis, probably as a result of immune complex deposition (see Chapter 67).

Cutaneous Responses to Bacterial Toxins (Toxic Shock Syndromes and Scarlet Fever)

The skin can respond to toxins elaborated during infections that take place at a distant site. An example is scarlet fever, which is characterized by rash and pharyngitis caused by certain strains of group A streptococci that elaborate an exotoxin called **erythrogenic factor** or **pyrogenic exotoxin**. The toxin spreads through the bloodstream and is responsible for the rash, enlarged papillae of the tongue (known as **strawberry tongue**), and desquamation of the skin on the extremities. Scarlet fever used to be a serious disease of childhood; the marked decrease in its severity over the last century has defied explanation.

Staphylococci cause two specific toxin-induced skin diseases: **scalded skin syndrome** and **toxic shock syndrome** (TSS; see Chapter 11). Staphylococcal scalded skin syndrome, a disease of infants, results from the action of a toxin, **exfoliatin**, that separates the epidermis by destroying the intercellular connections (desmosomes). The result resembles skin scalded with hot water.

The case of Mr. N. is a typical clinical presentation of TSS, which is caused by exotoxins produced by certain strains of *S. aureus.* TSS was first described in children in the early 1970s but became widely known in the early 1980s when young menstruating women using "superabsorbent tampons" developed the syndrome. Characteristically, patients develop hypotension, tachycardia, multiorgan dysfunction, and a diffuse red rash resembling sunburn. Patients require aggressive fluid resuscitation to maintain adequate blood pressure. TSST-1 has been implicated in menstrual cases. Today tampon-associated TSS is rare, and most cases of TSS are related to the production of enterotoxins, particularly type B, and follow a soft tissue infection, as illustrated in the case of Mr. N.

A similar syndrome also can occur in patients with severe and disseminated *S. pyogenes* infection and is referred to as streptococcal toxic shock syndrome (streptococcal TSS). In contrast to staphylococcal TSS, streptococcal TSS has been associated with necrotizing fasciitis and bacteremia. Interestingly, group A streptococcus produces a myriad of pyrogenic exotoxins that, like staphylococcal TSST-1 and enterotoxins, are superantigens that induce massive cytokine production by both lymphocytes and antigen-presenting cells such as monocytes and macrophages. Antibiotics that inhibit protein synthesis (e.g., clindamycin) block toxin production and enhance the efficacy of antibiotics that inhibit bacterial cell wall synthesis in animal models of TSS and in some retrospective clinical reviews.

Methicillin-Resistant *Staphylococcus aureus* Infections

Methicillin-resistant *S. aureus* (MRSA) strains have emerged over the last 30 years in hospitals throughout the world. Since 2000, community-acquired MRSA infections also have dramatically increased in most parts of the world and are associated with a variety of skin and soft tissue infections, including impetigo, cellulitis, furunculosis, necrotizing soft tissue infections, and TSS. In addition to the general increase in the prevalence of these strains, epidemics of MRSA soft tissue infections have occurred among wrestlers, football players, and prison inmates. Genetic evidence suggests that a higher percentage of MRSA strains possess potent toxins such as TSST-1, enterotoxins, and the Panton-Valentine leukocidin in comparison to methicillin-susceptible strains. Clearly, empiric treatment of presumed MRSA infections of any type may fail if nafcillin, dicloxacillin, or any of the cephalosporins are used. Thus, in patients who have systemic manifestations, or very aggressive soft tissue infections, empiric treatment should include an agent that currently is reliably active against MRSA, such as vancomycin, linezolid, or daptomycin.

CONCLUSION

The skin and its underlying soft tissues protect the body from hostile influences in the environment. Traumatic breaks, animal bites, or other skin diseases often facilitate the penetration of these barriers by infectious agents. Microorganisms also may lodge in the skin and soft tissues as the result of hematogenous or lymphatic dissemination. The resulting diseases are extraordinarily varied and caused by a wide variety of mechanisms. Because of the diverse etiologies of soft tissue infection, a careful history and physical examination are crucial. Obtaining appropriate samples from aspirates, biopsies, surgical debridement, or blood cultures is essential to establish a diagnosis and determine susceptibility of the causative microbes to antibiotics.

Suggested Readings

Bryant AE, Stevens DL. Gas gangrene and other clostridial infections. In: Longo DL, Fauci AS, Kasper DL, et al., eds. *Harrison's Principles of Internal Medicine*. 18th ed. New York: McGraw-Hill; 2011:Chapter 142.

Feingold DS, Hirschmann JV. Approach to the patient with skin or soft tissue infection. In: Gorbach SL, Bartlett JG, Blacklow NR, eds. *Infectious Diseases*. 3rd ed. Philadelphia, PA: WB Saunders; 2004:1150–1151.

Stevens DL, Bisno AL, Chambers HF, et al. Practice guidelines for the diagnosis and management of skin and soft-tissue infections. *Clin Infect Dis*. 2005; 41:1373–1406.

Swartz MN. Clinical practice: cellulitis. *N Engl J Med*. 2004:350;904–912.

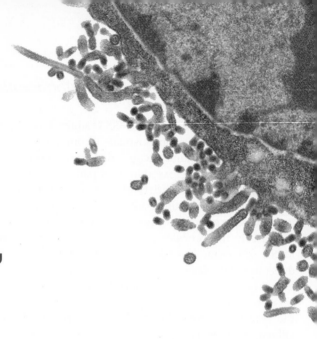

Chapter 65

Infections of the Bones, Joints, and Muscles

Joseph J. Nania

INFECTIONS of the bones, joints, and muscles are a diverse collection of diseases that have a number of common features. Organisms with a predilection for these sites vary by the age of the affected individual and share certain virulence determinants. Bone, joint, and muscle infections may develop as a consequence of either hematogenous dissemination or extension from a contiguous site. Complications of these infections can lead to local anatomic compromise and systemic spread. The emergence of antibiotic-resistant bacteria poses new challenges for the treatment of bone, joint, and muscle infections. The pathogenesis of each entity is discussed in this chapter, with an emphasis on microbial etiologies and comorbidities that lead to an increased risk of these infections by certain pathogens.

BONE INFECTIONS

Infections of the bones, or **osteomyelitis**, can result from bloodborne infections (hematogenous) or from the direct introduction of microorganisms from external (environmental) or contiguous sources (soft tissues or joints).

A special type of infection from contiguous sources occurs in the foot bones of persons with diabetes. The pathophysiology of the diseases, the types of infecting agents, and the treatments and prognoses vary among the infections.

CASE • O., a 15-year-old boy, sustained a blunt force injury to the lower part of his right thigh in a high school football game. The pain was so intense that he had to leave the game. Although it subsided later that night, the pain returned the next evening, accompanied by chills and a fever to 39.5°C. The following morning, O.'s parents took him to the family physician, who noted that O.'s lower right thigh was tender just above the knee. Minimal swelling and erythema were evident in the area of tenderness, and the knee joint was normal with a full range of motion. The physician noted several small boils on O.'s neck and chest. Some were scarred and crusted, and O. admitted to having squeezed them in the past 2 days. An x-ray of the right femur showed soft tissue swelling without any abnormalities of the bone.

This case raises several questions:

1. What is the most likely cause of O.'s infection?
2. How did the bacterium spread to the bone?
3. What are the complications of untreated osteomyelitis?

See Appendix for answers.

O. was diagnosed with acute hematogenous osteomyelitis. That diagnosis becomes even more plausible when the pathophysiology of the infection is understood. Several features of the history and physical examination of the patient point to the diagnosis:

• The trauma to the leg suffered in the football game damaged the distal femur and probably resulted in the rupture of small blood vessels and formation of hematoma

---

(or blood clot) in the bone. Disruption of the normal anatomical barriers made the bone more susceptible to infection.

- Manipulation of the boils by O. likely resulted in bacteremia, with *Staphylococcus aureus* being the most common infecting organism. Bloodborne *S. aureus* could have then seeded the traumatized bone and caused the infection.

- The history of chills and fever, as well as worsening pain and inflammation over the area of trauma, suggests that

O. developed an infection. The normal plain film of the leg did not exclude osteomyelitis because it usually takes several weeks for characteristic radiographic changes in bone to appear (periosteal proliferation or elevation, loss of bone cortex, and bone lysis). A radionuclide bone scan is more likely to be positive early in the disease because the technique measures inflammation, although not infallibly (Fig. 65-1A). Magnetic resonance imaging (MRI), which detects bone marrow edema early in the course of infection, is another useful early diagnostic tool (Fig. 65-1B).

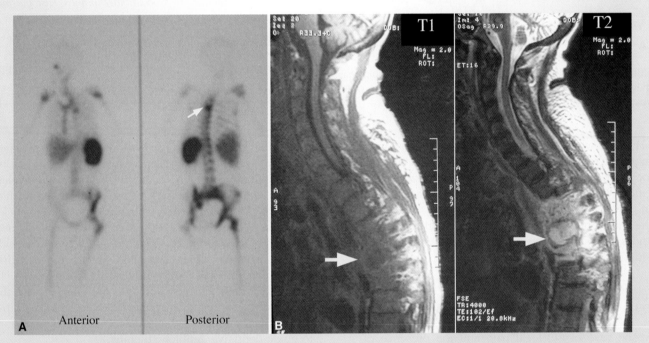

FIGURE 65-1. Vertebral osteomyelitis in an adult. A. Radionuclide bone scan shows retention of the tracer in a thoracic vertebra (*arrow*). Notice also the uptake in the pelvis and hip (also a result of osteomyelitis), the maxilla (caused by a dental abscess), and slight uptake in both shoulders (a result of inflammatory arthritis). The liver and spleen are routinely visualized with this technique. **B.** Magnetic resonance imaging scan of the thoracic spine of the same patient. In the T1 image (**left**), loss of bony structure in a vertebra is seen (*arrow*). In the T2 image (**right**), the high signal intensity owing to water molecules shows edema and infiltrate in the same vertebra.

Hematogenous Osteomyelitis
PATHOPHYSIOLOGY

Bone has a high rate of synthesis and resorption, two processes that depend on a rich vascular supply. **Hematogenous osteomyelitis** thus occurs primarily in childhood and adolescence, stages in life when long bones are growing rapidly. The most frequent sites of infection are the growing ends, or **metaphyses**, of long bones, where rapid bone growth and turnover occur. Osteomyelitis is most likely to develop when the bone has suffered trauma, with resultant disruption of blood vessels and hematoma formation.

The anatomy of the vascular supply of the metaphysis predisposes the area to infection. The capillaries from the nutrient arteries of bone make sharp loops close to the growth plate. They then expand to large sinusoidal vessels that connect with the venous network of the medullary cavity. The sudden increase in the diameter of those vessels slows blood flow and results in sludging of red blood cells (Fig. 65-2). Areas where sludging of blood cells occurs are ideal for the growth of bacteria because microclots form spontaneously in areas of slow blood flow. Clots retain bacteria and shield them from neutrophils, thus allowing the bacteria to proliferate. The result is inflammation, small areas of bone necrosis, and an acidic

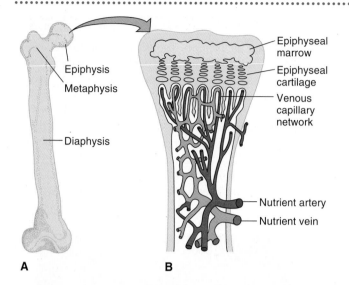

FIGURE 65-2. Structure of the femur. A. Femur showing epiphysis, metaphysis, and diaphysis. **B.** Schematic representation of the vascular supply of a long bone.

TABLE 65-1 Some Predisposing Causes and Etiologic Organisms Leading to Osteomyelitis

Predisposing Causes	Etiologic Organisms
Infancy	Group B streptococci
Unvaccinated child	*Haemophilus influenzae*
Sickle cell disease	*Salmonella* spp.
Immunosuppression	Opportunistic fungi, *Nocardia* spp., *Pseudomonas* spp.
Residing in an endemic area	*Coccidioides immitis*, *Histoplasma capsulatum*
Trauma to the jaw	*Actinomyces israelii*
Animal exposure	*Bartonella henselae*, *Brucella* spp.
Pulmonary tuberculosis	*Mycobacterium tuberculosis*

pH, all of which cause more tissue destruction and allow more bacterial growth. Endothelial cells in the capillary loops and sinusoids in the bone lack phagocytic properties, which also predisposes those areas to infection. In adults, hematogenous osteomyelitis often starts at the intervertebral disk, which has a rich blood supply, and spreads to adjacent vertebral bodies (see Fig. 65-1). Trauma also often precedes this type of infection.

DIAGNOSIS AND TREATMENT

In the case of O., local pain and the presence of systemic signs of infection suggested a serious disease, acute osteomyelitis, which usually calls for admission to the hospital for administration of parenteral antibiotics and often requires surgical drainage. Blood cultures, which are positive in about half of patients, should be obtained. When possible, a bone aspirate of the site of suspected infection should be attempted. The procedure has the potential to both make a microbiologic diagnosis and evaluate the need for immediate surgery to drain a bony abscess, as would be indicated by the yield of frank pus from a needle aspiration. With culture of both blood and material obtained from direct tissue sampling, the infecting organism is isolated in as many as 90% of cases.

Treatment should be initiated with antibiotics after obtaining cultures but before the return of results. Because about 90% of patients with this clinical presentation are infected with *S. aureus* (in children previously vaccinated against *Haemophilus influenzae*), a β-lactamase–resistant penicillin (such as nafcillin or oxacillin) or a first-generation cephalosporin (such as cefazolin) has historically been the treatment of choice. However, in places where **methicillin-resistant *S. aureus*** has become a common community-acquired pathogen, it is advisable to use vancomycin or clindamycin instead of, or in addition to, a β-lactam antibiotic until culture and sensitivity results are available.

In some circumstances, hematogenous osteomyelitis is more likely to be caused by an organism other than *S. aureus* (Table 65-1). For example, *Salmonella* species often cause infection in children with sickle cell disease; *Pseudomonas aeruginosa*, *Candida albicans*, and oral flora in injection drug users; and *Escherichia coli* and enterococci in adults with urinary tract obstruction. In such cases, or when blood cultures are negative and the patient does not respond appropriately to initial therapy, aspiration or biopsy of the bone for culture is important to guide definitive antibiotic therapy.

Treatment of acute hematogenous osteomyelitis requires high doses of antibiotics, usually administered parenterally, and long courses of therapy, traditionally in the range of 4 to 6 weeks. High serum levels of antibiotic are necessary to penetrate bone tissue, especially in areas of infection-induced necrotic bone that shield bacteria from host defenses. Outpatient administration of parenteral therapy has become a common practice that has been facilitated by the use of antibiotics with long serum half-lives, employment of **peripherally inserted central catheters (PICC lines)**, and increasing experience with and lower costs for the therapeutic approach. In addition, many children with hematogenous osteomyelitis can be successfully treated with an abbreviated course of parenteral therapy followed by high doses of an oral agent, presumably because of the excellent blood supply to the area of infection. However, such patients must be selected carefully and followed closely, preferably by someone with expertise in the practice.

If appropriate treatment is initiated early in the course of infection, before significant bone necrosis occurs, patients usually respond quickly, and cure can be achieved in more than 90% of cases. If fever and pain continue for longer than 48 hours after the initiation of treatment, surgical drainage of a subperiosteal collection or soft tissue abscess may be required. Computerized tomography (CT) and MRI are useful in demonstrating focal collections and in guiding the surgeon's approach should drainage be necessary. Persistent fever also may suggest a metastatic focus of infection, such as endocarditis or a visceral abscess.

Hematogenous Osteomyelitis at Various Ages

Infants

The clinical presentation of hematogenous osteomyelitis depends a great deal on the age of the patient. Osteomyelitis in an infant most commonly begins at the metaphysis of a long bone. The bones of an infant are soft, and the periosteum is loosely attached to the cortex. Therefore, infection originating in medullary bone can easily spread and rupture through the thin cortex into the subperiosteal space. **Subperiosteal abscesses** are common in this age group and lead to a stimulation of periosteal bone formation at an inappropriate site, as periosteal cells transform into osteoblasts. The new bone formation is disorganized and produces a weakened bone called an **involucrum** (Fig. 65-3).

Osteomyelitis in an infant can be a devastating disease because early in life the capillaries of the metaphysis extend into the epiphyseal growth plate. Infection can

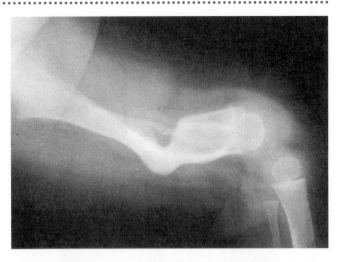

FIGURE 65-4. Deformity resulting from pathological fracture secondary to osteomyelitis.

spread by that route into the epiphysis and adversely affect growth of the bone. Consequently, osteomyelitis in an infant can be a destructive process resulting in permanent deformity of bone and abnormalities of growth (Fig. 65-4).

Children

In children between the age of 1 year and puberty, bone infection also occurs most frequently in long bones but is generally contained within the metaphysis. This pathophysiology is likely attributable to the thicker cortex and lack of transphyseal blood vessels in children of this age in contrast to infants. The periosteum also adheres more tightly to the cortex in this age group; thus, rupture of infection into the subperiosteal space and formation of involucrum is less likely. However, within the bone itself, pressure can increase and cause occlusion of arterioles and clot formation in the capillaries. The end result is often necrosis of bone, and in advanced cases, a **sequestrum** can form (Fig. 65-5). Tissue in a sequestrum is no longer in contact with the vasculature and acts essentially as a foreign body in which organisms can proliferate out of reach of both host defenses and antibiotics. Ultimately, the sequestrum must be resorbed (by the body) or removed surgically if the infection is to be cured. As children age, this complication is even more likely because the bone is more calcified and the periosteum even more tightly attached to bone.

Adults

Hematogenous osteomyelitis seen in adults most frequently involves the vertebral bodies. The reason for that predilection is uncertain but may stem from degenerative bony changes and vascular proliferation in the disk space between the vertebrae, which normally occur with age. The infection usually begins in the **disk space** and then spreads to the contiguous vertebrae. The radiographic finding of an abnormal disk space with erosion of the adjacent vertebral plates is highly suggestive of infection rather

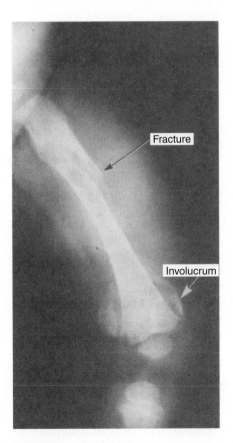

Fracture

Involucrum

FIGURE 65-3. Involucrum secondary to extensive periosteal reaction and fracture caused by weakened infected bone.

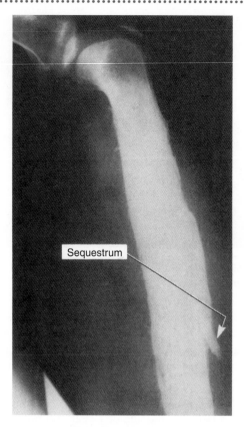

FIGURE 65-5. Radiograph showing changes in more advanced osteomyelitis with extensive bone lesions. A sequestrum is indicated.

than other causes, such as malignancy (Fig. 65-6). Frequent complications of vertebral osteomyelitis are **spinal epidural abscess**, which, if not treated appropriately, can cause irreversible loss of neurologic function, and **psoas abscess**, which often requires surgical drainage for cure.

S. aureus is the most common cause of vertebral osteomyelitis (presumably resulting from bacteremia from a mucocutaneous source), but enteric Gram-negative bacteria, viridans streptococci, *Mycobacterium tuberculosis*, and enterococci are also common etiologic agents.

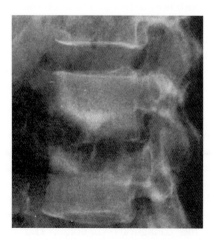

FIGURE 65-6. X-ray of the lumbar vertebrae showing destruction of bone associated with staphylococcal osteomyelitis.

These organisms may seed the disk space and adjacent vertebrae by hematogenous spread from primary infection in the bowel, gallbladder, or urinary tract, especially among persons over the age of 60 years with diverticular disease, obstructive uropathy, or other predisposing processes. Infection of vertebrae can also result from drainage of infected pelvic organs through pelvic veins into the complex, interconnected venous networks surrounding the spinal column known as Batson plexus.

Because the possible causes of vertebral osteomyelitis are numerous, it is imperative to obtain material from the infected area for culture (unless blood cultures rapidly yield causal organisms). Such cultures usually can be accomplished by closed aspiration or needle biopsy of the disk space under the guidance of fluoroscopy or CT scan. Vertebral osteomyelitis usually responds to medical therapy alone, but the neurologic status of the patient must be monitored closely because infection can spread from the vertebral body into the subdural or subarachnoid space through the rich venous and arterial plexus of the paravertebral circulation. The development of sensory or motor changes requires urgent surgical drainage to prevent irreversible neurologic damage.

Osteomyelitis Secondary to Contiguous Foci of Infection

Bone infection can result from the direct introduction of microorganisms from an external source or spread from a contiguous source. Penetrating trauma is an obvious cause of this type of infection. An additional common setting for contiguous bone infection is following insertion of orthopedic hardware, such as a joint prosthesis or bone fixation device (Fig. 65-7). These infections are difficult to eradicate because the bone has been traumatized (reducing the effectiveness of host defenses), and the foreign body acts as an avascular sanctuary for the persistence of bacteria. Bacteria, especially staphylococci, can grow and reside in biofilms on the surface of foreign bodies and are thus sheltered from antibiotics.

In the face of active infection, deciding whether to remove a fixation device or joint prosthesis to facilitate cure is often difficult and emotionally traumatic. On one hand, such a device may be necessary to achieve bony union or to allow ambulation or proper joint function; on the other hand, its presence may prevent cure of the infection. In some infections involving orthopedic prostheses, the devices can be salvaged, especially if the infection is caught early, the organism is exquisitely susceptible to antibiotics (as are streptococci), and there has not been loosening of the prosthesis. However, infections caused by *S. aureus*, Gram-negative bacilli, or fungi are infrequently cured without device removal. Treatment decisions require close interactions between surgeons and infectious diseases specialists to determine if and when removal is necessary and in the best overall interest of the patient.

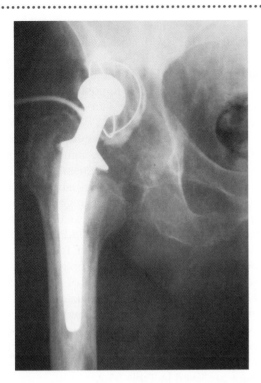

FIGURE 65-7. Osteomyelitis in bone with a prosthetic fixation device.

S. aureus is the organism that most commonly causes contiguous osteomyelitis, but the presence of a foreign body and the disruption of host defenses predispose to infection with other bacteria that are normally less pathogenic. The identity of the pathogen often reflects the circumstances of the trauma and the part of the body involved. Contamination of a wound by dirt or water often leads to infection with Gram-negative bacteria, including *P. aeruginosa*, whereas postoperative infections are frequently caused by *S. aureus*, the prototypical nosocomial pathogen. A wound may become contaminated with bacteria that are constituents of fecal flora, particularly in an incontinent patient with a hip fracture. Coagulase-negative staphylococci are more likely to cause infections in the presence of a prosthesis.

Osteomyelitis in Persons with Diabetes

A special category of osteomyelitis occurs in persons with diabetes as a consequence of the large vessel and microvascular disease and neuropathy that frequently complicate this condition. Skin and soft tissue ulcerations on the feet may go unnoticed because of **sensory neuropathy**, persist because of impaired host defenses, and ultimately penetrate into bone. The bone infections are more likely than others to be polymicrobial in nature. *S. aureus*, streptococci, enterococci, and Gram-negative bacteria are common pathogens, and anaerobic bacteria may be involved as well because of poorly oxygenated and necrotic tissue.

Bone infections in diabetic patients are especially difficult to treat owing to the poor vascular supply to necrotic bone. The most important determinant of successful therapy is adequate débridement of necrotic bone and soft tissue, with antibiotics serving an adjunctive role. It is especially important to determine the bacterial etiology of the infections because of the frequent involvement of inherently resistant organisms such as enterococci and *P. aeruginosa*. Results of surface cultures correlate poorly with those taken from bone and deep tissue and should not be used to guide therapy. In the absence of definitive culture results from bone or deep tissues, antibiotics must target a wide range of Gram-positive and Gram-negative bacteria, including anaerobic bacteria. Unfortunately, amputation is frequently the result of what may have started out as a trivial soft tissue infection of the foot, in spite of appropriate surgical and medical management. Good foot care is essential in preventing foot infections in diabetic patients.

Chronic Osteomyelitis

A serious complication of inadequately treated acute osteomyelitis is chronic osteomyelitis. Chronic osteomyelitis can remain dormant, and affected patients can be asymptomatic for years or even decades. Exacerbations are often associated with purulent drainage from a fistulous tract to the skin and may be accompanied by worsening pain, fever, and elevations in **C-reactive protein** and **erythrocyte sedimentation rate**. Antibiotic therapy often results in resolution of such episodes, and patients generally feel entirely well between them. However, over time, chronic osteomyelitis can cause progressive bone destruction. Thorough débridement of infected and necrotic bone along with adjunctive, often lifelong therapy may result in cure or prolonged suppression of the infection.

JOINT INFECTIONS
PATHOPHYSIOLOGY

A swollen, red, warm, painful joint in a patient with fever should raise suspicion of septic arthritis. In evaluating a patient presenting with arthritis, the physician must make three determinations. First, the physician must decide whether the joint inflammation is the result of infection. Noninfectious inflammatory joint disease can be caused by gout, pseudogout, rheumatoid arthritis or other connective tissue diseases, or viral infection, and these entities may be difficult to distinguish clinically from a bacterial process. Second, if infection appears likely, the physician must determine the pathophysiology of the infectious process. As with osteomyelitis, a joint can be seeded during the course of bacteremia from another primary focus, bacteria can be introduced directly into the joint by trauma or a surgical procedure, or bacteria can extend into the joint space from adjacent bone. Third, the physician must identify the infecting organism. Usually, all three determinations can be made by obtaining a complete history, performing a careful physical examination, and analyzing fluid obtained by aspiration of the joint.

The diagnosis of infection is supported by the finding of numerous white blood cells, predominantly neutrophils, in joint fluid, a positive Gram stain or culture of the fluid, and an absence of other potential causes for inflammation, such as crystals.

Synovial fluid consists of water, electrolytes, and other low molecular weight substances filtered from plasma, as well as components synthesized and secreted by synovial cells. Serum proteins are present in normal synovial fluid but in lower concentrations than in plasma. Because fibrinogen is absent, normal synovial fluid does not clot. The inflammatory reaction in synovial fluid is caused by the interaction of serum proteins, phagocytic host cells, and microorganisms.

The diagnosis of one type of joint disease does not preclude the presence of a second. Therefore, a joint deformed by arthritis can become infected with bacteria, particularly if that joint has recently been operated on or if steroids have been injected into it. The key to understanding the disease process is to obtain joint fluid for analysis and culture.

Infections of the joints can be caused by viruses, bacteria, and fungi. These etiologies can be differentiated by the clinical presentation of the patient and by the results of laboratory tests of the joint fluid. In general, bacterial infections are more common than the other types of infections and produce a higher number of white blood cells in the joint fluid, with a predominance of neutrophils. Some organisms, like *Neisseria gonorrhoeae*, *S. aureus*, streptococci, and several spirochetes have an unusual tropism for the joints. The reason for that predilection is unknown.

The frequency with which specific bacterial agents cause septic arthritis varies with age. Again, *S. aureus* is the most common overall cause and affects all age groups. *H. influenzae* type b, formerly the most frequent cause in children between the ages of 6 months and 3 years, has become uncommon since the introduction of an effective vaccine. In children less than 2 years of age, *Kingella kingae*, an oral commensal, is a frequent cause of septic arthritis. However, it is much more common in some areas of the world than in others and is generally more difficult to cultivate in the clinical microbiology laboratory than are other bacteria that cause arthritis. The gonococcus is the leading cause of septic arthritis in sexually active adults and accounts for 30 to 50% of hospital admissions for septic joints in adults less than 30 years of age.

The etiologic organism causing septic arthritis can be identified by Gram stain and culture of joint fluid. Even if the Gram stain is negative, antibiotic treatment should be started immediately after joint fluid and blood are obtained for culture to prevent continued infection and destruction of the structures in the joint. The relative frequencies in which organisms infect the joints in certain age groups are listed in Table 65-2.

TREATMENT

In addition to appropriate high-dose antibiotic therapy given parenterally, the infected synovial fluid should be drained. Drainage can be performed by repeated aspirations or by an open surgical procedure. Usually, aspiration is attempted first, and surgery is used only when

TABLE 65-2 Most Frequent Causes of Bacterial Arthritis by Age

Organism	Children			Adults
	Neonates	*2 mo to 2 y*	*3–10 y*	
Staphylococcus aureus	10–25%	25–50%	25–50%	25–75%
Streptococcus spp. (group A, viridans, microaerophilic, anaerobic, *S. pneumoniae*)	1–10%	10–25%	10–25%	10–25%
Group B streptococci	10–25%	Rare	Rare	1–10%
Kingella kingae	Rare	1–40%	Rare	Rare
Haemophilus influenzae type b[a]	Rare	Rare	Rare	Rare
Neisseria spp.	Rare	1–10%	10–25%	10–25%[b]
Gram-negative bacilli	5–15%	1–10%	1–10%	1–10%
Anaerobes	Rare	Rare	Rare	Rare
Other	1–10%	Rare	1–10%	Rare

[a]Occurs only in unvaccinated or undervaccinated children.
[b]Generally adults less than 30 years of age.

aspiration fails. Open drainage is always performed in septic arthritis of the hip joint and is required to prevent necrosis of the head of the femur, which can occur because the blood supply to that part of the bone is tenuous. Unlike the treatment of osteomyelitis, in which antibiotic levels achieved in infected bone are low, treatment of septic arthritis is facilitated by the ease with which most antibiotics penetrate synovial fluid and their slow efflux back into serum, resulting in synovial fluid concentrations of drug that exceed serum levels. Therefore, after patients with septic arthritis respond clinically to drainage and parenteral antibiotics, it is common practice to complete therapy with an equivalent oral agent. Total length of treatment for septic arthritis is generally 3 to 4 weeks.

MUSCLE INFECTIONS
PATHOPHYSIOLOGY

Symptoms of muscle aches and stiffness (**myalgia**) commonly occur as part of a viral syndrome. A classic example occurs in the convalescent phase of infection with influenza B in children and is characterized by sudden onset of severe bilateral calf pain, often called benign acute childhood myositis. Although common in viral infections, myalgias also are prominent features of infections of many causes, including bacterial infections (e.g., endocarditis and osteomyelitis), rickettsial infections, and parasitic infections. In most cases, infecting organisms are not present in muscular tissue. Rather, muscle involvement is indirect, resulting from the accelerated catabolism of skeletal muscle, part of the so-called acute phase response that accompanies sepsis and trauma. Catabolism is probably mediated by several products of macrophages (monokines), including **interleukin-1 (IL-1)** and **tumor necrosis factor (TNF)**. The systemic symptoms resulting from macrophage products are mediated by the increased synthesis of **prostaglandin E2**, which in turn activates muscle proteases. IL-1 and TNF also act on the hypothalamus, resulting in fever. These events explain why inhibitors of prostaglandin synthesis, like aspirin, help resolve both fever and muscle aches.

Although less common, direct infection of muscles can occur. Several of the more common causes of infectious myositis and their specific clinical presentations are listed in Table 65-3. Muscles may be invaded either from contiguous sites of infection (such as osteomyelitis) or by hematogenous spread from a distant focus. **Pyomyositis** is a purulent bacterial infection of the muscle. Trauma to the muscle, either by blunt or penetrating force, is thought to be an important factor in disease pathogenesis. In the case of blunt trauma, focal disruption of blood flow, at times with hematoma formation, provides a milieu conducive to abscess formation should seeding from bacteremia occur. Penetrating trauma, in distinction, leads to direct, deep muscular inoculation with skin flora or environmental organisms. Pyomyositis is most commonly caused by *S. aureus*, with methicillin-resistant strains causing a significant proportion of these

TABLE 65-3 Pathogenesis of Muscle Infections

Pathogenesis	Clinical Presentation	Principal Etiologies
Localized and spread from a contiguous site	Gas gangrene	*Clostridium perfringens*, occasionally other clostridial species
	Synergistic myositis or gangrene	Mixed infections with anaerobic bacteria and enteric bacteria
	Muscle abscesses	*Staphylococcus aureus*, group A streptococci
	Gram-negative bacteria	
	Miscellaneous	*Actinomyces* spp., *Nocardia* spp., *Mycobacterium* spp., fungi
Hematogenous spread	Bacterial	Groups A and B streptococci, *S. aureus*, Gram-negative bacteria
	Fungal	*Aspergillus* spp., *Candida* spp., *Coccidioides immitis*, *Histoplasma capsulatum*
	Mycobacterial	*Mycobacterium tuberculosis*, nontuberculous mycobacteria
	Parasitic	*Dracunculus medinensis*, *Trichinella spiralis*
	Viral	Coxsackievirus, echovirus

infections. Group A streptococcus is another less common but important cause owing to the occasional aggressive spread to adjacent tissues with potential for necrotizing tissue damage. Although perhaps more common in tropical climates, pyomyositis occurs in temperate climates as well. Clinical presentations of other types of muscle infections are so distinctive that they readily suggest the etiologic agent. For example, **crepitus**, the physical sign that indicates the presence of gas in muscle, suggests gas gangrene and myonecrosis secondary to *Clostridium perfringens* and other anaerobic bacteria. Generalized muscle pain and peripheral eosinophilia in a patient who has eaten undercooked pork should raise the possibility of trichinosis (see Chapter 55).

DIAGNOSIS AND TREATMENT

Myalgia due to viral or other systemic illness is usually suspected by the presence of other symptoms suggestive of the primary infection. For example, history of recent onset of cough, headache, and high fever should prompt testing for respiratory viral infections, such as influenza virus that would explain all symptoms including the muscle pain. Therapy of nonspecific myalgia is usually directed at symptom relief. Diagnosis of pyomyositis can be difficult and requires a high index of suspicion. Fever and focal musculoskeletal pain should prompt evaluation that usually requires imaging with CT or MRI to make the diagnosis. Infection of the deep pelvic musculature (e.g., the iliopsoas, gluteus, or piriformis) can be particularly problematic since pain emanating from this region is often poorly localized. Once a focal muscle abscess is identified, drainage should be attempted, either percutaneously with the guidance of radiographic imaging or by surgery. Extensive surgical débridement may be necessary if necrotic tissue is present. Antistaphylococcal antibiotics should be given empirically while awaiting the results of cultures.

CONCLUSION

Infections of the musculoskeletal system occur at all ages as a result of invasion of microorganisms from contiguous tissues, the bloodstream, or external sources. Although pain and constitutional symptoms are relatively nonspecific complaints of many ill patients, the presence of focal pain in a febrile patient should raise suspicion of an infection involving a bone, joint, or muscle. Careful physical examination in such patients will often reveal swelling, warmth, erythema, and reproducible focal pain of the musculoskeletal tissues. Radiologic studies are often helpful in supporting the diagnosis, and aspiration of affected sites is generally indicated to make a specific microbiologic diagnosis and speed recovery with antibiotic therapy. Given the need for urgent treatment before culture results are available, knowledge of the organisms commonly found at specific sites of infection and in various patient age groups is essential to guide the initiation of therapy.

Suggested Readings

Berbari EF, Steckelberg JM, Osmon DR. Osteomyelitis. In: Mandell GL, Bennett JE, Dolin R, eds. *Mandell, Douglas, and Bennett's Principles and Practice of Infectious Diseases*. 7th ed. Philadelphia, PA: Elsevier Churchill Livingstone; 2009:1457–1467.

Carrillo-Marquez MA, Hulten KG, Hammerman W, et al. USA300 is the predominant genotype causing *Staphylococcus aureus* septic arthritis in children. *Pediatr Infect Dis J.* 2009;28:1076–1080.

Davis JS. Management of bone and joint infections due to *Staphylococcus aureus*. *Intern Med J.* 2005;35(suppl 2):S79–S96. Review

Frank G, Mahoney HM, Eppes SC. Musculoskeletal infections in children. *Pediatr Clin North Am.* 2005;52:1083–1106.

Kaplan SL. Challenges in the evaluation and management of bone and joint infections and the role of new antibiotics for gram positive infections. *Adv Exp Med Biol.* 2009;634:111–120. Review.

Lew DP, Waldvogel FA. Osteomyelitis. *Lancet.* 2004;364:369–379.

Lipsky BA. Osteomyelitis of the foot in diabetic patients. *Clin Infect Dis.* 1997;25:1318–1326.

Ohl C. Infectious arthritis of native joints. In: Mandell GL, Bennett JE, Dolin R, eds. *Mandell, Douglas, and Bennett's Principles and Practice of Infectious Diseases*. 7th ed. Philadelphia, PA: Elsevier Churchill Livingstone; 2009:1443–1456.

Pannaraj PS, Hulten KG, Gonzalez BE, et al. Infective pyomyositis and myositis in children in the era of community-acquired, methicillin-resistant *Staphylococcus aureus* infection. *Clin Infect Dis.* 2006;43:953–960.

Pasternack MS, Schwartz MN. Myositis and Myonecrosis. In: Mandell GL, Bennett JE, Dolin R, eds. *Mandell, Douglas, and Bennett's Principles and Practice of Infectious Diseases*. 7th ed. Philadelphia, PA: Elsevier Churchill Livingstone; 2009:1313–1322.

Chapter **66**

Sepsis

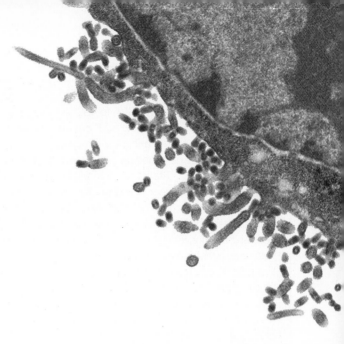

Suzanne F. Bradley

DESPITE IMPROVEMENTS in antibiotic therapy, sepsis is still the 10th leading cause of death among critically ill patients. Of the 750,000 cases of sepsis diagnosed in the United States annually, nearly one-third of patients will die. The following cases illustrate the different responses of two hosts to a disseminated infection.

CASE

Infection from a wound

Mr. D., a 48-year-old farmer, cut his thumb while working. The next morning the thumb was sore, and the skin surrounding the cut was red. Nevertheless, Mr. D. worked around the farm as usual and did not return home until well after dark. By that time, his thumb was swollen and throbbing, and oozing some yellow–white pus. Mr. D. noticed two red streaks going up the inside of his forearm, and he suddenly had a shaking chill and felt queasy. His wife drove him 17 miles to the county hospital. When they arrived at the emergency department, Mr. D.'s temperature was 39.7°C.

He was flushed and ill appearing, his pulse was 125 beats per minute, and his blood pressure was 100/60 mm Hg, much lower than his usual of 145/85 mm Hg. Blood cultures were drawn, and Mr. D. was started on intravenous fluids and an antibiotic active against staphylococci and streptococci. By morning, he was somewhat better, and by the following day, his symptoms had disappeared. His subsequent recovery and wound healing were uneventful. The blood cultures were found to be positive for *Staphylococcus aureus* on the second day of his illness.

CASE

Postsurgery infection

At 59 years of age, Mrs. J. underwent extensive pelvic surgery to remove a cervical carcinoma, including removal of all pelvic organs, removal of a segment of ileum to construct a new bladder, and a colostomy. At first, she seemed to be recovering well. During the evening of the third postoperative day, the nurse on the evening shift noticed that Mrs. J.'s respiratory rate had increased from 16 to 26 breaths per

minute. Mrs. J. said she did feel sick. She was not short of breath or in much pain, and her temperature was actually subnormal at 36.2°C.

The next morning Mrs. J. had some fever, 38.3°C, but she continued to feel fairly well. Her wound showed no sign of infection, and her abdomen was no more tender than expected. That afternoon, however, Mrs. J. was clearly in trouble. She was flushed, anxious, and restless; her blood

continued on page 672

pressure was down from 135/75 to 105/58 mm Hg, and her temperature was 39.2°C. Blood cultures were drawn, antibiotics were started, and intravenous fluids were rapidly infused to stabilize her blood pressure. Nevertheless, Mrs. J.'s condition worsened. The following morning, she was short of breath and had rales heard throughout her lungs. Intravenous fluids were decreased, and a vasopressor was required to maintain her blood pressure. She was moved to the intensive care unit for monitoring. To better assess her hemodynamic status, a catheter was inserted in the pulmonary artery via the jugular vein, right atrium, and right ventricle. Mrs. J. was found to have a cardiac output nearly double the normal for a resting adult of her size. However, her systemic vascular resistance was extremely low, which accounted for her low blood pressure despite the high cardiac output.

Over the next 24 hours, Mrs. J. continued to do poorly; her urine output was negligible, and she required mechanical ventilation to maintain oxygenation. The surgeon decided that reexploration of her abdomen was warranted because of persistent sepsis in the presence of broad-spectrum antimicrobial therapy. At surgery, the suture line attaching the ileum to the colon was found to be partially disrupted, with leakage of bowel contents, intense inflammation of the peritoneal cavity, and early abscess formation. Appropriate repairs were made and drains inserted. Thereafter, Mrs. J. recovered slowly but completely. Cultures of blood remained sterile.

These cases raise two questions:

1. How did Mr. D.'s clinical course differ from that of Mrs. J., and why was his response to infection less severe?
2. Why was an infecting organism not isolated from Mrs. J.?
3. Why did Mrs. J. not respond to antibiotic treatment as Mr. D. did?

See Appendix for answers.

DEFINITION

Sepsis is an ancient Greek word meaning, roughly, "putrefaction." Today, sepsis is a general clinical term that describes signs and symptoms of a generalized and severe inflammatory response. An infection can remain localized or it can spread with signs of generalized infection such as fever, abnormal white blood cell count, and abnormal clinical symptoms and signs. A classification scheme has been developed to characterize the various progressive stages of this generalized inflammatory response from **systemic inflammatory response syndrome** (**SIRS**) to **sepsis**, **severe sepsis**, **septic shock**, and **multiorgan dysfunction syndrome** (**MODS**). This classification reflects a progressive worsening of symptoms, inflammatory signs, and organ failure that frequently result in death (see the box titled "Clinical Syndromes Associated with Disseminated Infection"). Many investigators have searched in vain for a specific test (**biomarker**), but the diagnosis of sepsis is still based on clinical definitions.

ETIOLOGY

SIRS is generally referred to as sepsis when infection is the presumed or identified cause. When an infection is identified, the presence of bacteria in the bloodstream (**bacteremia**) is the most common cause, but **fungemia**, **viremia**, **parasitemia**, and microbial toxins also can lead to a generalized inflammatory response. Localized infections of the skin and the urinary, respiratory, and gastrointestinal tracts are the most frequent sources of bloodstream infection (**secondary bloodstream infection**). Occasionally, patients have bacteremia without an obvious source (**primary bloodstream infection**). Even when infection is strongly suspected as the cause of sepsis, extensive microbiological investigations for a

source may be negative. Sepsis can also occur in response to massive tissue injury and necrosis (burns), drugs, and chemical reactions.

All bloodstream infections do not lead to sepsis. Asymptomatic and transient low-grade bacteremia occurs in all of us on a daily basis following minor mucosal damage caused by toothbrushing or defecation, but those organisms are rapidly removed from the circulation and rarely ever cause us any harm. Why then does sepsis occur in some settings but not in others? The answer is that the risk of sepsis is complex and involves both microbial virulence factors and patient risk factors. Any microbe can lead to a systemic inflammatory response if it is present in the bloodstream in high enough numbers (**inoculum effect**). Some pathogens can cause sepsis more readily at low inoculum because they have virulence factors that facilitate host invasion and dissemination of infection (*Streptococcus pyogenes*), provoke an intense inflammatory response (pneumococci), or produce microbial toxins. The following defects in host defenses are also major risk factors for disseminated infection and sepsis:

- *Disruption or penetration of intact skin and mucosa:* Mucocutaneous barriers that limit the entry of pathogens can be breeched by devices, trauma, impairment of the blood supply, or drug effects. For example, drugs (chemotherapies) that damage rapidly dividing mucosal cells lining the mouth and gastrointestinal tract frequently cause ulcerations and make a portal of entry for pathogens. Necrotic tissue has no blood supply and can serve as a rich culture medium for microbes. Lack of blood supply to tissues also impedes the ability of host phagocytes, antibodies, and complements to defend against invasion.
- *Granulocytopenia and defective granulocyte function:* Neutrophils are the first line of defense against many

CLINICAL SYNDROMES ASSOCIATED WITH DISSEMINATED INFECTION

Systemic inflammatory response syndrome	Defined as having two or more of the following: • Fever • Elevated or low white blood cell count (leukocytosis or leukopenia) • Elevated heart rate (tachycardia) • Elevated respiratory rate (tachypnea)
Sepsis	SIRS, as defined above, plus confirmed infection
Severe sepsis	SIRS, as defined above, plus low blood pressure (hypotension) (Corrected by administration of fluids)
Septic shock	SIRS, as defined above, plus persistent hypotension (Aggressive fluid resuscitation not effective. Drugs to increase vascular tone required)
Multiorgan dysfunction syndrome	SIRS, as defined above, plus persistent hypotension leading to the following: • Evidence of clotting disorders or failure of renal, hepatic, cardiac, or cognitive function • Accumulation of products of metabolism that cannot be cleared (e.g., lactic acidosis)

bacteria as well as many fungi. Granulocytopenia that occurs following chemotherapy predisposes patients to many infections from their own normal flora (**endogenous infections**) or, less often, from the environment (**exogenous infection**). In poorly controlled diabetes mellitus, the number of granulocytes is normal, but adherence, chemotaxis, ingestion, oxidative burst, and killing are all impaired.

- *Complement defects*: Homozygous deficiencies in classical pathway components and in C3 are associated with bacteremia and sepsis in some affected patients. A rare defect in the alternative pathway, properdin deficiency, predisposes to fulminant sepsis with *Neisseria meningitidis*. Deficiencies in late components (C5 through C9) also create a susceptibility to neisserial infections, but those infections are apt to be less severe. Cirrhosis and severe burn injury are complement-deficient states because of decreased syntheses and increased complement; the result is impaired neutrophil chemotaxis. Premature infants comprise another complement-deficient group of patients with an increased incidence of sepsis.

- *Immune defects*: Loss of opsonic and bactericidal antibodies (humoral defects) and loss of the ability to activate macrophages in response to specific antigenic stimuli (cellular defects) predispose to sepsis. Humoral immune defects, as seen in B-cell malignancies; protein-losing states, as in burns; transplant recipients; and the late stages of AIDS are particularly associated with bacterial infections, including sepsis.

- *Splenic malfunction or absence:* Loss of the spleen creates a humoral immunodeficiency, particularly in primary antibody responses. Additionally, without the spleen, the body's ability to clear encapsulated bacteria from the blood is impaired. A person lacking a functioning spleen is susceptible to fulminant sepsis caused by bacteria such as *Streptococcus pneumoniae*, *Haemophilus influenzae*, and *N. meningitidis*. That person would have to be immunized and warned to seek emergent medical attention at the first sign of illness. Some people without a functioning spleen take antibiotics on a long-term basis in the hope of preventing an episode of severe infection.

- *Genetic predisposition:* Studies in mice and humans suggest that minor changes in some genes (genetic polymorphisms) may explain why some hosts are more susceptible to sepsis than others.

SPREAD AND MULTIPLICATION

Host Response: A Delicate Balance

Following the introduction of infection or tissue injury, high levels of **proinflammatory cytokines**—typically, **tumor necrosis factor-α** (**TNF-α**) and **interleukin** 1 (IL-1), IL-6, and IL-8, among others—are rapidly released, often within minutes. The proinflammatory cytokines are produced primarily by the **cellular innate immune system**. Secondary stimulation and release of other

TABLE 66-1 Putative Mediators of Sepsis

Mediator	Physiologic Effects
Tumor necrosis factor-α (TNF-α)	Mimics sepsis syndrome; margination of neutrophils is particularly striking after TNF-α administration.
Interleukin 1	Fever, increased adhesiveness of endothelial cells and leukocytes, endothelial procoagulant activity
Interleukins 2, 6, 8	Hypotension, capillary leak, decreased myocardial contractility, synthesis of "acute phase" proteins (e.g., fibrinogen) by the liver, leukocyte chemotaxis
Hageman factor (factor XII), tissue factor, factor X	Coagulation, fibrinolysis
Complement cascade	Neutrophil chemotaxis, neutrophil aggregation, capillary leak
Endorphins	Hypotension
Leukotrienes and thromboxane	Platelet aggregation, neutrophil adhesion, capillary leak, decreased myocardial contractility
Prostaglandins (especially E_2 and I_2)	Hypotension, neutrophil adhesion to endothelium, fever, muscle aches, muscle proteolysis
Bradykinin (via factor XII and kallikrein)	Hypotension, capillary leak
Serotonin	Pulmonary hypertension, capillary leak
Histamine	Hypotension, capillary leak
Platelet-activating factor (PAF)	Hypotension, capillary leak, platelet aggregation, leukocyte activation, decreased myocardial contractility
Phagocyte products—lysosomal proteins, oxygen, free radicals	Endothelial cell damage, capillary leak
Myocardial depressant factor	Decreased myocardial contractility
Endothelin 1	Vasoconstriction, especially in the kidney
Endothelial relaxing factor	Hypotension

inflammatory mediators, like cytokines, **prostaglandins**, **leukotrienes**, **toxic oxygen products**, **adhesion proteins**, and **proteases**, occurs so rapidly that it is often difficult to discern what factor is contributing to damage of tissues. Rapid activation of **plasma protein systems**, including the complement and coagulation cascades and the **kallikrein-kinin system**, also ensues (Table 66-1).

In the absence of an inflammatory response, the patient would die of overwhelming infection. However, an unopposed inflammatory process can also be detrimental. Fortunately, a **compensatory anti-inflammatory response syndrome** (**CARS**) typically follows the proinflammatory response in association with increasing levels of **anti-inflammatory cytokines** (e.g., IL-4, IL-10, IL-11, **transforming growth factor-β**). The levels of other anti-inflammatory factors, such as soluble TNF-receptors and IL-1 receptor antagonists, and stress hormones also rise following the proinflammatory response. Lymphocytes

of septic patients become hyporesponsive to infectious stimuli and enter a state of immunosuppression or **immunoparalysis** that contributes to an increased risk of secondary infection.

Thus, a complex and delicate balance of proinflammatory and anti-inflammatory responses occurs during sepsis. It is no longer thought that the chaotic dysregulated proinflammatory response is solely responsible for the severity of symptoms, organ system failure, and increased risk of death seen with sepsis; an unopposed anti-inflammatory response may also play a detrimental role.

How Does the Host Recognize Invasion by Microbes?

All infectious agents do not have the same ability to cause sepsis. Components of the cell walls of various microbes have varying abilities to stimulate the production of proinflammatory cytokine production. The cell wall components of Gram-negative bacilli, **lipopolysac-charide (LPS)** or **lipid A**, are among the most potent stimulators of cytokines. It is therefore not surprising that those organisms are closely associated with septic shock. Less-potent stimulators of cytokines have been found in the cell walls of Gram-positive bacteria (**lipoteichoic acid, peptidoglycan**), mycobacteria (**lipoarabinoman-nan**), and fungi (**mannan**).

The innate immune system is the first line of defense against invading microorganisms. Neutrophils, monocytes, macrophages, and dendritic cells recognize microbes and products of damaged host cells though the presence of **pattern recognition receptors (PRR)**. PRR may be located on extracellular surfaces or within endosomes of immune cells. PRR initiate the initial innate immune response and regulate the adaptive host response to infection or tissue injury.

The first PRR were first identified in fruit flies and called **toll receptors**. When similar molecules were identified in mammals, they were termed **toll-like receptors (TLRs)**. Other PRR important in sepsis include **nucleo-tide-oligomerization domain leucine-rich repeat (NOD-LRR)** and **cytoplasmic caspase activation and recruiting domain helicases**. **NOD-LRR** and helicases play an important role in the recognition of bacterial pep-tidoglycan and viral DNA respectively.

PRR on immune cells involved in sepsis recognize **pathogen-associated** (or microbial-associated) **molecular patterns (PAMPs)** and **danger-associated molecular patterns (DAMPs)**. PAMPs are conserved molecules present in all microbes and are not found in vertebrates. DAMPs are host tissue molecules (heat-shock proteins, hyaluronic acid, fibrinogen, biglycan, surfactant A, and high-mobility group box-1) that signal noninfectious consequences of sepsis such as damage related to hypoperfu-sion, ischemia, and reperfusion.

The characterization of 10 TLRs in man has been a major advance that begins to explain how various microbes and even drugs and tissue necrosis can interact with the innate immune system, leading to stimulation of cytokines and sepsis (Table 66-2). TLRs localized on the host cell surface recognize PAMPs that are present on the surface of the microbe, while endosomal TLRs pri-marily recognize microbial nucleic acids. It is clear that the limited numbers of TLRs cannot bind specifically to every microbe that a host will encounter in its lifetime, and overlap in PAMPs and pathogen recognition must occur. The binding sites for the TLRs and their ligands are, in fact, highly conserved with leucine-rich repeating motifs. Overlap in the TLR system is probably important so that the innate immune system can recognize a wide variety of existing and emerging pathogens. Redundancy in the TLR system also suggests that these molecules play a crucial role in host defense; recent discovery of specific TLR mutations and genetic polymorphisms for TNF-α and other cytokines have not necessarily been predictive of an increased risk of infection, sepsis, or poor outcome.

To bind with PAMPs and become activated, TLR must bind with accessory molecules or form dimers or heterodi-mers with other TLRs. TLR binding and activation results in recruitment of adaptor molecules (MyD88, TIRAP/MAL, TRAM, and TRIF) and initiation of multiple signal transduc-tion pathways that generate **nuclear factor κB** and **acti-vator protein 1** and result in a proinflammatory response.

HOW DOES DAMAGE IN SEPSIS OCCUR?

The cardiovascular system is the primary target and the initial manifestations are **hypotension** and **capillary leak** (Fig. 66-1). Hypotension and capillary leak can result in relative intravascular volume depletion with decreased perfusion, dysfunction, necrosis, and failure of vital organs (brain, lungs, kidney, liver, and gastrointesti-nal tract), impaired oxygen delivery, and accumulation of toxic metabolites (**lactic acidosis**).

Damage and organ failure are the consequence a complex interplay between the proinflammatory response, the coagulation cascade, and others. Neutrophils play a pivotal role in the development of organ failure. In the patient without sepsis, neutrophils rapidly arrive, contain, and kill the infection and then, just as rapidly, die by a process of programmed cell death called **apoptosis**. The proinflammatory response stimulates **apoptosis** and the generation of counterinflammatory mediators, leading to resolution of inflammation and minimization of local tissue damage.

However, in sepsis, neutrophil survival is prolonged and rates of apoptosis are reduced, leading to systematic activation of a large number of neutrophils that contrib-ute to organ failure. Neutrophil depletion studies in ani-mal models of sepsis have shown improved survival and reduced organ damage. However, neutrophil activation alone does not necessarily lead to organ failure.

Sepsis, neutrophil activation, and organ damage are also closely associated with the development of a procoagulant state called **disseminated intravascular coagulation (DIC)**. In sepsis, proinflammatory neutro-phil–endothelial cell interactions activate the coagulation cascade and inhibit fibrinolysis, leading to consumption of clotting factors, deposition of fibrin, and clot forma-tion within the microvasculature. Impaired organ func-tion, hemorrhage, and necrosis can ensue. Activation of the coagulation cascade is also associated with a positive feedback loop, stimulation of proinflammatory cytokine production, and further organ damage. In this fashion, both the proinflammatory response and procoagulant state contribute to the development of organ failure in sepsis.

The impact that sepsis has on the body is summa-rized in this list:

• *Vasculature*: Early dilation of the arteries (decreased **systemic vascular resistance**) and pooling in veins

TABLE 66-2 Toll-like Receptors and their Ligands

Receptor	TLR (+) Cells	Microbial Component	Microbial Origin	Synthetic Ligands/ Host Proteins
TLR1	All cells (forms TLR1–TLR2 heterodimers when receptor is engaged)	Triacyl lipopeptides Soluble factors	Bacteria/mycobacteria *Neisseria meningitidis*	
TLR2	Monocytes, dendritic, and NK cells	Lipoproteins/lipopeptides Lipoteichoic acid Phenol-soluble modulin Glycolipids Atypical lipopolysaccharide (LPS) Zymosan	Gram-positive bacteria Gram-positive bacteria Staphylococcus Spirochetes Leptospires, mouth flora Yeast	
TLR3	Dendritic and NK cells (endosomal location)	Viral RNA (double stranded)	Viruses	
TLR4	Macrophages, dendritic cells, endothelial cells (forms TLR4 dimers when receptor is engaged)	LPS + CD14 Fusion protein	Gram-negative bacteria Respiratory syncytial virus	Taxol (chemotherapy) Fibronectin Hyaluronan
TLR5	Monocytes, young dendritic cells, epithelial cells, NK and T cells	Flagellin	Flagellated bacteria	
TLR6	Primarily B cells, monocytes, and NK cells to a lesser degree (forms TLR2–TLR6 heterodimers when receptor is engaged)	Diacyl lipopeptides Lipoteichoic acid Zymosan	Mycoplasma Gram-positive bacteria Fungi	
TLR7	B cells and some dendritic cells (endosomal location)	Viral RNA (single stranded)	Viruses	Antivirals such as: Imidazoquinolines Loxoribine
TLR8	Primarily monocytes, NK and T cells (endosomal location)	Viral RNA (single stranded)	Viruses	Imidazoquinolines
TLR9	B cells, macrophages, neutrophils, NK cells, microglia, some dendritic cells (endosomal location)	CpG-containing DNA	Bacteria and viruses	
TLR10	B cells, dendritic cells	Unknown	Present uropathogenic bacteria	

NK cells, natural killer cells; TLR, toll-like receptor, CpG, cytidine–phosphate–guanosine.

(**increased venous capacitance**) lead to leakage of fluids into extravascular tissues associated with decline in blood pressure and increased cardiac work.

- *Heart*: Infection directly affects the ability of the heart to function as a pump by depressing **mitochondrial function** and **myocardial contractility**. Eventually, **stroke volume** is decreased to the point where a compensatory increase in heart rate (**tachycardia**) can no longer maintain the increase in **cardiac output**

needed to maintain blood pressure. Early in the course of sepsis, the combination of very low blood pressure (in adults, defined as <90 mm Hg systolic or >40 mm Hg below baseline) and high cardiac output has been termed **warm shock** because the patient is vasodilated with warm or even flushed skin. In some cases of late sepsis, cardiac output falls and peripheral vasodilation is replaced by vasoconstriction in an attempt to shunt blood to vital organs. The skin becomes pale and cold,

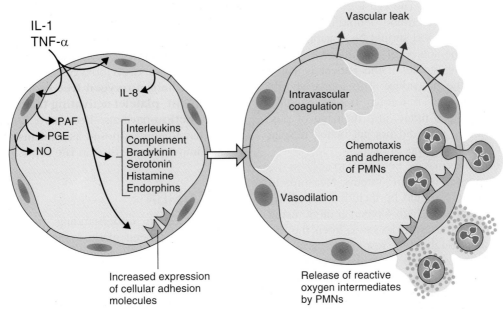

FIGURE 66-1. Vasculature effects in sepsis. The release of interleukin 1 (IL-1) and tumor necrosis factor-α (TNF-α) causes the outpouring of a number of cytokines and other effectors. In turn, that outpouring leads to intravascular coagulation, vasodilation, increased neutrophil adherence to vessel walls, and vascular leakage. (NO, nitric oxide; PAF, platelet-activating factor; PGE, prostaglandin E; PMN, polymorphonuclear leukocyte.)

the hands and feet are blue–purple in color, and the patient expires in **cold shock**.

- *Brain*: Hypotension, decreased perfusion of the brain, and direct effects of the infection itself can render patients confused, delirious, stuporous, or comatose.
- *Lung*: Capillary endothelial damage and leak may be enhanced by activated neutrophils that adhere to the pulmonary endothelium in large numbers, spewing oxygen radicals. Fluid exudes into the interstitium and alveolar spaces, the lung becomes soggy and stiff, and adequate gas exchange is impossible. This condition is called the **adult respiratory distress syndrome (ARDS)**. Oxygen must be pumped into the patient's lungs under pressure using a ventilator.
- *Kidney*: Hypotension and infection lead to **acute tubular necrosis** and renal failure. Dialysis is frequently required in septic patients to remove dangerous metabolites that accumulate.
- *Liver*: Necrosis of the liver and impaired gallbladder function frequently lead to jaundice and impairment of hepatic functions such as drug metabolism, production of albumin, and clotting factors. Lack of albumin contributes to leakage of fluid out of blood vessels into tissues (**edema**) and can contribute to further decline in intravascular blood pressure.
- *Gastrointestinal tract*: Hypotension can cause ischemia and necrosis of the bowel mucosa and wall leading to hemorrhage.
- *Endocrine and metabolic effects*: Sepsis is a **catabolic state**, with massive proteolysis, lipolysis, and glycogenolysis. Increased production of hormones (**cortisol,**

catecholamines, glucagon) is part of the normal **stress response** seen with sepsis. Increased levels of these hormones can also contribute to insulin resistance and elevated glucose levels (**hyperglycemia**). Hyperglycemia has been associated with impaired phagocytic functions and increased mortality in critically ill patients. Some patients cannot generate adequate stress responses; low levels of cortisol seen in sepsis are termed **relative adrenal insufficiency**. Oxygen metabolism is abnormal, with a high fraction of oxygen sent to the tissues returning to the heart unused. Impaired oxygen use results from some organs not being perfused or their cells being too metabolically impaired to use the oxygen delivered to them. Either way, in a low oxygen state, glycolysis by cells leads to the formation of pyruvic acid and the accumulation of lactic acid, resulting in **lactic acidosis**.

TREATMENT

Standardized goals for the treatment of sepsis within 6 hours of diagnosis have been recommended. Resuscitation with massive amounts of fluid to correct intravascular volume depletion, resolve hypotension, and improve perfusion is essential to preserve function of vital organs. If organ perfusion cannot be attained by fluids alone, then drugs that cause vasoconstriction and increase myocardial contractility (**vasopressors**) should be given. Broad-spectrum, primarily intravenous and bactericidal, antibiotics directed against the most likely pathogens should be administered within 1 hour of diagnosis of septic shock or severe sepsis. The cause of the infection should be determined to determine optimum treatment. At minimum, cultures of blood should be obtained prior to giving antibiotics. The source of the infection should be identified by imaging studies if the patient is stable enough to complete the procedure. The source should be controlled by removal of foreign bodies, surgical debridement of devitalized tissue, and drainage of pus, as illustrated by Mrs. J., who did not get better, despite antibiotics, until her abscess was drained.

Additional measures may be necessary to address the effects of sepsis on various organ systems. Measures to promote oxygen delivery should be included, supplying the patient with air that has a high oxygen content, using a ventilator or other mechanical device to keep the airways under pressure throughout the respiratory cycle, and transfusing to maintain adequate hemoglobin concentrations. In patients with severe renal failure, dialysis (**renal replacement therapy**) may be necessary. Hyperglycemia should be controlled by intravenous insulin infusions. Treatment with corticosteroids remains controversial, but it has been suggested in patients in whom volume resuscitation and vasopressors have not been effective. **Activated protein C** replacement has been shown to be of benefit in some trials and not others; its use is generally limited to patients at high risk of death without bleeding problems and other contraindications.

Newer treatments based on an understanding of cytokine biology have been disappointing. **Hyperimmune globulin** and **monoclonal antibodies** have been tried unsuccessfully as a strategy to inactivate specific proinflammatory mediators or to prevent binding to their receptors. It is thought that the cytokine cascade and its damage occur so quickly that therapeutic interventions cannot be given soon enough to impact the course of sepsis. Consequently, antibodies directed against TNF-α, IL-1, or their receptors have not been effective, nor have anti-inflammatory agents that antagonize the production of proinflammatory cytokines and prostaglandins, such as glucocorticoids and cyclooxygenase inhibitors. Similarly, strategies to inhibit **oxygen free radicals**, **bradykinin**, **complement**, **platelet-activating factor**, and **free radical production** have also been tried. Colony-stimulating factors have been proposed as a means of reversing the state of immunodepression in late sepsis.

CONCLUSION

Major strides in understanding the pathophysiology of sepsis have been made in just the past few years. Advances in technology and antimicrobial agents have greatly increased the options available to physicians who treat critically ill patients. Unfortunately, little impact has been made on the outcome of this most serious of infectious syndromes.

Suggested Readings

Abraham E, Singer M. Mechanisms of sepsis-induced organ dysfunction. *Crit Care Med.* 2007;35:2408–2416.

Cinel I, Opal SM. Molecular biology of inflammation and sepsis: a primer. *Crit Care Med.* 2009;37:291–304.

Dellinger RP, Levy MM, Carlet JM, et al. Surviving sepsis campaign: International guidelines for management of severe sepsis and septic shock: 2008. *Crit Care Med.* 2008; 36:296–327.

Leaver SK, Finney SJ, Burke-Gaffney A, et al. Sepsis since the discovery of Toll-like receptors: Disease concepts and therapeutic opportunities. *Crit Care Med.* 2007;35:1404–1410.

Lever A, Mackenzie I. Sepsis: definition, epidemiology, and diagnosis. *Br Med J.* 2007;335:879–883.

Remick DG. Pathophysiology of sepsis. *Am J Pathol.* 2007;170:1435–1444.

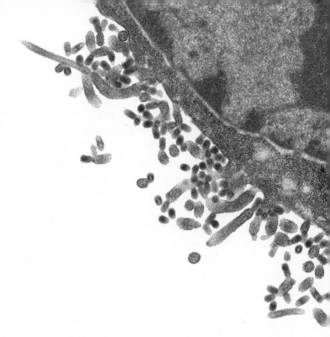

Chapter 67

Intravascular Infection

Rasmus V. Rasmussen, Adolf W. Karchmer, Niels E. Bruun, and Vance G. Fowler

MANY MICROORGANISMS gain entry to the intravascular space and are passively carried throughout the circulatory system, either suspended in plasma or within various cellular components of blood. Usually, entry of microorganisms into the circulation represents a brief phase of an infection centered primarily in another organ system. However, for some bacteria and protozoa, the primary site of infection is within the vascular system—that is, the cellular components of blood or the structural elements of the circulatory system. For example, *Plasmodium* species (the cause of malaria), *Babesia microti* (the cause of babesiosis), and *Bartonella bacilliformis* (the agent of Oroya fever) produce disease by invading or adhering to erythrocytes. Occasionally, microorganisms infect the endothelial surface of a specific component of the cardiovascular system. Intravascular infection of an artery is called **endarteritis**, of an endothelial site in the heart, **endocarditis**, and of the lumen of a vein, **phlebitis**.

Infective **phlebitis** occurs mainly by direct spread from an adjacent focus of infection or when intravascular foreign bodies (such as catheters) implanted in veins become infected. **Infective endarteritis** arises in an analogous manner and, on rare occasions, when congenital arterial anomalies (e.g., patent ductus arteriosus, coarctation of the aorta) or diseased arterial endothelium (e.g., atherosclerotic plaques) become infected during transient bacteremia. **Infective endocarditis**, with the exception of episodes that arise as a consequence of cardiac surgery or intracardiac instrumentation, results from seeding of endothelial sites by microorganisms that are transiently present in the circulation. Most vascular endothelial infections are caused by bacteria and, rarely, by fungi. Infective endocarditis is the prototype of spontaneously occurring intravascular endothelial infection and is the focus of this chapter. The term *endocarditis* will refer here to infective endocarditis.

ENDOCARDITIS

DEFINITIONS AND CLASSIFICATIONS

Infective endocarditis is an infection of the endocardial surface of the heart. Endocarditis is usually localized on the cardiac valves, but it can also occur on one of the **cordae tendineae** or on areas of the atrial or ventricular wall. Endocarditis has traditionally been classified according to the tempo of the clinical illness, for example, acute and subacute endocarditis. Patients presenting with markedly febrile, toxic courses lasting only days to several weeks have **acute endocarditis**. In contrast, patients with **subacute endocarditis** have lower fevers and illnesses marked by anorexia, weakness, and weight loss, and are symptomatic for longer than several weeks. However, a more contemporary and clinically relevant classification is based on the microbiological cause and the site of infection. This classification is more precise and has led to specific recommendations about therapy and prognosis. Examples are "α-hemolytic streptococcal native valve endocarditis" and "*Staphylococcus epidermidis* prosthetic aortic valve endocarditis."

EPIDEMIOLOGY

Over the past two decades, the incidence of endocarditis in developed countries has ranged from 2 to 8 cases per 100,000 persons each year. Endocarditis accounts for approximately 1 in 1,000 admissions to large general hospitals. The median

CASE • Mrs. Q., who at 75 years of age had a history of a systolic ejection heart murmur and mild aortic stenosis, hypertension, and diabetes, was admitted to the hospital because of 6 weeks of intermittent fevers, malaise, weakness, and loss of appetite. The day before admission, she noted her temperature was 41.2°C and discovered that she was 14 pounds below her usual weight.

On examination, Mrs. Q. was pale, her temperature was 38.1°C, heart rate 100 beats per minute, and blood pressure 150/90 mm Hg. Three small hemorrhages were noted on the right palpebral conjunctiva. The fundi were normal. She was edentulous. A grade III/VI systolic ejection murmur was heard at the base of the heart, suggesting aortic stenosis, and a grade I/VI brief, high-pitched decrescendo diastolic murmur was heard at the left sternal border, indicating aortic insufficiency. The spleen could not be palpated.

Laboratory tests revealed hemoglobin of 10.3 g/dL (normal is >12.1 g/dL), normal leukocyte count, C-reactive protein of 138 mg/L (normal is <10 mg/L), and creatinine level of 1.9 mg/dL (normal is <1.3 mg/dL). Urine analysis showed 25 to 30 red blood cells per high-power field but no white blood cells or casts. Chest x-ray did not show signs of pneumonia, but echocardiography demonstrated a bicuspid aortic valve with moderate stenosis, mild aortic insufficiency, and three 6- to 8-mm mobile elements consistent with vegetations. No other specific focus of infection was found. Six blood cultures obtained over 48 hours were all positive for *Streptococcus bovis*.

Treatment for subacute bacterial endocarditis was started with 3 million units of penicillin administered intravenously every 4 hours. On the sixth hospital day, Mrs. Q. was found unresponsive with a dilated left pupil. An emergency cranial CT scan revealed a large left parietal hematoma. Mrs. Q died on the eighth hospital day.

Autopsy confirmed vegetations on the aortic valve at the closure line. The valve was bicuspid and thickened. A Gram stain of the vegetation confirmed the presence of Gram-positive cocci. Small embolic infarcts were noted in the myocardium and in the spleen. Changes of focal glomerulonephritis and several small infarcts were found in both kidneys. Also noted was a massive subarachnoid and left parietal intracerebral hemorrhage from an apparent leaking aneurysm (a mycotic aneurysm or saclike dilatation, which results from growth of bacteria in the vessel wall).

This case raises several questions:

1. What underlying medical condition placed Mrs. Q. at risk for developing endocarditis?
2. What virulence factors elaborated by *S. bovis* contributed to endocarditis?
3. What is the significance of the urinalysis showing 25 to 30 red blood cells per high-power field?

See Appendix for answers.

---

age of patients with endocarditis has increased steadily since the preantibiotic era; in the 1920s, the median age was less than 30 years, whereas currently more than 50% of cases involve people older than 50 years of age.

The type of structural heart disease that serves as the predisposing factor for endocarditis also has changed. **Acute rheumatic fever** and subsequent rheumatic heart disease has declined in developed countries as a predisposing factor for endocarditis. The common predisposing factors for endocarditis are now **congenital cardiac defects** (especially bicuspid aortic valves, ventricular septal defects, tetralogy of Fallot, and patent ductus arteriosus), **degenerative valvular disease** (calcific valvular disease), and **mitral valve prolapse** with significant mitral regurgitation. In recent reports, about 20% of patients with endocarditis have infection on a prolapsing regurgitant mitral valve. **Prosthetic heart valves** also have become an important site for the establishment of endocarditis. Another area of concern is the increasing number of **cardiac rhythm management device (CRMD)** infections. The number of CRMDs implanted has increased by 49% from 1996 to 2003 and, in the same period, the number of CRMD infections has increased

3.1-fold. Accordingly, the rates of CRMD infections have increased faster than the implant rates, a development mainly driven by a sixfold increase in implantable cardioverter–defibrillator infections. Between 15 and 30% of patients with endocarditis do not have a prior valvular abnormality.

Endocarditis can affect older people for the following reasons:

- The age of the general population and therefore that of persons with degenerative valve disease has increased.
- Persons with congenital heart disease now live longer.
- Prosthetic valves to correct valve dysfunction are implanted more frequently in this age group.
- CRMD devices are implanted more frequently in the elderly.
- The precipitating circumstances for transient bacteremia resulting in endocarditis, such as genitourinary tract infections and manipulations, colonic pathology (benign polyps and malignancy), and health care–associated bacteremias (occurring both during hospitalization and among outpatients), are more common in the elderly.

However, injection drug use has also led to an increased incidence of endocarditis among younger persons.

Different structures are affected by infections in patients of different age groups. Endocarditis in persons who do not use injection drugs usually involves a previously abnormal **aortic** or **mitral valve**. In injection drug users, endocarditis can affect previously abnormal left heart valves, and in half the cases, it involves an apparently normal **tricuspid valve**.

ENCOUNTER

Endocarditis is caused by a large variety of microorganisms, but the most prevalent are staphylococci, streptococci, and enterococci (Table 67-1). In studies reporting cases occurring within the last decade, *Staphylococcus aureus* was found to be the most common causative organism, reflecting the interaction of its pathogenicity and the frequency of events leading to *S. aureus* bacteremia: health care–associated infections and injection drug use. Specific organisms show preferences for the type of valve infected (native or prosthetic) and the event or site causing the endocarditis-inciting bacteremia (e.g., dental source, injection drug use, or nosocomial infection).

The organisms that cause native valve endocarditis present as either acute or subacute infections. In acute endocarditis, *S. aureus* accounts for 60% of cases, with the rest caused by pneumococci, streptococci, or aerobic Gram-negative bacilli. In contrast, in subacute endocarditis, α-hemolytic and nonhemolytic streptococci cause 60% of these infections, with enterococci, coagulase-negative staphylococci, and fastidious Gram-negative rods causing the remainder. Among the streptococci causing subacute illness, *Streptococcus mitior*, *S. bovis*, *S. sanguis*, and *S. mutans* predominate and account for 70% of the isolates.

The organisms that cause infection among injection drug users vary depending on whether the infection involves the tricuspid valve (or occasionally the pulmonic valve) or the valves of the left heart. Among injection drug users, *S. aureus* causes 75% of right-sided endocarditis, whereas a broader range of organisms cause left-sided infection (*S. aureus*, 25%; streptococci, 15%; enterococci, 25%; fungi, 10%; and Gram-negative bacilli, 8%). *S. aureus* isolated from injection drug users with endocarditis are often resistant to methicillin. Advances in blood culture technology, molecular analysis (e.g., polymerase chain reaction [PCR]) of surgically removed vegetations, and serologic testing have led to the identification of a rickettsia, *Coxiella burnetii* (especially in Western Europe), and *Bartonella* species as infrequent but important causes of subacute endocarditis. Previously, endocarditis caused by these organisms was often classified as culture negative (i.e., unknown cause).

TABLE 67-1 Microbiology of Infective Endocarditis in Specific Populations at Risk[a]

Organism	Native Valve Endocarditis			Prosthetic Valve Endocarditis		
	Community Acquired (N = 683)	*Nosocomial* (N = 82)	*Injection Drug Users*[b] (N = 550)	≤2 mo (N = 161)	2–12 mo (N = 31)	>12 mo (N = 194)
Staphylococci	269 (39)	53 (65)	313 (57)	87 (55)	15 (48)	56 (29)
Staphylococcus aureus	240 (35)	45 (55)	313 (57)	36 (22)	4 (12)	34 (18)
Coagulase negative	29 (4)	8 (10)		51 (32)	11 (32)	22 (11)
Streptococci	228 (33)	6 (7)	50 (9)	5 (3)	3 (9)	61 (31)
Viridans	151 (22)					
Other	77 (11)					
Enterococci	57 (8)	13 (16)	55 (10)	13 (8)	4 (12)	22 (11)
HACEK[c]	22 (3)					11 (6)
Fungi	5 (1)	3 (4)	25 (5)	12 (7)	4 (12)	3 (1)
Other bacteria	63 (9)	5 (6)	91 (16)	32 (20)	3 (9)	25 (14)
Culture negative	38 (6)	2 (2)	16 (3)	7 (7)	2 (6)	16 (8)

[a]Data derived from large series reported from 1990 to 2004.
[b]Of 550 cases, 346 involved right-sided valves, largely tricuspid, and 77% of total cases were caused by *S. aureus*.
[c]HACEK, *Haemophilus*, *Actinobacillus*, *Cardiobacterium*, *Eikenella*, and *Kingella* species of bacteria; IE, infective endocarditis.

The microbiology of prosthetic valve endocarditis depends on the time after surgery when infection becomes symptomatic. In the first year after valve placement, many infections are nosocomial and often the result of perioperative wound contamination. As with other nosocomial infections, staphylococci cause more than 50% of endocarditis cases occurring in that first year, with Gram-negative rods, corynebacteria, and fungi each accounting for about 5%. Prosthetic valve endocarditis with symptoms beginning more than 1 year after valve surgery is almost always community acquired and occurs as a consequence of transient bacteremia similar to the pathophysiology of native valve endocarditis. Accordingly, streptococci, *S. aureus*, enterococci, and fastidious Gram-negative coccobacilli are the major causes of later-onset prosthetic valve endocarditis. However, coagulase-negative staphylococci remain an important cause of infections that involve prosthetic valves. In persons who have acquired endocarditis in the first year after valve replacement, 80% of coagulase-negative staphylococci are β-lactam antibiotic-resistant *S. epidermidis*, whereas in patients who become infected later, other staphylococcal species, often those that are β-lactam sensitive, are more common. This pattern suggests that late-onset staphylococcal prosthetic endocarditis is probably acquired as a consequence of transient bacteremia.

ENTRY, SPREAD, AND MULTIPLICATION

Transient bacteremia is a common event (see Chapter 66). It occurs when heavily colonized mucosal surfaces are traumatized and spontaneously when mucosal surfaces are breached (Table 67-2). For example, spontaneous bacteremia was documented in 10% of patients with severe gingival disease who were studied before undergoing a dental procedure. Despite the frequency of bacteremia and the broad spectrum of organisms that gain entry into the

TABLE 67-2 Frequency of Transient Bacteremia in Selected Settings

Event	Percentage of Patients with Bacteremia	Common Organisms Recovered
Oral Cavity		
Dental extraction	30–80	Streptococci, diphtheroids, *Staphylococcus epidermidis*
Tooth rocking	85	
Chewing paraffin	50	
Gingival surgery	30–85	
Airway		
Tonsillectomy	38	Streptococci, *Haemophilus* spp., diphtheroids
Bronchoscopy (rigid scope)	15	Streptococci, *S. epidermidis*, aerobic Gram-negative rods
Gastrointestinal Tract		
Upper gastrointestinal endoscopy	8–12	Streptococci, *S. epidermidis*, diphtheroids, *Neisseria* spp.
Colonoscopy	2–10	Aerobic Gram-negative rods, streptococci, *Bacteroides* spp.
Urinary Tract		
Urethral dilation	20–36	Aerobic Gram-negative rods, diphtheroids, streptococci
Cystoscopy	17	
Transurethral prostatic resection	10–45	
Genital Tract		
Parturition	0–5	Aerobic Gram-negative rods, streptococci
Intrauterine device insertion/removal		

Adapted from Everett ED, Hirschmann JV. Transient bacteremia and endocarditis prophylaxis. A review. *Medicine.* 1977;56:61–77; Murdoch DR et al. Clinical presentation, etiology, and outcome of infective endocarditis in the 21st century. *Arch Intern Med.* 2009;169:463–473.

circulation, endocarditis remains a relatively rare disease. Most cases of endocarditis begin at an endocardial lesion that allows bacteria to adhere to and invade the heart valve. Damage to the endothelium results in exposure of the underlying extracellular matrix and production of tissue factor, which triggers coagulation and formation of sterile vegetations (nonbacterial thrombotic endocarditis). Such sterile vegetations facilitate bacterial adherence and infection during transient bacteremia. The colonization of the lesion is followed by further bacterial growth with extension of the lesion, tissue damage, vegetative growth, and dissemination of septic emboli to visceral organs and the brain.

Inflammatory lesions of the endocardium also can promote endocarditis. In response to local inflammation, endothelial cells express β1 integrins. The cell-surface integrins bind plasma fibronectin, which allows bacteria to adhere to the endothelial surface using fibronectin-binding adhesins. Attachment of bacteria to host cells triggers bacterial internalization and intracellular replication, thus allowing the bacteria to escape host defenses. In response to this invasion, further inflammation develops, promoting vegetation enlargement.

Role of Nonbacterial Thrombotic Vegetations

Normal vascular endothelium is resistant to bacterial infection, as can be inferred from the relative infrequency of endocarditis involving normal heart valves as well as from the difficulty of inducing endocarditis in laboratory animals. Microscopic examination of the traumatized valve in experimental animal models of endocarditis reveals that intravenously injected bacteria initially adhere to aggregates of platelets and fibrin, the so-called **nonbacterial thrombotic vegetations**.

Several lines of evidence suggest that nonbacterial thrombotic vegetations play a prominent role in the development of endocarditis in humans. First, this type of vegetation is seen in persons with chronic disease and malignancy (marantic endocarditis) at the exact valve sites most commonly involved in infective endocarditis. Second, the cardiac abnormalities associated with endocarditis promote the formation of platelet–fibrin aggregates at these sites. Cardiac abnormalities that allow blood to flow from an area of very high pressure through a narrowing into a low-pressure reservoir (e.g., ventricular septal defects and mitral and aortic valve regurgitation) are commonly associated with endocarditis. That flow pattern results in a **Venturi effect**, in which a low-pressure area is formed immediately downstream and to the sides of the narrowed orifice. When combined with turbulent flow, the Venturi effect allows platelet–fibrin aggregates to form on the endothelium at the low-pressure side of regurgitant aortic or mitral valves and ventricular septal defects. Additionally, high-velocity jet streams of blood flowing through the regurgitant valves and septal defects injure the endothelium on the wall of the left atrium, the right ventricle, or

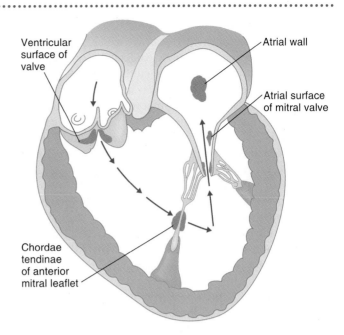

FIGURE 67-1. The location of endocarditic vegetations resulting from high-velocity regurgitant blood flow. The arrows indicate a high-velocity stream of blood. Regurgitant flow through the orifice of an incompetent aortic valve results in vegetations on the ventricular surface of the valve or on the chordae tendineae of the anterior mitral leaflet. Regurgitant flow across an incompetent mitral valve into the low-pressure left atrium allows vegetations to form on the atrial surface of the mitral valve (or at the site of jet stream impact on the atrial wall).

the chordae tendineae–anterior mitral valve leaflet. In turn, platelet–fibrin thrombi form at the sites of endothelial injury and serve as a niche for infective endocarditis (Fig. 67-1). Interestingly, cardiac lesions that result in low-pressure gradients (ostium secundum atrial septal defect) or low flow and reduced turbulence (chronic congestive heart failure) are rarely associated with infective endocarditis.

Microbial Virulence Factors

Although a broad array of bacteria gain entry into the circulation, only a limited number can produce endocarditis. To cause endocarditis, organisms must enter the circulation, survive host defenses, adhere to the thrombotic vegetation or valve endothelium, replicate on the valve surface, and promote further vegetation formation. For that sequence of events to culminate in endocarditis requires a complex interaction between infective agent, host defenses, endothelium, plasma components of the coagulation system, platelets, and host proteins. The precise molecular interactions vary among specific agents and are not completely understood. However, some elements of those interactions have been inferred by studies of organisms causing endocarditis and their capacity to do so in animal models.

Once they reach the cardiac valves, organisms capable of causing endocarditis that reach the cardiac valves must be resistant to the complement-mediated bactericidal activity of serum and escape phagocytosis and killing by neutrophils. Moreover, endocarditis-causing organisms must adhere to the thrombotic vegetation or the valve endothelium. Structures in the bacterial cell wall or extracellular polysaccharides have been implicated in interactions with host tissue receptors that result in the adherence of selected organisms. The common bacteria causing endocarditis, *S. mutans*, *S. sanguis*, *S. mitior*, and *S. bovis*, produce extracellular dextran, which mediates vigorous adherence of the organisms to platelet–fibrin aggregates on the heart valves. In addition, the capacity to produce dextran by streptococci isolated from blood cultures is strongly associated with endocarditis. Adherence of streptococci to fibrin also is facilitated by a bacterial protein, **FimA**, previously identified as an oral cavity adhesin. Furthermore, FimA is associated with the virulence of streptococcal strains in animal models of endocarditis. Cell wall **lipoteichoic acid** and a protein with major homology to the streptococcal oral adhesins may promote adherence of enterococci to platelet–fibrin aggregates.

Endocarditis-producing organisms, including *Enterococcus faecalis*, *S. aureus*, *S. mutans*, and *S. sanguis*, bind more vigorously to **fibronectin** than do organisms rarely implicated in the disease, suggesting a role for that host protein in mediating microbial adherence to cardiac valves. Binding of *S. aureus* and coagulase-negative staphylococci to fibronectin-coated foreign devices correlates with device infection and may initiate prosthetic valve infection as a consequence of bacteremia. Fibronectin is present on the surface of nonbacterial thrombotic vegetations and exposed as subendothelial matrix when the endothelium is injured. However, the protein is not present on normal intact endothelium.

Fibrinogen is both present in nonbacterial thrombotic vegetations and a key target for the adherence of *S. aureus*. The initial adherence is mediated through a fibrinogen-binding protein of the *S. aureus* cell surface (clumping factor) and may account for acute endocarditis without prior valvular disease. Interestingly, coagulase, which is used to identify *S. aureus* (vs. coagulase-negative species), does not promote adherence to thrombotic vegetations and is not a virulence factor associated with endocarditis. The explanation is that coagulase is secreted into the medium rather than being bound to the bacterial surface. *S. aureus* and streptococci possess surface components that recognize adhesive matrix molecules (MSCRAMM) that bind to extracellular matrix molecules acting as specific ligands, causing adherence of the organisms to thrombotic vegetations and injured endothelium (see Chapter 11).

After adherence to the valve, bacteria must survive and replicate if endocarditis is to occur. The virulence factors that initially favor bacterial survival are not well known. Fibronectin-binding proteins of *S. aureus* facilitate invasion of endothelial cells and subsequent production of tissue factor, a glycoprotein that acts as a procoagulant for thrombin formation. *S. epidermidis* and streptococci

also induce tissue factor activity, but by interactions with locally recruited monocytes. Growth and maturation of the vegetation and the resulting envelopment of the microorganisms aid in organism survival and replication, which ultimately leads to overt endocarditis.

Platelets activated by thrombin release low molecular weight, cationic, microbicidal proteins that kill some *S. aureus* and α-hemolytic streptococci. Resistance of adherent organisms to the platelet microbicidal proteins, termed thrombocidins, may be an important factor in progression from valvular adherence to endocarditis. A capsular polysaccharide expressed by coagulase-negative staphylococci may enhance their resistance to clearance by host defenses and thus facilitate development of prosthetic valve endocarditis by strains that contaminate the valve intraoperatively.

Vegetation formation and bacterial growth feed on each other. When a vegetation is colonized by bacteria, it tends to grow by continued deposition of platelets and fibrin. *S. aureus* and α-hemolytic streptococci promote platelet adhesion and aggregation and vegetation growth by complex unique and independent mechanisms unrelated to the elaboration of tissue factor and its procoagulant activity. Protected within the vegetation, bacterial proliferation proceeds unimpeded, leading to dense populations of organisms (10^8 to 10^9 bacteria per gram of tissue). The relative absence of phagocytic cells in vegetations is likely a factor that permits bacterial growth to continue without interruption. On the other hand, experimental data suggest that phagocytic cells limit infection at extracardiac intravascular sites and on the tricuspid valve (perhaps a reason why bacteremic infection of these sites is infrequent). When animals with experimental endocarditis are treated with anticoagulation or fibrinolytic therapy, the size of the vegetation is reduced. However, that strategy has not been translated to effective adjunctive therapy for endocarditis in humans.

DAMAGE

A **vegetation** is the cardinal pathologic feature of endocarditis (Figs. 67-2 and 67-3). Classically, vegetations occur along the line of valve closure on the low-pressure surface of the regurgitant valve or septal defect or at the site of a jet stream lesion. Vegetations vary in size from a few millimeters to a centimeter or larger and may be single or multiple. Microscopically, vegetations are a mass of fibrin, platelets, and clumps of bacteria; neutrophils are rare. Microorganisms deep in vegetations are often metabolically inactive, whereas the more superficial ones are actively proliferating. A broad array of symptoms and signs are associated with endocarditis (Table 67-3). The following events are the causes of those symptoms and signs:

- Persistent bacteremia
- Release of cytokines, resulting in constitutional symptoms

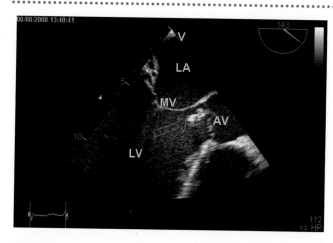

FIGURE 67-2. Transesophageal echocardiogram from a patient with nonhemolytic streptococcal native aortic valve endocarditis. A large vegetation is indicated with the *arrow*. LA, left atrium; LV, left ventricle; MV, mitral valve; AV, aorta valve; V, left side of the scanning picture.

- Tissue destruction by infecting organisms
- Fragmentation of vegetations into the circulation, causing peripheral **septic emboli** with resultant organ injury
- Induction of antibodies, which combine with bacterial antigens to form circulating immune complexes

Organisms proliferating near the surface of the vegetation are continuously shed into the blood. Although the number of organisms in the blood varies over time, endocarditis is characterized by **continuous bacteremia**. Bacteremia mediates the release of cytokines, resulting in the constitutional symptoms associated with endocarditis: fever, sweats, fatigue, anorexia, and weight loss.

Endocarditis is often complicated by intracardiac damage that involves distortion and destruction of valve leaflets (Figs. 67-4 and 67-5), rupture of chordae tendineae (Fig. 67-5) or, in the case of infected prosthetic valves, destruction of a valve leaflet, impaired mobility

TABLE 67-3 Symptoms and Signs Associated with Infective Endocarditis

Symptom	Frequency (%)	Sign	Frequency (%)
Fever >38°C	96	Fever	96
Weakness	50	Murmur	68
Sweats	30	Embolic event	35
Anorexia	50		
Weight loss	60	Osler nodes	3
Malaise	60	Petechiae	2
Myalgia, arthralgia	15	Janeway lesions	5
		Roth spots	2
Back pain	10	Stroke	20
Confusion	10	Splenomegaly	11
		Septic complications	20

of the valve mechanism, and paravalvular flow caused by dehiscence from the annulus. The resulting valvular dysfunction may precipitate congestive heart failure. Infection can extend beyond the valve leaflet into the annulus to cause a perivalvular abscess (Fig. 67-6).

Clinical clues to invasive infection include development or worsening of congestive heart failure (due to progressive valvular insufficiency or other causes of hemodynamic

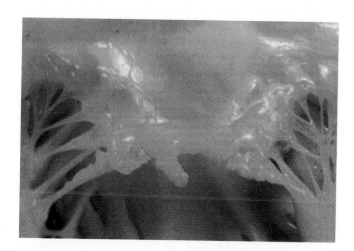

FIGURE 67-3. Preoperative picture of a vegetation on a heart valve from a patient with bacterial endocarditis.

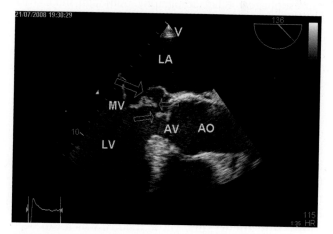

FIGURE 67-4. Transesophageal echocardiogram from a patient with *Streptococcus sanguis* native mitral and aorta valve endocarditis. *Small arrows* indicate vegetations on the anterior mitral valve leaflet and the aortic valve. *Large arrow* shows perforation of the anterior mitral valve leaflet. LA, left atrium; LV, left ventricle; MV, mitral valve; AV, aorta valve; AO, aorta; V, left side of the scanning picture.

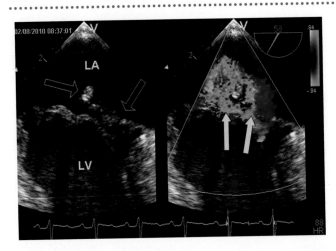

FIGURE 67-5. Transesophageal echocardiogram from a patient with nonhemolytic streptococcal native mitral valve endocarditis and prolapse of the anterior mitral valve leaflet with ruptured chordae tendineae. *Arrows* on the left side show a vegetation on the ruptured chordae tendineae and a perforation of the anterior leaflet. *Arrows* on the right side show a regurgitation jet through the prolapse and through the perforation. LA, left atrium; LV, left ventricle; V, left side of the scanning picture.

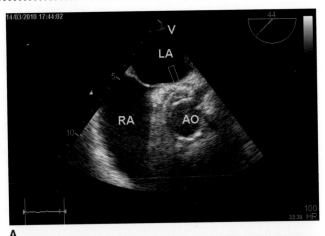

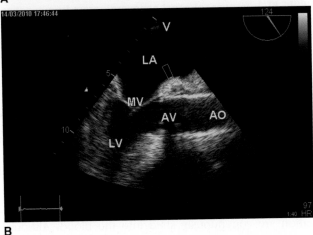

FIGURE 67-6. Transesophageal echocardiogram from a patient with β-hemolytic streptococcal endocarditis of a composite aorta graft. *Arrows* indicate an abscess in the wall between the graft and the left atrium in cross-sectional **(A)** and longitudinal **(B)** views. LA, left atrium; RA, right atrium; LV, left ventricle; MV, mitral valve; AO, aorta; V, left side of the scanning picture.

compromise such as fistulae, paravalvular leak, or dehiscence of a prosthetic valve), fever that persists for more than a week despite appropriate antimicrobial therapy or, more rarely, new electrocardiographic conduction changes primarily in aortic valve endocarditis (a consequence of the anatomic proximity to the mitral and aortic annuli of the atrioventricular conduction system, the bundle of His, and the bundle branches), and pericarditis (a consequence of infection extending into the pericardial space). Vegetations, valve function, hemodynamic status, and perivalvular–myocardial abscess are evaluated by transthoracic or transesophageal echocardiography. Although intracardiac complications can occur with all microbial causes of endocarditis, they are more common when virulent pyogenic bacteria are responsible or when infection involves prosthetic valves (particularly within the initial year after valve surgery). These complications, if not repaired surgically, are major causes of death from endocarditis.

Infection of remote sites often complicates endocarditis caused by pyogenic bacteria. Included among such complications are septic arthritis, vertebral osteomyelitis, and abscesses of virtually any organ system. Infection in the **vasa vasorum** of larger arteries and arteritis beginning at the site of arterial occlusion from septic emboli especially in patients with *S. aureus* endocarditis give rise to **mycotic aneurysms**. Those lesions, which can occur in any artery, are usually asymptomatic until they rupture (as in the case of Mrs. Q).

Although emboli are recognized in 25 to 35% of patients with endocarditis, occult lesions are present in up to 70% of patients. Arterial occlusion, infarction, and other secondary complications in virtually any organ can result from emboli. Emboli are most notable as a cause of

stroke, acute myocardial infarction, and abdominal, flank, and back pain resulting from intestinal, splenic, and renal infarction, respectively. In tricuspid valve endocarditis, septic pulmonary artery emboli with secondary pneumonia, lung abscess, or pyopneumothorax may occur. These complications are prominent components of *S. aureus* tricuspid valve endocarditis.

Circulating **immune complexes** that contain antigen from the causative organism are detectable in most patients. The concentration of these complexes correlates with prolonged duration of the disease, occurrence of extracardiac manifestations, and reduced serum complement concentration. Tissue injury mediated by deposition of circulating immune complexes occurs in the skin, choroid plexus, spleen, and synovium. Clinical findings such as **Osler nodes**, **petechiae**, **vasculitic purpura**, and arthralgia are caused by deposition of immune complexes in the skin, arterial wall, and synovium.

Glomerulonephritis is the best documented immune-mediated complication of endocarditis (see Chapter 12). Endocarditis is associated with a continuum of immune renal injury from focal embolic glomerulone-phritis (a lesion with few clinical consequences) to diffuse proliferative glomerulonephritis that results in an active urine sediment (i.e., containing erythrocytes and erythro-cyte casts) and is commonly associated with decreased creatinine clearance. In patients with prolonged episodes of subacute streptococcal endocarditis, circulating immune complexes, which form intravascularly under conditions of antibody excess, deposit in a subepithelial location along the glomerular basement membrane. Immunofluorescence studies reveal IgG and early complement components on the glomerular basement membrane in a lumpy distribu-tion (Fig. 67-7). Among patients with subacute endocar-ditis, glomerulonephritis is frequent, generally focal and mild, and remits with effective therapy of the infection. Acute staphylococcal endocarditis causes an immune-mediated glomerulonephritis as a consequence of antigen deposition at the glomerular basement membrane and activation of the alternative complement pathway. This type of lesion is found in more than 25% of patients with *S. aureus* endocarditis of less than 2 weeks duration.

DIAGNOSIS

The clinical presentation of endocarditis is variable and, although symptoms may be suggestive, they are mostly nonspecific. Therefore, establishing a diagnosis of endo-carditis depends primarily on blood cultures that yield microorganisms that commonly cause endocarditis and echocardiographic findings demonstrating characteristic lesions. A cardinal finding is documentation of persistent bacteremia through multiple positive blood cultures (at least three) for the same organisms over 24 to 48 hours. Blood cultures positive for organisms that commonly cause endocarditis should raise the possibility of the diag-nosis, even in the absence of other clinical findings. With-out prior antibiotic therapy, at least 95% of patients with endocarditis have positive blood cultures. In almost all cases, one of the initial two cultures is positive. Depend-ing on the susceptibility of the organism, administration of antibiotics during the preceding 2 weeks may significantly reduce the frequency of positive blood cultures. There-fore, to avoid false-negative results, blood cultures should be obtained before antibiotics are given. In approximately 5% of patients with endocarditis, blood cultures will remain sterile. By far, the most common cause of cul-ture-negative endocarditis is administration of antibiotics prior to obtaining blood cultures. For this reason, empiric antibiotics should be avoided whenever possible, and blood cultures (three sets are virtually always sufficient) should be obtained before antibiotics are initiated. In sta-ble patients with apparent culture-negative endocarditis, ongoing antibiotic therapy may be held for several days in an attempt to obtain a pathogen. Transthoracic echocardi-ography, often followed by transesophageal echocardiog-raphy in patients with a high suspicion of endocarditis, is a highly sensitive and specific approach to the identification

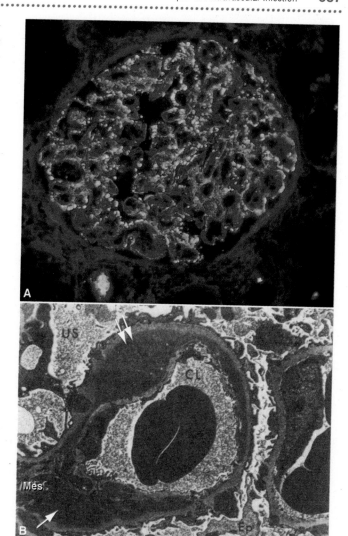

FIGURE 67-7. Immune complex glomerulonephritis. A. Immu-nofluorescence staining of a glomerulus with antibodies directed against C3 showing deposits in the capillary walls and the me-sangium. **B.** Electron micrograph of a glomerular tuft revealing electron-dense immune complex deposits in the mesangium (*single arrow*) and subendothelial capillary space (*double arrow*). The basement membrane splits to surround the subendothelial deposits, giving rise to the double-contoured appearance noted in part A. These deposits will be stained by fluorescently tagged antihuman IgG in a lumpy distribution. CL, capillary lumen; Ep, epithelial cell; Mes, mesangium; US, urinary (Bowman) space.

of vegetations on valves and intracardiac complications such as abscess formation, pseudoaneurysms, tissue per-foration, paravalvular leak, or dehiscence of a prosthetic valve. Although this approach is not suitable for screen-ing patients with little clinical evidence of endocarditis, it is mandatory in patients in whom the disease is highly suspected to confirm the diagnosis. Other laboratory tests that are frequently abnormal in patients with endocardi-tis—including hematocrit, C-reactive protein, urinalysis, circulating immune complex concentration, and rheuma-toid factor—are not helpful in making a specific diagnosis.

TREATMENT

Effective treatment for endocarditis requires identifying the causative agent and determining its antimicrobial susceptibility. That information enables the deployment of an effective antimicrobial regimen. Because host defenses are not very effective at inhibiting bacteria within vegetations, bactericidal antibiotics or combinations of antibiotics are required for optimal therapy. Antibiotics are administered parenterally to achieve high serum concentrations, which are necessary to penetrate the depths of relatively avascular vegetations. The reduced metabolic state of organisms deep in vegetations may render the bacteria difficult to eradicate and supports the use of prolonged antibiotic courses for most patients with infective endocarditis.

The increasing prevalence of enterococci that are resistant to penicillins, vancomycin, and the aminoglycosides (high-level resistance to streptomycin and gentamicin)—as well as staphylococci resistant to methicillin (also resistant to all semisynthetic penicillinase-resistant penicillins, cephalosporins, and carbapenems)—may result in endocarditis that is difficult to eradicate with antibiotics. Fungi and antibiotic-resistant Gram-negative rods also may cause endocarditis that is difficult to treat without surgical intervention. Surgery to excise valves infected by antibiotic-resistant organisms may help to resolve those infections. Additionally, the survival of patients with intracardiac complications, such as valve dysfunction that leads to congestive heart failure or perivalvular abscess, is greatly enhanced by surgery to debride sites of infection, restore anatomic defects, and replace a dysfunctional valve with a prosthesis.

PREVENTION

The value of prophylactic antibiotics to prevent endocarditis in patients at risk is uncertain because carefully controlled studies have never been performed. Although some animal studies support the use of antibiotic prophylaxis, it is now recognized that endocarditis more often is the result of exposure to transient bacteremia associated with routine daily activities such as tooth brushing, use of wooden toothpicks, or chewing food than to bacteremia during dental, gastrointestinal tract, or genitourinary tract procedures. In addition, antibiotic prophylaxis may prevent only an extremely small number of cases of endocarditis, and the risk of antibiotic-associated adverse events greatly exceeds the potential beneficial effects. Emphasis on improved oral health in patients with a high risk of the acquisition of endocarditis is therefore much more important to reduce the incidence of transient bacteremia causing endocarditis than the use of prophylactic antibiotics. As a consequence, the American Heart Association now only recommends prophylaxis for the following high-risk patients: (1) prosthetic heart valve recipients; (2) those with a history of previous endocarditis; (3) persons with unrepaired cyanotic congenital heart disease, completely repaired congenital heart disease with prosthetic material during the 6 months after the procedure, or repaired congenital heart disease with residual defects at the site or adjacent to the site of prosthetic material; or (4) cardiac transplant recipients who develop cardiac valvulopathy. Since these new recommendations represent a radical departure from previous guidelines, it is anticipated that some clinicians and patients will be more comfortable continuing previous practice. It may take several years before the new recommendations are accepted.

CONCLUSION

In spite of improvements in health care, endocarditis remains an important life-threatening infection with an incidence of 2 to 8 cases per 100,000 persons every year. The evolving epidemiology of the infection in the developed world reflects new predispositions in an aging, health care–supported population and new behavioral practices with attendant risks. *S. aureus* has become the predominant causative organism in many parts of the developed world. An understanding of the complex interactions of bacteria and host resulting in endocarditis is improved but still incomplete. Echocardiography is a cornerstone in diagnosis and patient assessment. Potent antibiotics for therapy and surgical intervention have improved survival rates, but challenges still exist. Prevention of morbidity, especially from emboli and ruptured mycotic aneurysms, remains an important objective. Endocarditis prophylaxis has become significantly more restricted.

Suggested Readings

Fowler VG, Bayer AS. Infective endocarditis. In: Goldman L, Ausiello D, eds. *Cecil Medicine*. 23rd ed. Philadelphia, PA: Saunders; 2008:537–547.

Karchmer AW. Infective endocarditis. In: Libby P, Bonow RO, Mann DL, Zipes DP, eds. *Heart Disease: A Textbook of Cardiovascular Medicine*. 6th ed. Philadelphia, PA: Saunders; 2008:1713–1738.

Li JS, Sexton DJ, Mick N, et al. Proposed modification to the Duke criteria for the diagnosis of infective endocarditis. *Clin Infect Dis*. 2000;30:633–638.

Moreillon P, Que Y-A, Bayer AS. Pathogenesis of streptococcal and staphylococcal endocarditis. *Infect Dis Clin North Am*. 2002;16:297–318.

Moreillon P, Que Y-A. Infective endocarditis. *Lancet*. 2004;363: 139–149.

Mylonakis E, Calderwood SB. Infective endocarditis in adults. *N Engl J Med*. 2001;345:1318–1330.

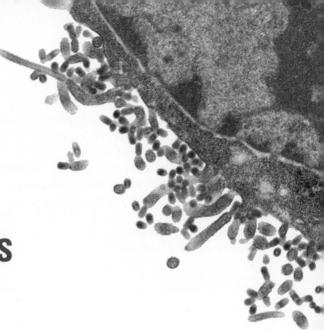

Chapter 68

Head and Neck Infections

Preeti N. Malani and Mark A. Zacharek

INFECTIONS of the head and neck occur most commonly when organisms spread from contiguous mucosal surfaces into soft tissue and interstitial spaces. Less often, infection results from hematogenous seeding of organisms from the bloodstream. Regardless of the route, clinical manifestations of head and neck infections primarily involve **inflammation**. The resultant swelling is often readily recognized, as when it causes facial cellulitis or it acutely affects a physiological function like swallowing or breathing.

The **air-filled cavities** of the head (sinuses, mastoids, middle ear) are lined by respiratory epithelium (Fig. 68-1). Infections of those spaces result when **normal drainage routes become obstructed**. The ciliated respiratory epithelium normally removes bacteria by trapping them in mucus and propelling the mucus out. When drainage is blocked, the epithelium cannot function normally. As aerobic bacteria reach their maximum growth, oxygen in the affected cavity becomes depleted, permitting anaerobes to grow. Bacteria release fragments of cell wall (such as lipopolysaccharide or murein subunits) that elicit a cytokine response, leading to more inflammation and obstruction. An intact immune system is essential for defense against and recovery from head and neck infection. Both cell-mediated and humoral immunity play critical roles. Patients who lack normal immune response (such as transplant recipients, cancer patients, those with HIV infection, or other immunodeficiencies) can present with infection atypically. These immunocompromised hosts are also susceptible to opportunistic infection from organisms that might not normally cause infection.

ENCOUNTER AND ENTRY

The common cold (**rhinitis**) and sore throats (**pharyngitis**) account for most head and neck infections (see Chapters 32 and 12, respectively, for more detail on those topics). Frequently, a more invasive infection follows a viral or streptococcal infection that disrupts the mucosal epithelium. Histological examination of respiratory mucosa during acute infection demonstrates loss of ciliated epithelial cells and thinning of the mucosal layer. The resulting loss of continuity allows bacteria to enter the underlying soft tissue (**cellulitis**) or overwhelm the defenses in the lymph nodes (**lymphadenitis**).

In **sinusitis**, the ostia can become blocked because of a viral upper respiratory infection or allergies, both of which produce **edema**. In the **middle ear**, eustachian tube dysfunction can occur congenitally (e.g., in infants with cleft palates), as a result of an upper respiratory tract infection, or secondary to allergies. Because the cavity of the middle ear is contiguous with the mastoid air cells, individuals with **acute otitis media** also have **mastoiditis**, an acute inflammatory reaction in the mastoid air cells.

The most common infections of the head and neck are listed in Table 68-1. The bacteria associated with the infections are mostly those isolated from the upper respiratory tract, including *Streptococcus pneumoniae, Haemophilus influenzae, Staphylococcus aureus, Streptococcus pyogenes,* and anaerobic bacteria. The six clinical cases presented in this chapter illustrate common manifestations of head and neck infections.

OTITIS MEDIA

Otitis media is among the most common infections seen by primary care providers. The majority of cases occur in

CASE • E., a 14-month-old girl, came down with the same "cold" that her older sister had had for the past 3 days. She became irritable, stopped taking her bottle, and developed a temperature of 39.8°C, prompting her mother to take her to the family's physician. In the office, the nurse used a tympanometer to measure the mobility of E.'s eardrum and told the mother that E. had an ear infection. On further otoscopic examination, the physician agreed and prescribed oral amoxicillin.

This case raises several questions:

1. Should E.'s sister be brought in and checked for an ear infection?
2. Should a culture be obtained before antibiotics are prescribed?
3. How can the physician be sure that amoxicillin is the right antibiotic for E.?
4. Could E. have complications of her ear infection?

See Appendix for answers.

children between 6 and 36 months of age, with an average child having two episodes per year during the first 3 years of life. Children are especially susceptible to otitis media for several reasons. One predisposing factor is that the medial orifice of the eustachian tube is more open in infancy than later in life. Supine feeding (giving a bottle at bedtime) permits reflux of pharyngeal contents into the lumen of the eustachian tubes, producing irritation that results in inflammation and occlusion. Additionally, the eustachian tube is shorter and more horizontal in young children, which allows reflux of nasopharyngeal organisms into the middle ear. Eustachian tube dysfunction is also facilitated by viral infections of the lymphoid tissue around the medial orifice (the adenoidal pad), such as those caused by respiratory syncytial virus, influenza A or B, or adenovirus. With inflammation and occlusion, normal upper respiratory flora can proliferate in the middle ear. The most common bacteria associated with otitis media are *S. pneumoniae*, *H. influenzae*, and *Moraxella catarrhalis*. Viral infections can promote bacterial replication in the middle ear by direct damage to the respiratory epithelium lining.

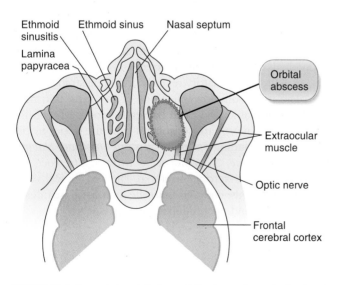

FIGURE 68-1. Superior axial view of the face through the level of the ethmoid sinus.

TABLE 68-1 Infections of the Head and Neck

Infections of Air-Filled Cavities

Otitis media (acute and chronic)

Sinusitis

Mastoiditis

Infections of Structures Contiguous to Air-Filled Cavities

Orbital cellulitis or abscess

Cavernous sinus thrombosis or thrombophlebitis

Lateral sinus thrombosis or thrombophlebitis

Cervical adenitis

Infections of Soft Tissues

Rhinitis

Pharyngitis, exudative and nonexudative

Conjunctivitis

Facial cellulitis

Abscess of canine fossa

Lymphadenitis

Oropharyngeal abscess

Paratonsillar Infection

Pterygomaxillary Infection

Lateral Neck Infection

Thyroiditis

Infections of Embryonic Remnants

Branchial cleft cellulitis or abscess

Thyroglossal duct cellulitis or abscess

DIAGNOSIS AND TREATMENT

The signs and symptoms of middle ear inflammation reflect the anatomy of the region. Early in the course, submucosal edema and hemorrhage lead to the outpouring of exudate into the middle ear space. As the cavity fills with fluid, the tympanic membrane becomes less mobile, resulting in a **conductive hearing loss**. Mobility can be measured by pneumatic otoscopy (changing the air pressure on the eardrum while looking at it) or by **tympanometry** (a technique that measures the compliance of the tympanic membrane). In a healthy ventilated ear, tension on the tympanic membrane varies with the pressure exerted on it. When fluid is present in the middle ear, the tympanic membrane cannot stretch with changes in pressure (poor compliance).

In **chronic otitis media**, the epithelium of the middle ear undergoes marked histological changes. Bacterial cell wall components and secreted toxins cause mucus-secreting cells to increase in number. Mucin is secreted into the middle ear, possibly in an effort to entrap and remove bacteria and inflammatory debris. The usual exit route for fluids, the eustachian tube, remains occluded. Accordingly, an essential part of treatment is fluid drainage. That can be accomplished indirectly by administering medications that restore eustachian tube function or directly by incising and placing a tube through the tympanic membrane (**myringotomy** and placement of **pressure equalization tubes**).

The middle ear can become infected with any of the bacteria present in the upper respiratory tract. In acute disease, the primary pathogens are pneumococci and nontypeable *H. influenzae* (together accounting for about 80% of infections overall). Antimicrobial drugs active against those two species have proven effective in the treatment of otitis media, alone or in combination with other measures. Thus, empirical treatment directed against the most common pathogens is justifiable in acute otitis media. However, several studies suggest that acute otitis media can resolve without antimicrobial medication. Some authorities advocate observation with limited antimicrobial use in older children. On the other hand, infants are almost always treated with antimicrobials because of an increased incidence of complications. Aspiration of the middle ear fluid (**tympanocentesis**) is not routinely performed for culture and susceptibility testing. Besides being a painful and risky procedure, the results do not significantly impact management because the microbiology is predictable in acute disease.

COMPLICATIONS

Although most ear infections treated with antimicrobial medications resolve without complications, chronic and recurrent episodes of otitis media can lead to infectious and noninfectious sequelae such as facial nerve paralysis, brain abscess, and epidural or subdural abscess. Some patients develop perforated tympanic membranes. In those cases, the associated pathogens occasionally include not only the upper respiratory flora but also Gram-negative bacilli, particularly *Pseudomonas aeruginosa* and *Proteus* species.

Another complication of otitis media is persistent middle ear fluid leading to conductive hearing loss. Uncorrected, the hearing loss can impact speech and language development. Children experiencing recurrent bouts of otitis media should be referred to an otolaryngologist for further evaluation. Some patients benefit from myringotomy and the surgical placement of pressure equalization tubes. In general, that procedure is considered when a patient has had recurrent episodes of acute otitis media (usually five to seven infections in a year), a persistent effusion lasting more than 12 weeks, and an associated conductive hearing loss. Prospective clinical studies demonstrate that children treated with tubes experience improved hearing and fewer recurrences of otitis media. Additionally, a child's nutritional status can improve along with quality of life parameters for parents and children. Like any surgical procedure, tube placement carries risk. Risks of tube placement include the development of chronic **otorrhea** (persistent drainage through the puncture site), tympanic membrane perforation, and, very rarely, ossicular chain injury and sensorineural hearing loss.

PREVENTION

Increasing antimicrobial resistance has encouraged novel approaches to the prevention of otitis media. In 2000, a capsule-protein conjugate vaccine against pneumococcal disease became available. The vaccine offers protection against the seven serotypes of *S. pneumoniae* responsible for a large portion of invasive and/or drug-resistant infections. In addition to excellent efficacy against invasive pneumococcal disease, the pneumococcal conjugate vaccine has demonstrated protection against acute otitis media caused by vaccine serotypes. In addition, the vaccine appears to be decreasing transmission of resistant pneumococcal strains within families by reducing upper respiratory tract colonization. In the United States, the original 7-valent pneumococcal conjugate vaccine has now been replaced by a 13-valent preparation. In other countries, including several European nations, a new vaccine containing 10 conjugated pneumococcal capsules with a nontypeable *H. influenzae* protein D conjugate is now being used. Annual influenza vaccination is now routinely offered to young children, particularly those less than 2 years of age. Theoretically, this also has a beneficial effect on otitis media.

ORBITAL CELLULITIS

Orbital cellulitis involves acute inflammation of the connective tissue of the eye socket and is a serious complication of acute sinusitis. The lateral borders of the ethmoid sinuses form the medial wall of the orbit, also known as the **lamina papyracea** (Latin for "paper thin"). Infection

CASE • B., a 13-year-old girl, has had ongoing problems with allergic rhinitis generally manifesting as a runny nose, watery eyes, and episodes of fullness in the front of her face. One morning, she awoke with headache, cough, and a foul taste in her mouth. Interpreting that as another episode of her allergies, B. took an antihistamine and some acetaminophen. The next morning, her headache had become severe and she was unable to open her left eye. Feeling terribly ill, she went to see her pediatrician, who noted marked erythema and swelling around B.'s eye and a slight exudate from the eyelids. B. had a temperature of 38.3°C and a heart rate of 120 beats per minute. When the doctor retracted B.'s eyelids, she found that the left eye was slightly deviated inferiorly and laterally and noted limitation in extraocular eye movements. She immediately referred B. to an otolaryngologist as she likely had a serious illness, orbital cellulitis.

This case raises several questions:

1. Why should B. see an otolaryngologist if the problem is with her eye?
2. How are B.'s allergies related to the development of orbital cellulitis?
3. Are antimicrobials necessary?

See Appendix for answers.

in the ethmoid sinus can erode through the lamina papyracea and enter the orbit. If the cellulitis becomes localized, an intraorbital but extraocular abscess, known as a **subperiosteal abscess**, can develop (see Fig. 68-1). By convention, orbital cellulitis is graded clinically based on the severity and extent of disease, ranging from preseptal cellulitis to cavernous sinus thrombosis. The approach to treatment varies with the extent of disease.

DIAGNOSIS

Clinical findings helped B.'s physician quickly recognize the disease. Because the superior and medial region of the orbit was affected, the eye was displaced inferiorly and laterally. Had she measured it, the physician would have found that the eyeball was proptotic (protruding out of the orbit). **Proptosis** is caused by the edema and inflammatory exudate in the orbit, literally making the cavity smaller and forcing the eye outward. Other signs of orbital cellulitis include limitation of extraocular eye muscles caused by the structures becoming edematous. In addition, stretching of the optic nerve can decrease visual acuity and can result in blindness.

TREATMENT AND PREVENTION

Because the source of orbital cellulitis is the sinus, treatment may require surgical drainage of the involved ethmoid. An external drainage procedure or an endoscopic transnasal decompression of the abscess can be performed to allow the globe to return to its normal position. Antimicrobials are also vital to treatment. As with other infections of the head and neck, bacteria associated with orbital cellulitis are from the oral and pharyngeal flora. More virulent infections, such as that experienced by B., are likely caused by *S. aureus*. Accordingly, clinicians should select antimicrobials active against *S. aureus* as well as members of the upper respiratory tract flora. Orbital cellulitis identified at an early stage (**preseptal cellulitis**) is usually treated with antimicrobials, steroids, and close observation. Surgical drainage is imperative with advanced disease.

FACIAL CELLULITIS
EPIDEMIOLOGY

Facial cellulitis in infants is almost exclusively caused by *H. influenzae* type b. Had R. been immunized with

CASE • R., a 14-month-old unvaccinated boy, awoke from his nap fussy, with a low-grade temperature and slight swelling of his right cheek. His mother thought R. might have bumped it with a bottle while feeding himself in the crib. That evening when she put R. to bed, he seemed improved but remained irritable. His right cheek was more swollen and had developed a slight purplish hue. Aside from a fever, he appeared well. The next morning, his temperature was 41.6°C, prompting his mother to take R. to the family doctor. The physician told her that R. would need hospitalization for parenteral antibiotics to treat **facial cellulitis**.

This cases raises two questions:

1. How did the bacteria get into R.'s cheek?
2. Why did R. need to receive intravenous antibiotics for cellulitis?

See Appendix for answers.

the conjugate *H. influenzae* vaccine, the disease could have been prevented. The pathogenesis is not entirely clear, but it is likely that minor facial trauma allows blood to seep into the soft tissues. When transient *H. influenzae* bacteremia occurs, the organisms seed and grow in the traumatized subcutaneous tissue using the extravasated red blood cells as a source of nutrition (*haemophilus* is Latin for "blood loving"). Because the soft tissue was seeded through the bloodstream, R. was at risk for other more serious complications of *H. influenzae* bacteremia, including meningitis, septic arthritis, and osteomyelitis.

DIAGNOSIS AND TREATMENT

Because *H. influenzae* does not make cell-damaging exotoxins, tissue inflammation is often minimal. At times, the distinction between a slight bruise on the face and cellulitis is difficult to make. The important clinical findings are fever and swelling out of proportion to the magnitude of facial trauma. R.'s physician suspected *H. influenzae* because of the typical purplish (not reddish) hue of the inflamed region and his knowledge that the family refused *H. influenzae* type b vaccine for religious reasons.

H. influenzae cellulitis resolves with the administration of appropriate antimicrobials. Because secondary diseases owing to *H. influenzae* are very serious, the usual treatment is to administer antibiotic therapy intravenously until the cellulitis has completely resolved.

OROPHARYNGEAL ABSCESS
DIAGNOSIS

Ms. J. had the typical symptoms of an oropharyngeal abscess. In her case, the most likely diagnosis was that of a **peritonsillar abscess**, as evidenced by examination of the oral cavity. The tonsils lie between the anterior and posterior pillars (mucosa that covers the palatoglossus and palatopharyngeus muscles, respectively; Fig. 68-2). The superior tonsillar poles overlie part of the superior pharyngeal constrictor muscle and the medial pterygoid muscle. Inflammation behind the tonsil adjacent to those structures causes their dysfunction. **Trismus**, the inability to open one's mouth, is caused by dysfunction of the medial pterygoid, and the inability to initiate swallowing results from dysfunction of the superior pharyngeal constrictor. Failure to elevate the palate results from edema, leading to a muffled, "hot potato" voice, even though the tongue is unaffected. Ms. J. could swallow because there was no mechanical obstruction to food entering her esophagus, but inflammation of the superior constrictor made it difficult to initiate the process. With peritonsillar abscess, the tonsil appears displaced, medially and downward. The uvula is deviated away from the involved tonsil. On palpation, the tonsil may feel fluctuant because of pus in the underlying fascial plane.

Group A streptococci are responsible for about half the cases of peritonsillar abscess. However, commensals are also frequently involved. The process begins as a cellulitis of the peritonsillar tissues, followed by local necrosis. The aerobic and anaerobic oral flora then gain access to the necrotic tissue. Such infections can progress quickly and result in deeper infection in areas such as the parapharyngeal space, retropharyngeal space, and even result in paravertebral infection.

TREATMENT

The primary therapy is surgical drainage. Antimicrobial drugs are also necessary and should include an agent active against common oropharyngeal flora as well as *S. aureus*. In most cases, the drug of choice is a semisynthetic penicillin resistant to staphylococcal β-lactamase. Patients allergic to penicillin can be treated with clindamycin.

CASE • Before going to bed one evening, Ms. J., a 19-year-old college student, noticed "a scratchy throat" with slight pain. Over the next 4 days, she had an increasingly sore throat and her right ear began to ache. She thought she had a fever and took some aspirin. On the sixth day of her illness, Ms. J. could barely open her mouth to eat breakfast. When she did get food into her mouth, it was difficult to swallow. Her roommate noted that her voice was of lower pitch and volume, as though she had something hot in her mouth. At the campus health clinic, the physician looked in Ms. J.'s mouth and then recommended hospitalization for additional tests and possibly surgery.

This case raises several questions:

1. Why did Ms. J.'s sore throat not go away by itself?
2. Why might she need surgery?
3. Does Ms. J.'s roommate have to worry about catching the illness?

See Appendix for answers.

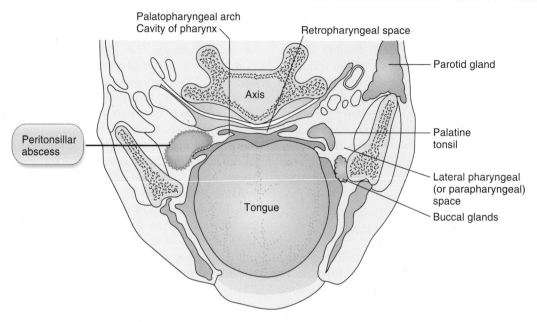

FIGURE 68-2. Axial view of the oropharynx through the level of the palatine tonsil.

CASE • C. was an active 9-year-old boy who returned from summer camp in good health. The next day, he awoke with the sensation that he had "something stuck" in his eye and conjunctival irritation. Later, C. developed blurred vision in the right eye, but his left eye felt fine. His mother took him to a physician when she noted that the inside of eyelids looked "bloody," and tears from that eye were blood tinged. The physician noted a tender, preauricular lymph node and a runny nose. After placing a patch over C.'s eye, the physician told the mother that C. had a "virus" and should improve in a few days.

This case raises two questions:

1. Could C.'s mother and father develop the eye infection?
2. Why did the physician not prescribe antibiotics for the infection?

See Appendix for answers.

CONJUNCTIVITIS

DIAGNOSIS

Conjunctivitis is a very common infection that physicians see primarily in children and young adults and must distinguish from more serious ocular conditions such as **keratitis** and **iritis**. Distinguishing features of keratitis include eye pain, photophobia, and impaired vision in addition to diffuse inflammation of the eye, a gritty irritation, and excessive lacrimation. When bacterial conjunctivitis occurs alone, the most common causative agents include nontypeable *H. influenzae*, adenovirus, pneumococcus, *M. catarrhalis*, and staphylococci.

Adenoviral and bacterial conjunctivitis can usually be distinguished clinically. Adenoviral disease is generally accompanied by upper respiratory symptoms. Also notable are hyperplasia of lymphoid follicles beneath the conjunctiva, hyperemia of the palpebral conjunctiva, and conjunctival hemorrhages on the globe. In many patients, adenoviral conjunctivitis is characterized by a diffuse

superficial keratitis that can result in transient blurring of the vision. Adenoviral keratoconjunctivitis is more commonly associated with preauricular lymphadenopathy. In C.'s case, a thorough history and physical examination enabled the physician to make the correct diagnosis.

Generally, organisms are introduced into the eye by direct contact with a carrier's hands. Rarely, the infecting agent is spread by respiratory droplets. Serious infections of the anterior portion of the eye are associated with herpes simplex virus, *P. aeruginosa* (contact lens wearers), and *Chlamydia trachomatis* (people in developing nations). In addition to the usual symptoms of conjunctivitis, herpes simplex virus and varicella-zoster virus cause vesicular lesions on the eyelid. Herpes simplex conjunctivitis progresses to keratitis in 50% of cases and is among the most common causes of severe corneal ulceration and acquired blindness in the United States. Because of the serious nature of herpes keratoconjunctivitis and the high risk of recurrence, patients must be referred to an ophthalmologist. Varicella-zoster conjunctivitis occurs in approximately 4% of children with chicken pox. Because the virus is delivered to the skin through the vascular compartment, vesicles present on the lateral aspect of the tip of the nose predict involvement of the eye and reflect involvement of the nasociliary branch of the first division of the trigeminal nerve. Thus, subsequent involvement of the anterior structures of the eye is inevitable.

TREATMENT

Symptomatic treatment of adenoviral conjunctivitis consists of removing exudates with saline-moistened cotton and patching to relieve pain. Antivirals active against adenovirus are not available. In patients with presumed bacterial conjunctivitis, application of an antimicrobial ointment four times a day improves the rate of resolution. Such ointments most often contain polymyxin and bacitracin.

Viral keratitis is treated with antivirals, either topically or systemically. Agents include idoxuridine, trifluorothymidine, vidarabine, acyclovir, and valacyclovir. Available data suggest that most herpetic corneal ulcers treated with trifluorothymidine applied every 1 to 2 hours resolve within 2 weeks. Close follow-up with an ophthalmologist is imperative.

Within 3 days, C.'s signs and symptoms were gone. The physician removed his eye patch, and no further treatment was needed. Had C. failed to improve, a reasonable approach would have been to reexamine the eye, looking for evidence of herpetic infection. If no herpes simplex virus was seen but exudate was still present, a trial of antibiotic ointment could have been administered.

CASE • Ms. M., an 18-year-old white college student, had lived in Minneapolis all her life. Six weeks after arriving at the University of Wisconsin, she experienced a mild sore throat and a low-grade temperature (37.8°C). While going to bed, she noted a small, slightly tender lump beneath the angle of her jaw. The next morning, the lump was the size of a walnut and more tender. She felt feverish, although her temperature was the same as the night before.

At the student health clinic, a physician told Ms. M. that she had cervical adenitis and that a throat culture and blood tests were needed to ascertain the bacterial agent of the infection (he suspected group A streptococcus) and determine the appropriate treatment. The blood tests were a complete blood count with differential and a screen for heterophile antibody.

This case raises several questions:

1. Is this a life-threatening illness?
2. Why did she need blood tests?
3. Should the physician prescribe antimicrobial drugs?

See Appendix for answers.

CERVICAL LYMPHADENITIS
ENCOUNTER AND ENTRY

Cervical adenitis, inflammation of the lymph nodes in the neck, can be caused by numerous infectious agents. Depending on the nature of the infecting agent in the lymph node, the influx of cells causing the swelling consists of neutrophils or histiocytes and lymphocytes. In general, bacterial infections result in necrosis of the center of the lymph node (**suppuration**). In contrast, viral infections of the cervical lymph nodes are rarely localized to one region, such as the neck; **lymphadenopathy** can be readily detected in other parts of the body.

DIAGNOSIS

Given the number of agents of this cervical adenitis, a physician's approach to a patient with the disease relies heavily on epidemiology. In certain parts of the world, infections with geographically restricted agents may occur (i.e., trypanosomiasis in tropical countries and *Pseudomonas pseudomallei* infection in Southeast Asia). Other important historical data include contact with animals (tularemia, plague, or cat scratch disease), immunization status (measles, rubella, or mumps), and exposure to tuberculosis.

Tuberculosis of the cervical lymph glands occurs in patients with pulmonary tuberculosis who inoculate the mouth through coughing. Rarely, it is acquired through the ingestion of milk contaminated with *Mycobacterium tuberculosis*. In the United States, most of *M. tuberculosis* infections (other than those in HIV-infected patients) occur in immigrants, Native Americans, and homeless individuals. In Ms. M.'s case, *M. tuberculosis* is unlikely on epidemiological grounds, and clinically the rapid onset of swelling is evidence against tuberculosis.

The major etiological agents that needed to be considered in Ms. M.'s case are group A streptococcus, *S. aureus*, and Epstein-Barr virus (EBV) infection. Clinically apparent primary infection with EBV usually causes sore throat, fever, and swelling in the neck. In addition, many patients experience headache, loss of appetite, malaise, and muscle aches. Extensive exudate in the posterior oral pharynx can be seen with EBV or with group A streptococcal infection. Because EBV infection does not localize to one side of the pharynx, clinical findings are generally bilateral. The test ordered by Ms. M.'s physician was a titer for **heterophile antibody**, which is present in about 90% of EBV cases. Another common, but nonspecific, finding is the demonstration of atypical lymphocytes on a complete blood count.

Most cases of bacterial cervical adenitis present with unilateral swelling of a single lymph node and minimal upper respiratory or constitutional complaints. The most common bacterial etiology for cervical adenitis is group

A streptococcus or *S. aureus*. Demonstration of group A streptococcus in the pharynx would impact the treatment plan because at least 10 days of antimicrobials are needed to prevent immune-mediated sequelae. Needle aspiration of the lymph node is a more definitive means of establishing the diagnosis.

CONCLUSION

Head and neck infections are among the most common diseases seen by primary care providers. Clinical history, physical exam, and an awareness of head and neck anatomy are essential for accurate diagnosis and management. Bacteria associated with infections in the head and neck regions are often commensals. Treatments for acute otitis media and sinusitis are major sources of antimicrobial use. Increasing antimicrobial resistance, especially against *S. pneumoniae*, can make treatment of such infections a challenge. Widespread use of conjugate pneumococcal vaccine appears to be beneficial in terms of preventing invasive pneumococcal infections as well as acute otitis media associated with vaccine strains.

Newer vaccines against nontypeable *H. influenzae* are under development and, if proven safe and effective, will likely offer further benefit in terms of preventing otitis media.

Suggested Readings

Benninger MS. Acute bacterial rhinosinusitis and otitis media: changes in pathogenicity following widespread use of pneumococcal conjugate vaccine. *Otolaryngol Head Neck Surg.* 2008;138:274–278.

Jansen AG, Hak E, Veenhoven RH, et al. Pneumococcal conjugate vaccines for preventing otitis media. *Cochrane Database Syst Rev.* 2009;15:CD001480.

Leibovitz E. The challenge of recalcitrant acute otitis media: pathogens, resistance, and treatment strategy. *Pediatr Infect Dis J.* 2007;26:S8–S11.

Prymula R, Schuerman L. 10-valent pneumonococcal nontypeable Haemophilus influenzae PD conjugate vaccine: Synflorix. *Expert Rev Vaccines.* 2009;8:1479–1500.

Rosenfeld RM, Andes D, Bhattacharyya N, et al. Clinical practice guideline: adult sinusitis. *Otolaryngol Head Neck Surg.* 2007;137:S1–S31.

Vieira F, Allen S, Stocks R, et al. Deep Neck Infection. *Otolaryngol Clin N Am.* 2008;41:459–483.

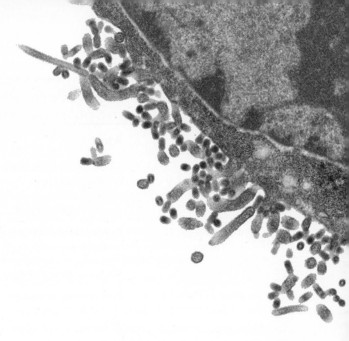

Chapter **69**

Sexually Transmitted Diseases

Jack Sobel and Jack Ebright

SEXUALLY TRANSMITTED DISEASES (STDs) are a broad but relatively well-defined group of infectious diseases, generally with acute manifestations that often progress to a chronic clinical picture. STDs rank among the most important of all infectious diseases with regard to the physical, psychological, and economic damage they cause to humans.

The agents of STDs are highly varied (Table 69-1); they include representatives of such different groups as the pyogenic cocci (gonococci), spirochetes (*Treponema pallidum* of syphilis), fastidious Gram-negative rods (*Haemophilus ducreyi* of chancroid), strict intracellular bacteria (*Chlamydia trachomatis*), viruses (herpes simplex viruses 1 and 2, human papillomaviruses [HPVs], and HIV), protozoa (*Trichomonas vaginalis*), and arthropods (scabies, pubic lice). There are other agents of STDs, but these are encountered less frequently in developed countries.

EPIDEMIOLOGY

The Magnitude of the Problem

Worldwide, nearly a million people acquire an STD, including the human immunodeficiency virus (HIV), every day, with the highest frequency among marginalized populations who have difficulty accessing health care services. Currently, more than 30 diseases are known to spread primarily through sexual activity. The socioeconomic costs are enormous, and the chronic medical conditions resulting from these infections include cervical cancer, liver disease, infertility, perinatal morbidity, childhood blindness, and chronic pelvic pain. Significantly, two of the Millennium Development Goals seek to address STD reduction. Goal 6 calls on nations to halt and begin to reverse the spread of HIV/AIDS by 2015. Goal 5 seeks to reduce maternal mortality by three quarters. Much progress with Goal 5 could be achieved by reducing pelvic inflammatory disease (PID), and life-threatening ectopic pregnancies, and by reducing transmission of HPV and subsequent risk of cervical cancer.

The United States has among the highest rates of STDs of any developed country in the world. At the beginning of the 21st century, more than 65 million people were living with an incurable STD, and an additional 15 million people were becoming infected with one or more STDs each year. Currently, approximately 19 million new infections occur each year in the United States, with a disproportionate number afflicting teenagers and minority populations (Table 69-2).

In 2008, 1,210,523 cases of sexually transmitted *C. trachomatis* infection were reported to the CDC, representing an increase of 9.2% compared with the rate in 2007. It is likely that at least some of the increase resulted from improved and increased screening for this infection. The rates in black women and men were 8 to 12 times higher than that in white women and men. Following a 74% decline in the rate of reported gonorrhea from 1975 to 1997, overall gonorrhea rates have plateaued over the past 11 years but remain well above the target of Healthy People 2010. In 2008, 336,742 cases were reported in the United States, only modestly decreased from that of 2007. Of ongoing great concern, adolescent girls, between the ages of 15 and 19 years, had the most Chlamydia and gonorrhea cases of any age group at 409,531. Both diseases impose enormous physical, emotional, and social costs, with an estimated US $1 billion annually spent to diagnose and treat gonorrhea alone. An estimated 50%

697

TABLE 69-1 Sexually Transmitted Diseases and Their Agents

Disease	Agent
Chlamydial infection	*Chlamydia trachomatis* (all biovars but L)
Gonorrhea	*Neisseria gonorrhoeae*
Genital herpes	Herpes simplex virus type II and type I
Warts, anogenital cancer	Human papillomavirus
Trichomoniasis	*Trichomonas vaginalis*
AIDS	HIV
Chancroid	*Haemophilus ducreyi*
Syphilis	*Treponema pallidum*
Lymphogranuloma venereum (LGV)	*C. trachomatis* (L biovars)
Granuloma inguinale	*Donovania granulomatis*
Candidiasis	*Candida albicans*
Bacterial vaginosis	*Gardnerella vaginalis*

TABLE 69-2 Dimensions of the STD Problem in the United States

STD	Reported New Cases or Estimates of Disease Burden
Chlamydial infection	1,210,523, 2008
Gonorrhea	336,742, 2008
Genital herpes	~45 million people currently infected
Papillomavirus infection	~20 million people currently infected[a]
Trichomoniasis	~9 million people currently infected
AIDS	42,655, 2007
Chancroid	25, 2008
Syphilis	13,500, 2008[b]
PID	~1 million, 2008

Note: Of all the STDs, only syphilis, gonorrhea, chlamydia, and AIDS are reportable in every state.
[a]50% of sexually active adults acquire HPV sometime in their lives.
[b]Primary or secondary syphilis.

of all preventable infertility among women is a result of infections with Chlamydia and gonorrhea. Compounding these problems is the increasing resistance of *Neisseria gonorrhoeae* to antibiotics for the past two decades. Chancroid, an STD that causes genital ulcer disease, has declined since 1987 but, along with syphilis, remains an important problem in certain geographic areas, such as the rural Southern United States and in inner cities, particularly among African Americans. In these settings, the cycle of infection reflects failure to diagnose and treat these diseases, a pattern that is driven by poverty and lack of access to health care. The rate of primary and secondary syphilis has increased each year since 2001, with 13,500 cases reported in 2008. Sixty-three percent of these cases occurred in men who have sex with men. Similarly, the number of congenital syphilis cases has increased from 339 in 2005 to 431 in 2008. The seroprevalence of genital herpes (HSV-2), on the other hand, has decreased from 21 to 17% over the past 20 years. An estimated 47 million North Americans are afflicted with genital herpes (HSV), 80% of whom are unaware of being infected.

Certain types of HPV infection have been recognized as the cause of cervical cancer. An estimated 27% of women in the United States are infected with genital HPV; the majority of these infections involve low-risk types associated with genital warts. Some, however, involve cervical dysplasias and cervical cancer. For reasons that are not understood but are likely to be linked to a functional immune system, only a small number of infected women progress to cervical cancer (15,000 per year), and one in three dies of this surgically treatable condition. Recently, two HPV type–specific vaccines have been approved for use in girls and women ages 11 to 26 years. The early studies showed protection against acquiring HPV infection and also from developing precancerous changes, indicating the potential for using a vaccine to prevent cervical cancer.

Population Dynamics

Efforts at prevention and control of STDs require an understanding of the factors that contribute to their spread and progression. Although STDs share a common mode of transmission, each of them presents unique challenges to diagnosis, therapy, and prevention. A large number of biological and social forces are also involved in the dynamics of STD transmission. To make sense of this multitude of variables, it is convenient to separate them according to a model proposed by May and Anderson, which states that the rate of movement of an STD throughout the population depends on (1) the **transmissibility** of the infectious agent, (2) the **rate of new partner acquisition** as well as the partners' sexual history, and (3) the **duration of infectiousness**. Each of the variables in this model is affected by biological, behavioral, and social risk factors.

The Transmissibility of the Agent (or Infectivity Rate)

The infectivity rate is defined as the risk of acquiring infection during a single contact with an infected partner. For each STD, the rate varies not only with the type of sexual activity but also the biologic properties of the infecting organism and, possibly, the immune status of the host. Behavioral factors, including drug and alcohol use, contraceptive practices, circumcision, and douching, also affect the infectivity rate. Consider HIV, which possesses specific surface molecules for attachment to host cell receptors found primarily on rectal epithelial cells as well as lymphocytes. Sexual behavior is an especially important factor in this instance since anal intercourse facilitates the spread of the virus. Several studies on risk-taking behavior among teenagers showed that risk-taking may be a characteristic of a subset of this population. Thus, smoking, alcohol and other substance abuse, a high number of sexual partners, and excessive automobile speeding are coassociated high-risk behaviors.

The Rate of New Partner Acquisition

The rate of new partner acquisition is defined as the number of new partners an individual has over a specified period of time. This parameter depends on the probability that any given partner may be infected. The greater the number of partners, the greater the chance that one of them is infected. Surveys indicate that most people have only a few sexual partners over their lifetime and that propagation of STD epidemics is actually attributable to a small number of individuals with a large number of sexual partners, referred to as the **core**. Thus, the number of sexual partners an individual has determines membership in the core. Common characteristics of STD core members include living in an urban environment, low socioeconomic status, age range between 15 and 30 years old, often minority ethnicity, and illicit drug use and prostitution. Sexual activity among core members sustains the diseases; sexual activity outside the core spreads the diseases.

Duration of Infectivity

The duration of infectivity is the length of time that an individual is capable of transmitting the infection. Included in this factor are biological characteristics of both the pathogen and the host. Some pathogens (e.g., chlamydiae) commonly cause asymptomatic disease; carriers of chlamydiae do not know they are infected and do not seek treatment. Thus, they remain able to transmit the disease. Antimicrobial sensitivity is also an important factor in duration of infectivity; if an agent is drug resistant, treatment will fail and the infective period will be increased.

The duration of infectivity also may depend upon patients' access to and use of health care as well as attitudes and behaviors of health care providers. Access to health care is affected by the location of the clinic, the speed with which care can be obtained, and the cost of the services. The likelihood that an individual will seek

TABLE 69-3 STD Complications Experienced Only by Women

Pelvic inflammatory disease
Infertility
Chronic pelvic pain
Ectopic pregnancy
Cervical cancer
Spontaneous abortion
Premature delivery
Congenital and neonatal infections of newborn

care is influenced by such factors as the stigma associated with using an STD facility, knowledge of the existence of the facility, and the perception of the quality of services provided. The availability of effective screening programs, **partner notification** systems, and effective treatment protocols as well as the willingness to change high-risk behavior also contributes to duration of infectivity.

Groups at Risk

The multiple, long-term, devastating consequences of STDs disproportionately affect women and infants (Table 69-3). STDs are especially prevalent among the young. In the United States, almost 50% of all STD cases occur in persons less than 25 years old. Sexually experienced teenagers are three times more likely to be diagnosed with PID than are 25- to 29-year-old women. Biological factors compound behavioral risk factors. Thus, features of the cervical anatomy of adolescents (primarily cervical ectopy) increase the likelihood of chlamydial or gonococcal infection and thereby the risk of PID.

The current STD epidemic in the United States also disproportionately affects minority groups. Both the incidence of STDs and long-term sequelae are consistently higher among nonwhites. This disparate impact has been observed for several decades. During the second half of the 1980s, syphilis increased enormously among low-income, inner-city heterosexuals and their children. In the 1980s, the incidence of gonorrhea decreased in whites of both sexes but increased in African Americans. A survey conducted from 1988 to 1994 showed that African American males were at least two times more likely than whites to be seropositive to herpes simplex virus type 2 (HSV-2). The difference between females was even greater.

ENCOUNTER AND ENTRY

Most of the STD-causing agents enter the body at local sites, through the mucosal or squamous epithelial layers of the cervix, urethra, rectum, oral pharynx or, to a lesser extent, the vagina. An exception is HIV. Although HIV is transmitted primarily by sexual contact, contaminated blood products or hypodermic needles are also a source of infection.

Nearly all the agents of STDs are relatively sensitive to chemical and physical factors and are practically never found free in the environment. Animal reservoirs are also unknown for most of these agents, thus the asymptomatic human carrier is the most frequent reservoir. The limited distribution of these agents makes these diseases theoretical candidates for eradication, but formidable medical, social, and behavioral obstacles lie in the way of achieving it.

SPREAD AND MULTIPLICATION

All the agents that cause STDs are able to resist the host's nonspecific defense mechanisms and are infectious, that is, they are able to attach to and enter tissue with relative ease. The fact that chronic manifestations of STDs are relatively frequent indicates that the agents often cause asymptomatic disease and are not easily eliminated by specific immune responses. The strategies employed to withstand antimicrobial defenses are varied and should be reviewed by reading the chapters on specific agents.

DAMAGE

The acute manifestations of the most frequent STDs fall into two groups: (1) **mucopurulent cervicitis and urethritis**, as in gonorrhea and chlamydial infection and (2) **genital ulcer disease**, as in syphilis, chancroid, and genital herpes.

With the exception of HIV, the STD-causing agents tend to cause primary lesions at or near the site of entry. It is not uncommon for these lesions to be so indolent as to go unnoticed or to be located at an anatomical site as to be invisible. As a consequence, diagnosis and treatment are often delayed, enabling the transmission and progression of the disease to continue.

The most serious consequences of STDs relate to their progression to chronic infections. These include

- **Pelvic inflammatory disease (PID)**, an ascending infection of the uterus and fallopian tubes most commonly caused by gonococci and chlamydia
- **Anogenital cancer**, including **cervical cancer**, caused by some HPV types
- Secondary and tertiary **syphilis**
- **Recurrent herpes** infection

Many of these chronic infections cause additional adverse sequelae, including

- **Fallopian tube scarring and adhesions** of surrounding tissues, resulting in **ectopic pregnancy**, **infertility**, and **chronic pelvic pain**
- **Congenital diseases** such as in syphilis, herpes, papillomatosis, and chlamydial infection

- **Increased risk of acquiring HIV**, due to genital ulcers (found in syphilis, chancroid, and herpes) or altered genital mucosa (found in gonorrhea and chlamydial infection)
- **Adverse outcomes of pregnancy** including premature termination, fetal wastage, low birth weight, and premature rupture of membranes

SELECTED SEXUALLY TRANSMITTED DISEASES
Pelvic Inflammatory Disease

PID, or **female upper reproductive tract infection**, is an ascending infection of the uterus, fallopian tubes, ovaries, and adjacent peritoneal linings. PID frequently results in severe, irreversible sequelae such as infertility, ectopic pregnancy, and chronic pelvic pain. A case of postchlamydial PID is described in Chapter 14.

Accurate data on the incidence and prevalence of PID have been difficult to obtain, because the clinical diagnosis of acute symptomatic disease is imprecise. In addition, approximately 60% of cases are subclinical, during which women experience no or only mild symptoms and do not seek medical care until late sequelae such as infertility or an ectopic pregnancy occurs. It is estimated that approximately 1 million women experience an episode of acute PID each year in the United States, and more than 100,000 become infertile each year as a result of the infection. The incidence of PID is particularly high among young, nonwhite, single, or divorced women from urban areas.

Pathobiology

The events that lead to PID are not well understood. It is likely that almost all cases involve the ascending spread of infection from the lower to the upper genital tract. A proportion of cases progress to develop chronic sequelae.

Most cases of PID are caused by the sexually transmitted organisms *N. gonorrhoeae* or *C. trachomatis* and follow cervicitis and urethritis. Other organisms implicated in the etiology of PID include *Mycoplasma hominis*, *Mycoplasma genitalium*, *Ureaplasma urealyticum*, and numerous aerobic and anaerobic bacteria such as *Escherichia coli* and *Prevotella* species. These bacteria are referred to as **endogenous** because they are often isolated from the lower genital tract in the absence of any disease. Little is known about the pathogenesis of these infections. Usually, a primary episode of gonococcal and chlamydial PID is followed by subsequent episodes of PID caused by the endogenous organisms. The pathogenesis of gonococcal and chlamydial PID probably includes nonspecific inflammatory responses to bacterial invasion that result in tissue damage, as well as the specific immune responses to gonococci or chlamydiae.

In addition, several anatomical factors appear to be important in the pathogenesis of gonococcal or chlamydial PID:

- Gonococcal or chlamydial cervical infection may damage the endocervical canal, break down the mucus plug in the endocervix, and allow these pathogens, as well as endogenous vaginal organisms, to ascend into the upper genital tract.
- Adolescent females have a larger **zone of ectopy** (extension of columnar epithelium from the endocervical canal to the ectocervix) than do older women. This area of ectopy, unprotected by cervical mucus, results in increased susceptibility to gonococcal and chlamydial infections because columnar cells are preferential sites of microbial attachment and invasion.

Other host defenses are probably useful in preventing centripetal spread of organisms. These include tubal ciliary movement (unidirectional toward the uterus), flow of mucus in the tubal lumen (toward the uterus), and myometrial contractions during menses (resulting in sloughing of the endometrium).

Several additional risk factors appear to be important in the pathogenesis of PID. **Oral contraceptives** may decrease the risk of chlamydial (but perhaps not gonococcal) PID, whereas intrauterine devices appear to increase the risk of PID within the first few months of placement. Vaginal douching also is associated with an increased risk. Most cases of gonococcal (and possibly chlamydial) PID occur during or near the end of menses; hormonal changes during the menstrual cycle may lead to changes in the cervical mucus plug, permitting passage of organisms, particularly when estrogen levels are high and progesterone levels are relatively low. The reflux of infected blood during menstrual uterine contractions may also provide a route of entry into the fallopian tubes.

Types of PID

Gonococcal PID Investigators studying the pathogenesis and epidemiology of gonococcal infections have found strain typing of *N. gonorrhoeae* to be very useful. Strain typing is based upon two methodologies: (1) defining the specific amino acid and nucleoside nutritional requirements of the isolate (auxotype) and (2) serotyping based upon another membrane protein known as porin, which can be divided into two classes, PorA and PorB, each of which is composed of many serovars. Interestingly, strain variation of *N. gonorrhoeae* based on porin classification appears to be associated with the likelihood of disease progression to PID or disseminated infection.

The pathophysiological changes that occur have been studied in fallopian tube explants exposed to gonococci (Chapter 14). In the presence of these organisms, motility of ciliated epithelial cells slows and ultimately ceases. Ciliated cells are selectively sloughed from the epithelial surface, apparently due to the toxic action of lipopolysaccharide or murein fragments. Gonococci attach to nonciliated epithelial cells via pili after which they are internalized, move to the basal portion of the cells, and exit into the subepithelium to cause inflammation.

Progressive mucosal cell damage and submucosal invasion are accompanied by a vigorous polymorphonuclear leukocyte response contributing to local inflammation, microabscess formation, and purulent exudate. Tissue damage appears to result especially from two components of the gonococcal cell surface: lipooligosaccharide (LOS) and peptidoglycan. The toxic portion of LOS almost certainly is the lipid A portion.

Chlamydial PID The steps in infection of chlamydial PID include attachment of the organisms to cells, probably via specific receptor–ligand interactions, but these steps have not been confirmed. The chlamydial major outer membrane protein appears to be involved in these interactions. The organisms actively induce uptake by stimulating endocytosis. Phagolysosomal fusion does not occur, probably owing to the function of ill-defined surface components of the **elementary bodies** (the infectious form of the organism). The chlamydia-containing phagosomes, referred to as **inclusions**, are visible in histologic preparations. Within the phagosomes, elementary bodies differentiate into **reticulate bodies** (the metabolic form of the organism). Ultimately, the reticulate bodies reorganize into new elementary bodies and, in time, are released from the host cell to infect adjacent cells. The life cycle of these organisms is described in detail in Chapter 27.

Chlamydial infections incite a greater mononuclear immune response than those caused by gonococci, but neutrophils are also seen, mainly in the early phases of the inflammatory response. The chronic sequelae of chlamydial disease may relate not only to the inflammatory response elicited but also to the incomplete immunity against reinfection.

Coinfections by Gonococci and Chlamydiae The high prevalence of gonococcal and chlamydial coinfection has prompted recommendations that patients with either infection be treated for both. Experimentally, simultaneous gonococcal infection facilitates chlamydial replication in cervical epithelia by about 100-fold. It has been proposed that stimulation of endocytosis in nonciliated epithelial cells by the first parasite leads to alterations in the surface structure of these cells, which allow ready uptake of the second parasite. Thus, one pathogen may facilitate the engulfment of the second one.

Bacterial Vaginosis and PID Bacterial vaginosis (**BV**), the most common vaginal infection worldwide, is an asymptomatic or symptomatic disruption of the normal vaginal flora characterized clinically by a malodorous vaginal discharge. The normally dominant colonizing lactobacilli (especially species that produce hydrogen peroxide) are markedly reduced, while a variety of species including *Gardnerella vaginalis*, *Atopobium vaginalae*, anaerobic streptococci, *Prevotella* species, and genital mycoplasmas increase in numbers. Several investigators have demonstrated an association of BV and PID independent of chlamydial and gonococcal infections.

HIV and STDs

The AIDS pandemic has focused attention on STDs for several reasons. The relationships between HIV infection and other STDs are complex and intriguing. They explain, in part, the global spread of the HIV epidemic and may provide insights into the pathogenesis of all sexually transmitted infections. Furthermore, these relationships have compelling implications in efforts to control HIV.

Aside from sexual behavior, the two obvious relationships between HIV infection and other STDs are (1) increased transmission of HIV due to other STDs and (2) alteration in the natural history, diagnosis, or response to therapy of other STDs in the presence of HIV infection.

The Bidirectional Interplay between HIV and STDs

The risk of HIV transmission is increased three- to five-fold in the presence of both the genital ulcer diseases (e.g., genital herpes and syphilis) and nonulcerative diseases such as gonorrhea and chlamydial infections as well as vaginal diseases including BV, candida vaginitis, and trichomonal vaginitis. HPV infection and anogenital warts do not appear to facilitate HIV transmission, perhaps because they do not usually cause breaks in the skin or mucous membranes.

The compromised immune system of patients with AIDS may result in more severe manifestations of other STDs. Mucocutaneous genital and perirectal herpes infections, for example, may cause extensive and persistent ulcers that can be more difficult to treat in HIV-positive than in HIV-negative patients. Molluscum contagiosum, a cutaneous poxvirus infection, is seen more often in HIV-infected persons and can cause extensive and disfiguring lesions. Kaposi sarcoma, a malignancy that is at least partially attributable to a sexually transmitted herpesvirus (human herpesvirus type 8), was one of the first AIDS-defining conditions recognized at the outset of the epidemic in the United States. Genital warts due to papillomavirus may be extensive and more likely associated with cervical dysplasia; and chancroid may be less responsive to treatment and heal more slowly in HIV-infected patients.

In the past, the potential significance of the bidirectional interplay between HIV infection and other STDs has not been fully appreciated. Because HIV coinfection prolongs infectivity and severity of certain STDs, and the same STDs facilitate transmission of HIV, the two infections amplify one another. The increases in HIV and STD incidence may well contribute to the rapid spread of HIV in some heterosexual populations and may represent "epidemiological synergy" between diseases that are linked by a common mode of transmission.

How Is the Transmission of HIV Enhanced by Other STDs?

It is likely that the inflammatory changes that accompany STDs facilitate HIV entry by altering the barrier function of the genital mucosal epithelium. In fact, HIV has been isolated directly from genital ulcers in both men and women. It is recognized that intercourse during menses increases risk of HIV transmission, therefore it is likely that mucosal irritation, friability, and bleeding may shorten the route to target cells and impair the function of natural defenses. These defenses normally include an intact mucus layer and tight junctions between epithelial cells. Ulcer-producing STDs provide an easy portal of entry for HIV, and all STDs with enhanced superficial inflammation provide inflammatory cells as targets for viral invasion and dissemination. Local inflammation, even in the absence of ulcer formation, also results in proinflammatory cytokine production, which can enhance local HIV replication.

Molecular interactions may also contribute to the pathogenesis of HIV infection and other STDs. For example, HSV may potentiate HIV infection by stimulating the expression of surface receptors needed for HIV attachment. Conversely, HIV gene products have been shown to be potent intracellular transactivating factors. These factors may enhance the growth of herpesvirus and HPV.

PREVENTION AND CONTROL

Prevention and control of STDs is a multifaceted problem. Depending upon the circumstances, the objective may be prevention of infection, transmission, disease, or disease progression. These objectives can be achieved through a number of approaches: effective vaccines, interruption of transmission and progression through behavioral interventions, and curative medical interventions. The tools necessary to achieve these objectives include information about the prevalence of known high-risk behaviors and corresponding effective behavioral interventions; safe, efficacious vaccines; diagnostic tests; effective therapeutics; an efficient network of health care facilities; and trained, effective health care professionals.

In reality, almost all of these tools are still far from being fully developed and available. For some STDs, medical therapy is either unavailable (e.g., viral diseases) or problematic (e.g., antimicrobial resistance). More encouraging, however, is the prevention of two STDs by means of vaccines, that is, for hepatitis B and HPV.

Development and use of inexpensive, simple, rapid diagnostic tests that are appropriate for resource-limited settings, such as inner cities (where the majority of STDs occur), is a fundamental component of STD prevention and control. Such tests are particularly important for diagnosis of STDs in women. In resource-limited settings, clinical algorithms (syndromic approach) based on recognition of symptoms and signs of STDs have been useful for diagnosis and treatment of urethritis and genital ulcer disease in men but are far less useful for diagnosis of STDs in women. The special requirements of resource-limited settings force us to conclude that useful diagnostics tests should be (1) inexpensive: provider cost less than US $1.00 per patient; (2) simple: no equipment and minimal training required; (3) rapid: results available before the patient leaves the clinic; (4) performed on convenient specimens: simple to collect, socioculturally acceptable, no separation or preparation needed; (5) able to utilize stable reagents: long shelf life, no refrigeration required; (6) packaged simply: functional, low cost; and (7) appropriately sensitive and specific: dependent, in part, on the potential morbidity and cost for undetected infection and the cost of the resulting treatment. Examples of diagnostic tests with the appropriate format are the occult fecal blood card and the urine glucose dipstick. Recently, progress has been made in developing methods to screen for sexually transmitted chlamydial infections using DNA amplification methods applied to samples of urine. In addition, we now have relatively easily performed and rapid assays for detecting HIV infection. Obviously, much more progress is needed in expanding the number of such tests and in reducing their cost.

Treatment of STDs would be greatly enhanced if we had safe, effective antimicrobial agents, which could be administered as single oral doses. Noncompliance is a formidable problem when treatment regimens involve multiple-dose therapy for prolonged periods, especially when treatment exceeds the duration of symptoms. Again, therapies should be inexpensive, have a long shelf life, have minimal side effects, and be safe for use during pregnancy. Theoretically, this approach should decrease the likelihood of antibiotic resistance. An example of such an advance is the recent development of azithromycin (an erythromycin-like macrolide antibiotic), a single-dose (although relatively expensive) treatment for chlamydial infection.

There is general consensus that prevention of sexually transmitted STDs, including HIV infection, will be facilitated by the development of safe and effective female-controlled **chemical barriers** called topical **microbicides**. A microbicide effective not only against the most common agents of STDs but also those of genital ulcers would have a substantial impact on HIV transmission. The male condom, which is very effective if used consistently and correctly, requires male partner cooperation and is too often not accepted or used. Just as hormonal contraceptives and intrauterine devices have dramatically enhanced women's ability to avoid unwanted pregnancy, effective female-controlled microbicides are urgently needed to enhance a woman's ability to avoid STDs. In addition, effective chemical barriers may reduce female-to-male as well as male-to-female transmission.

The ideal microbicide should be colorless, odorless, tasteless, stable, easy to store, fast acting, effective pre- and postcoitus, inexpensive, available without prescription, and safe for repeated use. Such microbicides could ideally be formulated with or without spermicidal activity. Noncontraceptive microbicides would be very useful for women who wish to become pregnant.

The role of the health care provider is an integral part of an STD prevention and control program. Currently, many medical school curricula lack focused STD training. Ideally, an integrated approach, including basic biomedical, clinical, epidemiological, and behavioral training, would be most effective.

CONCLUSION

In summary, the STD epidemic is a complex, multifaceted problem that mandates multifaceted approaches for prevention and control. Vaccines, diagnostics, therapeutics, health care delivery systems, and behavioral interventions will each play an important part in achieving these interrelated goals.

Suggested Readings

Centers for Disease Control and Prevention. Sexually transmitted diseases treatment guidelines 2006. *MMWR Morb Mortal Wkly Rep.* 2006;55 (No. RR 11):1–94.

Centers for Disease Control and Prevention. Sexually transmitted disease surveillance, 2008. Atlanta, GA: U.S. department of Health and Human Services; 2009.

Global Strategy for the prevention and control of sexually transmitted infections: 2006–2015: breaking the chain of transmission 2007. World Health Organization.

Lareau SM, Beigi RH. Pelvic inflammatory disease and tuboovarian abscess. *Infect Dis Clin N Am.* 2008;22:693–708.

Marrazzo JM, Handsfield HH, Sparling PF. *Neisseria gonorrhoeae.* In: Mandell, Douglas and Bennett, eds. *Principles and Practice of Infectious Diseases.* 7th ed. Philadelphia, PA: Churchill Livingston Elsevier; 2010:2753–2770.

Piper JM. Prevention of sexually transmitted infections in women. *Infect Dis Clin N Am.* 2008;22:619–635.

Stamm WE, Batteiger BE. *Chlamydia trachomatis* (Trachoma, perinatal infections, lymphogranuloma venereum, and other genital infections). In: Mandell, Douglas and Bennett, eds. *Principles and Practice of Infectious Diseases.* 7th ed. Philadelphia, PA: Churchill Livingston Elsevier; 2010:2443–2461.

Chapter 70

Infections of the Immunocompromised Patient

Michael A. Lane and Edgar Turner Overton

A PERSON is considered to be immunocompromised when suffering either from the disruption of specific defenses of a particular organ or system or from systemic abnormalities of humoral or cellular immunity. Often, it is possible to predict the general type of infection an immunocompromised patient is likely to acquire based on the component of the defense mechanisms that is disturbed. However, when the immune deficiency is general and profound, the patient could acquire one or several of a number of different infections.

Researchers have learned a great deal about the body's normal defense mechanisms by studying what happens when they become impaired. In fact, our knowledge of the relative importance of humoral and cellular immunity is derived from observing patients with immunodeficiencies. Thus, we note that persons with agammaglobulinemia are especially susceptible to extracellular bacteria that cause acute inflammation, whereas people with defects in cell-mediated immunity fall prey more readily to viruses, fungi, mycobacteria, and other intracellular agents of chronic diseases. Many of the major medical advances experienced, including bone marrow and organ transplantation, are made possible through the iatrogenic disruption of body defense systems. As a result, opportunistic infections have assumed immense importance in modern medicine. The practical need to understand the risk factors associated with defects in defenses against invading microorganisms cannot be overestimated.

Most infections acquired by immunocompromised patients are caused by commonly known pathogens. However, severe forms of immunocompromise open the door to infections by organisms not typically considered virulent, including many in the normal flora or in the environment. Unexpected extremes have been reached in scattered cases of infections of heart valves and other vital tissues transmitted by mushrooms (in their mycelial form) and colorless algae. This underscores how the definition of virulence must include not only the pathogenic properties of microorganisms but also the range of susceptibility of the patient.

This chapter recapitulates the consequences of risk factors mentioned throughout the book, presenting them according to the type of abnormality or defect in specific defense mechanisms.

Patients who have undergone bone marrow transplantation provide an extreme example of the profound disturbances of normal body defenses that can predispose to infection. For example, disruption of anatomic barriers by radiation and chemotherapy, resulting in skin and mucosal ulcerations, provides entry sites for invasive organisms. Severe neutropenia is characteristic of the period immediately following transplantation, and although granulocyte recovery begins in the third week after the procedure, qualitative defects remain for some time. Cellular immune function, which in the bone marrow recipient depends on donor macrophages and T cells, remains abnormal for several months. It is also compromised by the use of immunosuppressive therapy to treat graft-versus-host disease. Although IgG and IgM levels may return to normal after 45 months, B-cell function remains disturbed, and antibody levels to specific organisms, such as pneumococci, can remain depressed for years.

In the following sections, we review the disturbances in various body defense mechanisms and their consequences in affected individuals.

CASE • At 17 years of age, V. came to the hospital with fever and bruising and was eventually diagnosed with acute myelogenous leukemia (AML). Induction chemotherapy was initiated with cytarabine and daunorubicin to achieve remission of the AML. Seven days after the initiation of chemotherapy, V. developed burning mouth pain and white plaques. The mucosa subsequently sloughed off, leaving painful ulcers throughout her mouth.

With chemotherapy, V.'s AML went into remission, and **allogeneic** (nontwin) bone marrow transplantation was attempted in the hope of achieving a cure. Five days after transplantation, V. had no detectable circulating white blood cells, and 2 days thereafter, she became febrile. She denied any localizing signs or symptoms such as headache, cough, chest pain, abdominal pain, dysuria, or diarrhea. V. continued to complain of oral pain and difficulty swallowing as well as fatigue and malaise. Blood cultures taken at that time were positive for *Escherichia coli*. She responded well to antibiotics, and her temperature dropped rapidly.

Eight days later, V. again became febrile, and blood cultures were positive for *Candida albicans*. Although she was placed on antifungal therapy, she remained febrile for 4 days. However, her temperature rapidly dropped to normal after removal of a venous catheter that had been implanted in her subclavian vein for intravenous drug administration. Nineteen days posttransplantation, white blood cells started to appear in her circulation, indicating that the transplanted marrow had successfully engrafted and was beginning to function.

Thirty-one days after transplantation, V. complained of shortness of breath, and a chest radiograph showed a diffuse pneumonia. A lung biopsy revealed the presence of *Pneumocystis jiroveci*. Treatment with trimethoprim/sulfamethoxazole was started, and she slowly responded to therapy. She was discharged from the hospital 2 months after her transplantation, but 10 days later she developed a painful cutaneous herpes zoster infection. Following treatment, V. regained her health and remained well for the next 3 months, although she had developed mild chronic graft-versus-host disease. She returned again to the hospital 5 months after her transplantation, complaining of fever and shortness of breath. Physical examination and chest radiograph revealed a lobar pneumonia, and both blood and sputum cultures grew *Streptococcus pneumoniae*. She responded well to penicillin therapy and remained healthy thereafter.

This case raises several questions:

1. What risk factors predispose V. to the bacteremia with *E. coli*?
2. What risk factors predisposed V. to the fungemia with *C. albicans*?
3. What risk factors predisposed V. to the pneumonia with *P. jiroveci*?
4. What risk factors predisposed V. to the pneumonia and bacteremia with *S. pneumoniae*?

See Appendix for answers.

ABNORMALITIES OF HOST DEFENSE BARRIERS

The skin and mucous membranes provide an important barrier that prevents microbial invasion. The body's normal commensal flora also provides a barrier against infection. Those tissues not only serve as structural barriers preventing invasion by possible pathogens but also have other key antimicrobial factors preventing infection, including pH, temperature, local protective bacterial flora, and proteins with antimicrobial activity such as lysozyme. Disruption of local mechanical barriers can result from instrumentation (e.g., intravenous or urinary catheterization), surgery, drugs (including chemotherapeutic agents), or burns. Chemotherapeutic agents pose a specific problem because their antiproliferative properties have deleterious effects on tissues with a high turnover rate, such as the mucosal surfaces. That tissue damage gives infecting organisms a portal of entry into the body. Furthermore, the commensal flora resident at the entry site can also invade and cause infection. For example, breaching the skin with intravenous catheters can introduce *Staphylococcus epidermidis* into the bloodstream, with subsequent septicemia.

The consequences of immunological or biochemical impairment at the level of the integuments are less well understood. For example, it is not known with certainty if secreted IgA immunoglobulins or lysozyme contributes to resistance to infection. The suspicion is, however, that people with IgA deficiency are more prone to sinusitis, pneumonia, and gastrointestinal infections (e.g., giardiasis). Individuals with genetic defects in lysozyme have not been found.

Burns are an extreme example of the critical role of intact integument on resistance to infection. Among patients who survive the initial burn, infections are the leading cause of mortality. Necrotic skin tissue is an excellent culture medium for bacteria, thus increasing the size of the inoculum. In addition, the thermal injury itself leads to a poorly understood suppression of white blood cell function. It is not surprising that skin and subcutaneous tissue infections and septicemias with *Staphylococcus aureus* or *Pseudomonas aeruginosa* are major challenges in the management of patients with severe burns.

The normal bacterial flora can be disrupted by antibiotic treatment, which may in turn lead to superinfection by organisms resistant to the antibiotic being administered.

This happens particularly often in the intestine, sometimes as a result of a patient receiving an antibiotic to treat another infection. The antibiotic alters the normal flora of the gastrointestinal tract, allowing the overgrowth of resistant pathogens such as *Clostridium difficile*, which can cause severe diarrhea and toxic megacolon.

Some tissues possess additional local defense mechanisms. In the lungs, for example, the combination of mucous production by goblet cells and the ciliary activity of the respiratory epithelial cells traps microbes and carries them out of the lungs. Disruption of that disposal system predisposes to pneumonia. An extreme example is cystic fibrosis, a chronic hereditary condition characterized by the production of abnormally thick mucus. Cystic fibrosis patients experience recurrent pneumonia, and their lungs are often colonized by the opportunistic bacterium *P. aeruginosa*. Most patients are unable to clear the organism from the respiratory tract, causing repeated episodes of pneumonia, which may lead to respiratory failure and death.

INNATE IMMUNITY

Once the first line of defense is breached, the innate immune system assumes the critical role in checking the spread of invasive disease. This arm of the immune system is nonspecific and reacts rapidly (within the first 96 hours of infection) to the presence of foreign antigens. Complement activation occurs immediately and leads to the generation of soluble molecules that direct the innate immune response. Soluble mediators such as opsonins and chemoattractants recruit neutrophils, macrophages, and natural killer (NK) cells to the site of inflammation and infection.

The **neutrophil** is the key player of the innate immune response and kills pathogens either directly by phagocytosis or indirectly by recruitment of other cells through the release of cytokines. Defects in neutrophil activity, either qualitative or quantitative, predispose patients to infection with certain bacteria and fungi (Table 70-1). Examples of defects include a decreased number of phagocytic cells, impairment of their chemotactic response, and lowering of their ability to engulf and kill microorganisms.

Granulocytopenia, which is a decrease in the number of circulating neutrophils, clearly predisposes to infection. **Myelosuppressive cancer chemotherapy** is the most common cause of granulocytopenia in hospitals. Neutropenia also occurs in bone marrow failure caused by aplasia, autoimmune disease, hematological

TABLE 70-1 Common Causes of Compromised Immunity and Their Consequences

Impaired Function	Defect	Common Infecting Organisms	Sites Commonly Affected
Barrier	Damaged integument	Pyogenic cocci, enteric bacteria	Skin, subcutaneous connective tissue
	Loss of normal microbial flora	Pyogenic cocci, enteric bacteria, *Clostridium difficile*, *Candida albicans*	Skin, intestine
Phagocyte functions	Chemotactic dysfunction	*Staphylococcus aureus*, enteric bacteria	Skin, respiratory tract
	Neutropenia	*S. aureus*, enteric bacteria	Skin, respiratory tract
	Abnormal microbial killing	*S. aureus*, *Aspergillus* species	Skin, visceral abscesses
Humoral functions	Hypogammaglobulinemia	Pyogenic bacteria	Any site
	IgA deficiency	Pyogenic bacteria	Respiratory tract
	Lack of spleen	Pneumococcus, *Haemophilus influenzae*	Septicemia
	Complement deficiencies (early components)	Pyogenic bacteria	Bacteremia, meningitis
	Complement deficiencies (late components)	*Neisseria* species	Meningitis, arthritis
Cell-mediated immunity	Abnormal number or function of macrophages or T cells	Viruses, fungi, protozoa, intracellular bacteria	Any site

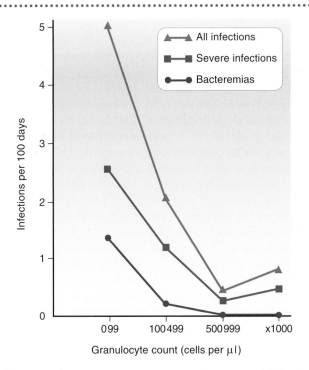

FIGURE 70-1. Relationship between the incidence of infection and the absolute neutrophil count in patients with acute leukemia. The incidence of infection rises as the neutrophil count decreases.

malignancy, or invasion of the bone marrow by a tumor. Serious infections, including bacteremia and invasive fungal infections, are a frequent and often life-threatening problem in neutropenic hosts. There is a direct correlation between the number of circulating neutrophils and the risk of infection. The rate of infection increases significantly as the number of neutrophils decreases (Fig. 70-1). Additionally, *the duration of neutropenia increases a person's risk to develop a severe infection not only from bacterial pathogens but also fungi and viruses.* Chemotherapy and radiation can disrupt the integrity of the skin and gastrointestinal tract, increasing the risk for these infections. The organisms responsible are usually derived from the patient's own flora, particularly that of the intestinal tract. Gram-negative enteric bacilli and staphylococci are the most common bacterial pathogens. Prolonged antibacterial therapy also predisposes to colonization by fungi. *Candida* and *Aspergillus* infections are the most important causes of fungal sepsis and mortality among patients taking antibacterial drugs for extended periods.

Chemotactic dysfunction of phagocytes is uncommon and usually congenital in origin. Defective neutrophil chemotaxis may result from inadequate signaling of the neutrophil, abnormalities of neutrophil receptors for chemoattractants, or disorders in cell locomotion. Patients with chemotactic dysfunction are at risk for recurrent cutaneous or deep abscesses due to *S. aureus*.

Abnormalities in microbial killing power are usually inherited disorders. Of the many disorders that have been described, the most common is **chronic granulomatous disease (CGD)**, a condition in which neutrophils fail to mount a respiratory burst during phagocytosis. The cause of CGD is a defect in the enzyme **NADPH oxidase** that results in hydrogen peroxide not being formed. Patients with the disorder are at risk of infection with **catalase-positive organisms**, especially *S. aureus*, fungi, and granuloma formation. Infections in these patients are usually localized to the respiratory tract, the skin, the liver, and the lymph nodes. The following organisms are the most commonly encountered pathogens in patients with CGD: *S. aureus*, *Burkholderia cepacia*, *Serratia marcescens*, *Nocardia* species, and *Aspergillus* species. Those organisms are relatively resistant to the **nonoxidative killing** mechanisms of neutrophils, which include antibacterial proteins and peptides stored in the **neutrophil-specific granules**. On the other hand, bacteria-like pneumococci and streptococci, which generate their own hydrogen peroxide but have no catalase, are likely to be killed by the defective neutrophils. CGD neutrophils contain the enzyme **myeloperoxidase**, which converts hydrogen peroxide made by the bacteria's metabolism to produce lethal radicals. Patients with CGD are given antibiotic prophylaxis with trimethoprim/sulfamethoxazole to prevent infections of bacterial pathogens, particularly *S. aureus*.

ADAPTIVE IMMUNITY

The **adaptive immune system** requires time to develop a functional response to invasive pathogens. That response is highly specific to the antigen of the invasive pathogen and is directed by antigen-specific lymphocytes. Adaptive immunity has both cellular and humoral components. **CD4+ T cells** have several important roles. CD4+ T cells are critical to antigen recognition. CD4+ T cells are also involved in the subsequent development of cellular immunity, which is key to the destruction of intracellular pathogens such as viruses, fungi, and mycobacteria. CD4+ T cells are also involved in the development of humoral immunity, which protects us from extracellular pathogens.

T cells play a critical role in the development of both the cellular and humoral components of the adaptive immune response. Once stimulated by antigen recognition, CD4+ T cells differentiate into Th1 or Th2 cells, which play an immunomodulator role. **Th1 cells** produce **interferon-γ** and **interleukin 2 (IL-2)**, which activate CD8+ T cells, macrophages, and NK cells to clear intracellular infections through lysis of infected cells. **Th2 cells** produce **IL-4, IL-5, and IL-10**, which cause differentiation of B cells and a highly specific antibody response against extracellular pathogens. Additionally, specialized populations of memory T and B cells develop as a result of the adaptive immune response. Those long-lived lymphocytes provide immunologic memory to respond rapidly to the re-presentation of the antigen that initially stimulated their development. The progressive depletion of CD4+ T cells in HIV infection and the development of opportunistic infections in AIDS exemplify the critical role of T cells in the maintenance of the adaptive immune response.

Abnormalities in Humoral Defense

The **humoral immune response** protects the host from extracellular bacteria that have evaded the cellular component of the innate immune system. The immediate response is carried out by the **complement** cascade, a nonspecific response leading to the production of nonspecific molecules that serve as opsonins and chemoattractants and effect bacteria lysis. The subsequent expansion of the B-cell population produces highly specific immunoglobulins that coat the extracellular microorganisms and lead to their clearance by the spleen. As stated previously, a subset of the B cells develops into memory cells to provide the host with long-term protection against subsequent infections.

Immunoglobulin deficiency can be congenital (e.g., **Bruton X-linked agammaglobulinemia**) or acquired (e.g., **common variable immunodeficiency**). Acquired hypogammaglobulinemia also arises as a result of conditions that lead to protein loss (e.g., nephrotic syndrome, intestinal lymphangiectasia), cancers of cells that make immunoglobulins (e.g., multiple myeloma, chronic lymphocytic leukemia), or burns. Defective B-lymphocyte function also occurs following bone marrow transplantation, as in V.'s case. The predominant infectious diseases seen in persons with immunoglobulin deficiencies are recurrent infections of the upper and lower respiratory tract caused by encapsulated bacteria, reflecting the important role of antibodies in opsonization of encapsulated bacteria such as *S. pneumoniae* and *Haemophilus influenzae*.

The rare cases of **complement deficiencies** are characterized by predisposition to infection with encapsulated bacteria. *Neisseria* species are a special problem for patients with *deficiencies of any of the late complement components (C6, C7, C8, or C9)* because complement-mediated lysis is required to kill those organisms. Many bacteria infect patients with defects earlier in the complement cascade. Most clinically significant complement deficiencies are congenitally acquired.

The **spleen** plays an important role in humoral immunity, both as a source of complement- and antibody-producing B cells and as the organ *primarily responsible for the removal of opsonized microbes from the bloodstream*. Defects in spleen function can result from splenectomy or diseases such as sickle cell anemia and put patients at risk of infection with encapsulated bacteria (e.g., pneumococci and *Haemophilus*). Bacterial infections can be fulminant in patients with splenic deficiency. Bacteremia and septic shock often result, and mortality is high unless patients receive appropriate therapy rapidly.

Disorders of Cell-Mediated Immunity

Defects in the function or number of macrophages and T lymphocytes lead to an increased risk of infection with intracellular bacteria as well as with viruses, fungi, and protozoa (see Table 70-1). Patients with defective cell-mediated immunity are divided into two groups, depending on whether the defect is congenital or acquired. Primary disorders of cell-mediated immunity are usually diagnosed in childhood, and patients usually die from opportunistic infections before adulthood. An example of this immunodeficiency is **severe combined immunodeficiency** (**SCID**), an inherited disease in which persons are born with no T cells but normal B-cell populations. The disease manifests early in life with failure to thrive, intestinal infections, and interstitial pneumonias caused by pathogens such as *P. jirovecii* (formerly *P. carinii*), *Candida* species, *Aspergillus* species, and viruses. Vaccination with live, attenuated viruses or bacille Calmette-Guérin vaccine could lead to possibly fatal disseminated infections. SCID patients should be given prophylactic therapy with trimethoprim/sulfamethoxazole for *P. carinii* and acyclovir to prevent herpetic infections.

Acquired defects in cell-mediated immunity are seen in an increasingly large population of patients treated in hospitals. The enormous success of transplant surgery is a consequence of the development of drugs (such as **cyclosporin** and **tacrolimus**) that prevent rejection of the transplanted organ and suppress the graft-versus-host response in bone marrow transplantation. However, those **immunosuppressive drugs** also interfere with normal cell-mediated immunity, putting transplantation patients are at increased risk of opportunistic infection. Some immunosuppressive drugs, especially **corticosteroids**, are used to treat various inflammatory diseases. Cell-mediated immunity is also disturbed in patients with lymphoma.

The most profound example of defective cell-mediated immunity occurs in AIDS patients. If untreated, HIV infection depletes CD4+ helper T cells, leading almost inevitably to death from uncontrolled opportunistic infection or malignancy. AIDS patients have profound disturbances of cell-mediated immunity, especially that mediated by cytotoxic lymphocytes and macrophages, and develop infections with eukaryotic agents (e.g., *P. jirovecii*), viruses (e.g., cytomegalovirus), and intracellular bacteria (e.g., mycobacteria).

MANAGEMENT OF INFECTION IN IMMUNOCOMPROMISED HOSTS: GENERAL CONSIDERATIONS

The presentation of infection in the immunocompromised patient can be subtle. Fever may be the only indication that the patient has an active infection, and the maximal temperature may be blunted by the level of immunosuppression. A thorough history and physical examination are crucial to effective management. History of previous infections and procedures and recent antibiotic and chemotherapeutic therapy should be assessed. In neutropenic patients, the physical examination may be unrevealing because inflammation associated with infection may not be evident without the presence of neutrophils. The physician should do a complete examination, paying particular attention to the oropharynx, sites of indwelling catheters, the perineum, scalp, and skin.

As with all patients, treatment of infections in the immunocompromised person should be directed against the specific infecting organism. However, defective host response heightens the risk of severe infection, and the need may be urgent to begin treatment presumptively, based on the most likely etiological possibilities. Knowing the type of immune defect, the likely resident microbial flora, the site and clinical features of the infection, and some epidemiological features often makes it possible to predict the likely infecting organism. For example, in granulocytopenic patients, broad-spectrum antibiotics with activity against both Gram-positive bacteria and Gram-negative bacteria (including those in the Enterobacteriaceae family) should be given at the first sign of infection, such as fever. Patients with decreased spleen function should be treated with drugs active against pneumococci and *H. influenzae*. A diffuse pneumonia involving most of the lung in a patient with AIDS is likely caused by *P. jirovecii*. However, that is not always the case, and in some patients, specifically identifying the causative organism is necessary to start appropriate treatment or avoid toxic therapy.

Therefore, whenever possible, specimens should be obtained before starting therapy for infections in immunocompromised patients. The clinician and the microbiology laboratory should coordinate to ensure the recovery and identification of opportunistic pathogens. Unless warned, the microbiological laboratory may consider *S. epidermidis* a contaminant from the skin and not report it.

It is particularly important to attempt to reverse the immune defect; whenever practical, iatrogenic causes should be eliminated. Catheters should be removed, or at least changed, and immunosuppressive drugs should be discontinued whenever possible. In some transplant recipients, it may even be necessary to allow the transplant to be rejected by suspending immunosuppressive therapy to permit an adequate host response to infection. In other cases, replacement therapy is beneficial. Passive administration of immunoglobulins decreases the incidence of infection in patients with hypogammaglobulinemia. In some patients with granulocytopenia, therapeutic administration of a synthetic **colony-stimulating factor** (e.g., **G-CSF**, or **filgrastim**) can stimulate the bone marrow to produce neutrophils. Alternatively, **granulocyte transfusions** have been used in some granulocytopenic patients with refractory Gram-negative bacterial infections.

Preventive measures are also important in the care of immunocompromised patients. Simple procedures such as care with use and insertion of catheters, careful hand washing, and appropriate isolation techniques may reduce the incidence of opportunistic infection acquired in hospitals. Some vaccines (e.g., against influenza virus or pneumococci) may be beneficial. It is essential to remember that live vaccines should be given with caution to immunocompromised patients, who can acquire severe disease even from attenuated viruses. Prophylactic antibiotics are rarely beneficial; major exceptions are the use of penicillin to prevent pneumococcal infections in children with sickle cell disease and the use of trimethoprim/sulfamethoxazole to prevent pneumocystic pneumonia in patients with severe defects in cell-mediated immunity.

CONCLUSION

The immune system is a complex system that protects us from many pathogens. The congenital absence or acquired loss of any component of the immune system can lead to immunodeficiency and the development of life-threatening infections. With improvements in chemotherapeutic agents for malignancies, greater success in transplantation, and prolonged survival of patients with congenital immune defects, the number of patients with compromised immune systems continues to expand. Immunocompromised patients are susceptible not only to pathogens encountered in normal hosts but also to opportunistic infections with less virulent organisms that are easily cleared by a functioning immune system. The key to successful management of these patients lies in the ability to recognize their immune deficits and the risks that those defects create. Once the defects are identified, immunocompromised patients can be treated appropriately by minimizing their level of immune deficiency when possible, giving prophylactic antimicrobial therapy when indicated, aggressively seeking diagnosis early with appropriate tests and procedures, and recognizing the importance of pathogens associated with specific defects.

Suggested Readings

Calandra T, Holland SM, eds. Infections in the immunocompromised host. In: Cohen J, Powderly WG, eds. *Infectious Diseases*. 2nd ed. St. Louis, MO: Mosby; 2004:1031–1194.

Donnelly JP, Blijlevens NMA, De Pauw BE. Infections in the immunocompromised host: general principles. In: Mandell GL, Bennett JE, Dolin R, eds. *Principles and Practice of Infectious Diseases*. 7th ed. New York: Churchill Livingstone; 2009:3 781–3792.

Holland SM, Gallin JI. Evaluation of the patient with suspected immunodeficiency. In: Mandell GL, Bennett JE, Dolin R, eds. *Principles and Practice of Infectious Diseases*. 7th ed. New York: Churchill Livingstone; 2009:167–178.

Piot P, Careal M. Global perspectives on HIV infection and AIDS. In: Mandell GL, Bennett JE, Dolin R, eds. *Principles and Practice of Infectious Diseases*. 7th ed. New York: Churchill Livingstone; 2009:1619–1634.

Rubin RH, Young LS. *Clinical Approach to Infection in the Compromised Host*. 4th ed. New York: Plenum; 2002.

Chapter 71

Acquired Immunodeficiency Syndrome

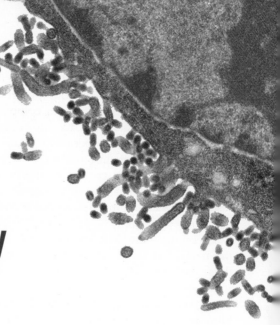

William G. Powderly

AS OF 2008, the World Health Organization estimated that approximately 33 million people were infected with human immunodeficiency virus (HIV), the causative agent of acquired immunodeficiency syndrome (AIDS). Of those, approximately over 1 million lived in North America. Worldwide, the number of new infections has averaged 3 million per year, and the number of deaths was approximately 2 million in 2008 alone. In many parts of sub-Saharan Africa, AIDS is the leading cause of death among young adults.

The impact of AIDS cannot be overemphasized. In 1995, the syndrome was the leading cause of death in the United States among men 20 to 45 years of age and was rapidly rising among women. Even with advances in therapy, it remains a major cause of mortality in some ethnic groups and urban areas. By 2002, more than 500,000 people had died of AIDS in the United States. Thanks to advances in treatment, deaths from AIDS declined sharply in the United States, from a peak of about 50,000 per year in 1995 to about 17,000 per year in 2008, even though the number of people living with HIV continued to rise. Unfortunately, only 10% of the people living with HIV worldwide have access to antiretroviral medications, and in many parts of Africa, AIDS is the leading cause of death among young adults.

AIDS is a constellation of clinical illnesses, primarily opportunistic infections and malignancies that can occur when HIV destroys the immune system. The syndrome is the final manifestation of an HIV infection that occurred many years previously (10 years on average). The continuous and relentless progression of HIV infection has been well characterized, and several methods are used to classify its stages. Chapter 38 describes the basic virology of HIV and the course of a typical HIV infection in terms of its progressive stages. This chapter focuses on one clinical case to describe the progression from HIV infection to AIDS, the manifestations of the syndrome, patient management, and preventive measures.

EARLY ACUTE HIV INFECTION

Mr. F.'s complaints and manifestations are nonspecific and common. His presentation is typical of many viral infections, including those caused by HIV, the Epstein-Barr virus, and cytomegalovirus (CMV). A clinician should consider the possibility of acute HIV infection if

CASE • Mr. F., a 26-year-old married bisexual man who worked as a hospital phlebotomist, was seen in his physician's office complaining of a 1-week history of fever, swollen lymph nodes, and headache. He stated that he had unprotected sexual contact with a new male partner 3 weeks previously. On examination, he had a red and inflamed pharynx, enlarged cervical lymph nodes, and a splotchy rash all over his body.

At this point, the case raises two questions:

1. Could Mr. F. have been infected with HIV?
2. Can HIV be diagnosed at the initial stage?

See Appendix for answers.

CASE • After counseling about the implications and possible outcome of HIV testing, Mr. F. had an HIV antibody test, which was negative. However, testing of his serum for p24 antigen was positive. He returned for a follow-up 6 weeks later. His symptoms had resolved completely and he felt well. Serological testing at the time revealed a positive **enzyme-linked immunosorbent assay** (ELISA) for HIV, signifying antibodies specific to HIV. A **Western blot** confirmed that result.

At this point, the case raises two questions:

3. How accurate are the tests for HIV?

4. Can Mr. F. be sure he is infected?

See Appendix for answers.

---

a patient presenting with the signs and symptoms of a viral infection is currently sexually active (especially a gay or bisexual man) or is an intravenous drug user. Mr. F. has three possible risk factors for HIV infection: he is a bisexual man, he has had multiple sex partners who may have been infected, and he is a hospital phlebotomist.

Acute illness occurs in 50 to 90% of persons 2 to 4 weeks after infection by HIV. In most cases, the only symptoms are mild fever and sore throat. A small subgroup may have fever, myalgias, lethargy, pharyngitis, arthralgias, lymphadenopathy, and a maculopapular rash of the trunk. Some patients have aseptic meningitis, and the headache that Mr. F. complained of may have been caused by mild meningeal irritation. The illness typically lasts 3 to 14 days, and complete recovery is the rule, even in patients with neurologic complications.

Antibodies against HIV are usually not detectable initially. However, various methods of detecting viral RNA in the blood have been developed. Although patients with acute HIV infection usually have high levels of viral RNA, follow-up serological testing is needed to confirm a diagnosis.

DIAGNOSTIC TESTS

Measurement of viral RNA by polymerase chain reaction (PCR) methodologies can detect HIV early in infection. However, because of its cost, a PCR test is not used to screen for infection unless the clinician suspects acute infection. Instead, HIV infection is typically diagnosed by detecting circulating antibodies to the virus. Unlike most antibody tests, in which the presence of specific antibodies signifies past infection with the agent in question, a positive HIV antibody test signifies current infection. Any individual who has HIV antibodies must be assumed to have active infection that can be transmitted to others. It is important, therefore, that individuals with positive HIV antibody tests receive counseling about the issues involved in transmission so that spread can be minimized.

Specific anti-HIV antibodies generally appear 6 to 12 weeks after infection. However, studies using PCR to test for specific HIV RNA have shown that in rare cases infected individuals do not develop antibodies for several months or years after exposure. Those unusual

individuals have false-negative serological tests for HIV. In addition, some patients in the terminal phases of AIDS have negative serological tests (presumably because of **severe B-cell dysfunction**). Fortunately, patients with advanced disease can usually be identified by other than serological means; however, B-cell dysfunction also complicates the serologic diagnosis of several of the opportunistic infections that occur in AIDS.

The most common method for testing for HIV antibodies is the ELISA. This test is performed by adding a sample of the patient's serum to small wells to which HIV antigens are bound. If antibodies are present, they will complex with the antigen. An anti-immunoglobulin antibody linked to an identifier enzyme is then added to bind to the complex. Although the ELISA is a highly sensitive test (>99%), it is not completely specific, and false-positive results occur. When screening a large population (such as all adults in the United States), *even a false-positive rate of less than 0.01% would mean that many uninfected individuals would be misidentified.* Consequently, positive ELISA results should be verified with a more specific test. In most laboratories, that test is an **immunoblot** (or "**Western blot**"), which detects antibodies to specific viral polypeptides. The Western blot is a sensitive and specific way to test for HIV antibodies; however, it is too time consuming and expensive to be used for primary screening purposes.

Rarely, some people exhibit nonspecific cross-reactivity in serological HIV tests and may be difficult to distinguish from patients with early HIV infection. The true pattern can usually be determined by repeating the Western blot after 3 or 4 months. By then, a person with true infection will usually have developed new antibodies to different epitopes (which show up in the Western blot), whereas those with nonspecific reactivity will have the same pattern as before. Waiting for repeat HIV tests can be a difficult time for patients, who will need counseling and support to help them understand the limitations of technology.

Other assays to determine the presence of HIV infection are available but are not always useful. The **p24 antigen** is the viral core protein produced by the *gag* gene, and its presence denotes active viral replication. High levels are seen in acute infection and it can be useful diagnostically in that circumstances. However, in established infection, the antigen is not detectable in the serum of all patients and thus is less useful.

HIV RNA PCR is widely used in clinical practice, most commonly to assess the need for and effectiveness of antiretroviral therapy. It is rarely used to screen for infection, although it is useful for cases of acute retroviral infection, prior to the development of a detectable, specific antibody response. HIV DNA PCR, which amplifies chromosomally integrated HIV provirus, is a highly sensitive and specific method of detecting early infection. It is most commonly used to identify HIV-infected infants born to HIV-positive mothers, for whom maternal antibodies could complicate serologic diagnostic tests. Although the DNA test becomes positive only slightly later than the HIV RNA PCR, the RNA test can occasionally become undetectable in established infection, even in the absence of antiretroviral therapy, and the DNA test does not. Both DNA and RNA PCR tests can give false-positive results in cases of laboratory cross-contamination. Therefore, follow-up serologic confirmation of a positive test is necessary. Additionally, genetic drift causes mismatch with the primers used in PCR assays and can give false-negative results, particularly in some HIV **clades** or clonally related groups. HIV can be cultured from lymphocytes of most infected individuals, but that test is technically difficult and is rarely used outside research settings.

HIV TRANSMISSION

Mr. F. has clearly seroconverted (from negative to positive) and is infected with HIV. How did he get his infection? HIV is transmitted primarily by direct inoculation of infected blood or body fluids into the host. Thus, the epidemiology of HIV mirrors that of viruses spread by that means (e.g., hepatitis B and C). *Most cases of HIV infection are acquired sexually*, and sexual practices associated with trauma, such as receptive anal intercourse, facilitate the spread of the virus. Other sexually transmitted diseases, especially genital ulcer diseases, are associated with an increased risk of HIV transmission, possibly because the epithelial barrier is breached by the ulcers. In the United States and other Western countries, HIV initially infected mainly homosexual men and was wrongly perceived as an exclusive disease of that community. However, in other parts of the world, sexual transmission of HIV is predominantly heterosexual. In the United States, the number of cases of HIV infection acquired by heterosexual contact has risen steadily. Some studies suggest that women are more easily infected than men, but transmission clearly occurs in both directions.

Contact with infected blood or blood products is another important form of transmission of HIV. Transmission through infected blood and blood products has considerably diminished since blood donor testing and treatment of plasma to inactivate the virus was instituted. However, that mode of transmission has not been eliminated completely. Because of the "window period" in early infection, blood donors with early HIV infection may not have developed HIV antibodies.

Bloodborne spread of HIV remains a considerable problem among intravenous drug users who share needles and syringes. Individuals who exchange sex for drugs may then infect their sexual partners. Infected women can infect their children in utero or intrapartum (**vertical transmission**). Additional risk of transmission occurs with breast-feeding. Without antiretroviral therapy for HIV infected mothers, between 13 and 40% of their infants will be infected with the virus. Antiretroviral therapy for HIV-infected pregnant women may substantially lower the risk of transmission to their babies—to less than 1%—under optimal circumstances. The reason all children with HIV-infected mothers are not infected is unknown, although it may be related, in part, to maternal immune responses to HIV and to the level of HIV circulating in the mother's blood.

HIV is also an occupational problem for health care workers. Exposure to HIV-infected blood, predominantly through needlestick injuries, is a potential hazard for health care workers. The risk of infection after such exposure is low; it is estimated that 1 in 300 such exposures leads to infection. Cases of AIDS resulting from needlestick injuries have been documented but can be prevented with rapid use of antiviral drugs. Transmission in the opposite direction (i.e., from an infected health care worker to a patient) has also been documented but is extremely uncommon. **Universal precautions** (assuming all blood or other fluids are potentially infected) are important to prevent transmission of HIV infection in health care settings.

Thus, Mr. F. could have been infected in a number of ways. He is a bisexual man with a recent new sexual partner, and he is a phlebotomist who may have had exposure to infected blood. Statistically, it is most likely that he acquired HIV from sexual contact.

When should people be tested for HIV infection? Persons with HIV disease seek medical attention at various stages of the disease. Many patients with early HIV infection do not seek medical attention and do not know they are infected until they develop AIDS. However, most patients are seen by a physician before they develop AIDS. Many want to be tested for HIV because they perceive that some aspect of their lifestyle puts them at risk. Others consult a physician with complaints that are not obviously caused by HIV disease, and the diagnosis is made when their physician counsels them to be tested for HIV. Currently, the U.S. Centers for Disease Control and Prevention recommend routine HIV screening of all adults, adolescents, and pregnant women in health care settings in the United States. The rationale is that infected individuals who do not know they are infected cannot avail themselves of advances in therapy that might extend their lives or cannot change behavior to protect others.

CASE • Mr. F. returned to his physician's office 2 weeks later to get the results of his antibody tests. When told he was HIV positive, he became anxious and asked, "Does that mean I have AIDS?"

At this point, the case raises two questions:

5. Will Mr. F. get AIDS?

6. What kind of lifestyle changes should Mr. F. consider making to minimize the risk of spreading the infection to others and to maintain his health as much as possible?

See Appendix for answers.

CONSEQUENCES OF BEING HIV POSITIVE

The period following a definitive diagnosis of HIV infection is a difficult time for a patient. Anxiety about the possibility of AIDS and concern about transmission of the virus to close family members are common reactions. Counseling patients is, therefore, important at that point. Patients should be taught how the virus is spread and educated fully about their duty to protect other people, especially their sexual contacts. Infected persons should be informed that abstinence from sexual intercourse is the only sure way of avoiding transmission. *Sexual practices that do not involve contact with semen or vaginal secretions are considered safe.* Condom use is essential if patients are going to continue to have sexual intercourse. Patients should be reassured that casual contact with others does not pose a risk of transmission.

The probability of progression to AIDS can be estimated by determining the degree of immunodeficiency. The most helpful measurement is the level of **T-lymphocyte** subsets. Because the **CD4+** (**T4** or **helper-inducer**) **T cells** are a specific target of HIV, measurement of the number and percentage of those cells in the circulation indicates the degree of immune impairment and thus the risk of developing AIDS. The normal CD4+ T-cell count in adults ranges from 800 to 2,000 cells/mm³. Progressive loss of the cells over time is the usual pattern of progressive HIV infection (Fig. 71-1). The probability of AIDS-related opportunistic infections rises sharply when a patient's CD4+ T-cell count falls below 200 cells/mm³, and the types of infections to which the individual is susceptible varies according to the degree of immunosuppression. The rate of decline of CD4+ T cells over time can also give important prognostic clues. In addition, the **viral load**, as reflected by measurements of the HIV plasma RNA, also provides important prognostic information, perhaps even more important than the CD4+ T-cell count. The higher the viral load in the plasma, the more rapid the progression of a patient to clinical AIDS or death.

Once HIV enters the body, it rapidly disseminates to many organs, especially the lymphoreticular system and the brain. Initial infection may, in fact, be associated with a profound, albeit temporary, loss of CD4+ T cells (and even opportunistic infections in occasional patients). With the appearance of a cellular immune response, the levels of viral RNA in the plasma decrease dramatically. However, active viral replication continues at a high rate

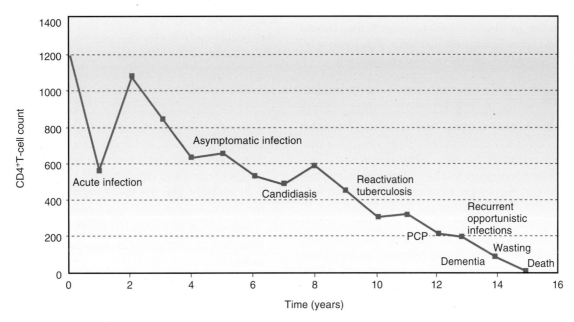

FIGURE 71-1. The natural history of HIV disease.

within lymph nodes. HIV infection is a state of immune activation with a high turnover of virus and of CD4+ T cells occurring on a daily basis until the body's reserve of lymphocytes is depleted. Pathologically, the lymph nodes are progressively destroyed at the same time, and ultimately the virus escapes the partial surveillance, and high plasma levels of virus are seen again as the disease progresses.

Symptoms or clinical illnesses that suggest immuno-deficiency also help identify patients who are likely to progress more rapidly to AIDS. Consequently, a careful history should be taken regarding fever, night sweats, unintentional weight loss, or unexplained diarrhea. The presence of *Candida* infection in the mouth (**thrush**) also indicates a poor prognosis. Despite those prognostic markers, precisely how quickly a particular patient will progress to AIDS cannot routinely be foretold. The mechanisms controlling the rate of progression are not well understood, and factors such as genetic variability (i.e., the host), host immune response, viral phenotype, and viral load are all potentially important factors.

Because most HIV-infected individuals develop progressive immunodeficiency, they should be assessed for occult infections that may become problematic later. Tuberculin skin testing and a chest radiograph should be performed when a patient has a history of a positive tuberculin skin test because the risk of reactivation tuberculosis is dramatically increased in HIV-infected persons. Patients who test positive to the skin test and thus do not have active tuberculosis should be treated prophylactically with isoniazid. Patients with positive serology for syphilis require antitreponemal therapy, particularly if neurosyphilis is suspected. Baseline **cytomegalovirus (CMV)** and *Toxoplasma gondii* antibody testing identifies persons at risk for reactivation disease by those agents. HIV-positive individuals are also candidates for vaccination against pneumococcal disease and annual immunization against influenza. Because patients are also at risk for hepatitis B, they should be tested for antibodies against that virus, and those who are negative should be offered vaccination against it.

PROGRESSION TO AIDS

Acute HIV infection is followed by a latent period during which infected individuals are asymptomatic and appear healthy. The duration of that period is variable, ranging from *several months to more than 15 years*; the median time is about 10 years. Although the period is referred to as asymptomatic, many patients in fact have complaints that are not obviously linked to HIV infection or to the associated immunodeficiency. For example, HIV-infected persons are particularly prone to skin complaints. The reason is unknown, but infection of the epidermal Langerhans cells may be a contributory factor. Many patients complain of excessively dry skin or pruritus, **seborrheic dermatitis with eczema folliculitis**, or **psoriasis**. Onset of severe psoriasis, eczema, or folliculitis in a previously healthy adult should raise the possibility of HIV infection. Furthermore, reactivation of **herpes zoster (shingles)**, as occurred with Mr. F., can also be a sentinel of HIV infection. Patients are also prone to recurrent **herpes simplex** infection, **molluscum contagiosum**, and drug eruptions. In addition, a type of skin cancer, cutaneous **Kaposi sarcoma**, may be the first manifestation of AIDS. It is characterized by blue–violet palpable, nonpruritic, painless lesions.

Patients in the latent stage of infection may also present with localized or generalized lymphatic enlargement, as Mr. F. did. **Painless generalized lymphadenopathy** is a common manifestation of HIV disease but *has no prognostic significance*. On the other hand, localized adenopathy or changes in already enlarged nodes can be early signs of infection or malignancy and should be investigated.

Recurrent mucocutaneous candidiasis(vaginal or oral in women, oral in men) and extensive oral aphthous ulcerations (canker sores) are common early manifestation of HIV infection. These conditions identify patients at increased risk of advancing to AIDS. **Hairy leukoplakia** (plaques of thickened mucosa on the tongue and elsewhere in the mouth) is caused by Epstein-Barr virus and also occurs early in HIV disease. Another feature of early HIV disease is the appearance of abnormal laboratory

---

CASE • Mr. F.'s CD4+ T-cell count was measured and found to be 600 cells/mm³. His plasma HIV RNA level was 43,000 copies/mL. He was otherwise completely well. His physician advised him that he had no evidence of significant immune impairment and should return for a checkup every 6 months for viral load and CD4+ T-cell measurement and clinical evaluation.

Unfortunately, Mr. F. did not keep his scheduled appointments. Four years passed before he returned to his physician's office complaining of a blistering rash on his left shoulder and upper torso. He also complained of sore throat and white spots in his mouth. Examination showed oral thrush; enlarged, nontender cervical, axillary, and inguinal lymph nodes; and a vesicular (blistering) rash in a dermatomal distribution consistent with shingles. Mr. F.'s CD4+ T-cell count was 280 cells/mm³.

At this point, the case raises two questions:

7. By ignoring his physician's advice and not having regular checkups, has Mr. F. caused himself irreparable harm?

8. What kind of treatment and management should Mr. F. receive?

See Appendix for answers.

findings. For instance, many infected individuals have isolated hematologic cytopenias, usually anemia, lymphopenia, or thrombocytopenia. Abnormalities in liver function tests, which are also common, are usually a result of previous or concurrent viral hepatitis.

The progressive loss of CD4[1] T cells and the oral *Candida* infection suggest that Mr. F.'s cell-mediated immunity has significantly diminished since his physician last saw him. Mr. F. does not yet have AIDS. However, the drop in CD4[1] T cells and the oral candidiasis are poor prognostic signs and an indication for starting specific antiretroviral treatment. Mr. F. should also start prophylactic therapy to prevent *Pneumocystis jiroveci* (*Pneumocystis carinii*) infection.

The status of patients in the natural progression of HIV infection is routinely assessed in three ways:

- Ongoing clinical evaluation for HIV- and AIDS-related conditions
- CD4+ T-cell count
- Quantification of HIV viral burden

HIV viral burden is typically measured in blood using a nucleic acid–based test, such as a PCR assay. Measurement of viral load has been shown to predict progression to AIDS and long-term survival. The decision to initiate antiretroviral therapy is usually based on one or more of the three standard assessments. Although when antiretroviral therapy should begin in early HIV infection is still a controversial question. In the past, the presence of an AIDS-defining illness, a CD4+ T-cell count less than 350 cells/mm^3, and pregnancy have been used as criteria for initiating therapy. With the increasing efficacy, tolerability, and availability of antiretroviral drugs, treatment is now being initiated at earlier stages of infection.

When antiretroviral therapy was in its infancy, only a few agents were available. Treatment with the first of these, **zidovudine (AZT)**, a nucleoside inhibitor of viral reverse transcriptase, as a single agent showed that the progression to AIDS could be modestly delayed, but certain indicators of HIV progression, such as CD4+ T-cell counts and viral burden, progress in spite of therapy after a few months. The progression of disease in spite of antiretroviral treatment results from the emergence of resistant HIV during therapy. In the case of AZT and other reverse transcriptase inhibitors, the mutations occur in the viral gene encoding the enzyme. Similarly, mutations within the protease gene are associated with resistance to protease inhibitors. The emergence of resistance can be prevented by combining several different antiretroviral agents that act at different steps of viral replication or that require distinct mutations to confer resistance (Fig. 71-2). Current therapeutic approaches involve two or three active drugs (e.g., two reverse transcriptase inhibitors and a protease inhibitor). Combination antiretroviral regimens typically induce long-lasting reductions in viral burden and increases in CD4+ T-cell counts, and the regimens have contributed to a very significant reduction in AIDS-related deaths in the United States and prolonged survival in patients who respond to treatment. These regimens are referred to as "**highly active antiretroviral therapy,**" or "**HAART.**"

Pneumocystic pneumonia (PCP) is a preventable disease. Prospective studies of HIV-positive patients have shown that at least one-third of patients with CD4+ T-cell counts less than 200 cells/mm^3 develop PCP within 3 years in the absence of prophylactic therapy. The risk is considerably greater if the patients are also symptomatic (i.e., have fever, night sweats, weight loss, or oral candidiasis). The risk of infection can be substantially reduced with prophylactic therapy such as trimethoprim/sulfamethoxazole. PCP is less clearly correlated with CD4+ T-cell counts in children. HIV-infected infants with CD4+ T-cell counts less than 1,500 cells/mm^3 should be considered candidates for prophylaxis.

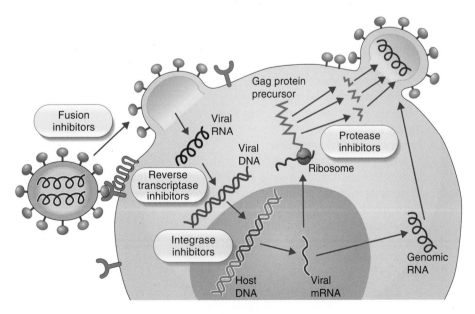

FIGURE 71-2. Possible sites of intervention in the inhibition of HIV replication.

CASE • Mr. F.'s physician prescribed combination antiretroviral therapy and trimethoprim/sulfamethoxazole tablets. When he broke out in an itchy rash 10 days later, Mr. F. stopped taking all his medications but did not inform his doctor. Six months later, he arrived at a local emergency department complaining of a 6-day history of gradually worsening dry cough and shortness of breath. His temperature was 40°C and a chest radiograph showed a diffuse bilateral interstitial pneumonia. Examination of fluid from bronchoalveolar lavage revealed *P. jiroveci*. Mr. F.'s infection had advanced to AIDS.

At this point, the case raises two questions:

9. What other infections might Mr. F. acquire?
10. Can any treatment help him avoid those infections at this stage?

See Appendix for answers.

CLINICAL MANIFESTATIONS OF AIDS

The signs and symptoms of PCP place Mr. F. in the category of AIDS patients, but any of a number of other opportunistic infections, singly or in groups, would lead to the same diagnosis. The box titled "AIDS-Defining Illnesses" (see below) indicates the major infections associated with AIDS, most of which are caused by intracellular agents usually controlled by cell-mediated immunity. These infections are often the result of endogenous reactivation of previously acquired organisms, rather than newly acquired infection.

Most AIDS-related infections do not occur until the CD4+ T-cell count falls below 200 cells/mm³. Kaposi sarcoma is the major exception to that rule because its occurrence seems to be independent of the underlying T-cell depletion, although it is more frequent at lower CD4+ T-cell counts. Reactivation tuberculosis, which is the most frequent presenting opportunistic infection worldwide, can also occur with CD4+ T-cell counts above 200 cells/mm³, but the risk of reactivation increases with progressive immunodeficiency. Infections in AIDS patients are characterized by a high density of organisms and disseminated disease, as well as infections with multiple organisms. The infections are rarely cured. Control of disease consequently requires prolonged acute therapy as well as long-term use of antimicrobial agents to prevent relapses.

AIDS-DEFINING ILLNESSES[a]

1. Multiple or recurrent bacterial infections (two in a 2-year period) affecting a child less than 13 years of age: septicemia, pneumonia, meningitis, bone or joint infection, or internal abscess caused by *Haemophilus influenzae*, streptococci, or other pyogenic bacteria
2. Candidiasis of the esophagus, trachea, bronchi, or lungs
3. Disseminated coccidioidomycosis
4. Extrapulmonary cryptococcosis
5. Chronic cryptosporidiosis, with diarrhea for more than 1 month
6. Cytomegalovirus infection
7. Mucocutaneous herpes simplex virus infection persisting for more than 1 month
8. HIV encephalopathy
9. Disseminated histoplasmosis
10. Isosporiasis, with diarrhea for more than 1 month
11. Kaposi sarcoma
12. Primary lymphoma of the brain
13. Non-Hodgkin lymphoma of B-cell or unknown phenotype, including Burkitt lymphoma
14. Lymphoid interstitial pneumonia affecting a child less than 13 years of age
15. Disseminated mycobacterial infection (not *Mycoplasma tuberculosis*)
16. Extrapulmonary tuberculosis
17. *Pneumocystis jiroveci (Pneumocystis carinii)* infection
18. Progressive multifocal leukoencephalopathy
19. Recurrent *Salmonella* infection
20. Toxoplasmosis of the brain

[a]Any of these diseases indicates a diagnosis of AIDS in the presence of laboratory evidence of HIV infection.

CASE • After the episode of pneumonia, Mr. F. made a complete recovery and was able to return to work. He took zidovudine, **lamivudine**, and **efavirenz** for his HIV and **trimethoprim/sulfamethoxazole** as prophylaxis for pneumocystic pneumonia. However, his plasma viral load remained high, and he admitted that he had not been taking his medications regularly. Mr. F. had no clinical problems for about a year until he went to his physician complaining of difficulty swallowing and diarrhea. His diarrhea was intermittent but could be as severe as 20 bouts of loose watery stools per day. On examining his mouth, the physician noticed multiple white plaques on his palate and tongue.

At this point, the case raises two questions:

11. Why did Mr. F. have difficulty swallowing?

12. What caused his diarrhea?

See Appendix for answers.

Lung Infections

Pneumonia caused by *P. jiroveci* is the most frequent opportunistic infection associated with AIDS and occurs in 25 to 60% of patients. The typical symptoms are **fever**, **cough**, and **shortness of breath**. PCP is treatable yet is associated with a mortality rate of 10 to 20% from irreversible respiratory failure.

An opportunistic infection such as PCP does not mean that patients will automatically develop multiple medical problems and soon die. The use of specific antiretroviral therapy and anti–*P. jiroveci* drugs has led to an improvement in the quality and length of life for AIDS patients. Many people are able to resume normal lives for long periods. In patients who achieve optimal responses to antiretroviral medications, there is usually significant reconstitution of cellular immune responses, with concomitant reduction in the risk of opportunistic infections for as long as the retroviral replication can be suppressed. Nevertheless, therapy is not curative, and long-term success is dependent on patients adhering to treatment. If patients cannot adhere to therapy or cannot tolerate side effects or pill burden, then treatment failure and the emergence of resistant virus can limit the success of antiretroviral regimens. Progressive deterioration with repeated episodes of infection is the outcome for patients with advanced HIV disease, if suppression of viral replication cannot be achieved.

Gastrointestinal Infections

Gastrointestinal problems are common in patients with AIDS. Candidiasis of the mouth and pharynx is almost universal in patients with profound immunodeficiency but is usually manageable. A substantial number of patients go on to develop esophageal candidiasis, which can cause pain and difficulty on swallowing, leading to considerable weight loss. Esophageal infection can also be caused by the herpes viruses, herpes simplex, and CMV, although they more typically involve other sites. Herpes simplex causes recurrent skin infections, especially perirectally, that can become resistant to therapy. CMV typically causes disseminated disease with viremia. Involvement of the colon can lead to severe abdominal pain and diarrhea. CMV infection of the eye presents as blurred vision and may lead to blindness. Diarrhea is a common problem in patients with advanced AIDS and may be severe and difficult to diagnose and treat. It can be caused by a large number of agents:

- CMV and other viruses
- Enteric Gram-negative bacteria such as *Salmonella* and *Shigella* species (with accompanying bacteremia)
- Nosocomial infections like *Clostridium difficile*
- Mycobacterial infection (especially the *Mycobacterium avium* complex) that affects the small bowel and colon and causes malabsorption and diarrhea
- Intestinal parasites such as *Giardia*, *Isospora*, and *Cryptosporidium* species and microsporidia

Malignancies such as Kaposi sarcoma or lymphoma involving the stomach or colon may also cause gastrointestinal symptoms. Furthermore, HIV itself may infect the cells of the gastrointestinal tract and cause an enteropathy leading to diarrhea.

Investigating intestinal distress in AIDS patients requires culturing stool for bacteria and examining it microscopically for parasites. If the examination does not give an answer, it may be necessary to perform invasive tests.

CASE • Mr. F., was found to have esophageal candidiasis and Salmonella infection. Following treatment, his symptoms resolved. His virus had now developed multiple mutations in the reverse transcriptase gene, and he was started on a new regimen. Unfortunately, he was not able to take his medications regularly. Two months later, he was admitted to the hospital with a high fever, cough, and shortness of breath. A chest radiograph showed a lobar pneumonia, and sputum cultures grew *Streptococcus pneumoniae*. He responded rapidly to penicillin treatment.

At this point, the case raises two questions:

13. What other agents of pneumonia is Mr. F. susceptible to?

14. Is he at risk for tuberculosis, and is it treatable?

See Appendix for answers.

CASE • On recovering from pneumonia, Mr. F. returned to work. He was restarted on antiretroviral therapy but again was unable to take it regularly. He went back to see his physician 4 months later when he developed high fever and headache. Although his examination was normal, the physician obtained a rapid test for cryptococcal antigen on the patient's serum. This test was positive, and the physician then recommended a spinal tap. The cell count and glucose and protein levels on the cerebrospinal fluid were normal, but an India ink smear of cerebrospinal fluid showed it to be packed with encapsulated yeast. Mr. F. responded well to antifungal treatment.

At this point, the case raises one questions:

15. Why did the physician perform a serum cryptococcal antigen test despite Mr. F.'s normal examination?

See Appendix for answer.

Mycobacterial and Fungal Infections

Although *P. jiroveci* is a frequent cause of pneumonia in AIDS patients, other causes must be considered, such as pneumococci, *Haemophilus influenzae*, and enteric Gram-negative rods. Tuberculosis is another important cause of pneumonia in AIDS, and it can disseminate widely to cause lymphadenitis, hepatitis, or meningitis.

Although most opportunistic infections occur during severe immunodeficiency, tuberculosis is an exception and can occur earlier, when the immune function of AIDS patients is only mildly impaired (i.e., in the "asymptomatic" phase). Consequently, *HIV infection should be considered in the event of pulmonary tuberculosis in previously healthy young adults or adolescents.* Infected patients can easily spread tuberculosis to household members and other close contacts. Indeed, the rise in incidence of tuberculosis in the United States that began in the late 1980s can be attributed largely to the spread of tuberculosis among HIV-infected persons and their close contacts. Fortunately, tuberculosis is treatable in patients with HIV infection and remains one of the few AIDS-associated opportunistic infections that does not require lifelong suppressive treatment after a prolonged course of curative therapy.

Disseminated infection with the *M. avium* complex is also common in AIDS. Although the MAC organism can cause pneumonia, it more typically causes disseminated disease, particularly in the lymphoreticular organs and the gastrointestinal tract. Typically, patients develop fever, night sweats, weight loss, and enlarged livers and spleens; some also develop diarrhea. Similar symptoms are seen in patients with disseminated fungal infection, such as **histoplasmosis**, which is common in patients from the Midwest and Latin America. Disseminated **coccidioidomycosis** is found in patients from the southwestern United States.

Infections of the Nervous System

Opportunistic infections can also cause neurological problems in AIDS patients. Fever and headache are the most common presentations of infection with the fungus *Cryptococcus neoformans*, which typically causes meningitis (see Chapter 48). Mr. F.'s case illustrates one of the major problems of treating such infections in a patient with AIDS. His spinal fluid was teeming with fungi, yet because of his immune defect, he was unable to mount an effective inflammatory response (which explains his normal cell count and glucose and protein levels).

Other opportunistic infections can affect the brain. Reactivation of infection with the parasite *T. gondii* typically causes a *multifocal infection in the brain.* Patients may present with headache, confusion, or seizures. Infection with another virus, the **JC virus**, causes a progressive and fatal encephalopathy (**progressive multifocal leukoencephalopathy**, or **PML**). CMV causes retinitis and occasionally encephalitis.

CASE • Mr. F. became increasingly concerned about his weight loss. In fact, on reviewing Mr. F.'s records, the physician found that his weight loss over the previous year was 90 lb, although Mr. F. reported he was eating fairly well. He continued to have difficulty adhering to antiretroviral therapy, and multiple mutations were detected in both the reverse transcriptase and protease genes. He also noted fevers, night sweats, and intermittent bouts of severe diarrhea.

At this point, the case raises a question:

16. What caused Mr. F.'s significant weight loss?

See Appendix for answer.

CASE • A few days later, Mr. F. returned to his physician with several purple–red skin lesions on his legs and trunk. The lesions were biopsied, and Kaposi sarcoma was diagnosed.

At this point, the case raises a question:

17. What is Kaposi sarcoma?

See Appendix for answer.

Direct Manifestations of HIV Itself

HIV itself can directly affect many organs of the body, such as the intestine and the kidney. **HIV nephropathy** is manifested by proteinuria, the nephrotic syndrome, and kidney failure and may respond to antiretroviral therapy. **Myopathy** and **myositis** both occur and may be related to HIV infection or the effects of drug therapy. **Cardiomyopathy** also occurs. One of the most distressing features of late AIDS is a **wasting syndrome** that is characterized by profound weight loss with concomitant loss of muscle mass. The pathogenesis of wasting syndrome in AIDS is unclear; however, it carries a grave prognosis and usually portends death.

Oncological Manifestations in Advanced AIDS

It is important to realize that the illnesses we associate with AIDS change in frequency and importance as therapies change. As physicians became more adept in treating and preventing infections like PCP, other infections (e.g., those caused by mycobacteria and CMV) assumed greater importance. Neurological manifestations of HIV in its later stages (discussed in the next section) and malignancies also assumed more importance. As patients live longer with profound immunodeficiency, malignancies are seen more frequently. The two most common HIV-associated malignancies are Kaposi sarcoma and lymphoma. However, as HIV-infected patients live longer as a result of effective antiviral treatment, other common cancers (e.g., lung cancer) are more frequently seen.

Kaposi sarcoma is associated with **human herpes virus 8**. It is most commonly seen in male homosexuals with HIV disease. Its occurrence is independent of underlying immunocompromise, although it behaves more aggressively and is more difficult to treat as the CD4+ T-cell count falls. In its mildest form, it may merely cause localized skin disease without significant morbidity. Severe cases of Kaposi sarcoma present with widely disseminated lesions; involve the lymph nodes, gastrointestinal tract, and lungs; and can be fatal.

Both Hodgkin disease and non-Hodgkin lymphoma occur more frequently in HIV-infected patients. The latter is an increasingly important problem. Involvement of the central nervous system is common and usually associated with poor prognosis. Epstein-Barr virus has been associated with most cases of central nervous system lymphoma, suggesting a probable role for this virus in the pathogenesis of this tumor.

Malignant transformation associated with human papillomavirus is also a significant concern in AIDS patients. Cervical cancer is more common in women with both HPV and HIV, and HPV-associated anal carcinoma is emerging as a serious problem among HIV-infected men who have sex with men.

Neurological Manifestations in Advanced AIDS

Although opportunistic infections and lymphomas can involve the nervous system in AIDS, by far the most common neurological problems are caused by HIV itself. HIV is a lentivirus and, like many others in that group, is neurotropic. Infection of the nervous system occurs early in the disease, probably soon after exposure. The presence of HIV in the nervous system has been documented by viral culture of brain tissue, in situ hybridization demonstrating viral DNA sequences, and electron micrographic identification of retroviral particles. Within the central nervous system, the virus resides predominantly in macrophages and cells derived from macrophages, although the pathogenesis of HIV-associated neuronal damage is unclear.

CASE • Mr. F. missed his next two appointments with his physician, and the next time he came to the office he was accompanied by his parents, who reported that he had become more forgetful and withdrawn. They informed the physician that Mr. F. had lost his job because he was constantly late and could not concentrate on tasks. When his physician examined him, Mr. F. appeared inattentive and, although he knew who and where he was, he had problems remembering simple commands. The physician ordered a computerized tomography (CT) scan of his head, which showed profound brain atrophy.

At this point, the case raises a question:

18. What is Mr. F.'s prognosis?

See Appendix for answer.

Manifestations of nervous system involvement can occur at any stage of HIV disease. Acute primary infection may be complicated by aseptic meningitis, encephalitis, myelitis, or inflammatory neuropathies such as Guillain-Barré syndrome. Later in HIV disease, patients may have peripheral neuropathies, both motor and sensory, or spinal cord syndromes, resembling subacute combined degeneration of the cord. The most common form of neurological disease, however, is HIV-associated encephalopathy, which leads to progressive dementia, as in the case of Mr. F.

In its earliest form, HIV dementia may consist of generalized mental slowing, difficulty concentrating, and forgetfulness, all of which must be differentiated from the depression that often accompanies HIV infection. In the later stages of HIV dementia, patients have profound deficits in cognitive, motor, and sensory functions and may be totally unable to care for themselves. CT scans of the brain often show considerable atrophy (Fig. 71-3). Severe dementia is almost inevitably fatal.

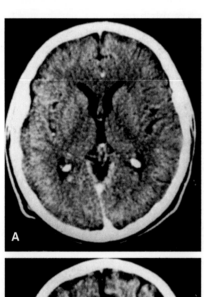

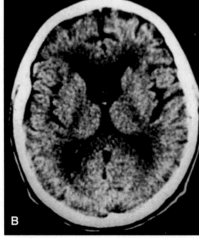

FIGURE 71-3. Computerized tomography (CT) scan of the brain of a patient with AIDS. A. Normal CT scan. **B.** Scan from the same patient 4 months later when he presented with mental slowing and confusion. Note the profound loss of brain substance and consequent enlargement of the fluid-filled ventricles.

> **CASE** • Two weeks later, Mr. F.'s parents called the physician to tell him that Mr. F. had died at home that day.

Outcome

Mr. F.'s outcome is typical of the usual course of untreated HIV infection. Although HIV disease is, as yet, incurable and fatal, its progression varies. With improved antiretroviral therapy and use of prophylactic antimicrobial therapy, HIV infection is increasingly a chronic disease in many patients. A case like Mr. F has become a rarity in the Western world. Modern antiretroviral therapy is potent and generally well tolerated, and even for patients infected with resistant virus, effective and durable options are increasingly available.

GENETIC AND DEVELOPMENTAL PREDISPOSITION TO AIDS

Would the course of Mr. F.'s illness have been different if he had been a female? Probably not, although some of the indicator diseases may have been different. As mentioned earlier, recurrent **vaginal candidiasis** may be a common and troublesome complaint in HIV-infected women. In addition, increasing evidence shows that human papillomavirus infection may behave more aggressively in persons with HIV infection. Consequently, **cancer of the uterine cervix** emerged as an important complication.

Host-specific genetic determinants that likely affect the rate of progression of disease in HIV infection are only beginning to be elucidated. In addition, differences may exist among patients regarding the toxicity of antiretroviral agents, depending on patients' genetic backgrounds. It should be noted that there are no indications that drug treatment is ineffective or harmful; thus, no person should go untreated because he or she belongs to a particular racial group or gender.

HIV infection in children follows a similar course, with progressive immunodeficiency, recurrent opportunistic infections, and neurological involvement. However, the pace of the disease can be much more rapid in infants. Transmission is usually vertical (i.e., acquired from the mother), and 13 to 40% of babies born to HIV-infected mothers acquire the infection. Combination antiretroviral therapy of HIV-infected mothers during the last two trimesters and during labor may reduce the transmission rate to less than 2%.

Most children with vertically acquired HIV infection have an indolent course with slow progression (8 or more years) to clinical disease; however, 15 to 20% of those children rapidly progress to symptomatic disease and death within 2 to 4 years after birth without medical intervention. In addition to their opportunistic infections, the infants fail to thrive (i.e., have abnormal growth rates), and many have developmental delays secondary to HIV brain infection. Recurrent bacterial infections (e.g., otitis, pneumonia) are common and are related to B-cell dysfunction. However, as with adults, antiretroviral treatment and prophylactic therapy for infection improve the quality and extent of life.

MANAGEMENT OF HIV-INFECTED PATIENTS

Management of the HIV-infected patient involves a long-term commitment from physicians and other members of the health care team not only to provide medical treatment and management but also to support and educate the patient and the family. Patients need to be alerted about symptoms that require prompt medical attention, such as changes in fever patterns or new onsets of cough or headache. Physicians must be prepared to deal with the many complaints that develop and distinguish those that herald important complications. Patients must be educated about the modes of transmission so that new cases can be prevented. In addition, the members of the health care team need to help the patient cope with the changing social dimensions of the disease. Confidentiality and maintenance of employment and insurance benefits are prime concerns. Family and friends also need support and education.

Antiretroviral therapy has changed HIV infection from an inevitably fatal condition to a chronic manageable disease. Starting antiretroviral therapy early in the disease has been shown to delay the progression of HIV infection. Even if given later in the disease, therapies can reverse immunodeficiency and significantly prolong survival. Potent agents have been developed that target several different points on the viral life cycle: CCR5 (coreceptor) binding, viral fusion, retroviral-specific DNA polymerase, integration into the host chromosome, and the viral protease (see Fig. 71-2). In a manner analogous to the therapy of tuberculosis, chemotherapy for HIV involves combinations of agents acting at different sites to achieve synergism and delay the emergence of resistant viruses. As with tuberculosis, failure to adhere to correct schedule of therapy often leads to drug resistance, as occurred in Mr. F's case. However, for most patients who are able to take treatment, long-term complications of living with HIV disease (cardiovascular, liver, and bone disease) cause more problems than AIDS itself.

PREVENTION

By far, the best approach to controlling AIDS is by the prevention of HIV transmission. Education of the general public, as well as targeted education of HIV-infected persons, can effect behavioral changes that limit the spread of the virus. These include the promotion of routine and regular screening of persons at risk for HIV infections, "safe sex" practices among persons who are already infected (e.g., promoting condom use), and elimination of "needle sharing" among intravenous drug users.

HAART therapy has also been shown to decrease the rate of HIV transmission, suggesting that earlier identification and treatment of HIV-infected persons is also a means of reducing the spread of infection.

Development of an effective vaccine would eliminate the future threat of the disease. However, development of an HIV vaccine has been hampered by many problems. One is an incomplete understanding of the host immune response to the virus; although many individuals develop neutralizing antibodies to HIV, their role in vivo is unclear. Thus, circulating antibodies effectively clear the bloodstream of infectious virus yet fail to prevent the progression of HIV infection. In addition, HIV shows great variability in its major antigens (Chapter 38). Finally, the evaluation of HIV vaccines for protective efficacy requires testing people at risk for infection and thus can raise ethical concerns. Even after vaccines are developed and applied, it may be decades before AIDS ceases to be a major problem.

Until vaccines are developed, education and behavioral changes, early identification of infected individuals, and antiretroviral treatment to reduce the viral burden remain the most effective ways of stemming the spread of HIV.

CONCLUSION

AIDS is a devastating disease that will continue to have a profound effect on society. Scientifically, it has enhanced our understanding of the human immune system. The practice of medicine has been irrevocably changed with the recognition of this new incurable disease. In Western society, the crisis has forced people to face issues such as the economics and inequity of health care delivery and discrimination in employment and insurance. In wealthier nations, the force of law and the success of HAART therapy have converted AIDS from an inevitably fatal disease to a chronic, but manageable, medical problem. In the underresourced, developing world, the sobering truth is that high mortality from AIDS will continue to be a fact of life in spite of the infusion of money, medicines, and technical support from donor countries. In many places in the world, the devastation caused by HIV will continue for the foreseeable future in spite of our best efforts to contain it.

Suggested Readings

Clumeck N, Powderly WG, eds. HIV and AIDS. In: Cohen J, Powderly WG, Opal S eds. *Infectious Diseases.* 3rd ed. London: Mosby; 2010:915–1052.

Coffey S, Bacon S, Volberding P. HIV InSite Knowledge Base. University of California–San Francisco and San Francisco General Hospital. Available at http://www.hivinsite.com/InSite?page=KB. Accessed July 20, 2010.

Dolin R, Masur H, Saag MS, eds. *AIDS Therapy.* 3rd ed. New York: Churchill Livingstone; 2008.

Panel on Antiretroviral Guidelines for Adults and Adolescents. Guidelines for the use of antiretroviral agents in HIV-1-infected adults and adolescents. Department of Health and Human Services. December 1, 2009; 1–161. Available at http://www.aidsinfo.nih.gov/ContentFiles/AdultandAdolescentGL.pdf. Accessed July 20, 2010.

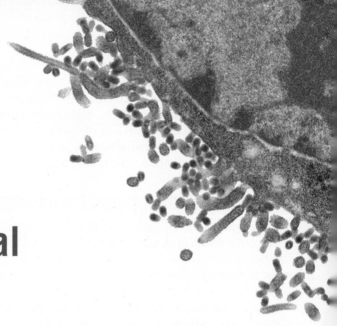

Chapter **72**

Congenital and Perinatal Infections

Roshni Mathew and Charles G. Prober

FETUSES and neonates are susceptible to a variety of infections unique to this period of development. Congenital (also called intrauterine or prenatal) infections are those that occur during fetal life and result from transplacental transmission from mother to fetus. Perinatal infections (those occurring during the first 4 weeks after birth) are contracted from the mother at birth or during the neonatal period, from either maternal or nonmaternal sources. Infections acquired in utero result from viral pathogens such as cytomegalovirus (CMV), herpes simplex virus (HSV), human immunodeficiency virus (HIV), parvovirus B19, rubella virus, and varicella-zoster virus (VZV), bacterial pathogens such as *Treponema pallidum*, and protozoal organisms such as *Toxoplasma gondii*. Infectious agents most commonly responsible for perinatal infections include group B streptococcus (GBS), Gram-negative enteric pathogens (especially *Escherichia coli*), *Listeria monocytogenes*, HSV, and hepatitis B virus (HBV).

SPECIAL IMMUNOLOGICAL PROBLEMS OF THE FETUS AND NEONATE

Fetuses and neonates are immunocompromised hosts. When compared with older children and adults, every component of their immune system (phagocytic system, natural killer [NK] cells, complement, B lymphocytes, and T lymphocytes) is deficient. The degree of deficiency is inversely related to gestational age and birth weight, although even term infants are immunologically naïve, compared to older children and adults.

Fortunately, the fetus is partially sheltered from infection by the fetal membranes and the placenta, which serve as barriers against many maternal microorganisms. Further protection is provided by the passive transport of considerable quantities of maternal immunoglobulins, largely of the IgG class. At term, the fetal concentration of IgG antibodies may be greater than that of the mother, as the placenta actively transports these molecules into the fetal circulation. Conversely, a baby born prematurely may not have received a full complement of maternal antibodies, further contributing to the increased risk of infection of premature infants. Some degree of protection is afforded by breast milk, which contains secretory IgA antibodies that reduce the likelihood that nursing infants will contract severe infection caused by certain pathogens.

DETERMINANTS OF FETAL INFECTION

The risk of transmission of infection and its subsequent consequences depend on the stage of pregnancy when the infection occurs. For example, maternal infection with *T. gondii* and rubella virus in the first trimester causes severe fetal consequences. Infection late in pregnancy with these organisms usually has no adverse effects on the fetus. In the case of CMV, the risk of transmission depends on whether the maternal infection was a primary infection or a recurrence. The approximate incidence of congenital infections in the United States caused by the four most common agents is summarized in Table 72-1.

DAMAGE

Three types of effects on the growing and developing fetus may result from intrauterine infection. First, intrauterine infection may interfere with normal

CASE

Congenital Infection

Baby L. was born at 37 weeks' gestation following an uneventful pregnancy to a 28-year-old healthy mother. On physical examination about 30 minutes after delivery, the baby weighed 2 kg (less than third percentile) and had a head circumference of 28 cm (less than third percentile). He was pale and had numerous nonblanching purple spots on his trunk, back, face, and extremities. His vital signs were normal, and his cardiopulmonary examination was unremarkable. He had an enlarged liver and spleen. A urine culture, obtained on the second day of life, was positive for cytomegalovirus (CMV), establishing the diagnosis of congenital CMV infection.

This baby presents clinical signs and symptoms typical of congenital infections, including intrauterine growth retardation and multisystem disease (including microcephaly, a rash compatible with hematologic problems, and hepatosplenomegaly). Notably, the symptoms of this infection were present at birth. Also characteristic of many intrauterine infections is the fact that the mother was asymptomatic during her pregnancy.

This case raises several questions:

1. How did Baby L. become infected inside the womb?
2. What are the signs and symptoms of intrauterine CMV infection?
3. What is the prognosis for Baby L.?
4. Could Baby L.'s mother have done anything to prevent her son's infection?

See Appendix for answers.

---

organogenesis, which may result in structural abnormalities in tissues and organs. For example, congenital rubella may cause cataracts and defects of the retina, **patent ductus arteriosus**, pulmonary artery stenosis, pulmonary valvular stenosis, or sensorineural deafness. Second, intrauterine infection may provide an intense inflammatory reaction that leads to tissue injury. For example, congenital CMV or *T. gondii* infections may cause **cerebritis**, which can lead to cerebral atrophy and intracranial calcifications. Third, direct placental infection may result in **placental insufficiency**. Inflammation, edema, and fibrosis associated with placental infection may compromise normal growth and development of the fetus, leading to low birth weight, premature birth, or fetal death.

Although the damage to fetal cells and organs occurs prenatally, the effects of the damage may not become clinically apparent until several months to years after birth. For example, deafness or intellectual impairment as a result of congenital CMV or rubella infection may not become evident until infected children have reached an age at which language or other cognitive skills can be evaluated reliably. In addition, certain tissue damage continues after birth in some congenital infections (such as CMV, rubella, and untreated syphilis) as the microbes continue to replicate after delivery.

Some of the most common clinical manifestations associated with congenital infections are listed in Table 72-2. Although certain malformations may suggest congenital infection caused by a specific pathogen, there is too much overlap between the patterns of abnormalities induced by each agent to allow definitive diagnoses to be made without laboratory confirmation.

DIAGNOSIS

Recognizing exposure of a pregnant woman to an infectious agent that may result in fetal or neonatal injury is important if documentation of infection might result in specific therapy or a recommendation to consider pregnancy termination. Detection of either IgM antibodies specific for the microbial agent or a rising titer of specific IgG antibodies in the mother's serum may be helpful in assessing the risk of congenital toxoplasmosis, CMV, HIV, rubella, or syphilis. Other specific tests, such as dark-field microscopy, antigen detection, or polymerase chain reaction (PCR), may be warranted under certain clinical circumstances. If maternal infection is strongly suspected, prenatal testing of amniotic fluid or fetal blood may be useful to determine whether fetal infection has occurred. Unfortunately, most agents that cause congenital infection produce minimal or no symptoms in

TABLE 72-1 Approximate Incidence of Congenital Infections in the United States

Agent	Incidence per 100,000 Births	Approximate Number of New Cases in the United States per Year
CMV	1,000	40,000
Toxoplasma gondii	10–100	400–4,000
Treponema pallidum	11	450
HIV	2.7	100

CMV, cytomegalovirus; HIV, human immunodeficiency virus.

TABLE 72-2 Common Manifestations of Congenital Infection

Prematurity

Intrauterine growth retardation

Congenital defects

  Abnormal head size

    Microcephaly

    Hydrocephalus

  Intracranial calcifications

    Periventricular

    Diffuse

  Eye abnormalities

    Chorioretinitis

    Cataracts

    Microphthalmia

  Hearing loss

  Hepatosplenomegaly

  Hematologic abnormalities

    Anemia

    Thrombocytopenia

  Bone lesions

  CSF inflammation

CSF, cerebrospinal fluid.

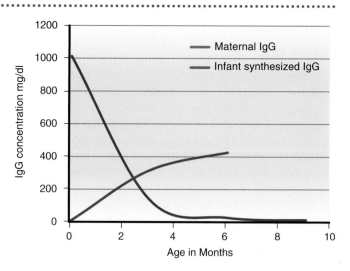

FIGURE 72-1. Maternal IgG in infant.

the mother and consequently arouse no suspicion until after the infant is born.

Attempts should be made to identify an infecting agent in symptomatic infants, such as the one presented in the case history. Serologic tests are of limited value in diagnosing congenitally infected neonates because IgG antibodies readily pass from mother to infant through the placenta. Therefore, the presence of such antibodies in the baby is not alone sufficient to diagnose intrauterine infection. Although not of immediate diagnostic utility, the serial assessment of serologic responses in an infant may support the diagnosis of congenital infection. Because the half-life of maternal IgG is approximately 20 days, most of the maternal IgG will have been lost after several months, and any IgG detectable in the baby after that time is most likely to be of infant origin (Fig. 72-1). Thus, in the congenitally infected baby, IgG antibody will remain the same or increase over time, whereas in an uninfected baby, specific antibodies of maternal origin will eventually disappear.

Maternal IgM antibodies, on the other hand, do not readily cross the placenta. Therefore, the presence of IgM antibodies specific for CMV, rubella virus, or *Toxoplasma* in a baby suggests that the baby has been infected. Unfortunately, IgM antibody assays are not well standardized, resulting in high rates of false-positive and false-negative tests.

The specific diagnostic evaluation of an infant with a possible congenital infection varies for different pathogens. For the diagnosis of congenital CMV, viral cultures of specimens from urine, saliva, pharynx, peripheral blood leukocytes, or any other body fluid can be done. Blood DNA or RNA PCR can detect HIV infection with excellent sensitivity and specificity. Diagnosis of rubella infection can be made by isolation of rubella virus in cultures from throat or nasal specimens or by detection of viral nucleic acid by PCR. Congenital syphilis can be evaluated by immunoassay to detect *T. pallidum* antigens in blood or by dark-field microscopy to identify *T. pallidum* from oral or skin lesions. Serology (IgG, IgM, and IgA) in a lab with expertise in *Toxoplasma* serology assay is the primary means of diagnosis of congenital toxoplasmosis. Peripheral blood leukocytes and cerebrospinal fluid (CSF) also can be assayed for *Toxoplasma* PCR in a reference laboratory.

TREATMENT

Penicillin G is effective in treating neonates congenitally infected with syphilis. Infants with congenital toxoplasmosis have been successfully treated with a combination of pyrimethamine and sulfadiazine. Use of ganciclovir for the treatment of congenital CMV may diminish hearing loss. There is no antiviral therapy for congenital rubella syndrome. Management of many types of congenital infection requires multidisciplinary supportive care.

TABLE 72-3 Congenital Infections

Pathogen	Clinical Manifestations	Diagnostic Tests	Treatment
CMV	Intrauterine growth retardation, hepatosplenomegaly, microcephaly, intracerebral calcifications, thrombocytopenia, purpuric skin lesions, sensorineural hearing loss	Culture of virus from specimens of urine, saliva, pharynx	Ganciclovir administered early may have some benefit in decreasing hearing loss
Rubella virus	Intrauterine growth retardation, hepatosplenomegaly, cataracts, chorioretinitis, sensorineural hearing loss, patent ductus arteriosus, pulmonary stenosis, purpuric skin lesions	Culture of virus from nasal or throat specimens, IgM antibody	No effective treatment
VZV	Congenital varicella syndrome manifests with limb hypoplasia, cutaneous scarring, ocular abnormalities	Physical examination findings and history of maternal infection	No effective treatment
Treponema pallidum	Hepatosplenomegaly, bone lesions, lymphadenopathy, snuffles, mucocutaneous lesions	Treponemal tests on serum, CSF nontreponemal test, dark-field microscopic examination for spirochetes	Penicillin
Toxoplasma gondii	Hepatosplenomegaly, lymphadenopathy, thrombocytopenia, microcephaly, cerebral calcifications, chorioretinitis	Serum IgM, IgG, and IgA, DNA PCR	Spiramycin for pregnant women with primary toxoplasma infection, pyrimethamine/sulfadiazine for infected infants
HSV (represents about 5% of HSV infections in newborn infants)	Skin lesions and scars, microcephaly, chorioretinitis, microphthalmia	Physical examination findings, culture of virus from mucosal surfaces	No effective treatment

CMV, cytomegalovirus; VZV, varicella-zoster virus; HSV, herpes simplex virus; CSF, cerebrospinal fluid; PCR, polymerase chain reaction.

PREVENTION

Appropriate immunization of the mother against rubella during childhood effectively prevents congenital rubella syndrome. While there were 20,000 reported cases of congenital rubella syndrome in the 1960s, there were no reported cases since 2004 in the United States. Routine prenatal serologic testing will detect syphilis in infected mothers, and treatment of the mother with penicillin more than 1 month prior to delivery will prevent most cases of congenital syphilis. Avoiding contact with cat litter boxes and consumption of undercooked meat will protect most susceptible pregnant women from contracting infection caused by *T. gondii*. Preventing congenital toxoplasmosis by treating acutely infected pregnant women with spiramycin followed by pyrimethamine and sulfonamide has been reported to decrease fetal mortality and improve long-term outcome. Meticulous hand washing will reduce the likelihood of contracting CMV

infection from exposure to secretions and body fluids of young children (frequently an older sibling) who may be excreting CMV.

Table 72-3 provides a summary of congenital infections.

PERINATALLY ACQUIRED INFECTION
DETERMINANTS OF NEONATAL INFECTION

Although neonates receive transplacental maternal antibodies, they are susceptible to organisms to which their mothers have not generated an immune response. In addition, they are unable to generate antibodies against certain types of antigens, particularly polysaccharides. Terminal components of the complement cascade, especially important for defense against Gram-negative enteric bacteria, are present at a concentration of less than 20% of

CASE

Perinatal Infection

C. is a 14-day-old baby brought to the emergency department with a 24-hour history of fever (38.9°C), poor feeding, lethargy, and irritability. The baby was born at term to a 22-year-old mother following an uneventful pregnancy. C. was discharged home with her mother 24 hours after delivery and had been well until the day prior to admission when the mother had to wake her for feeding. The baby then nursed only weakly and for a short period of time.

Evaluation in the emergency department revealed a white blood cell count of 24,000/mm³ with 68% segmented neutrophils, 20% bands, and 12% lymphocytes. Examination of the CSF revealed 230 white blood cells, 90% of which were neutrophils, a protein concentration of 830 mg/dL, and glucose concentration of 20 mg/dL. Gram-positive cocci in short chains were present on Gram stain of the CSF, and the culture grew group B streptococci. The baby was treated with ampicillin and gentamicin. After a difficult

hospital course characterized by apneic spells, seizures, and later, poor feeding, the baby was sent home following a 21-day course of antibiotics.

This baby was apparently healthy and normal at birth and developed acute symptoms suggestive of infection at 2 weeks of age. Thus, the infection was likely contracted during or after birth rather than before it. The presence of an inflammatory reaction and the recovery of pathogenic bacteria from CSF confirm the diagnosis of bacterial meningitis.

This case raises several questions:

1. To which infectious agents are newborns susceptible?
2. How do group B streptococci cause meningitis in newborn infants?
3. Could Baby C.'s mother have done anything to prevent her daughter's infection?

See Appendix for answers.

---

that found in older children and adults. Also, the neonatal cellular immune system is not completely functional as evidenced by decreased NK cell cytotoxicity and antibody-dependent cell-mediated cytotoxicity (ADCC). Phagocytic defenses are compromised by a smaller neutrophil storage pool, reduced capacity to adhere to endothelium and migrate to infectious foci, and variable deficiencies in ingestion and killing of microbes. Secretory IgA and other elements of mucosal immunity are not adequately developed until several weeks or more after birth. Thus, otherwise normal healthy neonates should be considered to be immunocompromised hosts. The immune system of a premature infant is even more compromised than that of a term infant. In addition, the mucoepithelial surfaces of chronically hospitalized premature neonates are colonized by multiresistant bacterial flora, often selected by their exposure to repeated courses of broad-spectrum antibiotics. Therefore, the risk of severe and life-threatening infections is substantially greater in premature babies than in term infants.

THE PATHOGENS: MICROBIAL AGENTS OF PERINATAL INFECTION

The most common types of bacteria that cause perinatally acquired infections are present in the maternal vaginal tract and include *E. coli* and other *Enterobacteriaceae*, group B streptococci, and *L. monocytogenes*. Other bacteria that are present in the baby's postnatal environment also may cause neonatal infection, including antibiotic-resistant Gram-negative enteric bacilli and, less frequently, *Staphylococcus aureus* and

coagulase-negative staphylococci. *Chlamydia trachomatis* and *Neisseria gonorrhoeae* may infect the ocular and respiratory mucous membranes during birth and cause neonatal conjunctivitis and systemic infection.

Several viruses are unique in their predilection for neonates. HSV and the enteroviruses can cause serious multiorgan system infection that may clinically resemble acute bacterial sepsis. Perinatal transmission of VZV also may result in overwhelming infection with multiorgan failure, when maternal varicella infection occurs within 5 days of delivery. This results from the virus readily crossing the placenta before protective maternal antibodies have been formed. HBV and HIV also may be transmitted perinatally, usually through exposure to infected maternal blood; infected babies usually are asymptomatic during the neonatal period. Respiratory syncytial virus and other respiratory viruses may cause nonspecific symptoms in neonates, including apnea. They also may cause mild-to-severe lower respiratory tract infections.

Candida albicans and other non-albicans species of *Candida* are increasingly important causes of perinatal infection, especially among prematurely born infants.

ENCOUNTER AND ENTRY

Babies are exposed to the agents causing perinatal infections in a variety of ways. Most bacteria responsible for infection during the first week of life colonize the maternal vaginal tract and are acquired by neonates as they pass through the birth canal. Within the first hours of life, babies become colonized with these organisms, particularly on their nasopharynx, skin, and around the umbilical stump; colonization of the neonatal gastrointestinal tract occurs more slowly. Babies also may be exposed at the time of delivery to bloodborne agents that do not readily cross the placenta. This is the most common mechanism of perinatal acquisition of HBV and HIV.

Many types of environmental factors can promote neonatal infection following exposure to viruses, bacteria, and fungi. During labor, many infants are evaluated for evidence of fetal distress by the application of monitoring devices to the fetal scalp. This procedure may result in direct inoculation of organisms resident in the maternal genital tract such as HSV and facilitate the translocation of organisms from the skin to the bloodstream. In addition, after the umbilical cord is severed, the healing stump provides a potential route for bacterial invasion. Many prematurely born newborns require intensive medical support such as endotracheal intubation with artificial ventilation, hyperalimentation, antibiotic therapy through intravenous catheters, and several other therapeutic or diagnostic procedures that are invasive or potentially injurious to the otherwise protective barriers of the skin and mucous membranes.

DAMAGE

The effect of perinatally acquired infections on the neonate is variable and depends on the specific pathogen, organs infected, and the degree of compromised immunity. Early clinical manifestations of infection are often nonspecific and may include poor feeding, lethargy, or irritability. Bacterial sepsis or meningitis can progress rapidly to severe neonatal illness or death within 12 to 24 hours. Even with timely, appropriate antibiotic therapy, the mortality of neonatal sepsis is between 10 and 40%, and significant neurological sequelae occur in 20 to 50% of survivors of neonatal meningitis.

The extent of involvement and the morbidity associated with perinatally acquired viral infections vary markedly. For example, HSV infection may involve a single organ such as the skin, with cutaneous vesicles being the only sign of infection, or it may cause multiorgan systemic infection involving the liver, central nervous system, and lungs and result in death or severe brain injury. In contrast, HBV is generally asymptomatic in neonates, but neonates infected with HBV are at very high risk (>90%) of becoming chronic carriers of HBV. Chronic HBV infection is associated with a high risk of hepatic cirrhosis or hepatocellular carcinoma in adulthood.

DIAGNOSIS

The diagnosis of a perinatally acquired infection depends on the recognition of suggestive symptoms and signs. Temperature instability, poor feeding, lethargy, or irritability may be the only presenting symptoms and signs of neonatal septicemia or meningitis, and these may be very subtle. Thus, the possibility of perinatal infection should be considered in neonates exhibiting even these nonspecific symptoms. Other, more specific signs, such as conjunctivitis or skin rash, may suggest a more focal infectious process.

Definitive diagnosis relies upon the detection of an etiological agent in infected body sites. However, the causative agents may not always be recovered by culture, sometimes because antimicrobial therapy is given before the collection of specimens or because specimens likely to reveal the organism cannot be easily obtained (e.g., lung, liver, or brain tissue). Detection of viral or bacterial antigens or nucleic acids in serum, urine, or CSF may reveal the causative agent. Antigen detection is available for group B streptococci, *E. coli* K1, HBV, and HIV. PCR has become a valuable diagnostic tool for enterovirus and HSV infections involving the central nervous system.

TREATMENT

The outcome of perinatal infections in babies is influenced by the type of pathogen, availability of specific antimicrobial therapy, severity of infection, and the presence of comorbidities. A variety of effective antimicrobial agents are available for the treatment of neonatal infections caused by most bacteria. In addition, antifungal agents may be effective in treating *Candida* infections. The antiviral agent acyclovir is useful in the therapy of neonates infected with HSV.

In general, antimicrobial treatment is most effective if initiated early after the onset of infection. Because identification of the specific pathogen is not immediate, selection of antimicrobial therapy usually is made empirically. The dosages and dosing intervals of drugs differ in neonates from those in older children or adults because neonates have decreased renal and hepatic elimination of most drugs and increased volumes of distribution of many drugs. Careful surveillance during therapy is necessary to ensure successful eradication of the infection and minimize potential antimicrobial toxicity.

PREVENTION

Because prematurely born infants are at greater risk of perinatal infection than full-term neonates, prevention of premature delivery would result in a significant reduction in the frequency of perinatal infections. Prematurely born babies often require prolonged hospital care and invasive medical interventions. Therefore, strict attention to infection control practices in the care of these vulnerable neonates (e.g., hand washing and equipment decontamination) also decreases the risk of infection.

Other potential preventive strategies are focused on the mother. For example, maternal immunization against tetanus provides protective transplacental antibodies to infants greater than 28 weeks' gestation, greatly reducing the potential for neonatal tetanus. Gestational screening for maternal HBV infection permits effective

TABLE 72-4 Perinatal Viral Infections

Pathogen	Clinical Manifestations	Diagnostic Tests	Treatment
HSV	Skin, eye, or mucous membrane vesicular lesions (SEM disease), encephalitis, disseminated infection involving particularly lungs and liver	Culture of virus and direct fluorescent antibody testing of skin lesions, DNA PCR in CSF, culture of virus from mucosal surfaces	Acyclovir
VZV	Generalized vesicular lesions	Culture of virus and direct fluorescent antibody testing of skin lesions, IgM antibody	Acyclovir
HIV	Usually asymptomatic at birth; if left untreated, can develop severe infections in the first few months of life	DNA or RNA PCR	Antiretroviral agents
HBV	Usually asymptomatic at birth	Hepatitis B surface antigen test and serology	Interferon alpha and lamivudine (used only in chronic HBV)

HIV, human immunodeficiency virus; VZV, varicella-zoster virus; HBV, hepatitis B virus; HSV, herpes simplex virus; CSF, cerebrospinal fluid; PCR, polymerase chain reaction.

immunoprophylaxis for the infant at birth. Detecting HIV infection in the mother would prompt institution of antiretroviral therapy and avoidance of breastfeeding, which both serve to reduce mother-to-child transmission of HIV. Intrapartum maternal administration of penicillin significantly reduces the risk of early-onset group B streptococcal disease in newborn infants.

Table 72-4 provides a summary of perinatal viral infections.

CONCLUSION

Congenital and perinatal infections are important causes of neonatal mortality and long-term morbidity. A variety of pathogens, including viruses, bacteria, fungi, and protozoa, can cause these infections. Immaturity of host defenses plays an important role in the pathogenesis of infections in newborn infants. Attention to their prevention through adherence to current recommendations for immunization, antibiotic prophylaxis, and infection control practices is incumbent upon health care providers. Recognition of these infections and the provision of appropriate therapy, when available, may ameliorate some of their important consequences.

Suggested Readings

Infections of the fetus and newborn (Section N). In: Long SS, Pickering LJ, Prober CG, eds. *Principles and Practice of Pediatric Infectious Diseases.* 3rd ed. Philadelphia, PA: Elsevier Health Sciences; 2008.

Remington JS, Klein JO, eds. *Infectious Diseases of the Fetus and Newborn Infant.* 6th ed. Philadelphia, PA: Elsevier Health Sciences; 2005.

Chapter **73**

Zoonoses

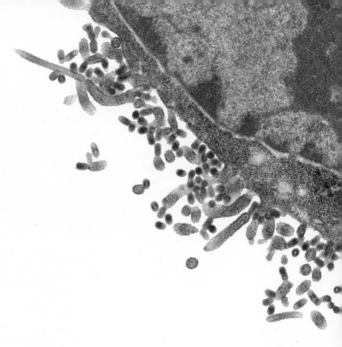

Daniel S. Shapiro

ZOONOSES are infections normally found in nonhuman vertebrates that are transmitted to humans. The diversity of zoonoses is extraordinary; they include viral (e.g., rabies), bacterial (e.g., anthrax), mycobacterial (e.g., bovine tuberculosis), fungal (e.g., some skin infections caused by dermatophytes), and parasitic (e.g., trichinellosis) infections, and even prion disease (the agent of bovine spongiform encephalopathy [BSE], or "mad cow disease," in cattle and variant Creutzfeldt-Jakob disease in humans). Some controversy surrounds what constitutes a zoonotic infection. For example, the numerous arthropodborne viral infections in which humans are bitten by an infected mosquito are not considered zoonoses by some experts but are by others. The term zoonosis is the singular of zoonoses.

In recent years, recognition of the importance of zoonotic infections has increased, partly because of the significant overlap of zoonoses within two areas of public health: emerging infectious diseases and potential agents of bioterrorism (Fig. 73-1). Thus, the potential for significant illness and death from zoonotic infections is of major concern. Both conventional public health and high-quality veterinary public health, which is not readily available in countries with limited resources, are essential in the recognition and control of zoonoses. Both types of public health strategies help to ensure a safe food supply for humans, which is important to human health and the economic vitality of countries that export food products or animals.

CONTACT BETWEEN HUMANS AND ANIMALS

The potential points of contact between humans and animals and humans and animal products are numerous (Table 73-1). Humans are in contact with animals as a result of occupational exposures, as in farming and veterinary medicine, and as a result of pet ownership. Less obvious, but of no less importance, is that our omnivorous diet puts us in contact with animal products during food preparation and ingestion.

Domestic Animals

The effect of a growing human population is of great importance in numerous threats to public health, including zoonotic infections. The tremendous number of animals with which humans have daily contact includes more than 100 million dogs and cats in the United States and huge numbers of cattle, pigs, goats, sheep, horses, chickens, and other domestic animals raised for food or their products (e.g., hides and fur). As the human population increases, so does the domestic animal population and the number of potential human–animal interactions. In addition, the need to dispose of the excrement of domestic animals poses substantial challenges. Large-scale factory farming includes hog farms that house many thousands of animals in a relatively small space and results in wastewater "lagoons" that have been implicated in the contamination of the environment with resistant bacteria. Broiler chickens in the United States are often raised in confinement pens that house between 10,000 and 20,000 birds, an arrangement that allows for economical production of

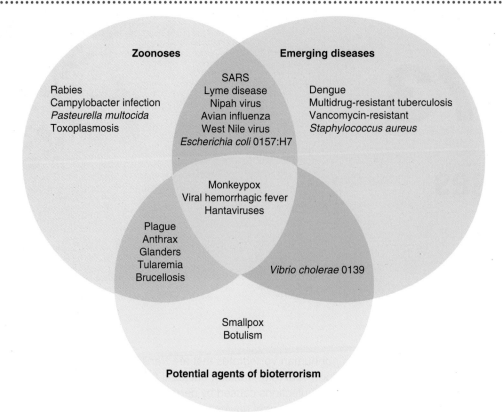

FIGURE 73-1. A schematic diagram of the interplay between zoonoses, emerging diseases, and potential agents of bioterrorism.

chickens but also creates an ideal environment for the spread of infectious agents between the birds.

Antibiotics in Feed

The practice of including antibiotics in animal feed, which results in selection of antibiotic-resistant bacteria that can be transmitted to humans, continues to be widely practiced in the United States. One recent estimate is that 27.5 million pounds of antibiotics are used for purposes that include growth promotion and disease prophylaxis in domestic animals, whereas 2 million pounds are used for veterinary therapeutic purposes. This awesome selective pressure enhances the risk of acquiring antibiotic-resistant organisms in humans.

Population Increase

The increase in the human population has resulted in people moving into areas where only wildlife had existed. The potential for exposure to zoonoses in those settings is significant, including diseases caused by direct contact with animals or their excreta and also diseases transmitted by arthropod vectors, such as Lyme disease. As humans enter new areas, the potential emerges for

exposure to pathogens that previously have not infected our species.

TRANSMISSION OF ZOONOTIC INFECTIONS TO HUMANS

Some zoonotic infections can be acquired by humans through many routes, as illustrated for tularemia in Figure 73-2. In most cases, however, a zoonosis can only be passed from an animal to a human through one of the six routes described in the following sections.

Direct Contact

Through **direct contact** with an animal or an animal product, a person can acquire various diseases, ranging from dermatophyte infections, which are common among veterinary assistants through contact with cat fur, to cutaneous anthrax, which is seen among workers handling contaminated animal hides (Table 73-2). Through **contact with urine**, sewer workers can acquire leptospirosis as a result of exposure to water that contains the urine of infected rats. Leptospirosis can also spread as a result of flooding and subsequent exposure to contaminated water.

TABLE 73-1 Contact Between Humans and Animals Documented to Result in the Transmission of Zoonoses

Type of Contact	Examples
Occupational	Animal groomer
	Butcher
	Cook
	Farmer
	Fisherman
	Furrier
	Hunter
	Laboratory animal caretaker
	Leather worker
	Pet store worker
	Sewer worker (contact with water contaminated by rat urine)
	Slaughterhouse worker
	Trapper
	Veterinarian
	Veterinary assistant
	Wildlife scientist (e.g., mammalogist)
	Woolsorter
	Zoo worker
Common activities	Camping
	Drinking milk
	Eating
	Owning a pet
	Preparing food
	Swimming
	Visiting a petting zoo or farm
Injuries	Animal bites
	Animal scratches
	Bites by ectoparasites (e.g., fleas, ticks)
	Fish fin injuries

Animal Bites or Scratches

Acquisition of infection through **animal bites or scratches** is a common mechanism of zoonotic infection (Table 73-3). For example, the bite of an infected dog, bat, wolf, fox, or other mammal can lead to rabies infection in humans. Bacterial infections also can be acquired by this mechanism, such as infection by *Pasteurella multocida* following the bite or scratch of a cat (typically) or a dog (less frequently).

Inhalation

Zoonotic infections can be acquired by **inhalation** of an infectious agent from the excreta of an animal, as occurs in the hantavirus pulmonary syndrome (HPS) (Table 73-4). Inhalation anthrax, which also is known as woolsorter's disease, is caused by inhaling spores of *Bacillus anthracis* present in the wool of sheep. This organism was used as an agent of bioterrorism when spores were sent in envelopes through the United States mail. That act resulted in a number of infections, both cutaneous and inhalation anthrax, and several deaths among individuals who were exposed to the spores, including postal workers in facilities that used mail-sorting machines.

Inhalation also is a means of acquiring the pneumonic form of plague. That infection can result from exposure to a person with pneumonic plague who generates an infectious aerosol of *Yersinia pestis* by coughing or sneezing. *Y. pestis* also can spread via inhalation through contact with infected cats or inhalation of an aerosol that has been engineered to serve as a weapon (see Chapter 57). Pulmonary tularemia has not been transmitted from person to person, but the disease can be acquired by individuals who work outside and mow over an infected animal or animal excreta, resulting in an infectious aerosol (see Fig. 73-2). In addition to pulmonary involvement, the aerosol can inoculate the conjunctiva.

Ingestion

Infections acquired through **ingestion** of undercooked meat or fish include trichinellosis, which results from eating undercooked pork contaminated by *Trichinella spiralis* (Table 73-5) and other less common *Trichinella* species. Drinking milk that has not been pasteurized, a process involving rapid heating and cooling, can cause human cases of bovine tuberculosis if the cows were infected with *Mycobacterium bovis*. Other common food-borne bacteria include *Salmonella* species and *Yersinia enterocolitica*.

Contamination of food at any step in the production process, from animal slaughter or milking to food preparation or storage, can result in human infection. Examples include outbreaks of *Escherichia coli* O157:H7 infection from contaminated ground beef used in hamburgers served at fast-food restaurants and large-scale outbreaks of salmonellosis among Inuit communities where people ate meat from a dead, rotting whale that had birds feeding on the carcass. An important concern for the consumption of beef is the transmission of variant Creutzfeldt-Jakob disease, a prion disease that epidemiologic and laboratory evidence has linked to cattle infected with BSE. In addition to the United Kingdom, where more than 100 people have been infected with variant Creutzfeldt-Jakob disease, France has had a large number of cases of BSE, and isolated cases have been detected in cattle in other European countries, Canada, and the United States.

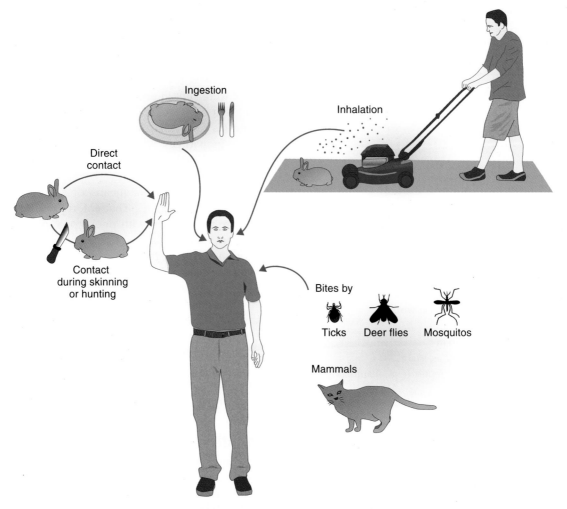

FIGURE 73-2. Means by which tularemia can be acquired.

Fecal–Oral Transmission

Acquisition of zoonotic infection by the **fecal–oral route** is quite common. *All vertebrates potentially can be infected by Salmonella species* and excrete the organism in their feces. Thus, contact with animal feces can result in human cases of salmonellosis. The risk of *Salmonella* infection is of particular importance to individuals who have pet reptiles, which commonly serve as carriers of salmonellosis and may excrete the organism intermittently in their feces, especially when stressed. Other possibilities include the many parasitic diseases for which an infective form appears in animal feces, such as the oocysts of *Toxoplasma gondii* in cat feces. Because *T. gondii* is an organism that may cause an infection that crosses the placenta and affects the fetus, pregnant women should avoid contact with cat feces and wear gloves if they must dispose of cat litter.

Another documented route of fecal–oral transmission is contaminated public water supplies. This mode of transmission includes the lack of a clean source of potable water in resource-poor countries and also problems with the treatment of water in countries with good public health infrastructures. In 1993 in Milwaukee, Wisconsin, approximately 400,000 people became infected with *Cryptosporidium* protozoa as a result of incomplete removal of the organisms by filtration of contaminated water.

Arthropod Bites

Many pathogens are transmitted to humans through the **bites of arthropods** (Table 73-6). Infection can occur as a result of mechanical transmission of the pathogen, as when an arthropod vector bites an infected animal and subsequently bites a human. With that form of

TABLE 73-2 Direct Skin Penetration

Disease	Organism Name	Group	Animal
Bacterial			
Anthrax[a,b]	*Bacillus anthracis*	Gram-positive aerobic spore-forming rods	Domestic mammals (herbivores)
Brucellosis[a,b]	*Brucella melitensis*	Gram-negative rods	Goats, sheep
	B. abortus		Cattle
	B. suis		Swine
	B. canis		Dogs
Erysipeloid	*Erysipelothrix rhusiopathiae*	Gram-positive rods	Swine, poultry, fish
Leptospirosis	*Leptospira interrogans*	Spirochete	Rodents, dogs, domestic animals
Glanders[a]	*Pseudomonas mallei*	Gram-negative rods	Equines
Tularemia[a–d]	*Francisella tularensis*	Gram-negative rods	Rabbits, rodents, cats
Viral			
Orf (contagious ecthyma)	Parapoxvirus	Poxvirus family	Sheep, goats
Vesicular stomatitis	Vesicular stomatitis virus	Rhabdovirus family	Cattle, horses
Parasitic			
Cutaneous larva migrans (creeping eruption)	*Ancylostoma caninum* (dog hookworm)	Nematode	Dogs, cats, carnivores
	Ancylostoma braziliense (dog and cat hookworm)	Nematode	Dogs, cats, carnivores
Fungal			
Dermatophytes	Zoophilic trichophyton, microsporum	Fungi	Dogs, cats, cattle, other mammals

Alternative portals:
[a]Inhalation.
[b]Ingestion.
[c]Arthropod vector.
[d]Animal bite.

transmission, no intervening stages of development in the life cycle of the pathogen take place within the arthropod. For example, transmission of *Francisella tularensis*, the etiologic agent of tularemia, can occur following the bite of a tick, deer fly, or (in parts of northern Europe) mosquito that has bitten an infected animal. In contrast, the life cycle of the parasite *Babesia microti* involves both a rodent host and a tick. After the introduction of sporozoites into the rodent host, the parasite differentiates into male and female gametes. After the gametes are ingested by the deer tick host as part of a blood meal from an infected rodent, the gametes unite, ultimately resulting in sporozoites. If a tick that contains sporozoites bites a human rather than a rodent, the sporozoites can be introduced into the human, who will become infected.

GLOBAL CONCERNS ABOUT ZOONOSES

The range of species a given pathogen can infect is known as the **host range** of the pathogen. For most

TABLE 73-3 Animal Bite or Scratch

Disease	Organism Name	Group	Animal
Bacterial			
Pasteurellosis[a,b]	*Pasteurella multocida*	Gram-negative rods	Cats, dogs, and wild mammals
Rat bite fever[a,c]	*Spirillum minor*	Spirochete	Rats and other rodents
	Streptobacillus moniliformis	Gram-negative rods	Rats, rodents, turkeys
Capnocytophaga canimorsus	*C. canimorsus*	Gram-negative rods	Dogs
Cat scratch disease[d]	*Bartonella henselae*	Gram-negative rods	Cats, dogs suspected
Viral			
Rabies	Rabies virus	Rhabdovirus family	Bats, skunks, foxes, opossums, some domestic mammals
Herpes B encephalomyelitis[d]	Cercopithecine herpesvirus 1	Herpesvirus family	Rhesus macaques
Fungal			
Blastomycosis	*Blastomyces dermatitidis*	Fungi	Dogs (very rare)

Alternative portal:
[a]Skin penetration.
[b]Inhalation.
[c]Ingestion.
[d]Conjunctival inoculation.

viruses, the host range is narrow; one exception is rabies virus, which can infect many species. A broad host range also is seen with the bacterial cause of tularemia, *F. tularensis*, which is able to infect more than 100 mammalian species. The capacity of a pathogen to make the "species jump" to humans is of great concern because the new (to humans) pathogen must be detected, identified, and rapidly contained, although the pathogenesis and epidemiology of the pathogen in its nonhuman host may be unknown (see the box titled "Newly Recognized Zoonosis Caused by a Change in the Environment").

Another major concern that must be quickly addressed is whether a new pathogen can spread efficiently from person to person. This capability varies dramatically among pathogens. For example, rabies virus, which has a broad host range and can be transmitted to humans from many animals, has rarely been transmitted from human to human and only by extraordinary means (e.g., corneal transplant or organ transplant). In contrast, human immunodeficiency virus-1, which has spread globally, appears to have been introduced into the human population from a single species, chimpanzees (*Pan troglodytes troglodytes*). A potential major public health concern is the introduction of avian strains of

influenza A (e.g., H5N1) into the human population in Asia. The new influenza virus strains could eventually develop into strains that are efficiently spread from person to person, resulting in a pandemic in which millions of people perish. The pandemic strain influenza A (H1N1) that emerged in 2009 has genetic sequences that indicate that swine were involved in its origin. Birds and pigs are two types of animals that have served as reservoir hosts for human cases of influenza A.

The host range and efficiency of spread of viral pathogens depend on the molecular biology of the virus and the human host. A virus (really a viral population) with a high frequency of mutation or recombination prompts concern that strains will be selected that are able to both make the species jump to humans and spread efficiently from person to person. For some pathogens, the reservoir host in nature may not experience symptoms of chronic infection. In contrast, the pathobiology of the infection in a host of a different species cannot be easily predicted.

EVALUATION FOR POSSIBLE ZOONOSES

When a patient presents to the physician with an illness, an animal exposure history should be obtained.

TABLE 73-4 Inhalation

Disease	Organism Name	Group	Animal Reservoir	Inhalant
Bacterial				
Anthrax[a,b] (woolsorter's disease)	*Bacillus anthracis*	Gram-positive aerobic spore-forming rods	Goats, sheep, cattle	Spores from wool, animal hides
Ornithosis (psittacosis)	*Chlamydophila psittaci*	*Chlamydia*	Parrots, turkeys, birds	Dried excreta from infected birds
Plague[c]	*Yersinia pestis*	Gram-negative rods	Rats, rodents, cats (contact with infected cats especially likely to result in pneumonic form of plague)	Respiratory contact with humans with pneumonic plague and infected cats
Q fever	*Coxiella burnetii*	*Rickettsia*	Domestic animals	Soil and fomites contaminated with animal excretions, especially placental products
Tuberculosis[d]	*Mycobacterium bovis*	Acid-fast bacillus	Domestic mammals	Contaminated respiratory secretions
Tularemia[a,b,e,f]	*Francisella tularensis*	Gram-negative rods	Wild rabbits, rodents, wild mammals, cats that hunt outdoors	Excreta or aerosolized small animals
Viral				
Lymphocytic choriomeningitis	Lymphocytic choriomeningitis virus	Arenavirus family	Mice, hamsters, other rodents	Infected aerosols
Hantavirus pulmonary syndrome	Sin Nombre virus and other viruses	Bunyavirus family	Mice, other rodents	Infected aerosols
Fungal				
Histoplasmosis	*Histoplasma capsulatum*	Fungi	Birds, bats	Microconidia from contaminated soil

Alternative portals:
[a]Skin penetration.
[b]Animal bite.
[c]Flea bite.
[d]Ingestion of milk.
[e]Ingestion of infected animal.
[f]Arthropod bite.

The specific animal or exposure can provide clues about the patient's diagnosis. Of equal importance is the public health impact of establishing a diagnosis of a zoonotic infection because many infections occur in clusters as a result of common exposure (e.g., a large foodborne outbreak). The need to consider bioterrorism or the need to take appropriate action to safeguard the population from a mosquitoborne illness is especially significant. Being able to establish a broad differential diagnosis on the basis of the type of animal to which an individual is exposed and to generate a list of the possible types of exposure once a zoonotic infection is diagnosed are essential tools for the health of the patient and the community.

TABLE 73-5 Ingestion

Disease	Organism Name	Group	Animal Reservoir	Ingestant (Contaminated Foodstuff)
Bacterial				
Brucellosis[a,b]	*Brucella melitensis, B. abortus, B. suis, B. canis*	Gram-negative rods	Goats, cattle	Dairy products
Campylobacter	*Campylobacter jejuni*	Gram-negative rods	Domestic mammals, fowl	Milk, water, meat, poultry
Listeriosis[a]	*Listeria monocytogenes*	Gram-positive rods	Domestic mammals, rodents, birds	Meat, cheese, vegetables
Salmonellosis	*Salmonella* species (not *S. typhi*)	Gram-negative rods	Fowl, domestic mammals, turtles	Milk, eggs, meat, poultry, shellfish
Tuberculosis[b]	*Mycobacterium bovis*	Acid-fast bacillus	Cattle	Milk
Yersiniosis	*Yersinia enterocolitica*	Gram-negative rods	Pigs, cattle	Milk (particularly unpasteurized milk), pig intestines
Helminthic				
Anisakiasis	*Anisakis simplex*	Nematode	Marine fish	Larvae in undercooked fish
Tapeworm infection	*Taenia saginata*	Cestode	Cattle	Larvae (cysticercus) in undercooked beef
	Taenia solium	Cestode	Pigs	Larvae (cysticercus) in undercooked pork
	Diphyllobothrium latum	Cestode	Fish	Larvae in raw fish
	Echinococcus	Cestode	Dogs, sheep, reindeer, caribou, wolves	Ova from infected dogs via the fecal–oral route
Trichinellosis	*Trichinella spiralis*	Nematode	Pigs, domestic mammals, wild mammals, rodents	Larval cysts
Visceral larva migrans	*Toxocara canis* (roundworm of dogs)	Nematode	Dogs	Ova in soil from infected dogs via the fecal–oral route
Protozoal				
Cryptosporidiosis	*Cryptosporidium*	—	Cattle	Oocysts in fecally contaminated water
Toxoplasmosis[c,d]	*Toxoplasma gondii*	—	Cats	Oocysts from cat feces, tissue cyst from uncooked meat
Other				
Variant Creutzfeldt-Jakob disease	—	Prion	Cattle	Beef

Alternative portals:
[a]Skin penetration.
[b]Inhalation.
[c]Transplacental.
[d]Organ transplantation.

TABLE 73-6 Selected Arthropod-Borne Diseases

Disease	Vector	Organism Name	Microbial Group	Animal Reservoir
Bacterial				
Lyme disease	Tick	*Borrelia burgdorferi*	Spirochete	Rodents, deer
Plague, bubonic[a]	Flea	*Yersinia pestis*	Gram-negative rods	Urban rats, rodents, cats that hunt outdoors
Relapsing fever	Tick	*Borrelia* species	Spirochete	Rodent, wild mammals
Tularemia[a–c]	Tick, biting flies, mosquitoes (northern Europe)	*Francisella tularensis*	Gram-negative rods	Wild rabbits, rodents, wild mammals, cats that hunt outdoors
Rocky Mountain spotted fever	Tick	*Rickettsia rickettsii*	Rickettsia	Wild rodents, dogs
Scrub typhus	Mite (chigger)	*Rickettsia tsutsugamushi*	Rickettsia	Wild rodents, rats
Murine typhus	Flea	*Rickettsia typhi*	Rickettsia	Rats, opossums
—	—	*Rickettsia felis*	Rickettsia	—
Rickettsialpox	Mite	*Rickettsia akari*	Rickettsia	Mice
Ehrlichiosis	Ticks	*Ehrlichia* species	Ehrlichia	Deer, elk, rodents, dogs
Viral				
Yellow fever	Mosquito	Flavivirus	Flavivirus family	Primates (sylvatic cycle)
Eastern equine encephalitis	Mosquito	Alphavirus	Togavirus family	Birds
Venezuelan equine encephalitis	Mosquito	Alphavirus	Togavirus family	Birds
Western equine encephalitis	Mosquito	Alphavirus	Togavirus family	Birds
West Nile	Mosquito	Flavivirus	Flavivirus family	Birds
St. Louis encephalitis	Mosquito	Flavivirus	Flavivirus family	Birds
California encephalitis	Mosquito	Bunyavirus	Bunyavirus family	Mammals, wild rodents
Rift Valley fever[a]	Mosquito	Bunyavirus	Bunyavirus family	Sheep, goats, cattle
Crimean-Congo hemorrhagic fever[a]	Tick	Bunyavirus	Bunyavirus family	Domestic mammals, rodents
Colorado tick fever	Tick	Orbivirus	Reovirus family	Rodents
Protozoal				
Babesiosis	Tick	*Babesia* species	—	Domestic and wild animals
Leishmaniasis (kala azar, cutaneous leishmaniasis)	Sandfly	*Leishmania* species	—	Dogs, foxes, rodents, wild mammals
American trypanosomiasis[b]	Reduviid bug (kissing bug)	*Trypanosoma cruzi*	—	Dogs, cats, opossums, armadillos, wild mammals
African sleeping sickness	Tsetse fly	*Trypanosoma* species	—	Cattle, wild animals

Alternative portals:
[a]Skin penetration.
[b]Ingestion.
[c]Inhalation.

NEWLY RECOGNIZED ZOONOSIS CAUSED BY A CHANGE IN THE ENVIRONMENT

In May 1993, an outbreak of unexplained respiratory illness occurred in the Four Corners region of the United States, an area of the southwest shared by New Mexico, Arizona, Colorado, and Utah. The outbreak was notable for a severe illness in previously healthy young adults. They suddenly developed acute respiratory distress, and approximately half of the infected persons died. Usual and unusual (e.g., pneumonia and plague, respectively) causes were excluded by appropriate testing.

An investigation to determine the cause and epidemiology of the outbreak was successful. Tissues from infected individuals were sent to the Centers for Disease Control and Prevention (CDC), where molecular virology studies demonstrated an association between the pulmonary syndrome and a previously unknown hantavirus. This association led to the designation hantavirus pulmonary syndrome (HPS) for the disease. Collection of rodents, the hosts of hantaviruses, was performed, and in November 1993, the virus that caused the outbreak, a previously unknown hantavirus, was isolated by the Special Pathogens Branch at CDC from tissue of a deer mouse *(Peromyscus maniculatus)* that had been trapped near the New Mexico home of a patient. Approximately 1,700 rodents representing various species were trapped and studied during the investigation, and approximately 30% of the deer mice tested showed evidence of the infection.

Because the convention for naming hantaviruses is to use the name of the location where the virus was first isolated, the HPS hantavirus was initially named Muerto Canyon virus. However, that area is sacred to the Navajo, and the name was subsequently changed to Sin Nombre virus. The virus is a member of the genus *Hantavirus*, family *Bunyaviridae*. Studies of archived tissue from patients who were ill with respiratory infections demonstrated that there had been cases of HPS before 1993.

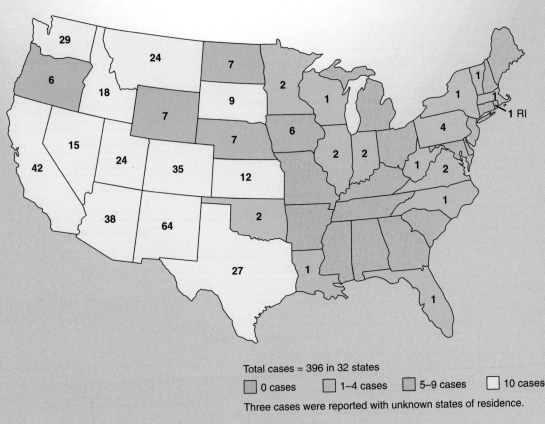

Total cases = 396 in 32 states

☐ 0 cases ☐ 1–4 cases ☐ 5–9 cases ☐ 10 cases

Three cases were reported with unknown states of residence.

FIGURE 73-3. Hantavirus pulmonary syndrome cases by state of residence, United States, May 1993 to July 2005.

(continued)

Why this outbreak occurred at the time and location it did was investigated by public health authorities. In 1993, the mouse population in the Four Corners area was unusually large. Following a drought that had plagued the area for several years, a marked increase in precipitation in early 1993 resulted in burgeoning plant growth. The availability of food for the deer mice increased dramatically, leading to an increase in their reproductive rate. At the time of the first cases of the outbreak, May 1993, 10 times as many mice inhabited the area as had been there a year earlier. The explosion in the mouse population led to a greater probability of mice interacting with humans, including the potential for human inhalation of virus from mouse excreta. According to the CDC, from May 1993 to July 2005, Sin Nombre virus caused 396 cases of severe respiratory disease with a mortality rate of 36%. The virus has been recognized in 32 states (Fig. 73-3).

The discovery of Sin Nombre virus as the cause of HPS spurred a great deal of research on it and related hantaviruses. Many hantaviruses have caused HPS in persons from Canada to South America. Fortunately, there is no evidence of person-to-person transmission of HPS, with the exception of HPS caused by Andes virus, a newly described hantavirus isolated in Argentina.

CONCLUSION

An awareness of zoonoses and their tremendous impact on human health—and the devastating potential of the introduction of new zoonotic agents into the human population—has led to increases in both surveillance for these agents and research in areas ranging from wildlife management to molecular biology. These efforts require the coordinated work of veterinarians, physicians, basic researchers, entomologists, and public health experts. Because many of the potential pathogens are found in developing countries that lack a public health infrastructure, the recognition of an outbreak of an established or novel pathogen may be delayed, with potentially disastrous consequences for the country of origin and also worldwide. Similarly, war often results in a breakdown in public health and an unwillingness to provide information by the government (or group) that is in power. These types of barriers are difficult, if not impossible, to overcome in the absence of the political will of the international community to recognize emerging zoonotic infections as a threat that knows no boundaries.

Suggested Readings

Brown C. Virchow revisited: emerging zoonoses. *ASM News.* 2003;69(10):493–497.

Chomel BB, Belotto A, Meslin F-X. Wildlife, exotic pets, and emerging zoonoses. *Emerg Inf Dis.* 2007;13(1):6–11.

Jones, KE, Patel NG, Levy MA, et al. Global trends in emerging infectious diseases. *Nature.* 2008;451(7181):990–993.

Smith GJD, Viaykrishna D, Bahl J, et al. Origins and evolutionary genomics of the 2009 swine-origin H1N1 influenza epidemic. *Nature.* 2009;459:1122–1125.

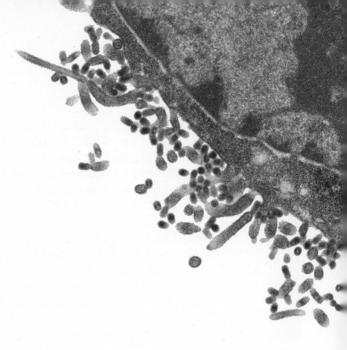

Chapter 74

Fever: A Clinical Sign of Infection

Suzanne F. Bradley

NOT ALL ELEVATIONS in body temperature are fever, nor are they necessarily caused by infection. An elevation of temperature that is a normal variant or reflects increased generation of body heat or an inability to dissipate it is called **hyperthermia**. An elevation of temperature caused by the release of inflammatory mediators in response to various foreign or exogenous stimuli is called **fever**. Although many people fear the complications of fever, it is a normal reaction to invasion by certain microorganisms and may actually play a beneficial role in the host response to infection. However, infection is only one of many causes of fever. Occasionally, the causes of prolonged temperature elevations may be difficult to diagnose. **Fever of unknown origin** (**FUO**) can be one of the greatest challenges for the infectious diseases consultant to solve.

WHAT IS NORMAL BODY TEMPERATURE?

Rigors (shivering), sweats, chills, flushing, tachycardia, lethargy, and increased warmth of skin have been recognized as signs and symptoms of disease since ancient times. Although crude mercury thermometers had been available for more than a century, the significance of increased body temperature and its association with the signs and symptoms of disease (fever) were not fully appreciated until 1871, when Carl Wunderlich reported his detailed studies of body temperature.

Generally, **normal body temperature** ranges from 36.3°C to 37.5°C (97.3°F to 99.5°F) in healthy humans. Body temperature normally fluctuates 1°C to 1.3°C (1.8°F to 2.4°F), with the lowest measurements noted between 2 and 8 AM and the highest between 4 and 9 PM. The daily, cyclic variation in temperature is called **diurnal variation**. Temperature measurements vary when measured at different body sites. Rectal temperature measurements are generally 0.8°C (1°F) higher than oral temperature measurements. Normal temperatures may be higher in females and lower in newborns and in the debilitated elderly. Therefore, the accepted "normal temperature" of 37°C (98.6°F), an average value, may have little clinical meaning for a given individual. Within these limitations, temperatures above 37.5°C (99.4°F) orally and 38.0°C

(100.4°F) rectally are generally accepted as abnormal in immunocompetent adults. Abnormal temperatures in newborns and the elderly may be lower. Mr. J's temperature at 38.9°C is definitely abnormal.

Every elevated temperature does not necessarily require evaluation for underlying disease. Normal elevations of body temperatures of 0.6°C to 0.8°C (1°F to 1.5°F) may be observed transiently in healthy persons after vigorous exercise or eating. A brief local increase in oral temperature measurements can occur after smoking, gum chewing, or drinking warm liquids. Following a self-limited febrile infection, some patients continue to take their temperatures even though their illnesses have resolved. A diary that details early morning and evening temperatures, measurements when the patient feels warm, and associated activities may be a helpful tool to determine whether a temperature is abnormal or merely reflects daily activities or normal diurnal variation.

NORMAL THERMOREGULATION

The main goal of thermoregulatory mechanisms is preservation of deep visceral or **core body temperatures** at levels that allow optimal function essential vital organs. As you have already seen, normal core body temperatures

• At 82 years of age, Mr. J. had been feeling well until he noted a significant decline in his vision, intermittent jaw pain, and headaches associated with night sweats. Over the following year, his symptoms extended to include anorexia, weight loss of 20 pounds, and occasional temperatures greater than 38.6°C. Examination revealed a decline in vision, mild anemia, and an erythrocyte sedimentation rate (ESR) of 129 mm/h (normal is 0 to 20 mm/h).

Mr. J. had no allergies and took no medications. He is a retired insurance salesman and had traveled throughout the United States. He lived with his wife, a dog, and a cat. His medical and family histories were unremarkable. He looked relatively well, but his clothes fit loosely. Physical examination was unremarkable except for a temperature of 38.9°C, a resting pulse of 105 beats per minute, and tenderness over the right temple. No sinus tenderness was elicited by palpation and the chest examination was normal.

The change in vision, anemia, anorexia, and elevated ESR were ascribed to "old age," and the jaw pain to poor dentition. He was treated with multiple antibiotics for sinusitis and bronchitis, although he denied productive cough or pain over his sinuses.

This case raises several questions:

1. Does Mr. J. have a fever?
2. Is his temperature elevation a danger to him?
3. Is his illness caused by infection?
4. How might Mr. J.'s physician begin to evaluate the potential causes of his symptoms?

See Appendix for answers.

---

are tightly regulated within a very narrow temperature (Fig. 74-1). Changes in peripheral or **shell body temperature** and core body temperature are perceived and carefully regulated via a network of **peripheral thermosensory neurons**.

Peripheral superficial thermosensory neurons are found primarily in the skin. These peripheral superficial sensors are primarily **cold sensitive**. Cold-sensitive neurons undergo rapid activation or depolarization of their membranes in response to significant shifts in shell

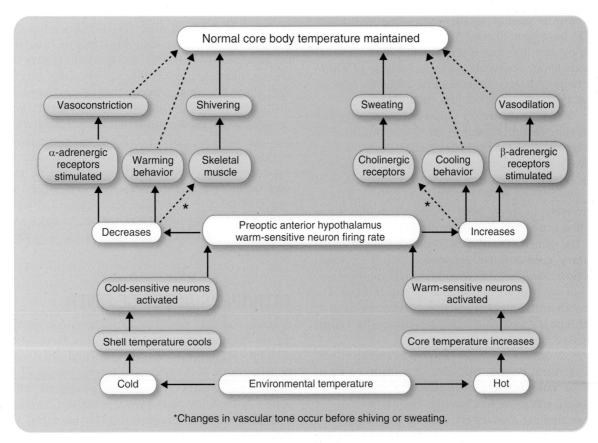

FIGURE 74-1. Thermoregulation in humans.

body temperature typically following contact with a cold environment. In contrast, **peripheral deep thermosensory neurons** are activated in response to significant changes in the body's deep (core) temperature. These deep sensory neurons are predominantly **warm sensitive** and are located in the viscera and large vessels.

Whether thermosensory neurons are cold sensitive or warm sensitive is determined by a **transient receptor potential (TRP) family** of ion channels. There are at least six different TRP channels that are independently activated by very narrow temperature thresholds ranging from very cold (≤ 17°C) to painfully hot (>52°C). Specific TRP channels have been associated with warm-sensitive (**TRPV1–4**) and cold-sensitive (**TRPM8, TRPA1**) peripheral thermosensory neurons. So distinct populations of thermosensory neurons may fire in response to different temperatures. Signals from these peripheral thermosensors are primarily transmitted through sensory neurons located in the ganglia of the dorsal root and trigeminal nerve to the dorsal spinal column, brainstem, and to the **preoptic anterior hypothalamus (POA)**.

The POA is the major thermoregulatory center in man. The POA receives thermal inputs from peripheral sensory neurons, monitors local temperatures within the brain, and regulates voluntary and involuntary responses that defend against body core temperatures that are too cool or too warm (Fig. 74-1).

In contrast with peripheral thermosensors that are activated only when there are significant changes in body temperature, the predominantly warm-sensitive neurons of the POA have been likened to a pacemaker that is constantly firing at a rate that is temperature dependent. At higher body temperatures, the increased activity of warm-sensitive neurons triggers defenses that inhibit the generation of heat and promote heat loss (**heat-defense**).

The initial **involuntary heat-defense** response results in skin **vasodilation** mediated by stimulation of β-adrenergic receptors of the sympathetic nervous system. If heat loss is insufficient, activation of the cholinergic receptors promote **sweating** and further dissipation of heat.

Conversely, at lower body temperatures, the lower activity of warm-sensitive neurons triggers defenses that increase the generation of heat (**cold-defense**). Initial **involuntary cold-defense responses** result in **vasoconstriction** mediated by stimulation of α-adrenergic receptors of the sympathetic nervous system. If initial heat gain is insufficient, further generation of heat can be generated through contraction of skeletal muscle (**shivering**) and increased catabolism.

The POA can also stimulate the cortex leading to perceptions of warm or cold that lead to **voluntary heat-defense** or **cold-defense responses**. A person who feels too cool will move to a warmer environment or put on warmer clothing. Conversely, cooling is accomplished through movement to a cooler environment and removal of excess clothing.

So, all thermoregulatory mechanisms are not driven by a single thermal set point to achieve normal core body temperature as had previously been assumed. The thermoregulatory system is much more complex. The activities of peripheral sensory neurons, the POA, and the sympathetic nervous system are regulated independently by different thermoeffector loops. Temperature thresholds determine when vasoconstriction/shivering and vasodilation/sweating occur, thus defining the lower and upper boundaries of normal body core temperature.

WHAT IS HYPERTHERMIA?

Dysregulation of normal thermoregulatory mechanisms leading to increased body temperature is termed **hyperthermia**. Patients with mild hyperthermia (**heat exhaustion**) may feel lethargic and thirsty and present with clammy skin and signs of mild dehydration. In patients with severe hyperthermia (**heat stroke**), high temperatures, delirium, coma, warm dry skin, signs of severe dehydration, organ failure, cardiac arrhythmias, and death may ensue. Treatment includes rehydration and immersion in cooling baths.

Persons with impairment of any aspect of thermoregulation may be at increased risk of hyperthermia. Elderly individuals or patients with cerebrovascular accidents, dementia, or other neuropsychiatric disorders may have impaired thermal perception. Conditions that impair mobility can prevent an individual from leaving a warm environment. Drugs with α-adrenergic activity can prevent vasodilatation, and drugs that increase fluid loss (diuretics) or have anticholinergic side effects (antipsychotics, antiemetics) can impede sweating. Patients with skin disorders that prevent them from sweating normally may be at risk for hyperthermia, as are those with cervical spinal cord injuries that have damaged the sympathetic nervous system, leading to dysregulated thermoregulatory responses. Endocrine disorders such as hyperthyroidism and pheochromocytoma or increased skeletal muscle activity as seen in generalized seizures can also lead to hyperthermia. None of those conditions was evident in the case of Mr. J., suggesting that the cause of his temperature elevation was fever, not hyperthermia.

PATHOPHYSIOLOGY OF FEVER

Fever is a normal physiologic phenomenon regulated by the central nervous system (CNS). Thus, fever differs in its pathophysiology from the dysregulated phenomenon of hyperthermia. Fever is caused by the release of **inflammatory mediators (endogenous pyrogens)** often stimulated by invading pathogens like bacteria, viruses, fungi, and parasites (see Chapter 6). The microbial products that elicit this response are generally microbial surface components (e.g., endotoxin, lipoteichoic acids, muramyl dipeptide, mannan) or exotoxins (staphylococcal toxic shock syndrome toxin 1). Antigen–antibody complexes can also stimulate endogenous pyrogen production.

Endogenous pyrogen activity has been attributed to several pyrogenic **cytokines**: interleukin 1 (IL-1), tumor necrosis factor (TNF), and IL-6. In addition, factors such as granulocyte-macrophage colony-stimulating factor, interferon-γ, IL-2, and others may indirectly cause fever by stimulating the production of those cytokines. The relative contributions of each cytokine to the febrile response are not clear. Many different cells contribute to the production of the mediators, but most are probably produced by monocytes and macrophages. Endogenous pyrogens presumably travel to the brain through the circulation, although TNF and IL-1 are usually not detected by assays of the blood in patients with overwhelming infection.

How circulating endogenous pyrogens produced in the peripheral blood interact with thermoregulatory centers in the brain such as the POA is not known. Three hypotheses, termed the **humoral hypotheses of fever induction**, are proposed. The large peptides that function as endogenous pyrogens may (1) interact directly with parts of the brain where the blood–brain barrier is incomplete, (2) bind directly to cytokine-specific receptors on brain endothelial cells, and/or (3) be actively transported across the blood–brain barrier.

There are structures in the CNS, termed **circumventricular organs**, that are highly vascular, but lack a blood–brain barrier, and whose cells are in contact with the cerebroventricular system. One circumventricular organ, the **organum vasculosum of the lamina terminalis (OVLT)**, is located in close proximity to the POA and appears to play a major role in the development of fever. Studies performed at cellular and molecular levels suggest that the OVLT functions as a sensor for endogenous pyrogens. The result of interactions of endogenous pyrogens with either the OVLT or brain endothelial cells is an increase in local levels of **prostaglandin E$_2$ (PGE$_2$)**. Local PGE$_2$ production activates prostaglandin receptors (subtype EP3) in the hypothalamus. Endogenous pyrogens may work by inhibiting warm-sensitive neurons in the POA, thus limiting heat loss and leading to an increase in the normal **thermoregulatory set point** in the hypothalamus. Essentially, the body's thermostat is turned up.

The POA also has other important functions including the secretion of hormones such as vasopressin and corticotropin-releasing hormone, regulation of blood flow (paraventricular nucleus), and the control of appetite (lateral hypothalamus). Those areas, in addition to the sleep/wake centers located in the hypothalamus and brainstem, account not only for the generation of fever but also for its associated symptoms of **anorexia** and **lethargy**.

The newly elevated thermoregulatory set point is maintained by a complex negative feedback loop. Endogenous pyrogen production leads to increased corticotropin-releasing, factor-mediated stimulation of the hypopituitary–adrenal axis. The **adrenal glucocorticoids** produced by this stimulation inhibit cytokine production and attenuate fever. Other factors with antiendogenous pyrogen activity, such as melanocyte-stimulating hormone and arginine vasopressin, may also be produced by the CNS. In addition, increased levels of the endogenous pyrogens themselves may downregulate their own production. When stimulated by cytokines, cells of target end organs may decrease their responsiveness to a specific mediator by downregulating the expression of the surface receptors or, in some instances, by shedding them. As a result, a patient who has reached the hypothetical thermoregulatory set point begins to sweat, and vessels dilate to dissipate excess heat. If the patient's temperature falls below the thermoregulatory set point, the cycle begins again with rigors, chills, and vasoconstriction to raise the body temperature. External means of cooling a patient with fever, such as using ice packs and cooling blankets, only further stimulate the body to reach its higher thermoregulatory set point. Frequent bouts of rigors and chills may be more uncomfortable to the patient than the fever itself.

To prevent recurrence of fever, the disease that causes the fever must be treated and the thermoregulatory set point lowered through the use of **antipyretic agents** (aspirin, nonsteroidal anti-inflammatory drugs, and acetaminophen) that inhibit endogenous pyrogen and PGE$_2$ production. In contrast to fever, hyperthermia is not mediated by endogenous pyrogens. Therefore, antipyretics are not effective in lowering the body temperature of patients with hyperthermia.

FEVER AS A BENEFICIAL HOST RESPONSE

In the last two centuries, fever has been perceived as a dangerous affliction to be eliminated by physician and layperson alike. However, until the 1800s and the advent of antipyretics, fever was seen as a potent ally, purging patients of the bad humors that caused disease. In fact, scientific evidence supports the concept that fever in the face of infection confers a survival advantage to the host. For example, numerous unrelated species of animals have evolved this mechanism as a common response to infection, and they each produce multiple cytokines with redundant endogenous pyrogen activity. Inhibiting fever in infected reptiles and fish results in increased mortality with infection. Similarly, humans with bacteremia or peritonitis who are unable to mount a febrile response are more likely to die than those who develop fever. Inhibition of the febrile response with antipyretics has been associated with prolonged shedding of rhinoviruses and delayed healing of varicella lesions.

Endogenous pyrogens not only cause fever but also influence the recruitment and function of many types of cells. Not unexpectedly, some of those cells function optimally at higher body temperatures. Thus, *phagocytosis and killing by neutrophils and macrophages are enhanced at elevated temperatures.* Antigen presentation by macrophages, helper T-cell–dependent antibody production, lymphocyte proliferation, cytotoxic T-cell function, and production of IFN-γ, IL-1, and IL-2 all increase at higher temperatures. Endogenous pyrogens also decrease the levels of trace metals (iron and zinc) that many bacteria require for growth. In addition, temperatures of 39°C to 41°C directly inhibit the growth of some bacteria (pneumococci, gonococci, *Treponema pallidum, Mycobacterium leprae*), fungi (*Sporothrix schenckii*), and some parasites in vitro. Motility, capsule formation, and cell wall formation may be inhibited, and antimicrobial susceptibility may increase at higher temperatures. Because many microorganisms prefer to grow at cooler temperatures, they may preferentially infect distal appendages. Local heating has been reported to be effective as a treatment of infection caused by chromomycosis, sporotrichosis, chancroid, and leishmaniasis.

In the past, physicians used artificial **fever therapy**, probably induced by infection with malaria, to treat leprosy, tumors, and other diseases. Recently, the artificial induction of fever in mammals has been shown to increase resistance to bacterial, fungal, and viral infections. In 1927, malarial therapy for neurosyphilis was sufficiently successful to earn its discoverer the Nobel Prize. In animal studies, injection of recombinant endogenous pyrogens before or within a few hours of infection has been shown to reduce mortality and sometimes the microbial load. Conversely, increased mortality has been seen when antibodies to endogenous pyrogens were given before some infections. Thus, evidence exists that fever may have a beneficial role in the host response to infection.

FEVER AS AN ADVERSE HOST RESPONSE

Unfortunately, the story of fever versus microbes is not as simple as hero versus villain. Excessive production of endogenous pyrogens may provoke the **sepsis syndrome** and result in necrosis of tissues, end-organ failure, shock, and even death. Monoclonal antibodies against TNF and its receptors, an antagonist of the IL-1 receptor, and other cytokine inhibitors appear to confer protection in animals, but subsequent studies in humans have shown less promise for their therapeutic use. Future therapies must aim to control excessive endogenous pyrogen production without loss of the beneficial effects of these cytokines.

Moderate fever alone is not dangerous and generally does not require medical intervention except for patient comfort. Although one could argue that inhibiting fever may be detrimental, it should be recognized that an increase in temperature of 1°C or more over 37°C leads to a 13% rise in oxygen consumption. Very high fevers (41°C or 106°F) considerably increase host metabolic demands and place substantial stress on the cardiovascular system, resulting in congestive heart failure and ischemia. Thus, decreasing body temperature is essential in some patients.

In the setting of very high fever, external cooling to rapidly reduce body temperature is appropriate when used in conjunction with antipyretics. Organ damage and death can theoretically occur when temperatures exceed 41.7°C (107°F). In the absence of serious underlying disease, such as in the case of Mr. J., low-grade fevers can be tolerated without adverse consequences.

Temperatures higher than 40°C (103°F) have been associated with generalized **seizures** in children. Children who have experienced seizures previously are likely to experience them again with high fevers, and there is little evidence that the early use of antipyretics and anticonvulsants is helpful in preventing further seizures. Fortunately, neurologic sequelae and resulting learning disabilities are very rare. Congenital malformations in the newborns of women who had high fevers while pregnant have also been reported.

EVALUATION OF ELEVATED TEMPERATURE

Elevated body temperature is a sign of possible disease. The temperature amplitude itself does not predict whether a patient has serious disease. Classic fever patterns, when present, may suggest specific diseases: Hodgkin disease (recurrent episodes, or Pel-Ebstein fever), malaria (fever every other day or every third day), yellow fever or dengue (saddleback or biphasic fever), or penicillin treatment of spirochetal diseases (Jarisch-Herxheimer reaction).

A careful clinical history, including present illness, past medical history, prescription and nonprescription medications, travel history, pets, family history, and review of systems, is essential to narrowing the diagnostic possibilities. A thorough physical examination looking for signs involving specific organ systems may further confirm or exclude clinical suspicions. How quickly the evaluation is performed and treatment initiated depends on the clinical status of the patient. A patient who appears clinically well can be evaluated and treated at a more leisurely pace than the patient who appears severely ill.

Infections are the most common causes of fever. Fortunately, the majority of infections encountered in routine practice get better with time, regardless of whether treatment is initiated. Malignancies, granulomatous diseases, vasculitis, autoimmune diseases, drug reactions, and other conditions may also present as febrile illnesses. Sometimes the etiology of fever defies easy diagnosis. This uncommon clinical syndrome, termed **fever of unknown (or undetermined) origin (FUO)** as demonstrated in the case of Mr. J., remains one of the greatest clinical challenges in medicine.

FEVERS OF UNKNOWN ORIGIN

Mr. J. had an FUO of longstanding duration. He looked relatively well, so it was not likely that he had an occult abscess, tuberculosis, or malignancy. His workup did not necessarily require hospitalization. Dismissing patient symptoms as normal consequences of aging is unwise. Declining vision, jaw pain, and ESR greater than 100 mm/h in an elderly man strongly suggests the diagnosis of **temporal arteritis**, a noninfectious inflammatory disease. An outpatient temporal artery biopsy revealed granulomas consistent with this diagnosis. With corticosteroid therapy, Mr. J.'s fever and jaw pain resolved, he regained weight, and his vision and anemia rapidly improved.

DEFINITION

A FUO is usually defined as the presence of temperatures higher than 38.3°C (101°F) noted on multiple occasions over a 3-week period. A possible etiology of that fever must not be evident following a reasonably intensive inpatient or outpatient diagnostic evaluation over a period of approximately 1 week. That definition excludes most self-limited causes of fever that usually resolve spontaneously or prolonged fevers that are diagnosed promptly.

The diseases that cause FUO usually are not rare or unusual but often are the *atypical presentation of common diseases*. Diagnosis is frequently delayed not because too few tests were ordered but because the physician overlooked significant clues to the diagnosis or misinterpreted their significance. Diagnosis may be particularly difficult in a patient who is either very young or very old and is unable to adequately perceive, interpret, and communicate symptoms. Repeated clarification of the history and reexamination of the patient can be extremely valuable. Each symptom, physical finding, and laboratory abnormality should be thoroughly evaluated and used to guide the judicious ordering of invasive or expensive diagnostic tests.

The spectrum of diseases responsible for FUOs changes with time as technological advances lead to improvements in diagnosis. The advent of computerized tomography, magnetic resonance imaging, and radionucleotide imaging has removed from the FUO category many patients with **abscesses**, **bacterial endocarditis**, and **collagen vascular diseases** (autoimmune or immune complex–mediated diseases) because those diseases are more easily diagnosed now than in the past.

Although physicians have become more successful in determining many causes of FUO, changes in the population result in new challenges. The spectrum of diseases causing FUO can vary in patients who are immunocompromised, including HIV-infected patients, transplant recipients, elderly persons, and those who develop FUO in the hospital. In general, infection remains the most common cause of FUO, followed by neoplasms, collagen vascular diseases, and granulomatous diseases (Table 74-1). Very rarely, patients will cause fever by injecting themselves with pyrogenic substances (fraudulent fever) or manipulate the temperature-measuring device to give the appearance of having fever (factitious fever).

TABLE 74-1 Differential Diagnosis of Fevers of Unknown Origin (FUO)

Category	Cases (%)
Infections	30–40
Abscesses (intra-abdominal)	—
Hepatic, biliary	—
Tuberculosis	—
Endocarditis	—
Cytomegalovirus infection	—
HIV infection	—
Malignancies	20–30
Hematologic	—
Leukemias (monocyte derived)	—
Lymphomas (Hodgkin disease, non-Hodgkin lymphoma)	—
Solid Tumors	—
Hypernephroma (renal)	—
Hepatoma (liver)	—
Collagen Vascular Diseases	9–29
Rheumatoid arthritis (Still disease)	—
Systemic lupus erythematosus	—
Rheumatic fever	—
Arteritis (temporal arteritis, polyarteritis nodosa)	—
Granulomatous Diseases	5–10
Sarcoidosis	—
Inflammatory bowel disease (Crohn disease)	—
Granulomatous hepatitis	—
Miscellaneous	10–20
Pulmonary embolus	—
Drug fever	—
Hematoma	—
Occupational (metal fume fever)	—
Periodic (familial Mediterranean fever)	—
Thermoregulatory disorders[a]	—

continued on page 746

TABLE 74-1 Differential Diagnosis of Fevers of Unknown Origin (FUO) (*continued*)

Category	Cases (%)
Cervical spinal cord injuries	—
Endocrine diseases (hyperthyroidism, Addison disease)	—
Congenital skin disorders	
Factitious or fraudulent fever[b]	
No Diagnosis	10–15

[a]Elevated body temperature in a thermoregulatory disorder is not fever but hyperthermia.
[b]Both types of fever are illusory; patients with factitious fever manipulate temperature-measuring devices, and patients with fraudulent fever inject themselves with pyrogenic substances.

TREATMENT

Even with improvements in diagnostic technology, 10% of FUO patients still defy diagnosis. Fortunately, most patients with undiagnosed FUO do well. More than 95% of patients under the age of 35 years spontaneously recover without therapy. In persons more than 65 years old, spontaneous resolution is rare, and usually a serious disease is ultimately discovered. Empiric trials of antitubercular therapy, corticosteroids, and anti-inflammatory agents may be tried in patients with persistent FUO but only if the patient's clinical condition is deteriorating rapidly and only after exhaustive attempts to make a diagnosis have failed.

CONCLUSION

It is important to interpret elevated body temperature measurements only after careful assessment of the patient. Not all elevated body temperatures are fever. The treatment of hyperthermia is different from that of fever. Some elevations of body temperature require treatment, others only careful observation. Fever may be a beneficial host response. The general rule is to treat the underlying cause, not just the elevated body temperature. Some etiologies of fever may be difficult to discern. A careful approach is essential for diagnosis, and empirical therapy should be used only as a last resort.

Suggested Readings

Cunha BA. Fever of unknown origin: Clinical overview of classic and current concepts. *Infect Dis Clin N Am.* 2007;867–915.

Mackowiak PA. Concepts of fever. *Arch Intern Med.* 1998;158:1870–1881.

Romanovsky AA. Thermoregulation: some concepts have changed. Functional architecture of the thermoregulatory system. *Am J Physiol Regul Integr Comp Physiol.* 2007;292:R37–R46.

Roth J, Rummel C, Barth SW, Gerstberger R, Hubschle T. Molecular aspects of fever and hyperthermia. *Neurologic Clin.* 2006;24:421–439.

Chapter 75

Health Care–Associated Infections

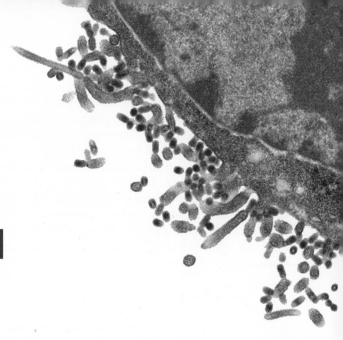

David R. Snydman and Shira Doron

AN INFECTION acquired during a hospital stay is called a **nosocomial infection** or **hospital-acquired infection**. Approximately 5% of patients develop infections while they are in hospitals. An infection resulting from intervention by a physician, in or out of a hospital, is known as an **iatrogenic infection**. **Health care–associated infection** is a broader term that includes those acquired at a nursing home or as a consequence of medical care received at home or other health care settings. Because of the complexity of medical care today with an increasing proportion being undertaken outside of the acute care hospital setting, the term **health care–associated infections** has recently been adopted as the standard terminology. **Health care–associated infections** can be extraordinarily costly in terms of morbidity and even mortality. Hospital stays are often prolonged in patients who acquire infections. It is estimated that about $5 billion is spent each year for the management of health care–associated infections in the United States.

Several factors related to hospitalization predispose patients to the risk of hospital-acquired infections. The most important factors are those that violate the host's own defenses. Invasive procedures produce **new portals of entry** for microorganisms from the patient's own flora or from the environment. Examples of invasion are the use of devices like endotracheal tubes, mechanical ventilators, bladder catheters, and intravenous or intra-arterial catheters as well as surgical procedures in general.

Broadly speaking, the incidence of a nosocomial infection is related to the severity of the underlying disease; that is, patients who have a high likelihood of dying during their hospitalizations also are most at risk of developing nosocomial infections. In contrast, patients admitted with less severe disease are less likely to acquire infections in the hospital. This underscores the need for improved management of the severely compromised patients. Unfortunately, it is estimated that only about one-third to one-half of nosocomial infections are preventable, even under the most favorable conditions.

AGENTS OF HEALTH CARE–ASSOCIATED INFECTIONS

Generally, the organisms that cause health care–associated infections are similar to those found elsewhere in the community. The most common causative agents may not be especially pathogenic; in fact, sometimes they are even less pathogenic than those that cause disease outside the hospital.

A salient example is the emergence of *Serratia marcescens* as a hospital-acquired pathogen. The bacterium was thought to be so benign that it was used in the 1950s to trace the movement of air in a subway system and to determine the movement of bacteria into the urethra through the catheter–meatal interface. This "nonpathogen" has become the source of significant nosocomial infections, although it rarely causes disease outside the hospital.

Like many pathogens associated with nosocomial infections, *S. marcescens* has acquired significant antibiotic resistance. Gram-negative bacterial strains that possess plasmid-mediated, multiple antibiotic resistance are commonly encountered in nosocomial infections. Plasmid transfer occurs among various strains of the same species and even among various genera. **Transfer of antibiotic resistance** has been demonstrated in the urine of patients with bladder catheters and on patients' skin. Presumably, transfer of antibiotic

747

resistance takes place in the gastrointestinal tract as well. Antibiotic-resistant pathogens have become so common that methicillin-resistant *Staphylococcus aureus* and aminoglycoside-resistant Gram-negative bacteria are regularly encountered in nosocomial infections. Examples of nosocomial pathogens are listed in Table 75-1. The list of pathogens that can cause health care–associated infections encompasses the agents of practically all infections. However, health care–associated infections generally have a greater degree of antibiotic resistance among both Gram-negative and Gram-positive organisms.

ENCOUNTER

A hospital is a microenvironment in which organisms can be transferred in many ways from one individual to another or from the hospital staff to patients (Fig. 75-1). Transmission between individuals can be direct by hand contact or indirect by inhalation, ingestion, or puncture through the integument. For example, methicillin-resistant staphylococci spread directly among patients or through hospital personnel. Tubercle bacilli

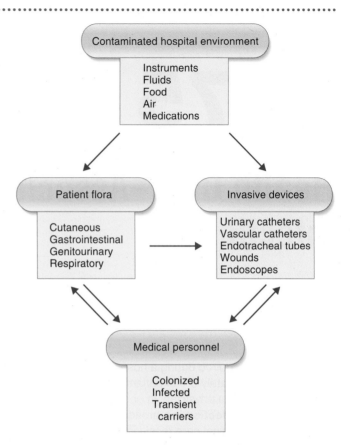

FIGURE 75-1. Sources of hospital-acquired infections. This figure demonstrates the common sources from which patients acquire infections in the hospital and the interaction between those sources.

TABLE 75-1 Common Hospital-Acquired Infections and Frequently Associated Organisms

Type of Infection	Most Common Organism
Surgical wounds	*Staphylococcus aureus*
	Escherichia coli
	Enterococcus spp.
Pneumonia	*Klebsiella pneumoniae*
	Pseudomonas aeruginosa
	S. aureus
	Enterobacter spp.
	E. coli
Intravenous catheter	*Staphylococcus epidermidis*
	S. aureus
	Enterococcus spp.
	Candida spp.
Urinary catheter	*E. coli*
	Enterococcus spp.
	P. aeruginosa
	Klebsiella spp.

(the agent of tuberculosis) are transmitted through aerosolization and inhalation. Viral agents, such as those of varicella zoster or influenza, can be spread through the air to susceptible immunocompromised individuals. Blood used for transfusions may be contaminated with hepatitis A, B, or C virus or human immunodeficiency virus (HIV). Food handlers may contaminate food eaten by patients, and physicians and nurses can introduce microorganisms into deeper tissues during operations or while dressing surgical or other wounds. Unusual epidemics can sometimes be traced to **specific carriers** among members of the hospital staff. For example, well-documented epidemics caused by group A streptococci have been attributed to carriers who had contact with patients in the operating room. In one epidemic, the organisms were located in the carrier's vagina and presumably were aerosolized through normal body movements.

Microorganisms that spread to patients may be **endemic** to the hospital environment. Notable examples include the fungi that cause aspergillosis, which may be present as more or less visible mildew on moist room walls or construction panels. Infections by exogenous organisms can also be acquired from improperly sterilized surgical instruments and even contaminated disinfectant solutions. Fortunately, those events are rare in most hospitals.

Patients acquire nosocomial infections as the result of breaks in their own defenses and from their inability to combat infection. Host defense breaks usually occur as the result of *invasive diagnostic or therapeutic interventions* that physicians perform on patients. Thus, the most common nosocomial infections affect the urinary tract because catheterization of the bladder is frequently used with bedridden patients. The commonly used bladder catheter bypasses the normal mucosal barriers and facilitates the entry of organisms that colonize the skin or the urinary introitus. Since Medicare will no longer pay hospitals for the increased cost of a nosocomial urinary tract infection, many hospitals have now developed policies limiting the use of bladder catheters to those patients in whom it is clearly essential, such as those whose bladders do not properly empty. The next most frequent types of nosocomial infections are surgical wound infections and respiratory tract infections, both of which result from invasive procedures as well.

ENTRY

Skin Penetration

The skin barrier is breached by intravenous catheters or devices used to measure intravascular pressure. *The longer devices stay in place, the higher the risk of both local infection and bacteremia.* That underscores the need for vigilance in the care of patients with indwelling devices, careful consideration of the necessity of these devices, and prompt removal of these devices when no longer necessary. National surveys conducted in the United States indicate that in the 1980s, with increased usage of venous catheters, the rate of nosocomial bacteremia almost doubled and the rate of *Staphylococcus epidermidis* infection tripled. In the authors' institution, 1 in 100 patients develops hospital-acquired bacteremia; half those cases result from the implantation of intravascular devices.

The role of the normal skin in protecting from microbial invasion is also evident in burn victims. Frequently, patients who have extensive second- or third-degree burns will become colonized with bacteria, especially *Pseudomonas aeruginosa*. Necrotizing lesions at the site of skin damage are accompanied by sepsis, the major cause of death in burn victims.

Inhalation

The most common cause of nosocomial pneumonia is the use of an **endotracheal tube**, a device that bypasses the normal epithelial defenses and allows the entry of organisms through aerosols. In the early 1960s, when mechanical ventilation of the lungs was being developed, epidemics of Gram-negative pneumonia occurred because nebulized mists contained bacteria-laden aerosols. An understanding of the problem prompted changes in ventilator design that have virtually eliminated the ventilator as a source of hospital-acquired pneumonia. Patients with endotracheal tubes still develop pneumonia, but now, the offending organisms tend to come from the patient's stomach or intestine to colonize the nasopharynx. From there, the bacteria can be aspirated into the lungs. As with any other devices, prompt removal is the best way to prevent infection. Today, guidelines mandate the use of sedation lightening and daily awakening protocols in order to assess a patient's readiness to wean from the ventilator. Other examples of nosocomial infections acquired by inhalation can be seen in hospital epidemics of influenza virus, respiratory syncytial virus, and varicella-zoster virus, which are particularly dangerous for immunocompromised patients.

Ingestion

Epidemics of nosocomial infection sometimes result from the ingestion of pathogenic bacteria. The organisms are often those associated with community-acquired infections, including those caused by *Salmonella* species, hepatitis A virus, and rotavirus, the latter being most frequent among neonates or infants. Epidemics of salmonellosis in hospitals usually result from eating foods contaminated during preparation. Another source of salmonellosis outbreaks is the use of contaminated carmine dye or other animal products for diagnostic purposes. *The gastrointestinal tract of hospitalized patients is a reservoir for antibiotic-resistant microorganisms* to which patients may be exposed in the environment. For example, vancomycin-resistant enterococci may be ingested from a contaminated environment, colonize patients, and then lead to a health care–associated infection, such as a bloodstream or urinary tract infection (see the cases presented later in the chapter).

Inanimate Environment

The complexity of a hospital environment provides innumerable opportunities for the encounter of patients with microorganisms. Some encounters are specific to the hospital environment and do not usually occur elsewhere. An example is the use of *contaminated intravenous solutions*, which have caused many epidemics. Contamination rarely takes place at the point of manufacture but more commonly occurs during the *handling of bottles and infusion lines*.

Instruments and dressings improperly sterilized before surgery also provide a possible source of infection. A separate technology has been developed to solve the problem of determining if autoclaves and sterilizing ovens perform their expected tasks. Thus, it is customary to insert a vial containing bacterial spores with the material to be autoclaved and to determine spore viability afterward. Deviance from established procedures can result in improper sterilization and in contamination of surgical or other wounds.

Environmental contamination can occur quite easily with organisms carried in the stool of patients, such as vancomycin-resistant enterococci or *Klebsiella pneumoniae* that harbor plasmids conferring resistance to late-generation cephalosporins, so-called extended-spectrum β-lactamase–producing organisms (ESBL), and even methicillin-resistant *S. aureus*, as well as other Gram-negatives such as *Enterobacter* species. Once the environment is contaminated, if hospital personnel do not pay attention to cleanliness and hand hygiene when making patient contacts, those organisms can be transmitted from the environment to the patient.

CONTROL AND PREVENTION

Control of nosocomial infections requires awareness by all health care professionals. Using **hand hygiene** techniques between patient contacts is a simple but much-neglected procedure. It has been estimated that only one-third of patient contacts are accompanied by appropriate hand hygiene. **Alcohol-based hand-rub** solutions are available to make it much easier for medical personnel to disinfect their hands before coming into contact with patients. Appropriate hand hygiene has become a focus for all hospitals and even licensing agencies because of its importance in decreasing transmission of microorganisms between hospital staff and patients. In our own institution, we have consistently demonstrated over the past year that hand hygiene compliance now exceeds 90% with the use of alcohol-based rubs. The use of **aseptic techniques** during surgical and other invasive procedures, as stressed in surgical training, is also a significant step in preventing infections. **Aseptic technique** involves not only aggressive hand cleaning and preparation of the site of the procedure but also the donning of a sterile gown, sterile gloves, a head covering, and a mask over the nose and mouth. During a procedure that requires aseptic technique, the sterility of the hands and gown as well as of the working field is maintained until the completion of the procedure.

Another control measure instituted by hospitals is the **infection control committee**, which is responsible for overseeing all aspects of infection control within the institution. The committee's oversight duties include supervising surveillance of hospital-acquired infections, establishing policies and procedures to prevent infections, and intervening when necessary in investigations of epidemics or other problems. Most hospitals have specific personnel, called **infection preventionists**, who are assigned these tasks and function as the "eyes and ears" of the committee. The practitioners, who are often trained as registered nurses, are responsible for tracing epidemics, monitoring infection rates, and determining the required level of isolation of patients. However, hospitals still have much to learn. Intense efforts are directed at reducing nosocomial infection rates despite the increasing number of immunocompromised patients and in devising effective means to prevent nosocomial pneumonias.

MODEL INFECTIONS
Nosocomial Urinary Tract Infection

The case of Mr. H. is a classic example of a nosocomial infection of the urinary tract. The use of bladder catheters for more than 1 or 2 days often results in contamination of the bladder, especially by fecal coliforms. Most catheters include an expandable collection bag for urine, thus making a closed system. Nonetheless, the risk of bacteriuria is cumulative and occurs at a rate of 5 to 8% of patients with catheters per day. The risk of bacteriuria is related to the skill of the person inserting the catheter, the sex and age of the patient, and the duration of catheterization.

CASE • At 67 years of age, Mr. H. underwent a transurethral prostatectomy for cancer of the prostate. Because of concern about postoperative bleeding from straining during urination, he had a catheter placed into the bladder. Three days later, Mr. H. developed a urinary tract infection with low-grade fever, some pain, and pyuria (white blood cells in the urine). Quantitative urine counts yielded 3×10^5 colonies of *Escherichia coli* per milliliter of urine. The organisms were resistant to all tested antibiotics except for the aminoglycosides. Within 2 days, Mr. H. developed bacteremia with hypotension and shock. Physicians were eventually able to control the bacteremia with gentamicin therapy. Fortunately, Mr. H. recovered completely and was discharged.

This case raises several questions:

1. How did Mr. H. acquire this infection?
2. What are the most likely organisms?
3. How can this scenario be prevented?

See Appendix for answers.

CASE • Ms. Z., an 82-year-old patient with rheumatic heart disease, underwent a mitral valve replacement and coronary artery bypass graft. Her postoperative course was complicated by bleeding in the mediastinum, which required more surgery. Subsequently, she recovered well and was discharged after 12 days. Three weeks later, Ms. Z. noticed some purulent drainage along the wound site on her chest. She continued to have pain but did not tell her family, assuming that the pain was related to her healing process. When she returned to see the surgeon 1 month later, she reported her pain and low-grade fever. The surgeon noted considerable drainage at the wound site. Probing the wound, he noticed a lot of pus.

Ms. Z. was hospitalized again. Cultures of the pus yielded *S. epidermidis*. Her wound was debrided (cleaned), which included the removal of the sternal wires and large portions of the sternal bone, and she was treated with intravenous vancomycin for 6 weeks while her chest was left open. At the end of that period, she required a plastic surgical device and a muscle flap to close the wound. She remained in the hospital for 2 months.

This case raises several questions:

1. How did Ms. Z develop her infection?
2. What are the most common organisms?
3. What is cost of such infections in morbidity?

See Appendix for answers.

Nosocomial Wound Infection

The case of Ms. Z. illustrates the problem of surgical wound infections and the serious impact they can have on patient recovery. Wound infections of the mediastinum complicate from 1 to 5% of open-heart surgeries. If the infection reaches deep portions of the chest, its effect can be extremely serious. Patients frequently require multiple surgical interventions with removal of devitalized bone, cartilage, and other tissue.

Surgical wound infections are the most costly of all nosocomial infections. Some are clearly preventable. Many are caused by *S. aureus*, but *S. epidermidis*, a normal skin commensal, is another significant pathogen. In the case of Ms. Z., the source of the infection was probably the **normal microbiota** on her skin. As with other infections, establishment of a surgical wound infection depends on the size of the inoculum, the pathogenic potential of the invading organisms, and the state of host defenses. All those factors should be taken into account before planning surgical treatment. When infection would be devastating to the patient's outcome—for instance, in an artificial hip implant—surgeons go to great lengths to prevent wound infections, such as using laminar airflow systems and prophylactic antibiotics.

Nosocomial Bacteremia

The case of Mr. S. is an example of primary bacteremia, which is defined as bacteremia that cannot be ascribed to another focus of infection. Primary bacteremia is frequently either the result of a contaminated intravenous line or associated with granulocytopenia.

Intravenous therapy provides many potential sources of contamination. The risk of intravenous catheter–related infection is generally influenced by the type of catheter and the duration of catheterization. In the example cited, the patient developed endocarditis, a rare but recognized complication. The usual pathogens of endocarditis are *S. aureus*, *S. epidermidis*, a variety of Gram-negative rods, or *Candida* species (see Table 75-1).

Another example of primary bacteremia is seen in leukemia and lymphoma patients who are granulocytopenic as a result of cancer chemotherapy. Typically, the source of the bacteremia is an intestinal pathogen, most often Gram-negative rods that translocate across the intestinal wall.

Nosocomial Pneumonia

Nosocomial pneumonia can be a devastating illness. Risk factors for development usually are the need for

CASE • Fifty-nine-year-old Mr. S. was hospitalized with acute myocardial infarction. His disease was so severe that he required a catheter to measure his cardiac pressure and output. After a week, he began to show signs of improvement and no longer required hemodynamic monitoring, but his catheter was left in place "just in case." Ten days after his infarction, Mr. S. developed fever, leukocytosis, and inflammation at the site of insertion of the catheter. Four blood cultures all revealed the presence of *S. aureus*. He was treated with intravenous antibiotics; however, a new cardiac murmur was noted 7 days into therapy. An echocardiogram revealed the development of a tricuspid valve vegetation. Mr. S. required 4 weeks of antibiotic therapy for his hospital-acquired, catheter-related endocarditis.

This case raises several questions:

1. From where did the organisms arise in Mr. S.'s infection?
2. How do the organisms enter the patient?
3. What is the best prevention for this type of infection?

See Appendix for answers.

CASE • Ms. I. was hospitalized for a stroke and required mechanical ventilation. After a few days, Ms. I appeared to be breathing on her own without difficulty, so her physicians attempted to remove the ventilator tube. Ms. I. then aspirated stomach contents, and over the next 24 to 48 hours, she developed a cough, was suctioned for purulent sputum, and had a pulmonary infiltrate on her chest X-ray. Culture of the sputum grew *Pseudomonas* *aeruginosa*. Treatment was initiated, and Ms. I. eventually recovered but not without a prolonged hospitalization.

This case raises several questions:

1. Where did the organisms arise?
2. What are the most common?
3. What preventive methods are there?

See Appendix for answers.

CASE • Dr. M. developed a needlestick injury while recapping a needle used on a patient who abused intravenous drugs. About 2 months later, Dr. M. developed arthralgias (joint pain), fatigue, malaise, and jaundice. Diagnosed as having hepatitis B, he lost 3 months of work but slowly recovered.

This case raises several questions:

1. What is the likelihood of transmission of HIV, hepatitis B virus (HBV), or hepatitis C virus (HCV) following needlestick?
2. What steps can be taken to prevent transmission?

See Appendix for answers.

mechanical ventilation, intubation, thoracoabdominal surgery, failure to be able to wean from a ventilator, and **older age**. The case of Ms. I. illustrates the role that intubation and aspiration play in the acquisition of organisms that cause nosocomial pneumonia. Often patients aspirate stomach or nasopharyngeal contents as a result of their debilitation. Infections acquired resulting from aspiration are frequently caused by organisms colonizing the back of the nasopharynx. Unfortunately, nosocomial pneumonia is difficult to prevent and is associated with the highest mortality rate among all hospital-acquired infections.

Nosocomial Bloodborne Disease

For decades, hepatitis B has been recognized as a nosocomial hazard for both health care workers and patients. Needlestick transmission is a recognized hazard, with rates of transmission approaching 25%. Blood transfusions constituted a major threat to patients before the early 1970s. Fortunately, the risk of transmission of hepatitis B virus (HBV) has been recognized, and using hepatitis B surface antigen screening has significantly reduced the bloodborne transmission of the virus.

The incidence of needlestick injuries has been significantly reduced by the practice of not recapping needles and the use of safety devices, which are now prevalent. For health care workers, needlestick transmission of hepatitis B is now infrequent because a vaccine is available to prevent transmission. Prior to the availability of vaccination, the rate of needlestick transmission of hepatitis

B was from 3 to 20%. However, needlestick transmission of hepatitis C and HIV still occurs at a rate of about 3%. For hepatitis C, no vaccination exists; thus, avoidance of needlestick is of the utmost importance. Current protocols try to treat early-onset hepatitis C virus infection to "revert" the infection. For HIV, needlestick transmission occurs in approximately 0.3% of needlestick injuries. There is evidence that use of antiretroviral agents within 8 hours of the needlestick can reduce the risk by about 60%.

CONCLUSION

Every physician encounters health care–associated infections. It is incumbent on the medical profession to minimize the occurrence of such infections by paying attention to isolation precautions, practicing scrupulous hand hygiene, and using safety devices when appropriate.

Suggested Readings

Aubrutyn E, Goldman DA, Scheckler WE, eds. *Saunders Infection Control Reference Service*. 2nd ed. Philadelphia, PA: W.B. Saunders Company; 2001.

Jarvis WR, ed. Bennett and Brachman's Hospital Infections. 5th ed. Philadelphia, PA: Lippincott Williams and Wilkins; 2007.

Martone WJ. Year 2000 objectives for preventing nosocomial infections: how do we get there? *Am J Med*. 1991;91(suppl 3B):39S–43S.

Mayhall CG. *Hospital Epidemiology and Infection Control*. 3rd ed. Baltimore, MD: Lipincott Williams & Wilkins; 2004.

Wenzel RP, ed. *Prevention and Control of Nosocomial Infections*. 4th ed. Baltimore, MD: Lippincott Williams & Wilkins; 2002.

Chapter 76

Foodborne Diseases

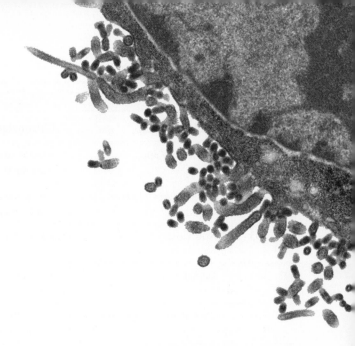

Christian B. Ramers

FOODBORNE infections are a significant public health problem. In the United States, these infections are a major cause of morbidity, although an infrequent cause of mortality. Illnesses caused by the nine most common foodborne pathogens in the United States have been tracked since 1996 by a surveillance network called the Foodborne Diseases Active Surveillance Network (FoodNet). In 2010, this network investigated 19,089 infections. Thus, it allows public health officials to estimate the nationwide burden of foodborne disease. Using these data, officials estimate approximately 1,000 outbreaks, 48 million illnesses, 128,000 hospitalizations, and 3,000 deaths annually due to foodborne illness in the United States. There have been some positive trends noted from 1996 to 2010. For example, there has been a decline in the incidence of six of the nine pathogens (*Listeria*, *Campylobacter*, *Escherichia coli* O157, *Shigella*, and *Yersinia*); however, no significant change has been observed in *Salmonella* infections since the start of active surveillance.

Public health interventions from the farm to the market to the dinner table have helped decrease the incidence of foodborne illness, but outbreaks continue to occur, highlighting the need for continued vigilance and investigative capacity.

A foodborne disease outbreak is defined by two criteria: (1) two or more persons must experience a similar illness, usually gastrointestinal, after ingestion of the same food and (2) epidemiological analysis must implicate the food as the source of the illness. However, exceptions to that definition exist. For some pathogens of public health significance, even a single case should prompt investigation. For example, one case of botulism constitutes an outbreak for the purposes of epidemiological investigation and control because of the high probability that other cases may be involved.

The most common diseases acquired by **ingestion of contaminated food** in the United States are those usually called **food poisoning**. A case of food poisoning results from the consumption of food contaminated with bacteria, bacterial toxins, parasites, viruses, or chemicals. Bacteria cause approximately 40% of the foodborne disease outbreaks in the United States for which an etiology can be determined; however, bacterial food poisoning is more likely to cause serious or life-threatening illness than viral or parasitic disease (Table 76-1). It should be noted that many foodborne disease outbreaks never have an etiology

confirmed, due mostly to the need for more expensive and sophisticated techniques to isolate individual viruses. This chapter discusses major food-poisoning illnesses that occur in the United States. The chapter is organized according to two main types of foodborne illnesses:

- **Intoxications caused by toxins made by pathogens**: In these cases, the organism does not have to be alive to cause disease, but rather it is the toxin, either preformed or manufactured inside the host that causes disease. Examples of causative bacteria are *Staphylococcus aureus*, *Clostridium botulinum*, *Bacillus cereus*, *Vibrio cholerae*, or *Clostridium perfringens*.

- **Intestinal invasive diseases**: In these cases, the organism itself typically causes inflammation and damage from invading the intestinal wall. The most common of these diseases is gastroenteritis caused by invasive organisms like *Salmonella* and *Campylobacter* species.

The distinction between foodborne illnesses caused by toxin-producing organisms and those caused by invasive pathogens is important clinically and epidemiologically. In general, **diseases caused by toxin-forming**

TABLE 76-1 Major Outbreaks of Foodborne Disease in the United States*a*

Year	Etiologic Agent	Circumstances
2008–2010	*Salmonella* spp.	Several large outbreaks (2008: fresh salsa; 2009: beef and peanut butter; 2010: eggs, ground turkey, strawberries)
2006	*Escherichia coli* O157: H7	One large outbreak in New Jersey, thought to be related to lettuce or green onion contamination
2002–2003	Norovirus	Multiple cruise ship outbreaks with very high attack rates disrupted operations for several cruise lines for weeks to months
1997, 2003	Hepatitis A	153 cases associated with eating frozen strawberries imported from Mexico and served in Michigan public schools
1996	*Cyclospora cayetanensis*	>40 individual outbreaks and >850 persons ill owing to contaminated raspberries imported from Guatemala and distributed nationwide
1996	Enterohemorrhagic *E. coli*	Juice and cider made with "dropped" apples harvested from the ground. Sixty-six illnesses and one death in western United States and Canada
1994	*Salmonella enteritidis*	Multistate outbreak caused by a national brand of ice cream contaminated at the factory; an estimated 224,000 persons became ill
1993	Enterohemorrhagic *E. coli*	>500 cases of hemorrhagic colitis associated with undercooked hamburgers served at 93 fast-food restaurants in several states (four children died)
1991	*Vibrio cholerae*	Four cases in nontravelers associated with tainted coconut milk imported from Thailand
1990	*Clostridium perfringens*	700 cases of food poisoning associated with beef and chicken tacos served in a Missouri prison
1988	*Campylobacter jejuni*	120 cases traced to raw milk served at a vacation Bible school in Kansas
1988	*Shigella sonnei*	3,175 illnesses among people who ate raw tofu salad at an outdoor music festival in Michigan (117 hospitalized)

*a*Selected from among ~500 outbreaks each year reported to the Centers for Disease Control and Prevention.

organisms like *S. aureus* have a short incubation period and are characterized by upper gastrointestinal complaints, such as nausea and vomiting. Since toxin is preformed before food is consumed, usually symptoms are related to the upper gastrointestinal tract with nausea and vomiting. Diarrhea is less frequent, and constitutional symptoms, including fever and chills, are uncommon. In contrast, **food poisonings caused by invasive organisms**—*Salmonella* species, for example—usually have a longer incubation period and are characterized by fever, chills, and lower gastrointestinal complaints. Diarrhea, often bloody or containing pus or mucus, is more prominent in invasive diseases than is nausea or vomiting. Therefore, ascertaining the type of food poisoning is generally a matter of determining whether the symptoms are more indicative of intoxication or invasion. Some overlap exists in this classification scheme, because organisms such as species of *Shigella* and *Salmonella* may have invasive properties as well as the ability to produce toxin.

In the United States, the most frequently recognized agents of bacterial food poisoning are generally limited to a dozen organisms (see Table 76-1). According to the FoodNet surveillance system, *Salmonella* infections are the most common cause of serious foodborne illness at an incidence rate of 17.6 per 100,000 population per year and comprise nearly half the reported cases of foodborne illness in 2010 (8,256 of 19,089 cases in the FoodNet network). That dominance is partly the result of the ease with which the infections are recognized as well as the awareness of physicians and the public. *Campylobacter* infections are the next most common, at an incidence of 13.6 per 100,000, followed by *Shigella*, *Cryptosporidium*, and *E. coli*. Other bacterial pathogens, such as *Yersinia*, *Vibrio*, and *Listeria*, as well as viruses such as hepatitis A and norovirus cause foodborne illness less frequently. Parasites and chemical agents acquired from food are the least frequent causes of foodborne disease. Of these infections, *Listeria* seems to be the most severe, requiring hospitalization in 89.6% of cases and death in 12.8%.

TABLE 76-2 Some Characteristics of Bacterial Food Poisoning

Organism	Mechanism	Incubation Period (h)	Vehicles	Features
Staphylococcus aureus	Heat-stable toxin	1–6	Ham, pastry, baked goods	Vomiting
Bacillus cereus	Heat-stable toxin	1–6	Fried rice	Vomiting
	Heat-labile toxin	8–24	Cream sauce	Diarrhea
Salmonella species	Invasion	16–48	Chicken, beef, eggs, milk	Fever, diarrhea
Campylobacter species	Invasion	16–48	Chicken, beef, milk	Fever, diarrhea
Vibrio parahaemolyticus	Invasion (toxin?)	16–72	Shellfish	Fever, diarrhea
Yersinia enterocolitica	Invasion (toxin?)	16–72	Milk, tofu	Diarrhea
Escherichia coli	Toxin	16–72	Salads	Diarrhea
	0157:H7 (verotoxin)	16–48	Beef	Fever, diarrhea
Clostridium perfringens	Toxin	8–12	Beef, poultry, gravy	Diarrhea

Features of the principal foodborne diseases are shown in Table 76-2.

It is important to note that **etiological patterns vary throughout the world**. Etiology depends on many factors, such as food preferences, awareness by physicians and the public, and laboratory capabilities. For example, in the United States, food poisoning by *Salmonella* and *Shigella* species represents about 70% of the outbreaks. In contrast, *C. perfringens* is implicated in more than 90% of the recognized foodborne illness in England and Wales. Japan has yet another etiological pattern, with *Vibrio parahaemolyticus* gastroenteritis representing more than 50% of reported outbreaks. For US citizens traveling abroad, the most common cause of traveler's diarrhea, which affects close to 50% of all travelers, is an enterotoxigenic strain of *E. coli* that is usually self-limited.

INTOXICATIONS
Staphylococcus aureus
CLINICAL FEATURES

Outbreaks of staphylococcal foodborne disease are characterized by explosive onset 1 to 6 hours after consuming contaminated food. Attack rates are usually quite high because very small quantities of staphylococcal enterotoxin can cause illness. In outbreaks involving single families and uniform doses of enterotoxin, virtually 100% of individuals are affected. The **staphylococcal enterotoxin is resistant to heat** and can remain in food after cooking, even though the causative organism has been killed.

Outbreaks from staphylococci can occur at any time of the year, but most are reported during the warm weather months. Staphylococci are so commonly present on the skin of healthy individuals that food preparation in almost any setting can result in transmission. Most outbreaks are reported from places where many people gather—for instance, in school cafeterias, group picnics, club dining halls, and restaurants. Many different foods have been implicated, including ham, canned beef, pork, or any salted meat and cream-filled cakes or pastries like cream puffs. Potato and macaroni salads are occasionally involved. Foods that have a high content of salt (ham) or sugar (custard) selectively favor the growth of staphylococci.

Foods that are involved in outbreaks have usually been cut, sliced, grated, mixed, or ground by workers who are carriers of enterotoxin-producing strains of staphylococci. Although animal carcasses may be contaminated before processing, competitive growth from other members of the normal microbiota usually limits the staphylococci. Therefore, transmission is from the food handler to the food product. Most commonly, the contaminated food has been allowed to sit at room temperature for some time before preparation or cooking, thus allowing the toxin to be produced in significant quantities.

DIAGNOSIS

The signs and symptoms of staphylococcal food poisoning are primarily profuse vomiting, nausea, and abdominal cramps, often followed by diarrhea. Notably, fever and other signs of abdominal pain or inflammation are absent, distinguishing it from appendicitis. In severe cases, blood may be observed in the vomitus or stool. Rarely, hypotension and marked prostration occur, but recovery is usually complete within 24 to 48 hours.

CASE • As the aircraft cruised at 35,000 ft, the cabin attendants passed out a lunch meal that included ham sandwiches. Two hours later, two-thirds of the passengers aboard the Boeing 747 jet developed nausea and vomiting. Diarrhea occurred in about one-third of those affected. The waiting lines for the toilets trailed down the aisle. As a result of this and similar epidemics, rules for serving the cockpit crew different meals went into effect.

This case raises several questions:

1. What was the most likely cause of the outbreak?

2. Is this more likely to represent an intestinal infection or an intoxication by a preformed toxin? Why?

3. How could one kind of meal have affected such a large number of individuals?

See Appendix for answers.

It was later discovered that two-thirds of the passengers on the flight were served ham sliced by a chef who had a pustular lesion on his hand. *S. aureus* was isolated from the lesion, and an identical strain was isolated from the ham. The passengers had ingested food contaminated with one of the many *S. aureus* toxins (see Chapter 11).

Staphylococcal food poisoning should be considered in anyone with severe vomiting, nausea, cramps, and some diarrhea. A history of ingesting meats of high salt or sugar content may be helpful. The best epidemiological clue, especially if many individuals are ill, is the short incubation period (1 to 6 hours). Of the bacterial foodborne diseases, only *B. cereus* has similar symptoms, with a short incubation period and a marked vomiting syndrome. However, because the *B. cereus* vomiting syndrome is closely associated with rice consumption, the epidemiological distinction can usually be made easily.

Diagnosis can be confirmed by culturing the suspected food, the skin or nose of the food handler, or, occasionally, the vomitus or stools of affected individuals. The recovered *S. aureus* may be typed either by phage or pulsed field gel electrophoresis to prove that the isolated strains are identical (see Chapter 11). Detection of staphylococcal enterotoxin is the ultimate means of making the diagnosis, but this is generally available only in specialized labs and not in routine clinical care.

Clostridium perfringens
CLINICAL FEATURES

C. perfringens food poisoning is generally characterized by watery diarrhea and severe cramping abdominal pain, usually without vomiting, beginning 8 to 24 hours after the suspected meal. Fever, chills, headache, or other signs of infection are usually not present. The illness lasts 24 hours or less. Rare fatalities have been recorded in debilitated or hospitalized patients who are victims of clostridial food poisoning.

The lengthy time between ingestion of suspected food and onset of symptoms, the clinical manifestations, and a high attack rate point to *C. perfringens* as the likely cause of the outbreak. *C. perfringens* food poisoning is thought to be a relatively common cause of foodborne disease in the United States. However, because the diagnosis is often difficult to establish due to the need to culture the organism anaerobically, reported cases probably represent a small fraction of the actual cases that occur.

Epidemics of *C. perfringens* are usually characterized by high attack rates. The incubation period in most outbreaks varies between 8 and 14 hours (median of 12 hours), but can be as long as 74 hours. For reasons that are not clear, more cases of *C. perfringens* food poisoning are reported in the fall and winter months. The nadir of reported cases occurs in the summer, in marked contrast to outbreaks of *Salmonella* and staphylococcal food poisoning. It may be that the kinds of food usually implicated in *C. perfringens* outbreaks, such as stews, are eaten less frequently in the summer.

Outbreaks caused by this organism are often reported from institutions and large gatherings. The latter is probably a reporting artifact, because only large groups recognize the illness as food poisoning. In the late 1940s, it was discovered that *C. perfringens* caused outbreaks of a severe and often lethal intestinal disease labeled **enteritis necroticans** that affected people in Germany and New Guinea (where it is termed pigbel, as discussed in the next section).

PATHOPHYSIOLOGY

Food poisoning from *C. perfringens* often occurs when dishes prepared with poultry, meat, or fish are cooked and then allowed to cool slowly without proper refrigeration for extended periods. Spores of the organisms present in the meat or fish resist the first heating and then germinate and grow in the unrefrigerated food. When the food is reheated, the already-multiplied bacteria form spores again. Illness occurs either when a large number of vegetative bacteria that survive reheating or a large number of spores are ingested with the food. Most commonly, ingested spores germinate in the intestine and release clostridial toxin in vivo.

The heat-labile protein enterotoxin has a molecular weight of approximately 34,000 Da. The clostridial toxin differs from cholera toxin in several respects. Its activity is maximal in the ileum and minimal in the duodenum, which is opposite to that of cholera toxin. Clostridial enterotoxin inhibits glucose transport, damages the intestinal epithelium, and causes protein loss into the intestinal lumen; no such effects are observed with cholera toxin. Recently, *C. perfringens* enterotoxin has been detected in the stools of affected individuals. Enterotoxin activity disappears quickly from the stool but can be measured in serum.

Immunity in *C. perfringens* intoxication is not well understood. One study has found that 65% of Americans and 84% of Brazilians have antienterotoxin activity in serum. In animal studies, enterotoxin antiserum blocks the action of the toxin on ligated rabbit loops. It is not known, however, if the presence of antibody in serum has any effect on toxin activity in the intestine.

Another disease rarely seen in the United States but caused by *C. perfringens* is enteritis necroticans (pigbel), which is characterized by high attack rates in children in New Guinea, coupled with a high mortality. Although enteritis necroticans and *C. perfringens* food poisoning are caused by the same organism, the two diseases are quite different. Outbreaks of pigbel have been clearly associated with the consumption of pork at large native feasts. At the feasts, improperly cooked pork was consumed in large quantities over 3 or 4 days.

As its name suggests, enteritis necroticans is a severe necrotizing disease of the small intestine. After a 24-hour incubation period, illness ensues with intense abdominal pain, bloody diarrhea, vomiting, and shock. The mortality rate is about 40%, usually as a result of intestinal perforation. The disease is caused by a toxin known as α-toxin, a 35-kDa protein unusually sensitive to proteases and thus rapidly inactivated by the intestinal enzyme trypsin. The disease usually affects people who eat large, high-protein meals that overwhelm the ability of the intestinal trypsin to neutralize the toxin.

CASE • A group of college dormitory residents sat down for a turkey feast at a nearby restaurant at 6 PM. They consumed turkey, giblets, gravy, and "all the fix-in's." At approximately 2 AM, the first of many of the group awoke with severe intestinal cramps and watery diarrhea. Most of the other students in the group became ill with similar symptoms at approximately 6 AM. Several students had to spend the night in the college infirmary. Fortunately, the wave of diarrhea resolved within 24 hours.

This case raises several questions:

1. What is the likely agent of this disease?
2. What is the pathophysiology of this type of diarrhea?
3. How could such an outbreak be prevented?

See Appendix for answers.

DIAGNOSIS

The diagnosis of *C. perfringens* food poisoning should be considered in any diarrheal illness characterized by abdominal pain and moderate to severe diarrhea, unaccompanied by fever and chills. Many individuals usually are involved in the outbreak; the suspected food is beef or chicken that has been stewed, roasted, or boiled and then allowed to stand without proper refrigeration. The incubation period is 8 to 14 hours; occasional outbreaks have incubation periods as short as 5 to 6 hours or as long as 22 hours.

A form of food poisoning caused by *B. cereus* may have similar symptoms and can only be ruled out by bacteriological study. Enterotoxigenic *E. coli* can also produce the symptoms associated with *C. perfringens* food poisoning, although low-grade fever is often present. *V. cholerae* produces more profuse diarrhea, which helps differentiate it from clostridial intoxication. *Salmonella* or *Campylobacter* infections are usually accompanied by fever, a longer incubation period, and more marked systemic signs.

Because *C. perfringens* can be isolated from normal stools, it is helpful to use an established serotyping schema to distinguish between the approximately 20 different serotypes. In an outbreak, the same serotype of *C. perfringens* should be recovered from all affected individuals and from the food they ate. If food specimens are not available, the diagnosis can be made by isolating organisms of the same serotype from the stool of most ill individuals but not from that of suitable controls. In the absence of either of those findings, culturing 10^5 or more organisms per gram of the suspected food is highly suggestive of the diagnosis.

Bacillus cereus
CLINICAL FEATURES

Food poisoning caused by *B. cereus* has two main clinical manifestations, diarrheal and emetic. The diarrheal form of the illness is characterized by a long incubation period, diarrhea (96%), abdominal cramps (75%), and vomiting (23%); fever is uncommon. The duration of disease ranges from 20 to 36 hours, with a median of 24 hours.

The predominant symptoms of the emetic form of the illness are vomiting (100%) and abdominal cramps (100%). Diarrhea is only present in one-third of affected individuals. The duration of the illness ranges from 8 to 10 hours, with a median of 9 hours. In both types of illness, the disease is usually mild and self-limited. The vomiting syndrome must be differentiated from *S. aureus* food poisoning. As stated earlier, the association with fried rice is epidemiologically useful in differentiating the two organisms.

B. cereus has been recognized as an increasingly significant cause of food poisoning since about 1970. Approximately 1% of all food-poisoning outbreaks in the United States are caused by the organism. Classically, this pathogen has been isolated from fried rice, although it can be found in other foods. Data from other countries are still generally sparse, so the incidence outside the United States is unknown.

The incubation period for the outbreaks of vomiting is usually 2 or 3 hours, whereas that for the diarrheal outbreaks is 6 to 14 hours. The clear-cut association between the vomiting syndrome and fried rice deserves emphasis. Most outbreaks of *B. cereus* vomiting syndrome in the United States and Great Britain implicate that dish as the vehicle. The diarrheal illness, however, has been caused by a variety of foods, including boiled beef, sausage, chicken soup, vanilla sauce, and puddings.

B. cereus is found in about 25% of foodstuffs sampled, including cream, pudding, meat, spices, dry potatoes, dry milk, spaghetti sauces, and rice. Contamination of food products generally occurs before they are cooked. The organisms grow if the food is maintained at 30°C to 50°C during preparation. Spores survive extreme temperatures and, when allowed to cool relatively slowly, germinate and multiply. No evidence exists that human carriage of the organism or other means of contamination play a role in transmission.

Contamination of rice by *B. cereus* is attributed to the practice common in Asian restaurants of allowing large portions of boiled rice to drain unrefrigerated to avoid clumping. The flash frying in the final preparation of certain rice dishes (e.g., fried rice) often does not raise the temperature sufficiently to destroy the preformed heat-stable toxin.

PATHOPHYSIOLOGY

Several **extracellular toxins** produced by strains of *B. cereus* may contribute to their virulence, including an enterotoxin that causes fluid accumulation in the rabbit intestine and stimulates the adenylate cyclase–cyclic adenosine monophosphate (cAMP) system in intestinal epithelial cells (see Chapter 9).

A second presumptive toxin has been isolated from a strain of *B. cereus* implicated in an outbreak of vomiting-type illness. Cell-free culture filtrates from that strain do not produce fluid accumulation in rabbit intestine, do not stimulate the adenyl cyclase–cAMP system, and only produce vomiting when fed to rhesus monkeys. This "vomiting toxin" is heat stable.

FOOD POISONING CAUSED BY INVASIVE ORGANISMS

Salmonella Gastroenteritis

This case of Mr. T. (below) underscores the invasive potential of several bacteria associated with food poisoning. Although many organisms are invasive, the most common agents are species of *Salmonella* and *Campylobacter*. Relatively uncommon invasive bacteria are *V. parahaemolyticus*, *Yersinia enterocolitica*, and a specific strain of *E. coli*. Invasiveness is generally associated with the presence of neutrophils in the stool and systemic signs such as fever, chills, myalgias, and headache. These organisms are discussed in more detail in Chapters 16 and 17.

Campylobacter jejuni

This small curved Gram-negative rod is found in a wide range of animals, including poultry, and typically causes human outbreaks of gastrointestinal illness after an incubation period of 3 days. Often, a prodromal illness comes first, composed of fever, chills, dizziness, rigors, and delirium, before any gastrointestinal symptoms. Abdominal cramping, pain, and voluminous diarrhea then follow, and about 10 to 15% of patients will have bloody diarrhea. Bacteremia may occur infrequently. The immune response against campylobacter infection may actually result in an autoimmune reaction against the host's own tissues, in the form of a reactive arthritis or even Guillain-Barré syndrome (immune-mediated polyneuropathy with ascending paralysis). In fact, nearly 30% of Guillain-Barré syndrome is felt be related to campylobacter infection.

Vibrio parahaemolyticus

Like *V. cholera*, *V. parahaemolyticus* is often associated with contaminated shellfish. The organism tends to behave as one of the invasive pathogens, rather than as a toxin-producing pathogen such as *V. cholera*.

Yersinia enterocolitica

Y. enterocolitica is a Gram-negative rod that has recently been implicated as a cause of food poisoning. Contaminated milk has been one well-documented source. The type of infection caused by the organism is generally invasive, although a heat-stable enterotoxin has been described. Tissue invasion, frequently mimicking acute appendicitis, is common in *Y. enterocolitica* infection. At surgery, the appendix of an infected patient may be normal, but the mesenteric lymph nodes surrounding the appendix will be markedly inflamed.

Escherichia coli

Although *E. coli* is part of the host's normal microbiota, some toxigenic and enteropathogenic strains are associated with food poisoning. Toxigenic *E. coli* occurs in about 50% of traveler's diarrhea (see Chapter 16). Travelers ingest the organisms in contaminated salads, raw fruits, and vegetables. This syndrome is usually associated with watery diarrhea; fever is less common. The organisms make both a heat-labile and heat-stable enterotoxin.

Another toxigenic strain of *E. coli* causes a syndrome of bloody diarrhea, generally without fever. The causative agent is a shiga toxin–producing strain of *E. coli* (serotype O157:H7). The mechanism of action of this toxin appears to be identical to that of *Shigella*, the agent of bacillary dysentery. A rare consequence of this illness in children is hemolytic–uremic syndrome, which can lead to severe kidney damage and hemolytic anemia and potentially death (see Chapter 17). The agent has been epidemiologically connected to poorly cooked hamburger or other poorly cooked beef products.

Listeria monocytogenes

Increasingly recognized as a foodborne pathogen, *Listeria monocytogenes* is a Gram-positive, motile rod that is relatively heat resistant; it withstands pasteurization of milk. It has a unique ability to withstand cold temperatures and may cause outbreaks despite adequate refrigeration. Elderly or immunosuppressed patients and pregnant women seem to have a slightly higher incidence of infection. The bacteria are widely distributed in nature and are found in the intestinal tracts of various animals and humans, as well as in sewage, soil, and water.

The syndromes usually associated with listeriosis include meningoencephalitis, cerebritis, rhomboencephalitis, bacteremia, or focal metastatic disease. Frequently, gastrointestinal symptoms such as diarrhea precede the bacteremic disease. The evidence that listeriosis is foodborne is accumulating from investigations of several recent epidemics. Contaminated coleslaw and raw and pasteurized milk have been implicated as vehicles for epidemic listeriosis. The source of sporadic *Listeria* infection is less well understood. Compared to other pathogens in this chapter, *Listeria* infections are the most severe, usually requiring hospitalization and often resulting in severe, fatal infections, with invasive and/or central nervous system consequences.

NONBACTERIAL FORMS OF FOOD POISONING

Several agents have gained attention as prominent causes of food poisoning in the past decade. Waterborne outbreaks of *Cryptosporidium parvum* have affected whole cities. In Milwaukee, Wisconsin, an estimated 350,000 cases of diarrhea resulted from contamination of the drinking water and other sources of potable water. Outbreaks of viral gastroenteritis have become very common, especially in crowded populations or those sharing common environmental conditions, such as cruise ships. Outbreaks of norovirus infections have had attack rates of more than 50% on some cruise ships, effectively requiring that the cruises be aborted, people brought to shore, and the ships decontaminated. However, the difficulty in eliminating the virus by cleaning and the very high attack rates in susceptible patients have made the norovirus a problematic organism. It is thought that food handlers excrete the virus and contaminate food during preparation. The incubation period is short and the attack rate quite high. Fortunately, patients recover after being ill with nausea, vomiting, and diarrhea for 24 to 72 hours.

TREATMENT

Because foodborne diseases are generally self-limited and, for the most part, toxin mediated, **antibiotics usually do not play a major role** in either therapy or prophylaxis. Occasionally, individuals with diseases caused by the more invasive pathogens like *Salmonella*, *Shigella*, *Listeria*, or *Campylobacter* require antibiotic therapy. Likewise, as in the case of traveler's diarrhea, a short course of oral antibiotics may be prudent to limit the duration

TABLE 76-3 Factors that Contributed to Foodborne Disease Outbreaks in the United States

Factor	Percentage Implicated[a]
Inadequate refrigeration	47
Food prepared too far in advance of service	21
Infected person with poor personal hygiene	21
Inadequate cooking	16
Inadequate holding temperature	16
Inadequate reheating	12
Contaminated raw ingredient	1
Cross-contamination	7
Dirty equipment	7

[a]Percentage values total more than 100% because more than one factor may contribute to one foodborne disease outbreak.

and severity of the illness. **Fluid replacement** is a major consideration in all foodborne illnesses.

CONTROL AND PREVENTION

The common theme that characterizes all foodborne illnesses is the improper handling of food before its consumption. A study of factors responsible for foodborne disease outbreaks in the United States over a 15-year period showed that inadequate refrigeration was the single most frequent factor (Table 76-3). Usually, other factors are also associated with a specific outbreak, such as advance preparation of food without adequate storage or improper reheating. To a lesser degree, contaminated equipment, cross-contamination, and poor personal hygiene of food preparation personnel contribute to outbreaks.

The ubiquity of *Salmonella* and *Campylobacter* species, *B. cereus*, and *C. perfringens* makes it mandatory that food be cooked properly and stored at low temperatures. Control of foodborne illnesses is based on the inhibition of bacterial growth, prevention of contamination after preparation, and destruction of potential pathogens with cooking. In general, foods should be heated to internal temperatures of 74°C, but lower temperatures for longer periods of time are also effective. (People should probably think twice before ordering steak tartare, sushi, or other uncooked or undercooked meat or fish.) Once cooked or processed, foods must be held at temperatures of 4.4°C or below.

Although those control measures are standard, many places where food preparation takes place do not abide by them. It is through diligent efforts of public health officials that reported outbreaks are investigated and food preparation techniques corrected. Therefore, recognition and reporting of foodborne illness becomes essential in the control of the problem. Education of the public, nurses, physicians, and eating establishment personnel is crucial to the control of foodborne illness. Carriage of most of the organisms considered in this chapter is not a problem, with the exception of staphylococci. Because staphylococcal carriage is necessary for the development of foodborne illness, food handlers must be educated to watch for boils and pustules.

CONCLUSION

Food poisoning caused by enterotoxins may occur after ingestion of preformed toxin in food or by production of toxin by organisms in the intestinal tract. Most cases of intoxication cause nausea, vomiting, or diarrhea; they do not typically cause fever. Some foodborne disease is associated with invasive intestinal pathogens such as *Salmonella* and *Listeria* species. These illnesses may present with gastrointestinal symptoms as well as inflammatory features, such as fever, and they may require treatment with antibiotics. Most foodborne illnesses occur because food is improperly handled and are preventable if food handlers are appropriately educated and observant of public health guidelines.

Suggested Readings

American Medical Association; American Nurses Association-American Nurses Foundation; Centers for Disease Control and Prevention; Center for Food Safety and Applied Nutrition, Food and Drug Administration; Food Safety and Inspection Service, US Department of Agriculture. Diagnosis and management of foodborne illnesses: a primer for physicians and other health care professionals. *MMWR Recomm Rep.* 2004;53(RR-4):1–33.

Boyce TG, Swadlow DL, Griffin PM. *Escherichia coli* 0157:H7 and the hemolytic uremic syndrome. *N Engl J Med.* 1995;333:364–368.

Centers for Disease Control and Prevention. Foodborne Disease Outbreaks. *Annual Summary.* 2006.

Doyle MP, ed. *Foodborne Bacterial Pathogens.* New York: Dekker; 1989.

FoodNet report 1996–2010. *MMWR Morb Mortal Wkly Rep.* 2011;60(22):749–755.

Hedberg CW, MacDonald KL, Osterholm MT. Changing epidemiology of food-borne disease: a Minnesota perspective. *Clin Inf Dis.* 1994;18:671–682.

Appendix A *Answers to Case Questions*

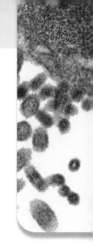

CHAPTER 11

Necrotizing Pneumonia and Purpura Fulminans

1. What was the source of the organisms that infected Mr. K.?

Staphylococcus aureus is a highly communicable bacterium. It is possible that Mr. K. carried the bacterium in his nose, and the organism made its way into his lungs from the nose. It is also possible that the original site of infection was a furuncle, with secondary infection of the nose and then lungs. Finally, it is also likely that this organism was acquired from any other source where other humans may have spread the organism to Mr. K. either by direct contact or aerosols. *S. aureus* can survive for extended periods of time on inanimate objects.

2. What might have contributed to development of the pulmonary abscess due to *S. aureus*?

The bacterium produces many cell surface virulence factors, collectively called MSCRAMMs. Many of these allow the bacterium to attach to host cells, but some including clumping factors allow the organism to wall itself off in abscesses. *S. aureus* also secretes coagulase that will allow it to form clots around itself. These factors and other cell surface factors, like protein A, provide protection from the host immune system.

3. What are the roles of the demonstrated exotoxins made by the causative bacteria?

S. aureus produces a variety of cytolysins (hemolysins) whose function is most likely to kill immune cells that invade locally in an attempt to clear the organism. These cytolysins are also potent agents for triggering inflammation by attracting neutrophils and macrophages. Superantigens, such as enterotoxin C in the case of Mr. K., dysregulate the immune system systemically, causing massive production of cytokines. These cytokines cause fever and hypotension (shock and death).

4. Why did Mr. K. die if the *S. aureus* did not invade his bloodstream?

There are at least two possibilities for this. First, lung congestion due to production of cytolysins could have caused breathing difficulties, resulting in death. Second and more likely, the production of the superantigen would result in that toxin gaining access to the bloodstream, causing superantigenicity, leading to cytokine production with consequent hypotension, shock, and death.

5. What does community-associated MRSA mean?

When originally described, methicillin resistant *S. aureus* (MRSA) was confined to hospital settings. In the 1990s, a group of researchers at the University of Chicago first described MRSA in children who had never been in hospitals. Thus, these children acquired their infections from the community rather than from hospitalized patients. Today, as many as 70% of hospital-associated *S. aureus* are MRSA, and as many as 30% of community strains are MRSA.

6. What is the appropriate antimicrobial and therapeutic approach?

The organism was shown to be resistant to methicillin (MRSA) but susceptible to clindamycin, trimethoprim/

sulfamethoxazole, tetracycline, linezolid, rifampin, and vancomycin. Vancomycin and rifampin are synergistic against MRSA. Vancomycin is a glycoprotein that inhibits cell wall synthesis by inhibiting the incorporation of newly synthesized precursors in the cell wall peptidoglycan, and rifampin inhibits RNA polymerase. Rifampin penetrates lung mucosal tissues extensively whereas vancomycin penetrates 25 to 50%. Clindamycin or linezolid should be considered to reduce production of exotoxins including superantigens, Panton-Valentine leukocidin, and α-toxin (in addition to their antimicrobial effects).

Soft Tissue Infection and Toxic Shock Syndrome

1. What was the source of the organisms that infected Ms. G.?

The organism was introduced into the knee during the arthroscopy. The source may have originated from the patient's skin, the surgeon, or the arthroscopic instruments (if they became contaminated or were inadequately sterilized). This bacterium was methicillin resistant, a feature of *S. aureus* that was distinctly unusual outside the hospital environment when the surgery was done. That suggests the infecting strain was probably acquired as a result of the surgery. It was therefore a medically related infection.

2. What contributed to the development of the subcutaneous abscess?

Because *S. aureus* is a pathogen that typically colonizes the skin, it is the most common cause of surgical wound infection. Any incision through the skin carries a risk of introducing *S. aureus* and creating an infection. For descriptions of the many virulence features that *S. aureus* has to prevent phagocytosis and killing by neutrophils and its adherence factors, see the chapter text.

3. Why is the incision site not highly inflamed?

Typically, the primary site in toxic shock syndrome (TSS) is a localized area where *S. aureus* are producing toxin but may not be creating much local damage. It is thought that there may be a local effect of the superantigen that reduces inflammation at the site of infection. Had this infection been caused by a non-toxin-producing strain of *S. aureus*, the patient would likely have presented with a fever and an obviously infected knee instead of TSS.

4. What properties of TSST-1 led to the patient's symptoms?

Toxic shock syndrome toxin 1 (TSST-1) is a superantigen. It activates a subclass of T cells that, as a result, may undergo apoptosis or trigger immune activation with the release of a cascade of cytokines. It is the latter that produces the clinical features of TSS.

5. What are the properties of the organism that prevented it from being cleared by nafcillin?

Resistance to all the semisynthetic antistaphylococcal penicillins (methicillin, oxacillin, nafcillin, and cloxacillin) results from alteration of the bacterial target of these antibiotics. Penicillin-binding proteins (PBPs or transpeptidases) are the targets of penicillins and cephalosporins that inhibit the cell wall synthesis function of these enzymes and cause cell death. When the native PBP is replaced by a variant

PBP2a (encoded by the *mecA* gene), this protein functions as the native PBP gene but does not bind antibiotics and continues to cross-link cell walls even in their presence. The *mecA* gene can be detected by a DNA probe or by testing the staphylococcal isolate for sensitivity to methicillin or oxacillin.

CHAPTER 12

1. **Streptococcal pharyngitis is a common self-limited disease. Why do physicians always treat this disease?**

    Although treatment of V.'s strep throat will shorten the period that she has symptoms, the real reason she was being treated with penicillin was to prevent the nonsuppurative sequela of acute rheumatic fever (ARF). Although ARF is a relatively rare complication, strep throat is a very common infection, and ARF was a major cause of rheumatic heart disease in the United States prior to the introduction of antibiotics. Antibiotic treatment also prevents the development of the rare local suppurative complications (e.g., pharyngeal abscesses), and it reduces the likelihood that V. will transmit her infection to other children.

2. **What bacterial process caused the rash?**

    The red rash with sandpaper texture is a manifestation of scarlet fever. Unlike a direct infection of the skin, such as cellulitis, this rash is caused by secreted streptococcal pyrogenic exotoxins (SpeA-C) that circulate in the bloodstream. The organisms that produced these exotoxins are contained in V.'s throat as a localized infection.

3. **Why were 2 days of antibiotics insufficient treatment, even though V. felt better?**

    The clinical signs and symptoms of strep throat may resolve shortly after initiation of antibiotic therapy. Several studies, however, have demonstrated that courses of penicillin shorter than 10 days are not enough to eradicate the organisms and to prevent an overly vigorous immune response. ARF cannot occur if a limited immune response is mounted against group A streptococci (GAS). An injection of long-acting penicillin compounds is an alternative that excludes the possibility of patient, or in the case of V. parental, nonadherence to therapy.

4. **Did the GAS directly spread to the heart and cause the damage to the heart valves?**

    No, the organisms were probably no longer present in V. The carditis of ARF is a consequence of an autoimmune attack on proteins in the tissues of the heart valves. Patients with ARF and scarred heart valves, however, will become more susceptible to endocarditis from bacteria that intermittently circulate in the bloodstream after minor traumas. Subsequent GAS infections can reactivate the carditis in patients who have had ARF, so they must remain on antibiotic prophylaxis for prolonged periods.

CHAPTER 13

1. **Where did Mr. P. acquire this organism? What host factors might have contributed to the pneumococcus gaining entry into his lungs?**

    There is no way to know from whom Mr. P. acquired pneumococcus, but it is certain that it came from a colonized human he had contacted in the recent past. The organism was likely transmitted to him by respiratory droplets, and he became colonized in the nasopharynx. Shortly thereafter, his lung became infected by

microaspiration of bacteria from his upper airway into his lower respiratory tract. The factors that contributed to pneumonia rather than continued asymptomatic carriage were his smoking and his recent viral infection. Both factors impede the clearance of inhaled particles by the mucociliary escalator, and both adversely affect the phagocytic function of alveolar macrophages.

2. **What possibilities should be considered if the initial antibiotic treatment was not effective in this case?**

    If the infection is very dense, the use of a rapidly bactericidal antibiotic can lead to the release of cell wall fragments that may increase the inflammatory response in the lungs. Antibiotic resistance is also a possible explanation for a poor response to therapy; however, that would be more likely if the patient had been treated with a penicillin or a macrolide, antibiotics to which resistance has emerged over the past few decades. Mr. P. was treated with a fluoroquinolone, levofloxacin, to which resistance is still relatively uncommon.

3. **If Mr. P.'s own immune response was not sufficient to control this infection, why might immunization have ameliorated or prevented these events?**

    Immunization provides the patient with type-specific antibodies against the 23 most common serotypes of pneumococcal capsule. With circulating antibodies against the infecting organism's capsule, the organisms in the alveoli would be opsonized with antibody and complement (by the classical pathway). With the influx of polymorphonuclear leukocytes into the alveoli, the bacteria would be rapidly ingested and killed, stopping the spread of infection.

CHAPTER 14
Pelvic Inflammatory Disease

1. **What test should be ordered for the cervical specimen? What will the stained preparation most likely reveal?**

    The presentation could be consistent with either gonococcal or chlamydial infection. A nucleic acid test for both pathogens could be sent on a single cervical swab. Alternatively, a culture for *Neisseria gonorrhoeae* could be plated at the bedside. A Gram stain is the most rapid diagnostic method, and this was reported in the case description. Intracellular Gram-negative diplococci were seen in association with neutrophils. This finding strongly suggests infection with gonococcus.

2. **Assuming that Ms. C. has PID, how did she acquire the infection?**

    Ms. C. would have acquired pelvic inflammatory disease by sexual contact with a male partner who was a carrier (probably asymptomatic) of *N. gonorrhoeae*.

3. **Is it significant that this patient has just finished her menses?**

    Yes. Spread of microorganisms from the cervix, through the uterus, to the fallopian tubes is most likely to occur at this point in the menstrual cycle because of the less resistant state of the cervical mucus.

4. **If the patient has PID, what other causative organisms, other than gonococci, should be considered?**

    Chlamydia trachomatis is another common cause of primary PID. After repeat cases, enteric bacteria and strict anaerobes may also be secondarily involved.

5. If the patient has PID, would the proper use of male condoms have prevented the infection? Could any other forms of birth control and/or disease prevention have prevented transmission?

Yes. A condom would have prevented transmission of the infection agent. Barrier precautions are the best means of prevention. Contraceptive jellies containing the spermicide non-oxynol-9 have some minor bactericidal effect, but protection against PID has not been demonstrated, and transmission of HIV may be increased with frequent use. Birth control pills are of no benefit in preventing transmission of infection.

6. What other benefits would Ms. C. realize if she and her partner used condoms consistently and correctly?

She would lower her risk of an unwanted pregnancy, and she would avoid the long-term complication of PID, including ectopic pregnancy, chronic pelvic pain, recurrent PID, and infertility.

CHAPTER 15

1. How did the two episodes of Ms. A.'s disease differ with regard to pathogenesis and the kind of bacteria involved?

The intra-abdominal infection resulting from the ruptured appendix followed a typical course. Initially, Ms. A. had acute inflammation with bacteremia. The blood culture was positive for *Escherichia coli*, and it is likely that an anaerobic blood culture was not ordered, or the *Bacteroides fragilis* may have been confined to the peritoneal cavity. The *E. coli* infection was resolved with cephalosporin treatment. *B. fragilis* persisted in the peritoneal cavity and induced a host response that led to abscess formation. The symptoms of this condition became evident in the 2nd week after the rupture.

2. Why did *B. fragilis* survive the first course of antibiotic treatment?

Bacteroidales species are resistant to many antibiotics. The cephalosporin used to treat the *E. coli* in the blood is ineffective against intestinally derived Bacteroidales. *Bacteroides* spp. have been shown to harbor many antibiotic resistance genes, many of which are contained on mobile genetic elements such as conjugative transposons or conjugative plasmids. This permits their transfer to other *Bacteroides* species and even to species of other genera. Antibiotics that were once effective against *Bacteroides*, such as clindamycin, are now ineffective in an increasing number of clinical strains.

3. Was Ms. A. treated properly? What could have been done to lessen the likelihood of abscess formation?

Ms. A. was not treated properly. When she presented with the ruptured appendix and colonic organisms were cultured from her peritoneal cavity, broad-spectrum antibiotics, including those active against both the facultative and the strict anaerobes, should have been administered. A drug targeting Bacteroidales species should have been given along with the cephalosporin therapy. Knowing that there was colonic spillage into the peritoneum, she could have been treated with a combination β-lactam–β-lactamase inhibitor, or a carbapenem like imipenem, or a β-lactam plus metronidazole.

A more rational antibiotic therapy would have decreased the likelihood of abscess formation.

4. How does *B. fragilis* facilitate intra-abdominal abscess formation?

Zwitterionic capsular polysaccharides of *B. fragilis* have been shown to induce the formation of intra-abdominal abscesses in experimental animal models. It is likely that many intestinal Bacteroidales species synthesize zwitterionic polysaccharides, which contain both positive and negative charges. The zwitterionic nature of the best studied *B. fragilis* capsular polysaccharide, polysaccharide A, is crucial to its ability to induce the formation of intra-abdominal abscesses. Zwitterionic polysaccharides interact with CD4+ T lymphocytes, setting in motion a series of immunological responses that lead to abscess formation.

CHAPTER 16

1. Why did the physician caring for Mr. D. think of cholera?

Three features of the clinical presentation created this suspicion. First, Mr. D. was seriously dehydrated because of the diarrhea. He was described as having "a rapid heart rate with a feeble pulse and low blood pressure," suggesting that the degree of dehydration was severe enough to affect his hemodynamic status and possibly lead to shock from hypovolemia. This is a rare occurrence in adults with ordinary diarrheal diseases but is common with cholera. Second, Mr. D. had recently traveled to South America where cholera occurs periodically among the local population. Third, Mr. D. used a medication that reduces his gastric acidity. This essentially lifts a barrier to passage of viable *Vibrio cholerae* to the small intestine and lowers the number of organisms that have to be ingested to cause disease. Mr. D. may have acquired a small but sufficient (for him) inoculum of *V. cholerae* in food or water that may have seemed reliable and sanitary to him.

2. Are all enteric bacteria capable of causing disease, or are some more frequently pathogenic than others? Which enteric pathogens cause diarrhea, and where do they come from?

Most enteric bacteria do not cause diarrheal disease. In fact, pathogenic *E. coli* in the human gastrointestinal (GI) tract are rare. A few strains of *E. coli* have picked up genes that encode pathogenic functions, such as toxin production, intimate adherence, and cellular invasion, probably by horizontal gene transfer or phage transduction from another microorganism. These are the ones responsible for various diarrheal diseases.

Table 16.1 is a list of common enteric bacteria that may cause disease. All the pathogens listed are inhabitants of the intestines of humans or animals. Thus, acquisition of infection can always be attributed to a fecal–oral route of transmission. Organisms that are acid sensitive and require very high inocula to establish infection generally require a vehicle such as food or water for transmission. Contamination of food sources or water supplies with raw sewage or animal feces may be to blame. By contrast, organisms that are acid resistant and establish infection at very low inocula can be acquired by direct contact with an infected individual (e.g., hand-to-hand-to-mouth) or transmitted on inanimate objects handled by an infected person (e.g., on fomites, like toys or pacifiers).

3. What are the clinical manifestations caused by enteric pathogens? Why do the organisms cause different intensity of symptoms in individuals?

Pathogens that produce enterotoxins or otherwise disrupt the absorptive function of the intestinal mucosal cells produce secretory diarrhea. The basis for these illnesses is electrolyte and water loss. Consequently, the principal clinical manifestations are watery, voluminous diarrhea; abdominal cramps; and nausea and vomiting (if the upper intestine or stomach is involved). Pathogens that attach to and invade the mucosa also induce a significant host inflammatory response. Diarrhea from *Campylobacter jejuni*, for example, a prominent foodborne pathogen around the world, may be as much a consequence of the inflammatory response as it is a consequence of any virulence factors produced by the microbe. Possible additional manifestations of such responses are fever, small stool volumes with mucus or blood, and abdominal pain.

In the case history of the D. family, it is likely that both Mr. and Mrs. D. ate and drank the same things. Why did he become ill with cholera while she did not? The major difference between the two hosts was probably their gastric acidity. Mr. D. was taking an antacid medication that rendered him more susceptible. It is also possible that acquired immunity might have played a role in Mrs. D.'s case because she was raised in Peru. Cholera tends to be less severe in adults from highly endemic regions (e.g., Southeast Asia and the Indian subcontinent) because they have been exposed frequently in childhood. The cholera morbidity in South America may not be sufficient to produce this effect.

4. What factors are involved in colonization? What factors are involved in causing symptoms?

V. cholerae has a pilus (TCP) that allows organisms to adhere to one another on the mucosal surface. Pathogenic *E. coli* has various fimbriae (or pili) that permit it to adhere to epithelial cells (e.g., bundle-forming pili in EAggEC, CFA in ETEC). Symptoms may be caused by toxins (e.g., cholera toxin, *E. coli* LT or ST) or by other direct interactions with cells that induce functional disturbances.

5. What is the proper therapy for watery diarrhea?

If the patient is in hypovolemic shock or impending shock, or if the patient is vomiting intractably, intravenous rehydration with correction of electrolyte losses may be necessary. However, most diarrheal illnesses, including cholera, can be treated with oral rehydration. Oral rehydration solutions generally contain sodium chloride and a simple sugar or carbohydrate that facilitates absorption via an unaffected pathway that links sodium ion absorption to glucose transport. Another important part of therapy is replacement of lost potassium and bicarbonate, ions that are also components of the World Health Organization rehydration formulation. Because illnesses with watery diarrhea are self-limited, antibiotics are rarely needed or used.

6. Can these diseases be prevented?

Public health measures and sanitation are of primary importance in prevention. From a public perspective, separating the disposal of human and animal feces from sources of food and water disrupts a critical cycle of transmission. Some pathogens, such as *C. jejuni* and enterohemorrhagic *E. coli* (EHEC), are present in raw meat or dairy products, so attention to proper food preparation is critical. In the case of personally transmitted

pathogens, such as *Shigella* species, hand washing may play an important role. In the case of Mr. D., cholera may never have developed if he had eaten only well-cooked foods and peeled fruits and vegetables and had drunk only boiled water. In the case of Baby D., it is unlikely that travel was involved, given the timing of the symptoms. Enteropathogenic *E. coli* (EPEC) infections often occur among infants in nurseries and day-care centers. Consequently, direct contact with other infants, caregivers, or fomites may be important. Because it is often difficult to control what goes into the mouth of a young child or infant, prevention is a significant challenge. Immunization against enteric diseases is an eventual goal but has not proven practical up to this point, except in the case of typhoid fever (see Chapter 17).

CHAPTER 17
Shigellae

1. What is the likely source of the shigellae?

The shigellae are human pathogens, and the only significant reservoir is in humans. Therefore, the source for this case was ultimately another individual. Shedding of shigellae in the stool may persist for several weeks after acute infection in an untreated individual. The mode of transmission was most likely direct contact between T. and an individual shedding shigellae in the stool, perhaps another child at day care. However, toddlers, more than any other age group, are likely to put objects into their mouths. It is possible that the source was a contaminated object.

2. How did these organisms enter into T.'s intestinal tract?

Shigellae are ingested most commonly on contaminated fingers or inanimate objects handled by an infected person. Occasionally, shigellae can be transmitted in food or water. Once ingested, the organism can transit the stomach unscathed because of its acid resistance. This accounts for the very low infectious inoculum and the modes of transmission that involve person-to-person spread.

3. What bacterial properties were involved in producing the bloody diarrhea?

The shigellae are able to invade the intestinal mucosa through M cells. They are then released into the lamina propria, where they invade intestinal epithelial cells through their basal surface. The bacteria are able to spread directly from cell to cell and induce a form of cell death called pyroptosis. This process involves the release of inflammatory cytokines that recruit neutrophils and macrophages into the area. Eventually, ulcers in the mucosa form; blood and inflammatory exudates are released into the lumen, accounting for the appearance of the stool.

4. How should this disease have been treated?

The fluid and antibiotic therapy given to T. was appropriate. Fluids are necessary because of the mild dehydration and the ongoing water loss associated with high fever. Antibiotics have been shown to reduce the duration of illness and to shorten the carriage state (thus preventing transmission to others after the acute illness resolves). In the United States, trimethoprim/sulfamethoxazole is the drug of choice. However, resistance to this agent is spreading around the world, and in most other countries, fluoroquinolones are more likely to be active.

Enterohemorrhagic *Escherichia coli*

1. What is the likely source of the organisms that caused these diseases?

Undercooked hamburger meat.

2. Why do only certain strains of *E. coli* cause the clinical manifestations seen in these cases?

The manifestations of enterohemorrhagic *E. coli* infection (EHEC) depend on the production of shigalike toxin. The gene for this toxin is carried on a bacteriophage on the bacterial chromosome. EHEC strains must carry this phage and also have the colonization factors that are required for attachment and effacement (like enteropathogenic *E. coli*).

3. By what mechanism does the responsible etiological agent cause these diseases?

Profuse bleeding in the colon is caused by the interaction of inflammatory cytokines and shigalike toxins, which damages blood vessels in the lamina propria. When the toxin is absorbed systemically, damage to small blood vessels in the kidney may trigger the hemolytic–uremic syndrome (HUS). Glomerular endothelial cell products (including von Willebrand factor, plasminogen activator inhibitor, prostacyclin, nitric oxide, and others) may mediate local pathophysiology leading to platelet thrombi, the characteristic feature of the disease.

4. What are the principal therapeutic concerns in such cases?

Antibiotics are usually avoided. Many antibiotics have the effect of inducing bacteriophages. Theoretically, this may increase the production of shigalike toxin and increase the risk of HUS. Patients with this illness, particular children, should be watched carefully for kidney damage. Dialysis is sometimes required.

Nontyphoidal *Salmonella* and Typhoid Fever

1. Do the same salmonellae cause diarrhea, dysentery, and typhoid fever?

Most Salmonella enteritis is caused by animal species and strains not fully adapted to humans. These strains cause gastroenteritis and may cause dysentery. *Salmonella typhi* is an exclusively human pathogen and is better adapted to invade and to persist in the human host than are the other salmonellae. The result is typhoid fever, a disease that is not a manifestation of infection with animal salmonellae in humans.

2. Can the epidemiology of typhoid fever be distinguished from that of other salmonelloses?

Because typhoid fever is caused by an exclusively human pathogen, cases can often be traced back to a human carrier, often a food handler. The animal Salmonella infections are generally associated with foods derived from infected animals, such as poultry, eggs, milk, and meat. These foodstuffs are generally contaminated from the farm, and they cause human infection when they are improperly handled or inadequately cooked.

3. Why were organs other than those of the digestive system involved in Ms. J.'s disease?

S. typhi causes a systemic infection with bacteremia. After the organisms penetrate through the intestinal mucosa, they are taken up by macrophages and dendritic cells and delivered to the spleen and liver. After a period of growth in these organs, there ensues a persistent and continuous second bacteremia that leads to invasion of the gallbladder and kidney and reinvasion of the gut mucosa, especially at the Peyer patches.

4. Why is it particularly important to treat cases of typhoid fever with antibiotics?

There are several concerns. First, reinvasion of the gut after the secondary bacteremia may cause more damage than the primary infection. Late in the course of typhoid fever, patients may develop intestinal perforations and fatal peritonitis. Second, invasion of other organs may result in catastrophic damage, including splenic rupture, hepatitis, or glomerulonephritis. Third, invasion of the gallbladder in an individual with stones may lead to a prolonged carrier state, adding to the human reservoir for further transmission.

CHAPTER 18

Pseudomonas Infection of an Immunocompromised Patient

1. What was the main predisposing factor for H.'s illness?

H.'s impaired host defenses, a consequence of his cancer and treatment, put him at increased risk for infection. Although it did not play a role in this case, an endotracheal tube or an indwelling catheter in the bladder or a vein increases risk by serving as a portal for infection.

2. Where did *P. aeruginosa* come from? How did it gain entry into H.'s bloodstream?

Infections in these patients are most often caused by the bacteria with which they are colonized. The gastrointestinal tract is the likely source of *P. aeruginosa* as chemotherapy may disrupt the gastrointestinal mucosa and serve as a portal of entry. Patients with severe defects in immunity, such as those induced by malignancies, diabetes, or chemotherapeutic or other immunosuppressive agents are at greatest risk from systemic pseudomonal infections. Neutropenia was a key factor in this case.

3. What caused the symptoms of the infection?

Pseudomonas species are Gram-negative bacteria with lipopolysaccharide (LPS). The lipid A component of LPS triggers a cascade of cytokines, which causes the symptoms and signs of sepsis.

4. What other sites could become infected in such a patient?

An endotracheal tube or an indwelling catheter in the bladder or a vein increases risk by serving as a portal for infection. The organisms can then disseminate to a variety of tissues (e.g., the skin) and cause metastatic infection if the bacteremia is not controlled.

Pseudomonas Infection of a Cystic Fibrosis Patient

1. How does the *P. aeruginosa* infection in Z.'s case differ from that of H.?

This patient has pneumonia but not disseminated infection with septic shock. In this case, the infection remains contained in the lungs. Also, the underlying predisposing condition, cystic fibrosis, is very different from H.'s neutropenia and immuno-compromised condition.

2. Is the strain of *Pseudomonas* that infects patients with cystic fibrosis the same that infects other people?

No. The *Pseudomonas* strains that infect cystic fibrosis patients tend to eventually emerge with distinguishing phenotypes including mucoidy, which promotes chronic colonization.

3. What was the route of entry of the organism in Z.'s case?

In this case, the organism was probably acquired orally or through aerosolization and may have temporarily colonized the upper airways before descending into the airways.

4. Would antibiotics help in Z.'s case?

Yes, they help to treat active pneumonia, but they do not fully eliminate the pathogen from the airway.

CHAPTER 19

1. How dangerous is whooping cough?

The most common serious complication of "whooping cough" is secondary bacterial pneumonia. However, the severe cough can also cause small hemorrhages in the brain and, together with the effect of some toxins, may cause younger children and infants to experience convulsions or other neurological symptoms requiring hospital care. Whooping cough may be life threatening in children with preexisting heart or lung disease.

2. Why was the physician sure of the diagnosis?

The rapid succession of hacking coughs that exhaust the patient's air, resulting in a huge gasping inhalation (or "whoop"), is characteristic of this disease. This is easy to recognize clinically after hearing it once.

3. Where did L. catch the "bug"?

It is most likely that L. acquired *Bordetella pertussis* from one of her three siblings or her grandfather who lived in the same household. All these individuals had "colds" recently, and because of partial immunity from prior vaccination (in the case of the siblings) or disease (in the case of the grandparent), their illness may not have expressed all the full-blown features of pertussis.

4. Will antibiotics make L. better?

Perhaps a bit. Antibiotics reduce the shedding of the organism from the patient's trachea. If given early enough in the course of illness, macrolides or tetracyclines may shorten the course of disease and lessen symptoms. However, these beneficial effects of treatment are not dramatic, because much of the damage to the airway will already have been done by the time that the patient comes to medical attention in most cases, and symptoms will improve only when this damage is repaired.

5. When can L. start getting her vaccinations?

As soon as she is no longer having fever, she should resume her normal childhood immunization schedule.

CHAPTER 20

1. What was the most likely source of the *C. difficile* that infected Mrs. T?

The *Clostridium difficile* was likely to have come from another infected patient in the same ward or hospital. Long-term stays in facilities such as nursing homes and hospitals lead to an increased number of patients carrying *C. difficile* in their colons. Most of these patients are asymptomatic carriers. However, if they undergo antibiotic treatment for a bacterial infection, *C. difficile* can grow to such an extent that it releases enough toxins to cause the diarrhea associated with the disease. The patient may also be colonized by *C. difficile* after the antibiotic treatment and then develop the disease. Transmission from patient to patient is thought to occur primarily via the hands of health care workers and by contaminated fomites and surfaces.

2. Is the history of previous treatment with cephalosporins and ampicillin pertinent to *C. difficile* infection?

Yes, ampicillin and cephalosporins are two of the antibiotic groups most often associated with *C. difficile* infection and development of diarrhea and pseudomembranous colitis.

3. Why was vancomycin not given at the initial occurrence of *C. difficile* infection?

To avoid the development of vancomycin-resistant strains of other Gram-positive pathogenic bacteria such as Enterococcus and Staphylococcus.

4. What was the likely source of bacteria for the relapse that occurred in the *C. difficile* infection?

Because spores are not killed by antibiotics, they are probably the means by which *C. difficile* can resist being killed by metronidazole treatment. While the vegetative bacteria present were killed by the antibiotic, some spores remained viable in the intestinal tract and were able to cause a recurrence of infection once the metronidazole treatment was halted. Alternatively, spores that are the infectious form that is transmitted to the patient after antibiotic treatment may have been reintroduced to Mrs. T.'s environment resulting in a new disease.

CHAPTER 21

1. How did Mrs. R. acquire *L. pneumophila*, and why was not anyone in her family or workplace also infected?

Although we cannot guess what specific exposure resulted in Mrs. R.'s infection, we can assume that she inhaled a water aerosol from the potable water system in the Florida hotel. This could have been from a faucet, shower, hot tub, decorative fountain, or evaporative cooling tower. It is likely that members of her family who accompanied her on the trip were also exposed but did not become ill. Mrs. R. probably developed Legionnaires disease after her exposure because of her age and her chronic smoking history. These factors impair the innate immune responses in resident macrophages in the lung. Her younger, nonsmoking family members were likely able to resist infection by any inhaled *L. pneumophila*.

2. Why was the diagnosis of Legionnaires disease initially overlooked in this case?

Legionnaires disease has few clinical features that are specific. In addition, the Gram stain and the sputum culture are usually not helpful. Because of the difficulty in making this diagnosis, most practice guidelines for the treatment of moderate or severe pneumonia call for a macrolide or fluoroquinolone in addition to a beta-lactam antibiotic in order to cover the patient for the possibility of Legionnaires disease. Had this been done at the time of Mrs. R.'s presentation, her course of illness may have been shorter and less severe.

3. Why did Mrs. R.'s pneumonia worsen during treatment with an antibiotic that kills *L. pneumophila* growing in bacteriological media?

Oral cephalosporins will kill *L. pneumophila* growing in culture, but they will be ineffective for therapy in infected patients. In this case, the patient worsened while taking an oral cephalosporin. The reason for this discordance is simple. Beta-lactam antibiotics penetrate poorly into living cells where most of the replication of *L. pneumophila* takes place. Antibiotics that are effective against this infection are ones that can cross eukaryotic membranes and enter cells. Some are even actively concentrated inside the cell. Macrolides, fluoroquinolones, and tetracyclines are reliably effective for treating Legionnaires disease.

CHAPTER 22

1. Was *H. pylori* the cause of this patient's 7-year bout of recurrent duodenal ulceration?

Helicobacter pylori–induced chronic gastritis is the most common cause of peptic ulcer disease in the United States. However, there are other etiological factors that can also lead to ulceration in the absence of infection. These include ingestion of aspirin or other nonsteroidal anti-inflammatory medications (NSAIDs), hyperacidity due to unrestrained gastrin production by a gastrin-secreting tumor (Zollinger-Ellison syndrome), Crohn disease, or gastric colonization by other rare microbial species (e.g., *Gastrospirillum*). In this case, the lack of a history of NSAID use or other abdominal symptoms associated with Crohn disease or Zollinger-Ellison syndrome (e.g., diarrhea) in conjunction with positive identification of *H. pylori* in the gastric mucosa makes it very likely that the patient's ulcer disease was due to colonization by *H. pylori*.

2. What features permit *H. pylori* to colonize the stomach when other bacteria cannot survive in this harsh environment?

H. pylori is a robust producer of urease, which catalyzes the hydrolysis of urea into ammonia and carbon dioxide, and ammonia production is an important survival mechanism for this organism within the acidic gastric environment. *H. pylori* also utilizes multiple polar flagella to facilitate locomotion through the mucus gel layer overlaying the gastric epithelium. Further, *H. pylori* possesses multiple chemotaxis systems to direct locomotion toward the mucus layer and gastric epithelium. Upon contact with the gastric epithelium, *H. pylori* utilizes a number of adhesins that allow for colonization amid gastric peristalsis.

3. What bacterial and/or host factors allow an infection with such high specificity for gastric epithelium to cause disease at an anatomically distinct site such as the duodenum?

Although the specific factors have not been entirely clarified, *H. pylori* infection results in down-regulation of somatostatin-producing D cells, which in turn leads to inappropriately elevated gastrin levels and enhanced gastric acid secretion. *H. pylori* can then populate regions of gastric metaplasia in the duodenum, establish infection, cause inflammation, and, in concert with elevated gastric acid levels, ultimately lead to ulceration at this site.

4. How can *H. pylori* infection be detected in patients with disease?

Several techniques can be used to diagnose *H. pylori*, and these can be classified as either invasive or noninvasive. Invasive methods require endoscopy with biopsy and include rapid urease tests, histologic techniques, and culture. Noninvasive tests include urea breath tests, which detect radioactive carbon dioxide in expired breath samples following ingestion of labeled urea. High values signify the presence of gastric urease activity, which is nearly always due to the presence of *H. pylori*. Another noninvasive test is serologic detection of *H. pylori*, which is based on measuring anti–*H. pylori* antibodies. Finally, the *H. pylori* stool antigen test can detect the presence of *H. pylori*–specific proteins in feces. Although none of the currently available diagnostic tests are completely reliable owing to differences in bacterial colonization density, many possess sufficiently high levels of accuracy so as to permit their widespread and singular use for initial diagnosis and/or confirmation of eradication.

5. How can *H. pylori* be eliminated from the stomach?

The stomach presents unique barriers to antibiotic efficacy that are usually not encountered within other anatomic niches of the human body. These include an acidic pH, peristalsis, active secretion, and a semipermeable mucous barrier overlaying the epithelium. Some antibiotics are less effective at lower pH (e.g., amoxicillin, clarithromycin), while other antibiotics (e.g., metronidazole) rapidly induce resistance in *H. pylori* strains, which decreases therapeutic efficacy. Many antibiotics exert only minimal bacteriostatic or bactericidal effects. Therefore, elimination of *H. pylori* requires multiple drugs for prolonged durations (10 to 14 days) to overcome these obstacles.

First-line therapy for *H. pylori* consists of a proton pump inhibitor (PPI) twice a day and clarithromycin and amoxicillin or metronidazole for at least 7 but preferably 10 days. If this regimen fails to eradicate the bacterium, the physician should initiate quadruple therapy, which consists of a PPI, bismuth subsalicylate, tetracycline, and metronidazole, for 14 days. Another appealing second-line regimen is sequential therapy consisting of 5 days of a PPI and amoxicillin followed by 5 days of triple therapy consisting of a PPI, clarithromycin, and metronidazole. Although successful eradication of *H. pylori* requires multiple medications, the absolute failure rate for treating the infection is very low, in part because of the multiplicity of treatment regimens available. For example, quadruple therapy achieves cure rates of approximately 90% in patients who have failed previous therapies and who are colonized with strains resistant to metronidazole and clarithromycin.

CHAPTER 23

1. How and when did Ms. A. most likely become infected with *Mycobacterium tuberculosis*?

Exposure most likely occurred years earlier when Ms. A. was on the AIDS ward in South Africa. At that time, she was exposed to patients with active, untreated tuberculosis who were coughing and thus creating aerosols of *M. tuberculosis* in droplet nuclei.

Ms. A. inhaled the droplet nuclei and developed a primary infection in the lung that resolved after she developed an immune response.

2. Why did it take so long for Ms. A. to develop active tuberculosis?

Until recently, her cellular immune response controlled the organism. When hypersensitivity against the organism created a cavity in her lung, her immune system lost control.

3. By what route did the tubercle bacilli most likely arrive at the apices of her lungs?

Organisms in aerosolized droplet nuclei were ingested by alveolar macrophages in the lower parts of the lung where the primary infection occurred. Some bacilli were then carried by the bloodstream and lymphatics (during the lymphohematogenous dissemination phase) to the well-aerated apices of the lungs where the bacilli grow more abundantly.

4. Which individuals are most likely to develop active TB from contact with Ms. A.?

Among the various persons with whom she has contact, the risk is greatest for the infants (<1 year of age) at the day-care center.

5. How would her illness have differed if she had had AIDS?

If she had had both AIDS and tuberculosis, the tuberculosis would have progressed more rapidly. She would have been more likely to have disseminated tuberculosis involving multiple organs, and she would not have developed cavities in the apices of her lungs. Pulmonary cavitation is due to a vigorous hypersensitivity reaction to the organisms that is impaired or absent in AIDS.

CHAPTER 24

1. Is it possible that this patient was not aware of having had a chancre before presenting with secondary syphilis?

Yes. The patient is a homosexual male and may have had a primary chancre in a location that was not visible or symptomatic (e.g., in the anal canal or rectum). Heterosexual males who are uncircumcised may occasionally overlook a painless chancre if it develops under the penile foreskin. Similarly, women with primary syphilis may have internal chancres that go unnoticed.

2. How did the spirochetes travel from the chancre to the patient's skin, lower lip, and lymph nodes?

After the initial chancre begins to heal, spirochetes disseminate in the bloodstream and then replicate in the lymph nodes, the liver, joints, muscles, skin, and mucous membranes distant from the site of the primary chancre. This process is often associated with fever but not frank sepsis. Because of the extent of organ involvement at this stage, the clinical features of secondary syphilis are highly variable.

3. Are the clinical features of secondary syphilis (rash, swollen lymph nodes, mucous membrane lesions) fully explained by spirochetes invading skin, lymph nodes, and lower lip? What host factors may be contributing to the disease process?

Secondary syphilis is associated with an abundance of spirochetes at the sites of involvement. Moist lesions will be teeming with live organisms. There is clearly an inflammatory response at the involved sites, but it is not clear what role the immune system plays in tissue damage at this point in the course.

4. Are the skin lesions and mouth lesions infective? Could another person acquire syphilis by touching them?

Yes. The secondary lesions are full of spirochetes, and they could infect another individual by touching, especially if there is a tiny break in the skin of the finger. Sexual contact with an individual with secondary lesions is extremely likely to transmit syphilis.

5. What will happen to this person's skin rash, lip lesion, and swollen lymph nodes if he is not promptly treated with antibiotics?

Secondary lesions eventually resolved on their own within weeks to months. A relapse of secondary manifestations may occur within the year that follows, or the infection may go into a prolonged latency and possibly reemerge many years later with manifestations of tertiary syphilis.

CHAPTER 25

1. How did Mr. G. acquire the infection? What is the likely significance of his vacationing in Nantucket in June? Is he likely to transmit the infection to anyone else?

Mr. G. was likely bitten by a deer tick that he acquired while hiking on Nantucket in June. Lyme disease is endemic to Nantucket, and June is a peak month for Lyme disease because it is when many nymphal-stage deer ticks feed. In addition to the summer peak, a second smaller peak of Lyme disease occurs in the fall, when adult ticks feed. Lyme disease is only acquired by a tick bite, and Mr. G. cannot transmit the infection to any other person.

2. What early clinical feature did Mr. G. exhibit that might have provided his physician with the best diagnostic hint that he had Lyme disease? Why was the diagnosis of Lyme disease overlooked when he saw a doctor while visiting Arizona?

Erythema migrans is a skin lesion that is characteristic of Lyme disease. However, in approximately 20% of cases, the rash is not apparent or is so mild as to be missed. Because Lyme disease is vanishingly rare in Arizona and because the diagnosis of Lyme disease is still largely a clinical one that requires the physician to actively entertain the possibility, it is not surprising that the patient was not diagnosed with Lyme disease in Arizona.

3. What feature(s) of the spirochete are responsible for Mr. G. suffering such diverse signs and symptoms, including headache, myalgia, facial droop, arthralgia, and arthritis?

The bacterium is highly motile, and many strains are capable of spreading to diverse tissues. Through complement evasion and antigenic variation, the spirochete can survive in many tissues, giving rise to the diverse signs and symptoms associated with Lyme disease.

4. Why was an immunoblot performed in addition to ELISA?

ELISA detects antibodies directed against *Borrelia burgdorferi* but has a significant false-positive rate, in part because the assay does not discriminate among different antibodies directed against different *B. burgdorferi* proteins. In contrast, immunoblotting allows for the specific detection of antibodies directed against defined *B. burgdorferi* proteins, and the Centers for Disease Control and Prevention has established criteria for interpreting immunoblots that have resulted in a much lower false-positive rate.

CHAPTER 26

1. Why did J. develop a different disease than M. when both were infected with the same organism, *B. henselae*?

M. was healthy and immunocompetent, and J. had AIDS. In immunocompetent individuals, the immune system responses vigorously to *Bartonella henselae* and responds by trapping the organisms within regional lymph nodes, surrounding them with a cellular infiltrate, and controlling their replication. In AIDS, the immune system is unable to contain the pathogen, and *B. henselae* spreads unimpeded through the blood to infect the skin, the liver, and possibly other sites.

2. Why did M. get well without treatment, while J. suffered a relapse despite treatment with an appropriate antibiotic?

M. has an intact immune system and can clear *B. henselae* with a vigorous immune response.

3. What was the source of the infection?

The family kitten was an asymptomatic carrier of *B. henselae*. M. acquired the infection by a cat scratch. It is not clear how J. acquired the infection, but the source was also likely the kitten.

4. By what route(s) did the organisms travel to the skin papule, the lymph nodes, and the pseudoneoplastic skin lesions?

In patient M., the skin papule occurred at the site of inoculation, probably a scratch from a kitten. Regional lymph nodes became infected and inflamed after the pathogen reached them via the regional lymphatics. In patient J., the site of inoculation was inapparent. Instead of causing a localized infection, the organism invaded the bloodstream, and the pseudoneoplastic skin lesions are metastatic infections that developed as a result of the bacteremia.

CHAPTER 27

1. What was the second antibiotic taken by Mr. C. and Ms. N., and why was it given?

The second antibiotic was azithromycin. Mr. C. was probably infected with both gonorrhea and chlamydiae at the time of his visit to the physician. Since more than 55% of men with gonorrhea have coexisting chlamydial infection, the Centers for Disease Control and Prevention recommends that every treatment for uncomplicated gonorrhea (a single intramuscular injection of ceftriaxone) be accompanied by a single dose of azithromycin for chlamydiae (since chlamydiae are not susceptible to ceftriaxone). Azithromycin is an attractive drug for chlamydial treatment for two reasons: (1) its long half-life provides sustained killing concentrations over the length of the slow chlamydial developmental cycle and (2) patient adherence is not an issue because the treatment requires only a single oral treatment of two 500-mg capsules rather than multiple pills over several days.

2. Why were nucleic acid amplification assays performed instead of culture on Ms. N.'s endocervical specimen?

Nucleic acid amplification tests are more sensitive and faster than culture, especially for chlamydiae. By amplifying the *Chlamydia trachomatis* plasmid DNA, the assays can detect as few as one to three elementary bodies (EBs). Chlamydial EBs, which are only 0.25 μm in diameter, cannot be recognized on Gram stain. They would appear as tiny, featureless red dots. Moreover,

because they are obligate intracellular bacteria, chlamydiae cannot be cultured on agar media. Culture of chlamydiae is done in epithelial cells, and cultivation takes at least 48 hours for growth. In addition, culture is expensive and is performed in only a few sophisticated hospital diagnostic laboratories that have tissue culture facilities (usually in clinical virology laboratories).

3. If Ms. N. had not heeded Mr. C.'s advice and sought medical attention, what might have been the consequences for her? What are the pathophysiological mechanisms of such sequelae?

Like most women with chlamydial cervicitis, Ms. N. was asymptomatic. Without appropriate azithromycin therapy, Ms. N. might have developed ascending infection and eventually pelvic inflammatory disease (PID)—endometritis and salpingitis. The pathophysiological mechanisms are likely immune mediated. Direct inoculation of a cultured Fallopian tube in vitro with *C. trachomatis* produces only mild salpingitis that heals with minimal scarring. However, in both patients and monkey models in vivo, the infection produces severe salpingitis, adhesions, scarring, and tubal occlusions. These observations support the belief that the immune response is an important component underlying the pathophysiology of the disease.

CHAPTER 28

1. What caused the rash, stupor, and gastrointestinal symptoms?

All the initial clinical manifestations of Rocky Mountain spotted fever are caused by the damage to infected endothelial cells and result tiny hemorrhages. In the skin, these hemorrhages produce that characteristic petechial rash. In the brain, the perivascular edema and hemorrhages may produce nonspecific neurological symptoms, such as stupor. Small hemorrhages and perivascular inflammation in the gastrointestinal tract may cause nausea, vomiting, and abdominal pain.

2. Why was the serological test for Rocky Mountain spotted fever negative in the hospital?

Patients with this infection typically develop symptoms before they have begun to produce antibodies against the pathogens. Serological tests become positive during convalescence, so they are not very useful for confirming an acute case.

3. Assuming that rickettsiae were circulating in the blood, why were the blood cultures negative?

Rickettsiae are obligately intracellular pathogens and will not grow in artificial media. They can be isolated in cell culture, but that is rarely attempted because it is difficult, time-consuming, and hazardous.

4. How did a girl from an eastern state get "Rocky Mountain" spotted fever?

Although Rocky Mountain spotted fever was first identified in the western United States, it is much more common in the eastern and southern states.

CHAPTER 29

1. How did B. acquire the organism?

Michelle acquired *Mycoplasma pneumoniae* infection through aerosol from her older brother. *M. pneumoniae* is a common cause of community-acquired respiratory infections and frequently linked to outbreaks in families and closed communities, such as military installations, schools, college dormitories, nursing homes, summer camps, health clinics, training facilities, and workplaces. Therefore, *M. pneumoniae* should be considered as the cause of unexplained respiratory illnesses as part of large outbreaks, especially among school-aged children and young adults, although all age groups are susceptible. Typically, rates of transmission are high with an incubation period of 2 to 3 weeks. Frequently, clusters of *M. pneumoniae* infections are characterized by a point-source outbreak.

2. What are distinguishing features of the organism and the treatment process?

M. pneumoniae does not have cell walls, requires sterol, and possesses one of the smallest genomes of any known self-replicating cell. Antibiotics that inhibit cell wall synthesis are of no therapeutic value, but those that inhibit protein and nucleic acid synthesis are effective. Treatment should include tetracyclines, macrolides, or quinolones and may have to be empirical because of a lack of standardized diagnostic tests and failures in microbiological culture. Early use of antibiotics will likely reduce the duration of signs and symptoms of illness. Delayed diagnosis or therapy can lead to serious consequences to the central nervous system, cardiovascular system, or joints or various multiorgan complications.

3. How can a definitive diagnosis of mycoplasmal infection be made?

Culture of throat, nasopharyngeal, or pleural specimens on specialized media may reveal small colonies in 10 to 28 days; the colonies can be visualized with a dissecting microscope. However, culture failures are frequent. PCR assays can be performed, and along with clinical signs and symptoms, results of commercially available serological tests can be useful in determining treatment modalities. Because of the lack of clinical criteria and widely available rapid diagnostic testing for *M. pneumoniae*, respiratory illnesses caused by this common bacterial pathogen are frequently overlooked.

CHAPTER 32
Outbreak of Poliomyelitis

1. What was the origin of the virus, and how did it spread among the students?

The virus was probably introduced into the private school by one or more of the day students who live at home. These students may have acquired the virus from other members of the community during their interactions such as in swimming classes. During outbreaks of poliomyelitis in the United States, swimming pools were often closed to prevent spread of the virus.

2. What caused the illness among the 17 students who complained of nonspecific signs and symptoms?

The symptoms of those 17 students were a consequence of poliovirus replication in the alimentary tract, establishment of a primary viremia, and systemic spread. These symptoms constitute the so-called minor illness or abortive poliomyelitis because the virus does not invade the central nervous system. Replication of the virus leads to an immune response and systemic "flulike" symptoms.

3. Why did the disease not spread to all of the students or to the community outside the school?

Students who had been previously immunized against poliovirus were protected from infection; those who had not been vaccinated were immunized by the outbreak. Assuming the rate of paralytic disease to be about 1% of infections, then it is likely that all of the unvaccinated students were infected; some of these had minor illness, but most did not display symptoms. By 1972, the date of this outbreak, most of the population of the United States had been immunized against poliovirus; as stated in the case, 95% of students at public schools had been vaccinated. As a result of immunization of the general population, the outbreak did not spread outside the private school.

4. How does poliovirus cause paralysis and other symptoms of disease?

The minor illness (flulike symptoms) is caused by viral replication in the alimentary tract and systemic effects of the immune response. In rare instances, the virus enters the spinal cord, where it replicates in motor neurons. When sufficient numbers of neurons that innervate a leg or arm muscle are destroyed, that limb becomes paralyzed.

5. What could have been done to halt further spread of poliovirus in the school?

The 3 weeks between the first and last cases was sufficient time to immunize all the students. Immunization should have been carried out immediately after the first case had been reported. Alternatively, the students could have been administered pooled human immunoglobulin, which would have provided passive protection against poliovirus.

Common Cold

1. What viruses can cause these symptoms?

Rhinoviruses are most frequently associated with the common cold, which includes the symptoms noted in this case. However, it is important to realize that the common cold syndrome also can be cause by infection with other viruses, including adenoviruses, coronaviruses, and metapneumoviruses.

2. How was the infection transmitted from the child to the mother?

The infection was most likely transmitted by contact with virus-laden respiratory secretions or by inhalation of virus-containing aerosols produced by sneezing, coughing, or speaking.

3. Will this infection induce immune responses that protect against future infections of the same type?

Rhinovirus infection will lead to a memory immune response that protects against future infections with the same viral serotype. However, because there are over 100 rhinovirus serotypes, the likelihood that a subsequent infection will be with the same viral serotype is remote.

CHAPTER 33
West Nile Virus

1. How and where did Mrs. K. become infected with West Nile virus?

It is most likely that she was bitten by an infected mosquito while gardening in her backyard. Many mosquitoes feed in the morning and evening. Therefore, being outside without protection against mosquito bites during those hours increases the likelihood of exposure and infection.

2. What was her most important risk factor for severe disease?

Age over 60 years is a risk factor for severe disease. Although it has been hypothesized that this may reflect a slower or less vigorous immune response in the elderly, that hypothesis has not been proven. The pattern of increased mortality in older individuals also has been observed for other flaviviruses that cause encephalitis.

3. How could this infection have been prevented?

No vaccine is currently available for West Nile virus, although several are in development. Insect repellent, wearing clothing that covers the body, and staying indoors or within a screened enclosure during the times mosquitoes are biting will prevent mosquito bites and thus infection. Elimination of mosquito breeding sites (e.g., old tires, buckets, pots, and other containers that fill with water) in her backyard and in the neighborhood will decrease the population of mosquitoes.

Yellow Fever Virus

1. How and where did Mr. W. become infected with yellow fever virus?

It is most likely that Mr. W. acquired infection while in the Amazon basin. Yellow fever virus is endemic in many forested regions of Brazil and Peru. Humans in those regions are exposed to forest-dwelling mosquitoes that maintain the jungle cycle of infection with monkeys as the vertebrate host. Humans infected in this way can introduce the virus into cities and urban populations of *Aedes aegypti*, leading to outbreaks of urban yellow fever with humans as the vertebrate host.

2. What was the reason for his bleeding disorder?

Yellow fever virus infects and irreversibly damages hepatocytes that are important for production of coagulation factors. In addition, yellow fever virus has been associated with more nonspecific causes of coagulation defects, such as platelet dysfunction, thrombocytopenia, and disseminated intravascular coagulation.

3. What could have been done to prevent this infection?

An attenuated strain of yellow fever virus, 17D, has been safely used for immunization since 1937. The 17D strain was attenuated by passage in chick embryo cells of the Asibi strain of the virus isolated in 1927 by inoculating a monkey with the blood of a patient from Ghana. The vaccine is licensed in the United States, is recommended for all travelers to endemic regions, and provides protection for at least 10 years after immunization.

CHAPTER 34
Measles Virus

1. Why was the diagnosis of measles not considered by B.'s physicians?

Exposure to natural measles is now rare in the United States because individuals who are not old enough to have had natural measles in childhood are now mostly vaccinated. It is important to note that the majority of younger physicians in developed countries are not familiar with the clinical presentation of measles due to high vaccination rates. Today, outbreaks of measles in the United States are almost always traced to imported cases from countries where infection is still endemic. Taking a careful travel and vaccination history is of paramount importance.

2. Is there a concern that he might transmit the infection to others?

Yes. Measles is transmissible 2 to 3 days before and for 4 days after the rash appears. Because measles is highly contagious to nonimmune individuals, substantial effort by public health authorities is required to identify persons exposed to an active case and to administer to such persons vaccine or measles immune globulin.

3. How could this illness be diagnosed as measles?

An experienced clinician can diagnose measles by its presentation. The three Cs (cough, coryza, and conjunctivitis) are followed by a maculopapular rash that spreads from the face downward and eventually becomes confluent. The appearance of classic Koplik spots in the mouth is virtually pathognomic for measles. If all these findings are present, the diagnosis is highly likely. However, since measles can produce unusual manifestations in partially immune or immunosuppressed individuals, laboratory diagnosis is necessary. Enzyme immunoassays demonstrating measles IgM or a fourfold increase in IgG antibodies is diagnostic. Isolation of measles virus is time-consuming and not widely available.

Respiratory Syncytial Virus

1. What was the role of N.'s sibling in this case?

The older sibling attended a child-care center, a known risk factor for acquisition of RSV. It is likely that the older sibling had been infected previously and was partially immune. Consequently, he may have acquired infection with only upper respiratory tract symptoms and transmitted the virus to his younger, more susceptible sibling.

2. What is the significance of hyperinflation with peribronchial thickening on the chest radiograph?

In bronchiolitis, the epithelia of the small airways are infected by RSV. The virus is cytotoxic for those cells, damages the epithelium, and induces an inflammatory host response. The result is narrowing of the airways with trapping of air in the pulmonary alveoli. Symptomatically, the situation causes expiratory wheezes. On the chest radiograph, the lungs may appear to be hyperinflated, and the inflammation around the small bronchi may be visualized as thickening of the walls of these passages.

3. Why did N.'s cough persist for 2 weeks after hospitalization?

RSV is cytotoxic to respiratory epithelial cells, with resultant damage to ciliary function. In addition, the host immune response plays an important role in the pathogenesis of RSV disease. Repair of respiratory epithelium after the resolution of viral replication can often require several weeks, hence the prolonged cough in the case of baby N. RSV is linked epidemiologically with asthma, although it is not clear whether infection with RSV increases a child's risk of developing asthma or whether RSV infection is more severe and thus more apparent in children who already have a genetic or physiological predisposition for this illness.

CHAPTER 35
A Bat Bite

1. Is this a "typical" case of rabies in the United States?

Yes, most indigenous human rabies cases in the United States are the result of exposure to bats.

2. What prophylaxis would Mr. B. have received had he gone to the emergency department immediately after he was bitten?

He would have received immediate basic wound care, administration of rabies immune globulin into the wound, and the first of four doses of cell-culture rabies vaccine. Unfortunately, in the case of Mr. B., he did not seek treatment after the bite, and prophylaxis was not administered.

3. What would have been the chances of success if Mr. B. had been provided with the appropriate prophylaxis against rabies?

If Mr. B. had received the recommended postexposure prophylaxis in a timely and appropriate manner, the chances for success would have been optimal. In fact, no such failures have occurred in the United States in more than two decades.

4. On average, how many cases of human rabies occur in the United States each year?

Dog rabies has been controlled in the United States. Consequently, on average, only one to three cases of human rabies are reported each year resulting from exposures to indigenous rabid wild animals or exposures occurring in countries with endemic rabies.

5. Approximately how many persons are vaccinated against rabies in the United States each year?

Although most are not truly exposed to the virus and are given needless prophylaxis, approximately 25,000 to 40,000 people are vaccinated each year.

6. Were Mr. B.'s symptoms characteristic of human rabies cases?

Yes, his symptoms were characteristic of rabies, starting with vague, prodromal symptoms, quickly progressing to an acute neurological phase and death. Focal numbness and pruritus at the site of the bite were early clues to the diagnosis.

A Dog Bite

1. Should Mrs. X. still be concerned about rabies exposure?

No, she should not be concerned. The decision not to vaccinate Mrs. X. was based on sound epidemiological principles—specifically, the absence of reported rabies cases in the main species affected in the region. This incident was a provoked bite by an otherwise healthy dog that is available for observation.

2. If the dog had not been found, would the treatment have been different?

No, the approach would not have been different if the dog had not been found, but the physician and public health department would need to explain the rationale and reassure the patient.

3. If this incident occurred outside the United States, would the protocol have been the same?

No, if this occurred in a country with dog rabies, such as China or India, the patient would require immediate basic wound care, administration of rabies immune globulin into the wound, and the first of four doses of cell-culture rabies vaccine.

CHAPTER 36

1. Why did the physician think P. would develop influenza, even though no laboratory tests supported the assumption?

The physician thought the symptoms of the 6-year-old brother described by the mother were consistent with influenza. Furthermore, the physician had seen many cases of clinical influenza during that week in January. Finally, the physician had been advised by the local health department of an influenza epidemic in the town. The incubation period of influenza is 1 to 2 days. Based on the timing of the disease experienced by his older brother, the 2-year-old was thought by the physician to be starting with disease symptoms.

2. What was the most likely drug the physician prescribed to the patient and other family members? Why did he not give the medication to the 6-year-old sibling?

The physician most likely prescribed a neuraminidase inhibitor for the young patient to inhibit the amplification of the virus. In the case of the mother, father, and the oldest sibling, the neuraminidase inhibitor would be an appropriate prophylactic drug to prevent the spread of disease to them. Because the 6-year-old brother already had full-fledged illness, giving the drug to him would not be of benefit (the maximum of virus replication occurs before the full spectrum of disease symptoms).

3. What should the physician have asked regarding all family members, and what should he have recommended the family do next year?

The physician did not ask whether anyone in the family had been vaccinated against influenza. To prevent influenza in the family, the physician should recommend that family members receive influenza vaccination in the fall to protect them against influenza during the following winter season.

CHAPTER 37
Rotavirus

1. How did M. acquire the virus?

Rotavirus is transmitted from person to person by the fecal–oral route. M. most likely acquired the infection either directly from a playmate or from a contaminated toy (fomite). It is also possible that she acquired the infection from an adult (e.g., a parent).

2. Is it significant that M.'s disease occurred in the spring?

Rotavirus infections occur seasonally in temperate climates, with peak illness during the winter. The rotavirus season may begin during the fall and extend into the spring.

3. Will M. ever have the same disease?

Reinfection with rotavirus is common. However, repeat infections are usually less severe and may even be asymptomatic. It is unlikely that M. will have a subsequent rotavirus infection of similar severity.

4. Why did the pediatrician suspect this etiological agent?

The pediatrician suspected rotavirus as an etiological agent based on the severity of the symptoms and the time of year that the illness occurred. It is likely that the pediatrician had recently been seeing many other patients with similar illnesses caused by rotavirus infection.

5. Could this illness have been prevented?

Two live attenuated rotavirus vaccines are licensed for use in the United States. These vaccines are most effective at preventing severe illness such as that requiring hospitalization.

Norovirus

1. How did Mr. S. acquire the virus?

Noroviruses are spread primarily by the fecal–oral route, but they also may be transmitted by aerosol following vomiting. Mr. S. could have acquired the infection in one of several ways on the cruise ship: (1) consumption of contaminated food or water, (2) contact with a fomite (contaminated inanimate object) on the ship, (3) direct contact with an ill or recovering traveler who did not wash his or her hands after defecation, and (4) exposure to an aerosol generated by a norovirus-infected person who was vomiting.

2. Why did the physician not perform any diagnostic tests?

Tests for norovirus infections are not routinely available. The clinical presentation and epidemiological factors in this case strongly suggest norovirus infection.

3. Why did the physician tell Mr. S. to use good hygiene practices at home and at work?

The primary means of transmission of norovirus infection is by the fecal–oral route, and the principal means of prevention is by using good hand washing practices. Although Mr. S. will be able to return to work after his symptoms resolve, he may continue to shed virus in his stool for up to 3 weeks. If he does not practice good hygiene, he could contaminate food in the restaurant and transmit the infection to his customers.

4. Will Mr. S. ever have the same disease again?

Yes, it is likely that Mr. S. will have the same disease again. Although short-term immunity to reinfection and disease caused by the same strain is observed following norovirus infection, reinfection and disease with that strain can occur 1 to 2 years later. Disease also can occur earlier with other unrelated norovirus strains.

CHAPTER 38

1. Was the presence of HIV antibodies in G.'s blood diagnostic of HIV infection?

The infant's positive HIV serology at birth may have been attributable to maternal antibodies transmitted transplacentally. Passively acquired maternal antibodies to HIV may persist until 15 months of age; thus, positive serology alone in young children does not mean that they are infected with the virus.

2. What was the basis of the initial diagnosis?

The diagnosis of AIDS in G. was based on his birth from a known HIV-infected mother and the absence of findings to suggest another cause for neonatal immunodeficiency.

3. How was the diagnosis confirmed?

The diagnosis was confirmed by finding HIV nucleic acid in the infant's blood. An earlier attempt to detect HIV RNA or proviral DNA would have facilitated an earlier diagnosis of HIV infection.

CHAPTER 39

1. What was the source of the virus that caused the disease?

The virus most likely was introduced into the office by a patient with an ocular adenovirus infection. During that patient's eye examination, instruments likely became contaminated. Inadequate instrument sterilization likely led to transfer of the virus to other patients. Virus was also transferred to work surfaces and, judging from the presence of the virus in the ophthalmologist's office, to the hands of the ophthalmologist as well. The virus found in the air conditioning filter suggests that some aerosolization of contaminated fluids occurred. Overall, infection control procedures seem to have been inadequate in this office.

2. Why did the disease resolve spontaneously?

Most adenovirus diseases, including epidemic keratoconjunctivitis, resolve spontaneously because of the vigorous immune response generated by the infection.

3. What measures helped prevent further spread of the disease?

In cases such as this where transmission occurs by the direct inoculation (meant literally) of virus, instruments are nearly always the culprits. Therefore, proper instrument sterilization and minimization of instrument use can prevent transmission.

4. Why were the medical personnel in the ophthalmologist's office not affected?

Transmission of epidemic keratoconjunctivitis is almost exclusively by direct inoculation of the eye. Office personnel did not have ocular contact with contaminated instruments, and apparently, ambient virus levels on surfaces were not high enough to result in casual transmission (e.g., by rubbing the eyes with contaminated fingers).

CHAPTER 40

1. How and when did Mr. M. acquire the HPV infection?

Penile warts are usually acquired by sexual contact. Because HPV infection can be subclinical for months and possibly years, one cannot state precisely when Mr. M. became infected.

2. Is Mrs. M. also infected, and what are the clinical implications?

Sexual contact is an efficient means to spread HPV, and it should be assumed that Mrs. M. has been exposed to the HPV present in Mr. M.'s warts. It is also possible that Mrs. M. was previously infected and spread it to him. Her immune response may have cleared the HPV although he still has the virus. She is at risk for cervical cancer if she shows abnormal pathology in cervical cells or has persistent high-risk HPV infection.

3. What, if any, laboratory tests should be performed on Mr. and Mrs. M.?

They should be examined, and any warts found should be treated. Cytological examination of the cervix such as a Pap test is indicated. This is currently the standard of care for all sexually active women. A highly sensitive nucleic acid–based test also might be considered.

4. If Mrs. M. has cervical warts, will they eventually result in cancer?

Presumably, this infection would be diagnosed by the presence of abnormal cells on a Pap smear or an HPV nucleic acid test followed by a biopsy. Depending on the degree of cellular abnormality, no further treatment may be indicated, and the patient may be followed with annual Pap exams. Most cervical infections resolve without treatment. If she develops high-grade dysplasia or cervical intraepithelial neoplasia (CIN), therapeutic intervention is warranted and should be effective.

5. How can Mr. M. and his wife be treated for the HPV infection?

Visible penile lesions should be treated; liquid nitrogen cryotherapy is commonly used. A topical agent such as imiquimod might be applied to treat subclinical lesions. Repeated testing of cervical specimens demonstrates that HPV infection of the cervix often resolves within a period of 1 to 3 years. Persistent high-risk HPV infection of the anogenital region and cervix is concerning and should be treated.

CHAPTER 41

1. What tests would be required to confirm Mr. H.'s suspicion that he has genital and oral herpes?

The history and clinical presentation probably would be sufficient to make the diagnosis of herpes simplex virus (HSV) infection. Definitive confirmation could be obtained by testing lesion specimens for the presence of HSV DNA by PCR or for specific reaction with anti-HSV antibodies or by isolating virus from oral and penile swabs in cultured cells and testing the infected cells for reactivity with anti-HSV antibodies.

2. Is it likely that Ms. C. would have engaged in sex when she had active herpetic lesions? If she had no lesions, how could she have transmitted herpes to Mr. H.?

It is unlikely that Ms. C. and Mr. H would have engaged in sex if she had had active lesions that were apparent to her or to Mr. H. It is possible for recurrences of viral replication to occur without the appearance of noticeable lesions. Transmission from one person to another can occur under those circumstances.

3. What are some of the more severe symptoms that can be associated with primary genital herpes?

Some of the complications of primary genital herpes, in addition to large and spreading mucocutaneous lesions, include meningitis, radiculitis, urinary retention, and constipation.

CHAPTER 42

Sore Throat and Swollen Glands in High School Cheerleader

1. How was her infection acquired?

Sally probably acquired this infection through intimate contact with an individual who had previously been infected with the causal virus.

2. What is noteworthy about Sally's symptoms and laboratory findings? Does her age together with her clinical presentation suggest a possible diagnosis?

Sally likely has a primary infection with EBV with clinical findings of a sore throat, fatigue, loss of appetite, and inflammation of her liver (infectious mononucleosis). Following the development of serological assays for EBV infections, epidemiological studies defined risk factors for early acquisition of EBV in the United States, which include lower socioeconomic status, crowded housing, and close contact with children. Those not infected in childhood more frequently develop symptomatic illness when the virus is acquired later in life. The clinical syndrome of acute infectious mononucleosis is associated with primary EBV infection, less frequently with CMV, and in rare cases toxoplasma infection. Thus, a clinical diagnosis together with minimal laboratory examination such as a complete blood count could establish the diagnosis of acute EBV infection with reasonable certainty, especially if a significant number (>10%) of atypical lymphocytes are detected in the peripheral blood smear. Additional testing for EBV-specific antibody responses will provide a definitive diagnosis.

3. How will the physician utilize the laboratory to confirm the diagnosis?

The physician will initially determine if Sally is producing heterophile antibodies that react against red blood cells of other species. These antibodies can be detected in the serum using a simple test commonly known as a monospot test. To confirm the diagnosis, the physician can obtain evidence of specific antibody responses to EBV by requesting EBV-specific serology, which includes testing for both IgM and IgG anti-EBV antibodies.

4. Will an antiviral drug alter her symptoms?

No. Although studies suggest that some antiviral agents can decrease shedding of EBV during acute infection, such therapy does not shorten the duration of illness, nor does therapy alter the characteristics of the persistent infection.

Betaherpesvirus Infection in Immunocompromised Renal Transplant Recipient

1. What factors could predispose Mr. K. to infection with either CMV or EBV?

Infection with CMV or EBV requires exposure to infectious virus. In this case, Mr. K. could have received a kidney allograft from an infected donor or infected blood products. Depending on the nature of the transplantation and the serological status of the recipient (past history of CMV or EBV infection), donors of blood products will be screened for evidence of CMV or EBV infection and, if positive, their blood products either will be depleted of white blood cells to limit transmission of CMV and EBV or provided to recipients with serological evidence of CMV and EBV infection. Immunosuppression does not predispose an individual to infection but can result in loss of immune control of virus replication, higher viral loads, and end-organ disease. In the post-transplant period, transplant recipients are given pharmacological agents to suppress T-lymphocyte allograft-specific responses to prevent rejection and preserve function of the transplanted organ.

2. Does the limited amount of information included in the case history provide clues to the possible cause of his illness?

Yes, the time of onset of his clinical disease is common for patients who develop CMV or EBV infections in the posttransplant period. Furthermore, his clinical illness resembles that seen in a nonimmunocompromised person with acute infection caused by either CMV or EBV.

3. What laboratory tests were used to make the diagnosis in this patient?

The diagnosis of CMV or EBV infection in transplant recipients is most often made by detection of viral nucleic acids by PCR or viral antigens in a clinical specimen such as the antigenemia test to detect CMV in peripheral blood or viral DNA in peripheral blood cells. Recovery of infectious virus is also used in some centers, although in most cases, this approach has been modified to allow rapid identification of virus in clinical specimens.

4. Is treatment with antiviral therapy indicated in this patient?

Yes, under most circumstances, this patient would receive an antiviral agent. Although CMV or EBV infection in such individuals can be self-limited, current diagnostic techniques cannot predict which individual patient will resolve the infection without therapy. In the case of EBV infection with symptoms and lymphadenopathy, it is likely that the transplant team would consider reducing the intensity of immunosuppressive therapy hoping that sufficient adaptive immunity will recover to control EBV replication and decrease the risk for the development of PTLD.

CHAPTER 43

1. By what route or routes might Mr. L. have become infected?

Although it cannot be concluded with certainty, it is likely that Mr. L. became infected with hepatitis B virus (HBV) by sharing needles with an HBV-infected chronic carrier. However, it is also possible that he contracted HBV sexually from his girlfriend.

2. What caused Mr. L.'s symptoms?

Mr. L. has acute hepatitis. That diagnosis is made by his symptoms of anorexia, nausea, and right-sided abdominal pain. He has increased levels of serum aminotransferases, bilirubin, and alkaline phosphatase. These findings indicate injury to hepatocytes. HBV infection does not result in hepatocyte injury. Instead, injury is caused by the antiviral response of cytotoxic T cells.

3. What was the significance of finding viral surface antigen but not antisurface antibodies?

Early in infection, the serum will contain HBsAg but not anti-HBs (see Fig. 43.5). This finding indicates active HBV infection of hepatocytes. Although HBsAg particles are not themselves infectious, only cells infected by HBV can make them, and such cells also make infectious virions. Therefore, the presence of circulating HBsAg also indicates that Mr. L. can transmit the virus to others (see answer to Question 6).

4. What follow-up tests will be required to determine his long-term prognosis?

Serum levels of HBsAg and anti-HBs should be monitored. If Mr. L. resolves his infection, HBsAg will become undetectable, and high titers of anti-HBs will develop. This serological response is associated with protection against reinfection by HBV. If HBsAg remains positive after 6 months, he would be considered to have a chronic HBV infection. Since it is also possible that Mr. L. was coinfected with hepatitis delta virus, he also should be tested for the presence of anti-HDAg IgG.

5. What treatment could be instituted?

The physician could not know with certainty whether Mr. L.'s immune response would be effective in clearing the viral infection. If Mr. L. does become chronically infected, the exact treatment will depend on several factors, including the ongoing severity of his symptoms and the extent of liver injury.

6. What advice can Mr. L. be given to avoid further transmission?

Mr. L. should be made aware that he can and will infect others unless he uses condoms during sex and does not share needles. In addition, he can no longer donate blood. His girlfriend should be tested for the presence of HBV. If her tests are negative, she should be vaccinated to prevent any future HBV infection.

CHAPTER 47

1. What is the main reason that the manifestations of pulmonary histoplasmosis were so different in the three patients?

The primary reason for the differences in manifestations relates to the host. The young boy was healthy and had a mild infection that his immune system could handle. The kidney transplant recipient was on immunosuppressive drugs and was unable to mount an effective cell-mediated immune response to *Histoplasma capsulatum*; therefore, she had extensive pulmonary infection that proved to be life threatening. The older man who had severe chronic obstructive pulmonary disease (COPD) had normal cell-mediated immunity but had severe structural damage to his lungs and was unable to eradicate *H. capsulatum* for that reason. This form of histoplasmosis is only seen in patients who have COPD.

2. What was the source of *H. capsulatum* that infected each patient? Can a discrete point source be found for most patients?

Most cases of histoplasmosis cannot be related to a discrete point source, but outbreaks continue to occur when groups take part in work-related or vacation-related activities that disperse the conidia of *H. capsulatum*. The likely source for the boy was the chicken coops he cleaned on his uncle's farm; they likely had accumulated bird excreta that allowed luxuriant growth of *H. capsulatum*. It is likely that the renal transplant recipient had reactivated a focus of *H. capsulatum* that she had acquired during childhood in the endemic area. She probably never knew that she had had histoplasmosis as a child. It is not clear when patients with chronic cavitary pulmonary histoplasmosis acquire the organism. It is likely that many are related to reactivation, but some may be from a recent exposure.

3. Why was therapy unique for each patient? Do most patients with histoplasmosis require treatment with an antifungal agent?

Most patients do not require therapy for acute histoplasmosis; indeed, most are not diagnosed as having a fungal infection at the time they are ill. Healthy hosts, unless infected with a very large number of organisms, are able to handle the infection when their CD4 cells become sensitized to Histoplasma antigens and activate their macrophages to kill the intracellular organisms. The transplant recipient, because of her immunosuppression, needed urgent therapy with intravenous amphotericin B, an agent that is cidal for *H. capsulatum*. In such a patient, in whom amphotericin B is necessary but risky because of its nephrotoxicity, a lipid formulation, which is less nephrotoxic, will be used, and therapy will be changed to oral itraconazole as soon as she has begun to respond. Chronic cavitary pulmonary histoplasmosis is a fatal disease if untreated, but it is chronic and can be treated with oral itraconazole quite well. Unfortunately, many of these patients die of respiratory insufficiency because of their severe COPD.

CHAPTER 48
Candidemia

1. What factors put Mrs. D. at risk for developing candidemia?

This woman had many risk factors for developing candidemia. She had a perforated colon, had been on broad-spectrum antibiotics, and had renal failure that required hemodialysis. In addition, she had a central venous catheter in place and was receiving parenteral nutrition through the catheter.

2. Where did the *C. albicans* come from?

Candida species are part of the normal flora of the gastrointestinal tract. The organism could have gained access to the blood at the time of the initial perforation of the colon. More likely, however, because the candidemia occurred 3 weeks later, the source of the candidemia was the central venous catheter. The catheter tip could have been seeded originally from the GI tract, or Candida could have colonized the catheter from the skin at the site of insertion or from the hub of the catheter as it was cared for.

3. What does the term "germ-tube positive" mean to the clinician?

The germ tube test is a rapid test that looks for the formation of an elongated bud arising out of the yeast cell when the cells are exposed to calf serum. This test differentiates *C. albicans* from most other Candida species. It is commonly used in clinical laboratories and reported to clinicians as germ-tube-positive yeast consistent with *C. albicans*.

Invasive Pulmonary Aspergillosis

1. Why was Mr. S. at risk for an opportunistic fungal infection?

The primary risk factor for invasive fungal infection in this patient was the prolonged and severe neutropenia induced by chemotherapy. Chemotherapeutic regimens often include corticosteroids that are another risk factor, and the use of broad-spectrum antibiotics also could have contributed to the development of a fungal infection in this patient.

2. Why did Mr. S. have pleuritic chest pain?

Aspergillus is an angioinvasive mold that invades through blood vessels, causing tissue infarction that can extend to the pleural surface and result in pleuritic chest pain.

3. How useful is a bronchoalveolar lavage showing septate hyphae?

In a highly immunosuppressed patient, the presence of septate hyphae in the bronchoalveolar lavage fluid is strongly suggestive of invasive fungal infection. Most often, this will be aspergillosis, but other molds have the same appearance, and only the culture will allow differentiation of the various organisms. In a patient who is not immunosuppressed and who has a low risk of invasive fungal infection, the presence of septate hyphae in bronchoalveolar lavage fluid usually means merely colonization or contamination, not invasive infection.

CHAPTER 49

1. Where did Mr. J. acquire the organism? Was it related to his dairy farming, raising Christmas trees, or keeping tropical fish?

This farmer most likely acquired sporotrichosis from planting and caring for Christmas trees. Seedlings frequently come wrapped in sphagnum moss, which is often contaminated with *Sporothrix schenckii*. The sharp needles on spruce and other evergreens inoculate the fungus into the subcutaneous tissues.

2. What other infections, besides sporotrichosis, were in the physician's differential diagnosis?

The physician wondered whether these lesions were due to *Mycobacterium marinum*, which is associated with injuries incurred in fish tanks; *Nocardia brasiliensis*, a soil organism; *Francisella tularensis*, often associated with rabbits; or less likely, an atypical staphylococcal infection.

3. Why was Mr. J. treated with itraconazole, which costs approximately 10 times more than the treatment long used for this infection, potassium iodide?

Although potassium iodide would likely be effective for this patient's lymphocutaneous sporotrichosis, it is difficult to administer. It is a liquid given with water or juice, beginning with 5 drops three times daily and increasing up to 40 to 50 drops three times daily, as tolerated by the patient. The side effects, which include metallic taste, salivary gland swelling, hypothyroidism, nausea and vomiting, fever, and rash, often result in the patient becoming noncompliant with taking the medication. Itraconazole in either the capsule formulation or the suspension is easier to administer.

CHAPTER 52
Malaria

1. Why did Ms. M.'s fevers occur in paroxysms (episodes) of shaking chills followed by fever and then drenching sweats?

During the course of malaria, the life cycles of the parasite in red blood cells becomes synchronized so that large crops of cells rupture to release merozoites at the same time. When that occurs, the parasite molecules responsible for inducing the inflammatory response become suddenly abundant in the blood. That causes the acute chills and fever, which resolve when the free merozoites are cleared from the bloodstream or enter other red blood cells. The sweat occurs when the hypothalamic thermal set point is lowered and the body must lose heat to bring the temperature down.

2. Why did she have dark urine?

Malaria induces red blood cell hemolysis. That occurs because of direct infection and destruction of cells to be sure, but more importantly, the infection also induces an autoimmune hemolysis that is responsible for most of the red blood cell loss.

3. Why did she develop edema of the lungs and an elevation of the serum creatinine?

Plasmodium falciparum is the species of malaria most likely to induce dysfunction of organs like the lung (edema), kidney (increased creatinine and decreased glomerular filtration rate), and brain (cerebral malaria) because the mature parasites make the parasitized red blood cells adhere to vascular endothelial. That stickiness impedes blood flow in capillary and small venular beds, causing ischemia and hemorrhage.

Acute Toxoplasmosis *Toxoplasma gondii*

1. How did Mr. H. acquire the infection?

Because the patient had no direct contact with cats, he likely acquired acute toxoplasmosis by eating raw lamb. It is very likely that all the other members of his family have also had this infection.

2. What was the purpose of the second serology?

The follow-up serology should show an increase in the amount of IgG antibody against *Toxoplasma gondii* in the patient's blood. This confirms that the infection is acute and recent and was not acquired in the remote past.

3. Why was the patient given no treatment?

If no organ damage is associated with acute toxoplasmosis, it is usually allowed to run its course. It is a self-limited infection, and treatment does not eliminate the probability that the organism will generate dormant cysts.

Leishmaniasis

1. How did Ms. Q. acquire the infection?

Leishmaniasis is acquired from the bite of a phlebotomine sand fly.

2. How would this case have evolved if Ms. Q. had not received treatment?

It depends on the species of Leishmania causing the skin ulcer. In the Americas, strains of *Leishmania mexicana* typically produce ulcers that heal spontaneously but slowly. In contrast, *L. braziliensis* infections can persist for years, only to recur in the nasal septum and turbinates many years later in a small percentage of patients. The latter infections should always be treated.

Chagas Disease *(Trypanosoma cruzi)*

1. What does the case reveal about Senhor R.'s past?

Senhor R. may be a well-to-do businessman now, but his childhood was probably spent in relative poverty. The bugs that transmit *Trypanosoma cruzi* typically live in cracks in the walls

of mud-brick houses or in thatched roofs. They emerge at night and bite residents of the houses while they sleep. Senhor R. must have originally come from a socioeconomic class that lives under these conditions.

2. Why were antiparasitic drugs not given?

The late phase of Chagas disease is thought to be immunologically mediated. Parasites are not to be found at this stage, and treatment is of no value.

African Sleeping Sickness *(Trypanosoma brucei)*

1. How did a parasite survive in Mr. B.'s blood for 8 months? Is he immunocompromised?

He need not be immunocompromised. African trypanosomes are able to undergo antigenic variation and vary their major surface protein to avoid an effective host immune response. Thus, complete clearance of the parasite is difficult and persistent in the bloodstream.

2. How would Mr. B.'s illness have been different if he had immigrated from South Africa rather than West Africa?

In contrast to the West African strains of sleeping sickness (*Trypanosoma gambiense*), the southeastern varieties (*Trypanosoma rhodesiense*) cause a much more acute illness, with fever and rapid progression to central nervous system disease over days to weeks.

Infection with Free-Living Amebas

1. How did amebas get into E.'s central nervous system?

Free-living amebae may proliferate in lake water when the temperature is persistently warm. The parasite is thought to enter the swimmer's central nervous system through the cribriform plate along the olfactory nerve tracts. Activities that facilitate contact between the water and this anatomical site (e.g., diving) can increase the risk of introducing the infection.

CHAPTER 53
Amebic Liver Abscess

1. Why were no amebas seen in Mr. A.'s stool?

In active amebic colitis, trophozoites may be difficult to find in the stool. The sensitivity of microscopy is improved by examining scrapings taken directly from colonic ulcers. Moreover, amebic liver abscess often occurs with no intestinal signs or symptoms. In such a case, cysts may be seen in the stool, but trophozoites would likely be absent. Nonmicroscopic diagnostic techniques may be useful in such cases. The stool *Entamoeba histolytica* antigen detection test (not used in this case) is sensitive and very specific. Instead, amebic serology was positive at a high titer in this patient, strongly suggesting that *E. histolytica* as the cause of the illness.

2. What was the role of steroids in this case?

Corticosteroids may have contributed to the exacerbation of a chronic ameba infection and permitted invasion of the parasite through the intestinal wall and into the portal circulation. As mentioned in the chapter text, humoral immunity is not effective in limiting ameba infection. However, cell-mediated immune responses may help to contain the infection, and these responses may have been blunted by corticosteroids.

Chronic Giardiasis

1. How did Mr. P. acquire *Giardia* infection?

In considering possible encounters with this pathogen, one must remember two facts about *G. lamblia*. First, it is a zoonosis. That is, animals are infected as easily as humans, and animal feces may be a source for human infection. Second, *G. lamblia* is usually acquired by drinking fecally contaminated water. Documented foodborne transmission of *G. lamblia* is rare, and person-to-person transmission is usually associated with exposure to infected children in day-care centers or with certain sexual activities. Given the patient's travel history, speculation centered on her recent backpacking trip. The patient was asked where she obtained drinking water on this trip and admitted to drinking untreated surface water. Surface streams, lakes, and even springs are often contaminated upstream with small mammal, bird and even human feces. It is always a mistake to assume that such water sources are free of *G. lamblia*, even when the water appears crystal clear.

2. What prompted the physician to check for a parasite rather than to culture for agents of bacterial gastroenteritis?

The patient's symptoms began 1 week after the backpacking trip, which was 2 months earlier. Therefore, the symptoms have persisted for at least 7 weeks. Most bacterial enteric infections (e.g., salmonellosis, shigellosis, campylobacteriosis) would surely have resolved over that period. The long duration of symptoms (more than 3 weeks) is more characteristic of a parasitic protozoal infection than a bacterial infection.

Cryptosporidiosis

1. How did Mr. W. acquire cryptosporidiosis?

Unless the patient is involved in a large outbreak, the source of cryptosporidium is usually unknown. Potential sources are similar to those of Giardia (see previous case) because cryptosporidium is also a zoonotic pathogen. Large waterborne outbreaks have occurred after contamination of municipal water systems and swimming pools. Direct contact with infected animals or humans is probably a less common mode of transmission.

2. What other significant pathogens might be seen on an acid-fast stain of the stool?

Another parasitic protozoa, *Cyclospora*, closely resembles *Cryptosporidium*. *Cyclospora* is also acid-fast and can be distinguished from cryptosporidia only on the basis of their larger diameter. In advanced AIDS patients, atypical mycobacteria (i.e., *M. avium-intracellulare*) may be seen on acid-fast stain of stool; however, those organisms are slender bacilli that would not be confused for the spherical protozoal oocysts.

3. Why was antiretroviral therapy given to control the diarrhea instead of an antiparasitic agent?

There is no satisfactory antiprotozoal therapy for persistent cryptosporidiosis. Nitazoxanide may reduce symptoms in infected children but does not appear to be helpful in immunocompromised patients. In AIDS, restoration of cell-mediated immunity by treating HIV infection appears to permit the patient to exercise some immunological control over the infection. These patients should be treated with hydrations, antimotility agents, and highly active antiretroviral therapy (HAART).

CHAPTER 54
Nematode Infection: Ascariasis

1. How did T. acquire the worms?

Worm eggs from other humans' feces mature in the soil. The mature eggs were ingested by the child, either directly by putting soiled hands in his mouth or indirectly by eating soil-contaminated fruits or vegetables.

2. Is T.'s case typical of *Ascaris* infections?

No. Most infections, with smaller worm burdens, are relatively asymptomatic. This case reflects a potential consequence of having a large worm burden—intestinal obstruction caused by a mass of worms.

Nematode Infection: Pinworm

1. What caused D.'s anal itching?

The female *Enterobius* worm resides in the rectum and deposits adherent eggs in the anal canal. The eggs are irritating and cause itching. Children's hands and fingernails become contaminated when they scratch, facilitating spread of the parasite.

2. Should her mother be concerned that D. may become reinfected after being treated?

Yes. Households with infected children often have significant contamination of the environment with pinworm eggs. In addition, other small children, and even adults, in the household can be infected. It is usually necessary to clean the child's room, wash the bedclothes, and treat the entire family to prevent reinfection.

Nematode Infection: Hookworm and Strongyloidiasis

1. How did these patients acquire adult helminths in their intestinal tracts?

Most often, these parasites are acquired when infectious helminth larvae in soil contact bare skin. These larvae are capable of penetrating normal skin, often the bare feet. The larvae enter the bloodstream in small venules and transit through the right side of the heart to the lungs. In the lungs, they enter airspaces and undergo further maturation. If the worm burden is high enough at this point, there may be cough and signs of pneumonia with eosinophilia. Eventually, the worms migrate up the bronchial tree to the trachea, where they pass around the epiglottis and are swallowed into the gastrointestinal tract. Adult worms attach to the mucosa of the small intestine. Infections with both male and female worms can result in the production of eggs, and eventually larvae, which may be deposited onto the ground in places where disposal of human feces is inadequate or nonexistent. Thus, the life cycle is completed.

2. Why did V. have anemia, while Ms. C. presented with recurrent Gram-negative sepsis?

Hookworms like *Ancylostoma duodenale* feed on blood. If the worm burden is large, the blood loss associated with worm feeding can be significant enough to produce anemia. However, intestinal hookworms do not invade beyond the intestinal mucosa, and the eggs they produce do not hatch into larvae within the intestinal tract. Thus, there are usually no other systemic manifestations. Adult female Strongyloides invade the intestinal mucosa to lay eggs. Consequently, multiple steps in larval maturation may occur before the parasite reaches the end of the intestinal tract, and some may mature into the filariform stage, the same stage that penetrates through the intact skin when the patient is initially infected. These larvae are invasive and can penetrate through the anal skin during defecation to complete the parasitic life cycle within a single host. Normally, this is a relatively rare event that does not significantly amplify the overall worm burden. However, an immunocompromised patient (such as a patient treated with corticosteroids) may experience a massive increase in worm burden, with symptoms of rash (of the anus and buttocks owing to worm penetration), cough (owing to passage through the lungs), and abdominal pain (owing to the massive increase in adult intestinal worms). The mass invasion of larvae from the lower gastrointestinal tract into the bloodstream is one cause of the recurrent episodes of Gram-negative bacteremia. Perforation of the adult females through the intestinal wall with subsequent peritonitis is another.

3. Can these patients transmit their infections to other people?

Hookworm infections are not transmissible because there is a period of maturation in the soil that must occur before the larvae become invasive. As mentioned in Question 1, patients with Strongyloides infection may have invasive larvae in their stool. Consequently, contact between a patient's stool and an uninfected person's skin can transmit the infection.

Intestinal Tapeworms

1. How could this infection have been prevented?

Because the infection was acquired by ingesting encysted larvae in undercooked beef, there are two important ways to prevent transmission of the disease to humans. First, cooking beef adequately will kill the incubating cysts and render the meat safe to eat. Second, beef can be cultivated without parasitic cysts. Cattle acquire the infection by exposure to human feces. Interrupting the contamination of grazing areas with human feces would prevent the cattle from ever becoming infected. Unfortunately, in the case of Mrs. N., avoiding exposure may not have been possible without creating a diplomatic incident. This illustrates the fact that health concerns may sometimes take a back seat to cultural sensitivity.

2. What would have happened to Mrs. N. had she been given no treatment?

Taenia saginata, the beef tapeworm, has no potential to produce encysted larvae in human tissues. Therefore, unlike the pork tapeworm, symptoms related to cysts in the brain or other tissues do not occur with intestinal beef tapeworm infection. This patient, left untreated, would likely have continued to pass tapeworm segments periodically, occasionally involuntarily. Some patients with tapeworms report vague GI discomfort, and some have allergic responses to the tapeworm (e.g., urticaria or "hives"). Eventually, the tapeworm head would become senescent and die, ending the infection.

CHAPTER 55
Trichinosis

1. How did Mr. Y. acquire this illness?

The patient ingested live *Trichinella spiralis* larvae embedded in the muscle of the pig from which the pork dish was made.

2. What caused Mr. Y.'s diarrhea and abdominal pain?

Penetration of the ingested larvae into the intestinal wall may cause diarrhea and abdominal pain in the early phase of the illness.

3. Why was his eosinophil count elevated?

T. spiralis is a helminth that invades tissues. The host responds to large pathogens (too big for conventional phagocytosis) by mounting a brisk eosinophilia. Other pathogens in this chapter that migrate through tissues do the same

4. How could the illness have been prevented?

If the pork had been adequately cooked to a sufficiently high temperature, the encysted larvae would have been killed before ingestion. The infection of the pig might have been prevented by heating its food also. The pig acquired trichinosis by ingesting a smaller animal (probably a rodent with trichinosis) in its food.

Pork Tapeworm and Cysticercosis

1. How did the two patients acquire their infections?

The Peace Corps volunteer, Ms. F., acquired an intestinal tapeworm by ingesting larvae in undercooked pork. At some point, the tapeworm segments were regurgitated into her stomach, where the eggs that they contain were induced by gastric acid to hatch into invasive larvae that penetrated the intestine and encysted in the patient's brain and other tissues. Ms. K., the Navajo woman, ingested echinococcal eggs from handling an animal that carried the tapeworm.

2. Why did Ms. F. have an intestinal tapeworm at some point but Ms. K. did not?

Taenia solium is a human tapeworm. Pigs never have the tapeworm but can develop cysticerci if they ingest eggs from the feces of a tapeworm-infected person. Humans with tapeworms may develop cysticerci by hatching of the eggs from their own tapeworm, or they can acquire cysticercosis by eating food contaminated with fecal material from tapeworm-infected food handlers. In contrast, *Echinococcus* is not a human tapeworm, and humans do not acquire intestinal infection. Cystic hydatid disease always results from accidental ingestion of echinococcal eggs from the feces of dogs or other canids, usually carried in abundance on their fur.

3. Can these patients be treated and cured?

Both patients can be treated. The drugs albendazole or praziquantel kill cysticerci. Echinococci can be treated with albendazole or, if the cyst is very large, by instillation of a parasiticidal agent into the cyst with a needle and evacuation of the contents.

Schistosomiasis

1. What caused the granulomatous changes associated with these infections?

Eggs released by the adult female parasite in the venules are transported through tissue to a hollow viscus where they exit the body, or they remain trapped in tissue where they degenerate. Antigens released from degenerating schistosome eggs induce granulomas. The granulomas eventually resolve with fibrosis and scarring.

2. Why was infection with *S. mansoni* associated with bleeding from the stomach, whereas *S. hematobium* was associated with blood in the urine?

The adult forms of *Schistosoma mansoni* reside in the mesenteric circulation. *S. mansoni* eggs may pass into the colon wall, possibly to be released into the lumen of the colon and subsequently excreted in the stool. Alternatively, they may be transported in the portal blood to the liver and form granulomas there. The persistent occurrence of granulomas in the portal tracts of the liver eventually leads to scarring and obstruction of the portal vessels in the liver. This obstruction results in increased pressure in the portal circulation and a tendency for collateral veins to dilate. This process typically occurs in the gastric, esophageal, and hemorrhoidal veins, which can connect the portal venous blood to the systemic venous circulation, bypassing the liver. Enlarged veins in these areas may be subject to bleeding, and hemorrhage from the gastric or esophageal veins may cause massive bleeding into the stomach, as was seen in the case of Ms. U.

In contrast, the adult worms of *S. hematobium* tend to reside in the venous plexus surrounding the bladder. The eggs of these parasites exit the body through the urine, although many eggs remain trapped in the bladder wall and in other parts of the urinary tract, where they produce granulomas and fibrosis. The long-term consequences are bleeding in the urine (hematuria) and obstruction of the urinary tract, with chronic recurrent urinary infection.

Skin- and Lymph-Dwelling Filaria Infections

1. Why did Mr. L. became blind, while Mr. J. developed swelling?

The filarial infections cause different manifestations, depending on whether the adult parasites dwell in the skin or in the lymphatic system. Those that dwell in the lymphatics tend to produce microfilaria that may degenerate and cause intermittent obstruction of lymph flow with swelling of the dependent extremity (e.g., *Wuchereria bancrofti* in Africa and the New World, and *Brugia malayi* in Asia). This was the manifestation seen in Mr. J.'s case. In contrast, in skin-dwelling filarial infection, such as onchocerciasis (Mr. L.'s case), microfilariae migrate under the skin and, when they degenerate, produce inflammatory changes there. If the adult worms reside in subcutaneous nodules in the upper part of the body or head, microfilariae may migrate into the anterior chamber of the eye. The repetitive inflammation associated with microfilarial degeneration in that location eventually leads to blindness.

2. How did these patients acquire the infections?

Lymph-dwelling filariae release their progeny microfilariae into the lymphatics, and they eventually circulate in the bloodstream. Consequently, the arthropod vectors for these infections are blood-sucking insects, mosquitoes. In contrast, the progeny of the skin-dwelling filariae remains. They are acquired by and transmitted by biting flies that cut into the dermis of the skin where the microfilariae are located. Thus, Mr. L. acquired infection from the bite of a deerfly, and Mr. J. acquired the infection from a mosquito bite.

CHAPTER 56

1. What features of Mr. I.'s case are characteristic of variant CJD?

At the age of 22 years, he is young for any of the other human prion diseases. The onset with psychiatric symptoms is typical and distinct for the onset of sporadic CJD. His evaluation included magnetic resonance imaging that showed high signal intensity in the pulvinar, which is characteristic of variant CJD. In addition, a tonsillar biopsy was positive for PrP^{Sc}, a finding that does not occur in other human prion diseases. Finally, he has the PrP^C codon 129 homozygosity for methionine, indicating that he belongs among the 30% of humans susceptible to variant CJD.

2. How and when did he acquire the disease?

Mr. I. acquired variant CJD by ingesting beef or beef products containing the bovine spongiform encephalopathy (BSE) PrP^{Sc}. Although it is not clear when this might have occurred, it is unlikely that he acquired variant CJD in the United States. He moved to Florida in 1992, and it is possible that he was previously exposed in Great Britain, when the BSE outbreak there was in full swing.

3. Should he be isolated to prevent transmission of the disease to others?

No. He should not be placed in isolation because only certain of his tissues (central nervous system, lymphatics) contain the pathological prion. Person-to-person transmission of variant CJD does not occur with normal contact. However, if he had a brain or tonsillar biopsy, one would assume that the instruments had become contaminated. They should be discarded after use rather than used in a subsequent surgery on another patient, because contaminated surgical instruments could be a vehicle for transmission of prion diseases.

4. What are his chances for recovery?

Unfortunately, Mr. I. will not survive.

CHAPTER 57

1. Why was anthrax considered early as a probable diagnosis in this case?

The physician who treated this patient was a skillful interpreter of Gram stains. He knew that the only community-acquired agent of meningitis associated with Gram-positive rods is *Listeria monocytogenes*, bacteria that are small and pleomorphic. In contrast to the appearance of *Listeria*, the organisms in the patient's Gram stain were large and rectangular, an appearance sometimes described as "boxcars." He recognized that the organisms were Gram stained as *Bacillus* species, and the only member of that genus ever found as a cause of meningitis is *B. anthracis*. So, it pays to know your basic microbiology.

2. Why was bioterrorism suspected?

No cases of anthrax had occurred in Florida for several decades. Past cases were cutaneous, not inhalational, anthrax. The patient had no apparent exposure to animals or animal products known to transmit the disease. There were no nearby facilities where anthrax is cultivated. Therefore, the most plausible explanation was exposure to deliberate release of anthrax spores. The accuracy of that interpretation of events became clear when anthrax-tainted mail began to appear in certain congressional offices and mailrooms in Washington, DC.

3. Why did antibiotic therapy fail to save Mr. O.'s life?

This patient received prompt and appropriate therapy with antibiotics. Unfortunately, the dissemination phase of anthrax proceeds very rapidly after the "flulike" prodrome, and large numbers of bacilli circulate in the blood, often seeding the meninges. As with other rapidly progressive bacterial infections, the infectious burden reaches a point at which the damage induced by the inflammatory response to the organisms is sufficient to bring about the patient's demise. The addition of agents to prevent the growth of the bacteria, or even kill them, can no longer prevent the inevitable outcome. Because it is difficult to know precisely when that limit has been reached in most infections, treatment is always offered with the hope that the critical, lethal burden is not already present.

CHAPTER 59

1. Were the cases reported in the two towns related?

The cases had similar clinical features. They had onsets at a particular time of the year (summer or early fall), and at least initially, they appeared to be isolated to a particular region in Connecticut. These observations strongly support the consideration that the illnesses have the same cause.

2. Did any other people in either town have similar symptoms?

After receiving phone calls from two concerned mothers, the investigators developed a case definition and were able to identify 51 similar cases in the immediate area.

3. Did the children have an infectious form of arthritis?

Yes. The investigators arrived at this conclusion using epidemiological data. That most of the cases began in the summer or early fall and most patients lived in wooded areas along lakes or streams suggested an arthropod-transmitted disease, possibly viral. However, many patients reported that the symptoms of arthritis were preceded by an unusual skin rash that started as a red spot and then spread to form a 6-inch ring. This feature was described in 1910 in Sweden and had been attributed to tick bites. Subsequently, investigators found that ticks were more abundant on the side of the Connecticut River where the cases occurred, and a prospective study of children with the rash showed that some went on to develop arthritis. Eventually, the etiological agent (a spirochete) was identified by examining the ticks and showing that patients had antibodies against the tick spirochetes.

4. What steps should epidemiologists take, and what principles should they apply to studying the reported cases, after discussions with the parents and local physicians?

The epidemiologists first establish a *case definition* to determine which individuals have the epidemic disease of interest. Next, they characterize the occurrence of the disease in terms of *person, place, and time*. Usually, this analysis allows them to generate *hypotheses* about the cause of the disease, whether it is likely to be transmissible, and if so, how it is transmitted. If the etiology of the disease is known, the epidemiologists may hypothesize about factors that increase the risk of illness, or if the disease is communicable, about a possible source of infection. Any of these hypotheses can be tested by conducting *case-control or cohort studies*, depending upon the specific circumstances.

CHAPTER 60
Candidiasis

1. What aspects of normal physiology prevent the development of thrush?

In most persons, *Candida* species cannot compete for nutrients with the commensal flora of the mouth. When the commensal flora is inhibited by antibiotics, yeast proliferates. The immune system provides an additional defense against *Candida* infections (see Question 2).

2. Should A. be evaluated for an immune deficiency?

In persons older than 6 months of age who are not receiving antibiotics, *Candida* infections are usually prevented by the combined efforts of neutrophils and T cells, which can activate phagocytes to greater potency. Had the patient not been receiving antibiotics, some deficiency of neutrophils or T cells (e.g., HIV infection) could have been considered. The patient does not require an evaluation of immune function if there are no other signs suggesting immunodeficiency.

Cholecystitis and Cholangitis

1. What risk factors contributed to the development of cholecystitis in Ms. F.?

The major risk factor for cholecystitis is cholelithiasis (gall stones), which can obstruct the drainage of bile and raise luminal pressure in the gallbladder. If cholelithiasis is not known to be present, then its risk factors are considered risk factors for cholecystitis. Obesity, female sex, age greater than 40 years, and premenopausal state are the most important risk factors for cholelithiasis.

2. What are the possible complications of this disease?

Cholecystitis can cause bacteremia, sepsis, necrosis of the gallbladder, and extension of the infection into the peritoneum. These are life-threatening complications, which means that cholecystitis should be considered a medical emergency.

Bacterial Overgrowth Syndrome

1. What is the underlying cause of the numbness and tingling experienced by Mr. O.?

Vitamin B_{12} is required for normal function of peripheral nerves. The absorption of the vitamin as a complex with intrinsic factor occurs in the ileum. Compromise of intestinal absorptive function thereby leads to vitamin B_{12} deficiency and resultant peripheral neuropathy.

2. What is the mechanism of the diarrhea that Mr. O. is experiencing?

Intestinal bacteria deconjugate bile acids; the deconjugated forms are toxic to the colonic mucosa, inducing a net secretory state. Thus, the abnormal presence of excess bacteria in the small bowel leads to bile acid enteropathy.

Amebic colitis

1. What placed Ms. T. at risk for amebiasis?

While amebiasis can be acquired in the United States, it is more likely that Ms. T. became infected during her work in Central

America, where *E. histolytica* is highly endemic. Eating food sold by street vendors (generally something to avoid to prevent traveler's diarrhea) may have placed her at substantially increased risk.

2. Why is it necessary to treat intestinal amebiasis with two different antibiotics?

In approximately half of all patients treated with nitroimidazole drugs like metronidazole, parasites persist in the intestine. To combat the remaining parasites, a nonabsorbable antibiotic like the aminoglycoside paromomycin is used to eradicate the luminal infection.

3. What might have happened if the biopsy had failed to reveal *E. histolytica*, and the patient had been started on immunosuppressive therapy instead?

It is important to recognize that it can be difficult to distinguish intestinal amebiasis from inflammatory bowel disease on clinical grounds alone. Occasionally, when patients with *E. histolytica* infections inadvertently receive immunosuppressive drugs like corticosteroids, their condition may worsen and lead to a condition known as toxic megacolon.

Giardiasis

1. How might the student have avoided infection?

People acquire *Giardia* infections by ingesting water contaminated with cysts. Cysts unfortunately are quite hardy and will survive in cold water. However, there are submicron filters that can remove cysts from drinking water. In addition, cysts will not survive boiling for several minutes (even at altitude).

2. Why was the diagnosis missed by O&P tests?

Giardiasis may be diagnosed by the direct microscopic identification of cysts or trophozoites in stool specimens. However, multiple tests are usually necessary (at least three stool specimens should be performed). Direct fluorescent antibody (DFA) tests identify cysts with high sensitivity and specificity, but this analysis requires a fluorescence microscope. Occasionally, sampling of small intestinal mucosa or fluid will reveal trophozoites, which may have been difficult to identify in stool.

Rotavirus Infection

1. How did A. become infected with rotavirus?

Rotavirus has a low infectious dose and is efficiently passed from person to person through fecal–oral transmission. Studies of child-care centers show that during the winter when rotavirus infections are most common, gross contamination of surfaces can occur, which can enhance transmission of the virus.

2. Is there a vaccine to prevent rotavirus disease?

Yes! There are now two rotavirus vaccines licensed for use in the United States: RotaTeq (Merck), an oral live pentavalent human–bovine reassortant vaccine, and Rotarix (GSK), an oral live-attenuated strain derived by serial passage and subsequent molecular modification of a human rotavirus isolate. Both vaccines are highly effective in reducing severe diarrheal illness, and neither vaccine has been associated with intussusception, which was observed with an earlier human–rhesus reassortant vaccine (RotaShield). Major programs are now under way to deploy these newer vaccines to developing countries to eliminate disease caused by this important diarrheal pathogen.

Hemolytic–Uremic Syndrome

1. What was the source of the *E. coli* that led to L.'s disease?

Shiga toxin–producing *E. coli* are commonly found in cattle herds in the United States, and unfortunately, the bacteria can find their way into the food chain. This occurrence is almost invariably the result of contamination with bovine manure, although the very small infectious dose (<100 organisms) means that the connection can be distant. In this case, the child most likely acquired the causal organism from ingesting a hamburger that was not adequately cooked (i.e., was not well done).

2. What is the basis for the renal manifestations of HUS?

Shiga toxin causes inhibition of protein synthesis in target cells, leading to cellular necrosis. In addition, the toxin activates proinflammatory and coagulation cascades. The glomeruli are frequent targets of the toxin owing to their high-level expression of the toxin receptor Gb3.

3. Should antibiotics have been administered to L.?

Although the question of whether or not antibiotics actually increase the risk of HUS has not been definitively resolved, it is clear that antibiotics currently available in the United States do not decrease the likelihood of this serious manifestation. Thus, antibiotics are not indicated for shiga toxin-producing *E. coli* infections.

Yersinia Infection

1. Why did the clinical manifestations of *Yersinia* infection differ in S. and I.?

Yersinia enterocolitica is a cause of inflammatory diarrhea, with a pathogenesis similar to that of shigellosis. In addition, *Yersinia* organisms that have invaded through the mucosa sometimes become lodged in GI tract lymphoid tissue, causing swelling of the terminal ileum, like that observed in I., or in the mesenteric lymph nodes. The pseudoappendicitis syndrome is thought to accompany inflammation of the terminal ileum, while mesenteric adenitis can lead to generalized abdominal pain and fever.

2. Describe the pathogenesis of the arthritis and rash that developed in Mr. D.?

Arthritis and rash commonly occur following *Yersinia* infection. Although the precise bacterial products remain a subject of controversy, it is agreed that these clinical manifestations result from immune responses elicited by some bacterial components that cross-react with host tissues.

CHAPTER 61
Bacterial and Viral Meningitis

1. Why did meningococcal meningitis, the etiology of Pvt. W.'s illness, produce alarm and warrant aggressive treatment and measures to prevent spread of infection, whereas viral aseptic meningitis, the etiology of Pvt. E.'s illness, did not require specific therapy?

Bacterial meningitis is a medical emergency because of the high morbidity and mortality associated with unrecognized and untreated disease. Empiric antibiotics likely to sterilize the cerebrospinal fluid (CSF) based on the probable organisms (considering the age and immune status of the host) should be started immediately, pending results of further microbiological testing. Viral meningitis may cause severe discomfort in affected patients, but it is predominantly a self-limited illness. Viral meningitis resolves without antimicrobial therapy and has minimal morbidity and mortality. *Neisseria meningitidis* causes outbreaks of epidemic bacterial meningitis. Close contacts of index patients should be treated with ciprofloxacin, rifampin, or ceftriaxone to eradicate nasopharyngeal carriage of the organism and prevent subsequent cases from occurring.

2. How do the CSF findings in Pvt. W.'s case (bacterial meningitis) compare with those in Pvt. E.'s case (viral meningitis)?

Bacterial meningitis is usually associated with a polymorphonuclear pleocytosis of hundreds to thousands of cells/mm³. Viral meningitis may be associated with polymorphonuclear pleocytosis in the first 24 hours of illness, but usually, fewer than 300 cells/mm³ are present, and a rapid shift to lymphocytic predominance occurs after the first 24 hours of illness. The CSF glucose is usually decreased in bacterial meningitis and normal in viral meningitis; the CSF protein is usually increased in bacterial meningitis and normal to mildly increased in viral meningitis.

Tuberculous Meningitis

1. What is the explanation for Ms. G.'s eye movement abnormalities?

In tuberculous meningitis, organisms spread throughout the subarachnoid space and become most prevalent in the basilar cisterns. An intense cell-mediated, delayed-type hypersensitivity reaction elicited by the organisms leads to the formation of granulomas in this area, which involves the region's cranial nerves and causes them to malfunction. In this case, the nerves affected were cranial nerves III and VI, which are located at the base of the brain. Those nerves have long courses and are frequently compromised by the presence of basilar exudates.

2. How do the CSF findings in tuberculous meningitis compare with those in viral and bacterial meningitis?

The degree of CSF pleocytosis seen in bacterial meningitis is similar to that seen in tuberculous meningitis, both of which are higher than that seen in viral meningitis. However, polymorphonuclear cells predominate in bacterial meningitis, whereas mononuclear cells predominate in tuberculous meningitis. CSF glucose levels are usually decreased in both bacterial and tuberculous meningitis, whereas they are usually normal in viral meningitis. CSF protein is usually increased in bacterial meningitis and even more markedly increased in tuberculous meningitis, whereas CSF protein is normal or only mildly elevated in viral meningitis.

3. Why are multiple drugs required for the treatment of tuberculous meningitis?

The emergence of drug-resistant strains of *Mycobacterium tuberculosis* in most parts of the world makes combination therapy with at least three and preferably four drugs with different mechanisms of action the standard of care for the treatment of active tuberculosis, particularly with involvement of the CNS. If the organism is isolated from the CSF (which may take up to 6 weeks), susceptibility testing should be performed to verify selection of the proper drug regimen for long-term therapy (usu-

ally 12 months). Steroids are used for treatment of CNS disease because the intense inflammatory response to the organism is a major component of neural dysfunction and damage to the brain and meninges.

HSV Encephalitis

1. What is the best single diagnostic method to establish a diagnosis of HSV encephalitis?

In the past, cerebral biopsy with virus isolation was the standard for the diagnosis of herpes simplex virus (HSV) encephalitis. However, this procedure has been replaced by detection of HSV DNA in the cerebrospinal fluid by polymerase chain reaction (PCR). If performed with optimal techniques in an experienced laboratory, specificity is 100% and sensitivity is 95%. However, recent reports indicate that HSV cerebrospinal fluid PCR performed within the first 48 hours of illness may have decreased sensitivity. A negative result should not be used to exclude the diagnosis in the appropriate clinical setting. HSV is rarely cultured from the CSF in patients with encephalitis. With widespread availability of the PCR test, brain biopsy is now rarely necessary to make the diagnosis of HSV encephalitis.

2. What is the prognosis for patients who survive HSV encephalitis?

Untreated HSV encephalitis is usually associated with severe focal encephalitis in adolescents and adults. Untreated, the disease carries a 70% mortality rate, and 97% of untreated survivors are left with permanent neurological deficits. Early recognition of HSV encephalitis is essential because the initiation of effective antiviral therapy (acyclovir) can significantly decrease the morbidity and mortality of the disease. In adults with HSV encephalitis, acyclovir has reduced mortality from 70 to 19% in comparison to placebo-treated patients. However, even in treated patients, neurological impairment is common, occurring in 40 to 60% of survivors. Outcome is related to the severity of disease at the time antiviral therapy is begun, hence the urgency to begin treatment as soon as the diagnosis is entertained. Neurological sequelae resulting from destruction of cerebral gray matter may result in personality changes, whereas involvement of the white matter may lead to significant residual paralysis.

Acute Abscess Caused by a Bacterial Infection

1. Why was antimicrobial therapy with both nafcillin and metronidazole continued even though no anaerobic bacteria grew from culture?

Acute abscesses in the CNS are frequently caused by a mixed bacterial flora consisting of strict and facultative anaerobes. The mixture of bacteria is similar to that found in the mouth or a parameningeal focus such as an infected middle ear, mastoid, or sinus. Because anaerobic bacteria are particularly difficult to culture, most patients should receive empiric therapy for anaerobes, regardless of the culture results.

2. What was the relationship between Ms. M.'s earache and the location of her brain abscess?

The patient's earache likely represented infection of the middle ear or mastoid, particularly with the history of recurrent ear infections. Veins that bridge the surrounding bony structures and the cerebral cortex may become infected (septic thrombophlebitis), leading to a decrease in local blood supply and providing a reservoir of bacteria. Brain abscess likely resulted from contiguous spread from the involved area (middle ear or mastoid), which is adjacent to the occipital lobe of the brain.

CHAPTER 62
Group A Streptococcal Pharyngitis

1. What common organisms cause pharyngitis?

Group A streptococcus, respiratory viruses, Epstein-Barr virus, and *Chlamydia pneumoniae* cause pharyngitis.

2. Why is it important to distinguish streptococcal pharyngitis from other forms of the disease?

Streptococcal pharyngitis can lead to pyogenic complications like peritonsillar and retropharyngeal abscesses and immunological complications like glomerulonephritis and rheumatic fever.

Acute Epiglottitis

1. Why was P. started on therapy for *H. influenzae* type B before culture results had returned?

Haemophilus influenzae type B is the most common cause of epiglottitis in children of this age group.

Laryngotracheitis

1. Why did the pediatrician suspect a viral pathogen?

In both children and adults, almost all cases of laryngotracheitis are caused by viruses, particularly the parainfluenza viruses. Rarely, *Staphylococcus aureus* as a cause has been reported in children, and *Moraxella catarrhalis* and *H. influenzae* in adults. Immunosuppressed patients, particularly those on steroids, may develop laryngitis due to *Candida albicans*.

Acute Tracheobronchitis

1. Do most cases of tracheobronchitis resolve on their own, or are antibiotics usually required?

Most cases of acute tracheobronchitis are viral in etiology and therefore do not require therapy. Studies have shown little to no benefit to administering antibiotics in immunocompetent patients without underlying structural lung disease.

Community-Acquired Pneumonia

1. How did the physician differentiate bronchitis from pneumonia?

Because the presenting signs and symptoms for bronchitis and pneumonia may be similar, the only way to truly differentiate is by chest radiography, usually a chest x-ray.

2. What organisms should a physician be concerned about when treating CAP?

Streptococcus pneumoniae is clearly the most important bacterial agent. *Mycoplasma pneumoniae*, *H. influenzae* (nontypeable), and *Chlamydia pneumoniae* are other common bacterial causes. It is important to consider *Legionella pneumophila* in older or immunocompromised patients, particularly smokers. Less commonly, viruses can cause pneumonia, including influenza, respiratory syncytial virus, parainfluenza, adenoviruses,

and others, but there are no effective empiric treatments for these pathogens.

Hospital-Acquired Pneumonia

1. How do most patients in the hospital contract pneumonia?

Microaspiration of bacteria from the oropharynx is felt to be the most common route of infection, although direct inoculation through an endotracheal tube is an important route of entry for mechanically ventilated patients.

2. Which patients are at increased risk for developing HAP?

Patients at increased risk are those with other chronic underlying illnesses (comorbidities); advanced age; poor nutrition; and a history of smoking, alcoholism, and intravenous drug use.

Subacute Pneumonias

1. Which organisms can cause cavitary lung lesions?

Anaerobic bacteria, *S. aureus*, *Klebsiella pneumoniae*, and mycobacteria are among the pathogens more frequently associated with lung cavitation.

Pneumonia in the Immunocompromised Patient

1. Which patients are at increased risk for developing *P. jiroveci* pneumonia (PCP)?

Primarily patients with HIV and CD4 lymphocyte counts less than 200 cells per mm^3.

CHAPTER 63
Acute Uncomplicated Cystitis

1. What is the most likely diagnosis in this woman?

The most likely diagnosis is acute uncomplicated cystitis.

2. What factors have contributed to this episode of infection?

Sexual intercourse, spermicide use, and genetic predisposition are contributing factors.

3. Should a urine specimen for culture be obtained?

A urine culture is not recommended routinely for all episodes of acute uncomplicated cystitis. A culture should be obtained if the presentation is atypical, the patient is pregnant, or there has been failure or early recurrence after therapy.

4. What is the optimal antimicrobial treatment of this episode?

Short-course (3 days) therapy with an effective antimicrobial is the optimal treatment.

5. What might prevent further episodes of infection?

To prevent further episodes of infection, the patient should avoid spermicide use. Prophylactic antimicrobials will prevent infections. Daily ingestion of cranberry juice can also decrease infections by about one-third.

Acute Uncomplicated Pyelonephritis

1. What is the most likely infecting organism, and what virulence factor is characteristic?

E. coli expressing the Pap G adhesin is the most likely infecting organism.

2. What initial investigations should be obtained to confirm the diagnosis and assess the clinical status of this woman?

Urinalysis, urine culture, blood cultures, peripheral leukocyte count, blood urea, and creatinine should be obtained.

3. What antimicrobial regimen should be initiated?

The patient should have antimicrobial therapy initiated intravenously. A switch to oral therapy can occur when the patient is stable and able to tolerate oral medication.

Complicated Urinary Tract Infection

1. Why is this man experiencing UTI?

The infections are the result of the patient's impaired bladder emptying because of neurological abnormalities from the spinal cord injury.

2. Why is the isolate resistant to some antimicrobials?

Prior antimicrobial therapy for recurrent urinary infection has promoted colonization with resistant organisms.

3. How will you select antimicrobial therapy to treat this infection?

The patient can be treated with oral therapy because he is clinically stable. The specific agent will be based on the susceptibilities of the *Klebsiella pneumoniae* strain isolated.

4. What additional management should be considered for this patient with complicated UTI and a recent increase in infection frequency?

Consider investigations such as measurement of postvoid residual urine, urodynamic studies to assess voiding, and urological studies to exclude bladder or renal stones.

Asymptomatic Bacteriuria

1. What is the diagnosis in this woman?

The diagnosis is asymptomatic bacteriuria.

2. What antimicrobial treatment should be given for the *E. coli* grown in the urine culture?

None. Treatment of asymptomatic bacteriuria in elderly nursing home residents is not recommended.

CHAPTER 64
Streptococcal Cellulitis

1. What risk factors predisposed Ms. W. to the development of cellulitis?

Ms. W. was placed at risk for development of cellulitis by minor trauma to the distal finger and either colonization with group A streptococcus or contact with a patient with group A streptococcal infection.

2. What virulence determinants are expressed by *S. pyogenes*?

S. pyogenes expresses hyaluronidase and several potent cytolysins or hemolysins such as streptolysin O or streptolysin S.

3. What antibiotic should have been administered at the time of the incision and drainage?

Group A streptococcus remains highly sensitive to penicillin, which remains the drug of choice. For more severe group

A streptococcal infections such as necrotizing fasciitis or toxic shock syndrome, clindamycin is often used in addition to penicillin due to its ability to shut off toxin production.

Staphylococcal Abscess

1. What was the source of the *S. aureus* in the case of Mr. C.?

Nasal colonization with *S. aureus* is common, and transfer to the skin occurs predominantly by the fingers. In this fashion, skin colonization occurs usually around hair follicles.

2. Should the physician suspect any underlying immune deficiency?

Patients with diabetes and immunocompromised individuals are at greatest risk. The greatest risk factor for recurrent furunculosis is nasal colonization.

3. What should be suspected if the infection fails to respond to β-lactam antibiotics?

Methicillin-resistant *S. aureus* (MRSA) has become common even among patients with no contact with hospitals or clinics. MRSA strains are resistant to beta-lactam antibiotics. For minor MRSA infections, trimethoprim/sulfamethoxazole, clindamycin, and tetracyclines have been useful, though resistance to these antibiotics has been reported. More severe infections should be treated with vancomycin.

Necrotizing Fasciitis

1. How does diabetes mellitus predispose to the development of skin infections?

Persons with diabetes mellitus are at increased risk for development of skin infections by compromised microvascular circulation, chronic fungal infections, and peripheral neuropathy.

2. Would antibiotics alone have been effective in eradicating this infection?

No. This case represents necrotizing skin and soft tissue infection caused by multiple microbes including aerobic, anaerobic, Gram-positive, and Gram-negative bacteria. In the face of tissue destruction, surgical intervention is required.

Ecthyma Gangrenosum

1. What alteration in host defense most directly contributed to the development of *P. aeruginosa* bacteremia in Mr. A.?

Mr. A.'s neutropenia likely was the single most important predisposing factor.

2. What is the pathogenesis of the skin lesions?

P. aeruginosa causes a venous vasculitis that results in cutaneous necrosis and the bluish-to-black hue of early cutaneous lesions.

3. Why was antibiotic therapy initiated prior to obtaining culture results?

Patients with ecthyma gangrenosum have bacteremia as a prerequisite to developing the metastatic cutaneous lesion. Prompt treatment of the bacteremia can be lifesaving.

Toxic Shock Syndrome

1. What conditions place persons at risk for the development of toxic shock syndrome?

Staphylococcal toxic shock syndrome (Staph TSS) was most commonly caused by TSST-1-producing strains colonizing the vaginal mucosa of women using tampons. Currently, postsurgical Staph TSS occurs with a frequency equivalent to that of menstrually related Staph TSS and may be caused by strains producing either TSST-1 or staphylococcal enterotoxin B.

2. What other organisms can cause this disease?

Group A streptococcus also can produce TSS.

3. How does TSST-1 cause shock and organ failure?

TSST-1, staphylococcal enterotoxin B, and several group A streptococcal pyrogenic exotoxins are superantigens that can simultaneously bind to MHC class II molecules expressed on macrophages and the V beta region of the T-lymphocyte receptor, leading to massive release of cytokines from both types of cells.

CHAPTER 65

1. What is the most likely cause of O.'s infection?

The most likely infecting organism is *Staphylococcus aureus*. Other causes of osteomyelitis in a child of this age include *Streptococcus pyogenes* (group A streptococcus). A major concern is the emergence of community-acquired methicillin *S. aureus* (MRSA). This organism is certainly possible in O.'s case.

2. How did the bacterium spread to the bone?

Osteomyelitis is most likely to develop when the bone has suffered trauma, such as a sports injury, with resultant disruption of blood vessels and hematoma formation. Areas where sludging of blood cells occurs are ideal for the growth of bacteria because microclots form spontaneously in areas of slow blood flow. O. most likely developed a transient bacteremia with *S. aureus* as a consequence of a localized skin infection. The organism then seeded the bone, resulting in osteomyelitis.

3. What are the complications of untreated osteomyelitis?

The principal complications are bony destruction and metastatic spread of infection to distant sites. This latter complication is especially worrisome with *S. aureus* because the organism has a predilection for vascular endothelium and can cause endocarditis.

CHAPTER 66
Sepsis from Wound Infections

1. How did Mr. D.'s clinical course differ from that of Mrs. J., and why was his response to infection less severe?

Mr. D. had severe sepsis with hypotension that only required treatment with intravenous fluids and antibiotics. In contrast, Mrs. J. had multiorgan system dysfunction (MODS). She had adult respiratory distress syndrome, acute renal failure, increased cardiac output, and persistent hypotension despite fluid replacement, adrenergic drugs, and antibiotics.

2. Why was an infecting organism not isolated from Mrs. J.?

Mrs. J. had a localized infection in her abdomen that had formed an abscess. This abscess was likely teeming with leukocytes and microorganisms, many of which were dead or fragmented. Recall that sepsis is induced by microbial products, such as cell wall fragments from Gram-positive bacteria or lipopolysaccharide from Gram-negative bacteria. Although

Mrs. J may have had transient or intermittent bacteremia associated with her abscess that was not detected by the blood cultures, we can safely assume that she had diffusion of bacterial products from the abscess into the bloodstream and that these microbial macromolecules triggered the cascade of events that led to sepsis. That is why drainage of the abscess was so important in resolving her septic episode.

3. Why did Mrs. J. not respond to antibiotic treatment as Mr. D. did?

Mrs. J. received prompt antibiotic therapy and intravenous fluids for presumed infection. The reasons that she may not have done well include the following:

- She may not have gotten the correct antibiotic treatment because the source of the infection was not evident. The sources of postoperative systemic inflammatory response syndrome (SIRS) in a postoperative patient are the so-called three Ws: wind, water, and wound. Early on, most patients have fever because noninfectious fluids accumulate in the lungs (wind). Urinary tract infections (water) in patients who have had a catheter placed in the bladder are the next most common source of SIRS. Wounds are considered relatively late in the course. Intravenous lines are also a potential source.
- Proinflammatory mediators are released rapidly. Even if she received the correct antibiotics, irreversible organ damage could have already occurred.
- Antibiotics do not treat necrotic tissue or leakage of colonic contents into the peritoneum that help drive the inflammatory response. Only when surgery was performed did she improve.
- Mrs. J. may have been more genetically predisposed to develop septic shock or MODS than Mr. D.

CHAPTER 67

1. What underlying medical condition placed Mrs. Q. at risk for developing endocarditis?

Mrs. Q. had aortic stenosis prior to the development of endocarditis. Cardiac abnormalities that allow blood to flow from a high-pressure area into a low-pressure area, like aortic stenosis, are associated with endocarditis. This flow pattern results in a Venturi effect, which allows platelet–fibrin aggregates to form on endothelial surfaces at the low-pressure side of the stenotic valve. These platelet–fibrin thrombi serve as a niche for infective endocarditis. Because *Streptococcus bovis* was the underlying cause of Mrs. Q.'s endocarditis, it is possible that she also had underlying colonic pathology, such as benign polyps or colon cancer.

2. What virulence factors elaborated by *S. bovis* contributed to endocarditis?

Organisms that cause endocarditis can adhere to thrombotic vegetations or valve endothelium. *S. bovis* produces extracellular dextran, which mediates adherence to platelet–fibrin aggregates. Endocarditis-causing organisms also promote the release of tissue factor, which leads to platelet aggregation and vegetation enlargement.

3. What is the significance of the urinalysis showing 25 to 30 red blood cells per high-power field?

Microscopic hematuria in persons with endocarditis is suggestive of glomerular nephritis. In those with prolonged episodes of subacute streptococcal endocarditis, such as Mrs. Q., circulating immune complexes, which form intravascularly under conditions of antibody excess, deposit in subepithelial locations along the glomerular basement membrane. These immune complexes can fix complement, leading to glomerular damage. This type of injury is pathologically distinct from emboli resulting from vegetation disruption. Mrs. Q. also had this complication of endocarditis, with large emboli noted in the myocardium and spleen.

CHAPTER 68
Otitis Media

1. Should E.'s sister be brought in and checked for an ear infection?

Acute otitis media is primarily a clinical diagnosis. Unless she is experiencing symptoms of otitis media, the sister does not need to be checked. Also, because the sister is older, observation might be pursued regardless of the clinical findings.

2. Should a culture be obtained before antibiotics are prescribed?

Tympanocentesis (aspiration of the middle ear fluid) is painful and poses more risk than benefit to patients. For this reason, it is not routinely performed for culture and susceptibility testing. Instead, antimicrobial agents that are effective against the most common otopathogens are selected empirically.

3. How can the physician be sure that amoxicillin is the right antibiotic for E.?

The primary pathogens associated with otitis media are pneumococci and nontypeable *Haemophilus influenzae*. Empiric use of antimicrobials active against these two species is a reasonable and effective approach.

4. Could E. have complications of her ear infection?

Most cases of otitis media that are treated with antimicrobials resolve without complication. However, patients experiencing recurrent or chronic infections may develop complications like facial nerve paralysis, epidural or subdural abscess, or brain abscess.

Orbital Cellulitis

1. Why should B. see an otolaryngologist if the problem is with her eye?

Orbital cellulitis is a complication of acute sinusitis. The lateral borders of the ethmoid sinuses form the medial orbital wall of the orbit. Infection in the ethmoid sinus may erode through the lamina papyracea and enter the orbit.

2. How are B.'s allergies related to the development of orbital cellulitis?

Patients with allergies develop edema of the natural ostia of the sinuses. This inflammation impedes drainage, resulting in bacterial overgrowth and infection.

3. Are antimicrobials necessary?

Orbital cellulitis must be treated with antimicrobials. The mildest forms can sometimes be treated with oral agents, but advanced disease requires parenteral therapy.

Facial Cellulitis

1. How did the bacteria get into R.'s cheek?

Minor facial trauma likely resulted in blood seeping into R.'s soft tissues. In a setting of transient *H. influenzae* bacteremia, the organisms can seed and grow in the traumatized subcutaneous tissue using the extravasated red blood cells as a source of nutrition.

2. Why did R. need to receive intravenous antibiotics for cellulitis?

Because secondary diseases due to *H. influenzae* are serious, the usual treatment is to administer antibiotics intravenously until the cellulitis has completely resolved. Fortunately, widespread use of an effective conjugate vaccine against *H. influenzae* type B has made this infection a rarity.

Oropharyngeal Abscess

1 & 2. Why did Ms. J.'s sore throat not go away by itself? Why might she need surgery?

Patients with peritonsillar abscess require surgical drainage to prevent spread and extension of infection. Most important is the potential to develop airway obstruction. Unchecked, infection can also spread along the fascial planes, resulting in life-threatening mediastinitis. Another potential complication involves rupture of the abscess and resultant aspiration of pus. Drainage can often be done at the patient's bedside.

3. Does Ms. J.'s roommate have to worry about catching the illness?

Although Group A streptococci is a commensal that can be spread with close contact, the correct setting is required to develop such an abscess. If the roommate were symptomatic, she should be examined and possibly cultured for group A streptococci.

Conjunctivitis

1. Could C.'s mother and father develop the eye infection?

Yes, J.'s mother and father could develop a similar infection. This infection is generally spread with direct inoculation by hand contact. Good hand hygiene practices can help limit spread among family members.

2. Why did the physician not prescribe antibiotics for the infection?

A viral infection is responsible for J.'s conjunctivitis. No effective antiviral treatments are available for this type of infection. Hence, antibiotics are not necessary for treatment. Patients will generally improve with symptomatic therapy within a few days.

Cervical Lymphadenitis

1. Is this a life-threatening illness?

No, this is most likely a viral adenitis related to Epstein-Barr virus ("mono"). Other considerations include bacterial infections, which are readily treatable with antimicrobials. The possibility of malignancy needs to be considered if the patient's symptoms do not resolve. In this case, the rapid clinical course strongly favors infection.

2. Why did she need blood tests?

The physician ordered blood tests to support a diagnosis of Epstein-Barr virus adenitis. In particular, a heterophile antibody titer is present in 90% of cases. Also, a complete blood count may contain atypical lymphocytes.

3. Should the physician prescribe antimicrobial drugs?

If Epstein-Barr virus adenitis is suspected, antimicrobials should not be given. Epstein-Barr virus infection does not respond to antibiotics. Additionally, patients can develop an immune-mediated rash to certain antibiotics in this setting.

CHAPTER 70

1. What risk factors predispose V. to the bacteremia with E. coli?

This patient unfortunately developed leukemia and was given chemotherapy to induce a remission from her malignancy. These antiproliferative medicines are nonspecific and affected all rapidly dividing cells, including the leukemic cells, the cells in her bone marrow, and the cells of the gastrointestinal (GI) mucosa. Without the protective GI mucosa, the normal flora of her GI tract was able to invade her tissues. Without neutrophils present, the innate immune system was unable to clear the bacteria, and she became bacteremic. In this case, E. coli has translocated across the GI mucosa and caused a systemic infection. V. also had a central venous catheter that could have served as an entry point for bacteria and required close monitoring for subtle signs of infection at the catheter insertion site.

2. What risk factors predisposed V. to the fungemia with C. albicans?

At this point in the patient's care, she had been neutropenic for 10 days and on antibiotics to fight her previous infection. The combination of prolonged neutropenia and use of antibiotics is a risk factor for the development of fungal infections. The presence of her central venous catheter became of greater concern as she remained febrile despite appropriate antifungal therapy. Candida species can cause fungemia in association with central venous catheters, and effective treatment requires not only antifungal therapy but also the removal of the central venous catheter.

3. What risk factors predisposed V. to the pneumonia with P. jiroveci?

In the 6 months after transplantation, V.'s cellular immunity provided inadequate protection against intracellular pathogens. This increased her risk for viral pathogens such as cytomegalovirus (CMV) and Epstein-Barr virus (EBV) as well as Pneumocystis jiroveci. Graft-versus-host disease could prolong the period of poor cellular immunity and increase V.'s risk for these pathogens as well as disease from fungal pathogens such as Aspergillus species.

4. What risk factors predisposed V. to the pneumonia and bacteremia with S. pneumoniae?

Although V. successfully engrafted the stem cell transplant, her adaptive immune system lacked normal function. Also, the history of graft-versus-host disease further suppressed her adaptive immunity. Because her adaptive immunity failed to provide adequate protection, she was at risk for pathogens such as

Haemophilus influenzae and Streptococcus pneumoniae from which people are normally protected by the humoral immune response.

CHAPTER 71

1. Could Mr. F. have been infected with HIV?

Yes, indeed. He has risk factors, and he has a clinical presentation that is compatible with acute HIV infection. He is at risk because he is bisexual and has had sexual relations with a new male partner within the past 3 weeks. He is also employed as a hospital phlebotomist, but the likelihood of occupational exposure is much less than that of sexual exposure. Mr. F's mononucleosis-like illness is typical of the acute retroviral syndrome that occurs a few weeks after HIV is acquired and generally resolves spontaneously as viral latency begins.

2. Can HIV be diagnosed at the initial stage?

He can be diagnosed but not with serological tests that detect antibody to HIV. At the acute retroviral stage, the virus can be detected with antigen based testes (e.g., p24) or nucleic acid-based tests such as PCR for viral RNA from a blood sample.

3. How accurate are the tests for HIV?

The common screening test for HIV is an enzyme-linked immunosorbent assay (ELISA). This test is usually positive 6 to 12 weeks after exposure to HIV; however, in some cases, the development of antibodies can be delayed leading to a false impression of negativity. False-positive tests occur rarely, so any positive ELISA test must be confirmed by using the more specific Western blot assay.

4. Can Mr. F. be sure he is infected?

Yes. A positive Western blot assay is definite evidence of HIV infection.

5. Will Mr. F. get AIDS?

If he does not receive any antiretroviral therapy, he will develop immunodeficiency and acquire an AIDS-defining condition. This process can take between a few months and 15 years (10 years on average). Effective treatment can prevent the progression to AIDS.

6. What kind of lifestyle changes should Mr. F. consider making to minimize the risk of spreading the infection to others and to maintain his health as much as possible?

To prevent further transmission of his virus, Mr. F. should be instructed to practice safe sex. This means engaging in no sexual activities that involve direct contact with semen or vaginal secretions. His wife and male sexual partners should be notified and be tested. Mr. F. will need regular medical follow-up to monitor the course of his disease and to intervene when appropriate.

7. By ignoring his physician's advice and not having regular checkups, has Mr. F. caused himself irreparable harm?

At this stage, his disease can still be treated. The decline in the number of CD4 lymphocytes may result in loss of certain specificities from the patient's repertoire. Thus, the immune system may be permanently weakened at some point, even if the viral infection is controlled.

8. What kind of treatment and management should Mr. F. receive?

Mr. F. should receive highly-active antiretroviral therapy (HAART) consisting of two or three antiretroviral agents that are active against his HIV virus. His CD4 count and viral load (by quantitative PCR) should be measured at regular intervals to assess his response, and he should be monitored for AIDS-related conditions.

9. What other infections might Mr. F. acquire?

An extensive list of AIDS-defining illnesses is presented in the printed text. Any of these illnesses could develop if the patient's CD4 cell count is low enough. See also Figure 71-1.

10. Can any treatment help him avoid those infections at this stage?

The best way to avoid opportunistic infections in AIDS is effective antiretroviral therapy to maintain a low (undetectable) viral load and to preserve the CD4 lymphocytes. When the lymphocyte count is very low, prophylactic treatment for *Pneumocytis jiroveci* is initiated. At lower counts, regimens to prevent recurrent candidiasis, *Mycobacterium avium* complex, and cytomegalovirus may be considered in some patients.

11. Why did Mr. F. have difficulty swallowing?

The white plaques in the mouth suggest a recurrence of candidiasis. At Mr. F's current stage of disease, he is at risk for extension of candida infection into the esophagus. This is the most likely explanation for his difficulty swallowing. Occasionally, herpes simplex or aphthous ulcers may also cause esophagitis.

12. What caused his diarrhea?

Persistent diarrhea in AIDS patients may be caused by viral infection (e.g., cytomegalovirus colitis), bacterial infection (e.g., such as *Salmonella* spp. or mycobacteria), or chronic protozoal infections (e.g., cryptosporidiosis). There are numerous potential causes.

13. What other agents of pneumonia is Mr. F. susceptible to?

Mr. F. has susceptibility to common bacterial agents of pneumonia, such as *S. pneumoniae* and *Haemophilus influenzae*. He is also susceptible to *Pneumocystis jiroveci*, *Mycobacterium tuberculosis*, and primary fungal infection of the lung.

14. Is he at risk for tuberculosis, and is it treatable?

Yes. Tuberculosis is one of the infections that can be cured in patients with AIDS if the patient is adherent to an effective course of chemotherapy.

15. Why did the physician perform a serum cryptococcal antigen test despite Mr. F.'s normal examination?

In AIDS patients, cryptococcal meningitis typically presents with fever and headache, but the classic physical signs of meningitis, for example, neck rigidity, may be absent because of the lack of a vigorous inflammatory response in the meninges. In fact, the spinal fluid may have no increase in the cell count in spite of numerous yeast forms circulating in the fluid. Because the lack of an inflammatory response allowed the pathogen to multiply to very large numbers, the serum cryptococcal antigen test is always positive in the spinal fluid and is almost always positive in the serum. A positive serum antigen test would dictate that a spinal tap for diagnosis and possibly to relieve spinal fluid pressure is essential.

16. What caused Mr. F.'s significant weight loss?

This could be the result of multiple opportunistic infection or it could be due to a wasting syndrome associated with HIV infection itself.

17. What is Kaposi sarcoma?

Kaposi sarcoma is a malignant neoplasm associated with human herpesvirus 8. It causes focal lesions in the skin, the digestive tract, and the respiratory tract. It may be fatal.

18. What is Mr. F.'s prognosis?

HIV encephalopathy is a progressive condition that responds poorly to therapy but occurs less frequently in patients who are on effective HAART. Mr. F. can expect progressive functional deterioration at this point, and as in the pre-HAART era, his survival is likely to be no more than 6 months. Mr. F can now be considered to have "end-stage" AIDS.

CHAPTER 72
Congenital Infection

1. How did Baby L. become infected inside the womb?

Baby L. developed congenital CMV infection as a result of in utero (vertical) transmission from his mother. The risk of developing congenital CMV is highest in infants born to mothers who have contracted primary CMV infection early in pregnancy.

2. What are the signs and symptoms of intrauterine CMV infection?

Most infants who develop congenital CMV are asymptomatic. The signs and symptoms of symptomatic congenital CMV include intrauterine growth retardation, microcephaly, intracerebral calcifications, sensorineural hearing loss, chorioretinitis, hepatosplenomegaly, thrombocytopenia, and purpuric skin lesions.

3. What is the prognosis for Baby L.?

Baby L. has symptomatic congenital CMV infection. More than half of symptomatic neonates develop intellectual disabilities, neurological abnormalities, sensorineural hearing loss, or retinitis. In contrast, less than 20% of infants with congenital CMV infections who are asymptomatic at birth develop central nervous system sequelae, the most common being progressive hearing loss.

4. Could Baby L.'s mother have done anything to prevent her son's infection?

About 40% of mothers who contract primary CMV infection during pregnancy transmit it to their infants in utero. Although meticulous hand washing can decrease the likelihood of CMV infection, particularly from young children at home, once acquired, there is nothing the mother could have done to prevent vertical transmission.

Perinatal Infection

1. To which infectious agents are newborns susceptible?

In comparison to older children and adults, neonates are relatively immunocompromised. They are susceptible to pathogens that constitute the microbiota of the maternal vaginal tract such as group B streptococci and *E. coli*. They are also susceptible to viruses such as enteroviruses and herpes simplex virus, perhaps in part due to relative immunocompromise and also because the rapidly proliferating cells and tissues of the newborn host may be more permissive for viral replication.

2. How do group B streptococci cause meningitis in newborn infants?

Group B streptococci use pili to bind mucosal surfaces. Following attachment, the bacteria invade the mucosa and enter the bloodstream. Capsular polysaccharides are major virulence factors of these organisms. Newborns do not generate high-titer antibody responses against bacterial polysaccharides, which allows group B streptococci to establish invasive infections such as bacteremia and meningitis.

3. Could Baby C.'s mother have done anything to prevent her daughter's infection?

Baby C. developed late-onset group B streptococcal infection. Although early-onset group B streptococcal disease, which occurs within 7 days of birth, has been significantly reduced by intrapartum antibiotic prophylaxis administered to colonized women, antibiotic prophylaxis does not reduce the likelihood of late-onset disease, which occurs after 7 days of age.

CHAPTER 74

1. Does Mr. J. have a fever?

Mr. J. does not have any of the conditions that would normally signal hyperthermia. In addition, he has evidence of an inflammatory disorder—the elevated erythrocyte sedimentation rate (ESR). The rapid sedimenting of his RBCs is caused by increased levels of fibrinogen in his blood. That increase is the result of a nonspecific response of the liver to produce fibrinogen and other acute phase substances in response to inflammatory mediators (cytokines). The presence of evidence for inflammation and an acute inflammatory response makes fever more likely than hyperthermia.

2. Is his temperature elevation a danger to him?

A temperature elevation to 38.9°C is a moderate fever that should be well tolerated by persons who have no obvious pulmonary, heart, or vascular disease. Mr. J. has tolerated the fever well.

3. Is his illness caused by infection?

Mr. J. has a noninfectious inflammatory disorder called temporal arteritis. The disorder occurs in elderly persons (usually males) and involves granulomatous inflammation of the branches of the carotid arteries. High fever and elevated ESR are common. Symptoms resulting from impaired flow through these arteries may also occur, including aching in the jaw with chewing, headache, and transient blindness in one eye.

4. How might Mr. J.'s physician begin to evaluate the potential causes of his symptoms?

Evaluation always begins with a thorough history and physical and documentation of the fever. Diagnosing Mr. J.'s condition

depends on recognizing the clinical features and performing a biopsy of the temporal artery.

CHAPTER 75
Nosocomial Urinary Tract Infection

1. How did Mr. H. acquire this infection?

The infection is a result of the use of an indwelling bladder catheter. Catheters may become infected in a variety of ways. Most commonly, microorganisms from the patient's perineum may ascend between the catheter and the urethral mucosa. Alternatively, the organism may be introduced into the drainage system at the time of insertion or by opening the drainage system once it has been placed.

2. What are the most likely organisms?

Enteric microorganisms such as *Escherichia coli*, *Enterococcus* spp., *Pseudomonas aeruginosa*, and *Klebsiella* spp. are most common. In patients who are on broad-spectrum antibiotics, *Candida* spp. infections may also occur.

3. How can this scenario be prevented?

The best way to prevent nosocomial urinary infections is to minimize the use of indwelling bladder catheters. These catheters should not be used for the sake of convenience and should be removed when there is no longer a medical indication for them.

Nosocomial Wound Infection

1. How did Ms. Z develop her infection?

It is most likely that the infecting organism was introduced into the wound during surgery.

2. What are the most common organisms?

Skin flora, such as *Staphylococcus aureus*, are the most common cause of surgical wound infection. When there are wires, prosthesis, or metal fixation devices inserted during surgery, coagulase-negative staphylococci are the prominent infection agents. Enterococci may also be involved.

3. What is the cost of such infections in morbidity?

Surgical wound infections are the most costly of all hospital-acquired infections to treat.

Nosocomial Bacteremia

1. From where did the organisms arise in Mr. S.'s infection?

The infectious organism, *Staphylococcus aureus*, was probably acquired from the patient's skin.

2. How do the organisms enter the patient?

The organism contaminated with catheter through the puncture site, either at the time of catheter placement or subsequently. If the patient has another site of infection that causes bacteremia, catheters may also become infected secondarily. This did not appear to be the case in Mr. S.'s infection.

3. What is the best prevention for this type of infection?

Long intravenous catheters that end in the central veins (e.g., superior vena cava) should be removed when they are no longer needed to avoid infection. Short intravenous catheters placed in peripheral veins should be removed after 72 hours and replaced at another site (if still needed).

Nosocomial Pneumonia

1. Where did the organisms arise?

The organisms arose in the patient upper respiratory tract and were aspirated into the lungs. Bacteria may also gain access to the lungs in an intubated patient when upper airway secretions leak around the endotracheal tube. Although Gram-negative organisms are not usually part of the upper respiratory tract flora, they become abundant in sick, hospitalized patients.

2. What are the most common organisms?

Klebsiella pneumoniae, Pseudomonas aeruginosa, Staphylococcus aureus, Enterobacter **spp.**, *Escherichia coli.*

3. What preventive methods are there?

It is critical to clean and sterilize tubing, circuitry, and humidification devices associated with the ventilator. In addition, personnel must practice good hand hygiene and careful technique when suctioning an intubated patient to avoid introducing potential pathogens. Avoiding mechanical intubation or removing the patient from the ventilator as soon as possible is the best way to avoid this complication. Elevating the head of the patient's bed may help to prevent stomach contents from being aspirated into the lungs. Good oral care to decrease the burden of bacteria in the mouth may help to decrease the chances of developing pneumonia as well.

Nosocomial Bloodborne Disease

1. What is the likelihood of transmission of HIV, HBV, or HCV following needlestick?

HIV—0.3% per injury
HBV—25% per injury (range: 6 to 30%)
HCV—1.8% per injury (range: 0 to 7%)

2. What steps can be taken to prevent transmission?

Health care workers are advised never to recap needles. Several devices are now available that serve to safely cover needles after they are used, and used needles should be discard in designated, puncture-proof containers. Health care workers should wear gloves when performing any needle procedure. All health care workers who are potentially exposed to patient body fluids should receive the full series of hepatitis B vaccine. Since there is no vaccine to prevent HIV, health care workers who have had a serious needlestick exposure from a patient with known HIV can promptly take a course of antiretroviral medications that will reduce the risk of transmission by 60%.

CHAPTER 76
Staphylococcus aureus

1. What was the most likely cause of the outbreak?

The outbreak was the result of preformed enterotoxin produced by *Staphylococcus aureus* in the food.

2. Is this more likely to represent an intestinal infection or an intoxication by a preformed toxin? Why?

This is almost certainly an intoxication due to the very short incubation period.

3. How could one kind of meal have affected such a large number of individuals?

Very small amounts of *S. aureus* enterotoxins can cause symptoms. Therefore, a contaminated food generally sickens everyone who eats it.

Clostridium perfringens

1. What is the likely agent of this disease?

Heat-labile protein enterotoxin of *Clostridium perfringens* is the likely agent.

2. What is the pathophysiology of this type of diarrhea?

This condition occurs when food is precooked and then reheated before serving. Clostridial spores that contaminate food of animal source resist the first heating and grow to large numbers in improperly cooked food. After reheating, the organisms are ingested as vegetative, toxin-producing bacteria or as heat-resistant spores. Ingested spores germinate in the intestine, releasing clostridial enterotoxin. The enterotoxin inhibits glucose transport, damages the intestinal epithelium, and causes protein loss into the intestinal lumen.

3. How could such an outbreak be prevented?

Food storage is the critical step in preventing clostridial food poisoning. To cause illness, the contaminating spores in the food must have the opportunity to grow between the first heating and the reheating. If foods are promptly refrigerated after cooking the first time, the amplification of the bacteria is inhibited.

Bacillus cereus

1. Which food is most likely to have contributed to this early-onset form of food poisoning?

Fried rice is the most likely food.

2. How could the food have become contaminated?

Rice is frequently contaminated with *Bacillus cereus* before cooking. The organisms can grow to dangerous numbers if cooked rice is allowed to drain at room temperature for prolonged periods before reheating, as in the preparation of fried rice.

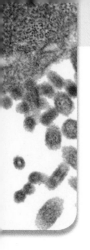

Appendix B *Quick Reference Summary Tables*

Main Pathogenic Bacteria

Organism	Gram Reaction, Morphology, Other Distinguishing Traits	Common Habitat and Mode of Encounter	Main Pathogenic Mechanism(s)	Typical Disease(s)	Relevant Chapters
Staphylococcus aureus	Positive, cocci in grapelike arrays	Nose, skin (carriers), breaks through skin and mucous membranes, ingestion of toxin-containing food	Acute inflammation and abscess formation involving many extracellular toxins (coagulase, leukocidin, catalase, toxic shock syndrome toxin, enterotoxins) and cell surface components (capsule, murein, teichoic acid, protein A, and other MSCRAMMS.)	Pyogenic infections and abscesses of many organs (e.g., subcutaneous tissue, bone marrow, endocardium), septicemia, toxic shock, food poisoning	11, 64, 65, 67, 76
Staphylococcus epidermidis	Positive, cocci in grapelike arrays	Skin, intestine (normal flora), breaks in skin and mucous membranes	Adherence and colonization of prostheses, intravenous devices via a slime layer	Infections of implanted devices, compromised patients	11, 67
Group A streptococci	Positive cocci in chains, β-hemolytic	Throat (carriers), breaks through skin and mucous membranes	Inflammation caused by surface components (M protein, lipoteichoic acids, hyaluronic acid, C5a peptidase, murein), extracellular enzymes (hemolysin, streptokinase, pyrogenic exotoxins); postsuppurative sequelae caused by as yet uncertain factors	Skin diseases (e.g., cellulitis, erysipelas, impetigo), tonsillitis, scarlet fever, septicemia, rheumatic fever, glomerulonephritis	12, 64
Other β-hemolytic streptococci	Positive (some normal flora), cocci in chains	Large intestine, vagina	Inflammation faciliated by resistance to phagocytosis (capsular polysaccharides)	Neonatal septicemia and meningitis	12, 72
α-Hemolytic streptococci	Positive (some normal flora), cocci in chains	Throat, intestine, genitourinary tract	Colonization of damaged heart valves caused by adhesion of organisms transiently in blood	Bacterial endocarditis, dental caries, abscesses	12, 67
Pneumococcus (*Streptococcus pneumoniae*)	Positive, diplococci, α-hemolytic	Throat (carriers), inhalation, hand contact	Inflammation facilitated by resistance to phagocytosis (capsule)	Pneumonia, empyema, meningitis, endocarditis, etc.	13, 62
Meningococcus (*Neisseria meningitidis*)	Gram-negative diplococci	Throat (carriers), inhalation, hand contact	Inflammation facilitated by resistance to phagocytosis (capsule), endotoxin	Septicemia, meningitis	14, 61
Gonococcus (*Neisseria gonorrhoeae*)	Gram-negative diplococci	Genital tract (carriers, some asymptomatic), contact with secretions	Inflammation caused by endotoxin, pili, and surface protein adhesins, IgA1 protease	Urethritis, salpingitis, pelvic inflammatory disease	14, 69

(continued on page 794)

Main Pathogenic Bacteria (continued)

Organism	Gram Reaction, Morphology, Other Distinguishing Traits	Common Habitat and Mode of Encounter	Main Pathogenic Mechanism(s)	Typical Disease(s)	Relevant Chapters
Haemophilus influenzae	Gram-negative, small rods, nutritionally fastidious	Throat (carriers), inhalation, hand contact	Inflammation facilitated by resistance to phagocytosis (capsule), endotoxin, IgA1 protease, pili, outer membrane protein	Meningitis (infants, 3 mo–2 y) with sequelae, respiratory infections, cellulitis	45, 58, 68
Bacteroides spp.	Gram-negative, rods, anaerobes	Intestine, vagina (normal flora)	Inflammation of sensitive sites after entry of organisms from intestinal, oral flora, Zwitterionic capsule	Abscesses (e.g., in peritoneum, lungs) often as part of mixed flora	15
Escherichia coli	Gram-negative, rods, many strains differing in pathogenic mechanisms (ETEC, EPEC, EHEC, etc.)[a]	Fecally contaminated bodies of water, foods; personal contact; ingestion	Various forms of diarrhea, dysentery caused by enterotoxins, endotoxin, shigalike toxins, adhesins; some of these factors also involved in urinary infection and other deep tissue infections	Secretory diarrhea (traveler's diarrhea), cystitis, septicemia, meningitis	16, 17, 60, 63, 72, 76
Shigella spp.	Gram-negative, rods, several species differing in pathogenicity	Fecally contaminated bodies of water, foods, personal contact, ingestion (small inoculum suffices)	Inflammation caused by invasion of small intestine mucosa helped by shiga toxin, adhesins	Dysentery (inflammatory disease)	17, 60
Klebsiella pneumoniae	Gram-negative, rods, heavily encapsulated	Usually, inhalation of oral contents	Inflammation facilitated by resistance to phagocytosis (capsule), perhaps endotoxin	Pneumonia, other inflammations in compromised patients	16, 62, 70
Proteus spp.	Gram-negative, rods, urea splitters (grow at high pH)	Probably fecal contamination from same individual	Inflammation, usually of urinary tract	Urinary tract inflammatory disease, associated with urinary calculi formation	16, 63
Vibrio cholerae	Gram-negative, rods, curved	Bodies of water, ingestion	Massive watery diarrhea caused by cholera toxin (ADP ribosylating), adhesins	Cholera (intense watery diarrhea)	16, 60
Salmonella spp.	Gram-negative, rods, species differing in pathogenicity (including S. typhi)	Fecally contaminated foods, personal contact, ingestion, most strains are zoonotic	Able to multiply in macrophages owing to largely unknown factors, diarrhea probably caused by toxins	Typhoid and related fevers, gastroenteritis, septicemia	17, 60
Pseudomonas aeruginosa	Gram-negative, rods, oxidative metabolism only (strict aerobes)	Water, soils, foods, inhalation, ingestion, penetration through breaks in epithelia	Toxins (toxin A [ADP ribosylating], elastase, exotoxin S, endotoxin), adhesins, alginate in cystic fibrosis	Pyogenic infection in burn patients, diabetics; lung infection in cystic fibrosis	18, 66, 70

Organism	Characteristics	Reservoir/Transmission	Virulence Factors	Disease	Chapter
Bordetella pertussis	Gram-negative, small rods, nutritionally fastidious	Throat (carriers), inhalation, hand contact	Pertussis toxin (ADP ribosylating), adenylate cyclase, tracheal cytotoxin, adhesins	Whooping cough	19, 62
Other enterics (*Enterobacter, Citrobacter, Serratia, Campylobacter, Yersinia*)	Gram-negative, rods	Usually fecal contamination, some derived from rodents	Virulence factors not well known but probably include endotoxins	Various forms of diarrhea, dysentery; some cause systemic disease and local inflammations	16, 60
Helicobacter pylori	Gram-negative, rods, spiral or coiled	Frequently found in stomach	Inflammation caused by uncharacterized factors, facilitated by CagA	Gastritis, perhaps gastric ulcers	22, 60
Clostridium difficile	Gram-positive, spore-forming rods, anaerobes	Intestine, spores persist in the environment and in the human colon	Toxin A (an enterotoxin) and toxin B (a cytotoxin)	Pseudomembranous colitis	20
Clostridium botulinum	Gram-positive, spore-forming rods, anaerobes	Soil, contaminated food, intestine, ingestion of preformed toxin (adult botulism)	Botulinum toxin	Botulism (flaccid paralysis), infant and wound botulism	20
Clostridium tetani	Gram-positive, spore-forming rods, anaerobes	Soil, contaminated food, intestine, punctures of skin, wounds	Tetanus toxin	Tetanus (spastic paralysis)	20
Clostridium perfringens and other spp.	Gram-positive, spore-forming rods, anaerobes	Soil, contaminated food, intestine, wound contamination, ingestion	Lecithinase (alpha-toxin), other hydrolytic enzymes	Myonecrosis, gas gangrene, food poisoning	20, 76
Legionella pneumophila	Gram-negative, small rods, nutritionally fastidious	Water (air conditioning, cooling systems, building water supplies), inhalation, ingestion	Intracellular infection is essential for virulence; alternates between a cell-invasive and vegetative intracellular phenotype.	Pneumonia, systemic infections rare	21
Mycobacterium tuberculosis and other spp.	Acid-fast (non-Gram-stainable), thin rods, slow growing	Human environment and secretions (*M. tuberculosis*), soil, waters (*M. avium-intracellulare*, etc.)	Chronic inflammation caused by bacterial persistence in macrophages, release of cytokines, adjuvant effect	Primary and secondary tuberculosis, *M. avium-intracellulare*, etc., typically infect AIDS patients	23, 62, 71
Mycobacterium leprae	Acid-fast (non-Gram-stainable), thin rods, slow growing	Human environment and secretions	Chronic inflammation caused by bacterial persistence in macrophages, release of cytokines	Tuberculoid and lepromatous leprosy	23

(*continued on page 796*)

Main Pathogenic Bacteria (*continued*)

Organism	Gram Reaction, Morphology, Other Distinguishing Traits	Common Habitat and Mode of Encounter	Main Pathogenic Mechanism(s)	Typical Disease(s)	Relevant Chapters
Treponema pallidum	Non-Gram-stainable, thin, helical rods; motile; not cultivable	Infected persons, acquired by intimate contact with human secretions	Chancre in first stage, acute inflammation in second, chronic inflammation and perhaps autoimmune-like sequelae in third, virulence factors not known	Syphilis	24, 69
Borrelia burgdorferi	Non-Gram-stainable, thin, helical rods	Wild animal reservoir, transmitted to humans via tick bite	Three stages of infection, vaguely reminiscent of syphilis, virulence factors not known, but some preference for attachment to brain gangliosides	Lyme disease	25
Bartonella benselae	Small, Gram-negative rods, nutritionally fastidious	Cat scratch or bite, lice, IV paraphernalia	Elicit granulomatous and suppurative response	Cat scratch disease, bacillary angiomatosis	26
Chlamydia trachomatis	Non-Gram-stainable, small organism in two forms (elementary [EB] and reticulate bodies [RB], strict intracellular parasite, not culturable extracellularly	Humans, direct contact with genital and other secretions containing EB	Inflammation caused by host cell destruction resulting from intracellular growth of RB	Genital infection with possible pelvic inflammatory disease, lymphogranuloma, pneumonia, neonatal conjunctivitis	27, 69
Rickettsia spp.	Non-Gram-stainable, small intracellular rods, strict intracellular parasite, not culturable extracellularly	Animal reservoirs, insect vectors, possibly human carriers in epidemic typhus	Damage to vascular endothelia caused by multiplication of the organisms, leakage of fluid leading to damage of vital organ function	Rocky Mountain spotted fever, various types of typhus, Q fever	28
Ehrlichia spp. and *Anaplasma* spp.	Small, Gram-negative rods, strict intracellular parasites	Ticks	Grow in white blood cells	Human monocytic ehrlichiosis, human granulocytic ehrlichiosis	28
Mycoplasma spp.	Small, non-Gram-stainable, lacking cell wall, some needing sterols for growth	Human carriers, animals, environment	Damage to respiratory epithelium, loss of ciliary function; perhaps caused by organism's metabolites, including hydrogen peroxide	Bronchopneumonia, especially in young adults, genital and intrauterine infections	29, 62

[a]EHEC, enterohemorrhagic *E. coli*; EPEC, enteropathogenic *E. coli*; ETEC, enterotoxigenic *E. coli*.

Main Pathogenic Viruses

This table is intended to review the main human viruses. Included are the agents of greatest medical relevance. Many of the viruses that cause relatively uncommon diseases are not included.

Virus	Group or Family	Nucleic Acid	Site of Genome Replication	Envelope	Capsid Symmetry	Disease(s) and Systems Involved	Relevant Chapters
Poliovirus	Picornaviruses	RNA(+)	Cytoplasm, on cellular membranes	No	Icosahedral	Gastrointestinal (GI) tract, anterior horn cells of the spinal cord	32
Coxsackie and other enteroviruses	Picornaviruses	RNA(+)	Cytoplasm, on cellular membranes	No	Icosahedral	GI tract, meninges, skin, heart	32, 61
Rhinoviruses	Picornaviruses	RNA(+)	Cytoplasm, on cellular membranes	No	Icosahedral	Upper respiratory tract (common cold)	32, 62
Hepatitis A	Hepatovirus (picornavirus)	RNA(+)	Cytoplasm	No	Icosahedral	Liver cells	32, 43
Severe acute respiratory syndrome	Coronaviruses	RNA(+)	Cytoplasm, on cellular membranes	Yes	Helical	Lower respiratory tract	32
Arboviruses	Togaviruses, flaviviruses,	RNA(+)	Cytoplasm, on cellular membranes	Yes	Icosahedral	Encephalitis, hemorrhagic fever	33, 61, 73
	Bunyaviruses (group includes hantaviruses)	RNA(−), 3 segments	Cytoplasm, on cellular membranes	Yes	Helical	Encephalitis, fever	33, 73
Rubella	Togaviruses	RNA(+)	Cytoplasm, on lysosome membranes	Yes	Icosahedral	Fever and rash, severe congenital infections	33, 72
Measles	Paramyxovirus	RNA(−)	Cytoplasm	Yes	Helical	Fever, rash, lower respiratory tract	34
Respiratory syncytial virus	Paramyxovirus	RNA(−)	Cytoplasm	Yes	Helical	Respiratory tract, bronchioles	34, 62
Rabies	Rhabdoviruses	RNA(−)	Cytoplasm	Yes	Helical	Peripheral and central nervous system	35, 73
Influenza	Orthomyxovirus	RNA(−), 8 segments	Nucleus	Yes	Helical	Upper and lower respiratory tracts	36, 62

(continued on page 798)

Main Pathogenic Viruses (*continued*)

Virus	Group or Family	Nucleic Acid	Site of Genome Replication	Envelope	Capsid Symmetry	Disease(s) and Systems Involved	Relevant Chapters
Rotavirus	Reoviruses	dsRNA, 11 segments	Cytoplasm	No	Icosahedral	GI tract, diarrhea and vomiting	37, 60
Norovirus	Calicivirus	ssRNA (+)	Unknown	No	Icosahedral	GI tract, diarrhea and vomiting	37, 60
HIV	Retroviruses	RNA (+), 2 copies	Nucleus	Yes	Icosahedral, helical nucleocapsid	AIDS: CD4+ lymphocytes depleted	38, 69, 71, 72
Parvovirus B19	Parvoviruses	ssDNA	Nucleus	No	Icosahedral	Bone marrow precursors	31
Hepatitis B	Hepadnavirus	dsDNA with some ssDNA	Nucleus	Yes	Multiple forms	Liver cells	43, 72
Adenovirus	Adenoviruses	dsDNA	Nucleus	No	Icosahedral	Respiratory and GI tract infections, conjunctivitis	39, 62
Papillomavirus	Papillomaviruses	dsDNA	Nucleus	No	Icosahedral	Stratified squamous epithelium, warts, cervical cancer	40, 69
Herpes simplex and varicella zoster	Herpesviruses	dsDNA	Nucleus	Yes	Icosahedral	Cold sores, genital herpes, chicken pox, shingles, latent in ganglionic neurons	41, 61, 69, 72
Epstein-Barr virus, cytomegalovirus, herpesvirus 6	Herpesviruses	dsDNA	Nucleus	Yes	Icosahedral	Mononucleosis, retinitis, colitis, congenital infections, erythema infectiosum, latent in B lymphocytes	42, 72
Smallpox	Poxvirus	dsDNA	Cytoplasm	Yes	"Brick-shaped" virion	Epidemic systemic illness with rash	57

Medically Important Fungi

Fungi	Name of Disease	Source	Geography	Organ Systems Involved	Clinical Features	Relevant Chapter
Systemic, Endemic Fungi						
Histoplasma capsulatum	Histoplasmosis	Soil, bird, and bat droppings	Ohio River Valley	Lungs, reticuloendothelial system, mucous membranes	Fever, chills, dry cough, weight loss, chronic pulmonary infiltrate with or without cavities	47
Blastomyces dermatitidis	Blastomycosis	Soil, decaying wood	Mississippi and St. Lawrence River valleys	Lungs, skin	Fever, chills, anorexia, fatigue, dry cough, patchy pulmonary infiltrates	47
Coccidioides immitis	Coccidioidomycosis	Desert soil	American Southwest, Central California, and Northern Mexico	Lungs, meninges, skin, bone	Valley fever with thin-walled lung cavities, chronic meningitis	47
Opportunistic Fungi						
Candida ssp.	Candidiasis	Normal flora	Cosmopolitan	Skin, mucous membranes, blood	Itchy red rash, thrush, vaginitis, esophagitis, IV catheter infections, endophthalmitis	48
Cryptococcus neoformans	Cryptococosis	Soil, bird droppings	Cosmopolitan	Lungs, meninges	Fever, chronic headache, stiff neck	48
Aspergillus ssp.	Aspergillosis	Ubiquitous in the environment	Cosmopolitan	Lungs, sinuses	Nodular lung disease with fever, pleuritic chest pain, cough, hemoptysis, or dyspnea	48
Zygomycetes	Mucormycosis	Ubiquitous in the environment	Cosmopolitan	Sinuses, lungs	Invasive sinusitis with pain, bone destruction	48
Pneumocystis jiroveci	Pneumocystis pneumonia	Reactivation of endogenous infection	Cosmopolitan	Lungs	Pulmonary infiltrates with fever, dyspnea	48
Subcutaneous and Cutaneous Fungi						
Sporotrix schenckii	Sporotrichosis	Soil, sphagnum moss, rose thorns, decaying wood and vegetation	Cosmopolitan	Skin, lymphatics	Discrete skin ulcers that appear along the distribution of lymphatics proximally from the extremities	49
Microsporum, Trichophyton, and *Epidermophyton* sp.	Dermatophytosis (tinea or "ringworm")	Soil, animals, humans	Cosmopolitan	Skin (superficial)	Itchy, scaly rash of scalp (tinea capitis), feet (tinea pedis) body (tinea corporis), crotch (tinea cruris), or nails (onychomycosis)	49

Major Bacteria

ENCAPSULATED BACTERIA OF MEDICAL IMPORTANCE

Genus and Species

1. Pneumococcus	6. *Staphylococcus aureus* (some strains)
2. Meningococcus	7. *Escherichia coli* (some strains)
3. *Haemophilus influenzae*	8. Gonococcus (some strains)
4. *Klebsiella pneumoniae*	9. *Bacteroides fragilis* (some strains)
5. *Streptococcus pyogenes* (some strains)	

MEDICALLY IMPORTANT STRICT ANAEROBES

Genus and Species

1. *Clostridium difficile*	6. *Bacteroides fragilis*
2. *C. botulinum*	7. Several other *Bacteroides*
3. *C. tetani*	8. *Actinomyces bovis*
4. *C. perfringens*	9. Some streptococci
5. Several other clostridia	10. Other members of the normal flora

TYPICALLY PYOGENIC (PUS-PRODUCING) BACTERIA

Genus and Species

1. *Staphylococcus aureus*	4. Gonococcus
2. *S. epidermidis*	5. *Pseudomonas aeruginosa*
3. *Streptococcus pyogenes*	6. Pneumococcus

MAJOR TOXINOGENIC ORGANISMS

Organism (Toxin and AB Organization Component)	Effect	Mechanism
Bacillus anthracis		
Anthrax toxin 2A + B	Required for other toxins	Receptor-binding domain
Protective antigen B		
Edema factor A	Edema	Adenylate cyclase
Lethal factor A	Pulmonary edema	Protease
Bordetella pertussis		
Adenylate cyclase	Inhibits, kills white cells	Adenylate cyclase, pore formation in membranes
Pertussis toxin AB5	Many hormonal effects	ADP ribosylation of G protein
Tracheal cytotoxin	Peptidoglycan fragment that kills cilia-bearing cells	Unknown
Campylobacter jejuni		
Enterotoxin AB5	Diarrhea	ADP ribosylates G protein
Clostridium botulinum		
Botulinum toxin AB	Neurotoxin	Inhibits synaptic vesicle fusion to the plasma membrane at the neuromuscular junction, flaccid paralysis
Clostridium difficile		
Toxin A	Fluid secretion, mucosal damage	Glucosylation of small GTP-binding proteins
Toxin B	Cytotoxin, mucosal damage	Glucosylation of small GTP-binding proteins (in conjunction with Toxin A)
Clostridia spp.		
α-toxin	Necrosis in gas gangrene, cytolytic, lethal	Phospholipase C (Lecithinase)
β-toxin	Necrotic enteritis	Unknown
Enterotoxin	Food poisoning, diarrhea	Cytotoxin, damages membranes
Clostridium tetani		
Tetanus toxin AB	Neurotoxin	Inhibits synaptic vesicle fusion with the plasma membrane nerve terminals at inhibitor synapses, spastic paralysis
Corynebacterium diphtheriae		
Diphtheria toxin AB	Kills cells	ADP ribosylates elongation factor 2
Escherichia coli (enterics)		
Heat-labile enterotoxin AB5	Diarrhea	Identical to cholera toxin
Cytotoxin	Hemorrhagic colitis	Like shiga toxin
Heat-stable enterotoxin	Diarrhea	Activates host guanylate cyclase
Legionella pneumophila		
Cytotoxin	Lyses cells	Unknown
Type IV secreted proteins	Inhibit endosome maturation	Interfere with Rab protein function

Organism (Toxin and AB Organization Component)	Effect	Mechanism
Listeria monocytogenes		
Listeriolysin	Membrane damage, allows release of ingested bacteria from endosomes into cytoplasm	Like streptolysin O
Pseudomonas aeruginosa		
Exotoxin A	Kills cells	Like diphtheria toxin
Type III cytotoxins	Modulate host cell physiology	Inhibit actin cytoskeleton
Salmonella		
Type III cytotoxins	Modulate host cell physiology	Alter actin cytoskeleton
Shigella dysenteriae		
Shiga toxin	Kills cells	Inactivates 60S ribosomes
Staphylococcus aureus		
α-toxin	Hemolytic, leukocytic, paralysis of smooth muscle	Pore-forming toxin
β-toxin	Cytolytic	Sphingomyelinase
δ-lysin	Cytolytic	Detergent-like action
Exfoliating toxin	Sloughing of skin ("scalded skin syndrome")	Protease
Superantigens		
Enterotoxins	Food poisoning (emesis, diarrhea)	Activate host antibody and cytokine synthesis by an antigen-independent mechanism
Toxic shock syndrome toxin	Fever, headache, arthralgia, neutropenia, rash	Activates host antibody and cytokine synthesis by an antigen-independent mechanism
Streptococcus pneumoniae		
Pneumolysin	Cytolysin	Similar to streptolysin O
Streptococcus pyogenes		
Streptolysin O	Cytolysin	Pore-forming toxin
Erythrogenic toxin (SpeA)	Fever, neutropenia, rash of scarlet fever	Mediated through IL-1
Vibrio cholerae		
Cholera toxin AB5	Diarrhea	Hormone-independent activation of adenyl cyclase
Yersinia enterocolitica		
Heat-stable enterotoxin	Diarrhea	Activates host guanylate cyclase
Type III cytotoxins	Modulate host cell physiology	Regulate actin cytoskeleton

ADP, adenosine diphosphate; GABA, gamma-aminobutyric acid; IL, interleukin.

Index

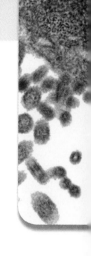

Note: Page numbers followed by 'f' indicate figures; those followed by 't' indicate tables; those followed by 'b' indicate boxes.